SILVA'S DIAGNOSTIC RENAL PATHOLOGY

THE KIDNEYS perform many vital functions, but their primary role as a filter of plasma, receiving approximately 25% of the cardiac output, makes them extremely susceptible to disease. These diseases often can only be diagnosed by renal biopsy, a complicated diagnostic procedure requiring that the pathologist integrate the findings of light microscopy, immunofluorescence, and electron microscopy. Because of the expertise required to practice renal pathology, many academic centers maintain a separately designated, specialized renal pathology laboratory for interpretation of medical renal diseases. This book covers all approaches and technical methods used by renal pathologists to diagnose a wide range of kidney diseases. Unlike most textbooks in the field, this book's level of coverage is situated midway between encyclopedic and superficial, with the needs of the practicing ("signing-out") pathologist in mind. While focusing on medical diseases of the kidney, the book also covers a full spectrum of renal tumors (both pediatric and adult). Its numerous diagnostic algorithms provide a simplified road map that directs the reader to the major patterns of interest. The text is illustrated with more than 1,000 photomicrographs and diagrams. The accompanying CD-ROM includes a supplemental set of images.

Xin J. Zhou, MD, is Drs. George & Anne Race Distinguished Professor of Pathology, director of renal pathology, and professor of internal medicine at the University of Texas Southwestern Medical Center, Dallas. Dr. Zhou has published extensively in the areas of renal diseases and has served on the editorial boards of several prestigious renal journals. Dr. Zhou is past president of the Chinese American Society of Nephrology.

Zoltan Laszik, MD, is associate professor of clinical pathology at the University of California at San Francisco School of Medicine. Dr. Laszik, a renowned renal pathologist, has published nearly 100 original papers and book chapters.

Tibor Nadasdy, MD, is professor of pathology and director of renal pathology at Ohio State University School of Medicine, Columbus. Dr. Nadasdy, an experienced academic renal pathologist, has published numerous original papers and book chapters in the fields of renal pathology and renal transplantation.

Vivette D. D'Agati, MD, is professor of pathology and director of renal pathology at Columbia University, College of Physicians and Surgeons, in New York. Dr. D'Agati has published more than 300 original articles and book chapters and coedited several renal pathology texts. She serves on the editorial boards of the major nephrology journals and has directed the Columbia University Renal Biopsy Course for more than two decades. She is past president of the Renal Pathology Society.

Fred G. Silva, MD, is executive vice-president/secretary-treasurer of the United States and Canadian Academy of Pathology, Augusta, Georgia. Dr. Silva is adjunct professor of pathology at Emory University and the Medical College of Georgia. He is formerly the Lloyd Rader Professor and chair of the department of pathology at the University of Oklahoma Health Sciences Center. Dr. Silva, a preeminent expert in renal pathology, has published hundreds of articles on subjects spanning the entire spectrum of renal pathology and coedited several renal pathology books.

SILVA'S DIAGNOSTIC
RENAL PATHOLOGY

Edited by

Xin J. Zhou
University of Texas Southwestern Medical Center

Zoltan Laszik
University of California at San Francisco School of Medicine

Tibor Nadasdy
Ohio State University Medical Center

Vivette D. D'Agati
Columbia University, College of Physicians and Surgeons

Fred G. Silva
United States and Canadian Academy of Pathology

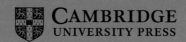

CAMBRIDGE UNIVERSITY PRESS

Cambridge, New York, Melbourne, Madrid, Cape Town, Singapore, São Paulo, Delhi

Cambridge University Press
32 Avenue of the Americas, New York, NY 10013-2473, USA

www.cambridge.org
Information on this title: www.cambridge.org/9780521877022

First published 2009

Printed in the United States of America

A catalog record for this publication is available from the British Library.

Library of Congress Cataloging in Publication Data

Silva's diagnostic renal pathology / edited by Xin J. Zhou … [et al.].
p. ; cm.
Includes bibliographical references and index.
ISBN 978-0-521-87702-2 (hardback)
1. Kidneys – Pathophysiology. 2. Kidneys – Diseases – Diagnosis. 3. Kidneys – Biopsy.
4. Kidneys – Diseases – Atlases. I. Zhou, Xin J., 1962– II. Silva, Fred G. III. Title: Diagnostic renal pathology.
[DNLM: 1. Biopsy – methods. 2. Kidney Diseases – pathology. 3. Kidney Diseases – classification.
4. Kidney Diseases – physiopathology. WJ 302 S5862009]

RC903.9.S55 2009
616.6′1075 – dc22   2008047233

ISBN 978-0-521-87702-2 hardback

ZHOU

To my loving wife, Jian Wang, and our wonderful children, Jason and Jaclyn

LASZIK

To my beautiful wife, Erika, and our wonderful children, Nandi, Laura, and Aron

NADASDY

To my wife, Gyongyi, and my daughters, Krisztina and Orsolya

D'AGATI

To my devoted husband, Edward Imperatore, and my loving children,

Edward and Paul, without whose constant support and encouragement

my academic career would not be possible

SILVA

To my lovely wife, Jean, and wonderful daughter, Lindsay

Contents

Contributors

MAHUL B. AMIN, MD
Department of Pathology and Laboratory Medicine,
Cedars-Sinai Medical Center, Los Angeles, California

PEDRAM ARGANI, MD
Department of Pathology, Johns Hopkins University
Medical Center, Baltimore, Maryland

STEVEN A. BIGLER, MD
Department of Pathology, University of Mississippi
Medical Center, Jackson, Mississippi

WILLIAM L. CLAPP, MD
Department of Pathology, University of Florida College
of Medicine, Gainesville, Florida

VIVETTE D. D'AGATI, MD
Department of Pathology, Columbia University, College
of Physicians and Surgeons, New York, New York

LUKAS HARAGSIM, MD
Department of Medicine, University of Oklahoma
Health Sciences Center, Oklahoma City, Oklahoma

RANDOLPH A. HENNIGAR, MD, PhD
Department of Pathology and Laboratory
Medicine, Emory University School of Medicine,
Atlanta, Georgia

GUILLERMO A. HERRERA, MD
Nephrocor, Bostwick Laboratories, Tempe, Arizona

MICHAEL D. HUGHSON, MD
Department of Pathology, University of Mississippi
Medical Center, Jackson, Mississippi

ZOLTAN G. LASZIK, MD, PhD
Department of Pathology, University of California at San
Francisco School of Medicine, San Francisco, California

GLEN S. MARKOWITZ, MD
Department of Pathology, Columbia University, College
of Physicians and Surgeons, New York, New York

SHANE M. MEEHAN, MD
Department of Pathology, University of Chicago,
Chicago, Illinois

GYONGYI NADASDY, MD
Department of Pathology, Ohio State University Medical
Center, Columbus, Ohio

TIBOR NADASDY, MD, PhD
Department of Pathology, Ohio State University Medical
Center, Columbus, Ohio

SAMIH H. NASR, MD
Department of Pathology, Columbia University, College
of Physicians and Surgeons, New York, New York

DINESH RAKHEJA, MD
Department of Pathology, University of Texas
Southwestern Medical Center, Dallas, Texas

THOMAS E. ROGERS, MD
Department of Pathology, University of Texas
Southwestern Medical Center, Dallas, Texas

ANJALI SATOSKAR, MD
Department of Pathology, Ohio State University Medical
Center, Columbus, Ohio

FRED G. SILVA, MD
United States and Canadian Academy of Pathology, Augusta, Georgia

MICHAEL B. STOKES, MD
Department of Pathology, Columbia University, College of Physicians and Surgeons, New York, New York

SATISH K. TICKOO, MD
Department of Pathology, Memorial Sloan-Kettering Cancer Center, New York, New York

ROBERT D. TOTO, MD
Department of Medicine, University of Texas Southwestern Medical Center, Dallas, Texas

JAMES A. TUMLIN, MD
Clinical Research Division, Southeast Renal Associates, Charlotte, North Carolina

ARTHUR G. WEINBERG, MD
Department of Pathology, University of Texas Southwestern Medical Center, Dallas, Texas

XIN J. ZHOU, MD
Department of Pathology, University of Texas Southwestern Medical Center, Dallas, Texas

Preface

"If you do not know the names of things, the knowledge of them is lost, too."

– Carl Linnaeus

Throughout our many combined years of teaching renal pathology, we have been impressed by the challenges to students learning the subject for the first time. There are many reasons why the study of renal pathology is considered difficult. First, there is insufficient knowledge of the normal histology/structure of the kidney. Second, one disease can manifest many different morphologic patterns, while a particular morphologic pattern can be produced by different diseases or etiologic factors. And finally, several different names (synonyms) have been applied to particular patterns or diseases. Yet, the many years of teaching have convinced us that there can be a systematic and orderly approach to the study of renal pathology. Therefore, a new book emphasizing an algorithmic, deductive approach to the interpretation of renal pathology seemed timely. This book organizes the various renal patterns and diseases in a standardized fashion, with emphasis on clinical–pathologic correlations. We have limited our inclusion of renal morphologic patterns to comparatively stable taxonomic groups covering the major diagnostic entities accepted by the published literature.

Standardized names and terminology are essential for communication among renal experts, whether they are clinicians or pathologists. The terminology used in this book is generally consistent with that used by most North American renal pathologists. Wherever possible, we have applied the widely recognized International Nomenclature of Disease (IND), a joint project of the Council for International Organization of Medical Sciences and the World Health Organization. The purpose is to ease communications and facilitate the storage and retrieval of medical information. As noted by the IND, a "few diseases have a single recognized name; most have several different…names. The principle objective of the IND is to provide…a single recommended name" (specific, unambiguous, self-descriptive, simple, and based on cause whenever feasible). It is meant to be a truly international language of disease. The importance of precise terminology and diagnostic criteria cannot be overstated.

The approach and classification used in this book are neither unique nor original. They are based on the "capture" of ideas from the many members of the Renal Pathology Society, Inc., and from major courses in the field, such as Medical Diseases of the Kidney, a postgraduate course held annually for more than 30 years by the Columbia University College of Physicians and Surgeons in New York City, under the direction of Dr. Vivette D'Agati. The approach to renal biopsy has been influenced enormously by Dr. Conrad L. Pirani, and it should come as no surprise that the editors of this book have either studied directly under him (V.D., F.G.S.) or been mentored directly by Dr. Pirani's student, Dr. Silva (X.J.Z., Z.L., and T.N.).

A useful classification (and the subsequent approach to diagnosis) should be based on the following requirements:

1. The classification should be clinically relevant and provide useful information to the clinician (about diagnosis, prognosis, identification of clinical subsets, optimal choice of therapy, evaluation of response to therapy, and future management).

2. It should be based on facts (reflecting the ideals of evidence-based medicine), be scientifically correct, and incorporate our current level of biologic understanding.

3. It should be relatively easy to use by pathologists throughout the world and be reproducible between observers.

The approach of *Silva's Diagnostic Renal Pathology*, which incorporates these principles, is morphologically based and designed for practicing anatomic (and renal) pathologists. By maintaining a high level of expertise in renal pathology, pathologists can ensure that the current trend of increasing use of renal biopsy for diagnosis and patient management will continue.

Many algorithms that collectively detail the clinical, laboratory, and pathologic patterns of renal disease have been included. These algorithms, based upon clinical and morphologic findings, will allow one to find the correct diagnosis. The algorithms provide a simplified road map that directs the reader to the major patterns of interest. To this end, we have adopted a combined "clinical and pathologic" classification scheme in this book. We have always found it ironic that most dictionaries, atlases, and textbooks require a priori that one knows what something is (e.g., what the diagnosis is and how to spell a particular word) in order to look it up and find the relevant entry. We hope that this book will eliminate that problem.

We believe that the approach in this book, neither final nor perfect, will allow the student to discover and categorize the type of renal involvement, correlate it with the clinical and laboratory findings, and determine the renal prognosis and optimal therapy. Of course, there are always "varieties" or "cross-overs" or "dual diseases," which render exact classification difficult. Nonetheless, a good description is always reliable. More atypical or unusual cases are likely to be referred for renal biopsy, because the clinically obvious cases (e.g., minimal change nephrotic syndrome in children, acute postinfectious glomerulonephritis, diabetic nephropathy with retinopathy) often are not biopsied unless they exhibit atypical features. In the end, it is the renal morphology interpreted in an informed clinical context that leads pathologists to an accurate diagnosis. Although this book is intended as a practical guide for the diagnostic pathologist with primary responsibility for renal biopsy interpretation, as "clinical biologists," we should not lose sight of the pathogenetic factors behind the morphology. Thus, we have included a short section on "Pathogenesis" in each of the chapters.

The authors each bring their own unique personal insights to their individual chapters. However, we have attempted to bind them together through a unanimity of purpose, as reflected in their similar styles and analytic approaches.

At each step, the renal pathologist is integrating knowledge about the light microscopy, fluorescence microscopy, electron microscopy, renal functional studies, urinalysis, systemic findings, medication history, serologies, and radiologic studies. It is this multidisciplinary approach that constitutes the most rewarding aspect of renal pathology. Despite the complexity of the subject material, we hope that the approach outlined in this book will provide a user-friendly guide into this fascinating field.

As our mentor, Dr. Conrad Pirani, often said, it is important that clinical nephrologists and pathologists work closely together for the good of the patient. The pathologist cannot function in isolation. The most difficult diagnostic dilemmas can usually be solved by combining the knowledge of clinician and pathologist on an individual case. As Dr. Pirani has stated in a renal biopsy textbook, "[s]tructure and function have finally met at the microscope." The pathologist and nephrologist can learn a great deal from each other by reviewing cases together over the multiheaded microscope.

Lastly, we would like to thank the renal patients, physicians, and pathologists without whom we would not have had the opportunity to collect these biopsy materials for teaching purposes. We thank them for providing us with such valuable illustrative cases. We, pathologists, strive to understand what we see and place it in a diagnostic context that guides the nephrologist toward more specific therapies. As better and more targeted therapies are developed, an accurate biopsy interpretation will become even more important. It is highly likely that the renal biopsy will continue to be cost-effective for all those we serve – our patients and our clinicians.

Renal Anatomy

William L. Clapp, MD

Knowledge of the elaborate structure of the kidney provides insight into its functions and facilitates an understanding of renal diseases. One cannot recognize what is abnormal in the kidney if one does not know what is normal. The following sections consider the macroanatomy, functional units, architectural organization, microanatomy, and basic functions of the kidney. Unless otherwise stated, the illustrations will emphasize the human kidney. For additional information, readers are referred to several detailed reviews [1–4].

GROSS ANATOMY

Location, Size, and Shape

The retroperitoneum is divided into fascia-enclosed compartments, including the anterior pararenal, perirenal, and posterior pararenal spaces. The kidneys lie within the perirenal space, which contains abundant fat and is enclosed by the anterior and posterior layers of renal fascia, known as Gerota's fascia. The kidneys extend from the twelfth thoracic to the third lumbar vertebrae with the right kidney slightly lower. Their position may be 2.5 cm lower in the erect than in the supine position and their craniocaudal movement during respiration may be up to 4 cm. The renal upper poles slant slightly toward the midline and the posterior. The hilar aspect of each kidney has an anteromedial orientation.

Each adult kidney weighs 125 to 170 g in men and 115 to 155 g in women. However, kidney weight correlates best with body surface area. Each kidney averages about 11 to 12 cm in length, 5 to 7.5 cm in width, and 2.5 to 3 cm in thickness. The left kidney is slightly larger than the right. As measured by magnetic resonance imaging (MRI), individual kidney volume averages 202 ± 36 ml for men and 154 ± 33 ml for women [5]. The estimated renal volume may vary with changes in blood pressure and intravascular volume. Known as bean-shaped organs, the posterior surface of each kidney is flatter whereas the anterior surface is more convex. The left kidney may have focal bulging of the lateral contour due to compression by the spleen. Located on the concave medial surface of each kidney is an aperture called the hilum through which pass branches of the renal artery and vein, lymphatics, nerves, and ureter. The hilum continues into a fat-filled cavity, the renal sinus, which contains the expanded portion of the ureter, the renal pelvis, and the calyces. A thin fibrous capsule surrounds the kidney. Within the renal sinus, the capsule does not enclose the columns of Bertin, allowing access between the cortical parenchyma and the sinus [6]. This continuity provides a route for tumor dissemination.

Blood Supply

After entering the hilar region, the main renal artery usually divides to form anterior and posterior divisions, which in turn, branch into segmental arteries that supply segmental regions of the parenchyma (Figure 1.1) [7]. The majority of the segmental arteries arise from the anterior division. No collateral circulation exists between the segmental arteries and their subsequent branches. Thus, they are considered end-arteries. Some so-called accessory arteries represent segmental arteries with an early origin from the main renal artery or aorta. Ligation of such a segmental artery in the belief that it is an accessory vessel will result in infarction of the corresponding parenchymal segment. Although the major intrarenal veins accompany the corresponding arteries, unlike the arteries, the veins form abundant anastomoses.

Form of Kidney

On the cut surface of a bisected kidney, the cortex (an outer region) and the medulla (an inner region) are revealed (Figure 1.2). The cortex has a more granular appearance due to the presence of glomeruli and convoluted tubules. The human kidney is a multipapillary type of mammalian kidney with the medulla containing striated conical structures called pyramids. The striated appearance reflects the parallel linear orientation of straight tubules (loops of Henle and collecting ducts). Each pyramid has a base situated at the corticomedullary junction and an apex extending into the renal sinus, forming a papilla. On the tip of each papilla, the area cribrosa, are twenty to seventy small openings that represent the distal ends of the collecting ducts (of Bellini). The cortex forms a 1 cm outer layer, covers the base of each pyramid, and extends down between pyramids forming the columns (septa) of Bertin. An enlarged column of Bertin may rarely be clinically mistaken for a renal tumor. Longitudinal light-colored striations, termed medullary rays, extend from the bases of the pyramids out into the cortex. Despite their name, the medullary rays are part of the cortex and formed by straight tubule segments (proximal straight tubules, thick ascending limbs, and collecting ducts).

A single pyramid with its surrounding cortex represents a renal lobe [8]. One lobe from a multipapillary kidney may be generally considered as equivalent to an entire unipapillary kidney, such as

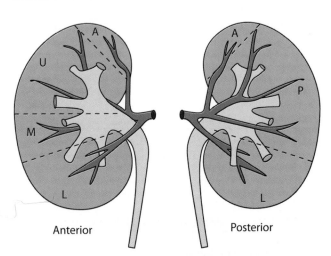

Anterior   Posterior

FIGURE 1.1: *Diagram of arterial supply of the kidney. The anterior division of the renal artery divides into segmental branches that supply the upper (U), middle (M), and lower (L) segments of the anterior surface. The apical (A) segment is usually supplied by a branch from the anterior division. The posterior division of the renal artery branches into segmental vessels that supply the posterior (P) and lower (L) segments of the posterior surface. (Modified from Graves FT. The anatomy of the intrarenal arteries and its application to segmental resection of the kidney.* Br J Surg *1954;42:132–9).*

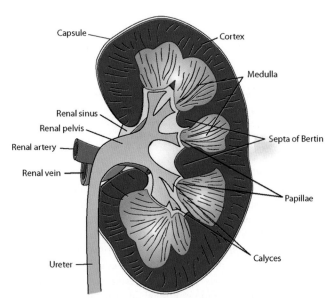

FIGURE 1.2: *Diagram of a bisected kidney showing major macroanatomic features. (Modified from Clapp WL, Croker BP. Kidney In: Mills SE, ed.* Histology for Pathologists. *3rd ed. Philadelphia: Lippincott Williams & Wilkins; 2007: 839–907.)*

those in a mouse or rat. The human kidney has an average of fourteen lobes, which are established by the twenty-eighth week of gestation. At this stage, deep surface clefts separate the lobes and fourteen calyces correspond with the same number of lobes. A process of lobar fusion during the embryologic development leads to coalescence of some pyramids and their papillae and remodeling of the corresponding calyces, reducing the number of papillae and calyces to between nine and eleven. Although the mature kidney eventually develops a smooth outer surface, a degree of persistent lobation is observed in some adult kidneys.

More lobar fusion occurs in the polar regions than in the midregion of the kidney, generating two types of pyramids (or papillae) (see Figure 1.2). Simple papillae occur mainly in the midregions, drain only one lobe, and have convex tips containing small, slit-like openings of the ducts of Bellini. Compound papillae are situated primarily in the polar regions, drain two or more adjacent fused lobes, and have flattened or concave tips with round, often gaping orifices of the ducts of Bellini. It is believed that the more open orifices of compound papillae are less capable of preventing intrarenal reflux, which may be associated with an increase in intrapelvic pressure and/or vesicoureteral reflux. This concept is supported by the observation that pyelonephritic scars associated with intrarenal reflux are found more commonly in the renal poles, where the compound papillae predominantly occur.

The renal pelvis is the saclike expansion of the upper ureter [9]. Outpouchings, the major calyces, extend from the pelvis and divide into the minor calyces, into which the papillae protrude. Elaborate extensions, termed fornices, extend from the minor calyces into the medulla. The smooth muscle within the walls of the calyces, pelvis, and ureter provides peristaltic contractions that facilitate urine movement toward the bladder.

NEPHRONS

The functional unit of the kidney is the nephron, which consists of the renal corpuscle (glomerulus and Bowman's capsule) connected to an elongated tubular component (proximal tubule, thin limbs, distal tubule), all of which are derived from the metanephric blastema. A transitional segment, the connecting tubule, joins the nephron components to a draining collecting duct, which is ureteric-bud derived. Although the collecting duct is not, strictly speaking, considered part of the nephron embryologically, practically the term nephron is used to include the nephron components and the collecting duct.

Nephron Number

Classically, it is stated there are 1 million nephrons per kidney. More recent stereological studies have revealed lower average nephron numbers, ranging from 600,000 to 800,000 per kidney. Moreover, such studies have shown that a large variation in nephron number per kidney exists among adults, from less than 500,000 to over 1,500,000 nephrons per kidney [10]. These studies have used glomerular number as a surrogate for nephron number. Nephron numbers are lower in individuals with a low birth weight, which may reflect intrauterine growth retardation or premature birth. A leading hypothesis is that a congenital deficit of nephrons associated with low birth weight predisposes individuals to acquired renal disease, including hypertension [11]. In fact,

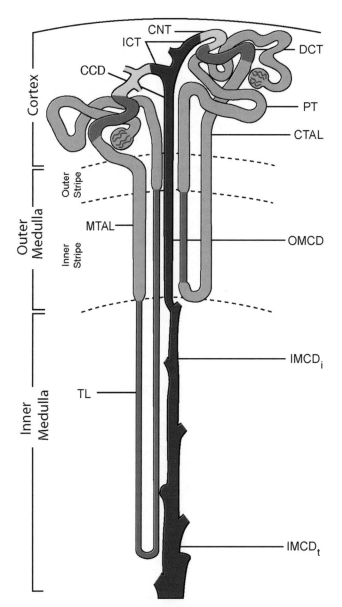

FIGURE 1.3: *Diagram depicting the segments of the nephron and the regions (zones) of the kidney. PT, proximal tubule; TL, thin limb; MTAL, medullary thick ascending limb; CTAL, cortical thick ascending limb; DCT, distal convoluted tubule; CNT, connecting tubule; ICT, initial collecting tubule; CCD, cortical collecting duct; OMCD, outer medullary collecting duct; $IMCD_i$, initial inner medullary collecting duct; $IMCD_t$, terminal inner medullary collecting duct. (Modified from Madsen KM, Tisher CC. Structural-functional relationships along the distal nephron. Am J Physiol 1986;250:F1–F15.)*

it has been reported that adults with a history of hypertension have fewer nephrons than matched normotensive controls [12].

Nephron Types

Nephrons are also classified by the length of their loop of Henle (Figure 1.3). Short-looped nephrons arise from superficial and midcortical glomeruli and form their bend within the outer medulla. Long-looped nephrons begin from juxtamedullary glomeruli and make their bend within the inner medulla. The short-looped nephrons are seven times more numerous than long-looped nephrons in the human kidney.

Nephrons are also classified as superficial, midcortical, or juxtamedullary, based on the position of their glomeruli in the cortex. Superficial nephrons have glomeruli located in the outer cortex, and they drain singly into a collecting duct. Juxtamedullary nephrons have glomeruli situated above the corticomedullary junction, and they empty into an arched arrangement of connecting segments called an arcade. Midcortical nephrons are located between the other two nephron types and most drain individually into a collecting duct.

ARCHITECTURE

The kidney has an intricate architecture that underlies its complex functions. The arrangement of nephron segments, vasculature, and interstitium provides for coordination (axial) of complex functions along the cortical–medullary axis, as well as integration (regional) of functions in a specific region of cortex or medulla.

Cortex

Cortical Labyrinth and Medullary Rays

In the cortex, the tubules are packed closely together with little interstitial space (Figure 1.4). Two architectural regions of the cortex – the cortical labyrinth and the medullary rays – can be distinguished (Figure 1.5) [13]. The cortical labyrinth is a continuous parenchymal zone that surrounds the regularly distributed medullary rays. The cortical labyrinth contains glomeruli, proximal and distal convoluted tubules, interlobular vessels and their branches, capillaries, and lymphatics. (Figure 1.6). The proximal convoluted tubules are the predominant component of the labyrinth.

The medullary rays contain the proximal and distal straight tubules and collecting ducts, all of which enter the medulla

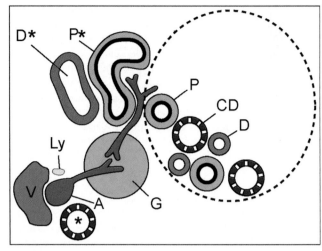

FIGURE 1.5: *Schematic drawing of architectural regions of the cortex. The cross section depicts a medullary ray (encircled by a dotted line), and the cortical labyrinth as a continuous zone (outside the dotted line). The medullary ray includes the proximal straight (P) and distal straight (D) tubules and collecting ducts (CD). The cortical labyrinth includes the glomeruli (G), proximal (P*) and distal (D*) convoluted tubules, arcades (*) of connecting tubules, arteries (A), veins (V), and lymphatics (Ly). (Modified from Kriz W, Kaissling B. Structural organization of the mammalian kidney. In: Seldin DW, Giebisch G, eds. The Kidney: Physiology and Pathophysiology. 3rd ed. Philadelphia: Lippincott Williams & Wilkins; 2000:587–654.)*

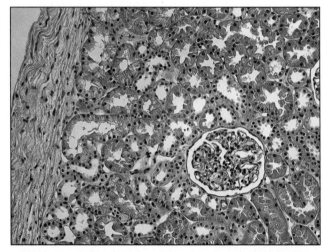

FIGURE 1.6: *Micrograph of outer cortex illustrating the cortical labyrinth. Proximal convoluted tubules are predominant. The renal capsule (left) is evident. (H&E, × 200.)*

(Figure 1.7). The distal straight tubules are the thick ascending limbs of Henle. Because of their perpendicular orientation to the corticomedullary junction, they are best identified in optimal longitudinal or cross-sections.

Renal Lobule

The renal cortex also can be partitioned into lobules. Most commonly, a renal lobule is considered as all the nephrons that

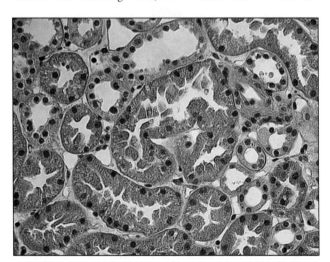

FIGURE 1.4: *Light micrograph of cortex showing compact back-to-back arrangement of tubules with minimal intervening interstitium. A few peritubular capillaries are evident. (H&E, × 400.)*

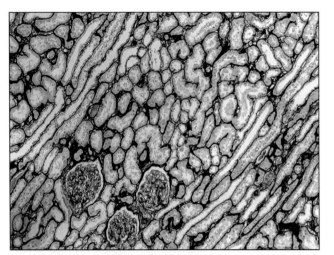

FIGURE 1.7: *Longitudinal section of cortex illustrating two linear arrangements of tubules representing medullary rays. The cortical labyrinth containing glomeruli and convoluted tubules is between the two medullary rays. (Methenamine silver, × 100.)*

surround and drain into the collecting ducts of a central positioned medullary ray. Another version proposes that the lobule consists of all the nephrons supplied by a central positioned interlobular artery. Adjacent renal lobules lack separating connective tissue septa and are difficult to demarcate histologically. Moreover, because there is no apparent structural–functional significance, the concept of the renal lobule is not favored.

Medulla

The location of the nephron segments at various levels in the medulla account for the division of the medulla into an outer and inner medulla. The relative tissue volumes for the cortex, outer medulla, and inner medulla are 70, 27, and 3 percent, respectively.

Outer Medulla

The outer medulla is subdivided into an outer and an inner stripe (see Figure 1.3). The outer stripe is relatively thin. It contains the terminal portion of the proximal straight tubules, the thick ascending limbs of Henle, and the collecting ducts. The thin limbs of Henle are not present in the outer stripe. Compared to the outer stripe, the inner stripe of the outer medulla is thicker. It contains thin descending limbs, thick ascending limbs, and collecting ducts. Proximal straight tubules do not enter the inner stripe.

Inner Medulla

The inner medulla tapers to form the papilla. The thin descending and the thin ascending limbs of Henle, and the collecting ducts are situated in the inner medulla (see Figure 1.3). Thick ascending limbs are absent in the inner medulla.

Algorithm for Architecture

Knowledge of the above architectural features allows one to determine the specific region or zone in sections of a kidney biopsy (Figure 1.8). The presence of glomeruli confirms the presence of cortex and more specifically, the cortical labyrinth. Proximal convoluted tubules are also a prominent marker of cortex and its labyrinth. A distinctive feature of proximal tubules, both convoluted and straight portions, is their periodic acid-Schiff (PAS)-positive luminal brush border. Profiles of proximal convoluted tubules are larger with more irregular or coiled (convoluted) contours than those of proximal straight tubules. The absence of convoluted portions but the presence of straight segments of

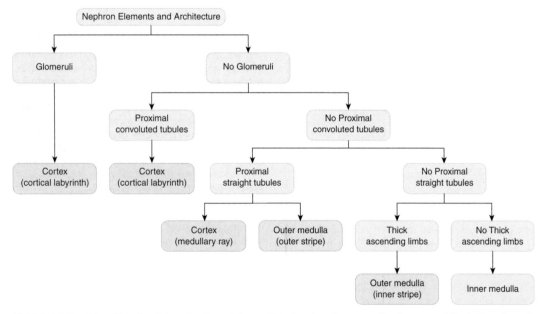

FIGURE 1.8: *Algorithm for determination of the architectural region or particular zone of the kidney based on the presence and/or absence of specific nephron components or segments.*

proximal tubules characterizes both the medullary rays of cortex and the outer stripe of the outer medulla. Although these two adjacent regions, cortex and outer stripe of outer medulla, can usually be differentiated by other tissue elements in the same section, it may be difficult near their transition. Proximal straight tubules are absent in both the inner stripe of the outer medulla and the inner medulla. However, the two regions can be distinguished by the presence of thick ascending limbs in the inner stripe of the outer medulla and their absence in the inner medulla. For example, a biopsy showing no glomeruli and no tubules with a brush border likely represents the medulla, and the presence of thick ascending limbs likely indicates the inner stripe of the outer medulla. Not uncommonly, different regions or zones are observed in a single renal biopsy.

PARENCHYMA

Knowledge of the four main components of the renal parenchyma – the vasculature, glomeruli, tubules, and interstitium – facilitates the morphologic evaluation of the kidney and an understanding of its diseases. Normal morphologic aspects and structural–functional relationships of these components are considered in the following sections. A standard nomenclature for these components exists [14].

Vasculature

Macrovasculature

The segmental arteries, branching from the anterior and posterior divisions of the main renal artery, divide to form the interlobar arteries. The interlobar arteries penetrate the parenchyma between the columns of Bertin and the pyramids. At the corticomedullary junction, the interlobar arteries give rise to the arcuate arteries, which curve along the base of the pyramids parallel to the kidney surface. From the arcuate arteries, the interlobular arteries arise and ascend within the cortical labyrinth between medullary rays. Similar to vessels elsewhere in the body, the arteries have three layers: an inner endothelial cell-lined intima, a media consisting of smooth muscle cells, and an outer collagenous adventitia. The media is separated from the intima by an internal elastic lamina. Some larger arteries have a thin external elastic lamina between the media and the adventitia. In all blood vessels, immunohistochemical studies for Factor VIII-related antigen, CD34 and CD31 stain endothelium, whereas the smooth muscle media stains with smooth muscle actin and vimentin antibodies.

Microvasculature

(Cortex). The regulation of hemodynamics in the kidney occurs, in large part, because of its intricate microvasculature (Figure 1.9) [15]. Arterioles have three layers, albeit thinner than arteries, but generally lack the internal and external elastic lamina. Arteries and arterioles have a nonfenestrated or continuous endothelium. The afferent arterioles branch off the interlobular arteries and supply the glomeruli. The angle of origin of the afferent arterioles from the interlobular arteries varies according to the area of the cortex. Afferent arterioles

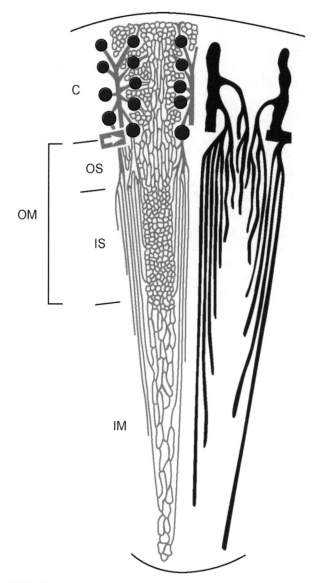

FIGURE 1.9: *Schematic of renal microvasculature. The arterial vessels, glomeruli, and capillaries are represented on the left side (red). An arcuate artery gives rise to an interlobular artery which ascends in the cortex and branches to form afferent arterioles which supply the glomeruli. The efferent arterioles of the superficial and midcortical glomeruli divide to form the peritubular capillaries of the cortical labyrinth and the medullary rays. The efferent arterioles of the juxtamedullary glomeruli descend into the medulla and form the descending vasa recta (DVR) which supply the adjacent capillary plexuses. The DVR traverse the inner stripe of the outer medulla within vascular bundles (shown as straight vessels). Note the prominent capillary network in the inner stripe of the outer medulla. The right side (blue) depicts the venous system. It may be superimposed on the arterial system (left). The ascending vasa recta (AVR) drain the medulla and empty into the interlobular and arcuate veins, which drain the cortex. The AVR from the inner medulla travel within the vascular bundles, whereas most AVR from the inner stripe travel between the bundles. (Modified from Kriz W, Kaissling B. Structural organization of the mammalian kidney. In: Seldin DW, Giebisch G, eds. The Kidney: Physiology and Pathophysiology. 3rd ed. Philadelphia: Lippincott Williams & Wilkins; 2000: 587–654.)*

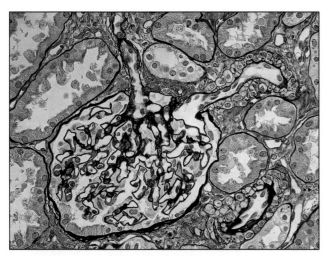

FIGURE 1.10: *Light micrograph of glomerulus depicting both afferent and efferent arterioles. The afferent arteriole (right) has a more prominent media of smooth muscle cells. (Methenamine silver, × 400.)*

supplying the superficial glomeruli arise at an acute angle; afferent arterioles to midcortical glomeruli travel transversely for the most part and those to juxtamedullary glomeruli tend to originate at a recurrent angle. The efferent arterioles drain the glomeruli, may loop partially around the glomerular tuft, and branch to form complex capillary networks that supply the cortical and medullary parenchyma. Thus, the blood supply to the renal parenchyma is postglomerular. At the vascular pole of the glomerulus, the afferent arteriole enters and the efferent arteriole exits (Figure 1.10) [16]. The afferent arteriole has a larger diameter than the efferent arteriole because of a larger lumen and thicker media. Within the media, the nuclei of smooth muscle cells are larger in the afferent arteriole. In contrast to the afferent arteriole, the efferent arteriole has a more continuous intraglomerular segment. At the glomerular tuft-exit, endothelial cells may bulge into the lumen of the efferent arteriole, reducing its diameter. These differences may be difficult to recognize since both the afferent and efferent arterioles of a glomerulus are seen only in fortuitous planes of section. However, the afferent arteriole may be identified by an observed connection to an interlobular artery or the presence of hyalinosis, which only involves the afferent arteriole in nondiabetics. The afferent arteriole can also be distinguished by the presence of intramural granular cells containing renin. In addition, the myosin heavy chain B isoform (MHC-B) is expressed in afferent, but not efferent arterioles [17]. The afferent and efferent arterioles regulate glomerular inflow and outflow resistance, respectively. For example, an increased afferent arteriolar tone prevents an elevated perfusion pressure being transmitted to the glomerular capillaries, preserving the glomerular filtration rate (GFR). In contrast, an increased efferent arteriolar tone maintains the GFR when the perfusion pressure is reduced.

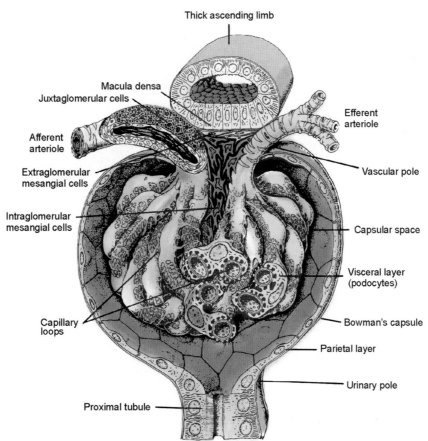

FIGURE 1.11: *Three-dimensional schematic drawing of the glomerulus. (Modified from Geneser F. Textbook of Histology. Philadelphia: Lea & Febiger; 1986.)*

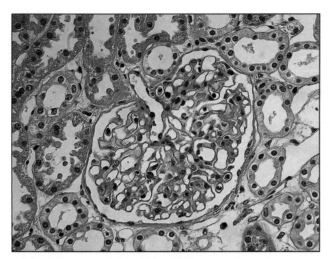

FIGURE 1.12:   Light micrograph of a glomerulus exhibiting a round configuration and filling Bowman's space. It shows normal cellularity and patent capillary lumens. (H&E, × 400).

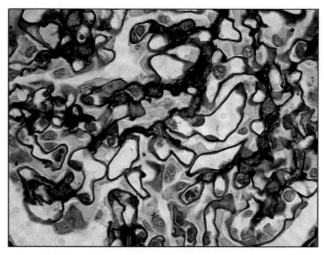

FIGURE 1.14:   Higher magnification light micrograph demonstrating thin glomerular basement membranes and narrow profiles of mesangial matrix. The glomerular cell types can be distinguished. (Methenamine silver, × 1,000).

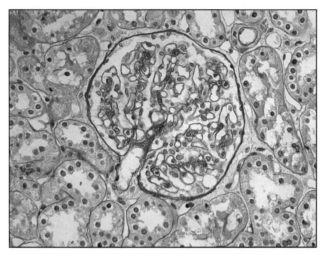

FIGURE 1.13:   Glomerulus showing delicate capillary loops and inconspicuous mesangium. (PAS, × 400.)

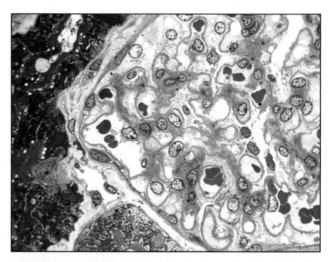

FIGURE 1.15:   Light micrograph of a glomerulus illustrating the intrinsic cell types: endothelial cells, mesangial cells, podocytes, and parietal epithelial cells. (1- um toluidine blue-stained Epon section, × 1,000.)

The efferent arterioles give rise to a complex postglomerular microcirculation (see Figure 1.9). Although gradations exist, three types of efferent arterioles may be distinguished. The superficial efferent arterioles branch into capillary networks that supply convoluted tubules of the outer cortical labyrinth. Efferent arterioles of midcortical glomeruli generate capillaries that supply the adjacent cortical labyrinths as well as the medullary rays in that region. Efferent arterioles from juxtamedullary glomeruli descend and supply the medulla. When compared to the efferent arterioles of superficial and midcortical glomeruli, those from juxtamedullary glomeruli have a larger diameter with thicker smooth muscle layers on cross section.

Of the total renal blood flow, 85 to 90 percent goes to the cortex. Convoluted tubules in the superficial cortex are perfused by capillaries arising from the efferent arterioles of their parent glomeruli. However, in the midcortex and inner cortex, there is a disassociation between the tubules and the origin of their supplying capillary network. Most tubules in the midcortex and inner cortex are perfused by capillaries from efferent arterioles of other glomeruli. In other words, the peritubular capillaries supplying a given nephron in the mid- or inner cortex are derived from several different efferent arterioles. As a result of glomerular filtration, the blood leaving the glomerulus in the efferent arterioles and entering the peritubular capillaries has a relatively high protein concentration, and thus an elevated oncotic pressure. Also, the flow of blood through two resistance vessels in series (afferent and efferent arterioles) leads to a decreased hydrostatic pressure within the peritubular capillaries. These physiologic factors favor the uptake of fluid reabsorbed from the proximal tubules into the peritubular capillaries.

(Medulla). The efferent arterioles of juxtamedullary glomeruli are the major source of blood supply to the medulla, which

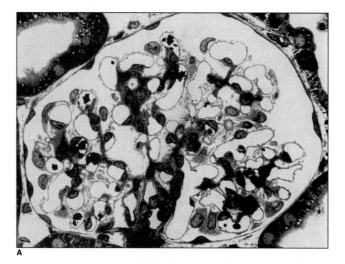

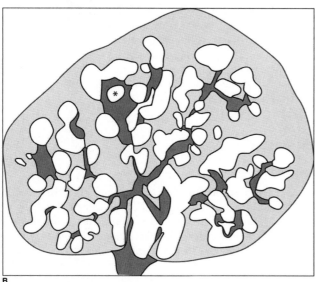

FIGURE 1.16: *Mesangial structure. A. Light micrograph of a rat glomerulus in a 0.5 um Epon section through the vascular pole. In the periphery, a "mesangial loop" (*), representing the complete enclosure of a capillary by mesangium, is observed. (× 960) B. Tracing of the glomerulus in A. showing the outline of the GBM around the capillaries and the mesangium (gray). Although on sections the mesangium may appear as islets separate from the main mesangial stalk at the vascular pole, three-dimensional studies have revealed there is continuity of the entire mesangium within a glomerulus. (× 430) (From Inkyo-Hayasaka K, Sakai T, Kobayashi N, et al. Three-dimensional analysis of the whole mesangium in the rat. Kidney Int 1996;50:672–83.)*

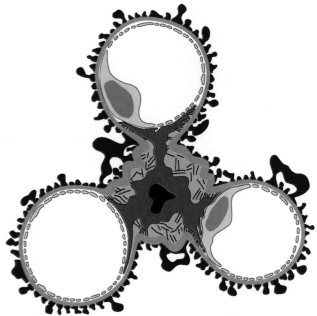

FIGURE 1.17: *Schematic illustrating the relationship between the glomerular capillaries, mesangium and GBM. The surrounding podocyte foot processes (dark brown) and the lining endothelium (light cytoplasm with blue nuclei) are illustrated. The mesangium consists of the central mesangial cell (medium brown cytoplasm and black nucleus) surrounded by the mesangial matrix (gray fibrillar texture). Note that the GBM encloses the mesangium and its attached capillaries. Two areas of the mesangium are shown: the juxtacapillary region adjacent to the capillary endothelium and the central axial region surrounded by the perimesangial GBM. Cytoplasmic processes of mesangial cells are connected to the GBM, directly or indirectly by microfibrils in the mesangial matrix. (Modified from Kriz W, Elger M, Lemley L, Sakai T. Structure of the glomerular mesangium: a biomechanical interpretation. Kidney Int. Suppl. 1990;30:S2–S9.)*

receives 10 to 15 percent of the total renal blood flow (see Figure 1.9). They extend downward and some early branches form a capillary network supplying tubules in the outer stripe of the outer medulla. However, most of the branches continue as the descending vasa recta organized into vascular bundles as they descend through the inner stripe of the outer medulla. At intervals, branches exit the bundles to form capillary plexuses supplying tubules between the bundles in the inner stripe. Descending vasa recta enter the inner medulla and their branches form capillary networks, which converge to form the ascending vasa recta.

Draining the inner medulla at various levels, the ascending vasa recta traverse the inner stripe within the vascular bundles. Some ascending venous recta, draining the inner stripe, ascend between the vascular bundles to the outer stripe. All the ascending vasa recta traverse the outer stripe as individual vessels, and finally empty into the interlobular or arcuate veins.

The descending vasa recta (DVR) display a continuous endothelium and are surrounded by pericytes that are immunoreactive for smooth muscle actin. The aquaporin-1 (AQP1) water channel and the facilitative urea transporter, UT-B, are expressed in the DVR. In contrast, the ascending vasa recta (AVR) have a highly fenestrated endothelium that is immunoreactive for the fenestrae protein PV-1. The counterflow arrangement of the DVR and AVR provides a countercurrent exchange of solutes and water in the medulla [18]. Solutes diffuse from the medulla into the DVR and as blood returns in the AVR, solutes diffuse into the interstitium. Water loss from the DVR, via AQP1, is shunted to the AVR. As a result, effective blood flow through the medulla is lowered and medullary hypertonicity is preserved, factors that facilitate urinary concentration.

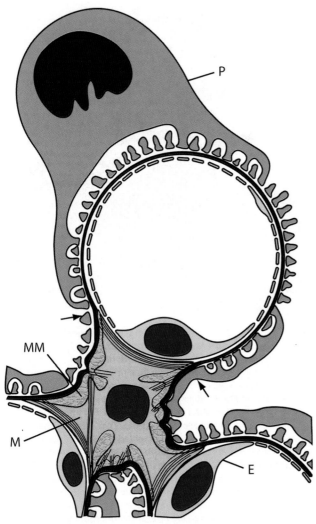

FIGURE 1.18: *Drawing of a glomerular capillary and the mesangium. In the center, a mesangial cell (M, yellow cytoplasm), is surrounded by mesangial matrix (MM, tan). Mesangial cell processes, containing microfilament bundles, extend to the GBM (black). The mesangial matrix is rich in microfibrils, which participate in connecting the mesangial cell processes to the GBM. The GBM surrounds the peripheral portion of the capillary, and at the "mesangial angles" (arrows), begins to cover the mesangium. The capillary endothelium (E) is fenestrated. The podocyte (P) foot processes overlie the entire GBM. (Modified from Reilly Jr RF, Bulger RE, Kriz W. Structural-functional relationships in the kidney. In: Schrier EW, ed.* Diseases of the Kidney & Urinary Tract. *8th ed. Philadelphia: Lippincott Williams & Wilkins;2007:2–53.)*

Lymphatics

Two lymphatic networks exist in the kidney: a deeper cortical system and a less extensive capsular network. Lymphatics originate as small vessels around the interlobular arteries and empty into arcuate and interlobar lymphatics, which drain into larger lymph vessels at the renal hilus. Valves are present in the interlobar and hilar lymphatics. Lymphatics are sparse to absent in the medulla. The less prominent lymphatics within the renal capsule drain into subcapsular lymphatic channels

that appear to communicate with the major lymphatics in the cortex.

The lymphatics are situated in the periarterial loose connective tissue but they are not prominent on routine histologic sections. Lymphatic vessels have a thin endothelial layer without an underlying basement membrane. The identification of lymphatics has been facilitated by the availability of markers of lymphatic endothelium including VEGFR-3, LYVE-1, Prox-1, and podoplanin. The lymphatics may serve as a route for the intrarenal distribution of hormones and inflammatory cells.

Nerves

The nerve supply to the kidney derives largely from the celiac plexus [19]. Nerve fibers, immunoreactive for neurofilament and S-100, accompany the arteries and arterioles in the cortex and outer medulla. There is prominent innervation of the juxtaglomerular apparatus. Nerve fibers escort the efferent arterioles and descending vasa recta until they lose their surrounding smooth muscle layer. Although the direct relationship of nerve terminals to tubules has been somewhat controversial, autoradiographic studies have provided evidence for the innervation of both proximal and distal convoluted tubules, and especially the thick ascending limb.

Glomerulus

General Features

The renal glomerulus (or corpuscle) is a tuft of interconnected capillaries, matrix, and specialized cells enclosed within Bowman's capsule (Figure 1.11). Rather than simply representing a cluster of capillaries, the glomerulus is one of the most intricate structures in the body. The capillaries are attached to a central supporting region termed the mesangium, which contains cells and surrounding matrix material. The capillaries are lined by a thin layer of endothelial cells contain an underlying basement membrane, and are covered by podocytes (epithelial cells) that form the visceral layer of Bowman's capsule. At the vascular pole where the afferent arteriole enters the glomerulus and the efferent arteriole exits, the visceral epithelium is continuous with the parietal epithelium lining Bowman's capsule. The glomerular tuft projects into Bowman's space, the cavity between the visceral and parietal epithelial layers. At the urinary pole, this space and the parietal epithelium continue into the lumen and epithelium of the proximal tubule. Thus, the glomerulus resembles a blind-pouched extension (Bowman's capsule) of the proximal tubule invaginated by a tuft of capillaries. Upon entering the tuft, the afferent arteriole divides into branches, which are arranged as lobules. Anastomoses exist between individual capillaries within a lobule as well as between lobules. This lobular arrangement is often inconspicuous in light microscopic sections. The efferent arteriole, formed by rejoined capillaries, is separated from the afferent arteriole only by the mesangium, and leaves the glomerulus at the vascular pole. In contrast to the afferent arteriole, the efferent arteriole has a more continuous intraglomerular segment.

The human glomerulus is round to oval with an average diameter of 200 μm. However, a significant degree of variation in

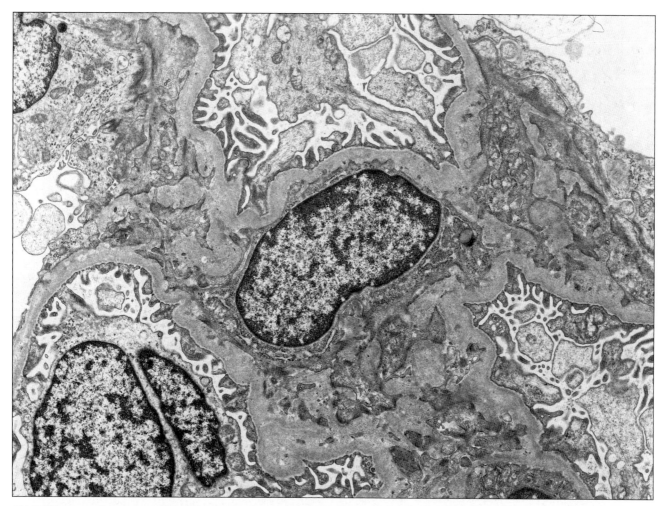

FIGURE 1.19: *Transmission electron micrograph showing glomerular mesangium. The central axial region of the mesangium is surrounded by the perimesangial GBM. Juxtacapillary regions where the capillary endothelium adjoins the mesangium are evident. Elongated processes from the central mesangial cell extend under the endothelium. Strands of mesangial matrix are present near the endothelial mesangial interface. (× 9,000, Courtesy of C.C. Tisher, MD.)*

individual glomerular volume exists in the normal human kidney. Although juxtaglomerular glomeruli have been traditionally reported to be larger than superficial glomeruli, recent stereological studies have found no size difference between these glomerular populations in the normal human kidney of young adults 20 to 30 years of age [20]. In the normal appearing kidneys of older adults, 50 to 70 years of age, mean glomerular volume in the superficial cortex was found to be 20 percent larger than in the juxtamedullary cortex [20]. This may reflect a degree of compensatory hypertrophy of the glomeruli in the superficial cortex, because, in this older age group, global glomerulosclerosis was greater in the superficial cortex when compared to the juxtaglomerular cortex.

An accurate assessment of glomerular cellularity requires histologic sections 2 to 4 μm thick (Figure 1.12). This avoids a misinterpretation of glomerular hypercellularity that may occur with increased section thickness. Generally, within a capillary lumen, there are no more than one to two endothelial cell nuclei and within the contiguous mesangial region, there are no more than three mesangial cell nuclei. Because greater numbers of cells may be seen near the vascular pole, where the intraglomerular and extraglomerular mesangial regions coa-

lesce (mesangial stalk), this area should be avoided when evaluating glomerular cellularity. In addition to hematoxylin and eosin (H & E) stained sections, the PAS and methenamine silver histochemical stains are commonly used to evaluate the renal parenchyma, especially the glomerulus. The PAS and especially the silver stains delineate the mesangial matrix and the glomerular basement membrane (GBM) (Figures 1.13 and 1.14). On thin sections, the capillary loops can be demarcated from the mesangium, and the endothelial cells, mesangial cells, and podocytes can be distinguished (Figure 1.15).

Sclerosis of an entire glomerulus (global glomerulosclerosis) may occur in normal kidneys as part of aging, and does not necessarily reflect renal disease [21,22]. Under the age of 40 years, it has been reported that 95 percent of normal kidneys should have less than 10 percent globally sclerotic glomeruli [21]. However, in this study, the mean percentage of glomerulosclerosis under the age of 40 years was 2.4 percent, appreciably less than the 10 percent value sometimes stated as the normal value in the literature. Another study demonstrated that the mean for globally sclerotic glomeruli was less than 3 percent in any age group less than 56 years [22]. In this study, the mean

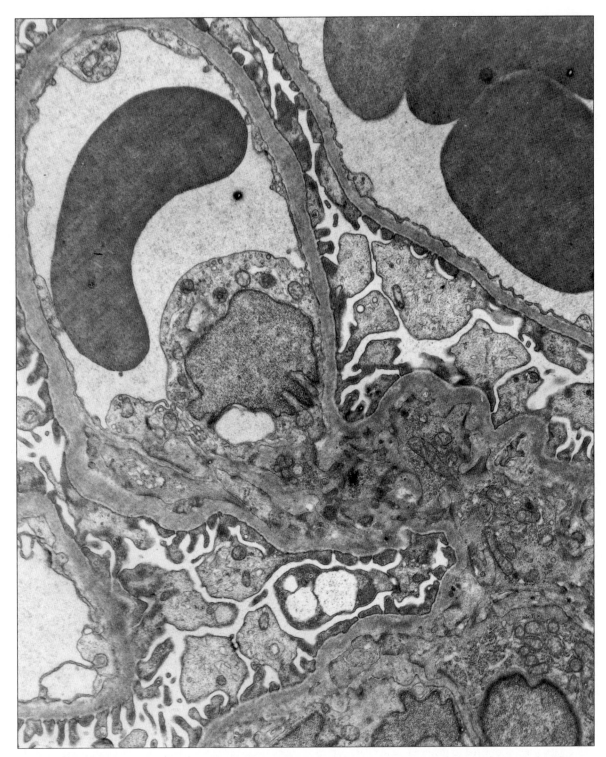

FIGURE 1.20: *Electron micrograph of glomerulus depicting capillary loop segments and portion of the mesangium. A endothelial cell nucleus overlies an irregular interface with the mesangium. (× 11,500, Courtesy of C.C. Tisher, MD.)*

percentage of global glomerulosclerosis in normal kidneys was: < 1 percent under the age of 20 years, 2 percent between 20 and 40 years, 7 percent between 40 and 60 years, and 11 percent between 60 to 80 years. The 90th percentile for global glomerulosclerosis may be generally estimated within a given patient by subtracting 10 from half the patient's age [22].

The mesangium represents the main stem of the glomerulus, providing a scaffold to which the capillaries are attached. The inner aspect of the capillary loop abuts the mesangium, whereas the peripheral portion of the loop bulges into Bowman's space. This peripheral portion, covered by the GBM and podocytes, is where filtration occurs. By light microscopy, this peripheral

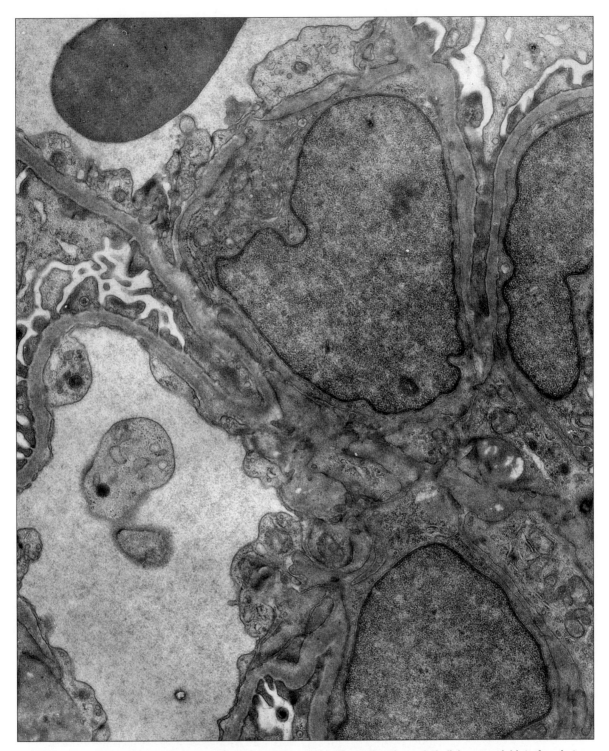

FIGURE 1.21: *Transmission electron micrograph of glomerulus illustrating the endothelial-mesangial interface in two capillary loops. The irregular interface on the left displays endothelium, mesangial cell processes and fragments of mesangial matrix. (× 10,000, Courtesy of C.C. Tisher, MD.)*

portion is often referred to as the glomerular capillary wall. By electron microscopy, the layers of the capillary wall can be distinguished: a fenestrated endothelium, the GBM, and the podocytes, all of which contribute to the filtration barrier.

Endothelial Cells

The inner surface of the glomerular capillaries is lined by a thin fenestrated endothelium. By light microscopy, the endothelial cells have indistinct wispy cytoplasm and oval, crescent-shaped

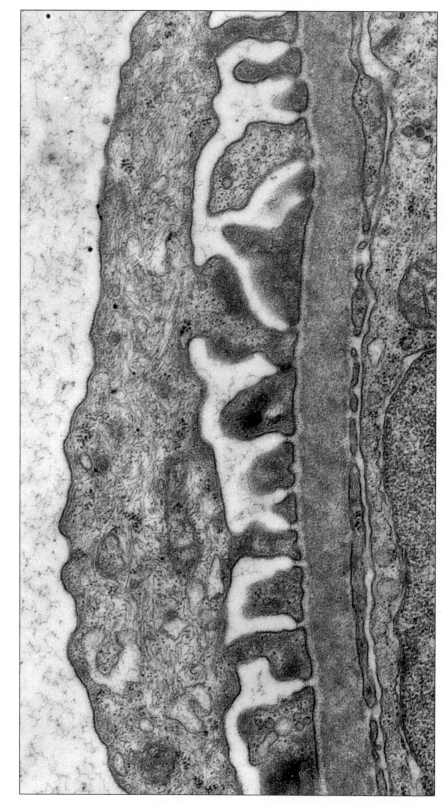

FIGURE 1.22:   Electron micrograph of glomerular capillary illustrating foot processes extending from a podocyte cytoplasmic process. The foot processes are embedded in the lamina rara externa of the GBM. Some slit diaphragms are observed connecting adjacent foot processes. The subpodocyte space underlies the cytoplasmic process that is giving off the foot processes. A thin fenestrated endothelium is present. (× 40,000, Courtesy of C.C. Tisher, MD.)

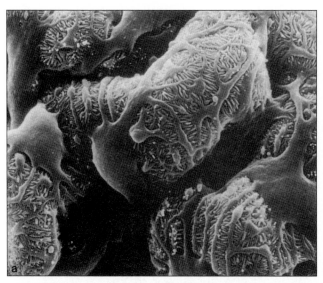

FIGURE 1.23: *Scanning electron micrograph of rat glomerulus demonstrating the elaborate podoctye cytoarchitecture. Mutiple primary processes extend from the cell body of the podocytes to wrap around the capillary loops. The primary processes divide into individual foot processes. (× 5,200) (From Kriz W, Hackenthal E, Nobiling R, et al. A role for podocyte to counteract capillary wall distention.* **Kidney Int** *1994;45:369–76.)*

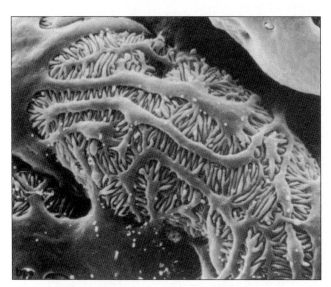

FIGURE 1.24: *Scanning electron micrograph illustrating the outer surface of a glomerular capillary loop from a rat kidney. The foot processes interdigitate with the foot processes of adjacent podocytes. Narrow slits, known as the filtration slit pores, are present between adjacent foot processes. (× 10,000) (From Kriz W, Hackenthal E, Nobiling R, et al. A role for podocyte to counteract capillary wall distention.* **Kidney Int** *1994;45:369–76.)*

or elongated nuclei. Their nuclei are situated within the capillary lumina, often adjacent to the mesangium (see Figures 1.14 and 1.15). The endothelium is perforated by round to oval fenestrae or pores measuring 70 to 100 nm in diameter. Traditionally, the glomerular endothelial fenestrae were believed to lack diaphragms, but thin diaphragms bridging across the fenestrae have been noted when modified fixation methods for electron microscopy are used. Moreover, glomerular endothelial cells have a glycocalyx surface layer which also fills the fenestrae forming "sieve plugs" [23,24]. Emerging evidence suggests this glycocalyx may be an important component of the filtration barrier. Polyanionic glycoproteins, including the sialoprotein podocalyxin, on the endothelial cells impart a negative surface charge. Nonfenestrated regions forming surface ridge-like structures are located near endothelial cell borders.

Glomerular endothelial cells produce molecules of the coagulation system, including von Willebrand factor and thrombomodulin. They synthesize the vasoactive molecules nitric oxide (NO), a vasodilator, and endothelin-1, a vasoconstrictor. Receptors for vascular endothelial growth factor (VEGF) are present on glomerular endothelial cells, and this molecule produced by podocytes is an important regulator of glomerular endothelial function. Both in vivo and in vitro studies have shown that VEGF induces fenestrae and increases the permeability of endothelial cells. Podocyte-derived VEGF plays an important role in the maintenance of glomerular endothelial differentiation and in the regulation of endothelial permeability [25].

Mesangium

To the student of the glomerulus, the mesangium has always appeared somewhat mysterious. The mesangium, composed of mesangial cells and a surrounding matrix, provides a branching scaffold for the glomerular capillaries. By light microscopy, mesangial cells can be identified by their central position within the mesangial matrix between capillary lumens (see Figures 1.14 and 1.15). In contrast to other glomerular cell types, mesangial cells have dark-staining nuclei. On histologic sections, the term "one mesangial area" is commonly used for the mesangium supporting the immediate adjacent (usually 1–3) capillary loops. As previously mentioned, normally there are fewer than three mesangial cell nuclei per mesangial area. The mesangial matrix is observed as a PAS- and silver-positive arborizing framework.

Three-dimensional analysis of the entire mesangium by ultrastructural reconstructions has demonstrated the mesangium as a continuous tree-like branching structure, without islets of mesangium, separated from the main mesangial tree [26]. These reconstruction studies showed the mesangium has three major trunks, each of which is connected to the vascular pole. Although the inner part (juxtamesangial) of a typical capillary loop is attached to the mesangium, the larger perimeter of the loop (peripheral part) projects into Bowman's space. However, the mesangial reconstruction studies revealed that some capillary loops may be completely surrounded by mesangium, forming so-called mesangial loops (Figures 1.16A) and (B).

The endothelium forms a continuous layer around the inner circumference of the glomerular capillary, but the GBM and podocyte layer do not completely encircle the capillary but enclose the mesangium between the capillaries (Figure 1.17). Thus, the GBM has a peripheral (pericapillary) segment and a perimesangial segment. The points where the GBM no longer encircles the capillary and begins to cover the mesangium are

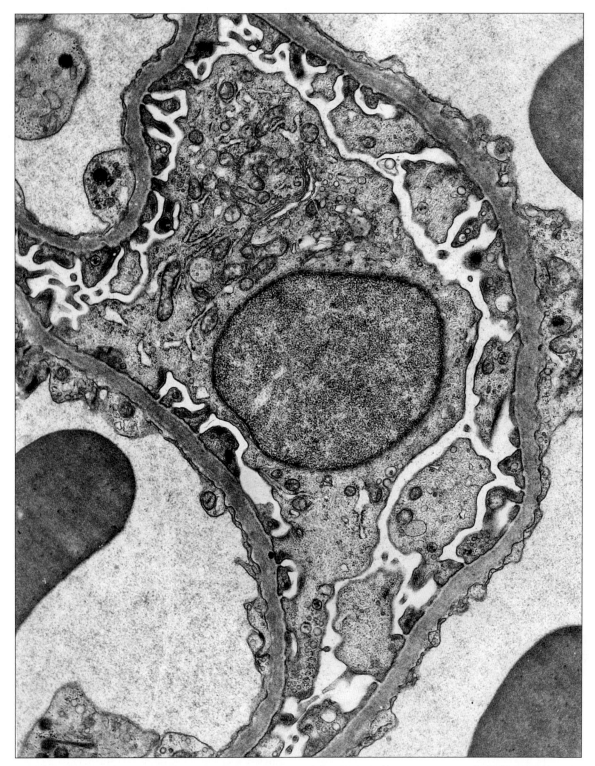

FIGURE 1.25: *Electron micrograph of glomerulus showing at least two capillary loop segments. A podocyte within Bowman's space is shown extending foot processes to each of the loops. Organelles, including mitochondria, vesicles, and a Golgi complex are evident in the podocyte cytoplasm. (× 9,000, Courtesy of C.C. Tisher, MD.)*

known as the "mesangial angles." Two general topographic areas within the mesangium can be distinguished: a juxtacapillary region bordering the capillary endothelium and a central axial region surrounded by the perimesangial GBM (Figure 1.18).

(Mesangial Cells). Mesangial cells are irregular in shape, with many elongated cytoplasmic processes that extend toward the endothelium and the perimesangial GBM (Figure 1.19). Near the endothelial interface, finger-like mesangial processes

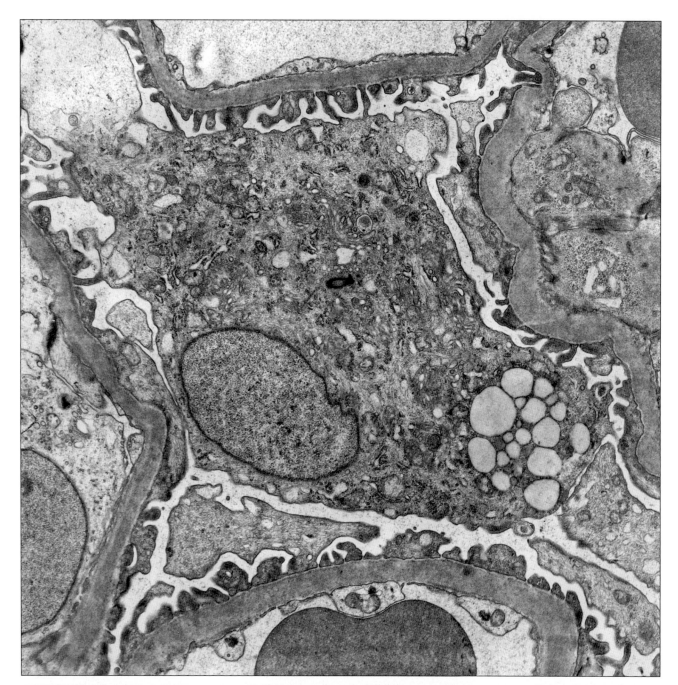

FIGURE 1.26: *Transmission electron micrograph demonstrating a podocyte with abundant cytoplasm containing an assortment of organelles, including endocytic vacuoles. Foot processes from the podocyte extend to four capillary loops. (× 8,600, Courtesy of C.C. Tisher, MD.)*

may extend a short distance into the narrow space between the endothelium and the GBM (Figures 1.20 and 2.21). In pathologic processes, these mesangial cell processes may insinuate between the endothelium and GBM for a considerable distance along the peripheral capillary wall (mesangial interposition). Bundles of microfilaments are prominent in the mesangial cell processes, which anchor to the mesangial angles of the GBM as well as the perimesangial GBM. In addition, the cellular processes connect to the GBM indirectly through extracellular microfibrils in the mesangial matrix. Several receptors of the

β-integrin family on mesangial cells likely mediate these attachments, via interaction with molecules, such as fibronectin, in the mesangial matrix. The mesangium is continuous with the extraglomerular mesangium, a part of the juxtaglomerular apparatus (JGA), along the glomerular stalk. The intraglomerular and extraglomerular mesangial cells (lacis or cells of Goormaghtigh) are similar and gap junctions exist between them. Interestingly, mesangial cells residing in the extraglomerular mesangial region may migrate and repopulate the intraglomerular mesangium upon glomerular injury [27].

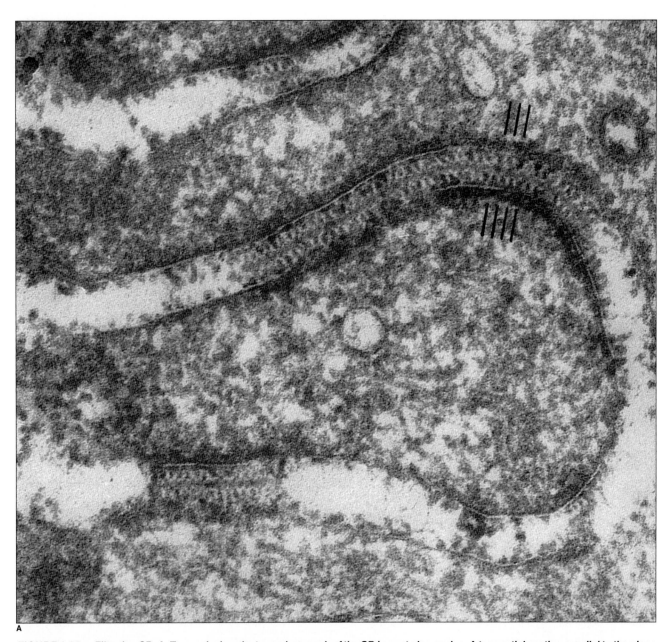

A

FIGURE 1.27: Filtration SD. A. Transmission electron micrograph of the SD in a rat glomerulus. A tangential section parallel to the plane of the GBM reveals cross-bridges extending across the space between two adjacent foot processes. A central filament appears as a longitudinal density in the space. In an area (marks), the cross-bridges appear to alternate on either side of the central filament giving the diaphragm a zipper-like appearance. × 153,000) B. Schematic diagram of the filtration slit diaphragm showing average dimensions of the pores between the cross-bridges, the cross-bridges and the central filament. The zipper-like substructure is evident in this model. (From Rodewald R, Karnovsky MJ. Porous substructure of the glomerular slit diaphragm in the rat and mouse. J Cell Biol 1974;60:423–33.)

Mesangial cells have similarities to modified smooth muscle cells or pericytes. They express contractile proteins such as myosin, α-actinin, and tropomyosin. Contraction as well as relaxation of mesangial cells has been documented, primarily in cultured mesangial cells. Because of these properties and their centrilobular or intercapillary location, mesangial cells are poised to participate in the regulation of glomerular filtration. This concept is attractive when one considers that mesangial cell processes connect to the GBM at two opposing mesangial angles of a single capillary, providing a possible bio-

mechanical advantage. Do mesangial cells have a dynamic or a static functional role in the control of glomerular filtration? [28]. Some studies suggest that dynamic (isotonic) mesangial cell contraction may alter capillary loop filtration by decreasing the filtration surface area. Others favor the idea that mesangial cell contraction is static (isometric) in nature, creating wall tension to counteract distending forces, resulting from the intra-capillary hydraulic pressure.

Mesangial cells have phagocytic capability and may play a role in the clearance of macromolecules, including immune

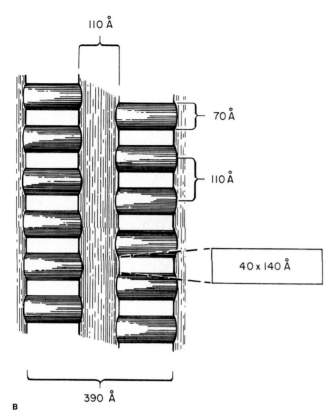

B

FIGURE 1.27: (continued)

complexes, from the mesangium. However, mesangial cells are not professional phagocytes, like blood-derived monocytes/macrophages. It is recognized that a small population (<10 percent) of cells in the mesangium of rodents are bone-marrow-derived macrophages and they play a role in immune responsiveness. The presence of such cells in the mesangium of human glomeruli remains to be clarified. Mesangial cells can respond to, as well as produce, a variety of molecules, including platelet-derived growth factor (PDGF), interleukin I and archidonic acid metabolites, which may play a role in the response to glomerular injury.

(Mesangial Matrix). The mesangial matrix fills the irregular spaces surrounding mesangial cells (see Figures 1.17 and 1.18). On electron microscopy, the mesangial matrix is slightly less electron-dense and more fibrillar than the GBM. The fibrillar character may be explained by the presence of abundant microfibrils, nonbranching structures, 10 to 12 nm in diameter and with a hollow core. The microfibrils, considered as "microtendons," connect the mesangial cell processes with the GBM. The proteins, fibrillin-1 and fibrillin-2, especially the former, are the major proteins of the microfibrils, but other associated proteins include microfibril-associated proteins (MAGP-1 and -2) and latent transforming growth factor-binding protein-1 (LTBP-1) [29,30]. Fibrillin-1-associated microfibrils have been shown to interact with perlecan, an intrinsic basement membrane protein. Elastin, a protein associated with the microfibrils of elastic fibers, is not present in the mesangium but is found in the

afferent and efferent arterioles. The mesangial matrix contains other proteins, including fibronectin, type IV collagen α-1 and α-2 chains (not α-3, α-4, or α-5 chains), type V collagen, and the proteoglycans perlecan and bamacan (but not agrin).

The interface between the capillary lumen and the adjacent mesangium is formed solely by the fenestrated endothelium, and may be considered somewhat leaky, giving rise to the belief that some plasma flow constantly seeps through the mesangial matrix. This notion is supported by studies, which show that injected small tracers, such as ferritin, rapidly enter the mesangium and appear in the mesangial matrix. Morphologic investigations have demonstrated spaces or "channels" in the matrix that lack surrounding membranes but do accumulate the tracers [31]. The pathways of flow through the mesangium and the exit routes are not well understood. Studies suggest the existence of at least three exit pathways of mesangial flow: filtration across the perimesangial GBM, contributing to the peripheral capillary wall ultrafiltrate in Bowman's space; fluid movement through mesangial channels into efferent segments of glomerular capillary loops; and flow through mesangial channels to the extraglomerular mesangial matrix of the JGA [32].

GBM

Unlike most basement membranes, the GBM is considerably thicker and situated between two cell layers, endothelial cells and podocytes. The GBM completely invests the endothelium of the peripheral capillary loops (pericapillary GBM) and the mesangium (perimesangial GBM) between loops. Although H&E- and PAS-stained histologic sections stain the GBM, the capillary luminal contents and endothelial and podocyte cytoplasm may also stain, making an evaluation of possible GBM abnormalities (thickening or irregularities) difficult. The silver stain reveals a sharper outline of the GBM since it is more specific for basement membranes (see Figure 1.14). On electron microscopy, the GBM consists of three layers: a central electron-dense layer, the lamina densa, and two surrounding thinner more electron-lucent layers, the lamina rara interna (between lamina densa and endothelium) and the lamina rara externa (between lamina densa and podocytes) (Figure 1.22). This trilaminar appearance is significantly less prominent in humans compared to rodents. In adults, the GBM has a mean thickness of 310–340 nm, and is significantly thicker in men than in women.

Like all basement membranes, the GBM is composed of glycoproteins and proteoglycans. The major glycoproteins of the GBM include type IV collagen, laminin, and entactin/nidogen. Proteoglycans of the GBM include agrin, perlecan, and type XVIII collagen, but the latter two localize primarily to the mesangial matrix. The unique character of the GBM is established by the intricate assembly of specific isoforms from the above protein families. Collagen type IV is the major component of the GBM [33,34]. Six chains, α1(IV) through α6(IV), represent the type IV collagen family. Three chains of collagen IV self-associate to form triple helical molecules termed protomers. Despite many possible combinations, the six chains form only three types of protomers, designated as α1.α1.α2(IV), α3.α4.α5(IV), and α5.α5.α6(IV). Protomers associate end-to-end at the carboxy terminal domains to form hexamers, and the amino terminal domains of four protomers bind side-to-side

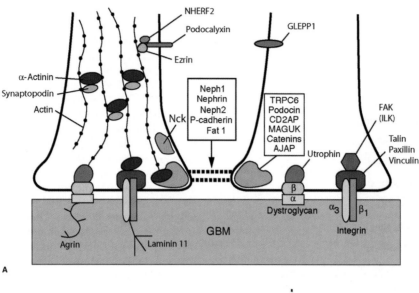

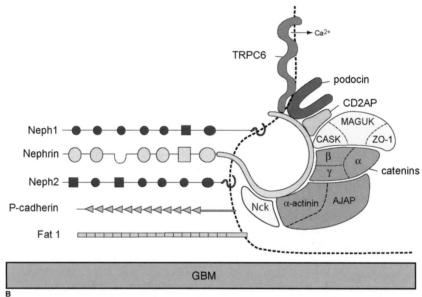

FIGURE 1.28: *Molecular components of the podocyte foot process. A. Diagram of the molecules and their interactions within the membrane domains of the podocyte. See the text for details. B. Schematic model of the filtration SD domain of the podocyte. The right side portrays the interactions of the nephrin-associated multiprotein complex within the foot process membrane and cytoplasm. The left side illustrates the molecules of the slit diaphragm itself, which bridges between adjacent foot processes. See the text for details. (Modified from Clapp WL, Croker BP. Kidney. In: Mills SE, ed. Histology for Pathologists, 3rd ed. Philadelphia: Lippincott Williams & Wilkins; 2007: 839–907.)*

to form tetramers. This assembly creates a polymerized network which serves as a scaffold for integration of other GBM molecules. Three sets of collagen IV networks form: the α1.α1.α2(IV)–α1.α1.α2(IV), the α3.α4.α5(IV)–α3.α4.α5(IV), and the α1.α1.α2(IV)–α5.α5.α6(IV) networks. The network of only α1/α2(IV) chains is present in nearly all basement membranes, whereas the network of only α3/α4/α5(IV) chains and the α1.α1.α2(IV)–α5.α5.α6(IV) network have a more restricted expression. The α3.α4.α5(IV)–α3.α4.α5(IV) network predominates in the adult GBM. The α1.α1.α2(IV)–α5.α5.α6(IV) net-

work is found in Bowman's capsule. Mutations of the genes encoding the α3, α4, and α5 (IV) chains cause Alport syndrome. Autoantibodies targeted to the carboxyterminal α3(IV) chain are responsible for anti-GBM disease.

Laminins represent a large family of heterotrimeric molecules composed of three chains: α, β, and γ. At least five different alpha, four beta, and three gamma chains exist, which can assemble in different combination to form distinct heterotrimers. Laminin- 521, containing the α5, β2, and γ1 chains, is the major laminin isoform in the adult GBM. Entactin (also called

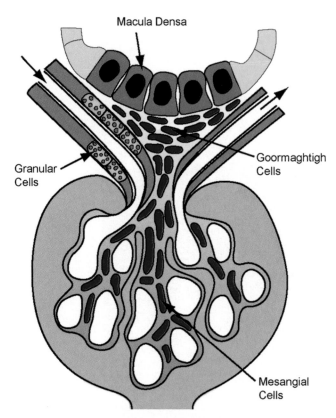

FIGURE 1.29: *Schematic of JGA depicting main components. (Modified from Kriz W, Kaissling B. Structural organization of the mammalian kidney. In: Seldin DW, Giebisch G, eds. **The Kidney: Physiology and Pathophysiology. 3rd ed. Philadelphia: Lippincott Williams & Wilkins; 2000:587–654.)*

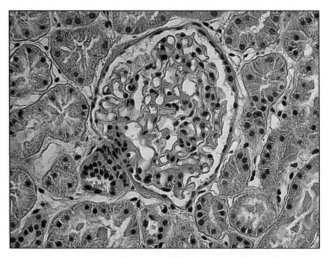

FIGURE 1.30: *Light micrograph of a prominent juxtaglomerular apparatus. Extraglomerular mesangial cells are observed. (H&E, × 400.)*

nidogen), a single chain protein, links the collagen IV and laminin networks. Proteoglycans consist of a core protein bound to one or more glycosaminoglycan (GAG) chains. The GAG chains contain either heparan sulfate or chondroitin sulfate.

Heparan sulfate proteoglycans (HSPG) include agrin, perlecan, and collagen XVIII, which are secreted into the extracellular matrix of organs. The major HSPG of the GBM is agrin. Perlecan and collagen XVIII are situated mainly in the mesangial matrix. Collagen XVIII is a nonfibrillar HSPG collagen. Endostatin, an antiangiogenic peptide, is situated within the carboxy terminal domain of collagen XVIII. Bamacan, a chondroitin sulfate proteoglycan, is present in the immature GBM, but disappears from the adult GBM, remaining in the mesangial matrix.

Podocytes

The podocyte (visceral epithelial cell) is the most complex and enigmatic cell in the kidney [35]. It is the largest cell in the glomerulus. By light microscopy, podocytes are positioned on the outside of the glomerular capillary wall often bulging into Bowman's space (see Figures 1.14 and 1.15). They have prominent nuclei and pale eosinophilic cytoplasm. Scanning electron microscopy has revealed their highly specialized cell structure (Figure 1.23). Podocytes have a prominent cell body, containing nuclei and organelles. The cell bodies give rise to long cytoplasmic primary processes, which branch, before surrounding the capillaries and dividing into foot processes. The cell body and primary processes of the podocyte are suspended within Bowman's space and not directly attached to the GBM. The foot processes from neighboring podocytes interdigitate with each other as they cover the capillary wall and contact the lamina rara externa of the GBM (Figure 1.24). Contrary to their name, the foot processes are slender and more finger-like rather than resembling a foot and its digits. A restricted area under the podocyte cell body, termed the subpodocyte space (SPS), has been reported to connect via narrow passages, termed subpodocyte exit pores (SEPs), with the main Bowman's space [36] (see Figure 1.22). The subpodocyte space covers up to two-thirds of the filtration barrier surface, and recent studies suggest that the solute and water movement across the SPS is a higher-resistance pathway than the parallel pathway across the barrier surface not covered by the SPS [37]. Moreover, this resistance across the SPS may be regulated by alterations of the SEPs [38].

By electron microscopy, the podocytes have abundant rough endoplasmic reticulum, a well-developed Golgi apparatus, and prominent lysosomes. The cell body and primary processes are rich in intermediate filaments, and microtubules (Figure 1.25). The foot processes contain a dense microfilament contractile apparatus, containing actin, myosin, α-actinin, talin, and vinculin, which connects to the intermediate filaments and microtubules of the primary processes. This arrangement of contractile proteins may allow the podocytes to stabilize the glomerular tuft and play a role in modifying the glomerular filtration surface. The foot processes from one podocyte may attach to multiple capillary loop segments (Figure 1.26). The GBM is synthesized mainly by the podocytes.

Adjacent foot processes near the GBM are separated by the filtration slit or pore, a space between 30 and 40 nm, bridged by a thin extracellular structure, the filtration slit diaphragm (SD). This diaphragm is observed as a thin line on electron microscopy. Based on detailed ultrastructural studies, Karnovsky and coworkers proposed an isoporous zipper-like structural model for

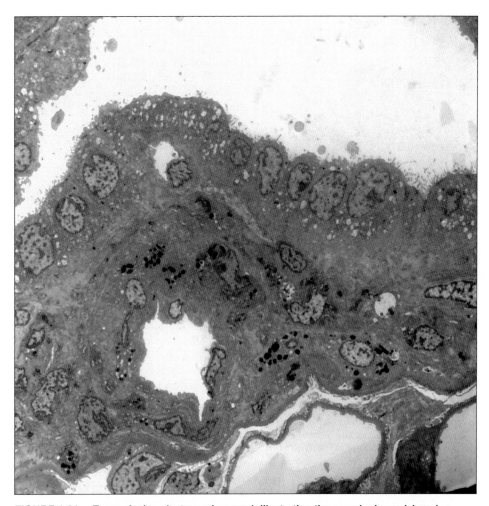

FIGURE 1.31:   Transmission electron micrograph illustrating the macula densa (above), a glomerular hilar arteriole, and a few glomerular capillary loops (below). Cells with cytoplasmic electron-dense granules (juxtaglomerular granular cells) are present in the wall of the arteriole and in the extraglomerular mesangial region. (× 3,200.)

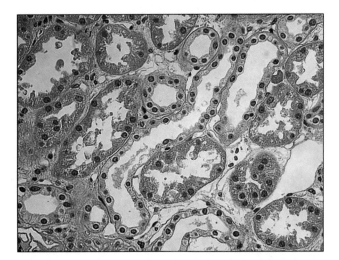

FIGURE 1.32:   Light micrograph of cortex illustrating proximal tubule and more distal nephron segments. The proximal tubular cells are taller, have more eosinophilic, cytoplasm, and lack sharp luminal borders compared to most distal nephron cells. (H&E, × 400.)

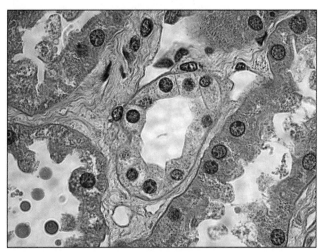

FIGURE 1.33:   Higher magnification micrograph of proximal tubules with eosinophilic columnar epithelium. Some cells show apical blebbing. In contrast, a collecting duct (center) diplays light cytoplasm, distinct lateral cell borders, and a smooth apical surface. (H&E, × 400.)

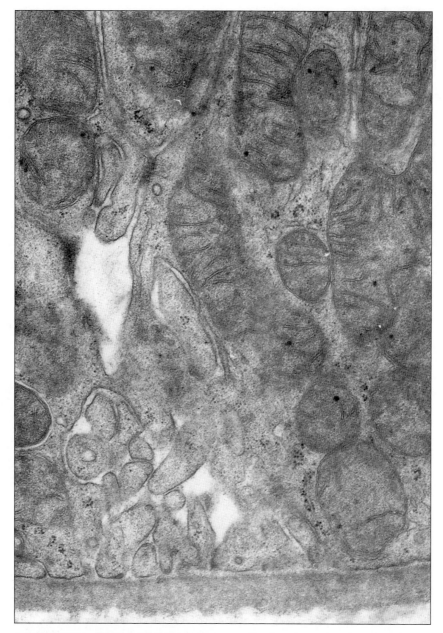

FIGURE 1.34: *Electron micrograph demonstrating basal cytoplasmic region of the proximal tubule. The prominent interdigitation of basolateral cellular processes is accompanied by the formation of intercellular spaces. Elongated mitochondria are present. (× 15,300 Courtesy of C.C. Tisher, MD.)*

the SD [39] (Figures 1.27A and B). In this model, a continuous central bar is connected to adjacent foot processes by regularly spaced cross-bridges, between which are the rectangular pores. The central bar corresponds to the central dot of the diaphragm occasionally observed on ultrastructural cross-sections at high magnification. Three-dimensional reconstruction studies by electron tomography showed the SD to consist of a network of winding strands, 30 to 35 nm long, which merge centrally into a longitudinal density [40]. The strands, creating a SD-thickness between 5 and 10 nm, surround pores that are of similar size or smaller than albumin molecules. These electron tomographic studies generally agree with the Karnovsky model to a remarkable

degree, although the pores appear somewhat more irregular than originally proposed. Although the SD shares similarities with both tight junctions and adherens junctions, it appears unique.

Podocytes, like other epithelial cells, are polarized with distinct membrane domains [41] (Figure 1.28A). The apical membrane domain, comprising a large surface area, is situated above the SD, whereas the basal membrane domain is located below it. The SD area, including the diaphragm itself as well as the adjacent foot process membrane and cytoplasm, is considered a highly specialized surface domain.

Our understanding of the podocyte and its SD was advanced with the identification of the protein nephrin, encoded by

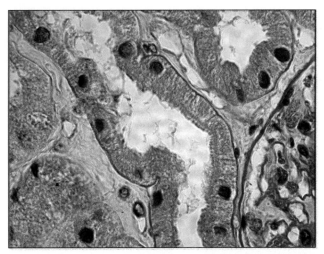

FIGURE 1.35: *Profile of proximal convoluted tubule adjacent to a glomerulus. The tubular cells display a distinct PAS-postive brush border on the lumenal surface. (PAS, × 1,000.)*

NPHS1, the gene mutated in congenital nephrotic syndrome of the Finnish type [42]. Nephrin, a transmembrane adhesion protein of the immunoglobulin superfamily, localizes to the SD. The lack of nephrin in the human congenital syndrome, or experimentally in mice, is characterized by loss of the SD, foot process effacement, and massive proteinuria. A burgeoning number of other proteins localize to the SD domain, where they interact with nephrin and other partners, forming an elaborate multiprotein complex (Figure 1.28B) [35,42]. Some proteins, such as members of the Neph family, are situated in the extracellular strands of the SD itself. Nephrin and Neph1 each form homodimers as well as heterodimeric interactions with each in the SD. Neph2 homodimerizes and forms heterodimers with nephrin, but not with Neph1. Other proteins localize to the podocyte plasma membrane or cytoplasm immediately adjacent to the SD. For example, members of the membrane-associated guanylate kinase (MAGUK) family of proteins, including MAGI-1, MAGI-2, CASK, and ZO-1 are present adjacent to the SD. These scaffolding proteins interconnect junctional membrane proteins to the actin cytoskeleton and various signaling cascades. Multiple adherens junction-associated proteins (AJAP), including α-actinin, IQGAP1, αII spectrin, and βII spectrin are partners in this expanding nephrin-associated complex.

The SD regulates actin cytoskeletal dynamics in the foot process [43]. For example, α-actinin, a protein in the SD domain interacts with synaptopodin, another actin-associated protein to facilitate the formation of long unbranched parallel actin filaments in differentiated podocytes. CD2AP, a cytoplasmic adaptor protein, likely connects nephrin to the actin cytoskeleton in podocytes, but also mediates nephrin signaling of the serine/threonine kinase AKT, which protects podocytes from apoptosis. Another signaling pathway linking nephrin with the actin cytoskeleton involves the Nck adaptor proteins [44,45]. The phosphorylation of tyrosine residues on the nephrin cytoplasmic domain results in the recruitment of Nck proteins (Nck1 and/or Nck2) to interact with nephrin, which in turn, induces actin polymerization.

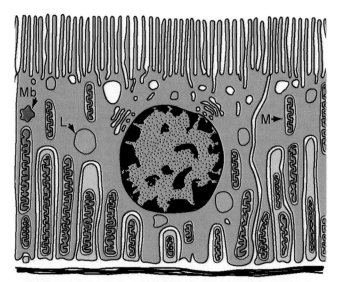

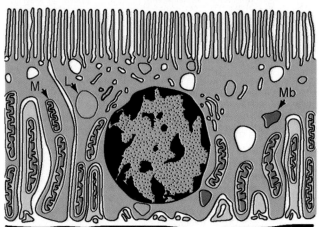

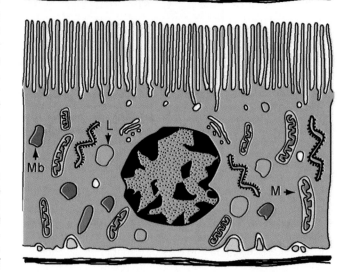

FIGURE 1.36: *Schematic drawing of the three segments of the proximal tubule: upper, S_1, middle, S_2; lower S_3. Interdigitating basolateral processes from adjacent cells are shaded lighter. M, mitochondrion, L, lysosome, Mb, microbody. (Modified from Maunsbach AB, Christensen EI. Functional ultrastructure of the proximal tubule. In: Windhager EE, ed.* Handbook of Physiology. Renal Physiology. *New York: Oxford University Press; 1992:41–107.*

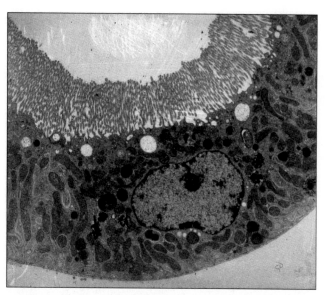

FIGURE 1.37: *Transmission electron micrograph illustrating an isolated perfused S_1 segment of the rabbit proximal tubule. The cells have a tall brush border of microvilli, an extensive endocytic-lysosomal apparatus, numerous mitochondria, and elaborate basolateral membrane invaginations. (× 9,000.)*

Mutations or deficiencies of genes encoding many of the proteins that comprise the SD domain, including nephrin, Nck1/2, Neph1, Fat1, podocin, CD2AP, α-actinin, and TRPC6, result in glomerular disease in humans and animals characterized by absent SDs, foot process effacement, and proteinuria [35,42]. Thus, the SD domain plays a crucial role in regulating the podocyte cytoskeleton, the maintenance of which is essential for a normal filtration barrier.

The podocyte basal membrane domain, the "sole" of the foot process, is inserted in the underlying GBM [35] (see Figure 1.28A). Integrins and dystroglycan, surface receptors in the basal membrane, anchor the foot processes by binding to their ligands in the GBM. The α3β1 integrin binds to type IV collagen, laminin, and nidogen (entactin), and dystroglycan binds to laminin, agrin, and perlecan. Adaptor molecules couple the integrins and dystroglycans to the actin cytoskeleton. The integrins bind the talin, paxillin, vinculin complex, and dystroglycan binds utrophin. Integrins also regulate actin dynamics in response to extracellular signals ("outside-in" signaling) through focal adhesion kinase (FAK) and integrin-linked kinase (ILK). The maintenance of foot process integrity requires an intact basal membrane domain.

The podocyte apical membrane domain, above the SD, is covered with a glycocalyx of negatively charged glycoproteins, including podocalyxin and GLEPP1 [35] (see 1.28A). Podocalyxin, essential for foot process stability, is linked to the actin cytoskeleton through a complex of ezrin, NHERF-1 and NHERF-2 (Na$^+$/H$^+$ exchanger-regulatory factor). The interactions involving GLEPP1, a receptor tyrosine phosphatase, remain to be resolved.

The mature podocyte is a terminally differentiated cell and generally does not replicate. By immunohistochemistry, podocytes express vimentin but are negative for cytokera-tins. Other markers of mature podocytes include CD10, podocalyxin, GLEPP1, nephrin, and other proteins of the filtration SD domain, and the Wilms tumor suppressor protein, WT1. Podocytes also express the cyclin-dependent kinase (CDK) inhibitors p27 and p57, which are involved in maintaining the cells in a quiescent state. In certain glomerular diseases, such as HIV nephropathy and the collapsing variant of focal segmental glomerulosclerosis, podocytes appear to reenter the cell cycle, showing decreased p27 and p57 but increased expression of p21, cyclin D and Ki-67 [46]. The involvement of podocytes in some glomerular diseases has been difficult to document because injured podocytes lose their markers of differentiation. Using the intermediate filament protein nestin as a podocyte marker that persists in glomerular disease, studies have reported podocytes represent a significant component of cellular crescents in severe glomerular disease [47,48].

Podocytes show nuclear immunoreactivity for WT1. Although WT1 has an essential role in early nephrogenesis, it also has an important role in podocyte maturation. Patients with the Denys-Drash syndrome (nephrotic syndrome, genital anomalies, and/or Wilms tumor) have WT1 mutations resulting in impaired podocyte and glomerular maturation [49]. VEGF, produced by podocytes, is necessary for the normal differentiation of endothelial and mesangial cells [50]. WT1, as a transcription factor, can regulate VEGF. In the WT1-mutated glomeruli of the Denys-Drash syndrome, podocyte expression of VEGF is dysregulated.

Glomerular Filtration Barrier

The glomerular capillary wall is believed to function as both a size- and charge-selective barrier. To pass through the capillary wall, a molecule must travel along an extracellular pathway through the endothelial fenestrae, the GBM, and the filtration SD. Despite several decades of research, the exact roles of the three layers of the glomerular capillary wall in filtration remain controversial and a critical area of investigation [51,52].

The permeability of the capillary wall to water and small molecules (hydraulic conductivity) is high, whereas its permeability to macromolecules, the size of albumin and larger, is low. Studies using mathematical modeling have concluded the GBM and filtration SD contribute equally to the total resistance to water filtration. Regarding macromolecules, such as albumin, the GBM has historically been considered the main barrier to filtration. However, the recent molecular and genetic dissection of the SD domain has shifted attention to the SD as the critical sieving layer.

The possible contribution of the glomerular endothelium to the filtration barrier has received little attention. However, emerging evidence suggests that the glycocalyx on glomerular endothelium contributes to the barrier toward macromolecules [53,54]. The GBM has been favored as the main structure responsible for the charge selectivity of the barrier. The high content of heparan sulfate proteoglycans (HSPG) endows the GBM with a negative charge. However, recent investigations have demonstrated that experimental removal of heparan sulfate from the GBM did not lead to increased

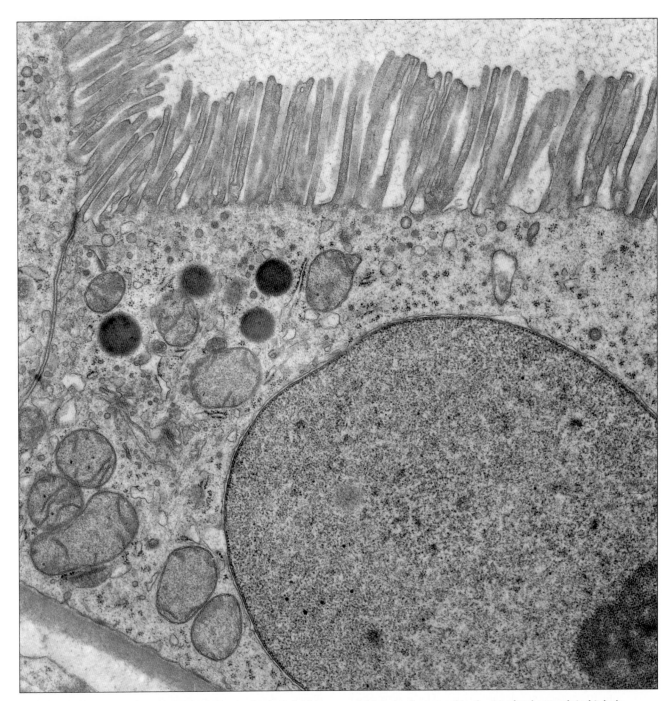

FIGURE 1.38: *Electron micrograph of the proximal straight (pars recta) tubule. Compared to the proximal convoluted tubule, the endocytic-lysosomal apparatus is less developed and the cytoplasmic organelles are less prominent. (× 11,600, Courtesy of C.C. Tisher, MD.)*

GBM permeability to protein [55]. Moreover, the removal of agrin, the principal HSPG in the GBM, led to a loss of GBM negative charge but did not alter the filtration barrier function in mice [56]. Thus, the roles of HSPGs and their negative charges in the GBM are not clear. On the other hand, there is recent evidence that an intact GBM does serve as a major barrier to protein permeability. The removal of the laminin chain β2 in the GBM led to albuminuria in mice that preceded filtration SD abnormalities and foot process effacement [57]. These results favor a view that the GBM serves as an important protein barrier and that an intact SD alone is not sufficient to prevent proteinuria. Mutations or deficiencies of genes encoding proteins of the SD domain, both in humans and mice, result in massive proteinuria, providing compelling genetic evidence for the important role of the SD in glomerular permeability [42]. Currently, the accumulated evidence

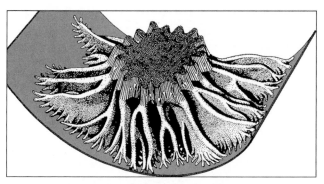

FIGURE 1.39: *Three-dimensional schematic of proximal convoluted tubule illustrating the basal and lateral cellular processes that interdigitate with those from adjacent cells. (Modified from Welling LW, Welling DJ. Shape of epithelial cells and intercellular channels in the rabbit proximal nephron.* **Kidney Int** *1976;9:385–94.)*

favors the SD as the key size-selective element in the filtration barrier.

A reasonable caveat regarding the laboratory research in this area is that the experimental creation of an abnormality in one component of the filtration barrier, whether the endothelium, the GBM or the podocyte SD, will likely induce an alteration in the other components. In summary, the capillary wall components do not operate independently but are linked in an integrative fashion to maintain normal glomerular filtration.

Parietal Podocytes

Investigations have identified cells lining Bowman's space, especially at the vascular pole, that have ultrastructural and immunophenotypical features of mature visceral podocytes that surround the capillaries [58]. These "parietal podocytes" may form apparent intercellular bridges with visceral podocytes. The origin and significance of the parietal podocytes are unclear.

Parietal Epithelial Cells

The main cell of the parietal layer directly lining Bowman's capsule is a flat squamous-like cell. The parietal epithelial cells express cytokeratin, cadherins, the transcription factor

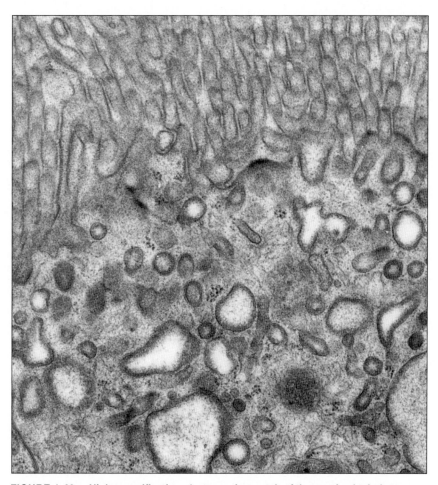

FIGURE 1.40: *High-magnification electron micrograph of the proximal tubule displaying the apical cytoplasmic region. Components of the endocytic-vacuolar apparatus, including coated vesicles, apical dense tubules, and endosomes lie beneath the surface microvilli. (× 18,500, Courtesy of C.C. Tisher, MD.)*

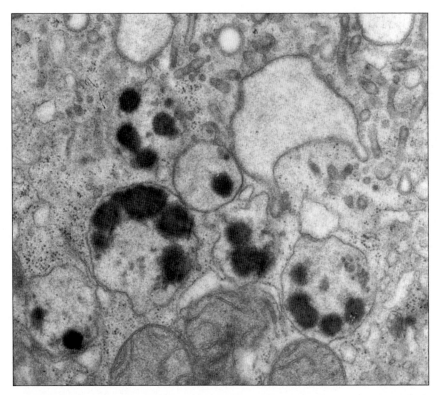

FIGURE 1.41: High-magnification transmission electron micrograph showing apical dense tubules, electron-lucent endosomes, and several lysosomes of the proximal tubule. The lysosomes are membrane-bound, and contain multiple dense homogenous bodies within a low density matrix. (× 19,000, Courtesy of C.C. Tisher, MD.)

Pax-2, but no podocyte markers. These cells have significant proliferative potential and are believed to participate in crescent formation associated with severe glomerular injury. The basement membrane of Bowman's capsule often has a lamellated appearance. In contrast to the GBM, the basement membrane of the capsule expresses the α6 chain of type IV collagen, which is part of the α1.α1.α2(IV)–α5.α5.α6(IV) network and bamacan, a chondroitin sulfate proteoglycan.

Peripolar Cells

The peripolar cell is situated between the visceral and parietal cell layers at the origin of the glomerular tuft in Bowman's space. These cells are rarely observed in human glomeruli. They are more commonly detected in sheep. By electron microscopy, the peripolar cell contains prominent electron-dense granules. Some believe they are a component of the juxtaglomerular apparatus and may have a secretory function but their relevance is undetermined.

JGA

The JGA is located at the vascular pole of the glomerulus and includes portions of afferent and efferent arterioles, the extraglomerular mesangium, and the macula densa (Figure 1.29) [59]. A prominent JGA may occasionally be observed in a normal glomerulus and should not be mistaken for a lesion such as focal segmental glomerulosclerosis. (Figure 1.30). Juxtaglomerular granular cells are distinctive renin-producing cells most abundant in the wall of the afferent arteriole (Figure 1.31). These cells may be observed in the wall of the efferent arteriole as well as in the extraglomerular mesangium. By electron microscopy, these cells contain myofilaments and attachment plaques, features of smooth muscles, and numerous cytoplasmic granules. The granules vary in shape and size and are membrane bound. Some smaller granules (protogranules) are rhomboid-shaped with a crystalline substructure and are believed to coalesce to form larger mature granules. A variety of studies have localized renin to these granules. Renin release occurs by exocytosis.

The extraglomerular mesangium (*lacis* or polar cushion) is situated between the afferent and efferent arterioles and adjacent to the macula densa. The extraglomerular mesangium is continuous with the intraglomerular mesangium. By electron microscopy, the extraglomerular mesangial cells (*lacis* or Goormaghtigh cells) are similar to mesangial cells within the glomerular tuft. Numerous gap junctions exist between the lacis, mesangial, and juxtaglomerular JG granular cells.

The macula densa (MD) is a plaque of specialized cells within the cortical thick ascending limb adjacent to the glomerular hilus. In contrast to adjacent cells in the thick ascending limb, the MD cells are taller and often protrude into the tubular lumen. By electron microscopy, they have apical nuclei, a Golgi apparatus on the

Type I

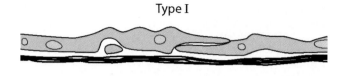

Type II

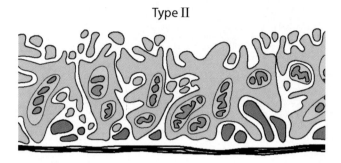

Type III

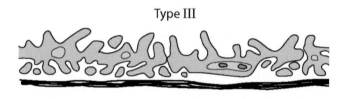

Type IV

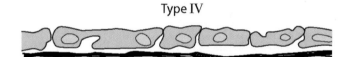

FIGURE 1.42: *Schematic representation of the four types of epithelium found in the thin limbs of Henle's loop. (Modified from Madsen KM, Nielsen S, Tisher CC. Anatomy of the Kidney. In: Brenner BM, ed. Brenner and Rector's The Kidney. 8th ed. Philadelphia: Saunders Elsevier; 2008:25–90.*

basal side of the nucleus, and basal cytoplasmic processes that interdigitate with those of extraglomerular mesangial cells. The width of the lateral intercellular spaces between MD cells varies. This is likely associated with their permeability to water. Compared to adjacent cells in the thick ascending limb, the MD cells express neuronal nitric oxide synthase (NOS) and the cyclooxygenase enzyme COX-2, but not the Tamm-Horsfall protein.

The topographic organization of the JGA is suited for intricate functional regulation of its integral components [60]. The JGA is involved in at least two major functions: the control of renin synthesis and release and the regulation of glomerular arteriolar flow and glomerular filtration. Renin secretion is controlled by several mechanisms. A baroreceptor mechanism involves decreased pressure or stretch within the wall of the afferent arteriole, resulting in renin secretion from the JG cells. Another mechanism involves a link between fluid delivered to the MD and the glomerular filtration rate, termed tubuloglomerular feedback. Several lines of evidence support the following: increased tubular sodium chloride delivery to the thick ascending limb results in solute uptake via a Na$^+$-K$^+$-2Cl$^-$ cotransporter on the luminal membrane of the MD cells. Sub-

sequent activation of the sodium pump leads to ATP hydrolysis in the MD cells, which release adenosine. Adenosine interacts with its receptors on extraglomerular mesangial cells, triggering an increase in cytosolic calcium. Gap junctions transmit the calcium flux to the adjacent afferent arteriole resulting in vasoconstriction, inhibition of renin release, and decreased glomerular filtration. Both nitric oxide (NO) and COX-2 generated prostaglandins influence the signaling between the MD and JG cells in the afferent arteriole.

Tubules

The tubular component of the nephron includes the proximal tubule, thin limbs of Henle's loop, thick ascending limb, distal convoluted tubule, and the collecting duct. These structurally and functionally distinct segments exhibit considerable cellular heterogeneity.

Proximal Tubule

At the urinary pole of the glomerulus, there is an abrupt transition from the flat parietal epithelium of Bowman's capsule to the columnar epithelium of the proximal tubule. The proximal tubule consists of an initial convoluted portion, the pars convoluta, and a straight portion, the pars recta. The convoluted portion forms several coils around its parent glomerulus in the cortex (cortical labyrinth) before continuing into the straight part located in the medullary ray. The human proximal tubule is 14 mm long. Because of its length and convoluted form, profiles of proximal convoluted tubules encompass the most surface area of any parenchymal component on histologic sections of the cortex. Proximal tubules are easily distinguished from other tubular segments on light microscopy (Figures 1.32 and 1.33). Their cells are cuboidal to columnar with eosinophilic granular cytoplasm and round nuclei in the center or near the base of the cells. Their lateral cell borders are indistinct due to extensive interdigitations of lateral cell processes with those from adjacent cells (Figure 1.34). An elaborate intercellular space compartment forms from these interdigitations. These lateral extensions and numerous elongated mitochondria result in vertical striations in the basal cytoplasm. Apical cytoplasmic vacuoles and granules correspond to a well-developed endocytic–lysosomal apparatus. There is a prominent PAS-positive luminal brush border composed of densely packed long microvilli (Figure 1.35). Compared to distal nephron segments, the lumens of proximal tubules are often collapsed after immersion fixation. On histologic sections, the brush border, apical cytoplasmic vacuoles, and basal striations are less prominent in the proximal straight tubules, which also have a less coiled outline. Proximal tubules show expression of cytokeratins 8 and 18 and cadherin-6, but no immunoreactivity for cytokeratins 7 or 34βE12 [61].

In several mammals, three distinct segments of the proximal tubule can be identified that have different morphologic and functional characteristics (Figure 1.36) [62,63]. However, there are differences among species. For example, in contrast to the rat and rabbit, no significant morphologic segmentation has been found in the mouse [64]. Although a convoluted and a

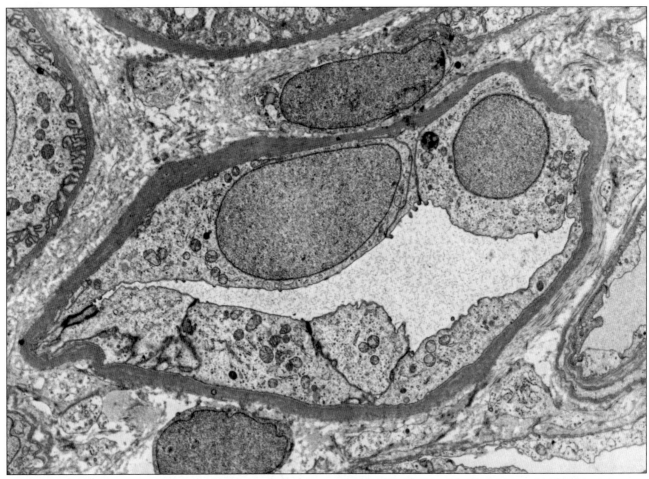

FIGURE 1.43: *Transmission electron micrograph of a thin descending limb. A few interdigitations of basolateral cellular processes are present. (× 5,100, Courtesy of C.C. Tisher, MD.)*

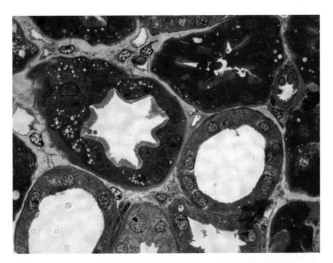

FIGURE 1.44: *Profiles of a proximal straight tubule (left) and a thick ascending limb (right) in the cortex. Both segments exhibit a dark-staining cytoplasm due, in large part, to abundant mitochondria. The cells of the proximal tubule are taller, contain small endocytic vacuoles, and have a brush border. Note the circular outline of the thick ascending limb lumen. (1 um toluidine blue-stained Epon section, × 1,000.)*

straight portion of the proximal tubule have been described in humans, the segmentation into three divisions has not been closely examined.

The three proximal tubule segments include the S_1, S_2, and S_3. The S_1 segment starts at the glomerulus and includes one-half to two-thirds of the pars convoluta. The S_2 represents the remainder of the pars convoluta and the initial pars recta. The S_3 segment corresponds to the remainder of the pars recta. Cells in the S_1 segment have extensive basolateral interdigitations, abundant elongated mitochondria, prominent endosomes and lysosomes, and a tall brush border (Figure 1.37). Cells in the S_2 segment cells are similar to those in S_1, however, their basolateral interdigitations, mitochondria, endocytotic organelles, and brush border are less prominent. The cells in S_3 are more cuboidal, have inconspicuous interdigitations, small mitochondria, and fewer endosomes (Figure 1.38). The length of the brush border varies among species but it is short in humans.

The proximal tubule is structured for immense reabsorption. It reabsorbs about 60 percent of the filtered Na^+Cl^- [65]. This transport occurs through the cells (transcellular) as well as between cells (paracellular). The paracellular route is a low-resistance pathway formed by the apical tight junction (zonula

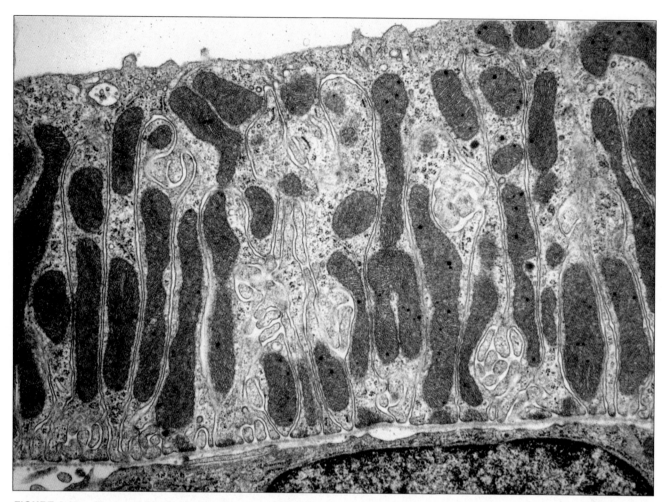

FIGURE 1.45: *Electron micrograph of a medullary thick ascending limb from a rat. Elongated mitochondria are surrounded by basolateral membrane invaginations, and extend nearly the entire thickness of the cell. These ultrastructural features are characteristic for epithelia involved in active ion transport. (× 13,000.)*

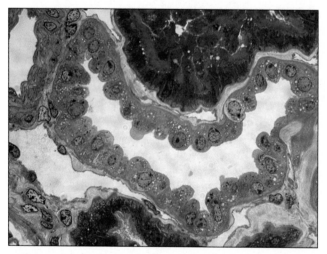

FIGURE 1.46: *Light micrograph of a distal convoluted tubule. Note the convoluted profile of the tubule. The nuclei are typically situated near the lumen. (1 um toluidine-stained Epon section, × 1,000.)*

occludens) and the lateral intercellular space. Transcellular sodium reabsorption in the proximal tubule is mediated primarily by the Na^+,K^+-ATPase (Na^+ pump) in the basolateral membrane. The $\alpha1\beta1$ heterodimer is the main Na^+,K^+-ATPase isozyme but $\alpha2$- and $\alpha3$-isoforms have been detected. This sodium pump-driven active transport of Na^+ out of the cell, and across the basolateral membrane, creates a lumen-to-cell concentration gradient for Na^+. The numerous mitochondria located in close proximity to the plasma membrane provide a source for the cellular energy required for active transport. The transport of Na^+ from the lumen into the proximal tubule down its concentration gradient is mediated by the Na^+/H^+ exchanger NHE3, expressed in the brush border. The reabsorption of chloride, bicarbonate, glucose, amino acids, and fluid is coupled to the transport of sodium. Extrusion of bicarbonate out across the basolateral membrane occurs by the Na^+/HCO_3^- cotransporter (NBC1). Aquaporin-1 (AQP1), present in both the apical and basolateral membranes mediates water permeability in the proximal tubule. An excellent correlation exists between the basolateral membrane surface area, the Na^+,K^+-ATPase activities in the basolateral membrane, and the capacity to transport sodium and other ions along

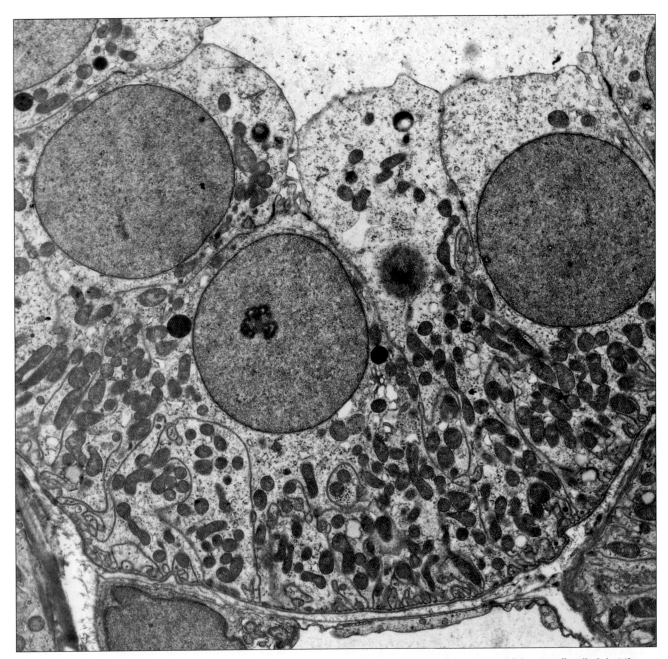

FIGURE 1.47: *Electron micrograph of distal convoluted tubule. The cells are similar to those in the thick ascending limb but they are taller and have nuclei closer to the lumen. (× 10,000, Courtesy of C.C. Tisher, MD.)*

the length of the proximal tubule (Figure 1.39) [66]. The intrinsic rates at which solutes and fluid are transported decrease along the proximal tubule from S_1 to S_3.

The prominent endocytotic–lysosomal apparatus in the proximal tubule is responsible for the reabsorption and degradation of albumin and low-molecular-weight proteins filtered by the glomerulus (Figure 1.40) [67]. Proteins are reabsorbed by receptor-mediated endocytosis, transferred to endosomes, and eventually delivered to lysosomes where they are degraded (Figure 1.41). The endosomes provide an acidic environment, which promotes segregation of the ligand–receptor complexes. Receptors are recycled back to the apical membrane via small

specialized structures termed apical dense tubules (see Figure 1.41). The lysosomal capacity for protein degradation decreases from the S_1 to the S_3 segment. Megalin and cubilin are multi-ligand receptors expressed throughout the endocytotic apparatus of the proximal tubule. These receptors operate independently but also interact as a dual complex to mediate the apical uptake of albumin and numerous other ligands, including low-molecular weight proteins, hormones, and vitamin-binding proteins. Recent studies have demonstrated a new pathway for lysosomal biogenesis in the proximal tubule, whereby lysosomal enzymes filtered by the glomerulus undergo megalin-mediated endocytosis and delivery to lysosomes where they are active [68].

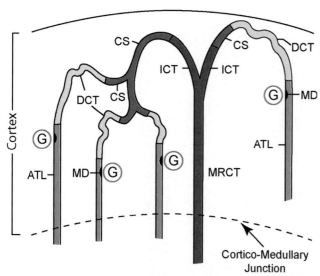

FIGURE 1.48: Diagram illustrating the anatomic variations of the connecting tubule joining the distal tubule to the collecting duct in different nephron types. See text for details. (G, glomerulus; ATL, ascending thick limb; MD, macula densa; DCT, distal convoluted tubule; CS, connecting segment; ICT, initial collecting tubule; MRCT, medullary ray collecting tubule.)

Thin Limbs of Henle's Loop

The entire tubular loop structure named after Henle may be considered to include the straight portion of the proximal tubule, the thin descending and thin ascending limbs, and the thick ascending limb. However, the eponymous designation of the loop is commonly used for primarily the descending thin limb (DTL) and the ascending thin limb (ATL). The abrupt transition from the proximal tubule to the DTL marks the border between the outer and inner stripes of the outer

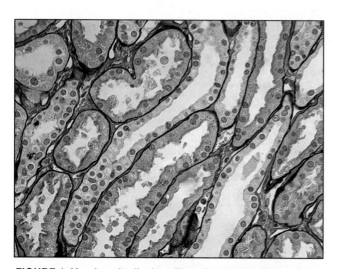

FIGURE 1.49: Longitudinal profiles of collecting ducts and proximal tubules in a medullary ray in the cortex. The collecting ducts have shorter, lighter staining cells with a relatively smooth luminal surface due the absence of a brush border. (Methenamine silver, × 400.)

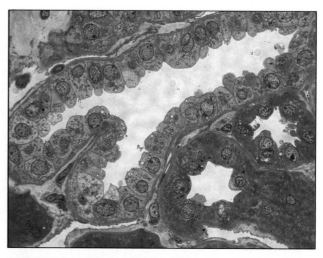

FIGURE 1.50: Micrograph of an initial cortical collecting duct showing a branched configuration. (1 um toluidine-blue stained Epon section, × 1,000.)

medulla (see Figure 1.3). Short-looped nephrons have only a short DTL, and not an ATL. Near the bend of the short loop, the DTL continues into the thick ascending limb. Long-looped nephrons have both a long DTL and a long ATL. The long DTL traverses the inner stripe of the outer medulla and enters the inner medulla. These long DTLs may have a tortuous course and the positions of their hairpin turns may vary [69]. The long ATL resides entirely within the inner medulla. At the boundary between the inner and outer medulla, the long ATL joins the thick ascending limb.

The flat, simple epithelium of the DTL and ATL observed by light microscopy belies their topographic, ultrastructural, and functional complexity. For example, most mammals, including humans, have a simple medulla characterized by vascular bundles containing only descending and ascending vasa recta but no thin limb segments. Complex medulla, formed in animals (mouse, rat) with a high urine concentrating ability, contain DTLs of short-looped nephrons incorporated within the vascular bundles with the vasa recta. Ultrastructural analysis has revealed four types of epithelia in thin limbs (Figure 1.42) [70]. It is not clear if four types exist in humans, but at least two types have been observed (Figure 1.43) [71]. Type I epithelium is found exclusively in short-looped nephrons covering the entire DTL. It is a very thin, simple epithelium with few cellular interdigitations and cell organelles. Type II epithelium forms the initial part of the DTL of long-looped nephrons in the outer medulla. This epithelium has taller cells, short microvilli, and more prominent organelles than in the other epithelial types. Type II leads into type III epithelium covering the DTL of long-loops in the inner medulla. Type III epithelium consists of simple cells with few organelles and no lateral interdigitations. Type IV epithelium forms the bends of the long loops and lines the entire ATL. It has low, flattened cells with few organelles, no microvilli but prominent lateral interdigitations. Thus, these epithelia are distributed as follows: Type I in the DTL of short loops, types II and III in the DTL of long loops, and type IV in the ATL of long loops.

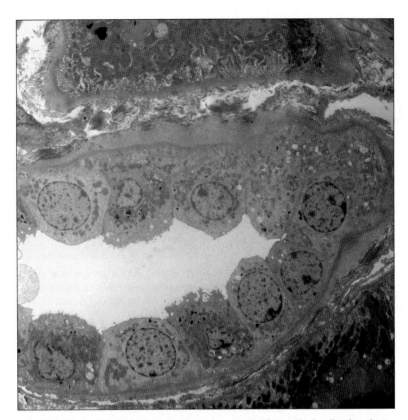

FIGURE 1.51:   Transmission electron micrograph of a cortical collecting duct. The majority of the lining cells are principal cells. However, some cells demonstrate a darker cytoplasm, abundant mitochondria, and apical projections characteristic for intercalated cells. (× 3,000.)

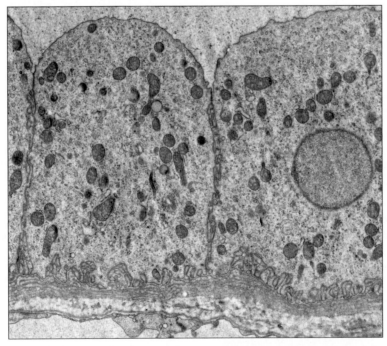

FIGURE 1.52:   Transmission electron micrograph of two principal cells of the cortical collecting duct. They have relatively few organelles, lack prominent basolateral membrane interdigitations, but display characteristic extensive infoldings of the basal plasma membrane. (× 10,000, Courtesy of C.C. Tisher, MD.)

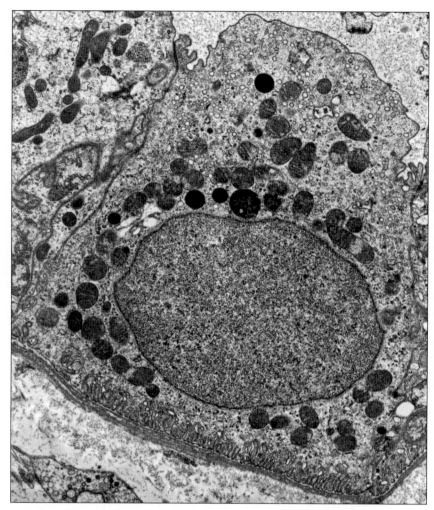

FIGURE 1.53: *Electron micrograph of intercalated cell of the cortical collecting duct. It has dense-staining cytoplasm and numerous mitochondria, warranting its other designation of "dark cell". There are numerous small vesicular structures in the apical cytoplasm. (× 11,500, Courtesy of C.C. Tisher, MD.)*

The thin limbs of Henle's loop are important for the urinary concentrating process, the detailed mechanisms of which have yet to be fully understood. Physiologic studies have shown that the DTL is permeable to water but has relative low permeability to sodium chloride, whereas the ATL is impermeable to water, but has high permeability to sodium chloride [65]. The aquaporin water channel protein AQP1 mediates water permeability in the DTL of long loops (type II epithelium). Interestingly, AQP1 is not expressed in the DTL of short loops (type I epithelium), but this segment does express the urea transporter UT-A2, which mediates urea secretion into the loop [72]. Expression of the chloride channel protein ClC-K1 exclusively in the ATL mediates the high chloride permeability of this segment.

The descending and ascending limbs of the loop establish a countercurrent multiplier mechanism in the medulla. The flow of fluid in opposite directions within the limbs of the loop creates an osmotic concentration gradient in the long axis of the medulla that surpasses that already present at each level along it. In brief, a hypertonic medullary interstitium concentrates sodium chloride in the DTL by extraction of water. The fluid entering the ATL has a higher sodium chloride concentration, resulting in solute reabsorption and dilution of the fluid in the ATL. However, little evidence exists for active Na^+Cl^- reabsorption by the ATL within the inner medulla. It is believed that active Na^+Cl^- reabsorption by the thick ascending limb in the outer medulla provides the energy source that drives the countercurrent multiplication system. Urea is recycled, whereby urea secreted into the DTL is returned to the collecting ducts where it is reabsorbed. Thus, the thin limb contributes to the maintenance of a hypertonic medullary interstitium, and delivers a dilute fluid to more distal tubular segments.

Distal Tubule

The distal tubule includes three distinct segments: the thick ascending limb (TAL), the macula densa (MD), and the distal convoluted tubule (DCT) (see Figure 1.3). The thick ascending limb in the cortex extends beyond the macula densa before

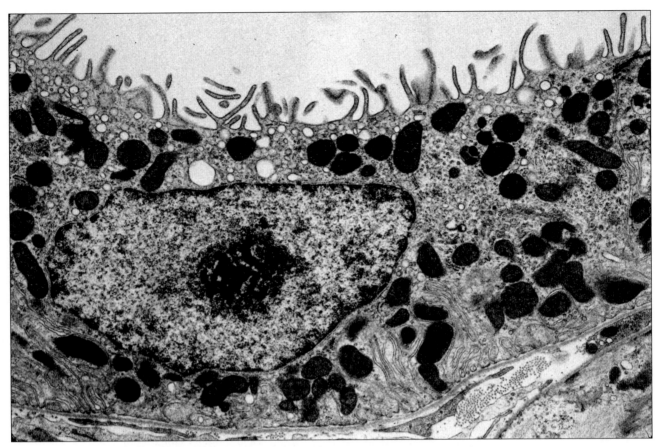

FIGURE 1.54: *Electron micrograph of a type A intercalated cell in the rat cortical collecting duct. Note the prominent vesicular structures in the apical cytoplasm and numerous microprojections on the luminal surface. (× 10,500, Courtesy of Dr. J. W. Verlander.)*

it forms an abrupt union with the distal convoluted tubule. The MD, as previously discussed (in "JGA" section), represents a specialized plaque of cells within the TAL.

(TAL). In short-looped nephrons, the conversion from the DTL to the thick ascending begins before the bend. As noted before, the short-looped nephrons have no ATL. In long-looped nephrons, the change from the thin ascending limb to the TAL marks the boundary between the inner medulla and the inner stripe of the outer medulla. By light microscopy, the TAL cells, like proximal tubular cells, have prominent eosinophilic cytoplasm, indistinct lateral borders due to extensive basolateral interdigitations, and basal striations due to abundant elongated mitochondria and the interdigitations (Figures 1.44 and 1.45). These morphologic features are typical for epithelial cells involved in active transport. However, compared to proximal tubular cells, TAL cells are more cuboidal, somewhat less eosinophilic, and lack a luminal brush border. Their nuclei tend to be near the apical region and produce a bulge into the lumen.

The TAL can be divided into medullary (MTAL) and cortical (CTAL) segments. As the TAL ascends into the cortex, there is a gradual decrease in cell height, basolateral membrane area, and size of the mitochondria [73]. This correlates with functional data demonstrating greater Na^+, K^+-ATPase activities and NaCl reabsorptive capacity in the MTAL. The TAL cells are immunoreac-tive for cytokeratins 8 and 18 and kidney-specific (Ksp) cadherin [61]. They synthesize Tamm-Horsfall protein and secrete it into the tubular lumen. The TAL is a critical component of the countercurrent multiplication system which generates an axial hypertonic gradient in the medulla, which is essential for urinary concentration. The TAL is known as the major diluting segment. Active reabsorption of NaCl by the TAL coupled with the water impermeability of this segment results in a hypertonic interstitium and delivery of a hypotonic fluid to more distal tubular segments. The hypertonic interstitium drives osmotic water reabsorption from the DTL. This reabsorbed water rapidly reenters the circulation via the vasa recta. The axial osmolarity gradient in the medulla facilitates water reabsorption by the collecting ducts resulting in concentration of the tubular fluid. The reabsorption of NaCl in the TAL is driven by the basolateral Na^+,K^+-ATPase and entry across the apical membrane is mediated by the Na^+-K^+-$2Cl^-$ cotransporter (BSC-1), which is the target of loop diuretics (for example, furosemide) [65].

(DCT). DCT commences beyond the MD in the cortex. It represents the terminal part of the distal tubule. Although the cells of the DCT are somewhat similar to those of the TAL, the DCT cells are taller, have nuclei closer to the lumen, and lack lateral interdigitations in the apical region between adjacent cells. By light microscopy, the DCT is easily distinguished from the proximal tubule. (Figures 1.46 and

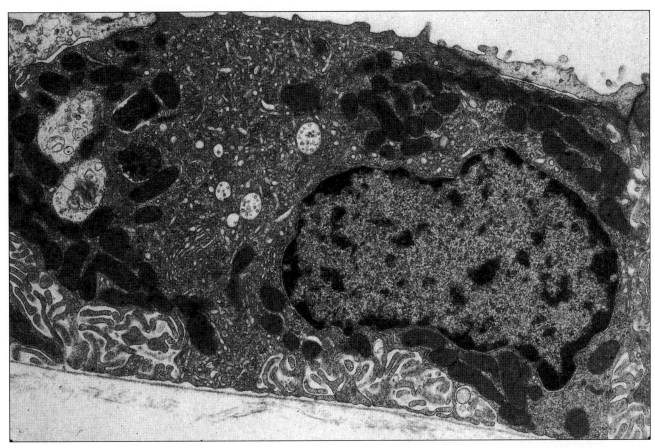

FIGURE 1.55: *Electron micrograph of a type B intercalated cell in the rat cortical collecting duct. Compared to the type A intercalated cell, the type B cell has a more dense cytoplasm and more mitochondria. The B cell has numerous small vesicles throughout the cytoplasm, but fewer vesicles immediately beneath the apical membrane. In contrast to type A cells, type B cells have a larger basolateral membrane area but a smaller apical membrane area. (× 10,500, Courtesy of Dr. J. W. Verlander.)*

1.47). Because the DCT is short, about 1 to 2 mm in length, fewer profiles of the DCT are observed on histologic sections. The DCTs typically display patent lumens and closely spaced nuclei. Also, the DCT cells are smaller, significantly less eosinophilic, and lack a well-developed brush border and apical endocytotic apparatus. The DCT expresses cytokeratins 8, 18, and 19 as well as Ksp-cadherin [61].

Similar to the TAL, the Na^+,K^+-ATPase in the basolateral membranes of the DCT drives solute reabsorption. In fact, biochemical studies have documented that the DCT has the highest Na^+,K^+-ATPase activity of any segment of the nephron. Entry of NaCl across the apical membrane of the DCT is mediated by the Na^+Cl^- cotransporter (NCC or TSC) [65]. NCC, the target of thiazide diuretics, is distinct from the cotransporter BSC-1, which is present in the TAL. Morphologic and physiologic studies indicate that the DCT, like the TAL, is relatively impermeable to water but responsible for the reabsorption of sodium chloride.

Connecting Tubule

The connecting tubule (CNT) is a transitional segment that joins the DCT with the collecting duct system (Figure 1.48). The CNTs of superficial nephrons empty directly into an initial collecting tubule, the first segment of the collecting duct system. In contrast, the CNTs of juxtamedullary nephrons and many midcortical nephrons join to form arched segments, termed arcades that ascend in the cortex before draining into an initial collecting tubule. In humans, most nephrons empty individually via single CNTs into the collecting tubules. Most species, including humans, contain different cell types in the CNT resulting from an intermingling of cells from the adjacent DCT and cortical collecting duct. The cell types include CNT cells, as well as intercalated, distal convoluted, and principal cells. The CNT cell is the most characteristic cell type of this segment. It is specific to the CNT. CNT cells have morphologic similarities to both DCT cells and principal cells of the cortical collecting duct. By electron microscopy, CNT cells exhibit basolateral interdigitations and also true infoldings of the basal membrane. Various subtypes of intercalated cells, similar to those in the cortical collecting duct, are present in the CNT and are likely involved in acid–base regulation. The principal cells in the CNT are similar to those in the cortical collecting duct and are involved in solute and water handling.

The CNT plays an important role in sodium reabsorption and potassium secretion, both regulated by aldosterone. In fact, the CNT has a greater capacity for Na^+ reabsorption and K^+ secretion than the cortical collecting duct [65]. The entry of Na^+ across the apical membrane occurs via the

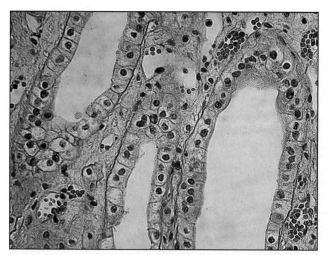

FIGURE 1.56: *Light micrograph demonstrating columnar cells of the terminal collecting ducts in the inner medulla. (H&E, × 400.)*

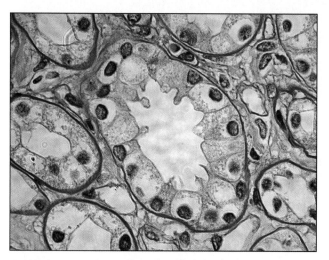

FIGURE 1.57: *Micrograph of inner medulla showing light cytoplasm and sharp lateral cell borders of collecting duct epithelium. (PAS, × 1,000.)*

amilioride-sensitive sodium channel (ENaC). The secretion of potassium is mediated by the K+ channel, ROMK, in the apical membrane. A portion of the CNT of superficial nephrons has been observed to lie adjacent to the afferent arteriole of its parent glomerulus. Physiologic studies have demonstrated that increased Na+ reabsorption in the CNT is associated with dilatation of the adjacent afferent arteriole [74]. This functional connection between the CNT and afferent arteriole has been called "connecting tubule glomerular feedback." Its significance remains to be detailed.

Collecting Duct

The collecting duct begins in the cortex and descends through the medulla to the papillary tip. It can be divided into three portions: the cortical collecting duct (CCD), the outer medullary collecting duct (OMCD), and the inner medullary collecting duct (IMCD). The diameter of the ducts increases from the CCD to the IMCD. Significant cellular heterogeneity exists along the collecting duct [75,76]

(Cortical Collecting Duct). CCD can be further separated into two successive segments: the initial collecting tubule and the medullary ray segment. By light microscopy, the epithelium of the CCD is composed of cuboidal cells with well-demarcated lateral cell borders and central round nuclei (Figures 1.49 and 1.50). In contrast to proximal tubules, they have open lumens, lack a brush border, and show positive immunoreactivity for pancytokeratin (AE 1/3), cytokeratin 7 and 34βE12 [61]. Cytokeratins 5/6, 17, and 29 as well as vimentin are restricted more to medullary collecting ducts. Compared to the TALs and DCTs, there is less immunoreactivity for Kspcadherin in collecting ducts. The CCD is composed of principal cells and intercalated cells (Figure 1.51). Principal cells are more numerous in the CCD. They have a pale cytoplasm due to relatively few organelles. By electron microscopy, principal cells have no interdigitations of lateral cell processes from adjacent cells, accounting for their distinct lateral cell borders on light microscopy (Figure 1.52). Prominent infoldings of the basal membrane render an accentuated clear appearance to the basal aspect of the cells. By scanning electron microscopy, principal cells have a smooth luminal surface with short microvilli and a single cilium.

Principal cells are involved in sodium reabsorption and potassium secretion [65]. Sodium entry into the cells is mediated by the amiloride-sensitive sodium channel, ENaC, situated in the apical membrane of principal cells throughout the entire collecting duct. ENaC activity is upregulated by both aldosterone and vasopressin. Potassium secretion largely occurs by the apical membrane ROMK potassium channel. The Na,+K+-ATPase mediates Na+ extrusion and K+ entry across the basolateral membrane. In the presence of elevated levels of the antidiuretic hormone vasopressin, the entire collecting duct becomes permeable to water. The principal cells are vasopressin-sensitive and responsible for water absorption. After vasopressin binds to its receptor on the basolateral membrane of principal cells, small apical cytoplasmic vesicles containing the aquaporin water channel AQP2 are shuttled to the apical membrane, which markedly increases water permeability. The presence of the water channel AQP3 and AQP4 in the basolateral membrane of the principal cells facilitates the exit of water into the interstitium, which results in a hypertonic urine. Thus, the principal cells play a critical role in urine concentration.

The intercalated cells are interspersed in the epithelium of the collecting duct. These specialized cells usually represent the minority cell type in tubular segments. Intercalated cells are most numerous in the CCD, where they may constitute 30 to 40 percent of the cells in some mammals. They are also present in the CNT, the OMCD, and the initial part of the IMCD. It is difficult to distinguish intercalated cells from principal cells on H&E paraffin sections, but intercalated cells can be identified by their dark-staining cytoplasm on toluidine blue-stained Epon sections. The presence of numerous mitochondria and a dense cytoplasm accounts for their dark appearance (Figure 1.53). All intercalated cells express high levels of carbonic anhydrase, the enzyme that catalyzes the

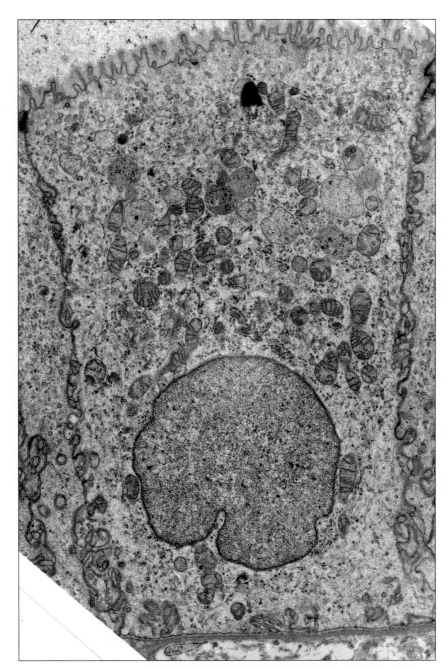

FIGURE 1.58: *Transmission electron micrograph of a cell in the inner medullary collecting duct. The tall cell has a basilar nucleus, relatively few organelles, and short stubby apical microvilli. (× 13,000, Courtesy of C.C. Tisher, MD.)*

interconversion of CO_2 to HCO_3^- suggesting they are involved in acid–base regulation.

Three subtypes of intercalated cells (ICs) have been characterized based on ultrastructural features and the subcellular localization of different transport proteins [77–81]. Moreover, combined structural–functional studies have supported the concept of cellular specificity underlying acid–base regulation. There are striking differences in the prevalence and distribution of the IC subtypes throughout the collecting duct (as well as the CNT) among mammalian species. On electron microscopy, type A ICs display prom-inent microprojections of the apical membrane and numer-ous vesicular structures in the apical cytoplasm (Figure 1.54). Compared to type A cells, type B ICs have a smaller apical membrane area, a small number of apical microprojections, and more mitochondria (Figure 1.55). In addition, type B ICs have fewer vesicles in the apical cytoplasm but more vesicles throughout the cytoplasm, and a larger basolateral membrane surface area. By scanning electron microscopy, type A cells have a convex luminal surface covered with complex microprojections called microplicae, whereas type B cells show a small angular luminal surface with small microvilli.

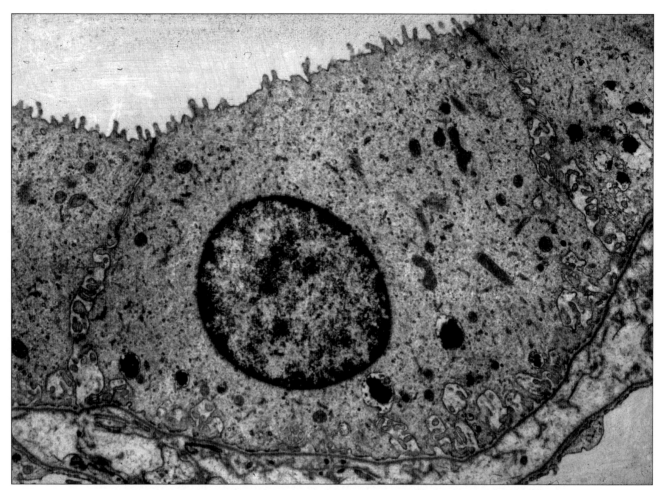

FIGURE 1.59: *Electron micrograph of an IMCD cell from the terminal segment of the rat inner medullary collecting duct. The cell is relatively tall, has few organelles and short apical microvilli. (× 10,000.)*

The third intercalated cell subtype, the non-A, non-B ICs, are larger than type A and type B ICs, have abundant mitochondria, and display prominent apical microprojections similar to those of type A cells.

Type A ICs are characterized by a proton pump H^+-ATPase in the apical membrane and a Cl^-/HCO_3^- exchanger, AE1, in the basolateral membrane. Type A ICs are responsible for H^+ secretion in the CCD. Hydrogen ions generated by cytosolic carbonic anhydrase are secreted by the apical H^+-ATPase and generated HCO_3^- is extruded across the basolateral membrane by AE1. Thus, type A ICs are responsible for H^+ secretion in the tubular segments where they are found. Type A ICs are present in the CNT, CCD, OMCD, and initial part of the IMCD.

Type B ICs are characterized by a Cl^-/HCO_3^- exchanger in the apical membrane and the proton pump H^+-ATPase in the basolateral membrane. The apical Cl^-/HCO_3^- exchanger is likely pendrin, a transporter not in the same protein family as AE1. Thus, type B ICs secrete HCO_3^- into the tubular lumen via pendrin and H^+ is extruded across the basolateral membrane by the H^+-ATPase. Type B ICs are found only in the CNT and CCD.

Type non-A, non-B ICs are defined based on the presence of pendrin, the Cl^-/HCO_3^- exchanger in the apical membrane, but also the presence of the proton pump H^+-ATPase in the apical membrane. It would seem that type non-A, non-B ICs may have the capacity of both HCO_3^- and H^+ apical secretion but this has not been resolved. Whether these cells found only in the CNT and CCD, represent a versatile cell type capable of secreting acid or base depending on the acid–base status, remains to be proven.

(OMCD). The collecting duct traverses the outer medulla without receiving tributaries. The OMCD is lined by principal cells and intercalated cells [76]. The principal cells in the OMCD are similar to those in the CCD, but are slightly taller and have fewer organelles and basal membrane infoldings. These cells in the OMCD are involved in Na^+ reabsorption via similar mechanisms as the principal cells in the CCD. However, little evidence exists for K^+ secretion by the principal cells of the OMCD.

Although they are taller with less dense cytoplasm than the type A cells in the CCD, the ICs of the OMCD are considered type A cells. Type B ICs are rare in the OMCD. These type A cells with their apical membrane H^+-ATPase and basolateral membrane Cl^-/HCO_3^- exchanger, AE1, are responsible for H^+ secretion in the OMCD. The OMCD is also an important site of potassium reabsorption, especially during dietary K^+

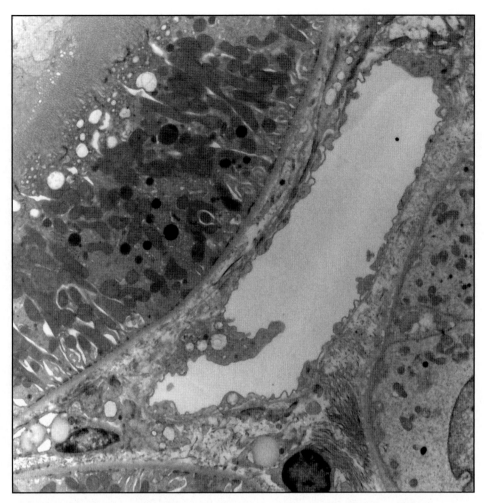

FIGURE 1.60: *Electron micrograph demonstrating an elongated profile of a peritubular capillary situated in the interstitium. Note its close proximity to a proximal tubule (left) and a collecting duct (right). (× 6,000.)*

restriction. This reabsorption is carried out in large part by the type A ICs, via apical membrane H^+-K^+-ATPase pumps. Both the gastric H^+-K^+-ATPase $\alpha 1$ and the colonic H^+-K^+-ATPase $\alpha 2$ isoforms have been immunolocalized to the apical aspect of the ICs. The principal cells also likely participate in K^+ reabsorption in this segment.

(IMCD). The IMCD is the terminal portion of the collecting duct. In this region, the ducts are fused, reflecting their branching embryologic origin from the ureteric bud. The inner medullary segments terminate as the ducts of Bellini, which open on the tip of the papilla, also called the area cribosa (Figure 1.56). There is often an abrupt transition between collecting ducts lined with cuboidal to low columnar cells to the ducts of Bellini, which are composed of taller columnar cells. By light microscopy, the IMCD cells show pale to clear cytoplasm and well-defined lateral cell borders (Figure 1.57).

Structural and functional heterogeneity exists along the IMCD [82]. It can be subdivided arbitrarily into three segments: the outer third ($IMCD_1$), middle third ($IMCD_2$), and inner third ($IMCD_3$). However, structural and functional studies support the existence of two distinct segments: an initial portion ($IMCD_i$), which mainly corresponds to the $IMCD_1$, and the terminal portion ($IMCD_t$), which includes most of the $IMCD_2$ and $IMCD_3$. The $IMCD_i$ consists mainly of principal cells that are similar to the principal cells in the OMCD. Intercalated cells, similar to the type A ICs in the OMCD, constitute about 10 percent of all cells in the $IMCD_i$ in some species. ICs are rare to absent in the $IMCD_i$ of humans. The $IMCD_t$ is composed of mainly one cell type, the IMCD cell. In contrast to principal cells, IMCD cells are taller with light staining cytoplasm containing numerous ribosomes, small lysosomes in the basal aspect, and fewer infoldings of the basal membrane (Figures 1.58 and 1.59). By scanning electron microscopy, the IMCD cells have more numerous small microvilli and lack a central cilium, which is characteristic of principal cells.

The IMCD plays an important role in urinary concentration. The reabsorption of water and urea in this segment results in the formation of a concentrated urine [83]. Water reabsorption is increased by vasopressin all along the collecting duct including the CCD, OMCD, and the IMCD. Both the $IMCD_i$ and $IMCD_t$ have a high water permeability in the presence of vasopressin. It is mediated by the aquaporin water channel AQP2 present in the

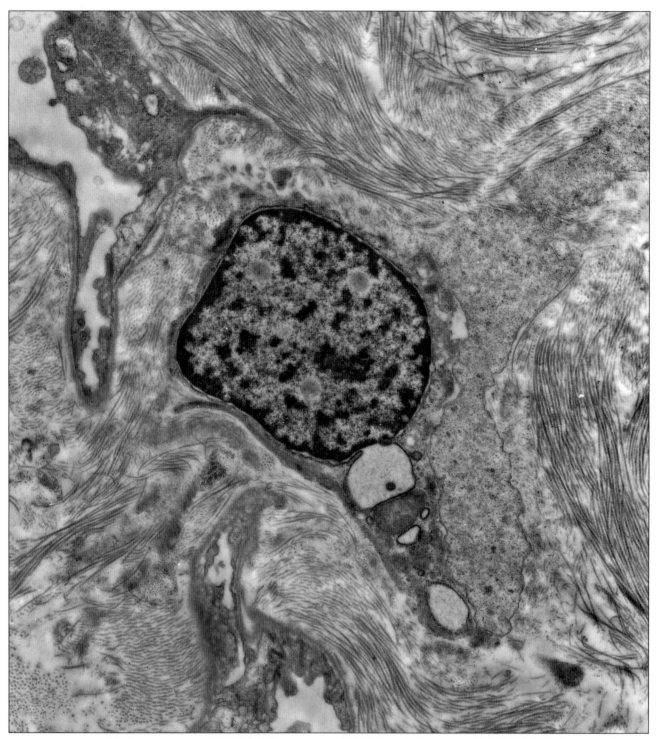

FIGURE 1.61: *Electron micrograph of an interstitial cell with an elongated cell process. It is situated between peritubular capillaries and surrounded by extracellular fibrils. (× 9,000, Courtesy of C.C. Tisher, MD.)*

apical membrane of principal cells (in CCD, OMCD, and IMCD$_i$) and IMCD cells (in IMCD$_t$). Urea is the solute most responsible for the osmolality gradient in the inner medulla. The urea permeabilities of the CCD, OMCD, and IMCD$_i$ are low. Vasopressin-dependent water reabsorption results in a high urea concentration in the lumen of these segments. Passive urea reab-

sorption occurs in the IMCD$_t$ mediated by the urea transporters UT-A1 and UT-A3 present in the IMCD cells. Vasopressin stimulates urea permeability in the IMCD$_t$ by upregulating the urea transporters. The lack of urea transporter expression in the collecting duct segments proximal to the IMCD$_t$ explains the low urea permeability in these segments. Although there is evidence

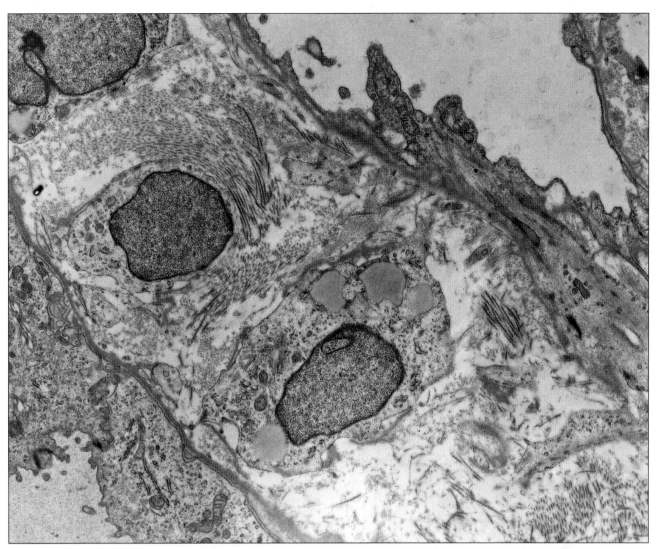

FIGURE 1.62: *Electron micrograph of medullary interstitium illustrating lipid-containing interstitial cells spanning the interstitial space between a thin limb of Henle (left) and a vasa rectum (right). (7,400, Courtesy of C.C. Tisher, MD.)*

that urine acidification occurs along the entire IMCD, the mechanisms have not been completely elucidated.

Interstitium

The interstitium of the kidney consists of an extracellular matrix and several types of interstitial cells [84].Values for the relative cortical interstitial volume in humans range from 5 to 20 percent, with a mean of 12 percent. The values increase with age. The cortical interstitium is divided into the peritubular interstitium and the periarterial connective tissue. In the normal cortex, the peritubular interstitium is inconspicuous and the tubules have a back-to-back architectural appearance. The peritubular capillaries are often inconspicuous on routine histologic sections (Figure 1.60). The periarterial connective tissue is a loose sheath around the intrarenal arteries and contains the lymphatic vessels. This sheath communicates with the peritubular interstitium. The periarterial connective tissue should not be misinterpreted as focal interstitial fibrosis. The

extracellular matrix of the interstitium consists of ground substance within a fibrillar reticulum. It contains proteoglycans, glycoproteins such as fibronectin, interstitial collagens (types I, III, and VI) and microfibrils. Fibroblasts, of which there are several subtypes, are the most numerous cells in the interstitium (Figure 1.61). Cortical peritubular fibroblasts have a stellate appearance, surround the tubules, and show immunoreactivity for ecto-5-nucleotidase (5-NT). A subset of the 5-NT-positive cortical fibroblasts is the erythropoietin-producing cells in the kidney. Dendritic cells of bone marrow origin represent another prevalent cell type in the cortical peritubular interstitium [85]. These dendritic cells (DCs), functioning as antigen-presenting cells in immune responses, include two main subpopulations: DCs of myeloid origin expressing BDCA-1 (blood DC antigen) and less frequent plasmacytoid DCs expressing BDCA-2.

The relative volume of the interstitium increases from the cortex to the tip of the medulla. Values reported for the medullary interstitial volume have been reported from 10 to 20 percent in the outer medulla to 30 to 40 percent at the papillary tip. This substantial amount of interstitium in the medulla should not be mistaken for interstitial fibrosis. The medullary interstitium has a gelatinous appearance on light microscopy. Although several types of interstitial cells exist in the medulla, the most distinctive are the lipid-laden cells, especially abundant in the inner medulla (Figure 1.62). These cells, often called renomedullary interstitial cells (RMICs), bridge the space between the thin limbs of Henle and the vasa recta. They have long cytoplasmic processes and prominent electron-dense lipid droplets. The lipid droplets contain prostaglandin precursors, phospholipids, and cholesterol. These substances produced by the RMICs are believed to contribute to an endocrine-like antihypertensive function that has been ascribed to the renal medulla [86].

REFERENCES

1. Madsen KM, Nielsen S, Tisher CC. Anatomy of the kidney. In: Brenner BM, ed. *Brenner and Rector's The Kidney*. 8th ed. Philadelphia, PA: Saunders Elsevier; 2008, pp. 25–90.
2. Reilly Jr, RF, Bulger RE, Kriz W. Structural-functional relationships in the kidney. In: Schrier EW, ed. *Diseases of the Kidney & Urinary Tract*. 8th ed. Philadelphia, PA: Lippincott Williams & Wilkins; 2007, pp. 2–53.
3. Bonsib SM. Renal Anatomy and Histology. In: Jennette JC, Olson JL, Schwartz MM, Silva FG, eds. *Heptinstall's Pathology of the Kidney*. 6th ed. Philadelphia, PA: Lippincott Williams & Wilkins; 2007, pp. 1–70.
4. Clapp WL, Croker BP. The Kidney. In: Mills SE, ed. *Histology for Pathologists*. 3rd ed. Philadelphia, PA: Lippincott Williams & Wilkins; 2007, pp. 839–907.
5. Cheong B, Muthupillai R, Rubin MF. Normal values for renal length and volume as measured by magnetic resonance imaging. *Clin J Am Soc Nephrol* 2007;2:38–45.
6. Bonsib SM, Gibson D, Mhoon M et al. Renal sinus involvement in renal cell carcinomas. *Am J Surg Pathol* 2000;24:451–8.
7. Graves FT. *Anatomical Studies for Renal and Intrarenal Surgery*. Bristol, England; Wright; 1986.
8. Hodson CJ. The renal parenchyma and its blood supply. *Curr Probl Diagn Radiol* 1978;7:5–32.
9. Schmidt-Nielsen B. The renal pelvis. *Kidney Int* 1987;31: 621–8.
10. Hoy WE, Hughson MD, Bertram JF et al. Nephron number, hypertension, renal disease, and renal failure. *J Am Soc Nephrol* 2005;16:2557–64.
11. Brenner BM, Garcia DL, Anderson S. Glomeruli and blood pressure: less of one, more of the other? *Am J Hypertens* 1988;1:335–47.
12. Keller G, Zimmer G, Mall G, et al. Nephron number in patients with primary hypertension. *N Eng J Med* 2003;348:101–8.
13. Kriz W, Kaissling B. Structural organization of the mammalian kidney. In: Seldin DW, Giebisch D, eds. *The Kidney: Physiology and Pathophysiology*. 3rd ed. Philadelphia: Lippincott Williams & Wilkins; 2000:587–654.
14. Kriz W, Bankir L. A standard nomenclature for structures of the kidney. *Kidney Int* 1988;33:1–7.
15. Lemly KV, Kriz W. Structure and function of the renal vasculature. In: Tisher CC, Brenner BM, eds. *Renal Pathology*. 2nd ed. Philadelphia, PA: JB Lippincott; 1994, pp. 981–1026.
16. Elger M, Sakai T, Kriz W. The vascular pole of the renal glomerulus of rat. *Advances Anat Embryol Cell Biol* 1998;139: 1–95.
17. Shiraishi M, Wang X, Walsh MP, et al. Myosin heavy chain expression in renal afferent and efferent arterioles: relationship to contractile kinetics and function. *FASEB J* 2003;17:2284–96.
18. Pallone TL, Turner MR, Edwards A, et al. Countercurrent exchange in the renal medulla. *Am J Physiol Regul Integr Comp Physiol* 2003;284:R1153–R1175.
19. Barajas L, Liu L, Powers K. Anatomy of the renal innervation: intrarenal aspects and ganglia of origin. *Can J Physiol Pharmacol* 1992;70:735–49.
20. Samuel T, Hoy WE, Douglas-Denton R, et al. Determinants of glomerular volume in different cortical zones of the human kidney. *J Am Soc Nephrol* 2005;16:3102–9.
21. Kaplan C, Pasternack B, Shah H, Gallo G. Age-related incidence of sclerotic glomeruli in human kidneys. *Am J Pathol* 1975;80:227–34.
22. Meleg Smith S, Hoy WE, Cobb L. Low incidence of glomerulosclerosis in normal kidneys. *Arch Pathol Lab Med* 1989;113:1253–5.
23. Rostgaard J, Qvortrup K. Sieve plugs in fenestrae of glomerular capillaries – site of the filtration barrier? *Cells Tissue Organs* 2002;170:132–8.
24. Hjalmarsson C, Johansson BR, Haraldsson B. Electron microscopic evaluation of the endothelial surface layer of glomerular capillaries. *Microvas Res* 2004;67:9–17.
25. Ballerman BJ. Glomerular endothelial cell differentiation. *Kidney Int* 2005;67:1668–71.
26. Inkyo-Hayasaka K, Sakai T, Kobayashi N, et al. Three-dimensional analysis of the whole mesangium in the rat. *Kidney Int* 1996;50:672–83.
27. Hugo C, Shankland SJ, Bowen-Pope DF, et al. Extraglomerular origin of the mesangial cell after injury. *J Clin Invest* 1997;100:786–94.
28. Kriz W, Elger M, Mundel P, et al. Structure-stabilizing forces in the glomerular tuft. *J Am Soc Nephol* 1995; 5:1731–9.
29. Sterzel RB, Hartner A, Schlotzer-Schrehardt U, et al. Elastic fiber proteins in the glomerular mesangium in vivo and in cell culture. *Kidney Int* 2000;58:1588–602.
30. Schaefer L, Mihalik D, Babelova A, et al. Regulation of fibrillin-1 by biglycan and decorin is important for tissue preservation in the kidney during pressure-induced injury. *Am J Pathol* 2004;165:383–96.
31. Makino H, Hironaka K, Shikata K, et al. Mesangial matrices act as mesangial channels to the juxtaglomerular zone. *Nephron* 1994;66:181–8.
32. Latta H, Fligiel S. Mesangial fenestrations, sieving, filtration, and flow. *Lab Invest* 1985;52:591–8.
33. Hudson BG, Tryggvason K, Sundaramoorthy M, et al. Alport's syndrome, Goodpasture's syndrome, and type IV collagen. *N Eng J Med* 2003;348:2543–56.
34. Hudson BG. The molecular basis of Goodpasture and Alport syndromes: beacons for the discovery of the collagen IV family. *J Am Soc Nephrol* 2004;15:2514–27.

35. Pavenstadt H, Kriz W, Kretzler M. Cell biology of the glomerular podocytes. *Physiol Rev* 2003;83:253–307.
36. Neal CR, Crook H, Bell E, et al. Three-dimensional reconstruction of glomeruli by electron microscopy reveals a distinct restrictive urinary subpodocyte space. *J Am Soc Nephrol* 2005;16:1223–35.
37. Salmon AHJ, Toma I, Sipos A, et al. Evidence for restriction of fluid and solute movement across the glomerular capillary wall by the subpodocyte space. *Am J Physiol Renal Physiol* 2007;293:F1777–F1786.
38. Neal CR, Muston PR, Njegovan D, et al. Glomerular filtration into the subpodocyte space is highly restricted under physiological perfusion conditions. *Am J Physiol Renal Physiol* 2007;293:F1787–F1798.
39. Rodewald R, Karnovsky MJ. Porous substructure of the glomerular slit diaphragm in the rat and mouse. *J Cell Biol* 1974;60:423–33.
40. Wartiovaara J, Ofverstedt L-G, Khoshnoodi J, et al. Nephrin strands contribute to a porous slit diaphragm scaffold as revealed by electron tomography. *J Clin Invest* 2004;114:1475–83.
41. Kerjaschki D. Caught flat-footed: podocyte damage and the molecular bases of focal glomerulosclerosis. *J Clin Invest* 2001;108:1583–7.
42. Patrakka J, Tryggvason K. Nephrin – a unique structural and signaling protein of the kidney filter. *Trends in Mol Med* 2007;13:396–403.
43. Faul C, Asanuma K, Yanagida-Asanuma E, et al. Actin up: regulation of podocyte structure and function by components of the actin cytoskeleton. *Trends Cell Biol* 2007;17:428–37.
44. Jones N, Blasutig IM, Eremina V, et al. Nck adaptor proteins link nephrin to the actin cytoskeleton of kidney podocytes. *Nature* 2006;440:818–23.
45. Verma R, Kovari I, Soofi A, et al. Nephrin ectodomain engagement results in Src kinase activation, nephrin phosphorylation, Nck recruitment, and actin polymerization. *J Clin Invest* 2006;116:1346–59.
46. Barisoni L, Kriz W, Mundel P, et al. The dysregulated podocye phenotype: a novel concept in the pathogenesis of collapsing idiopathic focal segmental glomerulosclerosis and HIV-associated nephropathy. *J Am Soc Nephrol* 1999;10:51–61.
47. Chen J, Boyle S, Zhao M, et al. Differential expression of the intermediate filament protein nestin during renal development and its localization in adult podocytes. *J Am Soc Nephrol* 2006;17:1283–91.
48. Thorner PS, Ho M, Eremina V, et al. Podocytes contribute to the formation of glomerular crescents. *J Am Soc Nephrol* 2008;19:495–502.
49. Schumacher VA, Jeruschke S, Eitner F, et al. Impaired glomerular maturation and lack of VEGF165b in Denys-Drash syndrome. *J Am Soc Nephrol* 2007;18:719–29.
50. Eremina V, Cui S, Gerber H, et al. Vascular endothelial growth factor A signaling in the podocyte-endothelial compartment is required for mesangial cell migration and survival. *J Am Soc Nephrol* 2006;17:724–35.
51. Deen WM. What determines glomerular capillary permeability? *J Clin Invest* 2004;114:1412–14.
52. Haraldsson B, Nystrom J, Deen WM. Properties of the glomerular barrier and mechanisms of proteinuria. *Physiol Rev* 2008;88:451–87.
53. Jeansson M, Haraldsson B. Morphological and functional evidence for an important role of the endothelial cell glycocalyx in the glomerular barrier. *Am J Physiol* 2006;290:F111–F116.
54. Singh A, Satchell SC, Neal CR, et al. Glomerular endothelial glycocalyx constitutes a barrier to protein permeability. *J Am Soc Nephrol* 2007;18:2885–93.
55. Wijnhoven TJM, Lensen JFM, Wismans RGP, et al. In vivo degradation of heparan sulfates in the glomerular basement membrane does not result in proteinuria. *J Am Soc Nephrol* 2007;18:823–32.
56. Harvey SJ, Jarad G, Cunningham J, et al. Disruption of glomerular basement membrane charge through podocyte-specific mutation of agrin does not alter glomerular permeability. *Am J Pathol* 2007;171:139–52.
57. Jarad G, Cunningham J, Shaw AS, et al. Proteinuria precedes podocyte abnormalities in *Lamb2*$^{-/-}$ mice, implicating the glomerular basement membrane as an albumin filter. *J Clin Invest* 2006;116:2272–9.
58. Bariety J, Mandet C, Hill GS, et al. Parietal podocytes in normal human glomeruli. *J Am Soc Nephrol* 2006;17:2770–80.
59. Barajas L, Salido EC, Smolens P, et al. Pathology of the juxtaglomerular apparatus including Bartter's syndrome. In: Tisher CC, Brenner BM, eds. *Renal Pathology.* 2nd ed. Philadelphia: JB Lippincott; 1994:948–78.
60. Schnermann J. The juxtaglomerular apparatus: From anatomical peculiarity to physiological relevance. *J Am Soc Nephrol* 2003;14:1681–94.
61. Skinnider BF, Folpe AL, Hennigar RA, et al. Distribution of cytokeratins and vimentin in adult renal neoplasms and normal renal tissue. *Am J Surg Pathol* 2005;29:747–54.
62. Maunsbach AB, Christensen EI. Functional ultrastructure of the proximal tubule. In: Windhager EE, ed. *Handbook of Physiology. Section 8: Renal Physiology.* New York: Oxford University Press; 1992, pp. 41–107.
63. Tisher CC, Bulger RE, Trump BF. Human renal ultrastructure. I. Proximal tubule of healthy individuals. *Lab Invest* 1966;15:1357–94.
64. Zhai XY, Birn H, Jensen KB, et al. Digital three-dimensional reconstruction and ultrastructure of the mouse proximal tubule. *J Am Soc Nephrol* 2003;14:611–19.
65. Mount DB, Yu ASL. Transport of inorganic solutes: sodium, chloride, potassium, magnesium, calcium, and phosphate. In: Brenner BM, ed. *Brenner & Rector's The Kidney.* 8th ed. Philadelphia, PA: Saunders; 2008, pp. 156–213.
66. Welling LW, Welling DJ. Shape of epithelial cells and intercellular channels in the rabbit proximal nephron. *Kidney Int* 1976;9:385–94.
67. Birn H, Christensen EI. Renal albumin absorption in physiology and pathology. *Kidney Int* 2006;69:440–9.
68. Nielsen R, Courtoy PJ, Jacobsen C, et al. Endocytosis provides a major alternative pathway for lysosomal biogenesis in kidney proximal tubular cells. *Proc Natl Acad Sci USA* 2007;104:5407–12.
69. Zhai X-Y, Thomsen JS, Birn H, et al. Three-dimensional reconstruction of the mouse nephron. *J Am Soc Nephrol* 2006;17:77–88.

70. Dieterich HJ, Barrett JM, Kriz W, et al. The ultrastructure of the thin limbs of the mouse kidney. *Anat Embryol* 1975;147:1–13.

71. Bulger RE, Tisher CC, Myers CH, et al. Human renal ultrastructure.II.The thin limb of Henle's loop and the interstitium in healthy individuals. *Lab Invest* 1967;16: 124–41.

72. Zhai X-Y, Fenton RA, Andreasen A, et al. Aquaporin-1 is not expressed in descending thin limbs of short-loop nephrons. *J Am Soc Nephrol* 2007;18:2937–44.

73. Kone BC, Madsen KM, Tisher CC. Ultrastructure of the thick ascending limb of Henle in the rat kidney. *Am J Anat* 1984;171;217–26.

74. Ren Y, Garvin JL, Liu R, et al. Crosstalk between the connecting tubule and the afferent arteriole regulates renal microcirculation. *Kidney Int* 2007;71:1116–21.

75. Myers CH, Bulger RE, Tisher CC, et al. Human renal ultrastructure. IV. Collecting duct of healthy individuals. *Lab Invest* 1966;15:1921–50.

76. Madsen KM, Tisher CC. Structural-functional relationships along the distal nephron. *Am J Physiol* 1986;250:F1–F15.

77. Verlander JW, Madsen KM, Tisher CC. Effect of acute respiratory acidosis on two populations of intercalated cells in the rat cortical collecting duct. *Am J Physiol* 1987;253: F1142–F1156.

78. Teng-umnuay P, Verlander JW, Yuan W, et al. Identification of distinct subpopulations of intercalated cells in the mouse collecting duct. *J Am Soc Nephrol* 1996;7:260–74.

79. Kim J, Kim Y-H, Cha J-H, et al. Intercalated cell subtypes in connecting tubule and cortical collecting duct of rat and mouse. *J Am Soc Nephrol* 1999;10:1–12.

80. Kim Y-H, Kwon T-H, Frische S, et al. Immunocytochemical localization of pendrin in intercalated cell subtypes in rat and mouse kidney. *Am J Physiol* 2002;283:F744–F754.

81. Wall SM. Recent advances in our understanding of intercalated cells. *Curr Opin Nephrol Hypertens* 2005;14:480–4.

82. Madsen KM, Clapp WL, Verlander JW. Structure and function of the inner medullary collecting duct. *Kidney Int* 1988;34:441–54.

83. Knepper MA, Hoffert JD, Packer RK, Fenton RA. Urine concentration and dilution. In: Brenner BM, ed. *Brenner and Rector's The Kidney*. 8th ed. Philadelphia, PA: Saunders Elsevier; 2008, pp. 308–29.

84. Lemley KV, Kriz W. Anatomy of the interstitium. *Kidney Int* 1991;39:370–81.

85. Woltman AM, de Fijter JW, Zuidwijk K, et al. Quantification of dendritic cell subsets in human renal tissue under normal and pathological conditions. *Kidney Int* 2007;71:1001–8.

86. Muirhead EE. Antihypertensive functions of the kidney. *Hypertension* 1980;2:444–64.

CHAPTER 2

Renal Biopsy: The Nephrologist's Viewpoint

Robert D. Toto, MD

INTRODUCTION

Kidney biopsy is an important procedure for diagnosing and managing kidney disease, and nephrologists are often called upon to determine the appropriateness of this procedure. In fact, it is probably the most important tool among the ones used in the management of patients with both acute and chronic kidney disease. However, very few patients with acute kidney failure and even (proportionally) fewer with chronic kidney disease (CKD) ever undergo biopsy. For example, annually more than 90,000 patients with the clinical diagnosis of diabetic nephropathy are initiated on dialysis, yet fewer than 10 percent undergo a kidney biopsy to confirm the diagnosis despite the fact that when kidney biopsy is performed in type 2 diabetes, up to two-thirds of cases reveal a histologic diagnosis other than diabetic nephropathy [1]. Moreover, when the clinical diagnosis is compared with the pathologic diagnosis in patients who undergo kidney biopsy for acute kidney failure, the clinical diagnosis is incorrect in at least 50 percent of cases [2–6]. Now, there are few noninvasive markers specific enough to correctly predict the morphologic diagnosis in most patients with kidney disease. Even in the future, accurate characteriza-tion of kidney disease by molecular methods that are guided by kidney biopsy will still be needed to achieve advances in the field of nephrology, for example, identification of genes or proteins utilizing in situ hybridization or microarray techniques that indicate the stage of kidney disease or predict clinical outcomes. This chapter discusses the indications, procedures, and compli-cations of kidney biopsy in the management of acute and chronic kidney disease.

IMPORTANCE OF UNDERSTANDING RENAL PATHOLOGY

All clinical nephrologists must have exposure to renal biopsy interpretation as part of their nephrology training. This is nec-essary to provide the nephrologist with an understanding of the value and limitation of careful examination of renal tissue in their patients. In most cases, even when the pathologic diagno-sis is clear, review of the biopsy with the renal pathologist coupled with the nephrologist's knowledge of the patient's clin-ical history and presentation can make a major difference in how the biopsy is interpreted. For example, in a transplant patient with evidence of allograft nephropathy, the decision to modify immunosuppression may depend on subtle findings shared directly by the pathologist with the nephrologist that might not occur based on the reading of a report. Thus, it should be emphasized that whenever possible, the nephrologist should review kidney biopsy specimens (side by side) with the pathologist. As Pirani said: "structure and function have finally met at the microscope" [7].

An important prerequisite for arriving at the correct pathologic diagnosis, which in turn aids the nephrologist in treatment consideration, is the provision of current and accurate clinical information to the nephropathologist. A concise clinical history, including family history of kidney disease and whether acute kidney injury or CKD is suspected, is important. In addition, a provision for a brief summary of key abnormal laboratory findings including urinalysis, serologic tests, and relevant imaging studies can make a difference not only in whether special stains or preparations are needed, but also in the final pathologic diagnosis rendered.

The ingredients necessary to provide an accurate diagnosis have been promulgated by the Renal Pathology Society and include the following: native kidney biopsies require examination by light microscopy, immunohistochemistry, and electron microscopy; support of a fully equipped anatomic pathology laboratory; technical expertise to process small fragments of tissue and to produce high-quality tissue sections; and the skills of a well-trained renal pathologist knowledgeable in renal pathology and renal medicine [8].

INDICATIONS

Clinical Decision Making

The decision to undertake a kidney biopsy should be based on careful assessment of the patient's clinical findings and expert knowledge of kidney disease and its consequences [9]. Kidney biopsy is currently done for three major reasons: (a) to establish the pathologic diagnosis, (b) to provide insight into treatment options, and (c) to provide prognostic information or gauge response to therapy. Patients, and when appropriate family members, must be informed by the nephrologist of the reasons, the risks, and the potential benefits of performing a kidney biopsy. In addition, the patient should be informed that in some cases (even with an adequate sample) a kidney biopsy may not provide a definitive diagnosis. The final decision to conduct a biopsy should, in most cases, be based on whether or not the biopsy will change the therapeutic plan. Therefore, biopsy should not be undertaken in patients who are unwilling to accept recommended therapies, such as immunosuppressive regimens. The benefits and risks of interventions should be clearly communicated to potential biopsy candidates.

Age is usually not a contraindication of renal biopsy. In elderly patients, nephrotic syndrome and systemic vasculitis are common reasons for conducting a kidney biopsy, and biopsy is generally safe in this population [10,11]. Children may also safely undergo kidney biopsy. However, in many young children with new-onset nephrotic syndrome, biopsy is often reserved for those who are unresponsive to high-dose oral corticosteroid treatment since minimal change disease or some variant thereof is the most common cause.

Kidney biopsy plays a critical role in the diagnosis, prognosis, initial treatment, and therapeutic response in patients with both acute and chronic kidney disease. In addition, a kidney biopsy may have important implications for short- and long-term cost-effectiveness of patient management. Several studies have shown that planned or ongoing therapeutic interventions were modified significantly after a diagnosis was obtained by kidney biopsy [2–6,12]. In addition, studies have documented the change in diagnosis and subsequent clinical decision making among patients with a variety of kidney diseases, including acute renal failure, nephrotic syndrome, systemic lupus erythematosus (SLE), diabetic kidney disease, and postrenal transplant evaluation [2,12–18]. Moreover, in some studies, it has been clearly shown that the renal biopsy was invaluable since the predictability of the renal histopathologic lesion based on clinical grounds was extremely poor (less than 50 percent accuracy). For example, in one prospective, single-center study of 276 native renal biopsies in 266 patients, changes in management as a direct result of the biopsy were confirmed in 86 percent of cases of nephrotic range proteinuria, 71 percent of cases of acute renal failure, 45 percent of cases of CKD. 32 percent of cases with hematuria and proteinuria, 12 percent of cases with nonnephrotic proteinuria alone, and 3 percent of cases with hematuria alone, with changes in management in 42 percent of cases overall [18]. In another 3-year prospective study of 80 patients, prebiopsy clinical diagnosis was changed in 44 percent of patients, prognosis changed in 57 percent of the patients, and therapy changed in 31 percent of the patients [2]. Taken together, these studies strongly suggest that when in doubt about the cause of acute or chronic kidney disease, a kidney biopsy should be performed whenever it is deemed safe by the treating physician.

Acute Kidney Injury

Native

The main indication for kidney biopsy in patients with acute kidney disease is whether a knowledge of the renal histology will make a significant difference in patient management. For example, a patient with suspected glomerulonephritis from a necrotizing vasculitis is at very high risk for rapidly progressive irreversible kidney failure. A biopsy in this situation will provide the critical information necessary to institute multifaceted immunosuppressive therapy that may be renal sparing and/or even life-saving. Moreover, a kidney biopsy can spare patients from unnecessary risks of immunosuppressive drugs and plasmapheresis if no inflammatory disease is present on kidney biopsy. Indications for biopsy in the setting of acute kidney injury (Table 2.1 and Figure 2.1) include new-onset proteinuria or hematuria, nephrotoxic injury from known or new suspected nephrotoxin, and absence of prerenal conditions. Importantly, syndromes that masquerade as another, such as SLE, necrotizing vasculitis, glomerulonephritis due to endocarditis, allergic interstitial nephritis, and cholesterol embolism syndrome, which may present as acute kidney injury, require a kidney biopsy to make a definitive diagnosis. Kidney biopsy is crucial because therapeutic interventions for suspected renal manifestations of these illnesses are potentially toxic and harmful. Thus, a tissue diagnosis is crucial before starting potentially

Table 2.1 Indications for Kidney Biopsy

Native

Acute kidney injury in the absence of prerenal cause
Rapidly progressive glomerulonephritis
Systemic lupus erythematosus
Diabetes mellitus
Suspected interstitial nephritis
Unexplained hematuria or proteinuria
New or known nephrotoxic injury (e.g., drug, chemical exposure)

Transplant

Acute rejection
Calcineurin inhibitor toxicity
Chronic rejection
Infections
Recurrent disease
De novo disease including drug-induced

dangerous immunosuppressive treatment in suspected cases of vasculitis, lupus nephritis, cholesterol embolism, and allergic interstitial nephritis.

Transplant

Biopsy of transplanted kidney for acute kidney injury is usually done to differentiate transplant rejection from calcineurin inhibitor toxicity, prerenal azotemia, acute tubular necrosis, or infections. However, it is also indicated for demonstration of recurrent disease (e.g., idiopathic focal segmental sclerosis) or de novo acute injury to the allograft such as from drugs or new glomerular or interstitial disease.

Chronic Kidney Disease

Native

General comments. The vast majority of patients with CKD, defined as kidney disease (imaging abnormalities, abnormal urine analysis, or an estimated glomerular filtration rate < 60 ml/min/ 1.73 m^2) present for 3 or more months, do not undergo kidney biopsy. The reasons for this include the fact that patients with CKD are frequently unrecognized in the community; there is therapeutic nihilism for treating advanced CKD and technical challenges particularly in obese patients whose prevalence in the general population has been increasing [9]. There is general

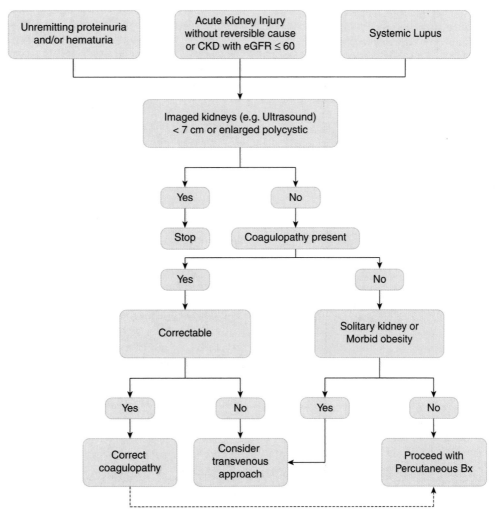

FIGURE 2.1: Renal biopsy algorithm.

consensus that kidney biopsy is a necessary procedure in patients with lupus who exhibit evidence of renal involvement (e.g., increased serum creatinine, abnormal urine sediment, or proteinuria). In contrast, there is no consensus on the need for kidney biopsy in a patient with asymptomatic proteinuria or microhematuria. Still, there are no widely accepted guidelines for when to perform a kidney biopsy, and the decision relies largely on clinical judgment (Figure 2.1). Further clinical decision-making studies and better noninvasive markers are needed to refine clinical practice. In general, a kidney biopsy is indicated in patients with CKD in whom (1) the diagnosis is uncertain based on clinical and laboratory data and (2) tissue diagnosis can provide evidence for an important therapeutic intervention. For example, a patient with CKD, proteinuria. and no clinical or serologic evidence of systemic disease may have a treatable form of glomerular disease such as idiopathic focal segmental glomerulosclerosis or IgA nephropathy, two common treatable causes of CKD.

Since the vast majority of patients with acute kidney injury and CKD in the United States do not undergo kidney biopsy, the precise cause of their kidney disease is uncertain. For example, more than 75 percent of new cases of end-stage kidney disease are attributed to either diabetes mellitus or hypertension, yet most of these patients have not had a kidney biopsy. Still, because many patients present to the nephrologist with advanced disease (and in some cases with small kidneys), biopsy is not performed. It is controversial whether all patients with kidney disease should have a kidney biopsy in order to characterize the disease. This is not a commonly accepted practice and needs to be debated.

Systemic lupus erythematosus. Kidney involvement in patients with SLE is common, occurring in 60 percent of patients. There has been substantial progress in understanding the disease process, and treatment is based largely on kidney biopsy for those with evidence of kidney disease as noted. The International Society of Nephrology and the Renal Pathology Society recently refined the World Heath Organization classification of kidney involvement in systemic lupus to better guide the therapy for this disorder [19,20].

Diabetes mellitus. Kidney biopsy is rarely performed in patients with longstanding diabetes who are detected to have kidney disease (e.g., elevated serum creatinine, albuminuria) [21]. However, kidney biopsy should be considered in diabetic patients who have persistent hematuria, lack of retinopathy (in type 1 diabetics), new-onset nephritic syndrome (worsening or new-onset hypertension, hematuria and deteriorating kidney function measured by serum creatinine), nephrotic syndrome, or rapidly deteriorating kidney function (e.g., doubling serum creatinine within a 3-month period), or normal hemoglobin A1C [1]. Whether this practice will change in the future is uncertain since the number of patients with type 2 diabetes and kidney disease, many of whom pose technical challenges because of accompanying obesity and concomitant medical comorbidities, is growing. Still, biopsy series of patients with type 2 diabetes and nephropathy frequently identify nondiabetic kidney diseases [22,23]. This dilemma has not been resolved by the nephrology community.

Proteinuria and hematuria. In general, kidney biopsy is indicated in all adult nondiabetic patients with new-onset nephrotic syndrome. This is because the differential diagnosis of nephrotic syndrome is too broad, and like most kidney diseases, noninvasive markers are not sufficiently specific or sensitive for predicting the etiology of nephrotic syndrome. The treatment and prognosis of nephrotic syndrome also vary considerably, providing strong indication for tissue diagnosis before initiation of therapy. Renal biopsy also provides important prognostic information to the patient. Persistent microhematuria (>3–5 RBC/ HPF) can be a harbinger of important progressive kidney diseases including IgA nephropathy and Fabry's disease. A kidney biopsy should be considered in such patients after a complete urologic workup to exclude malignancy or other urinary tract cause.

Transplant

Indications for biopsy in kidney transplant patients with slowly declining kidney function include allograft rejection, calcineurin inhibitor toxicity, and de novo renal disease. In addition, in recent years, viral infections, in particular the polyoma virus (BK) nephropathy, have been increasingly recognized as important causes of kidney disease in the transplant [24].

CONTRAINDICATIONS

Contraindications to kidney biopsy are relative, and a risk–benefit ratio of performing a renal biopsy should be conducted in every case. Table 2.2 illustrates relative contraindications to kidney biopsy. One of the relative contraindications is the patient's noncooperation. This may become evident only after the start of the procedure. Patients who are unable to cooperate with the biopsy procedure may be at increased risk for complications. This judgment must be made at the bedside by the treating nephrologist or radiologist performing the biopsy. Uncontrolled hypertension (blood pressure > 140/90 mmHg) is another common relative contraindication and has been reported to increase the risk for hemorrhage. In most cases, a kidney biopsy can be postponed until blood pressure is controlled. Patients with coagulopathy should not undergo biopsy until this is corrected. A normal partial thromboplastin time and international normalized ratio for prothrombin time should be ensured, and these may be corrected by transfusion. Intravenous infusion of desmopressin acetate dDAVP can be used to correct bleeding time or abnormal platelet function assay prior to biopsy [25]. In adults, small kidneys (e.g., < 8 cm) are often not biopsied because of the high likelihood of severe glomerular

Table 2.2 Relative Contraindications to Kidney Biopsy

Solitary kidney
Small kidneys (chronic kidney disease)
Polycystic kidney disease
Neoplasm
Vascular AV fistula
Uncooperative patient
Morbid obesity
Hydronephrosis
Coagulopathy
Uncontrolled hypertension

and interstitial scarring that is not amenable to current therapy (e.g., glucocorticoids, cyclosporine, alkylating agents).

COMPLICATIONS

Hemorrhage

In general, with proper evaluation and attention to coagulation parameters coupled with current imaging and tissue extraction tools, the complications of kidney biopsy are very low [5,26–29]. The most common complication of kidney biopsy is bleeding. With the available ultrasound and computed tomography equipment, even small hematomas can be detected. Studies indicate that only 1–2 percent of patients develop a hematoma, and only 0.1–1 percent develop an arteriovenous fistula. Surgical intervention is required in fewer than 1 percent of the patients, and mortality is less than 0.1 percent after biopsy, and these rates may be declining [5,26,30]. In one large retrospective review of complications related to percutaneous renal biopsy, poorly controlled hypertension, prolonged bleeding time, and elevated serum creatinine were identified as risk factors, and in multivariate analysis, those with serum creatinine greater than 5 mg/dl were 2.5 times more likely to have a complication [31]. It should be noted that in this study the cases were collected over a period of 20 years during which procedures and practice in conducting and monitoring percutaneous kidney biopsy had undergone changes.

Urinoma

A urinoma is defined as a collection of urine outside of the urinary tract. Urinoma is a rare complication of kidney biopsy that can occur with either native or transplant biopsy; however, as noted in the earlier section on hemorrhage, with better imaging methods, this complication has been almost completely eliminated. Urinoma may be evident by symptoms of fever, malaise, and abdominal discomfort and is often occult. Abscess formation, electrolyte disorders, and obstruction may occur. Computed tomography, cystography, and retrograde urethrography are helpful, as are pyelography (antegrade and retrograde) and renal scintigraphy [32]. The diagnosis is established by imaging a fluid collection followed by needle aspiration and measurement of simultaneous serum and fluid creatinine (or urea) concentration. An increased ratio of fluid to serum creatinine indicates the presence of urine. In most cases, it is not necessary to percutaneously drain these urinomas as they tend to resolve spontaneously.

Arteriovenous Fistula

Arteriovenous (AV) fistula is another rare complication that can be detected using color Doppler [33]. The precise incidence of this complication is unknown since it is not routinely looked for after biopsy. Bleeding from an AV fistula induced by percutaneous biopsy can occur days to weeks after the procedure. Therefore, patients should be counseled to contact their physician immediately in case of gross hematuria or new onset of severe back pain after biopsy. AV fistula can be closed by angiographic or surgical techniques.

Pain

Local pain after kidney biopsy is common and should be anticipated. It is usually mild and can be managed with short-term oral administration of analgesics including narcotics. Most patients do not have prolonged (more than 1 week) pain after kidney biopsy. In patients with chronic pain postbiopsy, further evaluation using ultrasound and color Doppler should be considered to rule out hematoma, urinoma, abscess, or fistula.

Infection

Infection is a very rare complication and is reported to occur in 0.2 percent of cases in large series, most of which were reported before the 1990s [26]. Due to availability of improved techniques, the likelihood of infection will be even lower. Indeed, infection has never occurred in the biopsies we conducted in the past 10 years.

PREBIOPSY EVALUATION

A complete history and physical examination should be performed on every patient before undergoing kidney biopsy. Kidney biopsy cannot be used as a substitute for a thorough clinical evaluation and workup. In addition, a history of bleeding diathesis and uncontrolled hypertension should be specifically asked about because they can increase risk of complications of this procedure. The examination should include a careful search for evidence of systemic disease including skin, funduscopic, neurologic, and gastrointestinal examinations. Laboratory data including prothrombin time, partial thromboplastin time and platelet count, and blood typing and hold should be done in every case. The extent of the additional laboratory work depends on the differential diagnosis and is beyond the scope of this chapter. However, blood and urine tests for kidney function, including a urine analysis and urine protein/creatinine ratio, are very helpful for biopsy interpretation. Serologic tests such as antinuclear antibodies, antineutrophil cytoplasmic antibodies, antiglomerular basement membrane antibodies, serum complement levels, hepatitis serologies, hemoglobin A1C, and serum and urine electrophoreses/immunofixation should be performed according to the history and examination.

TECHINIQUE OF PERCUTANEOUS BIOPSY

Native

Most percutaneous kidney biopsies are performed under ultrasound or computed tomography (CT) guidance by nephrologists or radiologists in an outpatient radiology suite or a nephrology office. However, in several instances, transjugular, laparoscopic, or an open surgical approach may be required to obtain kidney tissue [34,35]. After obtaining informed written consent, confirming that blood coagulation tests are normal, and blood is typed and cross-matched, the patient's vital signs should be recorded, an intravenous line placed, and the appropriate imaging method employed to visualize the kidneys. The patient should be informed that they will need to lie face down for 20–30 minutes, and a towel may be placed under the upper abdomen to assist in visualization of the kidney.

Imaging

Real-time imaging of the kidney during insertion of the biopsy needle is the preferred method for performing a percutaneous kidney biopsy. Several imaging tools can be used for kidney biopsy, including renal ultrasound with color Doppler, computed tomography, and magnetic resonance imaging (MRI) [36]. A major advantage of real-time ultrasound is the visualization of the biopsy needle as it passes through the skin and into the kidney [37]. Recent reports suggest low complication rates (especially hemorrhage) with combined use of ultrasound with color Doppler and 18-gauge biopsy needles [38]. As the kidney moves with respiration, imaging and marking the skin site for biopsy needle entry is typically performed while the patient is holding his/her breath. Patients should be trained to breathe steadily so that the depth of breath prior to holding is consistent at each pass with the biopsy needle. Repeated localization of the lower pole of the kidney after the patient has practiced the breathing ensures precise location of the kidney for biopsy.

Once skin is marked after imaging the kidney and identifying the lower pole of the kidney where the biopsy needle will be inserted, aseptic preparation of the skin and sterile field is employed to minimize the risk of infection. The skin and subcutaneous tissues are anesthetized and a small incision is made in the skin. The patient takes a breath and holds and the needle is positioned in the kidney. Kidney biopsy is usually performed using a spring-loaded, 18-gauge needle. A variety of these devices are available; in general these are easier to use than manual needles (e.g., Vim-Silverman) [37,39]. The choice of needle size can vary and is based on technical needs and the skill of the operator, but in general, an 18-gauge needle is a reasonable size for obtaining adequate tissue in most patients without increased risk of hemorrhage [30,37–39]. Three cores of tissue are obtained to provide an adequate sample for light, immunofluorescence, and electron microscopy. Whenever possible, demonstration of sufficient tissue including at least seven glomeruli should be ascertained at the bedside by visual inspection of the tissue core using a low-power dissecting microscope. When possible, a nephropathologist or technician can assist in this procedure. After biopsy, patients should be observed for complications, especially bleeding, for a minimum of 4 hours. During this observation period, vital signs including blood pressure and pulse rate should be measured frequently. In addition, patients should be specifically monitored for severe back, flank, or abdominal pain as well as gross hematuria. Serial hemoglobin and hematocrit should also be monitored. In some series, up to one-third of complications occur after 8 hours postbiopsy; therefore, some authors recommend a 24-hour observation period to reduce the risk of complications directly related to the procedure [31,34].

Kidney Transplant

The prebiopsy evaluation, imaging, and equipment needed for transplant biopsy are identical to those for native biopsy. However, because the transplanted kidney is in the pelvis, the patient does not have to lie prone. Also, breathing training is unnecessary because the excursion of the kidney with respiration is negligible or absent; therefore, transplant biopsy is generally an easier technique. Also, standard ultrasound is generally sufficient for marking and performing the biopsy because the transplanted kidney is extraperitoneal, relatively superficial, and often palpable on physical examination.

INTERPRETATION

This book is devoted to improving the understanding and utility of kidney biopsy in diagnosing and managing the kidney disease. It is critically important for the treating nephrologist to review the kidney biopsy findings with a skilled nephropathologist. In our experience, this interaction not only increases the likelihood that the patient will receive the best medical care but also serves to inform both the nephrologist and pathologist in each case. These interactions often bring into play important new information about the patient's presentation or condition and serve to confirm the pathological diagnosis and ultimately serve the patient's well-being. In particular, closer interaction during review of the kidney biopsy specimen can provide the nephrologist with a better sense of how to formulate and administer the optimal therapeutic plan for the patient.

Renal cortex is necessary in order to diagnose most known kidney diseases. However, there is no consensus on what constitutes an adequate supply of kidney tissue [8]. For some diffuse diseases such as membranous nephropathy or amyloidosis, a single glomerulus may be sufficient for diagnosis. On the other hand, focal diseases such as focal segmental glomerulosclerosis may be missed if only a few glomeruli are present in the sample [28]. The absolute number of glomeruli on the biopsy is less crucial than the ability to make the diagnosis. A number of studies have demonstrated safety and adequacy of tissue obtained with modern techniques including ultrasound imaging and spring-loaded biopsy needles [27,38–40].

LIMITATIONS

There are several limitations of kidney biopsy. First, not all patients are able or willing to undergo biopsy. Second, adequate tissue may not be obtained occasionally. Third, despite advances in morphologic methods, most kidney diagnoses are not made on the basis of a molecular cause and instead are necessarily descriptive. Fourth, though the biopsy is an invaluable tool for assisting in the management of patients with kidney disease, the test is not easily repeatable and often is not repeated after a course of therapy, which limits the ability of nephrologists, pathologists, and their patients to learn more about the healing process in the kidney and how to prognosticate the future. At the present time, the greatest limitation of kidney biopsy is the relative lack of use of this test in the majority of patients with kidney disease driven by the lack of better understanding of how to manage patients with different pathologic findings such as in diabetic nephropathy [22,23]. Finally, there is a need to identify better methods of providing definitive diagnosis with molecular markers that signify severity, reversibility, or predict response to standard and, in the future, novel therapeutics.

SUMMARY

In summary, kidney biopsy is an extremely important tool for diagnosing both acute and chronic kidney disease. Advances in imaging and other techniques for conducting kidney biopsy allow this procedure to be done safely with a high yield. Patient selection and standard techniques combined with an appropriate evaluation are important components of the biopsy procedure. Finally, interpretation of the biopsy by the pathologist–nephrologist team is optimal for providing the best patient care.

REFERENCES

1. Silva FG. Case 1 – Specialty Conference, Renal Pathology 2006; Available at: URL: www.uscap.org.
2. Turner MW, Hutchinson TA, Barre PE, Prichard S, Jothy S. A prospective study on the impact of the renal biopsy in clinical management. *Clin Nephrol* 1986 November; 26(5):217–21.
3. Appel GB, Silva FG, Pirani CL, Meltzer JI, Estes D. Renal involvement in systemic lupud erythematosus (SLE): a study of 56 patients emphasizing histologic classification. *Medicine (Baltimore)* 1978 September; 57(5):371–410.
4. Appel GB, Valeri A. The course and treatment of lupus nephritis. *Annu Rev Med* 1994; 45:525–37.
5. Appel GB. Renal Biopsy, how effective, what technique and how safe? *J Nephrol* 1993; 6:4.
6. Paone DB, Meyer LE. The effect of biopsy on therapy in renal disease. *Archives of Internal Medicine* 1981 July; 141(8): 1039–41.
7. Pirani C., Renal biopsy: An historical perspective. In: Silva, FG, D'Agati V, editors. *Renal Biopsy Interpretation*. New York: Churchill Livingstone; 1996, p. 1–19.
8. Walker PD, Cavallo T, Bonsib SM. Practice guidelines for the renal biopsy. *Mod Pathol* 2004; 17(12):1555–63.
9. K/DOQI : clinical practice guidelines for chronic kidney diseaseevaluation, classification, and stratification. *Am J Kidney Dis* 2002; 39(2 Suppl. 1):S1–266.
10. Modesto-Segonds A, Ah-Soune MF, Durand D, Suc JM. Renal biopsy in the elderly. *Am J Nephrol* 1993; 13(1): 27–34.
11. Donadio JV, Jr. Treatment and clinical outcome of glomerulonephritis in the elderly. *Contrib Nephrol* 1993; 105: 49–57.
12. Cohen AH, Nast CC, Adler SG, Kopple JD. Clinical utility of kidney biopsies in the diagnosis and management of renal disease. *Am J Nephrol* 1989; 9(4):309–15.
13. Al-Awwa IA, Hariharan, First MR. Importance of allograft biopsy in renal transplant recipients: correlation between clinical and histological diagnosis. *Am J Kidney Dis Nephrol* 1998; 31:S15.
14. Hommel E, Carstensen H, Skott P, Larsen S, Parving HH. Prevalence and causes of microscopic haematuria in type 1 (insulin- dependent) diabetic patients with persistent proteinuria. *Diabetologia* 1987; 30(8):627–30.
15. Jacobsen S, Starklint H, Petersen J et al. Prognostic value of renal biopsy and clinical variables in patients with lupus nephritis and normal serum creatinine. *Scandinavian Journal of Rheumatology* 1999; 28(5):288–99.
16. Marx BE, Marx M. Prediction in idiopathic membranous nephropathy. *Kidney Int* 1999; 56(2):666–73.
17. Matas AJ, Tellis VA, Sablay L, Quinn T, Soberman R, Veith FJ. The value of needle renal allograft biopsy. III. A prospective study. *Surgery* 1985; 98(5): 922–926.
18. Richards NT, Darby S, Howie AJ, Adu D, Michael J. Knowledge of renal histology alters patient management in over 40% of cases. *Nephrol Dial Transplant* 1994; 9(9): 1255–9.
19. Fine DM. Pharmacological therapy of lupus nephritis. *JAMA* 2005 June 22; 293(24):3053–60.
20. Schwartz MM. The pathology of lupus nephritis. *Semin Nephrol* 2007 January; 27(1):22–34.
21. Tuttle, K, editor. National Kidney Foundation. Clinical Practice Guidelines and Clinical Practice Recommendations for Diabetes and Chronic Kidney Disease. *Am J Kidney Dis* 2007; 49[2, Supplement 2]:S1–123.
22. Christensen PK, Larsen S, Horn T, Olsen S, Parving HH. Causes of albuminuria in patients with type 2 diabetes without diabetic retinopathy. *Kidney Int* 2000 October; 58(4):1719–31.
23. Gambara V, Mecca G, Remuzzi G, Bertani T. Heterogeneous nature of renal lesions in type II diabetes. *J Am Soc Nephrol* 1993; 3:1458–66.
24. Hirsch HH, Suthanthiran M. The natural history, risk factors and outcomes of polyomavirus BK-associated nephropathy after renal transplantation. *Nat Clin Pract Nephrol* 2006 May; 2(5):240–1.
25. Mannucci PM, Remuzzi G, Pusineri F et al. Deamino-8-d-arginine vasopressin shortens the bleeding time in uremia. *N Engl J Med* 1983 January 6; 308(1):8–12.
26. Parrish AE. Complications of percutaneous renal biopsy: a review of 37 years' experience. *Clin Nephrol* 1992 September; 38(3):135–41.
27. Doyle AJ, Gregory MC, Terreros DA. Percutaneous native renal biopsy: comparison of a 1.2-mm spring-driven system with a traditional 2-mm hand-driven system. *Am J Kidney Dis* 1994 April; 23(4):498–503.
28. Madaio MP. Renal biopsy. *Kidney Int* 1990; 38(3): 529–43.
29. Diaz-Buxo JA, Gotch FA, Folden TI et al. Peritoneal dialysis adequacy: a model to assess feasibility with various modalities. *Kidney Int* 1999; 55(6):2493–501.
30. Burstein DM, Korbet SM, Schwartz MM. The use of the automatic core biopsy system in percutaneous renal biopsies: a comparative study. *Am J Kidney Dis* 1993; 22(4): 545–52.
31. Whittier WL, Korbet SM. Timing of complications in percutaneous renal biopsy. *J Am Soc Nephrol* 2004; 15(1): 142–7.
32. Titton RL, Gervais DA, Hahn PF, Harisinghani MG, Arellano RS, Mueller PR. Urine leaks and urinomas: diagnosis and imaging-guided intervention. *Radiographics* 2003; 23(5): 1133–47.
33. Zubarev AV. Ultrasound of renal vessels. *Eur Radiol* 2001; 11(10):1902–15.

34. Whittier WL, Korbet SM. Renal biopsy: update. *Curr Opin Nephrol Hypertens* 2004; 13(6):661–5.

35. Mal F, Meyrier A, Callard P, Kleinknecht D, Altmann JJ, Beaugrand M. The diagnostic yield of transjugular renal biopsy. Experience in 200 cases. *Kidney Int* 1992; 41(2):445–9.

36. Ginsburg JC, Fransman SL, Singer MA, Cohanim M, Morrin PA. Use of computerized tomography to evaluate bleeding after renal biopsy. *Nephron* 1980; 26(5):240–3.

37. Wiseman DA, Hawkins R, Numerow LM, Taub KJ. Percutaneous renal biopsy utilizing real time, ultrasonic guidance and a semiautomated biopsy device. *Kidney Int* 1990 August; 38(2):347–9.

38. Hojs R. Kidney biopsy and power Doppler imaging. *Clin Nephrol* 2004; 62(5):351–4.

39. Mahoney MC, Racadio JM, Merhar GL, First MR. Safety and efficacy of kidney transplant biopsy: Tru-Cut needle vs sonographically guided Biopty gun. *AJR Am J Roentgenol* 1993; 160(2):325–6.

40. Mendelssohn DC, Cole EH. Outcomes of percutaneous kidney biopsy, including those of solitary native kidneys. *Am J Kidney Dis* 1995; 26:580–5.

CHAPTER 3

Algorithmic Approach to the Interpretation of Renal Biopsy

Xin J. Zhou MD, Zoltan Laszik MD, and Fred G. Silva MD

INTRODUCTION

The introduction of renal biopsy techniques in the early 1950s has revolutionized the study of renal diseases. Percutaneous renal biopsy has permitted not only the study of renal diseases in their early stages, but also the state of evolution of many diseases through sequential biopsies. In addition, obtaining a fresh renal tissue by a percutaneous biopsy has allowed the optimal use of immunofluorescence (IF) and transmission electron microscopy (EM), which have greatly enhanced our understanding of the pathogenesis and classification of renal diseases, and are an integral part of the routine diagnostic workup of renal biopsies [1,2].

The interpretation of renal biopsy is extremely challenging, but rewarding. Many factors contribute to the seemingly difficult field. First, one disease can have many different types of renal involvement. The classic example is systemic lupus erythematosus (SLE), which has numerous morphologic patterns of renal injury [3]. Second, a particular morphologic pattern can be associated with different disease processes with diverse etiologies, prognoses, and treatment. This is because the kidney reacts in a limited fashion, both clinically and morphologically, to a myriad of injurious agents. For instance, focal segmental glomerulosclerosis can represent just segmental scarring from any cause or denote a primary renal disease. Third, one specific pattern/disease can have several names/synonyms. For example, minimal change nephrotic syndrome or minimal change disease is also referred as nil disease, lipoid nephrosis, visceral epithelial cell disease, and podocytopathy. Finally, a lack of clear knowledge of the complex normal renal histology may add further difficulties to the task of renal biopsy interpretation. Indeed, one cannot know what is abnormal until one knows what is normal. In spite of all the difficulties, years of teaching have convinced us that there can be a systematic and ordered approach to the study and understanding of renal pathology. In this chapter, we propose an algorithmic approach to the overall evaluation of renal diseases that provides a basis for reaching an accurate and informative diagnosis that will, in turn, guide patient management.

The Renal Pathology Society has recommended that renal biopsies be processed only in laboratories that are proficient in the performance and interpretation of the tests [4]. Pathologists who interpret renal biopsies should have undergone formal training in renal pathology. They should have a thorough understanding of renal disease and good communication with the clinicians caring for the patients. It cannot be overemphasized that a single pathologist should be responsible for the interpretation and integration of all the renal biopsy findings in a given case including light, IF, and EM as well as data from laboratory studies and any other morphometric or immunohistochemical studies. Given the complexity of this discipline, it is strongly discouraged that a clinician be responsible for both the clinical and pathologic aspects of the patient workup.

APPROACH TO THE CLASSIFICATION OF RENAL DISEASES

Our understanding of renal diseases in general and renal pathology in particular were very limited in the first half of the twentieth century. What we knew about renal pathology was based almost exclusively on autopsy findings with advanced diseases [1]. The early classifications of renal diseases by Volhard and Fahr [5], and later by Addis [6], although useful, were inadequate and sometimes confusing. However, the pace of discovery soon quickened. In the 1950s, human renal tissues obtained by biopsy could be studied not only by light microscopy, but also by the new techniques of IF and electron microscopic examination. These advances ushered us into the modern era of nephrology and renal pathology.

A useful classification system should meet the following criteria: (a) be clinically significant, useful, and therapeutically relevant; (b) be based on pathogenesis within the limitations of our current knowledge; and (c) be relatively easy for all to use and morphologically reproducible [1]. Although the approach of practicing anatomic/renal pathologists is largely morphologically based, it is important to understand the morphology within the context of etiology and pathogenesis whenever possible. Currently, the most widely used and accepted classification is the one established by the collaborating Centre for the histological classification of Renal Diseases under the auspices of World Health Organization (WHO) and published in several atlases [7,8]. These books are dedicated, in part, to share the pathology-based information and to make sure that individuals throughout the world refer, in their diagnoses, the same entity (entities). Of course, with increasingly better and more specific therapies, the importance of renal diagnoses will become even greater.

There are several ways to classify renal diseases: (a) etiologic/pathogenetic, (b) clinical, (c) pathologic, and (d) immunohistochemical. A classification based on etiology and a deep understanding of disease pathogenesis would be preferable. Such a classification would give a specific cause (i.e., streptococcal infection) and lead to knowledge of fundamental biological processes underlying renal injury and repair (i.e., immune- or nonimmune-mediated). Unfortunately, this is not usually feasible because the precise etiologic agents are unknown for many renal diseases. Furthermore, recent advances have provided new evidence that ostensibly different classes of glomerulonephritis (for instance, immune versus nonimmune mediated glomerulonephritis) share fundamental biological underpinnings, irrespective of the etiological agent that initiates glomerular injury [9]. As the distinctions between immunity and inflammation continue to blur, it is inevitable that some earlier classification schemes require revision. In addition, with recent advances in podocyte biology, it becomes increasingly clear that a group of proteinuric glomerular diseases with diverse mor-

phologic phenotypes (i.e., minimal change disease, focal segmental glomerulosclerosis, diffuse mesangial sclerosis, and collapsing glomerulopathy) are all caused by podocyte damage or dysfunction. A classification for the so-called podocytopathies has been recently proposed [10]. Needless to say, an accurate and precise diagnosis has become increasingly more critical as we try to develop more etiology-specific and individualized therapies in the future.

A classification based on clinical syndrome such as nephrotic or nephritic syndrome can help to narrow the differential diagnosis to certain entities. However, an individual renal disease such as lupus nephritis may cause different clinical manifestations/syndromes in different patients. Conversely, a variety of different renal diseases with diverse etologies and prognoses may produce the same clinical syndrome. Thus, a clinical determination of a syndrome is not very precise in an individual patient. In most cases, a renal biopsy is required for a specific diagnosis. The common indications for renal biopsy have been discussed in Chapter 2.

A classification based primarily on morphologic patterns is not without shortcomings. Most morphologic patterns do not correspond to a single disease entity because the kidney can only manifest limited morphologic patterns to a wide variety of injuries. As discussed in Chapter 9, histologic patterns of renal thrombotic microangiopathy may be caused by hemolytic–uremic syndrome, thrombotic thrombocytopenic purpura, acute scleroderma, malignant hypertension, and cyclosporine A nephrotoxicity, to mention only a few. In contrast, any one disease may manifest itself with more than one morphologic pattern. However, given the shortcomings of other classification schemes, morphologic classification offers a simple, reproducible, and descriptive approach and represents the cornerstone of disease classification in nephrology.

A classification based on IF can separate renal diseases into two large categories: immune or nonimmune renal diseases. A few entities including IgA nephropathy or C1q nephropathy are defined by immunohistochemistry. In addition, this method of classification is currently the mainstay for crescentic glomerulonephritis that is divided into three types: (a) anti-GBM disease, (b) pauciimmune antineutrophil cytoplasmic antibodies (ANCA) glomerulonephritis, and (c) immune complex-mediated glomerulonephritis.

HANDLING AND PREPARATION OF RENAL BIOPSY SPECIMENS

Renal tissue is obtained either by a percutaneous needle biopsy or an open incision (wedge biopsy). In most instances, renal biopsy specimens are received as needle cores with fairly limited amount of tissue. Although wedge biopsy specimens are greater in size, they tend to contain only a superficial cortex, and therefore, lack juxtamedullary glomeruli and arcuate/subarcuate arteries [4,11].

Handling of Tissue

Renal biopsy specimens must be handled with great care in order to avoid introducing artifacts. The tissue should be kept moist with a small amount of cold normal saline solution during its handling. Manipulation of tissue is best achieved with a small wooden stick such as toothpick. Two cores of tissue are recommended whenever possible. Immediately after removal of tissue, the specimen should be examined by an experienced pathologist or a well-trained technologist with a hand magnifying glass, or under a dissecting microscope to identify the presence of glomeruli (which can be seen as red dots). The first core should be submitted for light microscopy and the second may be divided, cross-sectionally, for IF and EM. If direct glomerular visualization is unavailable, 1 mm cubes should be removed from the ends of both cores for EM. The remaining tissue can be cut in half by cross-sectioning. The larger two pieces should be submitted for light microscopy, and the two smaller pieces should be sent for IF. In the case of limited tissue, the clinical differential diagnosis may drive the division of material [4]. Since EM can often be performed on tissue reprocessed from paraffin-embedded material, in cases with limited tissue availability, saving specimens for light and IF microscopy is generally preferred.

Processing of specimens

Light Microscopy. Several fixatives have been used including 10 percent neutral-buffered formalin, alcoholic Bouin's, Duboscq-Brazil, among others. The simplest and most commonly used fixative is 10 percent buffered formalin, which has several advantages over other fixatives. It works well for all routine histological staining methods and many immunohistological methods including in situ hybridization. In addition, formalin fixed, paraffin-embedded tissue can be reprocessed for EM, if needed, with satisfactory quality. Although the newly developed fixative, RNA*later*, preserves RNA integrity in renal tissue during storage and processing, the renal morphology (both for light and IF microscopy) was negatively impacted [12]. Paraffin is the most commonly used embedding medium. Serial thin (2–3 μm) sections should be cut and mounted on consecutively numbered slides. In addition to H&E staining, several special stains including methenamine silver-periodic acid (Jones stain), Masson trichrome, and periodic acid-Schiff (PAS) should be routinely performed (Table 3.1).

IF Microscopy. Tissues for IF can be transported to the laboratory either fresh (on saline-soaked gauze) or in transport solution such as the Zeus medium. Serial sections should be cut at 3–4 μm in a cryostat. Direct IF method is used (except for C4d, which is determined by an indirect method). The fluorescein-labeled antibodies directed against human immunoglobulins, complements, fibrinogen, and albumin are applied to the frozen sections of kidney and examined under a fluorescent microscope. Table 3.2 summarizes the antigens that need to be routinely examined and their specific roles in the diagnosis of renal diseases. If needed, additional antibodies, such as collagen IV alpha chains in Alport's syndrome, can be stained. In the absence of appropriate tissue in the IF sample, paraffin-embedded sections may also be suitable for IF after treatment with proteolytic enzymes, as detailed elsewhere [13]. Photographic records should be kept for all positive findings because the fluorescence fades over time. IF is preferred by many nephropathologists because the use of dark-field microscopy produces a very high signal-to-noise ratio, which enables one to localize deposits accurately [4].

Table 3.1 Basic Stains Required for Light Microscopic Evaluation of Renal Biopsy

Stains	Specific Roles (Selected)
Hematoxylin and eosin (H&E)	*Glomerular:* exudative lesions *Tubular:* tubular epithelial damage *Interstitial:* edema; inflammation *Vascular:* inflammation
Periodic Acid-Schiff reaction	*Glomerular:* GBM thickening; capillary wall collapse; Bowman's capsule; hyalinosis; sclerosis; mesangial cellularity and matrix increase; mesangiolysis; endocapillary/extracapillary proliferation *Tubular:* tubular protein droplets; TBM thickening, tubulitis *Vascular:* hyaline arteriolosoclerosis
Methanamine-silver (Jones stain)	*Glomerular:* GBM spikes; double contours; breaks in GBM/Bowman's capsule *Tubular:* tubulitis *Interstitial:* fibrosis *Vascular:* internal elastic lamina
Masson trichrome	*Glomerular:* immune deposits; thrombi; fibrin; platelets *Tubular:* tubular atrophy *Interstitial:* fibrosis *Vascular:* thrombi

Table 3.2 Routine Antibody Panel for IF Microscopy

Immunoreactant	Specific Roles (Selected)
IgG	Immune complex disease, Anti-GBM disease
IgA	IgA nephropathy, Henoch-Scholein purpura, Liver disease, SLE
IgM	Waldenstrom's macroglobulinemia, Mixed cryoglogulinemia
C1q	C1q nephropathy, SLE
C3	Dense deposit disease, C3 mesangial GN, Resolving postinfections GN
Albumin	Distinguishing specific from nonspecific staining, Diabetes mellitus
Fibrinogen	Necrotizing lesions, Thrombotic microangiopathy, Crescents
Kappa & Lambda	Monoclonal immunoglobulin deposition disease, Amyloidosis
C4d (transplant)	Humoral rejection

Table 3.3 Glossaries of Descriptive Terms and Patterns of Glomerular Injury

Terms	Definitions
Related to Distribution	
Focal	Involving less than 50% of glomeruli by light microscopy
Diffuse	Involving 50% or more of glomeruli by light microscopy
Segmental	Involving a portion of the glomerular tuft
Global	Involving the entire glomerular tuft
Related to Structure	
Obsolescence	Total loss of normal glomerular architecture due to replacement by scarring (sclerosis)
Sclerosis	Increased collagenous extracellular matrix expanding the mesangium, occluding capillary lumina or forming adhesions to Bowman's capsule
Fibrinoid necrosis	Disruption of structure, with degeneration of local cells, extracellular matrix and the basement membrane, often associated with fibrin deposition
Lobular	Hypersegmentation of the normal lobular architecture of the normal glomerular capillary tuft due to intracapillary hypercellularity or significant mesangial expansions
Mesangiolysis	Dissolution or attenuation of mesangial matrix and degeneration of mesangial cells, often associated with glomerular capillary aneurysms
Mensangial Interposition	Extension of mensangial cells in the peripheral glomerular capillary walls in the space located between endothelial cells and glomerular basement membrane (subendothelial zone)
Hyalinosis	Accumulation of glassy, refractile acellular material/plasmatic insudation (PAS positive, methenamine-siver negative) which contains serum proteins, other glycoproteins and lipids
Glomerular capillary collapse	Retraction of glomerular tuft with closure of capillary lumina and wrinkling and thickening of glomerular capillary walls
Glomerular capillary aneurysm	Capillary lumen balloons out and appears ectatic due to degeneration of mesangial cell and matrix (mesangiolysis)
Wire-loops	Thickened glomerular capillary walls with a rigid appearance (wire-loop-like) due to the presence of large and confluent subendothelial immune deposits
Tram-tracking/GBM reduplication	Double contoured appearance of glomerular capillary walls on PAS/silver stains due to the presence of deposits and mesangial interposition between the endothelium and the original GBM with creation of a newer inner (subendothelial side) basement-membrane like material
Related to Cell Proliferation	
Mensangial hypercellularity	Presence of three or more mesangial and/or inflammatory cells per mesangial area away from the vascular pole in a section that is 2~3 μm in thickness (WHO definition)
Endocapillary hypercellularity	Increased cellularity within the confines of glomerular basement membranes composed of endothelial cells, mesangial cells and/or inflammatory cells, resulting in luminal narrowing or occlusion
Intracapillary hypercellularity	Hypercellularity present in both mesangium and endocapillaries
Crescent	The build-up of more than two layers of cells within Bowman's space caused by the proliferation of parietal cells, podocytes and infiltrating inflammatory cells, often with fibrin and collagen deposition. Crescents classified as cellular, fibrocellular and fibrous depending on the predominant component
Adhesion/synechia	Localized narrow bridges of connective tissue between glomerular tufts and Bowman's capsule
Membranoproliferative	Glomerular capillary wall thickening due to mesangial interposition and duplication of glomerular basement membranes
Related to Deposits	
Intramembranous	Within the glomerular basement membrane
Mesangial	Within the mesangial matrix
Subendothelial	Between the glomerular basement membrane and the endothelium
Subepithelial/epimembranous	Between the glomerular basement membrane and podocytes
Humps	Subepithelial electron-dense immune-type deposits with a cigar-or dome-like appearance

Table 3.4 Glossaries of Descriptive Terms and Patterns of Tubulointerstial and Vascular Injuries

Terms	Definitions
Tubules	
Tubilitis	Lymphocytes or other inflammatory cells infiltrating tubular epithelium
Tubular atrophy	Tubular involution/obsolescence due to ischemia, obstruction, toxic or inflammatory injury with different light microscopic appearances including classic atrophy, endocrine and thyroidization changes
Tubular casts	Various coagulated proteins and other elements in tubular lumens usually but not exclusively seen in distal nephron
Hydropic degeneration/ Osmotic nephrosis	Fine regular cytoplasmic vacuolization of the proximal tubules
Hyaline droplet	PAS/silver-positive protein reabsorption droplets because of increased protein loss by glomeruli
Fatty change	Finely vacuolated cytoplasm with clear vacuoles in the tubular epithelium in which the lipid has been dissolved out during preparation of paraffin sections
Hypokalemic change	Large irregular sized coarse clear vacuoles in the cytoplasm of tubular epithelial cells, especially the distal tubular cells
Intranuclear inclusions	Seen in nuclei with various morphology depending on etiology, often associated with viral infections (e.g. CMV, BK polyomavirus and adenovirus), can be observed in tubular epithelial cell regeneration and lead nephropathy
Interstitium	
Edema	Increased extracellular fluid in the interstitium resulting in increased spacing between tubules
Interstitial foam cells	Macrophages with cytoplasmic lipid-containing vacuoles
Inflammation	Infiltration of lymphocytes, plasma cells, and often eosinophils and netrophils with associated tubular injury
Fibrosis	Interstitial expansion by collagen
Granuloma	Collection of epithelioid histocytes with/without surrounding multinucleated giant cells and lymphocytes
Vessels	
Intimal thickening	Fibrous thickening of the intimal layer, usually in a concentric configuration and associated with varying degrees of luminal stenosis
Hyaline sclerosis	Accumulation of PAS-positive/silver-negative material in the intima and/or media resulting in a characteristic "glassy" acellular refractile change in small arteries and arterioles
Endothelialitis/endarteritis	Infiltration of mononuclear cells under arterial and arteriolar endothelium
Arteritis	Necrosis, fibrinoid degeneration and inflammation of arteries with leukocytoclasia and disruption of internal elastic lamina
Vasculitis	Necrosis, fibrinoid degeneration and leukocytoclastic inflammation of arteries, arterioles and veins

Immunoperoxidase (IP). When frozen tissue is not available or glomeruli are not present on frozen sections, IP staining on paraffin sections can also provide satisfactory results. In fact, it is a method of preference in some parts of the world such as Europe. Advantages of IP compared with IF are that (a) frozen tissue and expansive IF microscope attachment are not necessary, (b) sections are permanent, (c) no special arrangements for collection and storage of tissue in needed, and (d) the techniques can be applied retrospectively to renal biopsy specimens stored in paraffin for many years. The main disadvantage is that IP gives inconsistent results in many laboratories because of the presence of a high background despite of advances in antigen-retrieval techniques and applying of automated stainers [4]. In addition, it is less reliable for semiquantifying the intensity of various immunoglobulins and complements under immunoenzyme microscope. Generally speaking, the resolution of immunoenzyme microscopy is inferior to IF microscopy.

Electron Microscopy. For optimal results, the tissue for EM should be cut into fragments no larger than $1 \times 1 \times 1$ mm. The most widely used fixatives are 3 percent phosphate-buffered glutaraldehyde, or 2.5 percent glutaraldehyde in cacodylate buffer. Postfixation in 1 percent osmium tetroxide is recommended. If no glomeruli are present in the EM sample, tissue can be reprocessed from the paraffin block. Although the morphological preservation is suboptimal, it is generally satisfactory for the recognition of immune deposits and other significant alterations. It should be noted that plastic-embedded tissue is not suitable for IP studies.

Epon embedded, toluidine blue-stained, "thick" or "semithin" sections (1 μm) are examined under light microscope to choose the most appropriate area for subsequent ultrastructural examination. All tissues available should be examined by light microscopy since it is possible that focal lesions may present only in the tissue submitted for EM. Thin sections are then cut and stained with uranyl acetate and lead citrate. All renal

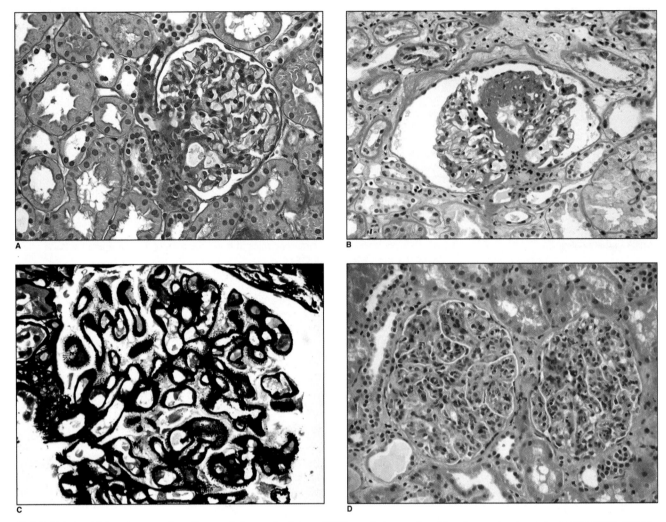

FIGURE 3.1: *Light microscopic patterns of glomerular injury. (A) Normal glomerulus. The glomerulus is normocellular with patent capillary lumina and single-contoured capillary walls (PAS; × 400.) (B) Focal segmental glomerulosclerosis. A peripheral segment is obliterated by increased mesangial matrix and hyalinosis (PAS; × 400.) (C) Membranous glomerulopathy. The glomerulus is normocellular with patent capillary lumina. The capillary walls are thickened with numerous spikes. In areas where the glomerular basement membranes are cut en face, the spikes give rise to a reticulated network (JMS stain; × 400.) (D) Acute diffuse proliferative (poststreptococcal) glomerulonephritis. The glomeruli are globally hypercellular with narrowed or obliterated capillary lumina due to the influx of leukocytes including numerous neutrophils. The glomerular capillary walls are delicate (H&E; × 200.)*

compartments should be evaluated under the electron microscope at low, medium, and high magnifications [1].

PATTERNS OF RENAL INJURY

Standardized names/terminology is essential for communication among clinicians and pathologists who deal with patients suffering from renal diseases. As elegantly stated by Carl Linnaeus, father of the biological binomial nomenclature, "If you do not know the names of things, the knowledge of them is lost too." Hence, one needs to gain familiarity with the patterns of renal injury and their definitions. The terminology used in this book is consistent with that used by most North American renal pathologists. When possible, we will use the widely recognized International Nomenclature of Diseases (IND), a joint project

for the Council for International Organization of Medical Sciences and the WHO. The purpose is to ease communications and facilitate the storage and retrieval of renal information. We have tried to limit our coverage of renal patterns of disease to stable "taxonomic groups" from the large amount of published works. The common terms used to describe histologic patterns of renal injury are summarized in Tables 3.3 and 3.4, and illustrated in Figures 3.1 to 3.3.

The best approach to achieve an accurate pathologic diagnosis is to recognize the patterns of injury found in each of the four compartments of the kidney. However, most of the patterns are not specific, diagnostic, or pathognomonic; therefore, knowledgeable and careful interpretation and integration of the sum of specific patterns of renal injury, the clinical syndrome, and laboratory data are needed to achieve an optimal and accurate diagnosis.

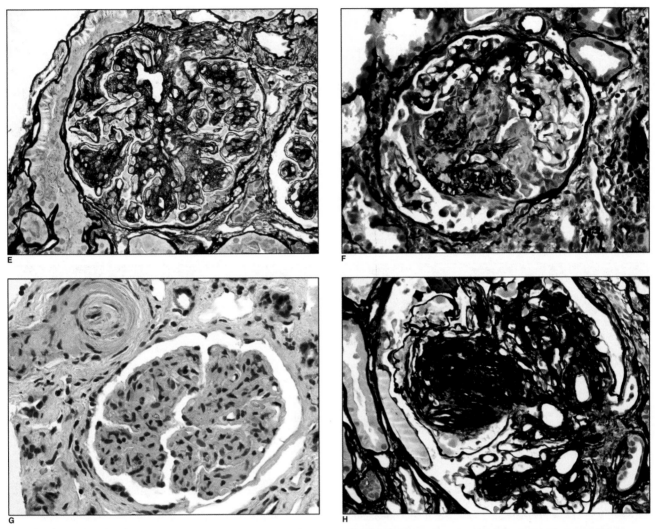

FIGURE 3.1: *(E) Membranoproliferative glomerulonephritis, type I. The glomerulus is hypercellular with an exaggerated lobular configuration and narrowed or obliterated capillary lumens. The glomerular capillary walls reveal extensive double contours with silver negative subendothelial deposits and interposed mesangial cells (JMS stain; × 400.) (F) Focal necrotizing ANCA glomerulonephritis. The glomerulus displays segmental necrosis with lysis of glomerular basement membranes and a small cellular crescent. The nonnecrotic segments are histologically unremarkable (JMS stain; × 400.) (G) Thrombotic microangiopathy. The glomerulus reveals marked endothelial swelling with obliterated capillary lumens. The arterioles show edematous intimal thickening and fibrinoid necrosis with fragmented red blood cells in the walls and obliteration of lumens (H&E × 400.) (H) Nodular diabetic glomerulosclerosis. The glomerulus reveals a large rounded mesangial region (Kimmelstiel-Wilson nodule) which is silver positive with lamination of mesangial matrix. The adjacent capillary lumens are still patent. A capsular drop lesion (acellular hyaline material interposed between Bowman's capsule and parietal epithelial cells) is also present (JMS stain; × 400.)*

APPROACH TO THE INTERPRETATION
OF GLOMERULAR DISEASES

Light Microscopy. A renal biopsy should be examined first at low power to evaluate the presence of relative proportion of renal cortex and medulla. The total number of glomeruli and the number of globally sclerotic glomeruli per section should be enumerated. This is best achieved on PAS or Methenamine-silver-stained sections. Up to 10 percent of the glomeruli may be globally sclerotic in normal individuals younger than 40 years [14]. When the number of globally sclerotic glomeruli exceeds the number calculated by the formula [(patient's age/2) – 10], patho-

logic glomerulosclerosis should be considered [15]. The glomeruli should be examined in detail at high power subsequently.

As illustrated in the algorithm (Figure 3.4), the first step in evaluating glomerular disease is to determine whether glomeruli are hypercellular or not. Glomerular hypercellularity can be divided into mesangial, endocapillary (with closure of glomerular capillary lumina) and extracapillary (i.e., crescents). It was believed in the past that the cellular crescents are a mixture of parietal epithelial cells, macrophages, and myofibroblasts. However, recent studies have shown that podocytes are an integral cellular component of cellular crescents [16]. In the absence of glomerular hypercellularity, one needs to examine the glomeruli

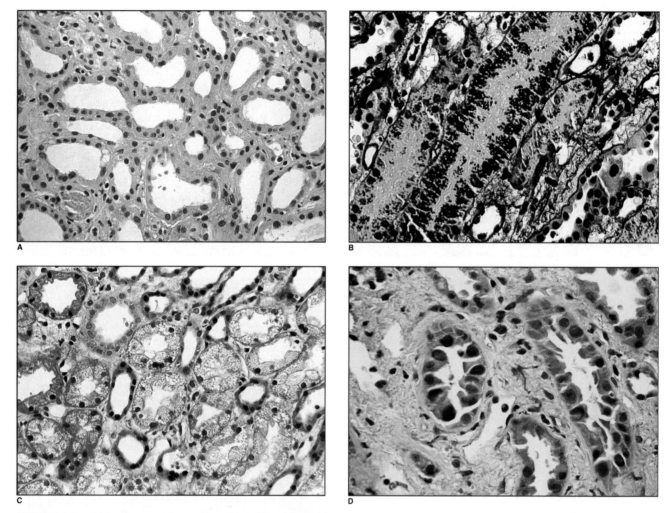

FIGURE 3.2: *Light microscopic patterns of tubulointerstitial injury. (A) Acute tubular necrosis. Many tubules are dilated with loss or thinning of epithelial cells (H&E × 400.) (B) Hyaline droplets. The proximal tubular epithelial cells show numerous silver-positive protein resorption droplets (JMS stain; × 400.) (C) Hydropic change (osmotic nephrosis). The cytoplasm of tubular epithelial cells show diffuse and fine vaculization (Trichrome stain; × 200.) (D) BK polyomavirus. Many tubular epithelial cells contain large basophilic nuclear inclusions with a ground-glass appearance (H&E × 400.)*

at high power to determine whether there are abnormalities in glomerular capillaries. The major categories of glomerular capillary abnormalities are: (a) capillary wall collapse, (b) capillary wall thickening, and (c) capillary occlusion. The glomerular lesions may be distributed in a focal or a diffuse manner in the kidney. The intraglomerular lesions may be segmental or global. It should be kept in mind that a sampling error may occur in a small renal biopsy which may result, therefore, in misjudging the extent of a focal lesion, or missing a segmental lesion.

IF Microscopy. Most primary glomerulonephritis and many secondary glomerular diseases are immunologic in nature, although little is known about the exact etiologic agents and triggering events in the individual patient [1,2,17]. As shown in Table 3.2, antibodies that are necessary in the evaluation of glomerular diseases include antibodies specific for IgG, IgA, IgM, C1q, C3, albumin, fibrin/fibrinogen, kappa, and lambda light chains. C4d should be stained in all allograft renal biopsies. The slides should be evaluated qualitatively and semiquan-titatively with an intensity score of 0 to 4+. In diseases such as IgA nephropathy/Henoch-Schonlein purpura and C1q nephropathy, the intensity of staining is critical as the diagnosis is based on the predominance/codominance of IgA and C1q, respectively, when compared with other immunoreactants. It is important to recognize autofluorescence. Arterial elastic fibers and lipid droplets are the most common materials that give rise to autofluorescence which appear yellow rather than the characteristic green fluorescence [18]. In addition, a modest background glomerular basement membrane (GBM) and tubular basement membrane (TBM) staining is frequently seen due to the use of a buffered transport medium [18].

Thus, in the evaluation of glomerular diseases by IF microscopy (Figure 3.5), the first step is to recognize whether or not the positive immunostaining is specific. With specific immunostaining, the pattern can be linear or granular. Glomerular staining is recognized as mesangial, capillary wall, or both. Nonspecific deposits are often observed in segmental or globally sclerotic glomeruli because there is plasma insudation or

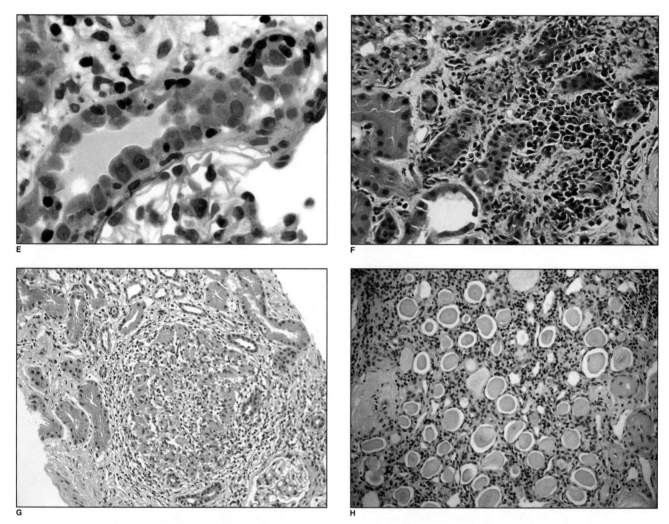

FIGURE 3.2: *(E) Tubulitis. There is moderate lymphocytic infiltration of the tubular epithelium coupled with tubular degeneration (H&E × 400.) (F) Acute interstitial nephritis. There is extensive interstitial inflammatory infiltrate composed of plasma cells, lymphocytes and numerous eosinophils, consistent with a drug-induced acute interstitial nephritis. There is also significant tubulitis (H &E × 400.) (G) Granulomatous interstitial nephritis secondary to sarcoidosis. There is a large noncaseating granuloma surrounded by significant inflammatory infiltrate (H &E × 200.) (H) Tubular atrophy ("thyroidization"). The tubules reveal very thin lining epithelium with uniform hyaline casts within the lumens resembling thyroid tissue, hence, the term thyroidization. There is also significant interstitial inflammation (H &E × 200.)*

leakage of serum proteins (generally albumin, IgM and C3) into sclerosed areas. Global linear staining along the GBMs and Bowman's capsule for IgG and albumin are frequently seen in diabetic nephropathy due to plasma proteins absorbed by thickened membranes. Common patterns of glomerular staining observed by IF are illustrated in Figure 3.6.

Electron Microscopy. Transmission EM is an essential part of the routine workup of a renal biopsy and provides useful diagnostic information in nearly half of native renal biopsies [1,19,20]. It is particularly useful in the following areas: (a) identification of deposits and their locations including discrete homogeneous electron dense immune-type deposits and deposits with organized substructure or other distinctive ultrastructural features, (b) evaluation of GBM alterations as seen in Alport's syndrome, (c) detection of cellular abnormalities such as foot process

effacement in conditions with heavy proteinuria, or swelling of endothelial cells in thrombotic microangiopathy. Of note, some diseases such as fibrillary or immunotactoid glomerulonephritis can only be diagnosed by EM [2,19,20].

Figure 3.7 introduces an algorithmic approach to the ultrastructural examination of renal biopsies. As illustrated, the initial step is to identify whether there are deposits. If present, the exact location of these deposits, either glomerular (i.e., subepithelial, intramembranous, mesangial, and subendothelial regions) or/and nonglomerular (i.e., tubules, interstitium, or vasculature) should be noted. If substructures (such as fibrils) are present, the thickness of the fibrils should be determined. It should be noted that the identification of various organized deposits require a study the renal tissue under high magnification (×30,000). In the absence of deposits, other abnormalities including GBM, visceral epithelial and endothelial cells should be carefully searched for.

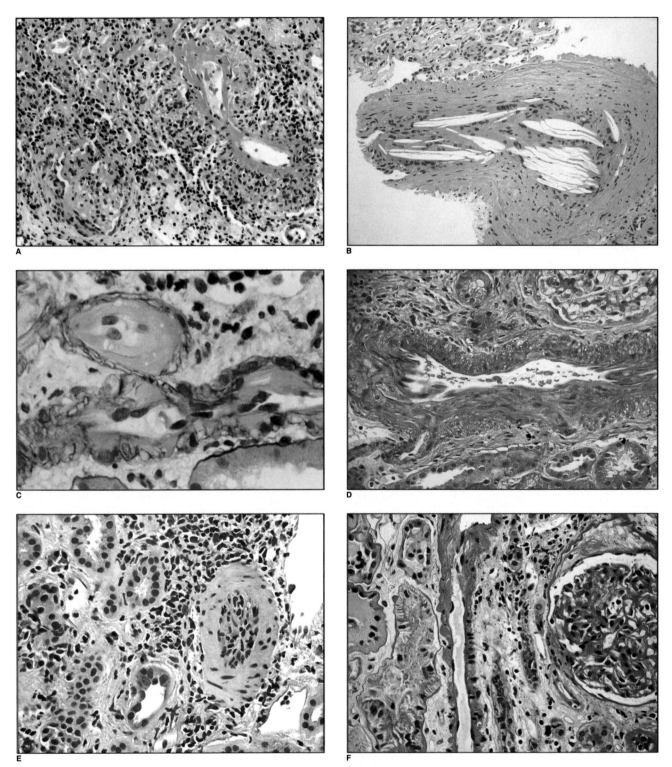

FIGURE 3.3: *Light microscopic patterns of vascular injury. (A) Necrotizing vasculitis. An interlobular artery reveals extensive fibrinoid necrosis with perivascular heavy inflammatory infiltrate (H &E × 200.) (B) Cholesterol embolus (Atheroembolus). The lumen of this interlobular artery is occluded by the marked multinucleated giant cell response to the atheroembolus (H &E × 400.) (C) Arteriolosclerosis. There is extensive hyalinosis in the arterioles (PAS; × 400.) (D) Arteriosclerosis (Arterial intimal fibrosis). The intima of this arcuate artery displays fibrous thickening and migration of medial muscle cells into the intima (Trichrome; × 400.) (E) Endarteritis. A small interlobular artery shows endothelial swelling with many lymphocytes in the subendothelial space. Mild tubulitis and interstitial inflammatory cell infiltration is also observed (H &E × 200.) (F) Nodular hyalinosis-chronic calcineurin inhibitor toxicity. A longitudinally sectioned arteriole reveals nodular hyalinosis in the outer media of the arteriolar wall. Mild glomerulitis and tubulitis are also present.*

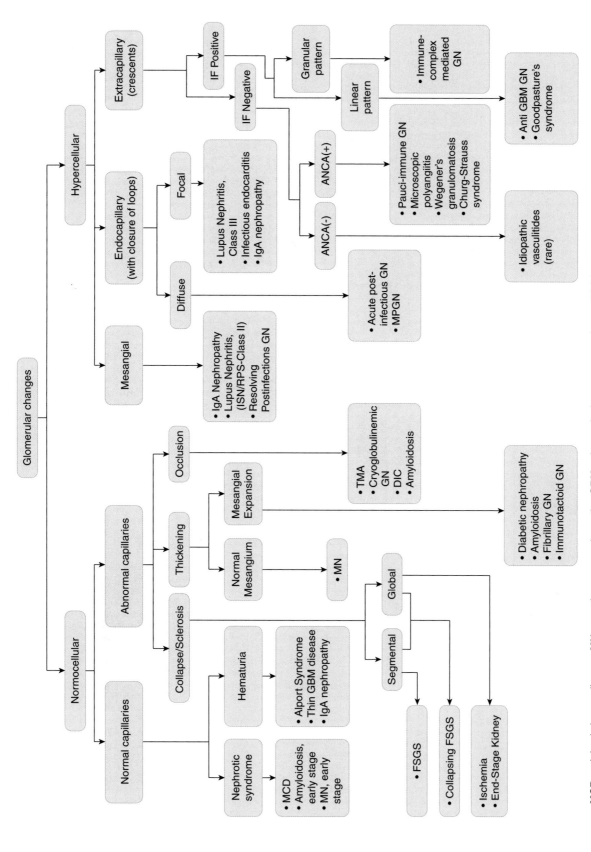

MCD: minimal change disease; **MN:** membranous nephropathy; **GBM:** glomerular basement membrane; **FSGS:** focal segmental glomerulosclerosis; **TMA:** thrombotic microangiopathy; **GN:** glomerulonephritis; **DIC:** disseminated intravascular coagulation; **ANCA:** anti-neutrophil cytoplasmic antibody; **MPGN:** membranoproliferative glomerulonephritis

FIGURE 3.4: *Algorithmic approach to the interpretation of glomerular injury by light microscopy.*

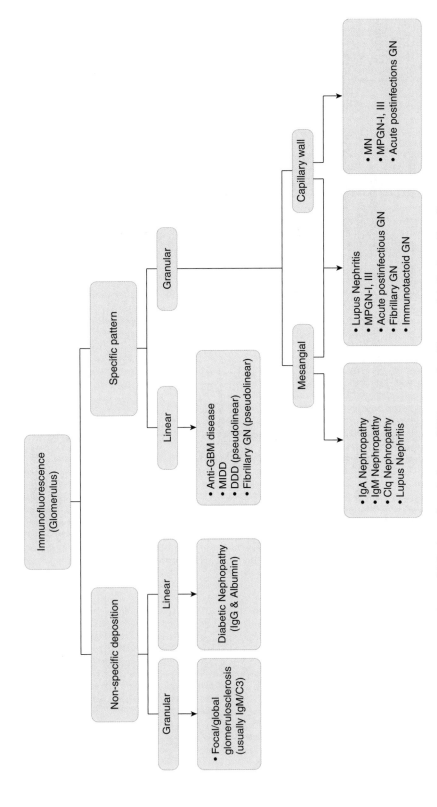

GBM: glomerular basement membrane; **DDD:** dense deposit disease; **MIDD:** monoclonal immunoglobulin deposition disease; **MPGN:** membranoproliferative glomerulonephritis; **MN:** membranous nephropathy

FIGURE 3.5: Alogrithmic approach to the interpretation of glomerular injury by IF microscopy.

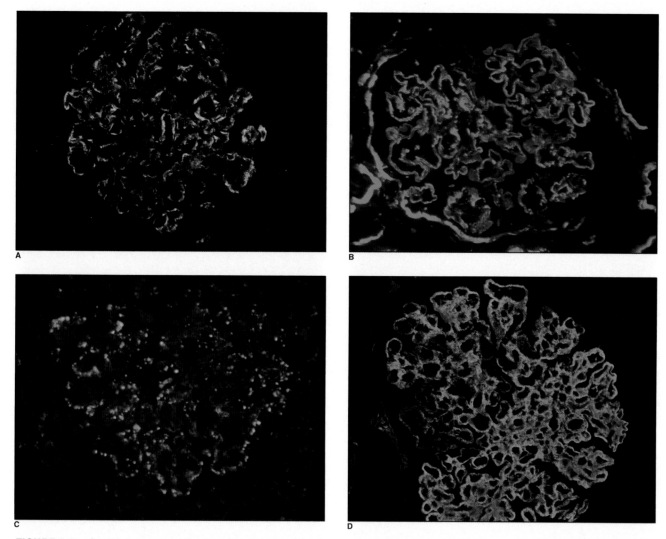

FIGURE 3.6: *Common patterns of glomerular staining by IF microscopy. (A) Membranoproliferative glomerulonephritis, type I. IF shows intense staining along the peripheral capillary walls for C3 (× 400.) (B) Dense deposit disease. IF with antiserum for C3 shows intense linear staining along the peripheral capillary walls, Bowman's capsule and focal tubular basement membranes. Scattered granular staining in the mesangium is also noted (× 400; courtesy of Dr. Tibor Nadasdy.) (C) Poststreptococcal glomerulonephritis. IF microscopy displays coarse granular staining of capillary walls and occasionally in the mesangial regions for C3 (courtesy of Dr. S. Bonsib) (× 400.) (D) Diffuse lupus nephritis. IF microscopy shows global strong granular staining along the capillary walls and in the mesangial regions for IgG (× 400.)*

It is noteworthy that not all electron dense deposits are immune complex in nature. Trapping of plasma proteins as seen in diabetes or segmental glomerulosclerosis can resemble immune type electron-dense deposits. In general, nonimmune complex deposits are slightly less electron dense. However, separation between the two also requires the incorporation of clinical information and light and IF microscopic findings [1,20]. The common patterns of ultrastructural changes are illustrated in Figure 3.8.

APPROACH TO THE INTERPRETATION OF TUBULAR DISEASES

Light Microscopy. As discussed in Chapter 1, the normal renal cortex is packed with tubules with little intervening intersti-

tium. Conversely, the tubules in the medulla are separated by varying amounts of interstitial tissue that is most prominent in the deep medulla [1,2]. Thus, it is difficult to determine if there is increased interstitium in the renal medulla, compared with the renal cortex where the tubules are normally back-to-back. Because of the intimate relationship between renal tubules and the continuous interstitium, it is often difficult to determine which compartment (i.e., tubular or interstitial) is primarily or initially involved by a disease process. In this situation, the term "tubulointerstitial nephritis/nephropathy" may be appropriate. For the interpretation of tubular diseases by light microscopy, the algorithm in Figure 3.9 should be followed. Based on the predominant tubular abnormality, the algorithm is divided into six branches: (a) tubular epithelial changes, (b) intraluminal material, (c) tubular atrophy, (d) tubulitis, (e) tubular basement

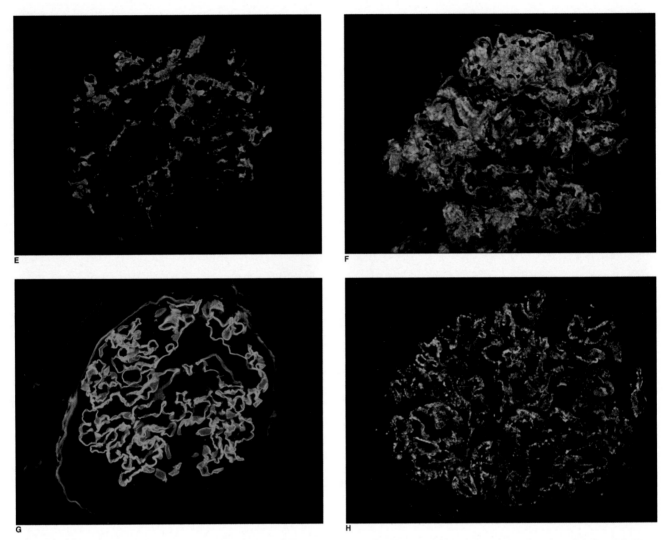

FIGURE 3.6: *(E) IgA nephropathy. IF microscopy for IgA reveals numerous bright mesangial deposits without significant deposits along the capillary walls (× 400.) (F) Fibrillary glomerulonephritis. IF microscopy shows pseudolinear or band-like staining along the capillary walls and intense contiguous mesangial staining for IgG (× 400.) (G) Anti-GBM disease. IF microscopy reveals intense linear staining along the capillary walls for IgG (× 400.) (H) Membranous glomerulonephritis. IF microscopy displays intense granular staining along the capillary walls for IgG (× 400.)*

membrane changes, and (f) other changes such as dysmorphic mitochondria of the tubular epithelial cells.

IF Microscopy. Although IF microscopy is not needed for the diagnosis of majority tubular diseases, it can, sometimes, be very useful for the diagnosis of certain tubular disorder such as primary antitubular basement membrane antibody nephritis. The algorithmic approach is illustrated in Figure 3.10. Similar to the evaluation of glomeruli, one needs first to decide whether the positive immunostaining in the TBMs or tubular epithelial cells is specific. Nonspecific linear TBM staining (generally for IgG and albumin) can be seen in diabetic nephropathy and atrophic tubules. Granular staining for albumin and some immunoglobulins (mainly IgA and IgG) may be found within the tubular epithelial cells, corresponding to intracytoplasmic protein resorption droplets. Most tubular casts often stain for several immunoglobulins, albumin, and fibrinogen. With specific immunostaining, the algorithm is divided into four branches: (a) linear TBM staining, (b) granular TBM staining, (c) granular tubular epithelial staining, and (d) staining of casts with monoclonal immunoglobulins.

APPROACH TO THE INTERPRETATION OF INTERSTITIAL DISEASES

Interstitial expansion is the most significant morphologic feature of interstitial disorders. In the interpretation of interstitial diseases by light microscopy, one needs first to determine whether a significant interstitial expansion is present. According to the type of cells and material expanding the interstitium, the algorithm shown in Figure 3.11 can be divided into four

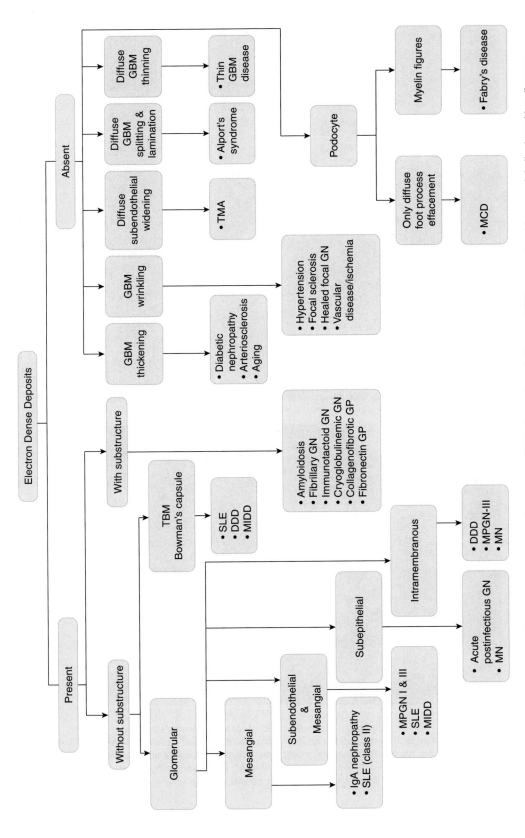

TBM: tubular basement membrane; **SLE:** systemic lupus erythematosus; **DDD:** dense deposit disease; **MIDD:** monoclonal immunoglobulin deposition disease; **MPGN:** membranoproliferative glomerulonephritis; **GBM:** glomerular basement membrane; **GN:** glomerulonephritis; **GP:** glomerulopathy; **MN:** membranous nephropathy; **TMA:** thrombotic microangiopathy; **MCD:** minimal change disease.

FIGURE 3.7: *Algorithmic approach to the interpretation of glomerular injury by EM.*

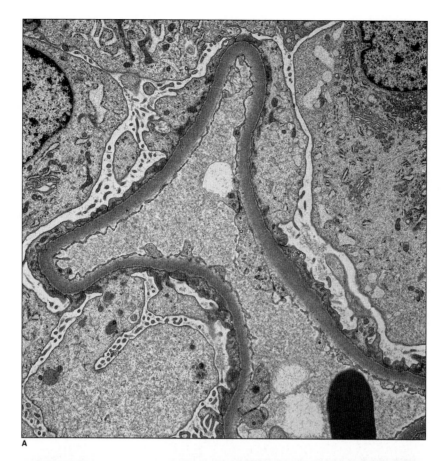

A

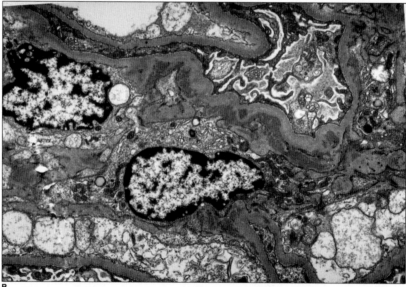

B

*FIGURE 3.8:   Common patterns observed on EM. (A) Minimal change disease.
Electron micrograph shows a patent capillary loop with fenestrated endothelium and
normal appearing glomerular basement membrane. The foot processes are entirely
effaced with hypertrophy of the podocyte cell bodies. (B) IgA nephropathy. Electron
micrograph reveals many paramesangial electron dense deposits.*

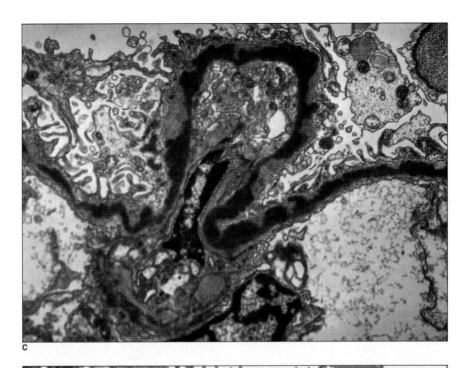

C

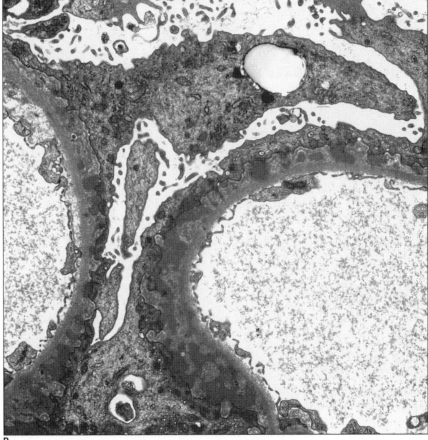

D

FIGURE 3.8: *(C) Dense deposit disease. Electron micrograph reveals fusiform thickening of the lamina densa by highly electron dense material alternating with thinned segments, giving rise the 'sausage-string'' appearance. (D) Membranous nephropathy. Electron micrograph reveals two potions of capillary loops with numerous subepithelial and intramembranous deposits with intervening spikes. There are diffuse foot process effacement and microvillous transformation of the podocytes.*

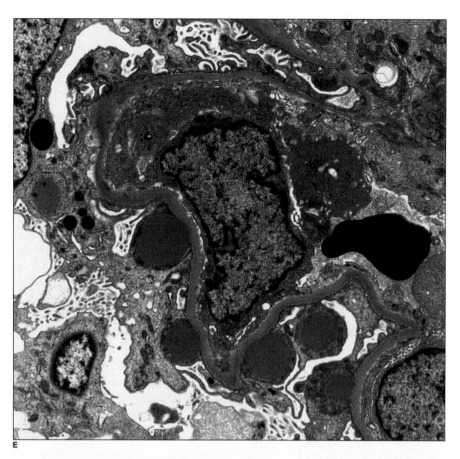

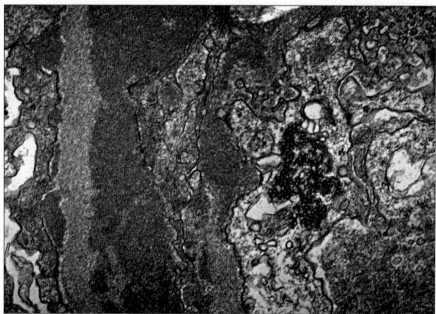

FIGURE 3.8:   (E) Acute postinfectious glomerulonephritis. Electron micrograph shows several large subepithelial electron dense deposits (humps). Significant foot process effacement is present. (F) Lupus IV with tubuloreticular structures. The glomerular endothelial cell contains a 24 nm interanastomosing tubular structure. Large subendothelial and subepithelial deposits are also noted.

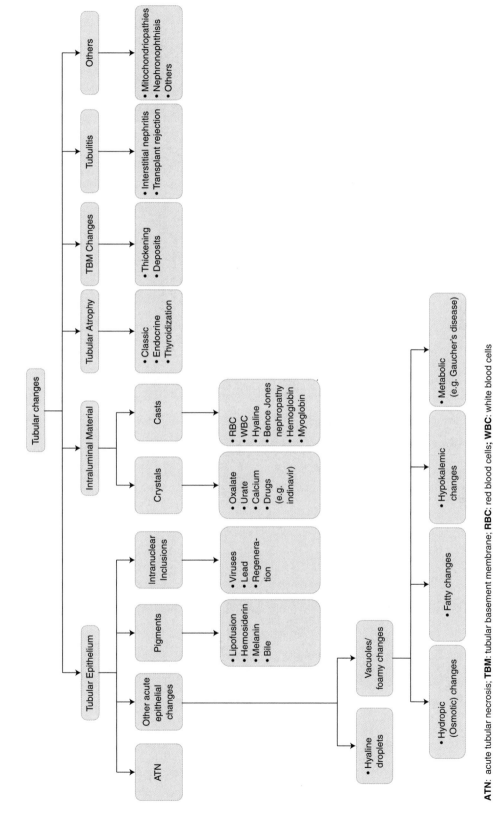

ATN: acute tubular necrosis; **TBM**: tubular basement membrane; **RBC**: red blood cells; **WBC**: white blood cells

FIGURE 3.9: Algorithmic approach to the interpretation of tubular diseases by light microscopy.

73

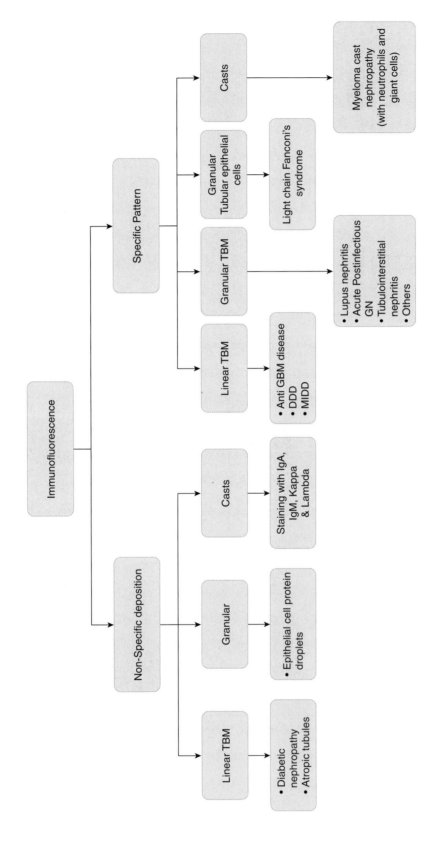

TBM: tubular basement membrane; **GBM:** glomerular basement membrane; **DDD:** dense deposit disease;
MIDD: monoclonal immunoglobulin deposition disease; **GN:** glomerulonephritis.

FIGURE 3.10: ***Algorithmic approach to the interpretation of tubular disease by IF microscopy.***

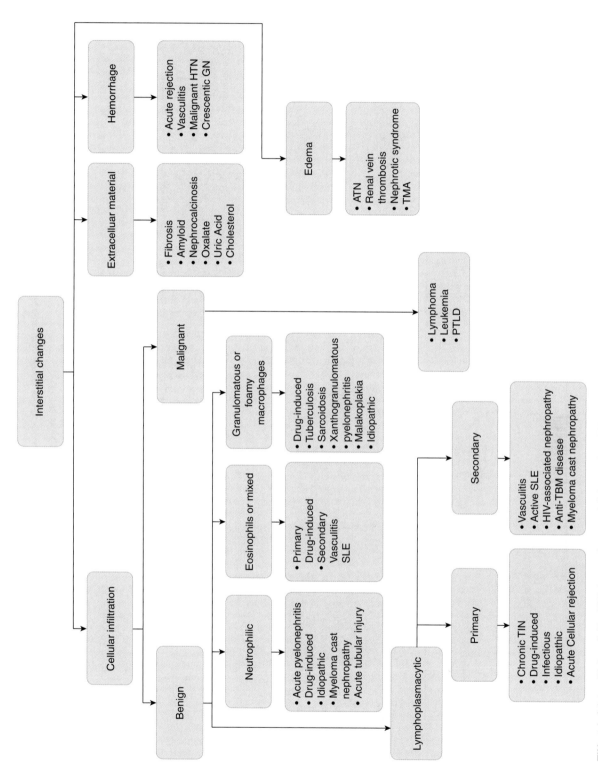

TIN: tubulointerstitial nephritis; HIV: human immunodeficiency virus; TBM: tubular basement membrane; SLE: systemic lupus erythematosus; PTLD: post-transplant lymphoproliferative disorder; HTN: hypertension; GN: glomerulonephritis; TMA: thrombotic microangiopathy; ATN: acute tubular necrosis

FIGURE 3.11:   Algorithmic approach to the interpretation of interstitial diseases by light microscopy.

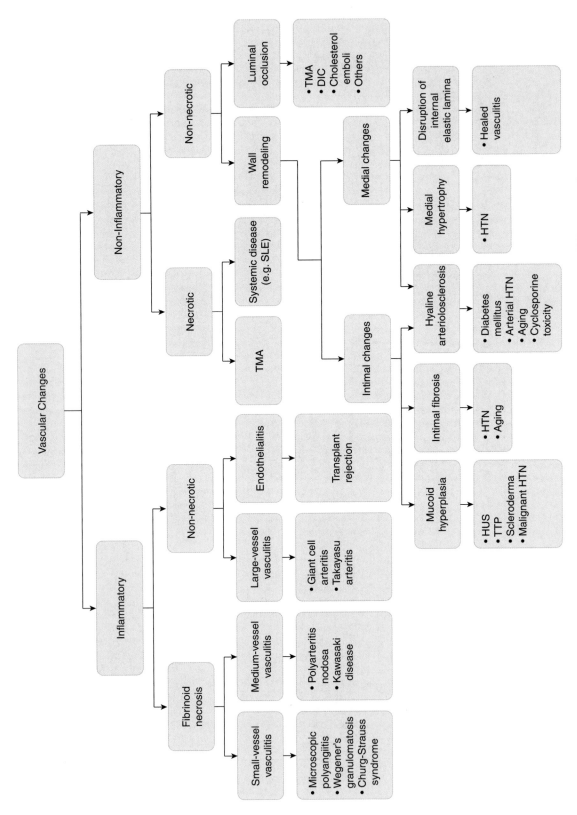

TMA: thrombotic microangiopathy; **HUS:** hemolytic uremic syndrome; **TTP:** thrombotic thrombocytopenic purpura; **HTN:** hypertension; **DIC:** disseminated intravascular coagulation; **SLE:** systemic lupus erythematosus

FIGURE 3.12: Algorithmic approach to the interpretation of vascular diseases by light microscopy.

major branches: (a) cellular infiltration, (b) extracellular/acellular material, (c) hemorrhage, and (d) edema. In the presence of cellular infiltration, it is critical to determine whether the infiltrating cells are benign or malignant. In the former situation, the predominant cellular composition (i.e., neutrophilic, lymphoplasmacytic, eosinophilic, or granulomatous) should be determined in order to further classify the interstitial disease.

It should be noted that diseases of the glomeruli, tubules, and blood vessels often involve interstitium, as such representing a "secondary" interstitial disease [2]. Therefore, the diagnosis of primary interstitial disease requires that (a) there is no significant pathology in other renal compartments sufficient to cause interstitial lesions, or (b) when disease is present in other compartments, the interstitial lesions should be caused by an unrelated pathogenetic mechanisms or the same mechanism affecting the interstitium and other renal compartments simultaneously [2]. Other important concepts include acute versus chronic interstitial nephritis. The separation of the two is not based on the type of infiltrating cellular components that are similar between the two, but rather based on the presence of interstitial edema or fibrosis. Thus, interstitial edema coupled with various leukocytic infiltration denotes acute interstitial nephritis whereas interstitial fibrosis (frequently associated with tubular atrophy) with various leukocytic infiltrate indicates chronic interstitial nephritis. However, precise distinction between the two might occasionally be challenging especially in cases with interstitial fibrosis due to preexistent renal disease.

APPROACH TO THE INTERPRETATION OF VASCULAR DISEASES

Based on light microscopy, renal vascular lesions can be divided into two broad categories: inflammatory and noninflammatory (Figure 3.12). Inflammation of the vessel wall is termed vasculitis that can affect any size vessels with different pathologic and clinical manifestations. The so-called primary vasculitis denotes vasculitis that is caused by neither major systemic rheumatologic disease nor direct invasion of vessel walls by infectious pathogens [21]. The primary vasculitis is typically characterized by leukocytic infiltration, karyorrhexis, and fibrinoid necrosis of the vascular walls. However, inflammation may be limited to the subendothelial space (termed endothelialitis) without fibrinoid necrosis as seen in acute T-cell mediated transplant rejection. Conversely, fibrinoid necrosis without inflammation can occur in a number of conditions including SLE, antiphospholipid antibody syndrome, and thrombotic microangiopathies.

Vascular lesions without inflammation and necrosis can be further divided into occlusive lesions and lesions associated with wall remodeling. An occlusive lesion denotes luminal obstruction by either platelet-fibrin thrombi or other type of emboli such as cholesterol clefts. Intimal changes may have different morphological and tinctorial appearances. For instance, mucoid hyperplasia stains pale by trichrome stain or PAS reaction whereas intimal fibrosis stains like collagen. In healed vasculitis, elastic stain may reveal disruption and fragmentation of the internal elastic lamina.

In general, vascular lesions do not need IF or EM for diagnosis.

RENAL BIOPSY SURGICAL PATHOLOGY REPORT

Currently no available technique/investigation can provide so much clinical relevant information (i.e., diagnosis, prognosis, therapy, and response to therapy) in such a timely and cost-effective fashion as renal biopsy. By integrating the observations made by light, IF, and EM with clinical and laboratory data, an accurate pathologic diagnosis can be made which, in turn, will determine the clinical course and guide the clinical management. A well-written and well-organized renal biopsy report is an essential component of the evaluation of renal biopsies. A complete report should contain the following parts in this order: (a) light microscopy findings, (b) IF findings, (c) EM findings, (d) diagnosis, and (e) comment, if appropriate [1]. In addition, renal transplant biopsy has a unique set of questions that need to be addressed differently from the native kidney biopsy (see Chapter 16). Tables 3.5 and 3.6 summarize the

Table 3.5 Components of Native Kidney Biopsy Pathology Report

Light Microscopy
- Presence and relative proportion of renal capsule, cortex, medulla, pelvic urothelial lining and others (i.e., skeletal muscle, liver, intestine)
- Total number of glomeruli and the number/percentage of globally sclerotic glomeruli if any
- Description of diagnostic morphologic lesions/changes/patterns in glomeruli, tubules, interstitium and vessels
- Description of important or relevant negative findings

Immunofluorscence Microscopy
- Total number of glomeruli and the number of globally sclerotic glomeruli if present
- Description of positive or negative results for each immunoglobulin and complement components in glomeruli
- Description of the location, stain pattern and intensity of the deposits in glomeruli
- Description of immunoreactants in tubulointerstitial compartment and vessels if present

Electron Microscopy
- Total number of glomeruli and the number of globally sclerotic glomeruli if present
- Description of glomerular abnormalities/changes
- Description of the location, number, size, appearance/ substructure of electron dense deposits if present
- Description of degree of foot process effacement
- Description of relative changes in tubulointerstitial and vascular components

Diagnosis
- Including morphologic pattern plus a particular pathogenic or clinicopathologic category of the disease (i.e., focal necrotizing and crescentic ANCA glomerulonephritis with 60% crescents)

Comment
- Clinicopathologic correlation
- List of differential diagnoses if necessary
- Pertinent histologic prognostic indicators
- Activity/chronicity indices of lupus nephritis

Table 3.6 Components of Renal Transplant Biopsy Surgical Pathology Report[a]

Light Microscopy
- Glomeruli: glomerulitis, fibrin thrombosis, double contours, and other glomerular lesions
- Tubules: tubular injury, inflammation (tubulitis), nuclear atypia/ inclusions
- Interstitium: nature and degree of cellular infiltrate (i.e., edema, activated mononuclear cell, malignant cells, leukocytes in peritubular capillaries)
- Vessels: endarteritis, myocyte necrosis, thrombi, nodular hyaline, intimal elastosis

Immunofluorscence Microscopy
- C4d staining in peritubular capillaries

Electron Microscopy
- Glomerular abnormalities
- Viral particles
- Peritubular capillary basement membrane multilayering

Diagnosis
- Including a particular pathologic or clinicopathologic category of disease (Banff Classification for Renal Transplant Pathology being the most widely used system)

Comment
- Clinicopathologic correlation
- List of differential diagnoses if necessary
- Pertinent histologic prognostic indicators

[a] This table only lists features specific for transplant pathology (refer to Chapter 16 for detail). However, all components described in Table 3.5 for native renal biopsy (if applicable) should be included in the report as well.

components of renal biopsy report. For transplant biopsy, the most widely used classification is the Banff schema [22].

CONCLUSIONS

Although the algorithmic approach offers an organizational schema to evaluate renal biopsies by light, IF, and EM, the proposed algorithms, by nature and necessity, are overly simplified and do not encompass all diagnostic entities. The same caveat applies to other algorithms throughout the book. In addition, biopsies with more than one disease process are not considered in these algorithms. Therefore, the readers are referred to the appropriate chapters in this book for detailed discussions on the morphological and clinical manifestations of specific entities and diagnostic nuances. The algorithms may be used as a convenient overview and effective guide into these detailed texts.

REFERENCES

1. Lajoie G, Silva FG. Approach to the interpretation of renal biopsy. In: Silva FG, D'Agati VD, Nadasdy T, eds. *Renal Biopsy Interpretation*. New York: Churchill Livingstone; 1996, pp. 31–70.

2. Jennette JC, Olson JL, Schwartz MM, Silva FG. Primer on the pathologic diagnosis of renal disease. In: Jennette JC, Olson JL, Schwartz MM, Silva FG, eds, *Hepstinstall's Pathology of the Kidney*. 6th ed. Philadelphia: Lippincott Williams & Wilkins; 2007: 97–123.

3. Weening JJ, D'Agati VD, Schwartz MM, et al. The classification of glomerulonephritis in systemic lupus erythematosus revised. *Kidney Int* 2004; 65:521–30.

4. Walker PD, Cavallo T, Bonsib SM. The ad hoc committee on renal biopsy guidelines of the renal pathology society: practice guidelines for renal biopsy. *Mod Pathol* 2004;17: 1555–63.

5. Volhard F, Fahr T. *Die Brightische Nierenkrankheit* 1914; Berlin: Springer.

6. Addis T. A clinical classification of Bright's disease. *JAMA* 1925; 35:163.

7. Churg J, Berstein J, Glassock RJ. *Renal Disease: Classification and Atlas of Glomerular Diseases*. 2nd ed. Tokyo:Igaku-Shoin; 1995.

8. Seshan SV, D'Agati, Appel GA, Churg J. *Renal Disease: Classification and Atlas of Tubulo-interstital and Vascular Diseases*. Philadelphis, PA: Williams & Wilkins; 1999.

9. Zecher D, Lakkis F. Declassifying glomerulonephritis. *J Am Soc Nephrol* 2007; 18: 1034–5.

10. Barisoni L, Schnaper HW, Kopp JB. A proposed taxonomy for the podocytopathies: a reassessment of the primary nephrotic diseases. *Clin J Am Soc Nephrol* 2007; 2: 529–42.

11. Lajoie G, Silva FG. Technical aspects of renal biopsy processing. In: Silva FG, D'Agati VD, Nadasdy T, eds. *Renal Biopsy Interpretation*. New York: Churchill Livingstone; 1996, pp. 423–35.

12. Roos-van Groningen MC, Eikmans M, Baelde HJ, De Heer E, Bruijn JA. Improvement of extraction and processing of RNA from renal biopsies. *Kidney Int* 2004; 65: 97–105.

13. Nasr SH, Galgano SJ, Markowitz GS, Stokes MB, D'Agati VD. IFon pronase-digested paraffin sections: a valuable salvage technique for renal biopsies. *Kidney Int* 2006; 70: 2148–51.

14. Kaplan C, Pasternack B, Shah H, Gallo G. Age-related incidence of sclerotic glomeruli in human kidneys. *Am J Pathol* 1975; 80: 227–34.

15. Smith SM, Hoy WE, Cobb L. Low incidence of glomerulosclerosis in normal kidneys. *Archives Pathol Lab Med* 1989; 113: 1253–5.

16. Thorner PS, Ho M, Eremina V, et al. Podocytes contribute to the formation of glomerular crescents. *J Am Soc Nephrol* 2008; 19: 495–502.

17. Johnson RJ, Floege J, Rennke HG, Feehally J. Introduction to glomerular disease: pathogenesis and classification. In: Feehally J, Floege J, Johnson RJ, eds. *Comprehensive Clinical Nephrology*, 3rd ed. Edinburgh: Mosby; 2007, pp. 181–91.

18. Bonsib SM. Differential diagnosis in nephropathology: an IF-driven approach. *Adv Anat Pathol* 2002; 9: 101–14.

19. Haas M. A reevaluation of routine electron microscopy in the examination of native renal biopsies. *J Am Soc Nephrol* 1997; 8: 70–6.

20. Silva FG, Pirani CL. Electron microscopic study of medical diseases of the kidney: update – 1988. *Mod Pathol* 1988; 1: 292–315.

21. Jennette JC, Falk RJ. Nosology of primary vasculitis. *Curr Opin Rheumatol* 2007; 19: 10–16.

22. Solez K, Colvin RB, Racusen LC, et al. Banff 07 classification of renal allograft pathology: updates and future directions. *Am J Transplant* 2008; 8: 753–60.

CHAPTER 4

Glomerular Diseases Associated with Nephrotic Syndrome and Proteinuria

Michael B. Stokes MD, Glen S. Markowitz MD, and Vivette D. D'Agati MD

INTRODUCTION

The normal kidney excretes <150 mg protein/day, comprising small amounts of filtered albumin and low molecular weight proteins, as well as Tamm Horsfall protein (uromodulin) secreted by the medullary thick ascending limb of Henle. Increased protein excretion may result from increased glomerular permeability, increased filtered protein load (e.g., due to increased synthesis of monoclonal immunoglobulin light chains in patients with dysproteinemia) or defective tubular reabsorption of normally filtered proteins due to tubulointerstitial disease. Persistent proteinuria in excess of 1 g/day generally reflects abnormal glomerular permeability. Severe defects in glomerular permeability give rise to heavy proteinuria and nephrotic syndrome. The nephrotic syndrome is defined as proteinuria >3.5 g/1.73 m² body surface area/24 hours (>40 mg/ m² body surface area/hour in children), hypoalbuminemia (serum albumin <3.5 g/dL), edema, and hyperlipidemia. A major systemic complication of the nephrotic syndrome is a hypercoagulable state, which may lead to vascular thromboses.

Causes of the Nephrotic Syndrome

The nephrotic syndrome is associated with diverse systemic diseases, including heredofamilial conditions, infections, toxins, autoimmune disease, malignancy, and metabolic disease. However, in most cases, the underlying cause is unknown (idiopathic nephrotic syndrome). Systemic diseases causing nephrotic syndrome, including diabetes mellitus, systemic lupus erythematosus (SLE), and dysproteinemia are discussed in other chapters, as are primary glomerular diseases that typically present with nephritic features (i.e. hematuria, renal insufficiency, fluid retention, and hypertension) in addition to nephrotic-range proteinuria, such as membranoproliferative glomerulonephritis, fibrillary glomerulonephritis, and immunoglobulin A (IgA) nephropathy.

This chapter focuses on the three most common patterns of glomerular injury associated with idiopathic nephrotic syndrome, namely minimal change disease (MCD), focal segmental glomerulosclerosis (FSGS), and membranous nephropathy (MN). An algorithm for the classification of these conditions based on the key renal biopsy findings is presented in Table 4.1. Secondary causes of these patterns, important clinicopathologic variants, and pathogenetic mechanisms are reviewed. Two other conditions that commonly present with the nephrotic syndrome – human immunodeficiency virus (HIV)-associated nephropathy (HIVAN) and C1q nephropathy–are also discussed. Finally, the major causes of nephrotic syndrome in the first year of life are reviewed.

Pathophysiology of Nephrotic Syndrome

The glomerular filtration barrier comprises cellular and extracellular structural elements including the glomerular basement membrane (GBM), endothelial cells, visceral epithelial cells (podocytes), and interposed slit diaphragms. Together these components restrict proteins on the basis of size and charge. The glomerular capillary wall has a net negative charge that derives from both heparan sulfate proteoglycans within the GBM and sialoproteins on the surface of glomerular endothelial cells and podocytes. Glomerular diseases manifesting the nephrotic syndrome are caused by defects in the glomerular filtration barrier. Disruption of the glomerular filtration barrier may result from diverse etiologies and pathogenetic mechanisms including genetic defects in podocyte proteins, circulating permeability factors, T lymphocyte abnormalities, immune complex deposition, glomerular inflammation, toxins, viral infections, stretch injury, and physicochemical alterations, such as occurring in diabetes mellitus and amyloidosis. These pathomechanisms are discussed in more detail in the various sections of Chapter 4.

In the nephrotic syndrome, hypoalbuminemia results from a combination of urinary loss of albumin, increased albumin catabolism in the kidney, and inadequate compensatory hepatic synthesis. [1]. Hypoalbuminemia and the resulting reduction in plasma oncotic pressure alter the balance of Starling forces, leading to net filtration of fluid into the interstitium and edema formation. Abnormal capillary leakiness in patients with the nephrotic syndrome may also result from the presence of a circulating vascular permeability factor or cytokine [2]. The resulting movement of water from the intravascular to the extravascular space causes hypovolemia and reduced renal perfusion. This in turn activates the sympathetic nervous system and the renin angiotensin system, promoting the release of aldosterone and secondary renal retention of water and sodium at the level of the distal nephron. Of interest, sodium retention occurs selectively in the ipsilateral kidney of rats with experimental nephrotic syndrome, suggesting important intrarenal mechanisms of sodium retention initiated by albuminuria. These include activation of sodium-potassium-adenosine triphosphatase (Na-K-ATPase) in the cortical collecting duct and induction of epithelial sodium channels, in part from hyperaldosteronism

Table 4.1 Algorithmic Classification of the Major Glomerular Disease Patterns Associated with Idiopathic Nephrotic Syndrome

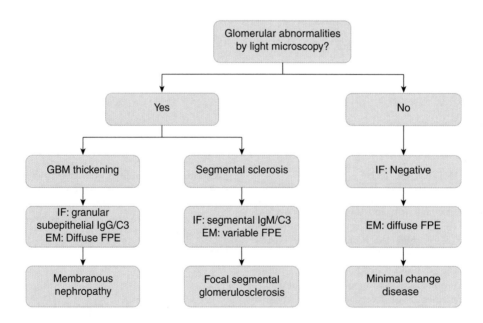

Abbreviations: **IF**, immunofluorescence microscopy; **EM**, electron microscopy; **FPE**, foot process effacement

[3,4]. A role for activation of the cortical Na/H exchanger (NHE3) at the level of the proximal tubule by increased albumin trafficking has also been identified [5].

Hyperlipidemia results from both overproduction and impaired catabolism of serum lipids. Because the severity of hyperlipidemia tends to correlate with the degree of hypoalbuminemia and both stimuli activate similar synthetic pathways in the liver, the reduced serum albumin is thought to promote increased hepatic synthesis of lipids and lipoproteins, leading to increased generation of low-density lipoproteins (LDL), apo A-1-rich high-density lipoproteins (HDL), and total cholesterol. Increases in very low-density lipoprotein (VLDL) are due in part to defective VLDL clearance through reduced VLDL receptor expression in nephrotic states [6]. Increase in lipoprotein (a) via increased hepatic synthesis is also thought to contribute to the atherogenic potential of the nephrotic syndrome.

The hypercoagulability of the nephrotic syndrome has complex pathomechanisms. These include increased hepatic synthesis of fibrinogen and numerous coagulation factors, including factors II, V, VII, VIII, X, and XIII. Platelet hyperaggregability and urinary losses of anticoagulation factors such as antithrombin III and plasminogen contribute to the increased thrombotic potential. Thrombosis often targets the renal vein, but may involve a variety of venous and arterial beds.

MINIMAL CHANGE DISEASE

Definition

Minimal change disease (MCD) is characterized clinically by nephrotic syndrome and pathologically by minimal or no glomerular alterations by light microscopy, the absence of glomerular immune deposits by immunofluorescence microscopy (IF), and the presence of foot process effacement by electron microscopy (EM).

Clinical Features

MCD may occur at any age but predominantly affects young children. MCD accounts for approximately 90 percent of cases of primary nephrotic syndrome in preadolescent children and less than 25 percent of cases in adults. In childhood MCD, the median age of onset is 2.5 years and 80 percent are <6 years of age. MCD is rare before 6 months of age.

Most cases of MCD are idiopathic. Secondary forms are more common in adults, accounting for up to 10 percent of cases (see "Secondary Causes of MCD"). There is a 2:1 male to female ratio in children that approaches unity in adulthood. Most patients present with full nephrotic syndrome, although asymptomatic subnephrotic proteinuria may be seen in cases that have undergone spontaneous partial remission. Hematuria and hypertension are typically absent in children and affect a minority of adults. Mild renal insufficiency is detected in less than one-third of children with MCD, reflecting reduced glomerular hydraulic conductivity due to obliteration of the filtration slit pores by effaced foot processes. Acute renal failure may be seen in older adults (see "MCD with Acute Renal Failure") but this complication is unusual in children with MCD, unless there is hypovolemic shock due to intravascular volume depletion from profound hypoalbuminemia or aggressive diuresis.

Approach to Interpretation

Gross Findings. Autopsies of patients with MCD reveal large, pale, and waxy kidneys, with a yellow color reflecting abundant lipid accumulation in proximal tubules (hence the older designation "lipoid nephrosis").

Light Microscopic Findings. Glomeruli display minimal or no histologic abnormalities (Figures 4.1 and 4.2) except for a slight increase in mesangial cellularity or matrix and mild swelling or prominence of the visceral epithelial cells. Globally sclerotic glomeruli may occur as a nonspecific finding (affecting up to 30 percent of glomeruli by 80 years of age) [7]. Proximal tubules may display intracytoplasmic protein resorption droplets (hyaline droplets) that are eosinophilic, periodic acid Schiff (PAS) positive, and trichrome red, and lipid resorption droplets that appear "empty" with these stains (Figure 4.3). Tubular atrophy, interstitial fibrosis, and interstitial inflammation are usually absent, except in older patients who may have age-related glomerular obsolescence and arteriosclerosis.

Immunofluorescence Findings. Typically, no glomerular immune deposits are seen. In some cases, there may be weak mesangial staining (1+ intensity) for IgM and C3.

Electron Microscopic Findings. There is extensive effacement of foot processes, usually involving >75 percent of the total glomerular capillary surface area (Figure 4.4). An exception is when partial remission has occurred by the time of the biopsy (either spontaneously or following therapy). Podocyte cell bodies frequently display microvillous transformation. A mild increase in mesangial cell number or matrix and rare small paramesangial electron densities representing trapped plasma proteins may be seen. Immune complex-type electron dense deposits are absent and glomerular basement membranes show no structural abnormalities. Proximal tubules may display intracellular electron-lucent lipid resorption droplets and electron-dense protein resorption droplets.

Etiology and Pathogenesis

The etiology of MCD is unknown. A role for abnormal T-cell function and immune dysregulation is supported by the high rate of response to steroids and the association with lymphoid malignancies, atopy, and other allergic conditions. Circulating "permeability factors" causing increased glomerular capillary wall permeability have been isolated from the serum, plasma, mononuclear cells, and urine of patients with MCD [8]. Puromycin aminonucleoside, a podocyte toxin, induces a MCD-like disease in experimental animals [9]. Animal models that overexpress interleukin (IL)-13 [10] or are exposed to lipopolysaccharide (LPS) [11] also develop MCD-like disease.

Treatment and Prognosis

Most children (95 percent) with MCD achieve remission of nephrotic syndrome within 8 weeks of starting corticosteroid therapy but adults may take longer to respond [12,13]. Relapses of nephrotic syndrome are common and may be persistent in 28 percent of adults [13]. Frequent relapsers may become steroid-dependent. Steroid-dependent nephrotic syndrome or frequent

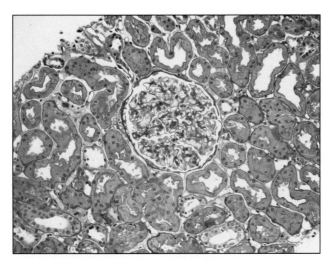

FIGURE 4.1: MC: Low-power magnification reveals no pathologic abnormalities (periodic acid-Schiff reaction (PAS, × 200).

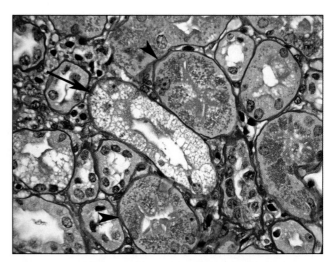

FIGURE 4.3: MCD. Tubules focally contain empty cytoplasmic vacuoles consistent with lipid droplets (arrow) and PAS positive protein droplets (arrow-head) (PAS, × 600).

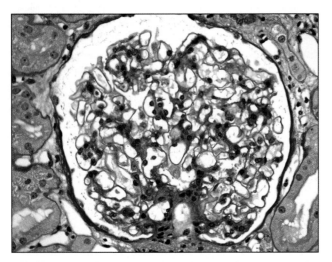

FIGURE 4.2: MCD. Glomerulus is of normal size and cellularity, with fully patent capillaries. The glomerular basement membranes appear normal in thickness, with a regular smooth texture (PAS, × 400).

relapsers may respond to other agents, including mycophenolate mofetil [13,14], chlorambucil, cyclophosphamide, levamisole, and cyclosporine[15], as may some of the 10 percent of MCD patients with steroid-resistant nephrotic syndrome. Progression to renal failure is rare in MCD and may be accompanied by lesions of FSGS on repeat biopsy [13]. In children with MCD, the presence of glomerular hypertrophy (glomerular area greater than 1.75 times that of age-matched controls) on initial biopsy may be a risk factor for subsequent evolution to FSGS [16].

Differential Diagnosis

Secondary causes of MCD are more common in adults, but even then only constitute a minority of cases (see "Secondary

Causes of MCD"). The major differential diagnosis is unsampled FSGS. This possibility should be considered (and additional tissue sections examined) if there is significant tubular atrophy, interstitial fibrosis and/or arteriosclerosis, particularly in children where arterionephrosclerosis due to aging and/or hypertension cannot be invoked. Particular attention should be directed at the tubular pole for evidence of glomerular tip lesion (GTL) as these entities share many clinical features (see "Morphologic Variants of FSGS") [17]. Autopsies of children dying with MCD have shown GTL, underscoring that these conditions may be confused due to sampling error in small biopsy specimens [18].

The possibility of genetic disease should be considered in patients who have a family history of nephrotic syndrome, disease onset within the first three months of life (see "Congenital Nephrotic Syndrome"), or steroid-resistant nephrotic syndrome. Genetic abnormalities in podocyte-expressed proteins (including podocin [19], TRPC6 [20], and dysferlin [21]) may all cause nephrotic syndrome with MCD phenotype. Up to 26 percent of children with steroid-resistant nephrotic syndrome (who may have either MCD or FSGS phenotype) may have genetic mutations in *NPHS2* encoding podocin [22]. In contrast to idiopathic MCD, genetic causes of nephrotic syndrome are usually steroid-resistant.

MCD may be superimposed on other glomerular conditions including mild lupus nephritis and IgA nephropathy (see "MCD with IgA Nephropathy"). The presence of C1q-dominant immune deposits (with or without IgG and other immunoglobulins) is diagnostic of C1q nephropathy (see "C1q Nephropathy").

MCD Variants

MCD with Acute Renal Failure

Definition. This variant is defined as acute renal failure occurring in the setting of MCD-induced nephrotic syndrome [13,23].

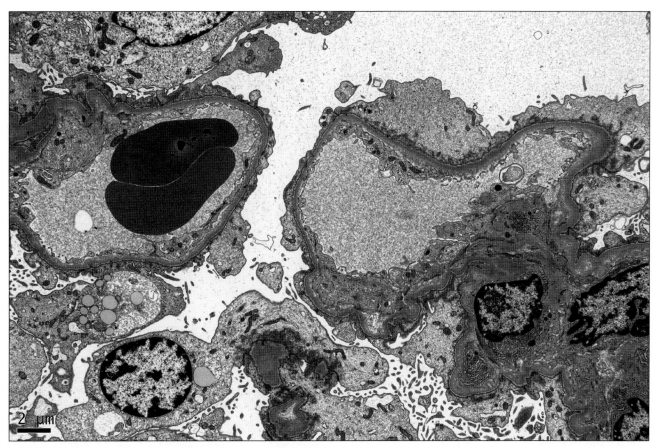

FIGURE 4.4: *MCD. Electron microscopy reveals diffuse foot process effacement over the entire capillary surface. Podocytes display focal lipid droplets. The glomerular basement membranes appear normal in thickness. There are no electron-dense deposits (electron microscopy, × 10,000).*

Clinical Features. This complication predominantly affects older adults who have severe nephrotic syndrome, massive edema, and a history of hypertension. Renal failure may be oliguric or nonoliguric.

Light Microscopic Findings. Biopsies show typical glomerular changes of MCD, accompanied by features of ischemic acute tubular necrosis in about 70 percent of cases; the remaining 30 percent display no significant tubulointerstitial findings by LM (Figure 4.5). Proximal tubular epithelium shows focal simplification with ectatic or irregular luminal profiles, flattened epithelium, attenuated or absent brush border, and enlarged regenerative nuclei with nucleoli (Figure 4.6). Increased tubular epithelial mitotic figures and apoptotic bodies may be seen. Cellular debris may shed into the tubular lumen but frank coagulation necrosis is not seen. Interstitial edema is common but usually this is mild and patchy. Arteriosclerosis is common, particularly in older individuals with a history of hypertension.

Immunofluorescence Findings. No immune deposits are seen.

Electron Microscopic Findings. Glomerular findings are similar to MCD. The proximal tubular cells appear simplified, with reduced apical microvilli, widening of the intercellular junc-

tions, reduced basolateral interdigitations, and fewer cytoplasmic organelles.

Etiology and Pathogenesis. Older age, heavier proteinuria, more severe hypoalbuminemia, systolic hypertension, and arteriosclerosis are risk factors. Arteriosclerosis presumably predisposes to acute renal failure by impairing compensatory response to the hemodynamic stresses of reduced renal perfusion associated with severe nephrotic syndrome.

Treatment and Prognosis. Most patients recover renal function within 5 to 7 weeks, as the nephrotic syndrome responds to immunosuppressive therapy and diuresis. However, a minority may develop irreversible renal failure.

MCD With Diffuse Mesangial Hypercellularity

Definition. Diffuse mesangial hypercellularity (DMH) is encountered in approximately 3 percent of pediatric cases of idiopathic nephrotic syndrome. DMH is defined as more than four mesangial cells per mesangial region affecting at least 80 percent of glomeruli in tissue sections of 2 to 3 μm in thickness according to the International Study of Kidney Diseases in Children (ISKDC) criteria [24]. The Southwest Pediatric Nephrology Study Group (SPNSG) defines DMH as involvement of more than 75 percent of glomeruli by mesangial

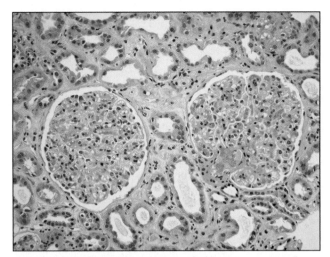

FIGURE 4.5: *MCD with acute renal failure. On low power, glomeruli appear normal. There is mild diffuse interstitial edema. Tubular epithelium shows diffuse simplification, with flattening of epithelium (H&E, × 200).*

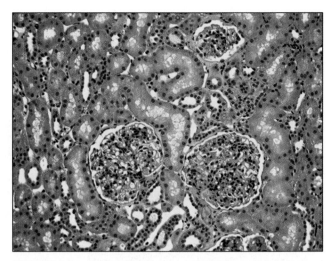

FIGURE 4.7: *MCD with diffuse mesangial hypercellularity. Low-power view shows diffuse and global mesangial hypercellularity. Tubules appear normal. (H&E, × 200).*

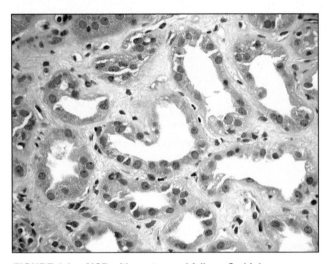

FIGURE 4.6: *MCD with acute renal failure. On high power, tubular epithelium shows loss of apical brush border. Nuclei are enlarged and nucleoli are visible. (H&E, × 400).*

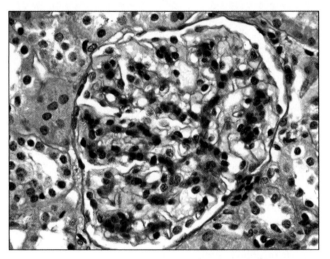

FIGURE 4.8: *MCD with diffuse mesangial hypercellularity. High-power view shows severe global mesangial hypercellularity, with more than six mesangial cells in some mesangial regions (PAS, × 400).*

hypercellularity that may be mild (three nuclei per mesangial area), moderate (four nuclei per mesangial area), or severe (five nuclei or more per mesangial area) [25].

Clinical Features. Patients with DMH are more likely to have hematuria (89 percent) and hypertension (46 percent) than patients with MCD [24]. Gross hematuria may be present.

Light Microscopic Findings. Mesangial hypercellularity ranges from mild to severe (Figures 4.7 and 4.8).

Immunofluorescence Findings. Glomeruli are usually negative for immune reactants. Mesangial staining for IgM and C3 may be seen in some cases [24].

Electron Microscopic Findings. Podocytes display diffuse effacement, similar to MCD (Figure 4.9). Small paramesangial electron-dense deposits are identified in up to 50 percent of cases.

Differential Diagnosis. This includes mesangial proliferative lupus nephritis, mild membranoproliferative glomerulonephritis, IgA nephropathy, C1q nephropathy, and the resolving phase of acute postinfectious glomerulonephritis. In children less than 1 year of age, the possibility of genetic disease should be excluded (see "Nephrotic Syndrome in the First Year of life").

Treatment and Prognosis. DMH may have a higher rate of initial steroid resistance than MCD but there is no significant difference in long-term outcome.

IgM Nephropathy

Definition. IgM nephropathy is defined by the presence of diffuse and global mesangial deposits of IgM in cases that otherwise resemble MCD [26]. Whether IgM nephropathy represents a distinct clinicopathologic entity is uncertain, reflecting

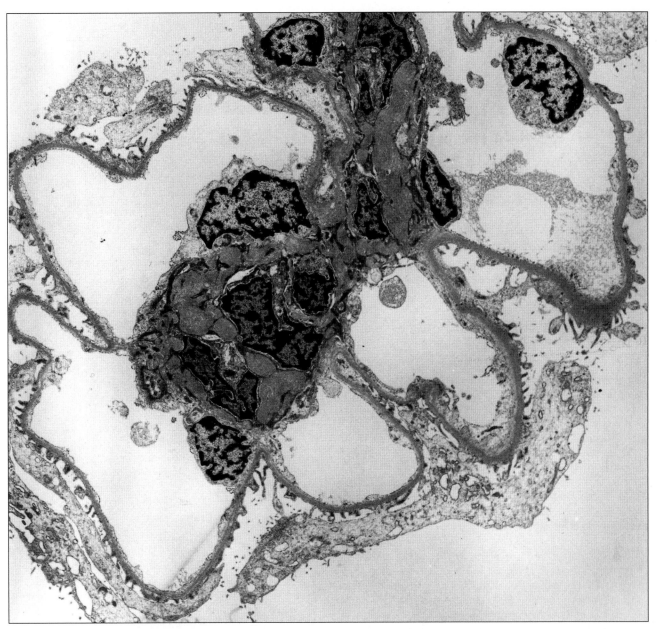

FIGURE 4.9: *MCD with diffuse mesangial hypercellularity. Electron microscopy reveals mesangial hypercellularity and diffuse foot process effacement. The glomerular basement membranes appear normal in thickness and there are no electron-dense deposits (Electron microscopy, × 4,000).*

different approaches to defining pathologic criteria such as intensity of IgM staining, mesangial hypercellularity, and mesangial electron-dense deposits. Weak immunofluorescence staining for IgM (without electron-dense deposits) is not uncommon in MCD. Therefore, the diagnosis of IgM nephropathy should be reserved for cases with ≥ 2+ (scale 0–3+) mesangial staining for IgM, irrespective of the degree of mesangial hypercellularity or the presence of mesangial electron-dense deposits.

Clinical Features. Both children and adults may be affected. Compared to MCD, hypertension [27]) and hematuria [28] may

be more common. Some patients may present with hematuria and minimal proteinuria [29].

Light Microscopic Findings. Glomeruli usually display no histologic abnormalities, although mesangial hypercellularity may occur [27].

Immunofluorescence Findings. Mesangial deposits of IgM exhibit 2+ or stronger intensity (Figure 4.10). Co-deposits of C3 are identified in 30 to 100 percent of the cases. Rarely, there may be trace to 1+ segmental mesangial costaining for IgG, IgA, and/or C1q.

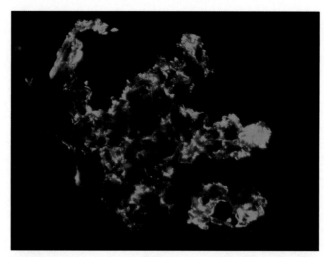

FIGURE 4.10: *IgM nephropathy. Immunofluorescence microscopy shows diffuse and global staining of mesangial areas for IgM (Immunofluorescence stain, × 400).*

Electron Microscopic Findings. There is extensive foot process effacement. Mesangial electron-dense deposits may be seen (Figure 4.11).

Differential Diagnosis. IgM nephropathy must be differentiated from IgA nephropathy, mesangial proliferative lupus nephritis, and the resolving phase of acute postinfectious glomerulonephritis. IgM nephropathy is distinguished by dominant mesangial staining for IgM (with/without C3) and the presence of severe foot process effacement in the setting of idiopathic nephrotic syndrome.

Etiology and Pathogenesis. Mesangial IgM staining probably represents nonspecific entrapment of circulating plasma proteins due to impaired mesangial clearance.

Treatment and Prognosis. There may be an increased incidence of initial steroid resistance and steroid dependence compared to MCD, ranging from 25 to 50 percent, but long-term renal prognosis is similar [26,27]. However, in one recent study, 50 percent of IgM nephropathy patients had hypertension, 36 percent developed renal insufficiency, and 23 percent reached end-stage renal failure.[29]. Similar to MCD, some cases of IgM nephropathy display FSGS on repeat biopsy [29,30].

MCD With IgA Nephropathy

Definition. This is defined by the presence of IgA dominant mesangial deposits and extensive foot process effacement, without peripheral capillary wall deposits, in patients with the nephrotic syndrome.

Clinical Features. Most reported cases are in children less than 10 years of age but this dual glomerulopathy may occur at any age [31]. The male to female ratio is 3:1. Nephrotic proteinuria is present in all patients, hematuria in 50 percent, and episodic gross hematuria (usually following upper respiratory tract infections) in 25 percent.

Light Microscopic Findings. Glomeruli display mild or no mesangial hypercellularity (Figure 4.12). Glomerular capillary lumens are patent, without evidence of endocapillary proliferation or segmental sclerosis. Red blood cells may be identified in the tubular lumens, reflecting the presence of hematuria.

Immunofluorescence Findings. There is dominant mesangial staining for IgA in a granular and diffuse pattern, with an intensity of 2+ or greater (Figure 4.13), often accompanied by staining for C3. Variable, less intense staining for IgG and IgM may be seen. C1q staining is typically absent.

Electron Microscopic Findings. Podocytes display diffuse foot process effacement and microvillous cytoplasmic projections (Figure 4.14). Mesangial electron-dense deposits are seen (Figure 4.15). No immune deposits are found in the subendothelial or subepithelial regions.

Differential Diagnosis. Pure IgA nephropathy presenting with nephrotic syndrome typically displays severe glomerular proliferative or sclerosing lesions and immune deposits involving the glomerular capillary walls.

Etiology and Pathogenesis. This entity probably represents the chance concurrence of two relatively common diseases of childhood, as evidenced by the asynchronous development of MCD and IgA nephropathy in some cases [31,32].

Treatment and Prognosis. Most patients have a prompt remission of nephrotic syndrome with steroid therapy, and the renal prognosis is excellent. Relapses and spontaneous remission of nephrotic syndrome have been described.

MCD Secondary to Drugs

Definition. This variant is defined as nephrotic syndrome with biopsy findings of MCD arising in the setting of drug use. The commonest drug association is with non-steroidal antiinflammatory drugs (NSAID) [33], but lithium, interferon, and pamidronate have also been implicated [34–38]. Remission of the nephrotic syndrome within weeks of withdrawal of the offending drug supports a drug effect.

Clinical Features. NSAID-induced MCD predominantly affects older adults (mean age: 65 years). The average duration of NSAID exposure prior to the development of nephrotic syndrome is 11 months but this complication may develop after several years [39]. Some patients present with nephrotic syndrome and acute renal failure. Hypersensitivity phenomena (fever, rash, and eosinophilia) affect fewer than 20 percent of patients, possibly reflecting the antiinflammatory properties of the NSAID.

Pathologic Findings. There is diffuse foot process effacement, similar to idiopathic MCD. Cases with acute renal failure may show either concomitant ischemic acute tubular necrosis (Figure 4.6) or acute interstitial nephritis, with interstitial edema, and a predominantly lymphocytic inflammatory infiltrate (Figure 4.16). Eosinophils are infrequent and tubulitis is usually mild.

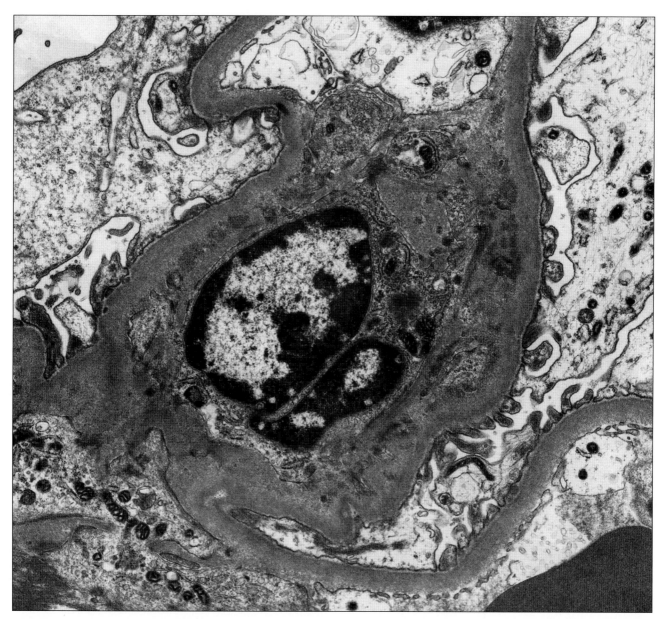

FIGURE 4.11: *IgM nephropathy. Electron microscopy reveals diffuse podocyte foot process effacement. Mesangial electron dense deposits are seen. (Electron microscopy × 10,000).*

Differential Diagnosis. The major differential diagnosis is idiopathic MCD. Features of acute interstitial nephritis support an allergic drug reaction whereas persistence of the nephrotic syndrome more than 8 weeks after discontinuing the drug (in the absence of steroid therapy) favors primary MCD.

Etiology and Pathogenesis. The mechanism of drug toxicity is unknown but the pathologic finding of diffuse foot process effacement suggests a role for direct podocyte injury. The acute interstitial nephritis component is presumably allergic in nature. Renal hypoperfusion related to hypoalbuminemia, and NSAID-induced inhibition of vasodilatory prostaglandins may contribute to the development of ischemic acute tubular injury.

Treatment and Prognosis. Proteinuria and renal insufficiency usually resolve within 2 to 8 weeks after discontinuation of the offending drug. Steroid therapy may hasten recovery. Future exposure to NSAID should be avoided.

Miscellaneous Secondary Causes of MCD

MCD may precede or occur simultaneously with the diagnosis of Hodgkin's disease and other hematologic malignancies including chronic myelogenous leukemia, acute myelogenous leukemia, angioimmunoblastic lymphadenopathy, angiotropic (intravascular) large cell lymphoma [40], mycosis fungoides, and T-cell leukemias. Support for a pathogenic association includes the response of the MCD to therapy directed to the

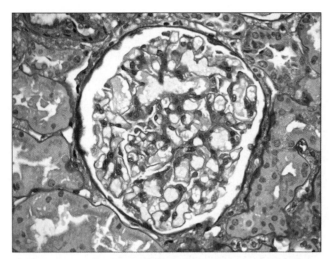

FIGURE 4.12:   Combined MCD/IgA nephropathy. High-power view shows mild segmental mesangial hypercellularity (PAS, × 400).

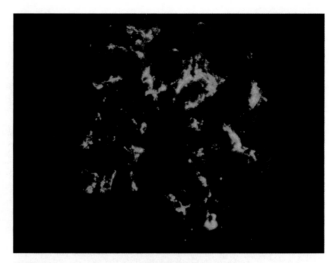

FIGURE 4.13:   Combined MCD/IgA nephropathy. Immunofluorescence microscopy shows diffuse and global staining of mesangial areas for IgA (Immunofluorescence stain, × 400).

Hodgkin's disease and the timing of recurrences of nephrotic syndrome with relapses of Hodgkin's disease.

MCD may also occur in association with thymoma, bee stings, food allergies, childhood immunizations, infectious mononucleosis, HIV infection, and SLE. A close temporal relationship between the inciting agent or disease and the development of the nephrotic syndrome supports a pathogenic role but coincidental occurrence may be impossible to exclude in an individual case. In SLE patients, the abrupt onset of nephrotic syndrome at the time of initial SLE diagnosis, or shortly thereafter, together with biopsy findings of minimal or no glomerular capillary wall immune deposits and diffuse podocyte foot process effacement suggest the possibility of a lupus-related podocytopathy [41].

FOCAL SEGMENTAL GLOMERULOSCLEROSIS

Introduction and Definitions

Focal segmental glomerulosclerosis (FSGS) is a pattern of glomerular injury characterized by segmental obliteration of the glomerular tuft by matrix accumulation (sclerosis) and/or hyaline, often with synechial attachment between the glomerular tuft and Bowman's capsule. Focal segmental glomerulosclerosis (FSGS) may result from diverse pathogenetic mechanisms including heritable mutations of podocyte proteins, viral infections, toxins, and medications (Table 4.2) [42]. FSGS may also be mediated by adaptive structural–functional responses to diverse insults in the setting of reduced or normal nephron numbers. Primary FSGS is a clinical–pathologic syndrome characterized by heavy proteinuria or nephrotic syndrome and biopsy findings of FSGS, in the absence of any known secondary cause.

Approach to Interpretation of FSGS

The diagnosis and clinical management of patients with FSGS is problematic for several reasons. Most importantly, FSGS is not a single disease but a clinical–pathologic syndrome resulting

from diverse etiologies and pathogenetic pathways. This inherent heterogeneity undoubtedly contributes to the clinical variability observed in studies of primary FSGS. Secondly, it may be impossible to exclude all the known secondary causes of FSGS due to incomplete clinical information. Moreover, exhaustive testing for all the known genetic causes of FSGS may not be feasible, given the low prevalence of the known causative mutations in patients with sporadic FSGS and the lack of testing facilities outside the research setting for some of these mutations. Thirdly, the pathologic diagnosis of FSGS is subject to sampling error. FSGS lesions may be missed in small biopsy specimens, or may have evolved to nondiagnostic global glomerulosclerosis lesions in the later stage of disease. Because early FSGS lesions predominantly affect juxtamedullary glomeruli, they may not be sampled in superficial renal cortical biopsy specimens.

Morphologic Variants and Classification of FSGS

FSGS lesions are morphologically heterogeneous, showing variable degrees of sclerosis and cellularity. The typical or "classic" FSGS lesion consists of segmental sclerosis with obliteration of the glomerular tuft by eosinophilic, PAS-reactive acellular matrix, and/or glassy, eosinophilic hyaline material (hyalinosis), usually with adhesion of the glomerular tuft to Bowman's capsule (Figures 4.17–4.20). Early FSGS lesions may consist solely of a synechial attachment between the glomerular tuft and Bowman's capsule (Figures 4.21 and 4.22), whereas more advanced lesions may show near-complete obliteration of glomerular capillaries, approaching global glomerulosclerosis. In addition to sclerosis and hyalinosis, FSGS lesions may show variable cellular features. This most commonly manifests as mild hypertrophy of visceral epithelial cells overlying the segmental sclerosis lesion (Figure 4.23). The spectrum of FSGS also includes lesion displaying segmental or global collapse of the capillary tuft without significant matrix increase (Figures 4.24–4.26). Collapsing lesions are typically accompanied by severe

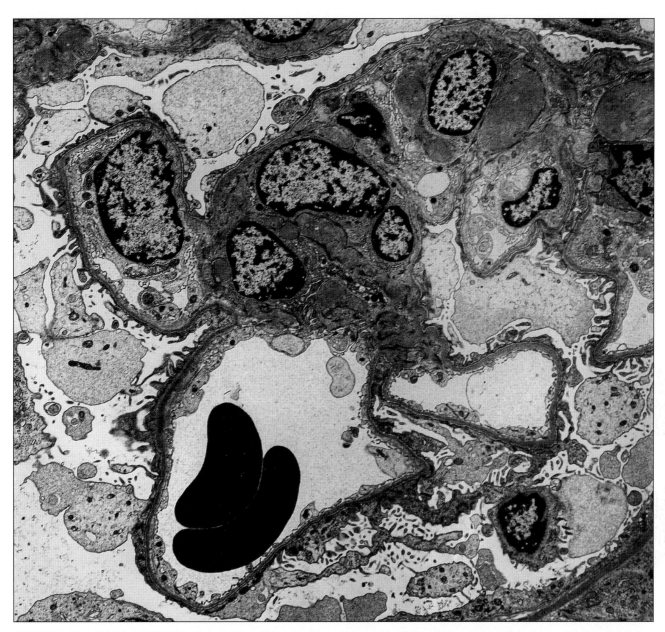

FIGURE 4.14: *Combined MCD/IgA nephropathy. Electron microscopy reveals diffuse foot process effacement without peripheral capillary wall immune deposits (Electron microscopy, × 3,000).*

epithelial cell hyperplasia in Bowman's space, mimicking a cellular crescent (Figure 4.25). Other FSGS lesions display expansion of the capillary tuft by endocapillary hypercellularity due to endothelial proliferation, foam cells and/or inflammatory cells, without features of capillary collapse (Figures 4.27 and 4.28). Segmental lesions may appear to prolapse into the lumen of the proximal tubule, with confluence of overlying epithelial cells and proximal tubular epithelial cells or synechial attachment to Bowman's capsule at the tubular pole (glomerular tip lesion) (Figures 4.29 and 4.30). Finally, FSGS lesions may localize predominantly to the vascular pole (perihilar FSGS) (Figure 4.31). Importantly, the spectrum of these morphologic lesions occur in both primary and secondary forms of FSGS, and different types of lesion may coexist in the same biopsy, or be seen in repeat biopsies from the same individual. The latter finding

suggests that morphologic variants of FSGS may represent stages in the evolution of glomerular lesions, rather than independent disease entities [43].

To standardize the pathologic diagnosis of FSGS variants, the Columbia Classification employs a systematic, hierarchical approach to define five mutually exclusive variants, namely collapsing (COLL), glomerular tip lesion (GTL), cellular (CELL), perihilar (PH), and not otherwise specified (NOS)[44]. This classification can be applied to both primary and secondary FSGS. Details of this schema are presented in Table 4.3 and an algorithmic approach to its use is provided in Table 4.4. The pathologic features of these variants are described in more detail in the section on "Primary FSGS." In brief, the finding of segmental or global capillary collapse with podocyte hypertrophy and hyperplasia in a single glomerulus

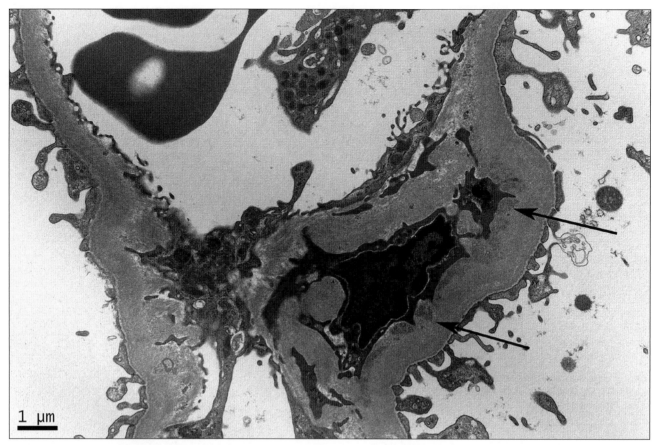

FIGURE 4.15: *Combined MCD/IgA nephropathy. Electron microscopy reveals small mesangial electron dense deposits (arrows) (Electron microscopy, × 3,000).*

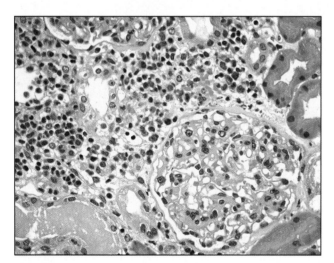

FIGURE 4.16: *MCD secondary to NSAID use. Glomerulus appears normal, consistent with minimal change disease. There is patchy interstitial edema and inflammation, consistent with associated acute interstitial nephritis (H&E, × 200).*

warrants a designation of COLL variant, regardless of findings in other glomeruli. In the absence of collapsing lesions, the finding of a single glomerular tip lesion defines GTL variant. CELL variant is defined by segmental endocapillary hypercellularity (with or without overlying extracapillary hypercellularity), without evidence of capillary collapse or tip lesion in any glomerulus. PH variant is diagnosed where >50 percent segmental lesions demonstrate perihilar involvement and no glomerulus shows capillary collapse. NOS variant is diagnosed, by default, when a biopsy does not meet criteria for any other variant. Schwartz et al. use the terms cellular FSGS and collapsing glomerulopathy interchangeably for cases that show either podocyte hyperplasia or endocapillary hypercellularity, with or without underlying capillary collapse, whereas the presence of capillary collapse distinguishes COLL variant from CELL variant in the Columbia Classification [45].

Some [17,46–48] but not all studies [43,45] have demonstrated significant clinical differences among the Columbia Classification variants when applied to cases of primary FSGS. The general clinical and pathologic characteristics of primary FSGS and its morphologic variants are discussed in the following sections.

Primary FSGS

Definition. Primary (idiopathic) FSGS is a clinical–pathologic syndrome characterized by nephrotic syndrome or heavy proteinuria with pathologic findings of FSGS, in the absence of any known secondary cause of FSGS.

Epidemiology and Clinical Presentation. The incidence of primary FSGS is influenced by age, sex, race/ethnicity, and

Table 4.2 Etiologic Classification of FSGS

Primary (Idiopathic) FSGS
? Mediated by yet unidentified circulating/permeability factor(s)

Secondary FSGS
1. Familial/genetic
   Mutations in nephrin
   Mutations in podocin
   Mutations in α-actinin-4
   Mutations in transient receptor potential cation 6 channel
     (TRPC6)
   Mutations in CD2-associated protein *(CD2AP)*
   Mutations in Wilms tumor-1 *(WT-1)*
   Mutations in phospholipase C epsilon-1 *(PLCE1)*
   Mutations in *SWI/SNF related, matrix associated, actin
     dependent regulator of chromatin, subfamily A-like
     protein 1 (SMARCAL1)* (Schimke immuno-osseous
     dysplasia)
   Mutations in mitochondrial proteins (mitochondrial cytopathies)
   Mutations in β4 integrin (Epidermolysis bullosa)
   Mutations in tetraspanin (Epidermolysis bullosa, deafness)
   Mutations in laminin β2 (Pierson syndrome)
2. Virus-associated
   HIV-1 ("HIV-associated nephropathy")
   Parvovirus B-19
   SV40
   CMV
3. Drug –induced
   Heroin ("Heroin nephropathy")
   Interferon-α
   Lithium
   Pamidronate
   Sirolimus
4. Mediated by Adaptive Structural–Functional Responses
Reduced Renal Mass
   Oligomeganephronia
   Unilateral renal agenesis
   Renal dysplasia
   Reflux nephropathy
   Sequela to cortical necrosis
   Surgical renal ablation
   Chronic allograft nephropathy
   Any advanced renal disease with reduction in functioning
     nephrons
Initially Normal Renal Mass
   Hypertension
   Atheroemboli or other acute vaso-occlusive processes
   Obesity
   Cyanotic congenital heart disease
   Sickle cell anemia

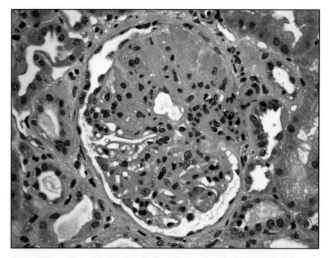

FIGURE 4.17: *FSGS. There is segmental obliteration of the glomerular tuft by acellular eosinophilic matrix (H&E, × 400).*

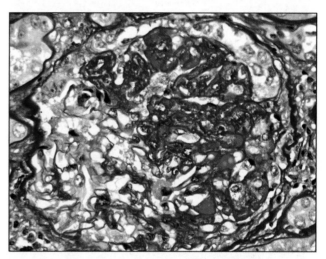

FIGURE 4.18: *FSGS. There is segmental obliteration of the glomerular tuft by sclerosis and hyalinosis, with synechial attachment of the glomerular tuft to Bowman's capsule (PAS, × 400).*

biopsy practice. Primary FSGS is slightly more common in males than females and is more common in black than white children [49]. In the United States, the incidence of primary FSGS in adults has increased over the past three decades [50] and is now the leading cause of primary nephrotic syndrome (35 to 58.5 percent) in some centers [50,51]. This increased incidence has been particularly striking in black adults [49–51] where FSGS now accounts for up to 64 percent of cases of primary nephrotic syndrome [51]. Primary FSGS accounts for 10 to 20 percent of idiopathic nephrotic syndrome in children and has emerged as an increasingly common cause of ESRD in the United States, par-

ticularly among African-Americans. This increased incidence probably reflects changing epidemiologic factors, rather than differences in biopsy practice or pathologic interpretation.

Nephrotic range proteinuria is found in 90 percent of children and 70 percent percent of adults [43,51,52]. Renal insufficiency is present in about 20 percent of children and 30 percent of adults. Hypertension is identified in approximately 30 percent of children and 45 percent of adults. Microhematuria affects approximately 55 percent of children and 45 percent of adults [51]. The relative frequency of the morphologic variants in primary FSGS is influenced by age and race/ethnicity. In all studies, NOS is the most common variant, ranging from 32 to 73 percent [43,46,48,53]. COLL variant exhibits black racial predominance whereas GTL variant predominantly affects Caucasian adults. CELL variant is rare in adults but may be more common in children, whereas GTL and PH variants are uncommon in children [43,53].

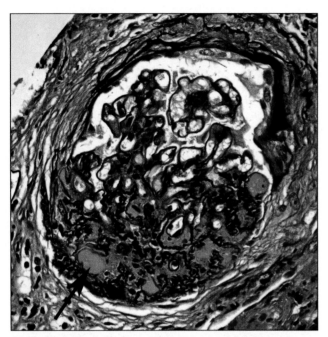

FIGURE 4.19: *FSGS. The segmental lesion shows argyrophilic (black) staining of matrix and pink staining of hyalinosis [Jones's methenamine silver (JMS), × 40].*

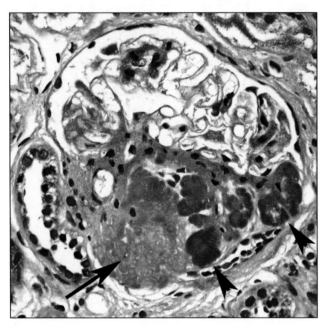

FIGURE 4.20: *FSGS. With trichrome stain, hyalinosis lesions stain red/orange (arrow-heads) whereas sclerosis stains blue (arrows) (Trichrome stain, × 400).*

In addition to black race, COLL variant in adults is associated with younger age, higher initial serum creatinine, heavier proteinuria, and lower serum albumin compared to the other FSGS variants [46,47]. In children, COLL variant is associated with higher initial blood pressure compared to CELL and NOS [53]. GTL variant usually presents with sudden onset of full nephrotic syndrome, similar to MCD [17] and has better initial

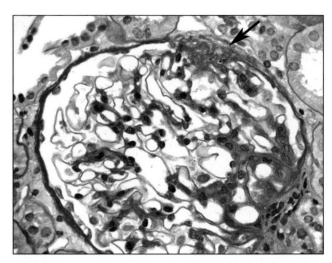

FIGURE 4.21: *An early lesion of FSGS consists of synechial attachment of the glomerular tuft to Bowman's capsule with small accumulation of matrix (arrow) (PAS, × 400).*

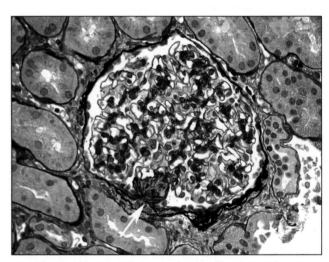

FIGURE 4.22: *FSGS. An early lesion consists of segmental hyalinosis with synechial attachment to Bowman's capsule (arrow) (JMS, × 200).*

renal function compared to COLL [17,46] and NOS variants. [48]. In a predominantly adult population, CELL variant showed heavier proteinuria, greater frequency of nephrotic syndrome, lower serum albumin, and a shorter interval from clinical onset of renal disease to biopsy compared to NOS [47]. In one study, PH variant had the lowest frequency of nephrotic syndrome (55 percent), highest frequency of hypertension (80 percent), and lowest initial serum creatinine [46]. Clinical features of NOS are closest to PH variant [46] with similar prevalence of hypertension (80 percent) but slightly more frequent nephrotic syndrome (67 percent). Cholesterol levels are similar in the different variants [17,46–48].

Light Microscopic Findings. COLL variant often shows diffuse glomerular involvement and severe tubulointerstitial injury (Figures 4.33 and 4.34). Glomeruli demonstrate segmental or

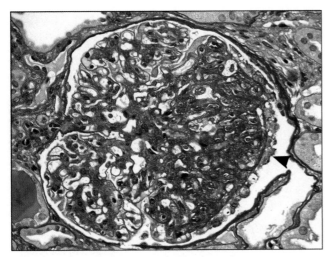

FIGURE 4.23: *FSGS. There is capping of visceral epithelial cells overlying the sclerotic tuft (arrowhead) (PAS, × 400).*

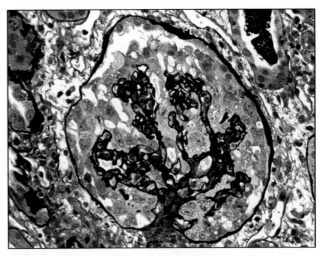

FIGURE 4.25: *Collapsing variant FSGS. Glomerulus shows global collapse of the capillary tuft. The marked hyperplasia of overlying epithelial cells resembles a cellular crescent. There is no discernible increase in matrix (JMS, × 400).*

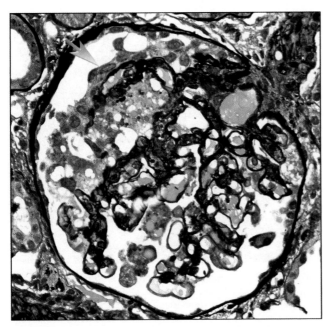

FIGURE 4.24: *Collapsing variant FSGS. Glomerulus shows segmental collapse of the capillary tuft (arrow) accompanied by hyperplasia and swelling of overlying epithelial cells. There is no discernible increase in matrix (JMS, × 400).*

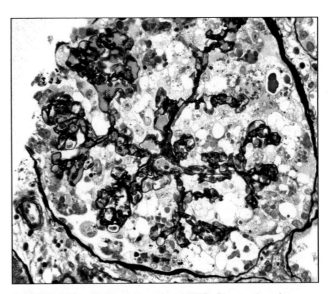

FIGURE 4.26: *Collapsing variant FSGS. Glomerulus shows global implosive collapse of the capillary tuft accompanied by marked hyperplasia and swelling of epithelial cells. There is no discernible increase in matrix (JMS, × 400).*

global occlusion of capillary lumina due to implosive wrinkling and collapse of the glomerular basement membranes, best seen with PAS or JMS stain (Figures 4.24–4.26 and 4.32). There is usually little if any increase in intracapillary or mesangial matrix. Epithelial cell hyperplasia is usually striking (Figures 4.25 and 4.26) and may include prominent intracytoplasmic protein resorption droplets, lipid droplets, and coarse vacuoles (Figure 4.32). Large vesicular nuclei with frequent nucleoli are common, and binucleate nuclei and rare mitotic figures may be identified. Proximal tubules frequently show severe degenerative and regenerative changes, including epithelial simplification, loss of apical brush border, enlarged nuclei, and

prominent nucleoli. Abundant cytoplasmic protein resorption droplets are commonly encountered (Figure 4.33). Increased interstitial fibrosis and tubular microcyst formation are also common (Figure 4.34).

GTL variant is characterized by segmental lesions in the peripheral tuft (tip domain), accompanied by confluence of podocytes with parietal or tubular epithelial cells, or synechia formation at the tubular pole (Figures 4.30, 4.31, 4.35, and 4.36A). Tip lesions are usually cellular and contain endocapillary foam cells (Figures 4.30, 4.35, and 4.36A), but may also contain hyalinosis. Tip lesions may appear to prolapse into the proximal tubule (Figure 4.31). As the lesion evolves,

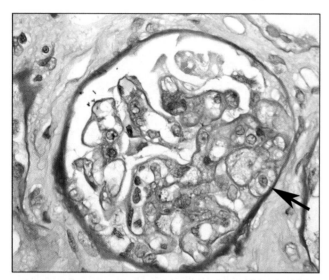

FIGURE 4.27: Cellular FSGS. There is segmental endocapillary hypercellularity with foam cells leading to expansion of the glomerular tuft (arrows). There is no evidence of capillary collapse (PAS, × 200).

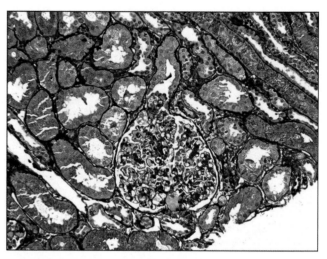

FIGURE 4.29: Glomerular tip lesion. There is a segmental cellular lesion at the origin of the proximal tubule (tip domain). There is no significant tubular atrophy or interstitial fibrosis (JMS, × 100).

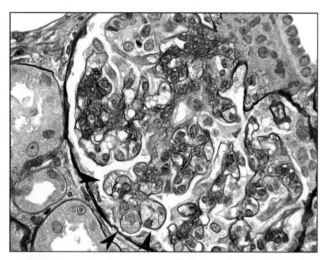

FIGURE 4.28: Cellular FSGS. There is segmental obliteration of capillary lumina by foam cells and mononuclear inflammatory cells (arrows) (JMS, × 400).

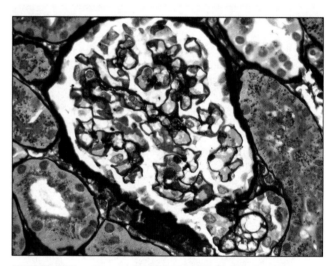

FIGURE 4.30: Glomerular tip lesion. On high power, a segmental cellular lesion with endocapillary foam cells is prolapsing into the proximal tubule lumen. Overlying visceral epithelial cells are confluent with proximal tubular epithelial cells (JMS, × 400).

segmental sclerosis is seen at the tip domain (Figure 4.36B). In most primary GTL cases, other segmental lesions that lack features of tip lesion may occur, either in the same glomerulus or in other glomeruli, but perihilar lesions are rare [17]. "Classic" FSGS lesions are more common in repeat biopsies of GTL, suggesting they may reflect evolution of tip lesions. Chronic tubulointerstitial injury is generally minimal [17] despite the older age of these patients compared to other FSGS subgroups [46].

CELL variant is characterized by focal and segmental glomerular hypercellularity, mimicking focal proliferative glomerulonephritis (Figures 4.27 and 4.28). The increased cellularity comprises endothelial cells, foam cells and occasional neutrophils. Segmental lesions predominantly affect the peripheral tuft but lack the defining characteristics of GTL. The affected segments have an expanded appearance that contrasts with the implosive, collapsed lesions in COLL variant. Importantly, cellular FSGS lesions are also commonly present in both COLL and GTL variants. Therefore, additional tissue sectioning to rule out these variants is necessary in biopsies of apparent CELL variant. Perihilar involvement by cellular lesions is rare.

In the PH variant, >50 percent of segmental lesions (which may be either cellular or sclerosing) involve the perihilar segment, and no collapsing lesions are identified in any glomerulus (Figure 4.37). There is often arteriolar hyalinosis, which may be contiguous with perihilar hyalinosis. Podocyte hypertrophy and hyperplasia are unusual, but glomerulomegaly is common. Other glomeruli may show "classic" FSGS lesions and/or global glomerulosclerosis.

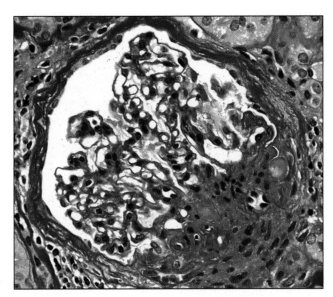

FIGURE 4.31: *Perihilar FSGS. The perihilar segment is obliterated by increased matrix and hyalinosis (PAS, × 400).*

NOS variant demonstrates "classic" FSGS lesions, consisting of segmental solidification of the glomerular tuft by relatively acellular collagenous matrix, which stains pink with H&E stain (Figure 4.17) and is PAS positive (Figure 4.18). Hyalinosis, or plasmatic insudation, consists of accumulation beneath the glomerular basement membrane of amorphous glassy material that is eosinophilic, PAS-positive, nonargyrophilic, and trichrome red (Figures 4.19 and 4.20). Clear lipid vacuoles may be present in the hyaline material. Adhesions or synechiae to Bowman's capsule are common (Figures 4.21 and 4.22). Visceral epithelial cells appear swollen and may form a cellular "cap" or have a "cobble-stone" appearance over the affected segment (Figure 4.38). Unaffected lobules may show mild swelling of the podocytes. Early in the disease, the segmental lesions have a predilection for the juxtamedullary glomeruli. In NOS variant, glomerulosclerosis and chronic tubulointerstitial injury are not particularly severe, supporting that this variant is not always an advanced phase of the other variants [46].

Mesangial hypercellularity may be encountered in any of the above FSGS variants. This finding appears to be more common in children with FSGS than in adults and is associated with a shorter time from clinical presentation to biopsy [52]. The degree of patchy tubular atrophy and interstitial fibrosis is generally commensurate with the severity and distribution of the glomerular sclerosis (Figures 4.39 and 4.40). Proximal tubules frequently contain intracellular lipid and protein resorption droplets. Interstitial foam cells, either as isolated cells or in aggregates, reflect long-standing proteinuria (Figure 4.41). In cases with severe unremitting nephrotic syndrome, tubules may display degenerative and regenerative changes, including epithelial simplification and enlarged hyperchromatic nuclei and nucleoli.

Immunofluorescence Findings. Segmental lesions often stain for IgM and C3 (Figure 4.42). The nonsclerotic glomerular segments may have mesangial positivity for IgM in some cases.

Electron Microscopic Findings. There is usually extensive effacement of foot processes overlying the segmental lesions and involving >50 percent of the glomerular capillary surface in nonsclerotic capillaries (Figure 4.43). Podocytes may be hypertrophied and display increased organellar content, focal microvillous transformation, and loss of primary processes. Where podocytes are detached from the sclerosing segment, an intervening accumulation of lamellated neomembrane material is seen (Figure 4.43). Segmental intracapillary foam cells may be present, particularly in GTL and CELL variants (Figure 4.44). In COLL variant, segmental accordion-like corrugation of GBMs may be seen, accompanied by overlying podocyte hypertrophy with abundant cytoplasmic electron dense protein dropets (Figure 4.45).

Differential Diagnosis. Secondary causes of FSGS are listed in Table 4.2. FSGS must be distinguished from the scarring that occurs in chronic glomerulonephritides, such as lupus nephritis, acute postinfectious glomerulonephritis, IgA nephropathy, or membranous glomerulonephritis. These diagnoses may be suggested by the clinical history and findings of residual immune complex deposits by IF and EM. Scarring of pauci-immune focal segmental necrotizing and crescentic glomerulonephritis is suggested by findings of focal rupture of Bowman's capsule and subcapsular fibrous proliferations, best seen with PAS or silver stain. Underlying Alport's syndrome, Fabry's disease, and mitochondriopathies may be diagnosed if electron microscopy shows characteristic defining features of these entities. Secondary FSGS may also occur superimposed on many other glomerulopathies as they progress to chronicity, particularly in the setting of structural–functional adaptation to glomerular hyperfiltration (see "Secondary FSGS Mediated by Adaptive Structural–Functional Responses").

Etiology and Pathogenesis. By definition, the nature of podocyte injury is unknown for primary FSGS but recent experimental evidence points to a critical pathogenic role for either direct loss of podocytes (podocytopenia) or functional podocytopenia in all forms of FSGS [54]. Podocyte injury may be related to heritable mutations, causing aberrant function of podocyte-expressed proteins, or exogenous injuries, such as toxins, viral infections, or physical stress. Injury directed to or inherent within the podocyte leads to podocyte detachment and apoptosis. Recruitment of parietal epithelial cells may contribute to the increased cellularity seen in some FSGS variants (notably the COLL, CELL, and GTL variants).

Genetic abnormalities leading to loss of podocyte protein function were first identified in rare familial forms of FSGS, and subsequently in some cases of sporadic FSGS, particularly in children (Table 4.2). Nephrin is a major structural component of the slit diaphragm and autosomal recessive mutations in the nephrin gene (*NPHS1*) are the principal cause of congenital nephrotic syndrome (discussed in more detail in the section on "Nephrotic Syndrome in the First Year of Life") [55]. Podocin is a slit diaphragm protein that recruits nephrin and CD2-associated protein (CD2AP) to lipid rafts in the slit diaphragm. Mutations in the podocin gene (*NPHS2*) are a major cause of autosomal recessive FSGS in early childhood, presenting with steroid-resistant nephrotic syndrome and rapid progression to

Table 4.3 Defining Characteristics of FSGS variants in the Columbia Classification

Variant	Inclusion Criteria	Exclusion Criteria
FSGS (NOS)	At least 1 glomerulus with segmental increase in matrix obliterating the capillary lumina. There may be segmental glomerular capillary wall collapse without overlying podocyte hyperplasia.	Exclude perihilar, cellular, tip, and collapsing variants
Perihilar variant	At least 1 glomerulus with perihilar hyalinosis, with or without sclerosis. Greater than 50% of glomeruli with segmental lesions must have perihilar sclerosis and/or hyalinosis.	Exclude cellular, tip, and collapsing variants
Cellular variant	At least 1 glomerulus with segmental endocapillary hypercellularity occluding lumina, with or without foam cells and karyorrhexis.	Exclude tip and collapsing variants
Tip variant	At least 1 segmental lesion involving the tip domain (outer 25% of tuft next to origin of proximal tubule). The tubular pole must be identified in the defining lesion.	Exclude collapsing variant
	The lesion must have either an adhesion or confluence of podocytes with parietal or tubular cells at the tubular lumen or neck. The tip lesion may be cellular or sclerosing.	
Collapsing variant	At least 1 glomerulus with segmental or global collapse and overlying podocyte hypertrophy and hyperplasia.	None

renal failure [17,20]. Mutations in the genes for alpha-actinin-4 [55] or transient receptor potential cation channel 6 (*TRPC6*) [20] have each been identified in approximately 4 percent of families with autosomal dominant FSGS but are rare in sporadic FSGS. Alpha-actinin-4 stabilizes the podocyte cytoskeleton structure while TRPC6 is an ion channel that may have roles in mechanosensation and regulating calcium entry. Haplo-insufficiency for CD2AP, a nephrin-associated protein, may increase susceptibility to FSGS [56] while mutations in the phospholipase C epsilon-1 gene (*PLCE1*) have been identified in children with early-onset nephrotic syndrome, associated with either diffuse mesangial sclerosis or FSGS phenotype [57,58].

Mutations in the gene Wilms tumor-1 (*WT-1*) occur in Denys Drash syndrome (presenting with infantile nephrotic syndrome and diffuse mesangial sclerosis) and Frasier syndrome (which presents with later onset of renal disease and FSGS). Mutations of *WT-1* and the gene for laminin β2 (*LAMB2*) have been linked to isolated diffuse mesangial sclerosis and some cases of sporadic steroid-resistant nephrotic syndrome with FSGS phenotype [22]. Combined mutations of two or more podocyte genes may contribute to the clinical and pathologic diversity of human FSGS [59]. A pattern of FSGS may also be associated with defective synthesis of GBM type IV collagen (in Alport syndrome), heritable mutations of mitochondrial genes (mitochondriopathies), and nail-patella syndrome.

Experimental toxic models of podocyte injury with MCD and FSGS phenotypes include puromycin and adriamycin. These agents mediate podocyte injury via generation of reactive oxygen species and induction of apoptosis. The association of FSGS with use of pamidronate, interferon, and lithium, and with intracytoplasmic light chain crystallization in some patients with dysproteinemia, also support a pathogenic role for direct podocyte injury. Infection of tubular epithelial cells and podocytes by HIV has been implicated in the pathogenesis

of FSGS lesions in HIV-associated nephropathy (HIVAN) (see section on "HIVAN").

A potential role for immunological factors in the pathogenesis of FSGS is supported by the identification of circulating glomerular permeability factors, possibly cytokines, in some patients [60,61]. Increased permeability factor activity correlates with the recurrence of nephrotic syndrome posttransplantation in some patients with idiopathic FSGS [62] but this has also been reported in some patients with genetic forms of FSGS, suggesting that it may serve as a cofactor for proteinuria in susceptible individuals.

An abnormal "dysregulated" podocyte phenotype has been shown by immunohistochemical staining, particularly in the COLL and CELL variants of FSGS. This aberrant phenotype recapitulates the phenotype of immature or developing glomeruli, with loss of mature podocyte markers [such as synaptopodin, podocalyxin, WT1, glomerular epithelial protein-1, C3b receptor, common acute lymphoblastic leukemia antigen, complement receptor 1, and vimentin [63,64]. Podocytes may show aberrant expression of cytokeratin and the monocyte/macrophage marker CD68 [64] and evidence of proliferation and/or apoptosis [63] including expression of Ki-67 [63] and reduction of the cyclin kinase inhibitors p27 and p57, consistent with reentry into the cell cycle [65].

Clinical Course, Prognosis, Treatment, and Clinical Correlation

A critical first step in the management of patients with FSGS is to exclude secondary causes to the best extent possible, because secondary FSGS is generally refractory to immunosuppressive therapy. Initial therapy for primary FSGS consists of a prolonged course (3 to 9 months) of steroid therapy. Steroid-resistant patients may respond to cyclophosphamide, cyclosporine, or mycophenolate mofetil. The combination of cyclosporine

Table 4.4 Algorithmic Approach to Diagnosing FSGS Variants Using the Columbia Classification

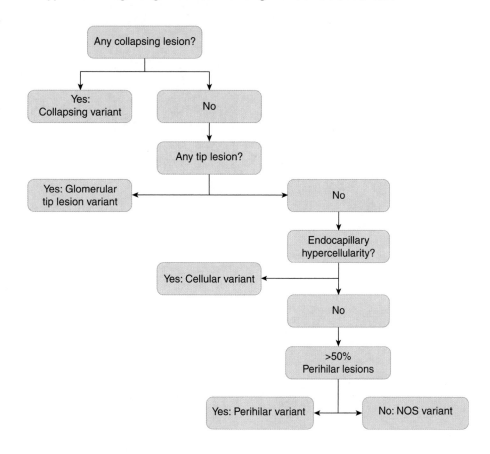

and prednisone in individuals with steroid-resistant FSGS is associated with reduction in proteinuria and preservation of renal function [66]. ACE inhibitors or angiotensin II receptor antagonists are often used to reduce proteinuria and may be used alone in patients with subnephrotic proteinuria.

The principal prognostic features in primary FSGS are initial serum creatinine, severity of proteinuria and remission response to therapy. Proteinuria >3.5 g/day is associated with higher rate of progression to end-stage renal disease (ESRD) compared to subnephrotic proteinuria (where the 10-year survival is >80 percent). Remission of nephrotic syndrome is associated with better outcomes [45]. Outcome is generally worse in blacks than whites, possibly reflecting heavier proteinuria, worse renal insufficiency, and the higher frequency of collapsing variant FSGS. The main pathologic predictors of poor outcome are degree of interstitial fibrosis and collapsing FSGS.

In most studies, COLL variant had the lowest rates of remission and poorest renal survival [46 47] whereas GTL variant had the best renal survival [46,48] and/or rate of remissions [17,47]. CELL variant showed intermediate response to immunosuppressive therapy and renal outcomes compared to GTL, NOS, and COLL [47]. Primary PH displayed low rates of complete and partial remission (around 10 percent for each) but good renal survival (89 percent at 1 year and 75 percent at 3 years), despite the fact that most patients did not receive steroid therapy [46]. Among NOS patients, complete remission

rate was low (13 percent) and renal survival at 3 years was 65 percent [46]. In a study from The Netherlands of predominantly Caucasian adults (age >16 years), the five-year renal survival was 55 percent for PH variant, 63 percent for NOS variant, and 78 percent for GTL variant [48]. However, two studies reported that renal outcomes were not significantly different among the pathologic variants after controlling for remission response [43,45].

The prognostic implications of diffuse mesangial hypercellularity are uncertain. Historical studies in pediatric cases of FSGS with diffuse mesangial hypercellularity described a higher rate of progression to renal insufficiency [67] or no significant difference in outcomes [52,68]. In one study of pediatric patients using the Columbia Classification, mesangial hypercellularity was not a risk for subsequent development of chronic renal failure [43].

Primary FSGS recurs in the renal allograft in up to 40 percent of patients. Recurrences are more common in children, in patients who progressed rapidly to ESRD, and in patients with recurrence in a previous allograft. The earliest pathologic findings consist of normal glomeruli by LM with extensive foot process effacement by EM, resembling MCD. Segmental lesions (often with cellular or collapsing features) develop several weeks to months later. Recurrent FSGS may respond to plasmapheresis, possibly via elimination of a pathogenic circulating permeability factor. Differences in recurrence rate among

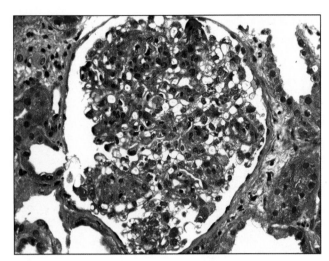

FIGURE 4.32: Collapsing FSGS. The hyperplastic podocytes contain numerous intracytoplasmic, red protein resorption droplets (Trichrome stain, × 400).

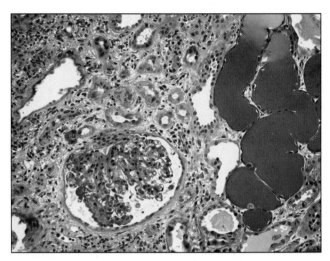

FIGURE 4.34: Collapsing FSGS. There is diffuse interstitial fibrosis (blue staining) and tubular microcyst formation (Trichrome, × 100).

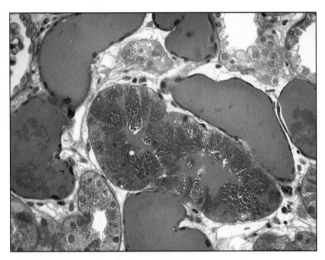

FIGURE 4.33: Collapsing FSGS. Tubules contain numerous cytoplasmic protein resorption droplets. Adjacent tubules show focal ectasia with attentuation of epithelial lining (PAS, ×100).

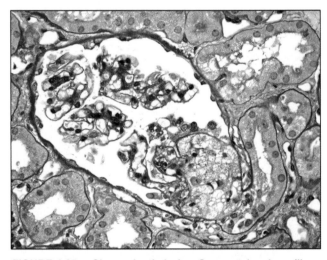

FIGURE 4.35: Glomerular tip lesion. Segmental endocapillary foam cells are seen at the origin of the proximal tubule (PAS, × 400).

the morphologic variants of primary FSGS have not yet been established.

Secondary FSGS Mediated By Adaptive Structural–Functional Responses

Definition. This is defined as postadaptive FSGS associated with either a reduced number of functioning nephrons or hemodynamic stress on an initially normal nephron population.

Clinical Features. Associations include morbid obesity, hypertensive nephrosclerosis, solitary kidney, sickle cell disease, reflux nephropathy, cyanotic congenital heart disease, and any advanced renal disease leading to significant loss of functioning nephrons. Despite heavy proteinuria, full nephrotic syndrome is

generally absent and serum albumin levels are typically in the normal range [69].

Obesity-related glomerulopathy (ORG) is associated with all grades of obesity (body mass index [BMI] ≥ 30.0). In the early stages of ORG, the glomerular filtration rate may be abnormally high (>120 mL/min) [70]. Hypertensive nephrosclerosis is more common in older patients with a history of long-standing hypertension, sometimes associated with atherosclerotic vascular disease. Importantly, these patients tend to have renal insufficiency prior to the onset of nephrotic proteinuria.

Light Microscopic Findings. Glomerular hypertrophy (glomerulomegaly) is a consistent finding in ORG (Figure 4.46A). Glomerular hypertrophy is best assessed in a plane of section that transects the hilus of the glomerulus. The measured glomerular area exceeds 1.5 times normal. Hypertrophied

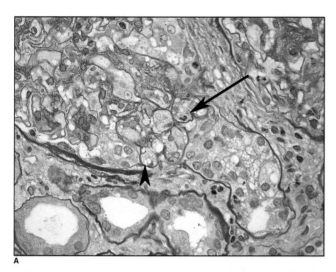
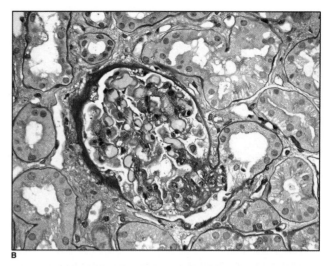

FIGURE 4.36: *Glomerular tip lesion. (A) A cellular lesion at the origin of the proximal tubule displays endocapillary foam cells (arrowhead) and mononuclear inflammatory cells (arrow) (PAS, × 600); (B) There is segmental sclerosis at the tip domain, with synechial attachment to Bowman's capsule at the point of transition to the proximal tubular basement membrane (PAS, × 400).*

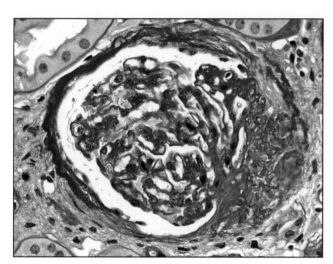

FIGURE 4.37: *Perihilar FSGS. The perihilar segment is obliterated by increased matrix and hyalinosis (PAS, × 400).*

FIGURE 4.38: *FSGS (NOS). There is segmental obliteration of the glomerular tuft with sclerosis and hyalinosis (arrows), and segmental capping of overlying epithelial cells, some of which contain cytoplasmic protein resorption droplets (PAS, × 400).*

glomeruli can be easily recognized because they usually fill the visual field when examined with a 40× objective lens (Figures 4.46A,B). Segmental sclerosis and hyalinosis lesions are seen in enlarged glomeruli (Figure 4.46C). In secondary FSGS resulting from loss of renal mass, there is usually extensive global glomerulosclerosis with corresponding tubular atrophy and interstitial fibrosis. Perihilar segmental sclerosis lesions are common, whereas podocyte hypertrophy and hyperplasia are infrequent. Thus, most cases would be classified as PH variant.

In hypertensive arterionephrosclerosis, prominent arteriolar hyalinosis and arteriosclerosis are common (Figure 4.47). Glomerulosclerosis predominantly affects the outer cortex and may be accompanied by subcapsular scars. FSGS lesions are often predominantly perihilar in location (Figure 4.48) but cellular and collapsing FSGS lesions may occur in the setting of acute ischemia (e.g., due to cholesterol embolization). Atubular glomeruli are commonly identified in the subcapsular region. These

display cystic dilatation of Bowman's space with a shrunken tuft that may be partially resorbed into Bowman's capsule (Figure 4.49). Chronic tubulointerstitial disease is invariably present. Ischemic atrophic tubules may resemble endocrine glands ("endocrine tubular atrophy").

Immunofluorescence Findings. Focal and segmental glomerular staining for IgM and C3 is seen in lesions of segmental sclerosis.

Electron Microscopic Findings. The degree of foot process effacement generally affects less than 50 percent of the total glomerular capillary surface area (Figure 4.50). However, because of sample variability and disease variation this criterion alone does not reliably distinguish primary from secondary FSGS.

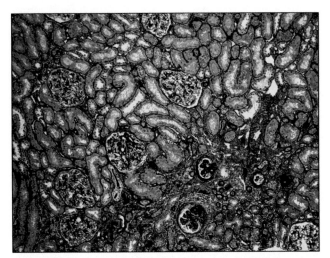

FIGURE 4.39: *Early FSGS shows mild patchy interstitial fibrosis and tubular atrophy (JMS, × 100).*

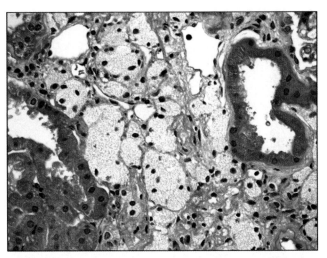

FIGURE 4.41: *FSGS. Numerous interstitial foam cells are seen. The patient had several year's duration of proteinuria prior to biopsy (Trichrome, × 400).*

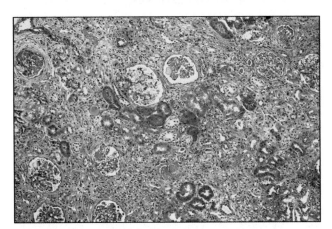

FIGURE 4.40: *Advanced FSGS. Trichrome stain shows severe diffuse interstitial fibrosis and tubular atrophy (Trichrome, × 100).*

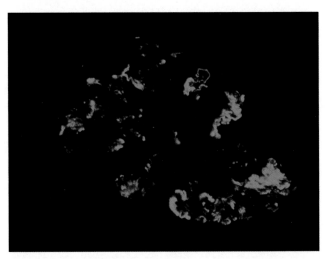

FIGURE 4.42: *FSGS. By immunofluorescence, there is segmental staining for C3 corresponding to a segmental lesion of sclerosis and hyalinosis (Immunofluorescence microscopy, × 400).*

In hypertensive arterionephrosclerosis, there may be ischemic-type wrinkling and thickening of the glomerular basement membranes.

Etiology and Pathogenesis. Secondary FSGS may be mediated by increased glomerular capillary pressures and flow rates as part of an adaptive response to the reduced number of functioning nephrons or other hemodynamic stresses. Increased wall tension causes mechanical strain on the connection between the podocyte foot process and the glomerular basement membrane, leading to local dilatation of capillaries and podocyte stretch. Severe and prolonged tension causes progressive podocyte cell body attenuation, pseudocyst formation, and detachment from the glomerular basement membrane. Podocyte detachment exposes bare patches of glomerular basement membrane that may form synechial attachment to Bowman's capsule, permitting misdirected flow of filtrate, obliteration of the tubular pole and microcystic dilatation of Bowman's capsule. These synechiae form the nidus for segmental sclerosis lesions to develop.

In hypertensive arterionephrosclerosis, elevated glomerular capillary pressure is associated with systemic hypertension and the adaptive response to loss of functioning nephrons. In ORG, the increased body mass relative to kidney mass is associated with increased glomerular filtration rate and increased renal plasma flow. Hypoxia related to sleep apnea activates the sympathetic nervous system, thereby stimulating the renin–angiotensin system and glomerular hypertension. In addition, hyperlipidemia and secretion of hormones and cytokines from adipose tissue may contribute to renal injury in ORG [71].

Treatment and Prognosis. Treatment of secondary FSGS depends on the underlying condition. Steroids are uniformly ineffective in secondary FSGS and may aggravate underlying diabetes or obesity. Reduction of glomerular capillary pressures via ACE inhibition, angiotensin II receptor antagonists, and a

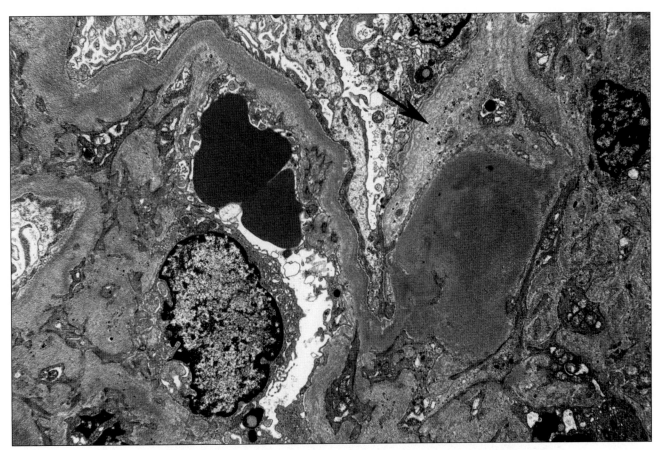

FIGURE 4.43: *FSGS. Electron microscopy shows segmental inframembranous electron dense material, consistent with hyaline. Overlying podocytes are focally detached. There is a layer of lamellated material between the detached podocyte and the glomerular basement membrane (arrow) (Electron microscopy, × 6,000).*

low protein diet, may reduce proteinuria and slow progression. Correction of the underlying process, such as surgical repair of congenital heart disease, weight loss, and sleep apnea therapy may be beneficial.

Differential Diagnosis. The main differential diagnosis is primary FSGS. A diagnosis of hypertensive arterionephrosclerosis is favored if there is a history of longstanding hypertension and renal insufficiency preceding the development of proteinuria, accompanied by pathologic findings of prominent vascular disease, glomerular hypertrophy, predominantly perihilar segmental lesions, and mild foot process effacement. In the obese patient, the presence of full nephrotic syndrome and finding of extensive foot process effacement should suggest a diagnosis of primary FSGS.

HIV-Associated Nephropathy

Definition. This is defined as secondary FSGS related to HIV infection. Most cases display features of collapsing variant FSGS [72].

Clinical Features. HIV-associated nephropathy (HIVAN) predominantly affects individuals of African descent (>90 percent). It is most common in male intravenous drug abusers (IVDU) but occurs in both sexes and with any HIV risk factor.

The incidence of HIVAN has risen steadily over the last two decades. Presenting features include heavy or severe proteinuria with hypoalbuminemia and renal insufficiency. Hypercholesterolemia and edema are uncommon, perhaps reflecting reduced hepatic synthesis of lipoproteins and cachexia in AIDS patients. Hypertension is relatively uncommon. Kidneys may be enlarged and echogenic.

Light Microscopic Findings. These are similar to collapsing variant FSGS (Figures 4.24–4.26, 4.32–4.34, 4.45, and 4.51). Collapsing lesions may coexist with nonspecific global glomerulosclerosis and NOS lesions. Tubular microcysts (Figure 4.52) are found in, up to 40 percent of cases and these may contribute to the enlarged kidneys and increased echogenicity, even in patients with end-stage renal failure. FSGS without collapsing features (NOS variant) has become more common in HIV patients in recent years, probably due the effect of highly active antiretroviral therapy (HAART) on HIV viral load.

Immunofluorescence Findings. Diffuse mesangial staining for IgM and C3 are common in HIVAN.

Electron Microscopic Findings. Abundant endothelial tubuloreticular inclusions (TRI) are common in HIVAN. Tubuloreticular inclusions (TRI) consist of 24-nm interanastomosing

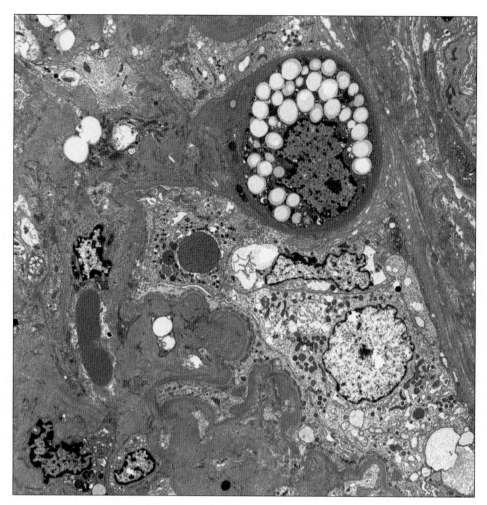

FIGURE 4.44: *FSGS. Electron microscopy shows segmental obliteration of a capillary lumen by foam cells (Electron microscopy, × 20,000).*

tubular structures located within dilated cisternae of the endoplasmic reticulum [72] Figure 4.53). TRI are most common in glomerular endothelial cells but may also be seen in arterial or interstitial capillary endothelial cells, and in infiltrating leukocytes. TRI are less frequently seen in the modern era of HAART, perhaps due to the reduced viral burden. The TRI are not diagnostic of HIV infection as these are also commonly seen in SLE patients and following interferon therapy. Less frequent ultrastructural findings include nuclear bodies within tubular and interstitial cells, granular–fibrillar transformation of the tubular nuclei, and confronting cylindrical cisternae.

Differential Diagnosis. This includes primary FSGS and other secondary causes of collapsing variant FSGS [73]. HIV serologies may help distinguish these entities. Other forms of glomerular disease in HIV infected patients are discussed in the section "Other Glomerular Diseases in HIV Patients."

Etiology and Pathogenesis. Experimental evidence supports a role for direct viral infection of tubular epithelial cells and podocytes in the pathogenesis of HIVAN. The kidney may be a reservoir for HIV infection in susceptible individuals. Mice transgenic for the noninfectious HIV genome (with a deletion

of gag and pol, but expressing the HIV regulatory genes) develop morphologic features of FSGS, supporting a role for viral gene expression in the kidney. Cross-renal transplantation experiments between transgenic mouse kidneys and nontransgenic littermates have revealed that the renal phenotype is dependent upon renal transgene expression. The failure of normal kidneys to develop nephropathy when transplanted into HIV transgenic mice argues strongly against a systemic cytokine effect [74].

Treatment and Prognosis. Rapid progression to renal failure is common. Early in the AIDS epidemic, the mean time to dialysis was < 2 months. In the modern era, the use of HAART has reduced viral load and improved renal survival. Following HAART therapy, there may be dramatic improvement in the renal biopsy findings, with reversal of tubular microcysts [75].

Other Glomerular Diseases in HIV Patients

Other glomerular and tubulointerstitial lesions are associated with proteinuria in HIV-infected patients. Children, in particular, may display diffuse mesangial hypercellularity or MCD, without collapsing FSGS. These patients typically display

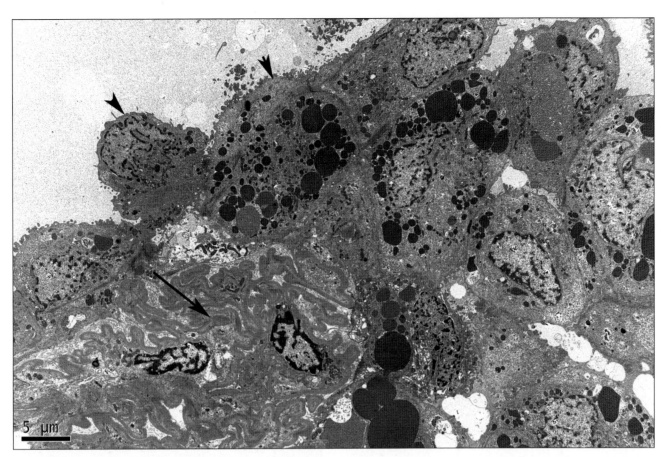

FIGURE 4 45: *Collapsing variant FSGS. Electron microscopy shows segmental wrinkling of glomerular basement membranes and collapse of capillary lumina (arrow). Overlying podocytes are swollen and show diffuse foot process effacement and prominent electron-dense inclusions consistent with protein resorption droplets (arrow-heads) (Electron microscopy, × 3,000).*

normal renal function, without the rapid course to renal failure that characterizes the collapsing form of HIVAN.

Immune complex-mediated glomerulonephritis [membrano-proliferative glomerulonephritis (type 1 or type 3) or membranous glomerulonephritis] may be seen in proteinuric patients with HIV infection, particularly in Caucasians [76] and those with hepatitis C virus (HCV) coinfection [77,78]. Similar lesions have also been described in HIV-infected African patients without HCV infection [79]. There may be overlapping features of HIVAN in some cases [78]. IgA nephropathy has been reported in both HIV-infected blacks and whites and may be associated with IgA-containing cryoglobulins. Immune deposits eluted from the glomeruli of some of these patients have shown specificity for HIV envelope or core proteins, supporting a pathogenic role for HIV infection. Other glomerular lesions occurring in HIV-infected patients include lupus-like glomerulonephritis, immunotactoid glomerulonephritis, acute postinfectious glomerulonephritis, and thrombotic microangiopathy.

C1q NEPHROPATHY

Definition

C1q nephropathy (C1qN) is a controversial entity that is defined by its distinctive immunopathologic features. C1qN

was initially described by Jennette and Hipp in 1985 as a glomerular disease with dominant or codominant IF staining for C1q in a predominantly mesangial distribution, occurring in the absence of evidence of SLE [80]. Similar to lupus nephritis, light microscopic findings ranged from normal-appearing glomeruli to mesangial proliferation to focal or diffuse endocapillary proliferation. By IF, C1q deposits were accompanied by equal or less intense staining for C3, IgG, and IgM. EM confirmed the presence of mesangial deposits, infrequently accompanied by subendothelial or subepithelial deposits. Endothelial tubuloreticular inclusions (TRIs) were not identified in any case. All 15 patients had negative antinuclear antibody serologies, normal serum complements, and no clinical evidence of SLE. Patients presented in the second or third decade of life with nephrotic range proteinuria, relatively intact renal function, and in some cases, hematuria.

Subsequent reports have offered a different interpretation of C1qN [81,82]. Iskandar et al. described 15 pediatric patients with C1qN (age 2–16 years), 9 of whom were fully nephrotic and were steroid-resistant or steroid-dependent prior to undergoing renal biopsy [82]. Similar to the previous study C1q dominant or codominant staining was present, EM revealed mesangial deposits in the absence of TRIs, and SLE was clinically excluded. In contrast to the previous study, light microscopy revealed either normal-appearing glomeruli (analogous

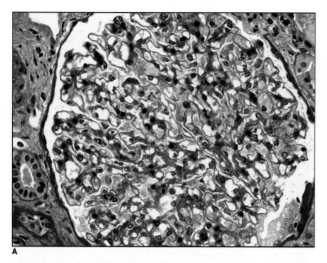

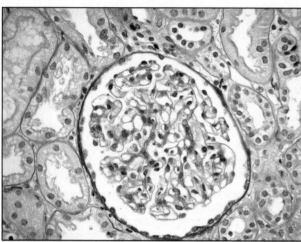

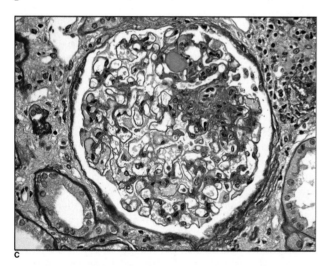

FIGURE 4.46: Secondary FSGS associated with obesity. (A) The glomerulus is enlarged and shows patent capillary lumen and normal-appearing basement membranes. (PAS, × 400); (B) By comparison, a normal glomerulus occupies less than half the visual field at the same magnification. (PAS, × 400); (C) The glomerulus is enlarged and shows segmental sclerosis and hyalinosis. In this plane of section, the relationship of the segmental lesion to the hilar region cannot be determined. (PAS, × 400).

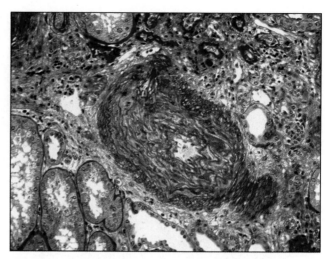

FIGURE 4.47: Secondary FSGS related to hypertensive arterionephrosclerosis. Arterial vessels show moderate to severe intimal fibrosis and medial hyperplasia (PAS, × 200).

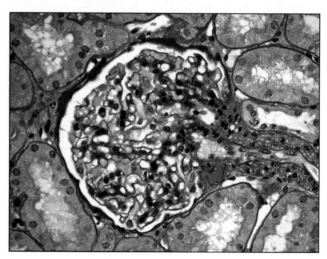

FIGURE 4.48: Secondary FSGS related to hypertensive arterionephrosclerosis. A small segmental hyalinosis lesion is seen in the perihilar region (PAS, × 200).

to MCD) or FSGS, in some cases accompanied by mesangial hypercellularity. A larger report in 2003 [81] similarly described nineteen patients with C1qN. In this study, the mean age was 24.2 years (range 3–42 years) and clinical presentation included nephrotic range proteinuria (78.9 percent), nephrotic syndrome (50 percent), and renal insufficiency (27.8 percent). Renal biopsy revealed FSGS in seventeen patients and MCD in two patients, with all biopsies exhibiting dominant or codominant staining for C1q by IF. In all cases, EM confirmed the presence of mesangial deposits. The mean degree of foot process effacement was 51 percent.

Three recent pediatric studies applied a similar definition of C1qN and found a predominance of FSGS and MCD. A study on 12 children with C1qN in Slovenia revealed FSGS in six patients, MCD in four patients, and focal glomerulonephritis in two patients [83]. A series of twenty children with C1qN from Memphis, Tennessee included eight children with

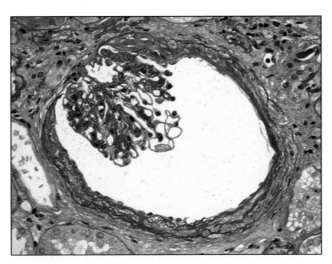

FIGURE 4.49: *Secondary FSGS related to hypertensive arterionephrosclerosis. An atubular glomerulus shows retraction of the glomerular tuft and periglomerular fibrosis (PAS, × 400).*

FSGS and six with MCD [84]. The remaining children had either mesangial proliferation or globally sclerotic glomeruli in the absence of segmental lesions. A series of thirty children with C1qN in Japan included twenty-two with MCD, two

with FSGS, and six with mesangial proliferative glomerulonephritis [85].

At present, the definition of C1qN remains controversial, with some reports continuing to define C1qN as a proliferative glomerulonephritis that resembles "seronegative lupus nephritis" and others suggesting that it represents a form of podocytopathy (FSGS or MCD) [82,83]. Based on the balance of evidence and the experience from our institution [81], we feel that most cases of C1qN fall within the spectrum of primary FSGS.

Clinical Features

C1qN is mainly seen in children and young adults. Similar to other forms of FSGS, C1qN typically presents with nephrotic range proteinuria, often associated with full nephrotic syndrome. Renal insufficiency and hematuria are present at the time of diagnosis in less than half of cases.

Light Microscopic Findings

In most cases, light microscopy reveals FSGS. Less frequently, glomeruli exhibit no abnormalities by light microscopy, akin to MCD. With either FSGS or normal-appearing glomeruli, mild mesangial hypercellularity may be encountered. Histologic

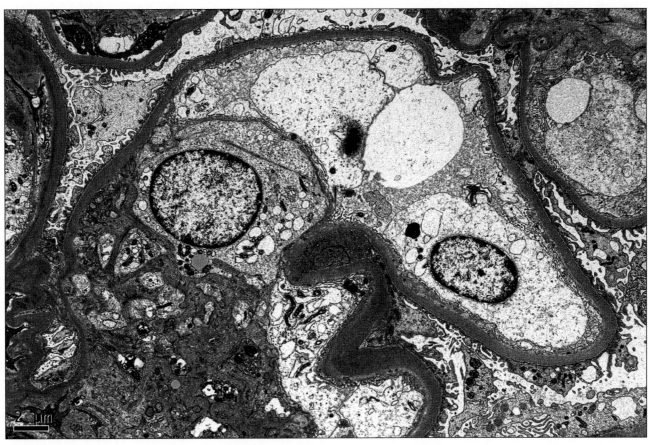

FIGURE 4.50: *Secondary FSGS associated with obesity. Electron microscopy shows mostly intact podocyte foot processes overlying a non-sclerotic capillary loop (Electron microscopy, × 5,000).*

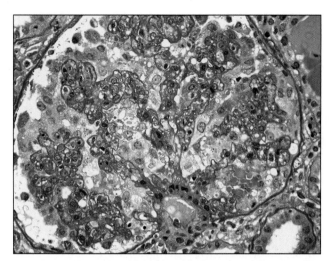

FIGURE 4.51: *HIV-associated nephropathy. Glomerulus shows global retraction of the capillary tuft accompanied by hyperplasia and swelling of overlying epithelial cells, many of which contain prominent PAS positive protein resorption droplets (PAS, × 400).*

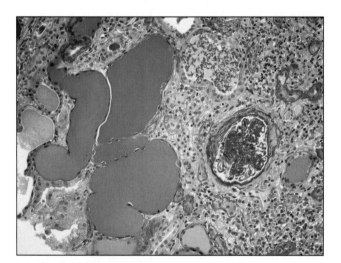

FIGURE 4.52: *HIV-associated nephropathy. Tubules display microcystic dilatation (PAS, × 100).*

variants of FSGS have been described in C1qN, including COLL or CELL variants [81,83].

Immunofluorescence Findings

Glomeruli display dominant or codominant mesangial positivity for C1q, with frequent costaining for IgG, IgM, IgA, and/or C3 (Figure 4.54). Small amounts of peripheral capillary wall staining may also be seen.

Electron Microscopic Findings

Mesangial electron dense deposits are identified in most, if not all, patients with C1q (Figure 4.55). Peripheral capillary wall deposits tend to be sparse and endothelial TRI should not be present. If endothelial TRI are seen, a diagnosis of lupus neph-

ritis or HIVAN should be carefully excluded. In the majority of cases, particularly patients with more severe proteinuria, moderate to marked foot process effacement is noted.

Differential Diagnosis

A diagnosis of C1qN requires exclusion of lupus nephritis and membranoproliferative glomerulonephritis, both of which typically exhibit C1q positivity. One report has suggested that hypocomplementemia should cast significant doubt on a potential diagnosis of C1qN [81].

Etiology and Pathogenesis

C1qN remains a poorly understood entity, with theories on etiology and pathogenesis dependent on whether it is viewed as an immune complex glomerulonephritis or an entity in the MCD-FSGS spectrum. Because C1qN is not accompanied by hypocomplementemia or evidence of systemic autoimmune or infectious disease, it has been speculated that C1q may become fixed to immunoglobulin that becomes trapped nonspecifically in the mesangium in the course of glomerular proteinuria [81]. In this way, the mesangial deposition of C1q might be the result of defective clearing of plasma proteins in the setting of podocytopathy rather than true immune complex-mediated disease. In the minority of cases of C1qN that more closely resemble a proliferative glomerulonephritis, an alternative explanation that involves immune-complex deposition with subsequent complement activation appears more likely.

Treatment and Prognosis

In the majority of studies, patients with C1qN have been treated with steroids. In the pediatric population, many of the patients only underwent biopsy after a period of steroid-dependence or steroid-resistance. Given that children with nephrotic syndrome are commonly treated with steroids prior to undergoing renal biopsy, it is difficult to draw firm conclusions about overall steroid responsivity. Multiple pediatric studies have described poor outcomes in children who present with nephrotic syndrome [83–85]. In the initial report by Jennette and Hipp [81], which included young adults, none of the nine patients treated with steroids achieved remission of proteinuria. In contrast, better outcomes were seen in the largest series that included young adults [81]. Twelve of sixteen patients with available follow-up received treatment with corticosteroids (five also received cyclosporine) and over a mean follow-up of 27.1 months, 75 percent had stable renal function [81]. Follow-up evaluation of proteinuria was available in thirteen patients, among whom one had complete and six had partial remission [81]. These outcome data are not unlike patients reported for primary FSGS.

MEMBRANOUS NEPHROPATHY

Primary (Idiopathic) Membranous Nephropathy

Definition. The defining features of membranous nephropathy (MN) are proteinuria associated with a spectrum of

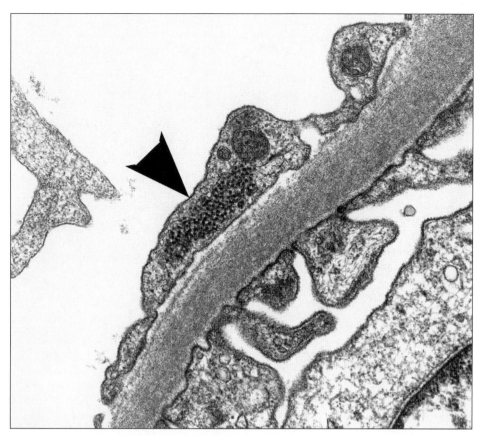

FIGURE 4.53: *HIV-associated nephropathy. Electron microscopy shows an endothelial tubuloreticular inclusion within an endothelial cell (arrowhead) (Electron microscopy, × 30,000).*

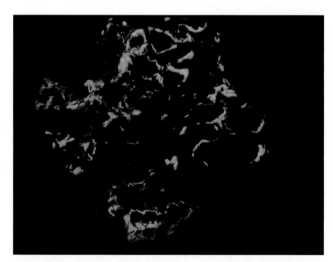

FIGURE 4.54: *C1q nephropathy. Immunofluorescence microscopy shows diffuse mesangial and segmental capillary wall staining for C1q, some of which have a "comma" shape appearance. (Immunofluorescence stain, × 400).*

glomerular capillary wall alterations resulting from the formation of subepithelial immune deposits.

Clinical Features. MN occurs at all ages but is most commonly diagnosed in the fourth and fifth decades of life [88,89]. Most cases (60 to 80 percent) are idiopathic. Secondary causes include autoimmune disease, neoplasia, infection, and exposure to certain therapeutic agents.

MN comprises only a small fraction of cases of nephrotic syndrome in infants and children, where the majority of cases of MN are secondary. MN becomes more prevalent during the second decade of life and is the most common etiology of nephrotic syndrome in Caucasian adults. Among adults, secondary forms of MN are most common in individuals above the age of 60 years. MN is more common in males, with a M:F ratio of 2:1.

Nephrotic syndrome is present in 75 percent of patients with MN [86]. The majority of patients have normal renal function and normal blood pressure at presentation [86]. Microscopic hematuria is present in approximately 50 percent. Gross hematuria is extremely unusual and should suggest the possibility of an additional disease process, either within the kidney or elsewhere in the genitourinary tract. Hypocomplementemia is rare in primary MN and should suggest the possibility of secondary MN due to SLE.

Light Microscopic Findings. Glomeruli range from normal in size to enlarged and typically appear normocellular. The predominant finding by light microscopy is thickening of the glomerular capillary wall (Figure 4.56). With the PAS and silver stains, GBM spikes are usually seen projecting into the urinary space (Figures 4.57 and 4.58). There may also be internal vacuolizations of the GBM. Trichrome staining often reveals

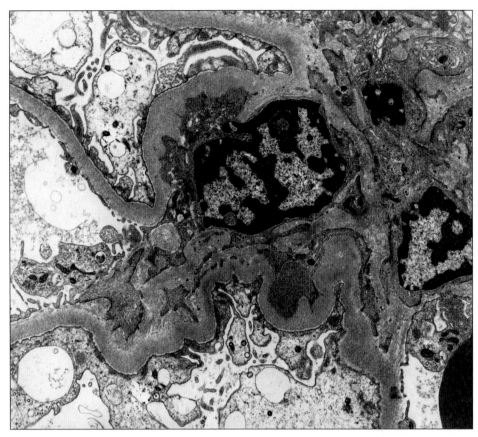

FIGURE 4.55: *C1q nephropathy. Electron microscopy reveals reveals mesangial electron-dense deposits. Podocytes show diffuse foot process effacement (Electron microscopy, × 10,000).*

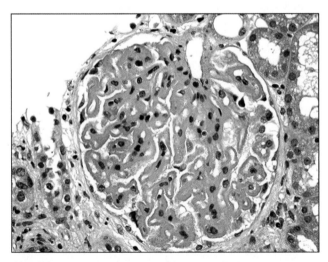

FIGURE 4.56: *Membranous nephropathy. By light microscopy, glomerulus exhibits global thickening of the glomerular basement membrane, in the absence of evidence of cellular proliferation (H&E, × 400).*

subepithelial fuchsinophilic deposits. Of note, a minority of cases of MN exhibit no glomerular abnormalities by light microscopy, particularly early in their course.

Mild mesangial hypercellularity may be seen in MN, but prominent mesangial proliferation, endocapillary proliferation,

GBM duplication with mesangial interposition (i.e., "membranoproliferative features"), fibrinoid necrosis, and crescent formation should suggest either a secondary form of disease or a superimposed disease process. Occasional glomeruli may exhibit intracapillary fibrin thrombi, probably reflecting the hypercoagulable state associated with nephrotic syndrome and MN. In such cases, the possibility of renal vein thrombosis should be considered.

Proximal tubules typically contain lipid and protein resorption droplets. In patients with more severe or unremitting proteinuria, tubular degenerative changes may develop. In time, chronic irreversible tubulointerstitial scarring may occur. The degree of tubular atrophy and interstitial fibrosis is an important prognostic marker. Mild interstitial inflammation is often present and is not associated with significant tubulitis. Interstitial foam cells are commonly encountered in cases of MN with longstanding proteinuria. Vessels may display arteriosclerosis and arteriolosclerosis with hyalinosis.

Findings of FSGS are encountered in a subset of cases of MN (MN–FSGS) [87,88]. Patients with MN–FSGS have a higher incidence of hypertension, microscopic hematuria, and nephrotic syndrome. Pathologic evaluation typically reveals more extensive tubular atrophy, interstitial fibrosis, and arteriosclerosis. The prognosis for renal survival is significantly better in MN than in MN–FSGS. In the majority of cases, the finding of segmental sclerosis represents a marker of chronicity in the

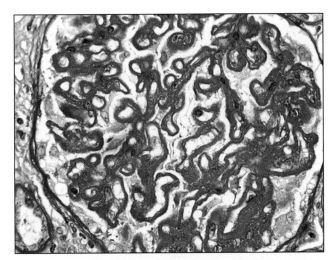

FIGURE 4.57: Membranous nephropathy. *The periodic acid Schiff stain demonstrates global thickening of the GBM with spike formation. Swelling of visceral epithelial cells is noted (PAS, × 600).*

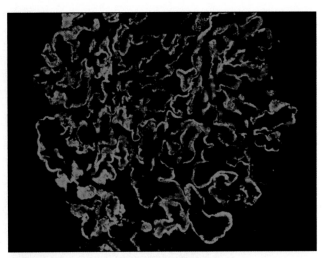

FIGURE 4.59: Membranous nephropathy. *Immunofluorescence staining for IgG reveals granular global positivity in a capillary wall (subepithelial) distribution (IgG, × 400).*

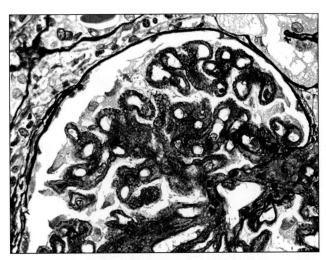

FIGURE 4.58: Membranous nephropathy. *Global GBM spikes and vacuolizations are best seen with the Jones methenamine silver stain. The pink material between the spikes represents immune deposits (JMS, × 600).*

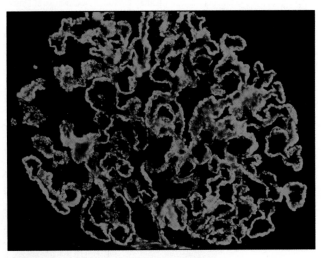

FIGURE 4.60: Membranous nephropathy. *Immunofluorescence staining for IgG reveals large, coarse granular subepithelial deposits (IgG, × 400).*

setting of MN. In rare cases, the clinical history, minimal chronicity, early stage of MN, and visceral epithelial changes typical of FSGS suggests an overlap of two separate disease processes [89].

Crescents are rarely seen in biopsies with MN and when present, typically involve a minority of glomeruli. When crescents are encountered, the possibilities of membranous lupus nephritis, superimposed ANCA-associated necrotizing and crescentic glomerulonephritis [90] or superimposed anti-GBM disease [91–93] should be considered.

Immunofluorescence Findings. Immunofluorescence reveals granular global subepithelial deposits that stain strongest for IgG (Figures 4.59 and 4.60). Staining for C3 is usually present

but is less intense than for IgG. Staining for C1, IgM, or IgA is uncommon in primary MN. Mesangial, subendothelial, tubular basement membrane, interstitial, and vessel deposits are not typically encountered in MN and strongly favor a secondary form of disease, most commonly membranous lupus nephritis. However, rare cases of apparent idiopathic MN with tubular basement membrane and Bowman's capsular deposits have been reported [94].

Electron Microscopic Findings. The hallmark of membranous nephropathy is the presence of subepithelial electron dense deposits. These deposits go through a series of stages of incorporation into the GBM, as originally described by Ehrenreich and Churg [95]. Stage 1 MN is defined by the presence of sparse small subepithelial electron dense deposits, without

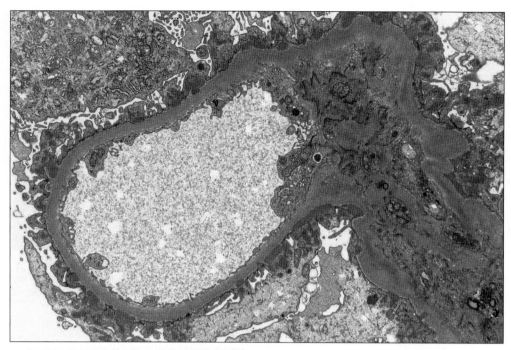

FIGURE 4.61: Membranous nephropathy. Stage 1 MN is characterized by small, interspersed subepithelial electron dense deposits, without significant intervening spike formation (Electron microscopy, × 10,000).

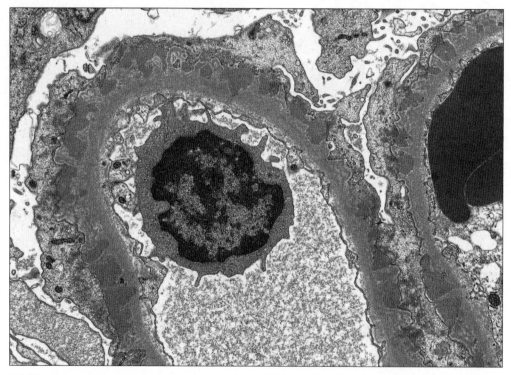

FIGURE 4.62: Membranous nephropathy. In stage 2 MN, the subepithelial deposits appear confluent with intervening GBM spikes. There is complete effacement of visceral epithelial cell foot processes (Electron microscopy, × 5,000).

GBM thickening or spike formation (Figure 4.61). Stage 2 is characterized by more extensive subepithelial deposits with intervening projections of the GBM that form "spikes" (Figure 4.62). By stage 3, the combination of GBM spikes and overlying neomembrane formation completely surrounds the deposits (Figure 4.63). These changes correspond to the vacuolization of the GBM noted by light microscopy. In many cases, the deposits in stage 3 appear electron lucent due to partial

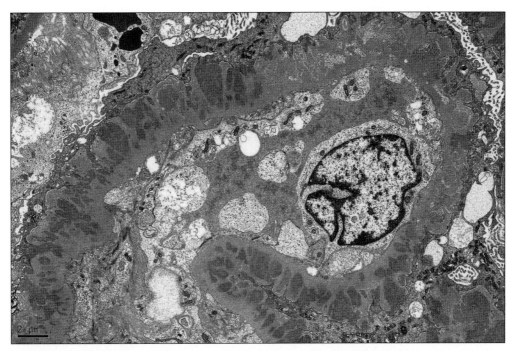

FIGURE 4.63: *Membranous nephropathy. Stage 3 MN is characterized by subepithelial deposits with intervening GBM spikes and overlying neomembrane formation. In the upper right portion of the image, some of the subepithelial deposits appear electron lucent, consistent with partial resorption (Electron microscopy, × 5,000).*

resorption. Stage 4 is characterized by irregular thickening of the GBM; the majority of deposits appear electron lucent due to resorption. In some cases of stage 4, electron-dense deposits are no longer seen and immunofluorescence is weak or negative. In all stages of MN, overlying foot processes show diffuse effacement (Figures 4.61–4.63).

The Ehrenreich & Churg stages provide a framework for understanding and uniform reporting of MN but these stages do not correlate with degree of proteinuria or prognosis. Furthermore, transformation between MN stages may be associated with either an increase or decrease in proteinuria and multiple stages of MN may overlap in the same biopsy specimen. However, the finding of "heterogeneous deposits", defined by the presence of multiple phases of asynchronous deposits, may be associated with a worse prognosis [96].

Rare cases of membranous nephropathy exhibit a distinct ultrastructural appearance in which the deposits form microspherical structures with a diameter of 80–100 nm (Figure 4.64) [97]. The significance of these peculiar structures is unknown.

Differential Diagnosis of Membranous Nephropathy

Some cases of MN may pathologically resemble acute postinfectious glomerulonephritis (APIGN), membranoproliferative glomerulonephritis (MPGN), or hereditary nephritis at the ultrastructural level. Patients with APIGN and MPGN generally have a history of hypocomplementemia and present with nephritic features, in addition to proteinuria. The subepithelial deposits in APIGN are generally larger than those seen in MN, have a hump-like configuration, and stain predominantly for C3, not IgG. Stage 3 MN may mimic MPGN; however, the

presence of mesangial and subendothelial deposits, in addition to intramembranous deposits, favors MPGN. Stage 4 MN may mimic hereditary nephritis, particularly when electron-dense deposits are no longer visible and there is extensive remodeling of the GBM. However, hereditary nephritis is usually associated with a history of longstanding hematuria, often with a family history of renal disease, and electron microscopy typically shows GBM thinning in addition to lamellation.

Secondary Forms of Membranous Nephropathy

Most cases of MN are diagnosed between 16 and 60 years of age and within this age group, 80 percent of cases represent primary disease [98]. Secondary etiologies of MN can be divided into four categories: autoimmune, drug-induced, infection-related, and neoplasia-associated forms of disease. Data compiled from nine large series on MN reveals a 23 percent prevalence of secondary forms of MN [98]. The highest prevalence of secondary MN is found in children < 16 years of age and adults > 60 years of age. Among children, the most frequent secondary causes of MN are SLE, HBV infection, and congenital syphilis. Among adults > 60 years of age, the majority of cases of secondary MN are drug-induced or associated with neoplasia.

The classic autoimmune disease associated with MN is SLE. A more complete review of membranous lupus nephritis is discussed in Chapter 7. MN is associated with rheumatoid arthritis (RA) as well as two agents utilized in the treatment of RA, gold and penicillamine.[99] MN also is seen in patients with mixed connective tissue disease, Sjogren's syndrome, sarcoidosis, Grave's disease [100], and Hashimoto's thyroiditis.

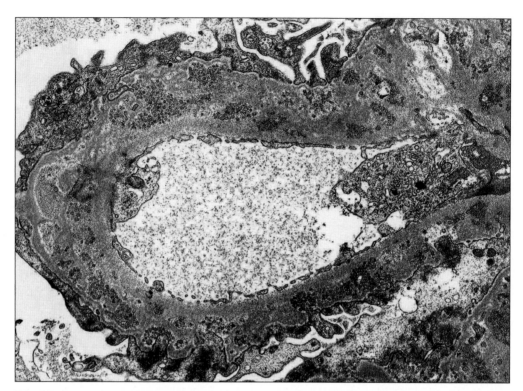

FIGURE 4.64:   Membranous nephropathy. A minority of cases of MN have subepithelial deposits which exhibit a distinctive microspherical substructure (Electron microscopy, × 10,000).

The best-documented forms of drug-induced MN have involved mercury, gold, and penicillamine. MN also has been associated with multiple NSAIDs, and rarely with COX-2 inhibitors [101] and captopril [102].

The most common infections associated with MN are the hepatitis B and C viruses. HBV-associated MN is a common secondary form of MN, particularly in children. Hepatitis B antigens, such as HBsAg and HBeAg, can be identified within the subepithelial immune complex deposits [103] and a reduction in proteinuria is seen following treatment of HBV with lamivudine [104]. HCV infection is more commonly associated with membranoproliferative glomerulonephritis than with MN, but HCV-associated MN is well-documented [105]. In contrast to HBV, HCV-associated antigens and antibodies have not been convincingly identified within the subepithelial immune complex deposits. Other infections that have been described in association with MN include syphilis and multiple parasites.

The majority of patients with neoplasia-associated MN have epithelial maligancies, although lymphoproliferative disorders and benigns neoplasms have also rarely been reported [106,107]. In a recent review of 240 patients with MN from 11 centers in Paris, France [108], 24 patients (10 percent) were found to have a malignancy at the time of diagnosis of MN or within one year, and more than half of tumors were asymptomatic. Twenty of the 24 cases were carcinomas (83.3 percent), most commonly of lung (eight patients), prostate (five patients), and stomach (two patients). While the overall incidence of malignancy in MN was 10 percent, the incidence among patients over the age of 64 was 24.7 percent [111], similar to another study showing a 19.4 percent incidence of malignancy in patients with MN who are over the age of 60 years [98].

Advanced age and a history of extensive tobacco use (i.e., greater than 20 pack-years) were the two factors most predictive of underlying malignancy [108]. Nine of the twelve patients with cancer remission had a complete or partial remission of nephrotic range proteinuria. Based on these studies, 6–10 percent of adult patients presenting with MN are likely to have an underlying malignancy, most commonly originating in the lung, breast, genitourinary, or GI tract [98,108]. Resection of the tumor may lead to remission of the nephrotic syndrome [106,108]. Search for underlying malignancy is particularly important in patients with MN who are older than 60 years or have a history of significant tobacco use [98,108]. Membranous nephropathy is also associated with sickle cell anemia and graft-versus-host disease [109].

Pathology of Secondary MN. Findings that favor membranous lupus nephritis over primary MN include mesangial, subendothelial, tubulointerstitial, and vessel wall deposits, "full house" immunostaining (IgG, IgM, IgA, C3, and C1), endothelial tubuloreticular inclusions, and significant mesangial and/or endocapillary hypercellularity [110] (Figure 4.65). Many of these findings, such as mesangial and subendothelial deposits, "full house" immunostaining, and mesangial hypercellularity, are also seen in other secondary forms of MN, including MN related to hepatitis B virus (HBV) infection [103,111].

Multiple studies have attempted to use staining for subclasses of IgG to differentiate primary and secondary forms of MN. In primary MN, there is typically dominant staining for IgG4 [112–114]. Staining for IgG1 is also commonly seen, while staining for IgG2 and IgG3 is typically absent or of minimal intensity [112–114]. In contrast, staining for all subclasses of IgG (IgG1, IgG2, IgG3, and IgG4) is common in membranous lupus nephritis but staining for IgG4 is seen least frequently and is of lowest intensity [113,114]. In malignancy-associated MN, staining for IgG1, IgG2, and IgG4 is most common and is of greatest intensity, but low intensity staining for IgG3 may also be encountered [112]. Due to the frequent overlap of IgG subclass staining in idiopathic MN, malignancy-associated MN, and membranous lupus nephritis, staining for IgG subclasses is mainly a research tool that is not widely employed in diagnostic renal pathology.

Etiology and Pathogenesis of MN

The classic animal model of membranous nephropathy is passive Heymann nephritis (PHN). Rats injected with fractionated renal cortex develop MN [115] and subsequent passive transfer of antibodies into naïve rats of the same species produces MN. The fractionated renal cortex (Fx1A) is enriched in proximal tubular brush border (PT-BB) antigens. Subsequent study has shown that the critical component of Fx1A in PHN is Gp330/megalin. Injection of Gp330 alone induces PHN whereas injection of Gp330-depleted Fx1A does not. Moreover, Gp330 localizes to the subepithelial deposits of PHN, consistent with in situ subepithelial antigen-antibody complex formation [116].

Gp330/megalin, referred to as the "Heymann antigen," is expressed in rat PT-BB and the clathrin-coated pits of visceral epithelial cells [117]. In humans, megalin has been identified in PT-BB but is not present in glomeruli or in the subepithelial deposits of MN.

Megalin has multiple apolipoprotein ligands including apo B & E. Megalin's normal role includes uptake of lipoproteins, a process that can be blocked by the presence of antimegalin antibodies [118]. In the setting of PHN, apolipoproteins B & E are present with the immune complex deposits, and reactive oxygen species may promote peroxidation of these apolipoproteins with subsequent adduct formation on GBM matrix proteins [119].

The development of proteinuria in PHN is complement-dependent and involves the formation of C5b-C9, the membrane attack complex (MAC). MAC inserts into the podocyte membrane causing sublytic injury, leading to synthesis of proteases, oxidants, extracellular matrix, and TGF-β [120,121]. Depletion of C6 or C8 inhibits the production of MAC and proteinuria, without affecting the formation of subepithelial deposits. [122,123] MAC formation in MN is thought to involve both the classical and alternative complement pathways. The presence of IgG within the deposits contributes to classical pathway activation. Although IgG4 deposits predominate in MN [112–114]. IgG4, unlike IgG1 and IgG3, has minimal ability to fix complement. In the normal state, complement regulatory proteins (CRP) are present in podocytes and inhibit complement activation via the alternative pathway. In the setting of MN, there is diminished CRP function, leading to alternative pathway activation and MAC formation. In support of this concept, antibodies against Crry, a rat CRP, have been identified in PHN [124,125]. Depletion of anti-Crry antibodies ameliorates proteinuria in PHN without disrupting subepithelial deposit formation [124]. Given the lack of leukocyte infiltration in MN and the geographic separation of the deposits from the circulation (by the GBM), MN appears to induce podocyte injury in a leukocyte-independent manner.

In 2002, Debiec and colleagues identified the first human Heymann antigen in a child who presented with congenital nephrotic syndrome [126]. Renal biopsy revealed MN with staining of GBM and PT-BB for neutral endopeptidase (NEP), associated with the presence of transplacentally transmitted maternal anti-NEP antibodies. Subsequently, the child's mother was found to be NEP-deficient. NEP is a zinc-dependent metalloproteinase that is expressed in podocytes, PT-BB, and vascular smooth muscle. Due to enzymatic redundancy, the absence of NEP is associated with a normal phenotype in mice and humans [126,127]. Two additional families with antenatal MN due to maternal NEP deficiency have been reported, suggesting that antenatal MN may result from fetomaternal allosensitization, analogous to Rhesus incompatibility [126,127]. The search for additional "human Heymann antigens" continues.

Patients with secondary MN may have evidence of circulating immune complexes with antibodies directed to nonvisceral epithelial cell antigens. For instance, HBsAg has been identified within the subepithelial immune complex deposits in patients with HBV infection [128]. The mechanism by which patients with secondary forms of MN develop subepithelial deposits may involve dissociation of circulating antigen–antibody immune complexes (particularly small, low-avidity cationic immune complexes) that traverse the GBM and reform in the subepithelial region.

Prognosis and Treatment

The first consideration in the management of membranous nephropathy is to exclude secondary causes of disease. Identification and treatment of a secondary etiology of MN, for instance HBV infection, is associated with an excellent outcome if the inciting antigenic stimulus can be effectively eliminated, and may avoid the unnecessary use of immunosuppressive agents. The 10-year prognosis of untreated primary MN is for one-third of patients to enter remission, one-third to have persistent proteinuria, and one-third to develop ESRD. Because of the high rate of spontaneous remission and slowly progressive course, studies on the treatment of MN need to include large numbers of patients and many years of therapy before significant differences can be detected. Studies utilizing steroid therapy for MN have produced equivocal results that have been unable to establish their effectiveness [129,130]. In contrast, combined regimens utilizing steroids and cytotoxic agents (i.e., chlorambucil or cyclophosphamide) have proven effective, albeit with a greater risk of toxicity [131]. Cyclosporine has also been used with success in the treatment of MN, although there is a high rate of relapse following discontinuation of therapy [132, 133]. Additional agents that have been used to treat MN include rituximab [134] and mycophenolate mofetil [135].

Prognostic factors can be used to determine which patients are most likely to benefit from aggressive therapy. Clinical factors that have been associated with a poor prognosis include male sex, increased age, higher levels of proteinuria, persistence of proteinuria, and renal insufficiency [86,136]. Children with MN and patients with subnephrotic proteinuria generally have a favorable prognosis. Pathologic findings which may portend a poor prognosis include tubular atrophy and interstitial fibrosis, glomerular lesions of segmental sclerosis [87,88] and the degree of complement deposition noted by immunofluorescence [136,137].

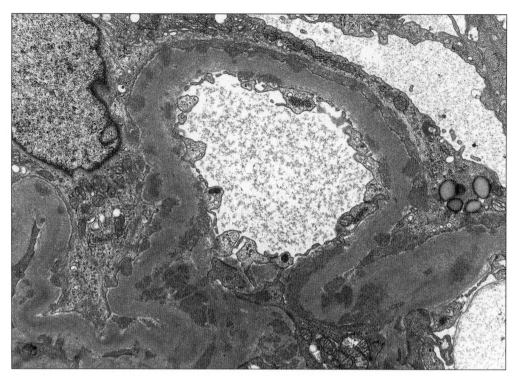

FIGURE 4.65: *Membranous nephropathy. In additional to global subepithelial deposits, electron microscopy this case of MN reveals mesangial and subendothelial deposits and endothelial tubuloreticular inclusions. These findings strongly favor a secondary form of MN. Upon further evaluation, the patient was found to have systemic lupus erythematosus. (Electron microscopy, × 5,000).*

Variants of Membranous Nephropathy

Combined Membranous Nephropathy and IgA Nephropathy

A minority of cases of MN exhibit mesangial deposits that stain dominantly for IgA [140]. When this finding is encountered, and staining for IgG is in a subepithelial distribution that spares the mesangium, the findings are best characterized as coexistent MN and IgA nephropathy. This dual glomerulopathy likely represents the chance superimposition of two distinct disease entities. More than 20 cases of coexistent MN and IgA nephropathy have been reported in the literature. The majority of patients presented with hematuria and proteinuria and despite the presence of two separate disease processes, poor renal outcomes have not been noted. Settings where this disease combination has been described include patients with HBV infection, patients of Asian descent, and in the renal allograft where recurrent IgA nephropathy and de novo MN are common occurrences [138].

Membranous Nephropathy with Renal Vein Thrombosis

Among patients with the nephrotic syndrome, individuals with MN and a serum albumin less than 2.0 g/dL are at the highest risk to develop renal vein thrombosis (RVT) [139]. While most reports describe an incidence of RVT in MN of less than 10 percent, studies that carefully evaluate all patients reveal a high incidence of asymptomatic, small RVTs. Pathologic changes seen on renal biopsy that suggest RVT include vascular con-gestion of glomerular or interstitial capillaries, disproportionate interstitial edema and subsequent fibrosis, and vascular thrombosis [140]. The treatment of RVT includes anticoagulants and in select cases, thrombolytic therapy [141].

Membranous Nephropathy Superimposed on Diabetic Nephropathy

Membranous nephropathy is the most common form of glomerular disease to occur superimposed on diabetic glomerulosclerosis (DGS). Clinical presentations include proteinuria in the absence of retinopathy, full nephrotic syndrome, and proteinuria out of proportion to the duration of diabetes mellitus. The diagnosis of MN in the setting of DGS is made difficult by the fact that DGS is also associated with GBM thickening by light microscopy and exhibits linear staining of the GBM for IgG by immunofluorescence. Careful examination of the IF staining reveals both linear and granular staining of the GBM for IgG, and EM reveals subepithelial deposits and basement membrane spikes emanating from a thickened GBM in MN with DGS.

Membranous Nephropathy in the Renal Allograft

Three different forms of MN may be encountered in the renal allograft. Approximately 75 percent of cases of MN in the allograft represent de novo disease [142]. MN is the most common form of de novo glomerular disease seen in the renal allograft and typically presents greater than one-year posttransplantation with either subnephrotic proteinuria or, less commonly, full nephrotic syndrome [143]. Recurrent MN is less common than de novo disease and tends to occur in the first year posttransplantation with an aggressive initial course and a high incidence of nephrotic syndrome. Among patients with MN, the incidence of recurrence in the allograft is 10–20 percent, depending on screening for proteinuria. The prognosis of de novo MN is better than recurrent MN although in both cases the prognosis is mainly dependent on whether acute or chronic rejections are present.

Interestingly, there have been two documented cases of donor-transmitted MN [144,145]. In one case, immunofluorescence revealed deposits of significant intensity at 11 days and again at 4 weeks posttransplantation, with a marked diminution in intensity at 7 weeks [145]. The patient expired due to metastatic carcinoma 20 months posttransplantation. At autopsy, ultrastructural evaluation of the allograft revealed electron-lucencies within the GBM, consistent with resorbed deposits. The other patient had no further biopsies but remained at a baseline creatinine of 1.2 mg/dL 34 months posttransplantation [144].

NEPHROTIC SYNDROME IN THE FIRST YEAR OF LIFE

Introduction

By convention, nephrotic syndrome in the first year of life is classified as either congenital nephrotic syndrome (CNS), which manifests in utero or in the first 3 months, or infantile nephrotic syndrome, which presents between 4 months and 1 year of age [146]. In contrast with nephrotic syndrome occurring in older subjects, where the etiology is usually unknown, most cases of nephrotic syndrome in the first year of life are related to genetic mutations of glomerular proteins, including nephrin (*NPHS1* gene), podocin (*NPHS2*), phospholipase C epsilon-1 (*PLCE-1*), Wilms tumor suppressor protein (*WT1*), and laminin β2 (*LAMB2*) (see Table 4.5) [58, 147]. These genetic conditions may be familial or sporadic and may be accompanied by extrarenal manifestations, including Wilms tumor, Denys Drash syndrome, Frasier syndrome, and Pierson syndrome.

The clinical and renal pathologic manifestations of the different genetic forms of CNS and infantile nephrotic syndrome are nonspecific. Podocytes typically display diffuse foot process effacement with variable additional findings, including tubular cysts, mesangial hypercellularity, mesangial sclerosis, and FSGS. This section focuses on Finnish-type CNS and diffuse mesangial sclerosis (DMS), the major causes of CNS and infantile nephrotic syndrome, respectively. Other causes of CNS and infantile nephrotic syndrome are listed in Table 4.6.

Finnish Type Congenital Nephrotic Syndrome

Definition. Congenital nephrotic syndrome of the Finnish type (CNF) is defined as CNS due to heritable *NPHS1* mutations [148]. CNF is inherited in an autosomal recessive pattern. CNF was first described in, and most commonly affects individuals of Finnish descent but also occurs in other ethnic groups. In the Finnish population, the disease incidence is 1.2 in 10,000 live births and the estimated gene carrier frequency is 1 in 200. The estimated incidence in North America is 1 in 50,000.

Clinical Features. CNF presents with severe, unremitting nephrotic syndrome at birth or developing within the first 3 months of life. Elevated alpha-fetoprotein levels may be detected in the maternal serum or the amniotic fluid by 16 to 18 weeks of gestation, reflecting fetal proteinuria. There is an increased incidence of premature birth, low birth weight, malpresentations, and postural deformities, such as contractures of the knees and elbows, which likely are related to the abnormally large placenta (placental/fetal weight ratio commonly exceeds 0.25).

Patients have proteinuria at birth and all develop nephrotic syndrome before the age of 3 months. Proteinuria ranges from 1 to 6 g/day and serum albumin levels are extremely low, usually less than 0.5 g/dL. Other features include microhematuria and signs of tubular dysfunction, including aminoaciduria and glycosuria. The presence of severe ascites may cause dyspnea. With disease progression, proteinuria becomes less selective. Hypogammaglobulinemia due to urinary losses predisposes to infection. Although renal function is usually normal at birth, there is a progressive decline in the glomerular filtration rate over the first 3 to 4 years of life.

Gross Findings. At autopsy, the kidneys are enlarged and pale, with smooth, swollen cortices. The ratio of kidney to body weight at birth usually exceeds twice normal. The kidney enlargement likely relates to tubular dilatation and interstitial edema. Minute cortical cysts may be seen.

Light Microscopic Findings. The most common feature is focal dilatation of proximal tubules forming microcysts, which are present in up to 75 percent of cases (Figure 4.66). Cysts begin in the deep cortex and spread to the outer cortex over time. The outer medulla is usually spared. Cysts may contain proteinaceous eosinophilic casts or appear empty (Figure 4.67). The epithelium lining the cyst is flattened and atrophic. Proximal tubules may contain intracytoplasmic protein and lipid resorption droplets (Figure 4.67).

There are no pathognomonic glomerular findings. Glomeruli often appear normal but may show mesangial hypercellularity or increased matrix (Figures 4.68 and 4.69). The number of infantile glomeruli is usually consistent with gestational age but

Table 4.5 Major Genetic Causes of Nephrotic Syndrome^a

Genetic Defect	Mode of Inheritance	Chromosomal Location
NPHS1	AR	19q13.1
NPHS2	AR	1q25-31
PLCE1	AR	10q23-24
LAMB2	AR	3p21
WT1	AD	11p13
TRPC6	AD	11q21-22
Alpha actinin 4	AD	19q13

Abbreviations: NPHS1, nephrin; NPHS2, podocin; PLCE1, phospholipase C epsilon-1; LAMB2, laminin beta 2; WT1, Wilms tumor-1; TRPC6, transient receptor potential cation channel 6; AR, autosomal recessive; AD, autosomal dominant.

^{a} Most present in the first year of life, with pathologic findings of focal segmental glomerulosclerosis (FSGS) or diffuse mesangial sclerosis (DMS).

Table 4.6 Causes of Nephrotic Syndrome (NS) in the First Year After Birth

***Congenital nephrotic syndrome (CNS):* presenting at birth or before 3 months of age**
Common
    CNS Finnish type (*NPHS1* mutations)
    CNS French type (diffuse mesangial sclerosis, +/− *WT-1* mutations)
    CNS associated with other mutations (*NPHS2, LAMB2, PLCE1)*
Less common
    Congenital infections (syphilis, toxoplasmosis, HIV, cytomegalovirus)
Rare
    Primary MCD, FSGS, membranous nephropathy
    Congenital membranous nephropathy
    Congenital epidermolysis bullosa (β-4-integrin gene mutation)
    Congenital SLE

***Infantile nephrotic syndrome:* presenting between 4 to 12 months**
Diffuse mesangial sclerosis
    Isolated (most cases)
        (Some have *PLCE1, WT-1, LAMB2, NPHS* mutations)
Syndromic DMS
    Denys Drash syndrome (*WT-1* mutations)
    Frasier syndrome (*WT-1* mutations)
    Pierson syndrome (*LAMB2* mutations)
Steroid-resistant nephrotic syndrome (NPHS2 mutations)
Other conditions
    Idiopathic MCD, FSGS, membranous glomerulopathy, HIVAN, hemolytic uremic syndrome, lupus nephritis, alpha-1-antitrypsin deficiency, mercury poisoning

Abbreviations: NPHS1, nephrin; NPHS2, podocin; PLCE1, phospholipase C epsilon-1; LAMB2, laminin beta 2; WT1, Wilms tumor-1; TRPC6, transient receptor potential cation channel 6; MCD, minimal change disease; FSGS, focal segmental glomerulosclerosis; HIV, human immunodeficiency virus.

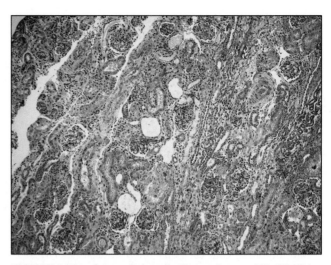

FIGURE 4.66: *Congenital nephrotic syndrome of the Finnish type. Low power view of a biopsy from a 2-week old infant shows focal microcysts. (PAS, × 100).*

may be increased compared to normal age-matched controls (Figure 4.70). Rarely, CNF manifests a pattern of DMS [58]. As the disease progresses, FSGS and global glomerulosclerosis are common (Figure 4.71) [149]. Podocyte hypertrophy and segmental small crescents may be observed. With progression to renal failure, there is increasing global glomerulosclerosis, tubular atrophy, and interstitial fibrosis, accompanied by a sparse mononuclear inflammatory cell infiltrate (Figure 4.72). Arterioles may show fibrinoid necrosis in infants who develop accelerated hypertension but vascular lesions are otherwise rare.

Immunofluorescence Findings. IgM and C3 may be seen in FSGS lesions. Tubular epithelium protein resorption droplets stain for albumin and immunoglobulins.

Electron Microscopic Findings. The nonsclerotic glomeruli display extensive effacement of the podocyte foot processes, similar to MCD (Figure 4.73). Podocytes may display cytoplasmic swelling and microvillous transformation. Glomerular basement membranes may show lamellation of the lamina densa, resembling hereditary nephritis of the Alport syndrome type. Slit diaphragms are anatomically absent (Figure 4.74).

Differential Diagnosis. CNF accounts for up to 75 percent of CNS and DMS for about 10 percent of cases. CNF typically has an earlier onset (*in utero* or at birth) compared to DMS (several weeks to 12 months of age). Thus, CNF is often associated with an abnormally large placenta, premature delivery, and low birth weight. Severe hypertension and rapid progression to renal failure are more typical of DMS. The pathologic findings in CNF and DMS may overlap and neither entity has pathognomonic findings. Although tubular cysts are commonly present in CNF, these may also occur as a nonspecific finding in DMS. Moreover, some cases of CNF manifest DMS [58]. FSGS lesions occur in both conditions. Although slit diaphragms are absent in most cases of CNF, identification of these structures may be difficult when foot processes are effaced. Absent or altered glomerular nephrin immunostaining, while characteristic, has also been described in other proteinuric glomerular diseases and is therefore not specific for CNF [150].

While CNF is the most common cause of CNS in the Finnish population, other genetic abnormalities may be more common in other populations. In one study of non-Scandinavian families with CNS, *NPHS1*, and *NPHS2* mutations were equally common (39.1 percent), whereas *WT-1* and *LAMB2* mutations were identified in 2.2 and 4.4 percent of families, respectively [58]. CNS has also been associated with triallelic mutations in *NPHS1* and *NPHS2* [59], and *PLCE1* mutations [147]. Except for *LAMB2*, these mutations more commonly present with infantile nephrotic syndrome and therefore these are discussed in "Diffuse Mesangial Sclerosis."

Less common causes of CNS include congenital infections (syphilis, toxoplasmosis, and cytomegalovirus) and congenital SLE. Renal biopsies in these conditions may display either minimal glomerular changes (resembling MCD), mesangial proliferation, membranous glomerulopathy, or diffuse proliferative glomerulonephritis [151]. Congenital membranous glomerulopathy has been linked to maternal neutral endopeptidase deficiency [126,127] (see "Membranous Nephropathy"). The immunofluorescence and electron microscopic findings of glomerular subepithelial immune deposits distinguish membranous nephropathy from CNF. CNS with biopsy findings of

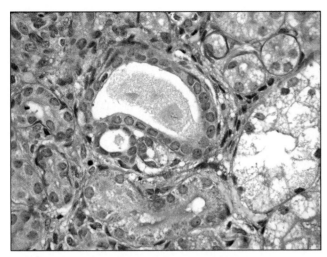

FIGURE 4.67: *Congenital nephrotic syndrome of the Finnish type. High power view of a tubular cyst containing a proteinaceous cast. The adjacent tubule on the right displays clear cytoplasm consistent with lipid resorption droplets. (PAS, × 600).*

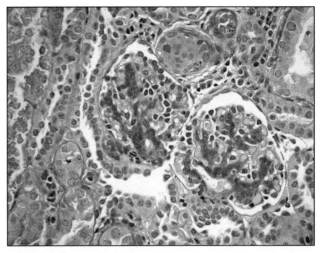

FIGURE 4.69: *Congenital nephrotic syndrome of the Finnish type. Two glomeruli display mild mesangial hypercellularity and prominent podocyte nuclei (PAS, × 600).*

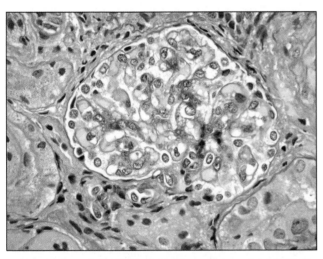

FIGURE 4.68: *Congenital nephrotic syndrome of the Finnish type. Glomerulus from a 2-week old infant shows patent capillary lumina and mild mesangial hypercellularity. (PAS, × 600).*

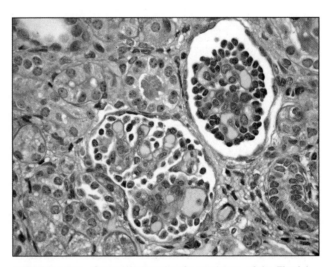

FIGURE 4.70: *Congenital nephrotic syndrome of the Finnish type. Immature glomerulus on the right displays prominent podocyte nuclei. The more mature glomerulus on the left shows mild mesangial hypercellularity (PAS, × 600).*

FSGS has been reported in a case of epidermolysis bullosa caused by mutations of β-4-integrin expressed on podocytes [152].

Other causes of nephrotic syndrome seen in older children and adults, such as primary MCD, membranous nephropathy and primary FSGS, are exceedingly rare before 3 months of age.

Etiology and Pathogenesis. CNF is caused by mutations in the *NPHS1* gene located on chromosome 19 (19q13) [148]. The gene product, nephrin, is the major structural protein of the filtration slit diaphragm. At least 59 different *NPHS1* mutations have been identified in CNF, including deletions, insertions, splice-site mutations, and nonsense mutations, resulting in frameshifts or premature stop codons. Many of these mutations result in a truncated molecule that lacks the intracellular and transmembrane domains. In the Finnish population, two nonsense mutations (Fin major and Fin minor) account for 94 per-

cent *NPHS1* mutations; however, these mutations are rare in non-Scandinavian populations.

Treatment and Prognosis. Treatment of secondary infectious causes of CNS usually results in complete remission of nephrotic syndrome. The genetic forms of CNS show no response to steroids or any other immunosuppressive therapy and the prognosis is usually poor. Many patients die before the age of 1 year due to infectious complications, reflecting the marked reduction in plasma immunoglobulin IgG. Other complications include growth retardation, delayed motor and mental development, thromboses, hypothyroidism due to urinary loss of thyroid-binding globulin, vitamin D deficiency and iron deficiency. In patients who survive, ESRD usually ensues by 4 to 8 years of age.

Clinical management consists of control of edema with oral diuretics and albumin infusions, replacement of thyroid hormones, iron, and vitamin D, and anticoagulation to prevent

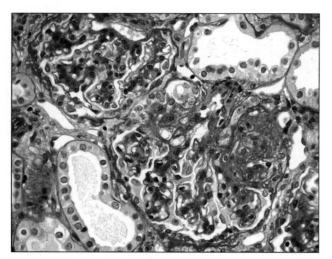

FIGURE 4.71: *Congenital nephrotic syndrome of the Finnish type. Nephrectomy from a 4 year-old child shows segmental glomerulosclerosis in the glomerulus on the right (PAS, × 400).*

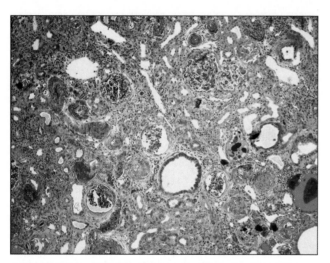

FIGURE 4.72: *Congenital nephrotic syndrome of the Finnish type. Nephrectomy from a 4 year-old child shows widespread tubulo-interstitial scarring with tubular microcysts (Trichrome, × 100).*

thromboembolic complications. Double nephrectomy is recommended within the first year or two of life, followed by dialysis until the child is old enough for renal transplantation (usually between the ages of 2 and 3 years). This approach mitigates the risk of infection and growth retardation associated with unremitting severe nephrotic syndrome.

Recurrence of nephrotic syndrome posttransplantation has been reported in 20 percent of Finnish patients with CNF with Fin-major/Fin-minor genotype [153]. Recurrence of nephrotic syndrome may occur immediately following transplantation. The sole pathologic finding consists of diffuse foot process effacement. Some cases of recurrent nephrotic syndrome may be mediated by autoantibodies to nephrin, causing immunologic destruction of the slit diaphragm [156]. Other cases are associated with presence a circulating glomerular permeability

factor [154]. Graft survival in recurrent CNF is generally poor, although some cases may respond to increased immunosuppressive therapy [154].

Diffuse Mesangial Sclerosis

Definition. Diffuse mesangial sclerosis (DMS) is a clinical–pathologic condition characterized by severe nephrotic syndrome, usually presenting within the first year of life, with pathologic findings of diffuse mesangial sclerosis [155]. DMS is usually an isolated sporadic condition but may be related to heritable mutations of *WT-1* (with or without Denys-Drash syndrome or Frasier syndrome) [156], *LAMB2* (with or without Pierson syndrome or ocular abnormalities) [153,154], or *PLCE1* [57,147]. Other, as yet identified genetic mutations are likely involved in apparently sporadic DMS.

Clinical Features. Nephrotic syndrome develops after birth, usually between 4 and 12 months of age (50 percent of cases). However, DMS also accounts for approximately 10 percent of cases of CNS ("French-type CNS") [146]. The remaining cases of DMS usually present before 2 years of age [159].

In contrast to CNF, placental abnormalities, premature delivery, and low birth weight are usually absent in DMS, reflecting the fact that proteinuria develops after birth. The majority of patients present with renal insufficiency and marked hypertension. Rapid progression to ESRD ensues, usually within 1 to 3 months.

Denys-Drash syndrome comprises DMS, male pseudohermaphroditism (46XY genotype), nephrogenic rests and an increased incidence of Wilms' tumor [156]. Patients display either ambiguous external genitalia or normal-appearing female external genitalia. The internal genital organs may be hypoplastic, dysplastic, or normal-appearing. Patients present with nephrotic syndrome within the first year of life, with rapid progression to ESRD.

Frasier syndrome is characterized by male pseudohermaphroditism (XY genotype), fully feminized external genitalia, streak gonads, and later onset of a more slowly progressive glomerulopathy with pathologic features of FSGS [157]. Frasier's syndrome carries an increased risk of developing gonadoblastoma, not Wilms tumor. ESRD develops in adolescence of early adulthood.

Light Microscopic Findings. Glomeruli display diffuse mesangial matrix increase, with or without increased mesangial hypercellularity (Figure 4.75). Shrunken, sclerotic glomeruli surrounded by a corona of hypertrophied podocytes are common (Figures 4.76), as are immature glomeruli. Podocyte hypertrophy and hyperplasia may resemble a cellular crescent (Figure 4.77). The mesangial sclerosis has a reticulated, spongy texture, which is best appreciated with silver stains (Figure 4.78). As the disease progresses, FSGS lesions, tubular atrophy, interstitial fibrosis, and interstitial inflammation become more prominent. Pathologic abnormalities are zonally distributed, being more severe in the outer cortex and milder in the inner cortex (Figure 4.79). Nephrogenic rests may be seen. In Denys-Drash syndrome there is an increased incidence of Wilms tumor, which is bilateral in 25 percent of cases.

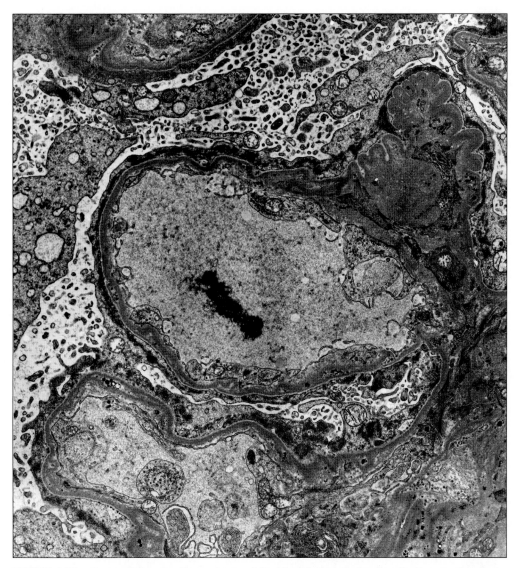

FIGURE 4.73: *Congenital nephrotic syndrome of the Finnish type. Podocytes display complete foot process effacement and microvillous cytoplasmic projections. (Electron photomicrograph, × 4,000).*

Immunofluorescence Findings. Segmental staining for IgM, C3, and C1 may be seen in sclerotic glomeruli.

Electron Microscopic Findings. Diffuse podocyte foot process effacement is typically seen. Mesangial matrix is increased. Glomerular basement membranes may be thickened and have a basket-weave/lamellated appearance. Small electron dense deposits may be seen, probably reflecting insudated plasma proteins (hyaline).

Etiology, Pathogenesis, and Differential Diagnosis. Most cases of DMS are idiopathic but some are related to mutations of *WT-1*, *PLCE-1* [(57,148], *LAMB2* [153,14], and *NPHS1* genes [58].

Mutations in *WT1*, located on chromosome 11p13, have been identified in more than 90 percent of patients with Denys-Drash syndrome but only rarely in patients with isolated

DMS. The *WT1* gene product is a zinc finger transcription factor that controls genes involved in maintaining cellular proliferation and switches on genes involved in blastemal differentiation. Dysregulation of these functions due to *WT1* mutations leads to uncontrolled proliferation and abnormal differentiation, including ambiguous genitalia and sexual dysmorphism. There is loss of expression of WT-1 seen in normal mature podocytes and increased expression of another transcription factor, PAX2, which is normally restricted to parietal cells in mature kidney. These abnormalities likely contribute to the synthesis of abnormal glomerular basement membrane and mesangial matrix during glomerular development, resulting in the DMS phenotype.

More than 60 different *WT1* mutations have been identified. In Denys-Drash syndrome, two *WT1* mutations occur, the first of which leads to the development of dysgenetic gonads, glomerulopathy, and nephrogenic rests. The second, postzygotic mutation occurs in nephrogenic rests, resulting in loss of

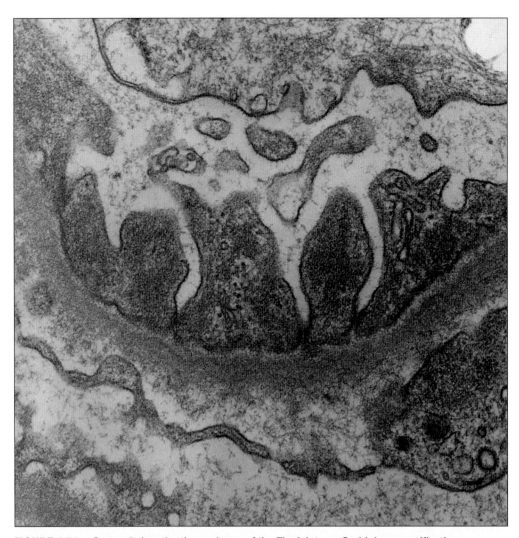

FIGURE 4.74: *Congenital nephrotic syndrome of the Finnish type. On higher magnification, no slit-diaphragms are visible between adjacent podocyte foot processes. (Electron photomicrograph, × 25,000).*

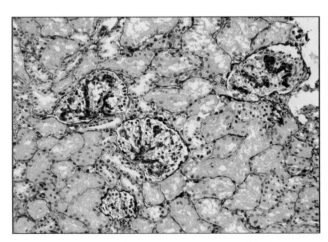

FIGURE 4.75: *Diffuse mesangial sclerosis. At an early stage, glomeruli show mild diffuse global mesangial matrix expansion. The tubulo-interstitial compartment appears normal (PAS, × 100).*

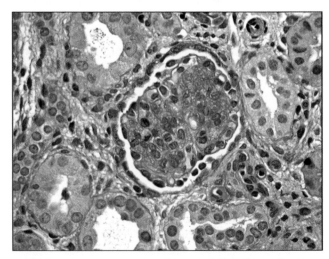

FIGURE 4.76: *Diffuse mesangial sclerosis. There is global mesangial expansion with accumulation of acellular matrix, surrounded by a corona of hypertrophied podocytes (PAS, × 600).*

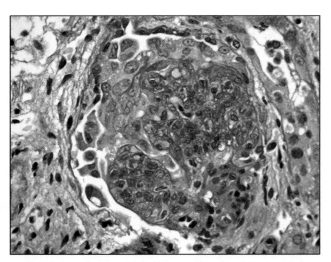

FIGURE 4.77: *Diffuse mesangial sclerosis. Visceral epithelial cells are swollen and hyperplastic, forming a pseudocrescent (PAS, × 600).*

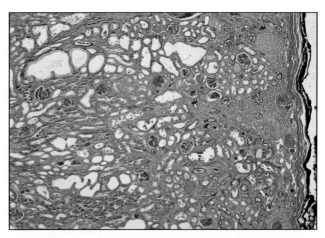

FIGURE 4.79: *Diffuse mesangial sclerosis. A nephrectomy specimen shows zonal distribution of pathologic changes. The subcapsular cortex (to the right) shows severe tubular atrophy and interstitial fibrosis. The mid-portion of the cortex (to the left) shows less severe changes (Trichrome, × 40).*

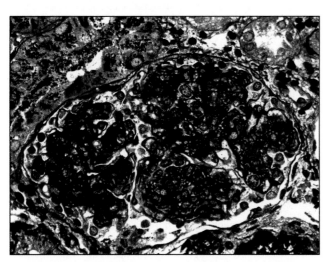

FIGURE 4.78: *Diffuse mesangial sclerosis. Even at a later stage, the mesangial matrix has a reticulated appearance with silver stains. There also appears to be increased mesangial cellularity (JMS, × 600).*

heterozygosity and development of Wilms tumors. Frasier syndrome, on the other hand, is associated with a heterozygous mutation in a splicing region (intron) of *WT1*, leading to altered ratios of *WT1* isoforms, rather than a mutant product [157].

The *PLCE1* gene, located on chromosome 10q, encodes one of a family of phospholipase C enzymes (PLCε1). Recently, Hinke et al. identified novel *PLCE1* mutations in fourteen patients from seven families with isolated early-onset nephrotic syndrome, eight of whom presented before 1 year of age (including 1 with CNS) [57]. None of these patients had extrarenal manifestations and the majority progressed to ESRD by 5 years of age. Renal biopsies were performed in ten patients, of which seven showed DMS (associated with homozygous truncating mutations), two showed FSGS (associated with a nontruncating missense mutation), and one had both DMS and

FSGS [58]. In a larger study of forty children from thirty-five families with isolated DMS, truncating *PLCE1* mutations were discovered in ten families (28.6 percent) and *WT1* mutations in three families (8.5 percent) [147].

PLCε1 is a signalling protein for many G protein-coupled receptors, including angiotensin II. PLCε1 localizes to the cytoplasm of the podocyte cell body and is highly expressed during the early capillary loop stage of development, suggesting that DMS associated with *PLCE1* mutations involves glomerular developmental arrest at this stage [57].

Laminin β2 is a major glycoprotein component of the glomerular basement membrane that is also expressed in other basement membranes, notably the intraocular muscles and lens, and in neuromuscular synapses. Mutations in the *LAMB2* gene leading to loss of laminin β2 expression were first described in infants with Pierson syndrome. Pierson syndrome is characterized by CNS due to DMS, early-onset renal failure, and severe eye abnormalities, including nonreactive narrowing of the pupils (microcoria) [158]. This severe phenotype is associated with biallelic truncating mutations, leading to complete loss of laminin β2 expression. Patients with CNS and nontruncating (missense) *LAMB2* mutations may display a milder variant of Pierson syndrome or isolated CNS, with slower progression to renal failure [159]. CNS due to *LAMB2* mutations may have biopsy findings of DMS or FSGS. Presumably, DMS results from abnormal laminin β2 expression in developing glomeruli.

Treatment and Prognosis. The therapeutic management is similar to that described above for CNF. Patients are usually not responsive to immunosuppressive therapy and are managed supportively until bilateral nephrectomy, followed by dialysis and renal transplantation, can be performed (usually between the ages of 2 and 3 years). However, two children with DMS, both with truncating mutations in *PLCE1*, responded to treatment with steroids and/or cyclosporine [57]. Unlike CNF, recurrence of nephrotic syndrome post transplantation has not been described in DMS.

Karyotyping is recommended in all DMS patients to rule out male pseudohermaphroditism. All patients with infantile nephrotic syndrome and biopsy findings of DMS or FSGS, and patients with steroid-resistant nephrotic syndrome who demonstrate rapid progression to ESRD, should be tested for *WT1*, *NPHS1*, and *NPHS2* mutations. Testing for *LAMB* and *PLCE1* mutations is not yet available outside the research setting. Those with *WT1* mutations need to be followed with repeated evaluation of the kidney and gonads for early detection of Wilms tumor and gonadoblastoma.

REFERENCES

1. Bernard DB. Extrarenal complications of the nephrotic syndrome. *Kidney Int* 1988; 33: 1184–1202.
2. Rostoker G, Behar A, Lagrue G. Vascular hyperpermeability in nephrotic edema. *Nephron* 2000; 85: 194–200.
3. Deschenes G, Gonin S, Zolty E, Cheval L, et al. Increased synthesis and avp unresponsiveness of Na,K-ATPase in collecting duct from nephrotic rats. *J Am Soc Nephrol* 2001; 12: 2241–2252.
4. Kim SW, Wang W, Nielsen J, Praetorius J, et al. Increased expression and apical targeting of renal ENaC subunits in puromycin aminonucleoside-induced nephrotic syndrome in rats. *Am J Physiol Renal Physiol* 2004; 286: F922–935.
5. Klisic J, Zhang J, Nief V, Reyes L, et al. Albumin regulates the Na+/H+ exchanger 3 in OKP cells. *J Am Soc Nephrol* 2003; 14: 3008–3016.
6. Kaysen GA, de Sain-van der Velden MG. New insights into lipid metabolism in the nephrotic syndrome. *Kidney Int Suppl* 1999; 71: S18–21.
7. Smith SM, Hoy WE, Cobb L. Low incidence of glomerulosclerosis in normal kidneys. *Arch Pathol Lab Med* 1989; 113: 1253–1255.
8. Savin VJ. Mechanisms of proteinuria in noninflammatory glomerular diseases. *Am J Kidney Dis* 1993; 21: 347–362.
9. Pinto JA, Brewer DB. Combined light and electron-microscope morphometric studies of acute puromycin aminonucleoside nephropathy in rats. *J Pathol* 1975; 116: 149–164.
10. Lai KW, Wei CL, Tan LK, Tan PH, et al. Overexpression of interleukin-13 induces minimal-change-like nephropathy in rats. *J Am Soc Nephrol* 2007; 18: 1476–1485.
11. Reiser J, von Gersdorff G, Loos M, Oh J, et al. Induction of B7-1 in podocytes is associated with nephrotic syndrome. *J Clin Invest* 2004; 113: 1390–1397.
12. Nolasco F, Cameron JS, Hicks J, Ogg CS, et al. Adult-onset nephrotic syndrome with minimal changes: response to corticosteroids and cyclophosphamide. *Proc Eur Dial Transplant Assoc Eur Ren Assoc* 1985; 21: 588–593.
13. Waldman M, Crew R, Valeri A, Busch J, et al. Adult minimal-change disease: clinical characteristics, treatment, and outcomes. *Clin J Am Soc Nephrol* 2007; 2: 445–453.
14. Bagga A, Hari P, Moudgil A, Jordan SC. Mycophenolate mofetil and prednisolone therapy in children with steroid-dependent nephrotic syndrome. *Am J Kidney Dis* 2003; 42: 1114–1120.
15. Durkan AM, Hodson EM, Willis NS, Craig JC. Immunosuppressive agents in childhood nephrotic syndrome: a meta-analysis of randomized controlled trials. *Kidney Int* 2001; 59: 1919–1927.
16. Fogo A, Hawkins EP, Berry PL, Glick AD, et al. Glomerular hypertrophy in minimal change disease predicts subsequent progression to focal glomerular sclerosis. *Kidney Int* 1990; 38: 115–123.
17. Stokes MB, Markowitz GS, Lin J, Valeri AM, et al. Glomerular tip lesion: a distinct entity within the minimal change disease/focal segmental glomerulosclerosis spectrum. *Kidney Int* 2004; 65: 1690–1702.
18. Haas M, Yousefzadeh N. Glomerular tip lesion in minimal change nephropathy: a study of autopsies before 1950. *Am J Kidney Dis* 2002; 39: 1168–1175.
19. Weber S, Gribouval O, Esquivel EL, Moriniere V, et al. NPHS2 mutation analysis shows genetic heterogeneity of steroid-resistant nephrotic syndrome and low post-transplant recurrence. *Kidney Int* 2004; 66: 571–579.
20. Winn MP, Conlon PJ, Lynn KL, Farrington MK, et al. A mutation in the TRPC6 cation channel causes familial focal segmental glomerulosclerosis. *Science* 2005; 308: 1801–1804.
21. Izzedine H, Brocheriou I, Eymard B, Le Charpentier M, et al. Loss of podocyte dysferlin expression is associated with minimal change nephropathy. *Am J Kidney Dis* 2006; 48: 143–150.
22. Ruf RG, Lichtenberger A, Karle SM, Haas JP, et al. Patients with mutations in NPHS2 (podocin) do not respond to standard steroid treatment of nephrotic syndrome. *J Am Soc Nephrol* 2004; 15: 722–732.
23. Jennette JC, Falk RJ. Adult minimal change glomerulopathy with acute renal failure. *Am J Kidney Dis* 1990; 16: 432–437.
24. Primary nephrotic syndrome in children: clinical significance of histopathologic variants of minimal change and of diffuse mesangial hypercellularity. A Report of the International Study of Kidney Disease in Children. *Kidney Int* 1981; 20: 765–771.
25. Childhood nephrotic syndrome associated with diffuse mesangial hypercellularity. A report of the Southwest Pediatric Nephrology Study Group. *Kidney Int* 1983; 24: 87–94.
26. Cohen AH, Border WA, Glassock RJ. Nephrotic syndrome with glomerular mesangial IgM deposits. *Lab Invest* 1978; 38: 610–619.
27. Al-Eisa A, Carter JE, Lirenman DS, Magil AB. Childhood IgM nephropathy: comparison with minimal change disease. *Nephron* 1996; 72: 37–43.
28. Tejani A, Nicastri AD. Mesangial IgM nephropathy. *Nephron* 1983; 35: 1–5.
29. Myllymaki J, Saha H, Mustonen J, Helin H, et al. IgM nephropathy: clinical picture and long-term prognosis. *Am J Kidney Dis* 2003; 41: 343–350.
30. Zeis PM, Kavazarakis E, Nakopoulou L, Moustaki M, et al. Glomerulopathy with mesangial IgM deposits: long-term follow-up of 64 children. *Pediatr Int* 2001; 43: 287–292.
31. Clive DM, Galvanek EG, Silva FG. Mesangial immunoglobulin A deposits in minimal change nephrotic syndrome: a report of an older patient and review of the literature. *Am J Nephrol* 1990; 10: 31–36.
32. Association of IgA nephropathy with steroid-responsive nephrotic syndrome. A report of the Southwest Pediatric

Nephrology Study Group. *Am J Kidney Dis* 1985; 5: 157–164.

33. Warren GV, Korbet SM, Schwartz MM, Lewis EJ. Minimal change glomerulopathy associated with nonsteroidal antiinflammatory drugs. *Am J Kidney Dis* 1989; 13: 127–130.

34. Barri YM, Munshi NC, Sukumalchantra S, Abulezz SR, et al. Podocyte injury associated glomerulopathies induced by pamidronate. *Kidney Int* 2004; 65: 634–641.

35. Kleinknecht D. Interstitial nephritis, the nephrotic syndrome, and chronic renal failure secondary to nonsteroidal antiinflammatory drugs. *Semin Nephrol* 1995; 15: 228–235.

36. Tam VK, Green J, Schwieger J, Cohen AH. Nephrotic syndrome and renal insufficiency associated with lithium therapy. *Am J Kidney Dis* 1996; 27: 715–720.

37. Dizer U, Beker CM, Yavuz I, Ortatatli M, et al. Minimal change disease in a patient receiving IFN-alpha therapy for chronic hepatitis C virus infection. *J Interferon Cytokine Res* 2003; 23: 51–54.

38. Nakao K, Sugiyama H, Makino E, Matsuura H, et al. Minimal change nephrotic syndrome developing during postoperative interferon-beta therapy for malignant melanoma. *Nephron* 2002; 90: 498–500.

39. Pirani CL, Valeri A, D'Agati V, Appel GB. Renal toxicity of nonsteroidal antiinflammatory drugs. *Contrib Nephrol* 1987; 55: 159–175.

40. D'Agati V, Sablay LB, Knowles DM, Walter L. Angiotropic large cell lymphoma (intravascular malignant lymphomatosis) of the kidney: presentation as minimal change disease. *Hum Pathol* 1989; 20: 263–268.

41. Hertig A, Droz D, Lesavre P, Grunfeld JP, et al. SLE and idiopathic nephrotic syndrome: coincidence or not? *Am J Kidney Dis* 2002; 40: 1179–1184.

42. D'Agati V. The many masks of focal segmental glomerulosclerosis. *Kidney Int* 1994; 46: 1223–1241.

43. Paik KH, Lee BH, Cho HY, Kang HG, et al. Primary focal segmental glomerular sclerosis in children: clinical course and prognosis. *Pediatr Nephrol* 2007; 22: 389–395.

44. D'Agati VD, Fogo AB, Bruijn JA, Jennette JC. Pathologic classification of focal segmental glomerulosclerosis: a working proposal. *Am J Kidney Dis* 2004; 43: 368–382.

45. Chun MJ, Korbet SM, Schwartz MM, Lewis EJ. Focal segmental glomerulosclerosis in nephrotic adults: presentation, prognosis, and response to therapy of the histologic variants. *J Am Soc Nephrol* 2004; 15: 2169–2177.

46. Thomas DB, Franceschini N, Hogan SL, Ten Holder S, et al. Clinical and pathologic characteristics of focal segmental glomerulosclerosis pathologic variants. *Kidney Int* 2006; 69: 920–926.

47. Stokes MB, Valeri AM, Markowitz GS, D'Agati VD. Cellular focal segmental glomerulosclerosis: Clinical and pathologic features. *Kidney Int* 2006; 70: 1783–1792.

48. Deegens JK, Steenbergen EJ, Borm GF, Wetzels JF. Pathological variants of focal segmental glomerulosclerosis in an adult Dutch population epidemiology and outcome. *Nephrol Dial Transplant* 2008; 23: 186–192.

49. Ingulli E, Tejani A. Racial differences in the incidence and renal outcome of idiopathic focal segmental glomerulosclerosis in children. *Pediatr Nephrol* 1991; 5: 393–397.

50. Haas M, Meehan SM, Karrison TG, Spargo BH. Changing etiologies of unexplained adult nephrotic syndrome: a comparison of renal biopsy findings from 1976–1979 and 1995–1997. *Am J Kidney Dis* 1997;30: 621–631.

51. Korbet SM. Primary focal segmental glomerulosclerosis. *J Am Soc Nephrol* 1998; 9: 1333–1340.

52. Yoshikawa N, Ito H, Akamatsu R, Matsuyama S, et al. Focal segmental glomerulosclerosis with and without nephrotic syndrome in children. *J Pediatr* 1986; 109: 65–70.

53. Silverstein D, Craver R. Presenting features and short-term outcome according to pathologic variant in childhood primary focal segmental glomerulosclerosis. *Clinical JASN* 2007; 2: 700–707.

54. Shankland SJ. The podocyte's response to injury: role in proteinuria and glomerulosclerosis. *Kidney Int* 2006; 69: 2131–2147.

55. Kaplan JM, Kim SH, North KN, Rennke H, et al. Mutations in ACTN4, encoding alpha-actinin-4, cause familial focal segmental glomerulosclerosis. *Nat Genet* 2000; 24: 251–256.

56. Kim JM, Wu H, Green G, Winkler CA, et al. CD2-associated protein haploinsufficiency is linked to glomerular disease susceptibility. *Science* 2003; 300: 1298–1300.

57. Hinkes B, Wiggins RC, Gbadegesin R, Vlangos CN, et al. Positional cloning uncovers mutations in PLCE1 responsible for a nephrotic syndrome variant that may be reversible. *Nat Genet* 2006; 38: 1397–1405.

58. Hinkes BG, Mucha B, Vlangos CN, Gbadegesin R, et al. Nephrotic syndrome in the first year of life: two thirds of cases are caused by mutations in 4 genes (NPHS1, NPHS2, WT1, and LAMB2). *Pediatrics* 2007; 119: e907–919.

59. Koziell A, Grech V, Hussain S, Lee G, et al. Genotype/phenotype correlations of NPHS1 and NPHS2 mutations in nephrotic syndrome advocate a functional inter-relationship in glomerular filtration. *Hum Mol Genet* 2002; 11: 379–388.

60. Savin VJ, Sharma R, Sharma M, McCarthy ET, et al. Circulating factor associated with increased glomerular permeability to albumin in recurrent focal segmental glomerulosclerosis. *N Engl J Med* 1996; 334: 878–883.

61. Le Berre L, Godfrin Y, Lafond-Puyet L, Perretto S, et al. Effect of plasma fractions from patients with focal and segmental glomerulosclerosis on rat proteinuria. *Kidney Int* 2000; 58: 2502–2511.

62. Cattran D, Neogi T, Sharma R, McCarthy ET, et al. Serial estimates of serum permeability activity and clinical correlates in patients with native kidney focal segmental glomerulosclerosis. *J Am Soc Nephrol* 2003; 14: 448–453.

63. Barisoni L, Kriz W, Mundel P, D'Agati V. The dysregulated podocyte phenotype: a novel concept in the pathogenesis of collapsing idiopathic focal segmental glomerulosclerosis and HIV-associated nephropathy. *J Am Soc Nephrol* 1999; 10: 51–61.

64. Bariety J, Nochy D, Mandet C, Jacquot C, et al. Podocytes undergo phenotypic changes and express macrophagic-associated markers in idiopathic collapsing glomerulopathy. *Kidney Int* 1998; 53: 918–925.

65. Shankland SJ, Eitner F, Hudkins KL, Goodpaster T, et al. Differential expression of cyclin-dependent kinase

inhibitors in human glomerular disease: role in podocyte proliferation and maturation. *Kidney Int* 2000; 58: 674–683.

66. Cattran DC, Appel GB, Hebert LA, Hunsicker LG, et al. A randomized trial of cyclosporine in patients with steroid-resistant focal segmental glomerulosclerosis. North America Nephrotic Syndrome Study Group. *Kidney Int* 1999; 56: 2220–2226.

67. Schoeneman MJ, Bennett B, Greifer I. The natural history of focal segmental glomerulosclerosis with and without mesangial hypercellularity in children. *Clin Nephrol* 1978; 9: 45–54.

68. Focal segmental glomerulosclerosis in children with idiopathic nephrotic syndrome. A report of the Southwest Pediatric Nephrology Study Group. *Kidney Int* 1985; 27: 442–449.

69. Praga M, Morales E, Herrero JC, Perez Campos A, et al. Absence of hypoalbuminemia despite massive proteinuria in focal segmental glomerulosclerosis secondary to hyperfiltration. *Am J Kidney Dis* 1999; 33: 52–58.

70. Kambham N, Markowitz GS, Valeri AM, Lin J, et al. Obesity-related glomerulopathy: an emerging epidemic. *Kidney Int* 2001; 59: 1498–1509.

71. Wolf G. After all those fat years: renal consequences of obesity. *Nephrol Dial Transplant* 2003; 18: 2471–2474.

72. D'Agati V, Suh JI, Carbone L, Cheng JT, et al. Pathology of HIV-associated nephropathy: a detailed morphologic and comparative study. *Kidney Int* 1989; 35: 1358–1370.

73. Albaqumi M, Soos TJ, Barisoni L, Nelson PJ. Collapsing glomerulopathy. *J Am Soc Nephrol* 2006; 17: 2854–2863.

74. Bruggeman LA, Dikman S, Meng C, Quaggin SE, et al. Nephropathy in human immunodeficiency virus-1 transgenic mice is due to renal transgene expression. *J Clin Invest* 1997; 100: 84–92.

75. Winston JA, Bruggeman LA, Ross MD, Jacobson J, et al. Nephropathy and establishment of a renal reservoir of HIV type 1 during primary infection. *N Engl J Med* 2001; 344: 1979–1984.

76. Monga G, Mazzucco G, Boldorini R, Cristina S, et al. Renal changes in patients with acquired immunodeficiency syndrome: a post-mortem study on an unselected population in northwestern Italy. *Mod Pathol* 1997; 10: 159–167.

77. Cheng JT, Anderson HL, Jr., Markowitz GS, Appel GB, et al. Hepatitis C virus-associated glomerular disease in patients with human immunodeficiency virus coinfection. *J Am Soc Nephrol* 1999; 10: 1566–1574.

78. Stokes MB, Chawla H, Brody RI, Kumar A, et al. Immune complex glomerulonephritis in patients coinfected with human immunodeficiency virus and hepatitis C virus. *Am J Kidney Dis* 1997; 29: 514–525.

79. Gerntholtz TE, Goetsch SJ, Katz I. HIV-related nephropathy: a South African perspective. *Kidney Int* 2006; 69: 1885–1891.

80. Jennette JC, Hipp CG. C1q nephropathy: a distinct pathologic entity usually causing nephrotic syndrome. *Am J Kidney Dis* 1985; 6: 103–110.

81. Markowitz GS, Schwimmer JA, Stokes MB, Nasr S, et al. C1q nephropathy: a variant of focal segmental glomerulosclerosis. *Kidney Int* 2003; 64: 1232–1240.

82. Iskandar SS, Browning MC, Lorentz WB. C1q nephropathy: a pediatric clinicopathologic study. *Am J Kidney Dis* 1991; 18: 459–465.

83. Kersnik Levart T, Kenda RB, Avgustin Cavic M, Ferluga D, et al. C1Q nephropathy in children. *Pediatr Nephrol* 2005; 20: 1756–1761.

84. Lau KK, Gaber LW, Delos Santos NM, Wyatt RJ. C1q nephropathy: features at presentation and outcome. *Pediatr Nephrol* 2005; 20: 744–749.

85. Fukuma Y, Hisano S, Segawa Y, Niimi K, et al. Clinicopathologic correlation of C1q nephropathy in children. *Am J Kidney Dis* 2006; 47: 412–418.

86. Cattran DC, Pei Y, Greenwood CM, Ponticelli C, et al. Validation of a predictive model of idiopathic membranous nephropathy: its clinical and research implications. *Kidney Int* 1997; 51: 901–907.

87. Wakai S, Magil AB. Focal glomerulosclerosis in idiopathic membranous glomerulonephritis. *Kidney Int* 1992; 41: 428–434.

88. Dumoulin A, Hill GS, Montseny JJ, Meyrier A. Clinical and morphological prognostic factors in membranous nephropathy: significance of focal segmental glomerulosclerosis. *Am J Kidney Dis* 2003; 41: 38–48.

89. Kambham N, Markowitz GS, Slater LM, D'Agati VD. An 18-year-old female with acute onset of nephrotic syndrome. *Am J Kidney Dis* 2000; 36: 441–446.

90. Tse WY, Howie AJ, Adu D, Savage CO, et al. Association of vasculitic glomerulonephritis with membranous nephropathy: a report of 10 cases. *Nephrol Dial Transplant* 1997; 12: 1017–1027.

91. Pettersson E, Tornroth T, Miettinen A. Simultaneous antiglomerular basement membrane and membranous glomerulonephritis: case report and literature review. *Clinical immunology and immunopathology* 1984; 31: 171–180.

92. Nasr SH, Ilamathi ME, Markowitz GS, D'Agati VD. A dual pattern of immunofluorescence positivity. *Am J Kidney Dis* 2003; 42: 419–426.

93. Klassen J, Elwood C, Grossberg AL, Milgrom F, et al. Evolution of membranous nephropathy into antiglomerular-basement-membrane glomerulonephritis. *N Engl J Med* 1974; 290: 1340–1344.

94. Markowitz GS, Kambham N, Maruyama S, Appel GB, et al. Membranous glomerulopathy with Bowman's capsular and tubular basement membrane deposits. *Clin Nephrol* 2000; 54: 478–486.

95. Ehrenreich T, and Churg G. Pathology of membranous nephropathy. In: SC S (ed). *Pathology Annual*. Appleton-Century-Crofts: New York, 1968.

96. Yoshimoto K, Yokoyama H, Wada T, Furuichi K, et al. Pathologic findings of initial biopsies reflect the outcomes of membranous nephropathy. *Kidney Int* 2004; 65: 148–153.

97. Kowalewska J, Smith KD, Hudkins KL, Chang A, et al. Membranous glomerulopathy with spherules: an uncommon variant with obscure pathogenesis. *Am J Kidney Dis* 2006; 47: 983–992.

98. Glassock RJ. Secondary membranous glomerulonephritis. *Nephrol Dial Transplant* 1992; 7 Suppl 1: 64–71.

99. Honkanen E, Tornroth T, Pettersson E, Skrifvars B. Membranous glomerulonephritis in rheumatoid arthritis not related to gold or D-penicillamine therapy: a report of four cases and review of the literature. *Clin Nephrol* 1987; 27: 87–93.

100. Becker BA, Fenves AZ, Breslau NA. Membranous glomerulonephritis associated with Graves' disease. *Am J Kidney Dis* 1999; 33: 369–373.

101. Markowitz GS, Falkowitz DC, Isom R, Zaki M, et al. Membranous glomerulopathy and acute interstitial nephritis following treatment with celecoxib. *Clin Nephrol* 2003; 59: 137–142.

102. Bailey RR. Captopril-induced membranous nephropathy. *N Z Med J* 1992; 105: 22.

103. Lai FM, To KF, Wang AY, Choi PC, et al. Hepatitis B virus-related nephropathy and lupus nephritis: morphologic similarities of two clinical entities. *Mod Pathol* 2000; 13: 166–172.

104. Tang S, Lai FM, Lui YH, Tang CS, et al. Lamivudine in hepatitis B-associated membranous nephropathy. *Kidney Int* 2005; 68: 1750–1758.

105. Uchiyama-Tanaka Y, Mori Y, Kishimoto N, Nose A, et al. Membranous glomerulonephritis associated with hepatitis C virus infection: case report and literature review. *Clin Nephrol* 2004; 61: 144–150.

106. Eagen JW. Glomerulopathies of neoplasia. *Kidney Int* 1977; 11: 297–303.

107. Burstein DM, Korbet SM, Schwartz MM. Membranous glomerulonephritis and malignancy. *Am J Kidney Dis* 1993; 22: 5–10.

108. Lefaucheur C, Stengel B, Nochy D, Martel P, et al. Membranous nephropathy and cancer: Epidemiologic evidence and determinants of high-risk cancer association. *Kidney Int* 2006; 70: 1510–1517.

109. Lin J, Markowitz GS, Nicolaides M, Hesdorffer CS, et al. Membranous glomerulopathy associated with graft-versus-host disease following allogeneic stem cell transplantation. Report of two cases and review of the literature. *Am J Nephrol* 2001; 21: 351–356.

110. Jennette JC, Iskandar SS, Dalldorf FG. Pathologic differentiation between lupus and nonlupus membranous glomerulopathy. *Kidney Int* 1983; 24: 377–385.

111. Honig C, Mouradian JA, Montoliu J, Susin M, et al. Mesangial electron-dense deposits in membranous nephropathy. *Lab Invest* 1980; 42: 427–432.

112. Ohtani H, Wakui H, Komatsuda A, Okuyama S, et al. Distribution of glomerular IgG subclass deposits in malignancy-associated membranous nephropathy. *Nephrol Dial Transplant* 2004; 19: 574–579.

113. Kuroki A, Shibata T, Honda H, Totsuka D, et al. Glomerular and serum IgG subclasses in diffuse proliferative lupus nephritis, membranous lupus nephritis, and idiopathic membranous nephropathy. *Intern Med* 2002; 41: 936–942.

114. Doi T, Mayumi M, Kanatsu K, Suehiro F, et al. Distribution of IgG subclasses in membranous nephropathy. *Clin Exp Immunol* 1984; 58: 57–62.

115. Heymann W, Hackel DB, Harwood S, Wilson SG, et al. Production of nephrotic syndrome in rats by Freund's adjuvants and rat kidney suspensions. *Proceedings of the Society for Experimental Biology and Medicine Society for Experimental Biology and Medicine (New York)* 1959; 100: 660–664.

116. Kerjaschki D, Farquhar MG. The pathogenic antigen of Heymann nephritis is a membrane glycoprotein of the renal proximal tubule brush border. *Proc Natl Acad Sci USA* 1982; 79: 5557–5561.

117. Kerjaschki D, Farquhar MG. Immunocytochemical localization of the Heymann nephritis antigen (GP330) in glomerular epithelial cells of normal Lewis rats. *J Exp Med* 1983; 157: 667–686.

118. Kerjaschki D, Exner M, Ullrich R, Susani M, et al. Pathogenic antibodies inhibit the binding of apolipoproteins to megalin/gp330 in passive Heymann nephritis. *J Clin Invest* 1997; 100: 2303–2309.

119. Exner M, Susani M, Witztum JL, Hovorka A, et al. Lipoproteins accumulate in immune deposits and are modified by lipid peroxidation in passive Heymann nephritis. *The Am J Pathol* 1996; 149: 1313–1320.

120. Nangaku M, Shankland SJ, Couser WG. Cellular response to injury in membranous nephropathy. *J Am Soc Nephrol* 2005; 16: 1195–1204.

121. Couser WG. Mediation of immune glomerular injury. *J Am Soc Nephrol* 1990; 1: 13–29.

122. Cybulsky AV, Rennke HG, Feintzeig ID, Salant DJ. Complement-induced glomerular epithelial cell injury. Role of the membrane attack complex in rat membranous nephropathy. *J Clin Invest* 1986; 77: 1096–1107.

123. Baker PJ, Ochi RF, Schulze M, Johnson RJ, et al. Depletion of C6 prevents development of proteinuria in experimental membranous nephropathy in rats. *Am J Pathol* 1989; 135: 185–194.

124. Schiller B, He C, Salant DJ, Lim A, et al. Inhibition of complement regulation is key to the pathogenesis of active Heymann nephritis. *J Exp Med* 1998; 188: 1353–1358.

125. Quigg RJ, Holers VM, Morgan BP, Sneed AE, 3rd. Crry and CD59 regulate complement in rat glomerular epithelial cells and are inhibited by the nephritogenic antibody of passive Heymann nephritis. *J Immunol* 1995; 154: 3437–3443.

126. Debiec H, Guigonis V, Mougenot B, Decobert F, et al. Antenatal membranous glomerulonephritis due to antineutral endopeptidase antibodies. *N Engl J Med* 2002; 346: 2053–2060.

127. Debiec H, Nauta J, Coulet F, van der Burg M, et al. Role of truncating mutations in MME gene in fetomaternal alloimmunisation and antenatal glomerulopathies. *Lancet* 2004; 364: 1252–1259.

128. Lai FM, Lai KN, Tam JS, Lui SF, et al. Primary glomerulonephritis with detectable glomerular hepatitis B virus antigens. *Am J Surg Pathol* 1994; 18: 175–186.

129. Muirhead N. Management of idiopathic membranous nephropathy: evidence-based recommendations. *Kidney Int Suppl* 1999; 70: S47–55.

130. Cattran DC, Delmore T, Roscoe J, Cole E, et al. A randomized controlled trial of prednisone in patients with idiopathic membranous nephropathy. *N Engl J Med* 1989; 320: 210–215.

131. Ponticelli C, Zucchelli P, Passerini P, Cesana B, et al. A 10-year follow-up of a randomized study with methylprednisolone and chlorambucil in membranous nephropathy. *Kidney Int* 1995; 48: 1600–1604.

132. Cattran DC, Greenwood C, Ritchie S, Bernstein K, et al. A controlled trial of cyclosporine in patients with progressive membranous nephropathy. Canadian Glomerulonephritis Study Group. *Kidney Int* 1995; 47: 1130–1135.

133. Cattran DC, Appel GB, Hebert LA, Hunsicker LG, et al. Cyclosporine in patients with steroid-resistant membranous nephropathy: a randomized trial. *Kidney Int* 2001; 59: 1484–1490.

134. Fervenza FC, Cosio FG, Erickson SB, Specks U, et al. Rituximab treatment of idiopathic membranous nephropathy. *Kidney Int* 2008 Jan;73(1):117–25.

135. Branten AJ, du Buf-Vereijken PW, Vervloet M, Wetzels JF. Mycophenolate mofetil in idiopathic membranous nephropathy: a clinical trial with comparison to a historic control group treated with cyclophosphamide. *Am J Kidney Dis* 2007; 50: 248–256.

136. Wehrmann M, Bohle A, Bogenschutz O, Eissele R, et al. Long-term prognosis of chronic idiopathic membranous glomerulonephritis. An analysis of 334 cases with particular regard to tubulo-interstitial changes. *Clin Nephrol* 1989; 31: 67–76.

137. Troyanov S, Wall CA, Miller JA, Scholey JW, et al. Focal and segmental glomerulosclerosis: definition and relevance of a partial remission. *J Am Soc Nephrol* 2005; 16: 1061–1068.

138. Stokes MB, Alpers CE. Combined membranous nephropathy and IgA nephropathy. *Am J Kidney Dis* 1998; 32: 649–656.

139. Llach F, Papper S, Massry SG. The clinical spectrum of renal vein thrombosis: acute and chronic. *Am J Med* 1980; 69: 819–827.

140. Rosenmann E, Pollak VE, Pirani CL. Renal vein thrombosis in the adult: a clinical and pathologic study based on renal biopsies. *Medicine (Baltimore)* 1968; 47: 269–335.

141. Markowitz GS, Brignol F, Burns ER, Koenigsberg M, et al. Renal vein thrombosis treated with thrombolytic therapy: case report and brief review. *Am J Kidney Dis* 1995; 25: 801–806.

142. Ramos EL. Recurrent diseases in the renal allograft. *J Am Soc Nephrol* 1991; 2: 109–121.

143. Truong L, Gelfand J, D'Agati V, Tomaszewski J, et al. De novo membranous glomerulonephropathy in renal allografts: a report of ten cases and review of the literature. *Am J Kidney Dis* 1989; 14: 131–144.

144. Parker SM, Pullman JM, Khauli RB. Successful transplantation of a kidney with early membranous nephropathy. *Urology* 1995; 46: 870–872.

145. Nakazawa K, Shimojo H, Komiyama Y, Itoh N, et al. Preexisting membranous nephropathy in allograft kidney. *Nephron* 1999; 81: 76–80.

146. Habib R. Nephrotic syndrome in the 1st year of life. *Pediatr Nephrol* 1993; 7: 347–353.

147. Gbadegesin R, Hinkes BG, Hoskins BE, Vlangos CN, et al. Mutations in PLCE1 are a Major Cause of Isolated Diffuse Mesangial Sclerosis (IDMS). *Nephrol Dial Transplant* 2007.

148. Kestila M, Lenkkeri U, Mannikko M, Lamerdin J, et al. Positionally cloned gene for a novel glomerular protein–nephrin–is mutated in congenital nephrotic syndrome. *Mol Cell* 1998; 1: 575–582.

149. Kuusniemi AM, Merenmies J, Lahdenkari AT, Holmberg C, et al. Glomerular sclerosis in kidneys with congenital nephrotic syndrome (NPHS1). *Kidney Int* 2006; 70: 1423–1431.

150. Benigni A, Gagliardini E, Tomasoni S, Abbate M, et al. Selective impairment of gene expression and assembly of nephrin in human diabetic nephropathy. *Kidney Int* 2004; 65: 2193–2200.

151. Dudley J, Fenton T, Unsworth J, Chambers T, et al. Systemic lupus erythematosus presenting as congenital nephrotic syndrome. *Pediatr Nephrol* 1996; 10: 752–755.

152. Kambham N, Tanji N, Seigle RL, Markowitz GS, et al. Congenital focal segmental glomerulosclerosis associated with beta4 integrin mutation and epidermolysis bullosa. *Am J Kidney Dis* 2000; 36: 190–196.

153. Wang SX, Ahola H, Palmen T, Solin ML, et al. Recurrence of nephrotic syndrome after transplantation in CNF is due to autoantibodies to nephrin. *Exp Nephrol* 2001; 9: 327–331.

154. Srivastava T, Garola RE, Kestila M, Tryggvason K, et al. Recurrence of proteinuria following renal transplantation in congenital nephrotic syndrome of the Finnish type. *Pediatr Nephrol* 2006; 21: 711–718.

155. Habib R, Gubler MC, Antignac C, Gagnadoux MF. Diffuse mesangial sclerosis: a congenital glomerulopathy with nephrotic syndrome. *Adv Nephrol Necker Hosp* 1993; 22: 43–57.

156. Habib R, Loirat C, Gubler MC, Niaudet P, et al. The nephropathy associated with male pseudohermaphroditism and Wilms' tumor (Drash syndrome): a distinctive glomerular lesion–report of 10 cases. *Clin Nephrol* 1985; 24: 269–278.

157. Denamur E, Bocquet N, Mougenot B, Da Silva F, et al. Mother-to-child transmitted WT1 splice-site mutation is responsible for distinct glomerular diseases. *J Am Soc Nephrol* 1999; 10: 2219–2223.

158. Zenker M, Aigner T, Wendler O, Tralau T, et al. Human laminin beta2 deficiency causes congenital nephrosis with mesangial sclerosis and distinct eye abnormalities. *Hum Mol Genet* 2004; 13: 2625–2632.

159. Hasselbacher K, Wiggins RC, Matejas V, Hinkes BG, et al. Recessive missense mutations in LAMB2 expand the clinical spectrum of LAMB2-associated disorders. *Kidney Int* 2006; 70: 1008–1012.

CHAPTER 5

Glomerular Diseases Associated Primarily with Asymptomatic or Gross Hematuria

Randolph A. Hennigar, MD, James A. Tumlin, MD

INTRODUCTION

Hematuria is classified as either gross or microscopic and may be isolated, transient, recurrent, persistent, symptomatic, or asymptomatic. Gross hematuria (macrohematuria) is defined as the visible appearance of blood in the urine. Microscopic hematuria (microhematuria) utilizes urine microscopy for diagnosis and may be defined as the presence of as few as 2–10 red blood cells (RBCs) per high-power field. Hematuria can be further subclassified as either glomerular or nonglomerular in origin, with the incidence of nonglomerular forms far exceeding that of glomerular hematuria. Microhematuria by itself is most often asymptomatic and incidental with associations ranging from rigorous exercise to cancer. Subsequently, the workup for hematuria can be extensive depending on the patient's age, gender, medical history, and clinical presentation. The presence of RBC casts, dysmorphic RBCs, and proteinuria on urinalysis argue for a glomerular source. The current chapter discusses glomerulopathies that are the most common glomerular diseases associated with isolated hematuria: IgA nephropathy, Henoch-Schonlein purpura, hereditary nephritis (Alport syndrome), thin basement membrane nephropathy, and loin pain hematuria syndrome.

The algorithm shown in Figure 5.1 depicts the basic workup of a patient with hematuria. Once the hematuria is defined as glomerular in origin, then consideration is given to the clinical differential diagnoses listed in Table 5.1. The histologic algorithm shown in Figure 5.2 is then applied as a basic approach to narrow the clinical differential.

IgA NEPHROPATHY

Introduction

IgA nephropathy (IgAN) or Berger's disease was first described in 1968 [1]. Although IgAN is classically thought of as a hematuric disease, all twenty-five of the original patients had moderate proteinuria in addition to recurrent hematuria. About half of the patients also reported bouts of gross hematuria "usually following an episode of acute sore throat." Dr. Liliane Striker, a protégé of Berger, recalls the light microscopy in detail: "The histologic findings ranged from focal and segmental lesions with occasional areas of necrosis to small intracapillary thrombosis, synechiae, and areas of hyalinosis. There was also a mild increase in the number of mesangial cells" [2]. According

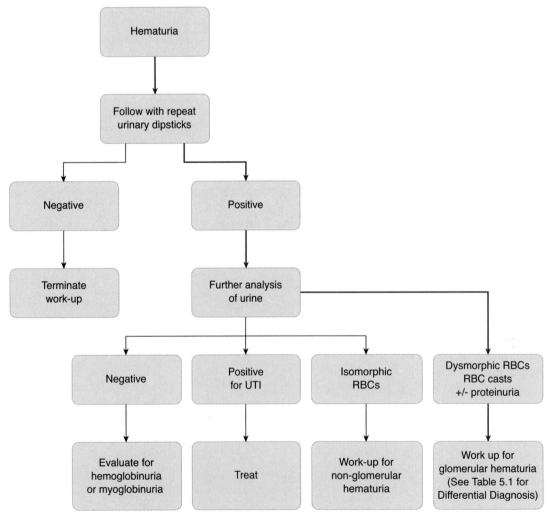

FIGURE 5.1:   Basic approach to assess the patient presenting with hematuria.

Table 5.1 Clinical Differential Diagnosis of Glomerular Hematuria

I. Glomerulopathies Associated Predominantly with Hematuria
Primary IgA nephropathy
Thin basement membrane nephropathy
Alport's disease (hereditary nephritis)
Loin pain hematuria syndrome

II. Glomerulonephritis (GN) Associated Predominantly with Hematuria and Proteinuria or Acute Nephritic Syndrome
Primary IgA nephropathy
Alport's disease (hereditary nephritis)
Nail-patella syndrome
Acute postinfectious GN
Infectious GN
Idiopathic membranoproliferative GN
ANCA-mediated disease
Anti-GBM or Goodpasture's disease

III. Other Systemic Diseases Associated with Glomerular Hematuria
Henoch-Schonlein purpura
Systemic lupus erythematosus
Essential mixed cryoglobulinemia
Thrombotic microangiopathies

IV. Disorders Associated with Glomerular IgA Deposition (Secondary IgA Nephropathy)
Hepatobiliary: chronic liver disease, cirrhosis
Gastrointestinal: ulcerative colitis, Crohn's disease, and celiac disease
Infectious: HIV, hepatitis B, *Staph. aureus* (methicillin-resistant), *Helicobacter*, and *Mycobacterium*
Integumentary: psoriasis, erythema nodosum, and dermatitis herpetiformis
Respiratory: cystic fibrosis, idiopathic interstitial pneumonia, and chronic obstructive bronchiolitis
Neoplastic: renal cell carcinoma, monoclonal IgA gammopathies, mycosis fungoides, lymphoma, Hodgkin's disease, and lung cancer
Systemic and inherited diseases: ankylosing spondylitis, sarcoidosis, Behcet's disease, Reiter's syndrome, Fabry disease, and thin basement membrane nephropathy

Table 5.2 Relative Prevalence of IgA Nephropathy Worldwide (A Partial List)

High	Low
China	United Kingdom
Japan	United States
Singapore	Canada
Hong Kong	Polynesians of New Zealand
Australia	Africa (and people of African descent)
Finland	
France	
Southern Europe	
Native Americans of New Mexico	
Aborigines of Australia	

Modified from Donadio and Grande [6].

to Striker, the biopsies consistently showed strong mesangial immunofluorescence for IgA and to a lesser extent for IgG and C3. Electron microscopy revealed mesangial dense deposits occurring mainly along the periphery of the mesangium. Soon after the original article, a second report by Berger recapitulated his earlier findings in an additional fifty-five patients [3]. Since then, IgAN has emerged as the most common form of glomerulonephritis (GN) in the world [4,5].

Epidemiology and Clinical Presentation

Table 5.2 lists the prevalence of IgAN in selected countries, regions, and ethnic groups worldwide (6). Although IgAN is prevalent in all ethnic groups, China, Japan and Singapore have some of the highest recorded incidences. About half of all new cases of GN and about 40 percent of all end-stage renal disease (ESRD) in Japan are attributed to IgAN. Indeed, prevalence rates are high along the western Pacific Rim and in Southeast Asia, and comparatively lower in the United Kingdom and North America. IgAN accounts for about 10 and 30 percent of GN in the United States and Western Europe, respectively [7]. Patients of African descent have significantly reduced frequency compared to other populations. Differences in screening and diagnostic approaches play a role in determining prevalence of IgAN. For example, Japan and Singapore have effective screening programs for hematuria that contribute to a higher incidence of IgAN. Nevertheless, certain populations appear to have a genetic predisposition to the development of the disease.

Primary IgAN most commonly presents in the second and third decades but can occur at all ages. It is a male predominant disease with a male:female ratio reaching as high as 6:1 in the United States and northern Europe. The disease can present in any number of ways including (1) gross hematuria, (2) asymptomatic microscopic hematuria and proteinuria, (3) acute nephritic syndrome with hypertension and renal insufficiency [including rapidly progressive GN (RPGN)], (4) nephrotic syndrome, (5) mixed nephritic–nephrotic syndrome, and (6) chronic renal failure. At least 75 percent of patients with IgAN present with hematuria. About 95 percent develop hematuria at some point in their disease. Emancipator [8] estimates that at least 50 percent of patients exhibit episodic gross hematuria, about three-fourths of whom are estimated to also have underlying persistent or recurrent microhematuria. Accordingly, fewer than 50 percent of patients develop persistent or intermittent microhematuria without any history of macrohematuria. Most patients with IgAN also present with proteinuria that is usually mild, whereas 5–10 percent of patients have nephrotic-range proteinuria or nephrotic syndrome. On average, about 30 percent of adults have hypertension at the time of biopsy.

The clinical presentation of primary IgAN is variable and clearly influenced by age and ethnicity. Pediatric and young patients present with painless macroscopic hematuria concurrent with onset of a viral pharyngitis, gastroenteritis, or pneumonia. In the Western Hemisphere, nearly twice as many children than adults with IgAN develop gross hematuria (about 80 vs. 45 percent, respectively). In contrast, the incidence of macrohematuria in

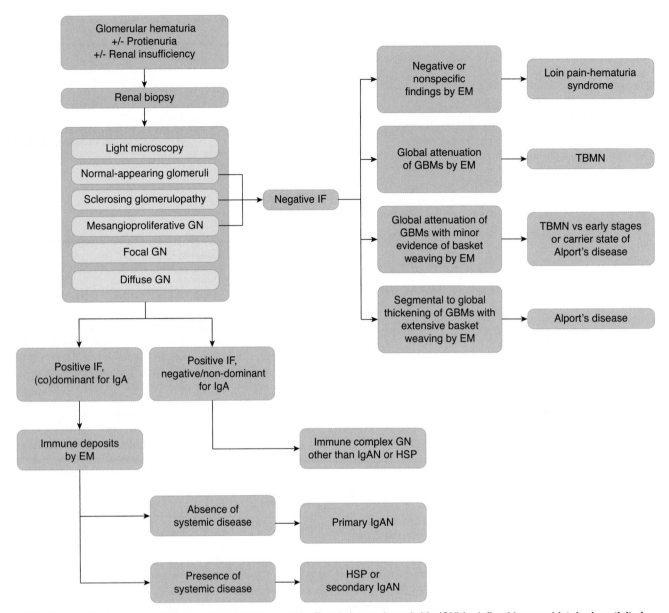

FIGURE 5.2: Histologic algorithm for glomerular hematuria. Focal glomerulonephritis (GN) is defined here as histologic activity in fewer than 50 percent of glomeruli, whereas diffuse GN is defined as histologic activity in 50 percent or greater of glomeruli (EM, electron microscopy; IF, immunofluorescence microscopy; IgAN, IgA nephropathy; HSP, Henoch-Schonlein purpura; GBMs, glomerular basement membranes; TBMN, thin basement membrane nephropathy).

children and adults is nearly the same in many regions of the Eastern Hemisphere (about 40 percent). Although macrohematuria is the most frequent initial presentation in younger patients in Western countries, as many as 20 percent of children may manifest their disease as asymptomatic microscopic hematuria with or without proteinuria [9]. Older patients (>40 years of age) tend to present with abnormal urinary sediment and proteinuria without signs of infection. Older patients are also inclined to show microscopic rather than gross hematuria, although a few studies report a higher than expected frequency of macrohematuria in older age groups [10]. IgAN in patients older than 50 years of age is associated with increased incidence of hypertension, slightly higher degrees of proteinuria, and lower creatinine clearance (CrCl), find-

ings that are just as likely related to older age than the disease itself. Onset of disease in Asian patients is more often heralded by microscopic hematuria and mild proteinuria than in Americans and Europeans, who present more frequently with gross hematuria. About 30–40 percent of patients with IgAN present with gross hematuria and renal dysfunction, including transient renal failure [11]. Renal dysfunction is more common in patients with macroscopic than microscopic hematuria, and worsening of renal function correlates with longer duration of gross hematuria. Acute renal failure is usually attributed to acute tubular necrosis in the setting of macroscopic hematuria (i.e., tubular obstruction with RBC casts) or acute necrotizing/crescentic GN, or both.

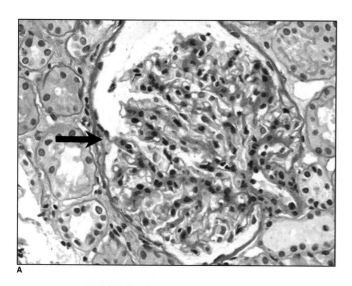

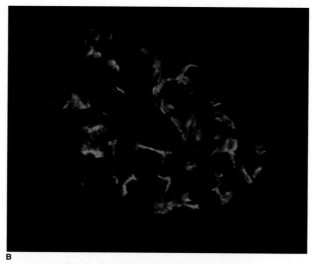

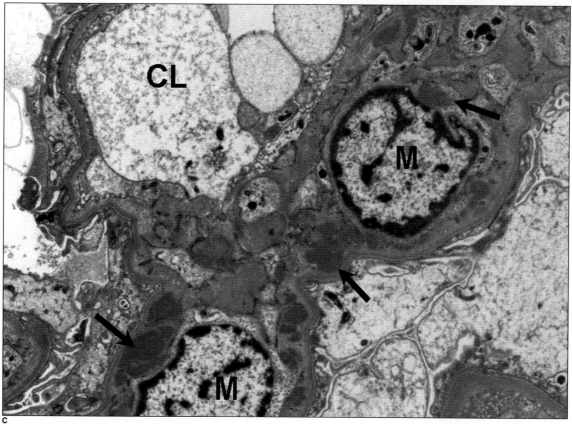

FIGURE 5.3: *"Classic" IgA nephropathy. (A) In most instances, glomeruli exhibit mild degrees of mesangial hypercellularity and matrix increase, as seen by light microscopy. The arrow delineates a small adhesion of tuft to Bowman's capsule [Periodic acid Schiff (PAS) stain, original magnification: × 400]. (B) Immunofluorescence for IgA occurs in a mesangial pattern (original magnification: × 400). (C) Electron microscopy detects granular "immune-type" dense deposits (arrows) in the mesangium (M). The capillary loop (CL) is devoid of dense deposits [Uranyl acetate-lead citrate (UA-LC) stain, original magnification: × 3,500].*

Approach to Interpretation

Light Microscopy

The diagnosis of primary IgAN is confirmed by kidney biopsy (Figure 5.2). In many instances, the biopsy reveals a "classic" form of the disease manifested as a mesangiopathic process characterized by mesangial proliferation by light microscopy, dominant or codominant mesangial IgA by immunofluorescence microscopy, and mesangial immune deposits by electron microscopy (Figure 5.3). The extent of mesangial cellularity and mesangial matrix increase is variable. Mesangial hypercellularity may be mild, moderate, or marked and is more often

Table 5.3 Comparison of the Haas and SMK Lee Classifications for Primary IgA Nephropathy

Haas subclass I *The minimal histologic lesion:* No more than minimal mesangial hypercellularity. No histologic activity or segmental glomerulosclerosis.	**Lee grade I** Similar to Haas subclass I but requires that tubulointerstitial scarring and inflammation be absent.
Haas subclass II *Focal segmental glomerulosclerosis-like:* Resembles primary focal sclerosis with no more than minimal mesangial hypercellularity. No histologic activity.	**Lee grade II** *Focal segmental mesangial hypercellularity and matrix increase:* Rare small crescents allowed. Requires that interstitial scarring and inflammation be absent.
Haas subclass III *Focal proliferative GN:* The presence of mesangial hypercellularity, endocapillary proliferation, cellular crescents, necrosis or any combination thereof in <50% of glomeruli. Lesions may be segmental or global. Includes cases of mild focal and segmental mesangial proliferative GN.	**Lee grade III** *Diffuse mesangial hypercellularity and matrix increase with focal and segmental "variation":* Occasional small crescents and tuft adhesions allowed. Focal interstitial edema and infiltrate occasionally present.
Haas subclass IV *Diffuse proliferative GN:* The presence of mesangial hypercellularity, endocapillary proliferation and cellular crescents in >50% of glomeruli. Lesions may be segmental or global.	**Lee grade IV** *Marked diffuse mesangial hypercellularity and matrix increase:* Cellular crescents allowed in up to 45% of glomeruli. Segmental to global glomerulosclerosis frequent. Tubulointerstitial scarring, interstitial inflammation, and interstitial foam cells allowed.
Haas subclass V *Advanced chronic glomerulopathy:* ≥ 40% glomerular obsolescence and/or ≥ 40% cortical tubular atrophy or loss.	**Lee grade V** "Similar to IV but more severe." >45% cellular crescents. Severe tubulointerstitial scarring or interstitial inflammation.

segmental than global in distribution. In some instances, mesangial proliferation is nominal and results in bland-appearing glomeruli by light microscopy. On the other hand, there are cases showing overt histologic activity in glomeruli, either in the form of endocapillary proliferation, cellular/fibrocellular crescents, fibrinoid necrosis, karyorrhexis, or any combination thereof. Such changes are usually accompanied by varying degrees of mesangial hypercellularity and matrix increase. Diffuse or florid mesangial proliferation by itself is seen only occasionally.

Although IgAN is commonly perceived as a mesangiopathic disease, glomerular lesions outside of the mesangium are relatively frequent (Figure 5.4). For example, the overall incidence of endocapillary proliferation in IgAN is estimated between 20 and 25 percent [8]. Endocapillary proliferation by itself occurs infrequently in IgAN, and in the vast majority of cases, it is accompanied by impingement of increased mesangial cells and matrix upon capillary lumina (Figure 5.4A). It is usually focal, segmental, and mild (Figure 5.4B). Diffuse or global endocapillary proliferation is infrequent. Extracapillary proliferation in the form of cellular or fibrocellular crescents occurs in about 10–35 percent of patients with primary IgAN (Figure 5.4C) [12–15]. They tend to be focal and noncircumferential (Figures 5.4A,D), rather than diffuse and fulminate (Figure 5.4C). Fewer than 2 percent of patients exhibit diffuse crescentic disease (greater than 50 percent crescents on initial biopsy). Crescents are sometimes accompanied by acute necrotizing lesions (i.e., fibrinoid necrosis) (Figure 5.4D). An estimated one in ten biopsies from patients with IgAN exhibits acute necrotizing GN

[16]. These lesions tend to be focal and segmental, and are accompanied by karyorrhexis and cellular crescents. A pure or florid acute necrotizing GN is uncommon in IgAN and warrants investigation of possible underlying antineutrophil cytoplasmic antibodies (ANCA) [17].

For years after the first descriptions of IgAN, a failure to achieve a representative nomenclature slowed the understanding of the natural history of specific subtypes of IgA and blocked development of class-specific therapies. In an attempt to address this problem, Lee and colleagues borrowed the Meadow's classification of Henoch-Schonlein purpura and modified it for IgAN (Table 5.3) [18,19]. Although the criteria are somewhat rigid, Lee's classification has certain practicalities that are still used in some quarters today. A more contemporary and versatile classification was introduced by Hass in 1997 (Table 5.3) [20]. The earlier classification of Lee et al. and the WHO classification for lupus nephritis served as the foundation for the Haas classification. In this classification, patients are divided into five subclasses based on the degree of mesangial cell proliferation, extent of glomerulosclerosis, and the quantity of extra- or endocapillary proliferation. Cases where the biopsy shows only minimal increase in mesangial cellularity are assigned to class I (Figures 5.5A,B). Class II lesions essentially represent examples of class I but with additional features of focal segmental glomerular sclerosis (FSGS) (Figures 5.5C,D). Class III disease, or focal proliferative IgAN, is characterized by increased mesangial hypercellularity, endocapillary proliferation, and/or cellular/fibrocellular crescents in fewer than 50 percent of glomeruli (Figure 5.6). Similar lesions in greater than

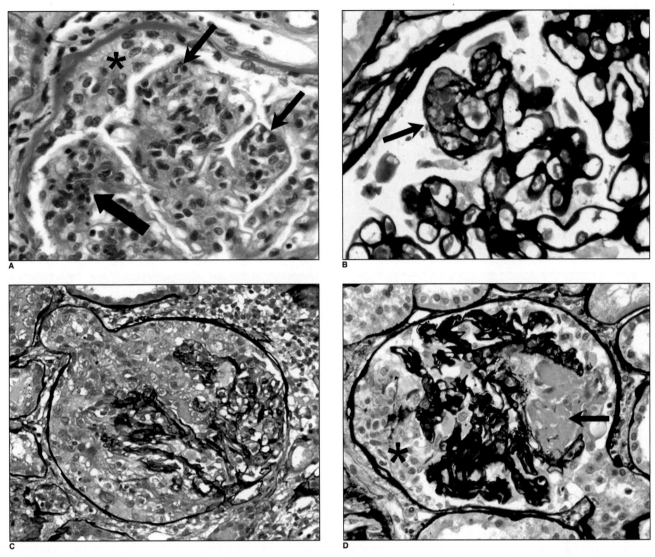

FIGURE 5.4: *Histologic activity in IgAN. (A) Endocapillary proliferation (smaller arrows) is characterized by occlusion of glomerular capillary loops by infiltrating mononuclear inflammatory cells and endothelial cell swelling and proliferation. It is usually associated with varying degrees of mesangial proliferation (larger arrow). The asterisk (*) marks a small cellular crescent. Cellular crescents are often accompanied by endocapillary and mesangial proliferation in IgAN [hematoxylin and eosin (H&E) stain, original magnification: × 400]. (B) Endocapillary proliferation in IgAN is usually limited to smaller, segmental lesions (arrow) [Jones' methenamine silver (JMS) stain, original magnification: × 600]. (C) A large cellular crescent fills Bowman's space and compresses the glomerular tuft (JMS stain, original magnification: × 400). (D) Crescentic lesions (*) may be associated with segmental fibrinoid necrosis (arrow) (JMS stain, original magnification: × 400).*

50 percent of glomeruli push the patient into class IV, or diffuse proliferative IgAN (Figures 5.7–5.9). Membranoproliferative forms of IgAN fall into this category, as well (Figure 5.10). Class V, or chronic sclerosing IgAN, encompasses those cases where ≥40 percent of glomeruli are globally sclerotic and/or where tubular atrophy approximates 40 percent or greater (Figure 5.11). Table 5.3 compares the specific criteria for both the Lee and Haas classifications.

The prevalence of Haas class I among biopsied cases of IgAN ranges from 10 to 50 percent (Figures 5.5A,B) [21]. Class I may progress to other classes analogous to lupus nephritis but with far less frequency. The prevalence of FSGS-like IgAN (Haas class II) varies but is generally 10 percent or less [21].

FSGS-like IgAN contrasts with idiopathic FSGS in showing a significantly lower incidence in African-Americans [22]. The diagnosis can be made on a single glomerulus showing segmental sclerosis. Adhesions of tuft to Bowman's capsule with synechiae are frequent, similar to primary FSGS (Figures 5.5C,D). Mesangial proliferation is nominal; endocapillary proliferation and cellular crescents are absent. Extracapillary proliferation may be present in the form of mild visceral epithelial cell hyperplasia and hypertrophy overlying areas of segmental sclerosis, also similar to primary FSGS. About one-third of biopsied patients with IgAN exhibit focal proliferative forms of IgAN (Haas class III) (Figure 5.6) [21]. Morphologies within class III include: (1) "relatively mild" focal and segmental

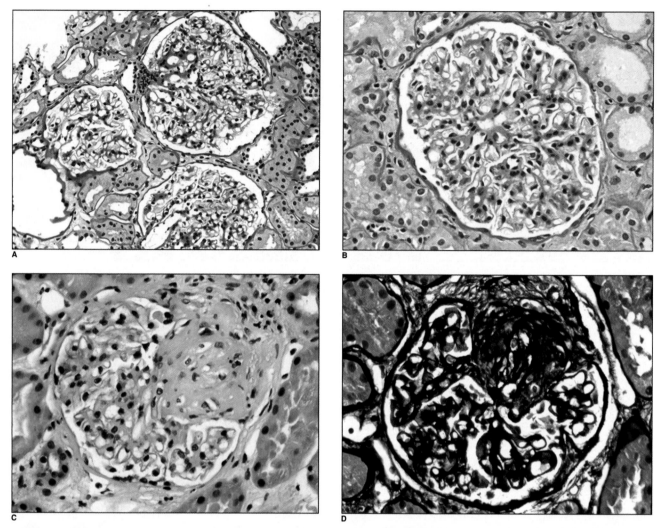

FIGURE 5.5: *Glomerular histology of Haas class I and II lesions. (A) Class I is characterized by glomeruli that are normal or nearly normal in appearance by light microscopy (PAS stain, original magnification: × 200). (B) In class I, glomeruli may exhibit mild mesangial prominence with mild increase in mesangial matrix but minimal increase in mesangial cells (PAS stain, original magnification: × 400). (C) Focal segmental glomerular sclerosis (FSGS)-like IgAN (Class II) resembles class I disease, but shows additional evidence of segmental glomerular sclerosis with adhesion of the scarred tuft segment to Bowman's capsule. Mesangial hypercellularity is nominal, similar to class I (H&E stain, original magnification: × 400). (D) Silver staining of the same glomerulus depicted in (C) (JMS stain, original magnification: × 400).*

mesangioproliferative GN (Figure 5.6A); (2) focal GN with segmental endocapillary proliferation with or without cellular crescents (Figure 5.6C); (3) focal GN with focal and segmental glomerulosclerosis; and (4) focal crescentic GN (Figure 5.6D). Haas class IV IgAN is found in 10–30 percent of biopsied cohorts [21]. Diffuse proliferative IgAN is equally diverse in its morphology (Figures 5.7–5.9). Lesions may range from diffuse mesangial hypercellularity without any other indicators of histologic activity (Figure 5.7), to fulminate acute necrotizing and crescentic GN (Figure 5.9). It should be noted that quantitation of crescents includes fibrocellular crescents and excludes sclerosed glomeruli. The criteria for Haas class V (advanced chronic glomerulopathy) is based solely on the extent of glomerular and tubulointerstitial scarring (≥40 percent), regardless of histologic activity (Figure 5.11). These cases account for 5–40 percent of IgAN.

Tubulointerstitial scarring (interstitial fibrosis and tubular atrophy) may be seen at any stage of IgAN. In class I disease, its presence is usually attributed to hypertension, although changes of hypertensive nephrosclerosis can occur at any stage of the disease. In FSGS-like IgAN, the extent of tubulointerstitial scarring is usually commensurate with the degree of glomerulosclerosis and maybe accompanied by a mild nonspecific chronic interstitial inflammatory infiltrate. The degree of tubulointerstitial scarring in higher grades of IgAN (Haas classes III and IV) is dependent upon several factors: (1) the progression of glomerular injury to glomerulosclerosis secondary to deposition of nephritogenic IgA; (2) the extent of active interstitial inflammation; and (3) the presence of other underlying diseases such as hypertension, infection, kidney stones, or a concomitant GN. In our experience, IgAN with highly active glomerular lesions (endocapillary proliferation, crescents, and/or segmental fibrinoid necrosis in ≥10 percent of glomeruli) are often accompanied by varying degrees of acute and chronic tubulointerstitial nephritis with prominent eosinophils. If left untreated, these cases will progress to ESRD within 3 years [23]. RBC casts are commonly seen and may correlate with transient renal failure (Figure 5.12).

Immunofluorescence Microscopy

The key diagnostic feature of IgAN is the demonstration of IgA deposition in glomerular mesangium by immunofluorescence microscopy (Figures 5.3B and 5.13A). IgA should be the dominant or at least codominant immunoglobulin in order to make the diagnosis of IgAN. Codeposition of C3 is common with IgG and less common with IgM (Figures 5.13B,C). C1q is infrequent but when present warrants suspicion of a secondary IgAN or possibly lupus nephritis. Immunofluorescence for C4 is rare. The deposition of κ and/or λ light chains is extremely variable. Both light chains are usually present but λ tends to immunofluoresce more brightly than κ (Figure 5.13D). This feature of λ immunofluorescence can be helpful sometimes in cases where the diagnosis of IgAN may be confounded by codominant immunoglobulins depositing along with IgA. The prevalence of λ-IgA does not represent a monoclonal proliferation. Mesangial immunofluorescence for fibrinogen is present in most cases of IgAN, which is consistent with studies reporting an affinity of IgA for fibrinogen.

Extension of IgA immunofluorescence into peripheral capillary loops is a marker of immune complex deposition outside of the mesangium and usually associated with more proliferative forms of the disease (Figure 5.14). Granular immunofluorescence for IgA along capillary loops in a pattern suggestive of membranous glomerulopathy is atypical for primary IgAN and probably represents either a secondary or an unrelated process, particularly hepatitis B–associated GN. Finally, glomerular deposition of IgA by itself may occur in apparently healthy asymptomatic individuals; the significance of these deposits is unclear [24].

Electron Microscopy

Electron microscopy is not required to make the diagnosis of IgAN but is utilized nonetheless to confirm the presence of granular electron-dense immune deposits in the mesangium (Figure 5.3C). Mesangial deposits may be sparse or abundant and associated with varying degrees of mesangial matrix increase. Sparsely distributed deposits tend to be small and aggregate along the periphery of the mesangium, just underneath the overlying basement membrane (paramesangium) or adjacent to the capillary lumina (Figure 5.15). Small deposits may be hard to detect and can be missed altogether if they are of lighter density. When abundant, immune deposits usually extend from the periphery deeper into the mesangial stalk where they are embedded in increased matrix material (Figure 5.16).

Although IgA deposition in glomerular mesangium is the hallmark of IgAN, the incidence of concomitant immune complex deposition along glomerular capillary walls is estimated in about 50 percent of cases [25]. Subendothelial immune deposits may be found in as many as 55 percent of IgAN patients, [26],

whereas they are uncommon in our biopsy population. They are usually small, elongated, and associated with mild subendothelial widening of capillary walls (Figure 5.17A). It is noteworthy that paramesangial immune deposits adjacent to the glomerular capillary loops maybe misinterpreted as subendothelial deposits. Membranoproliferative forms of IgAN exhibit larger subendothelial deposits that are sometimes accompanied by mesangial cell interposition and reduplication of glomerular basement membranes (GBMs) (Figure 5.17B). Subepithelial immune deposits tend to be small and infrequent (Figure 5.18). The presence of numerous subepithelial deposits is atypical for primary or secondary IgAN and implies a superimposed or unrelated immune complex–mediated process.

A number of GBM alterations have been described in IgAN with segmental attenuation being the most common. Other findings include: segmental reduplication or splitting of the lamina densa ("basket weaving") with alternating GBM thickening and attenuation similar to Alport's disease; segmental erosion of the external portions of the lamina densa; occasional gaps or "lysis" along GBMs; outward "spike-like" projections not associated with subepithelial dense deposits; and a few other miscellaneous findings [27–29].

Differential Diagnosis

Since IgAN is a hematuric disease, a thorough clinical differential includes a complete list of extrarenal and renal diseases that exhibit hematuria, which goes beyond the scope of this chapter. Instead, Figure 5.1 shows a basic algorithm leading up to glomerular hematuria. Table 5.1 continues with the clinical differential diagnosis of glomerular hematuria. Narrowing the differential down to IgAN on clinical grounds is an acuminous exercise that again goes beyond the scope of the book. Nevertheless, the clinician is responsible for ruling out as many mimickers as possible. The pathologist usually provides the lynchpin, since the kidney biopsy represents the gold standard for the diagnosis of IgAN.

The diagnosis does not always end with the simple detection of IgA, however. Ample amounts of IgA can deposit in the setting of any number of other diseases, which can confound interpretation. For instance, mesangial deposits of IgA are sometimes encountered in minimal change disease [30]. These cases are usually classified and treated as minimal change disease and not IgAN. The immune deposits are perceived as incidental since they have nominal impact on presentation, progression, outcome, or treatment [31]. On the other hand, some studies describe "minimal change disease with IgA deposits" where patients are symptomatic for both diseases and do not readily respond to steroids [32]. Such cases may represent mixed lesions, where a podocytopathy is superimposed upon primary IgAN. In another example, prodigious amounts of IgA may deposit in infectious or postinfectious GN associated with methicillin-resistant forms of *Staphylococcus aureus* and *epidermidis*, and therefore mimics IgAN [33–35]. These cases are usually characterized by positive cultures, hypocomplementemia, and subepithelial "humps," which help to reveal their infectious nature and distinguish them from primary IgAN.

IgAN can collide with a whole host of other diseases including thin basement membrane nephropathy, diabetes mellitus, ANCA-associated diseases (Figure 5.19), anti-GBM disease,

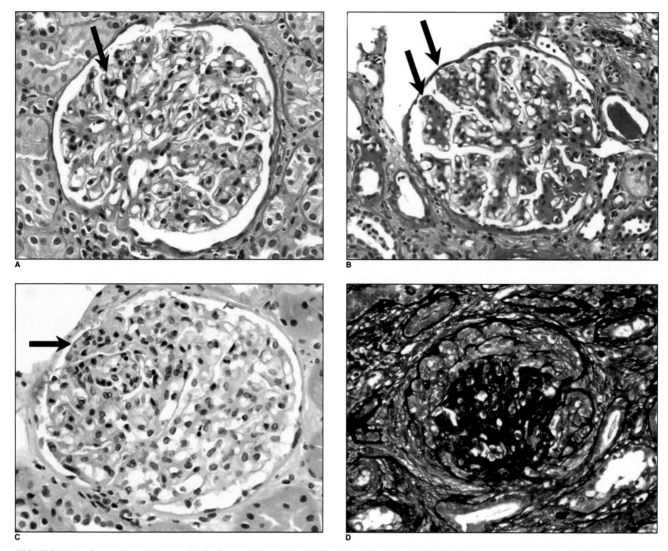

FIGURE 5.6: *Examples of glomerular lesions of Haas class III (focal proliferative IgAN). (A,B) The appearance of mild (A) to moderate (B) segmental mesangial hypercellularity and matrix increase (arrows) in fewer than 50 percent of glomeruli, places the biopsy into the category of focal proliferative IgAN (Haas class III) (PAS stain). (C) Endocapillary proliferation, when present, is usually segmental in distribution (arrow) (H&E stain). (D) A fulminate cellular crescent compresses the glomerular tuft in a case of focal crescentic IgAN (JMS stain, original magnification: × 400).*

antiphospholipid antibody syndrome, and hemolytic uremic syndrome, among others. In certain instances, there is a reasonable degree of suspicion that the "collision" is not fortuitous and that the presence of IgA is either directly or indirectly related to the other disease, especially if abrogation of the latter eliminates the former. For this and other reasons, such cases are often classified as secondary IgAN. The bottom of Table 5.1 lists the more commonly recognized associations and excludes diseases where the "association" with IgAN is restricted to a single case report. Exclusion of other diseases is a necessary step in establishing a diagnosis of primary IgAN. Consequently, the differential diagnosis of IgAN includes its secondary forms.

Certain generalizations can be made about secondary IgAN. The majority of cases are subclinical and benign. The depositing IgA is often nonnephritogenic and the failure to activate complement probably renders many cases clinically irrelevant.

Clinical manifestations, when present, are usually mild and limited to asymptomatic microscopic hematuria with or without mild proteinuria. Some patients with mild clinical activity may eventually develop renal insufficiency. However, clinically aggressive disease with gross hematuria, nephrotic syndrome, or RPGN is uncommon. The histology of secondary IgAN is usually unremarkable or shows only a mild mesangioproliferative process. Progression to glomerular sclerosis is infrequent. Histologic activity is rare. Immunofluorescence microscopy reveals dominant IgA deposition in a mesangial pattern with a lesser incidence of IgG codominance than in primary IgAN. C3 deposition also occurs to a lesser degree in secondary versus primary IgAN. Immune deposits detected by electron microscopy are usually restricted to the mesangium. Therapy for secondary IgAN is similar to other secondary GNs, that is, successful treatment of the underlying disease tends to

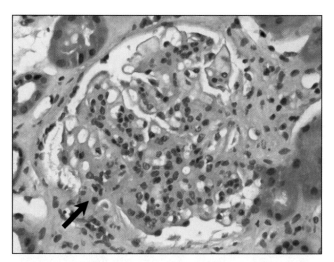

FIGURE 5.7: *Diffuse proliferative IgAN (Haas class IV). The extent of mesangial proliferation varies in diffuse proliferative IgAN. This case shows marked global mesangial hypercellularity and matrix increase with adhesion of the tuft to Bowman's capsule and early segmental sclerosis (arrow) (H&E stain, original magnification: × 400).*

ameliorate the GN. On the other hand, therapies specifically targeting the GN should be considered in instances of secondary IgAN with aggressive features.

Cirrhosis is the most common cause of secondary IgAN [36]. About 40–45 percent of patients with cirrhosis exhibit (co)dominant deposition of IgA in glomeruli [8]. Secondary deposition of IgA in cirrhosis occurs regardless of the etiology but is most prevalent in the alcoholic form. Like most secondary forms of IgAN, the vast majority of patients with cirrhosis-associated IgAN have little or no clinical manifestations of renal disease. Unlike primary IgAN and other secondary forms, there is a greater frequency of MPGN and MPGN-like lesions, as well as nodular glomerulosclerosis reminiscent of diabetic nephropathy (Figure 5.20). These lesions can sometimes be quite aggressive. Mesangial deposition of IgG and C1q occurs more frequently in cirrhosis-associated IgAN, in contrast to other secondary forms of IgAN. Of note, significant immunofluorescence for IgM may suggest codeposition of cryoglobulin, which sometimes binds to circulating IgA immune complexes in cirrhosis.

Etiology and Pathogenesis

Etiology

The cause of primary IgAN is unknown. Table 5.4 lists most of the suspected etiologic agents. The association between onset of IgAN with pharyngitis, gastroenteritis or pneumonia implies linkage to infectious agents. Antibodies to a wide variety of viral and bacterial agents have been detected in sera from IgAN patients. However, attempts to link IgAN to viral infection are inconsistent and controversial. Bacterial antigens have been identified in both the sera and the glomeruli of patients. Antigen derived from *Haemophilus parainfluenzae* is detected in the

mesangium of about one-third of patients, whereas antigen derived from *Staph. aureus* cell envelope colocalizes with glomerular IgA deposits in about 70 percent of patients [37]. The data are convincing but require further investigation and development. Other exogenous reagents thought to be involved in the etiology of IgAN include a variety of dietary substances. IgA antibodies to gliadin, a constituent of gluten, are occasionally encountered in IgAN. The results suggest a role for gluten intolerance in IgAN, but the concept has yet to reach fruition. Although a great deal of attention has focused on exogenous moieties, endogenous antigens have also been investigated including fibronectin and IgA itself.

Genetic Susceptibility

The ethnic clustering of IgAN suggests genetic factors. A role for genetics was bolstered further by the discovery of more than 100 families exhibiting inheritance patterns for IgAN [38,39]. The genetic transmission of IgAN appears to follow an autosomal dominant pattern of inheritance with incomplete penetrance and does not adhere to the laws of classic Mendelian inheritance. The reason, in all likelihood, is that primary IgAN is a complex polygenic disease. No single gene has yet been identified as the "IgA nephropathy gene" and no universal genetic event renders a patient susceptible to IgAN. Yet, the mere deposition of IgA in glomeruli does not cause significant pathology unless the patient is genetically susceptible. Accordingly, a number of susceptibility genes are identified for IgAN. Table 5.5 lists many but not all of them. Not surprisingly, many of these polymorphisms are inconsistent across kindreds and ethnic groups. For example, T-cell receptor Cα (TCR Cα) is a candidate susceptibility gene in Chinese, but not Japanese subpopulations. Such inconsistencies support the notion that multiple genes are involved and that molecular etiologies of IgAN vary worldwide. The molecular pathogenesis of IgAN is confounded further by environmental factors affecting expression of the multiple genes involved.

One of the more interesting gene polymorphisms occurs at the 6q22-23 locus, which has been termed the *IGAN1* gene [40]. The linkage of polymorphisms in *IGAN1* to the phenotype was highly statistically significant (LOD score >5.0) and linked to a staggering 60 percent of kindred members spanning two continents. The *IGAN1* locus harbors hundreds of genes that require further investigation to determine which are relevant to the pathogenesis of familial IgAN. Subsequently, the European IgA Nephropathy Consortium identified other multiplex families and found two loci other than *IGAN1*, associated with the development of IgAN [41]. The loci are located at 4q26-31 and 17q12-22 and contain several compelling genes including those encoding transient receptor potential channel 3, interleukin-2, interleukin-21, histone deacetylase 5, and granulin.

Background

Human IgA is subclassified into IgA1 and IgA2. Unlike IgA2, IgA1 is heavily glycosylated and is about 8 percent carbohydrate. The IgA1 molecule is both *N*- and *O*-glycosylated, which distinguishes it from the vast majority of serum proteins including IgA2 and other immunoglobulins (Figure 5.21). Both IgA1 and IgA2 exist as monomeric (mIgA) or polymeric (pIgA) forms. Although the definition of pIgA varies, we define it here as the

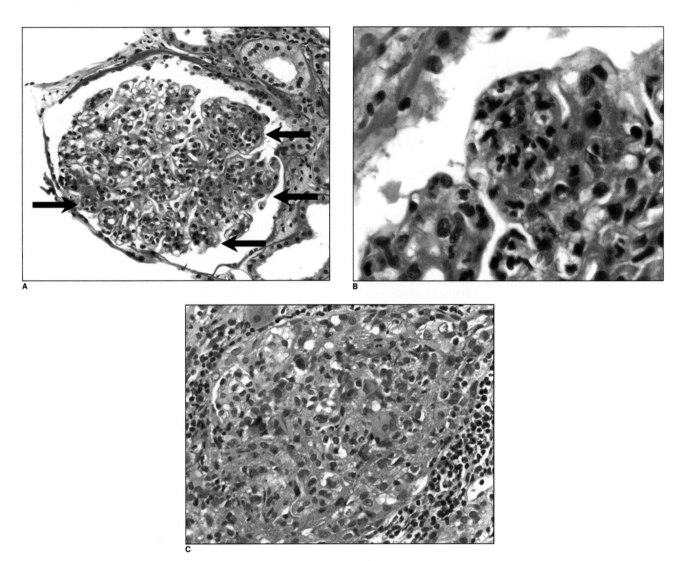

FIGURE 5.8: *Endocapillary proliferation in diffuse proliferative IgAN (Haas class IV). (A) Segmental endocapillary proliferation (arrows) is present on a background of mesangial proliferation (PAS stain, original magnification: × 400). (B) Higher magnification of (A) reveals a neutrophilic exudate as part of the proliferative process (PAS stain, original magnification: × 600). (C) Global endocapillary proliferation, as shown here, is infrequent in IgAN. The glomerulus is markedly hypercellular as a result of mesangial proliferation, endothelial cell swelling, and infiltrating polymorphonuclear and mononuclear inflammatory cells, all of which occlude the capillary loops and obliterate glomerular detail. These changes are accompanied by mild extracapillary proliferation, as well (H&E stain, original magnification: × 400).*

binding of two or more mIgA via J chains and consider dimeric IgA as the most common form of pIgA. Plasma cells in mucosa serve as the primary source of pIgA1 and pIgA2. Apparently, γδ T-cells play a major role in regulating mucosal production of IgA through the secretion of TGF-β. Although the mucosa produces mostly pIgA, serum or systemic IgA is derived predominantly from the bone marrow and is mainly mIgA1. Although mucosal pIgA and serum mIgA are under different control mechanisms, there is a complex "mucosa–bone marrow axis" that promotes cross talk between both compartments and facilitates oral tolerance. Here, antigen-specific T-cells derived from the mucosa migrate to the systemic immune compartments (bone marrow, spleen, and tonsillar tissue) and suppress potential systemic immune responses to mucosally derived antigens. This mechanism is important in preventing adverse sys-

temic reactions against food and commensal bacteria and keeps any immune response localized to the gut.

Pathogenesis of Primary IgAN

The pathophysiologic mechanisms of primary IgAN are mainly speculative and extremely complex. It is a multifactorial, polygenic disease that apparently exhibits gene–environment interaction. IgAN is also characterized by a wide variety of atypical immunologic events. The manner in which these genetic, environmental, and immunological events culminate into IgAN is unknown. Nevertheless, what follows is an attempt to summarize the most salient findings and integrate them into a plausible explanation about the pathogenesis of IgAN. Figure 5.22 collates these findings along an overly simplified pathway. A more detailed summary about the pathogenesis of primary IgAN is reviewed by Barrat et al. [42].

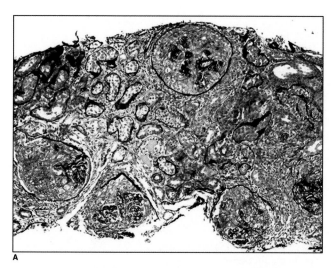

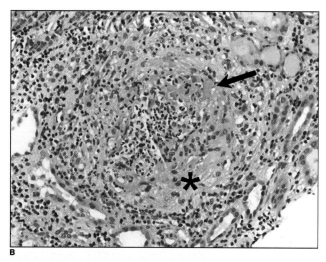

FIGURE 5.9: *Extracapillary proliferation in diffuse proliferative IgAN (Haas class IV). (A) Diffuse crescentic IgAN is uncommon in IgAN and is usually accompanied by significant tubulointerstitial damage, as shown (JMS stain, original magnification: × 200). (B) Crescentic IgAN can sometimes present with an additional component of acute necrotizing GN. Here, the glomerular tuft is heavily infiltrated by neutrophils and surrounded by a cellular crescent (*), which in turn is surrounded by an acute and chronic inflammatory infiltrate. The arrow points to early fibrinoid necrosis (H&E stain, original magnification: × 400).*

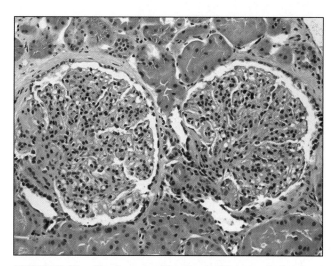

FIGURE 5.10: *Membranoproliferative IgAN accounts for about 5 percent of cases. Marked global mesangial proliferation and increased mesangial matrix impart a lobular appearance to the glomeruli. Capillary loops are variably thickened (H&E stain, original magnification: × 200).*

Primary IgAN is classified as an immune complex–mediated process based on historical data. Both circulating and in situ models of immune complex formation have been incriminated. The earliest notion was that IgA-containing immune complexes (IgAICs) were formed in the circulation and then deposited passively in mesangium. Consideration was subsequently given to the possibility that IgA might react with planted antigens or neoantigens in the mesangium (in situ formation), which would explain why certain patients with IgAN do not harbor circulating IgAICs. Acquired autoimmunity has also been proposed. Arguments pro and con exist for each mechanism and have been neither proven nor disproved. Newer paradigms are emerging, however.

Increased serum levels of IgA are not solely responsible for IgAN, as evidenced by the fact that a significant proportion of primary IgAN patients do not exhibit this finding and a significant percentage of patients with elevated serum IgA levels do not exhibit IgAN. Accordingly, there must be certain features about IgA that render it nephritogenic. Data strongly suggest that pIgA1 is the predominant form comprising IgA complexes depositing in the mesangium [43–45]. The observation that pIgA1 is the predominant isoform eluted from renal biopsies from IgAN patients, [46], as well as the high rate of recurrence of IgAN among kidney transplant recipients, implies that defects in IgA processing are central to the disease. The finding that pIgA complexes will completely resolve following transplantation into non-IgAN patients suggests that formation of polymeric complexes occurs in the plasma as opposed to de novo synthesis within the kidney [47]. Thus, the pIgA1 depositing in mesangium is derived from the circulation.

The implication has long been that the primary source of nephritogenic pIgA1 is altered or disrupted mucosa. Specifically, increased mucosal permeability leads to altered mucosal immunity and subsequent escape of pIgA1 into the circulation. However, IgAN patients exhibit decreased populations of pIgA1-secreting plasma cells in mucosa and increased populations of pIgA1-secreting plasma cells in bone marrow [48,49]. The latter finding is unexpected since bone marrow normally produces mIgA, not pIgA, and implies disruption of the mucosa–bone marrow axis and a breakdown of oral tolerance. The appearance of phenotypically mucosal IgA in the bone marrow might be blamed on mucosally activated CD4+ T-cells harboring abnormal homing signals and recently discovered in the sera of IgAN patients [50]. These cells have a potential to traffic to the systemic effector sites like the bone marrow and activate rather than suppress B-cells. Meanwhile, other data show that γδ T-cells are also significantly increased in the circulation of IgAN patients as compared to controls [51]. γδ

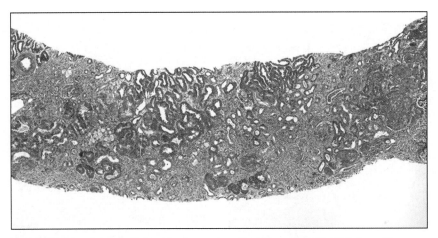

FIGURE 5.11: *Advanced chronic glomerulopathy (Haas class V). Staining with Masson's trichrome (MAS) imparts blue coloration to the fibrotic areas. At least 50–60 percent of the renal cortex is scarred (original magnification: × 50).*

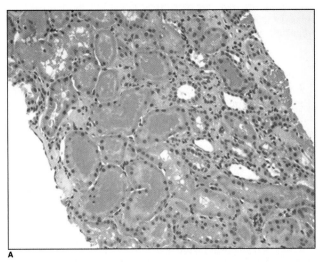
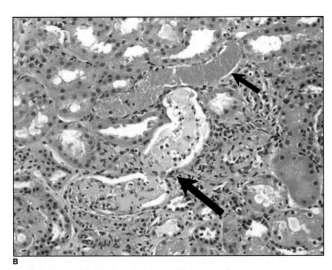

A   B

FIGURE 5.12: *Red blood cell (RBC) casts and acute renal failure in IgAN. (A) Occlusion of tubules by RBCs is common in IgAN. (B) RBC casts may be accompanied by changes of acute tubular necrosis. The larger arrow depicts a tubule containing necrotic epithelium and hyaline material, whereas the smaller arrow points to an RBC cast. Mild interstitial inflammation is also present (H&E stain, original magnification: × 200).*

T-cells normally predominate in mucosal tissue where they are responsible for the switching of naïve B-cells to IgA-secreting plasma cells. When activated, the circulating $\gamma\delta$ T-cells secrete large amounts of TGF-β in IgAN patients but not controls; TGF-β is one of the most potent cytokines promoting IgA class switching on B-cells. Theoretically, the signal also reaches CD4-primed B-cells in the bone marrow and promotes the switch there. Thus, it appears that the source of pIgA1 depositing in mesangium in IgAN is not mucosal but systemic, especially the bone marrow. In all likelihood, sensitization to mucosally derived antigens serves as the stimulus for the translocation process.

Another interesting feature of pIgA1 in IgAN is the aberrant glycosylation of its hinge region. There is an apparent failure to "cap" the O-linked core GalNAc residues with galactose (Gal) and/or sialic acid (NeuNAc), thereby leaving the GalNAc residue exposed [52,53]. The result is "Gal-deficient" O-glyco-

forms of pIgA1 that predominate in IgAN. The aberration may be attributable in part to a functional defect of β1→3 galactosyltransferase in B-cells, since peripheral B-cells of IgAN show inherently reduced activity of β1→3 galactosyltransferase [54].

Altered glycosylation of serum pIgA1 results in self-aggregation of the immunoglobulin to form circulating macromolecular complexes. Gal-deficient pIgA1 may subvert surveillance mechanisms performed by the monocyte–phagocytic system, resulting in decreased clearance of the immunoglobulin and thereby sustaining its serum concentration. Macromolecular aggregates are admixed with immune complexes in the form of IgG and IgA, which seem to recognize underglycosylated IgA as neoantigen. The aggregated complexes are bound and taken up by mesangial cells via IgA-binding receptors, which have a strong affinity for Gal-deficient IgA [52,55]. Transferrin receptor (CD71) may play a major role in capturing and

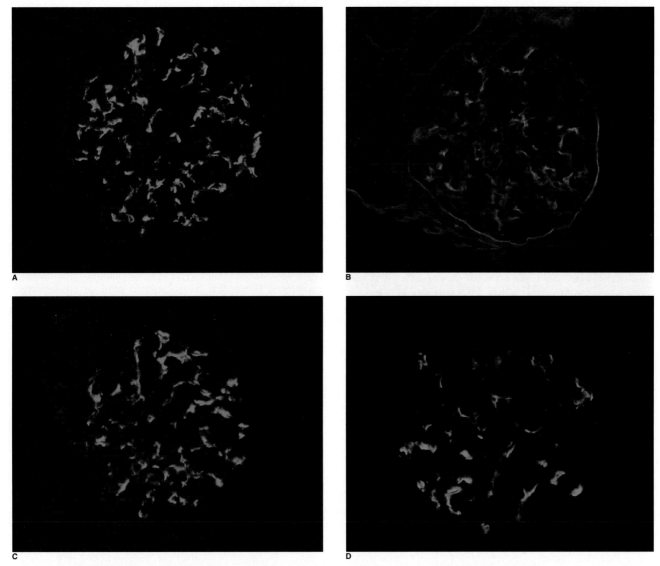

FIGURE 5.13: *Mesangial immunofluorescence in IgAN. (A) Immunofluorescence for IgA is confined predominantly to mesangium. Diagnostic criteria for IgAN require that the staining intensity for IgA is either brighter than (dominant) or equal to (codominant) that of IgG or IgM. (B) More often than not, immunofluorescence for IgG is weaker than IgA [c.f., (A)]. (C) Immunofluorescence for C3 often colocalizes with IgA in the mesangium. (D) Immunofluorescence for lambda light chain also colocalizes to mesangium (original magnification: × 400).*

internalizing IgA in primary IgAN [56,57]. Mesangial uptake is promoted further by size-dependent trapping, reduction of anionic electrostatic charge of IgA secondary to reduced sialylation, and an affinity for underglycosylated IgA1 for fibronectin. Aggregates of pIgA1 maybe joined in the mesangium by serum pIgA–FcαRI (CD89) complexes shed from myeloid cells, as well as the IgA–fibronectin complexes formed in situ.

In response to receptor binding and internalization of macromolecular complexes, mesangial cells activate and respond by proliferating and secreting matrix material. The process is accompanied by local activation of the alternative and/or mannose-binding lectin (MBL) pathways, rather than classical complement pathway, and glomerulonephritis ensues [58]. The alternative pathway is activated in about 75 percent of IgAN patients and the lectin pathway in about 25 percent [59]. There is also correlation between lectin pathway activation and increased histologic activity (including crescentic GN) and chronicity in renal biopsies from IgAN patients. Moreover, experimental data imply that the extent of glomerular inflammatory infiltrate in IgAN is directly proportional to the amount of macromolecular IgA1 deposited and inversely proportional to the degree of *O*-glycosylation [55]. It should be noted that the scenario above unfolds in genetically susceptible patients as a matter of course.

Pathogenesis of Secondary IgAN

The pathogenesis of secondary IgAN is perplexing. pIgA1 is the predominant immunoglobulin depositing in glomeruli, similar to primary IgAN. There is a paucity of evidence, however, to support a role for aberrant glycosylation of pIgA1 in secondary IgAN. Hypoglycosylated pIgA has been documented only in rare instances [60,61]. In contrast to primary IgAN, high levels of serum pIgA1 levels appear to be instrumental in the etiology of secondary IgAN, given that more than 90 percent of patients with cirrhosis have elevated serum pIgA1 [36], the source of which is unclear. Liver damage results in significant decrease in the number of available asialoglycoprotein receptor (ASGP-R) on hepatocytes and Fc R on Kupffer cells, which normally function to clear and catabolize circulating IgA and IgA-immune complexes. Consequently, loss or reduction of these receptors in the setting of abnormal IgA overproduction

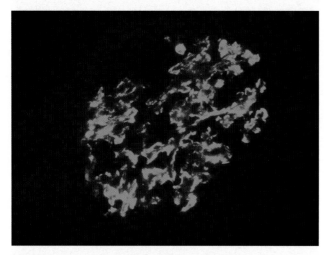

FIGURE 5.14: Immunofluorescence for IgA in membranoproliferative IgAN. Staining extends beyond the mesangium into glomerular capillary loops (original magnification: × 400).

leads to increased concentrations of serum IgA and therefore, a predisposition to glomerular deposition [62,63]. Another mechanism evokes portal shunting as a means of detouring a significant proportion of serum IgA around the liver and thereby avoiding degradation.

Perhaps the key to understanding the pathogenesis of secondary IgAN may lie in the nature of the IgAICs. For example, serum levels of pIgA are typically increased in inflammatory bowel disease (IBD), as they are in cirrhosis. Altered immunity results in antibody formation against normal intestinal flora. Sensitization to dietary peptides, bacterial and other antigens occurs, and may result in circulating immune complexes in both IBD and some cases of primary IgAN [64,65]. Indeed, circulating IgA-antigliadin antibodies are present in a significant percentage of patients with primary IgAN. It is tempting to speculate that the IgAICs depositing in most forms of secondary IgAN consist mainly of true immune complexes, whereas those of primary IgAN consist predominantly of self-aggregated (macromolecular) underglycosylated IgA admixed with immune complexes. Given that nonaggregated pIgA or appropriately glycosylated pIgA are less nephritogenic than macromolecular Gal-deficient pIgA1, this might explain the differences in the natural history of primary versus secondary IgAN.

Natural History

Earlier, primary IgAN was generally regarded as a relatively benign form of glomerulonephritis. The insidious nature of the disease became evident when follow-up studies revealed that as many as 50 percent of patients eventually developed ESRD. More detailed analyses of IgAN patients indicated a highly variable course ranging from patients with intermittent hematuria

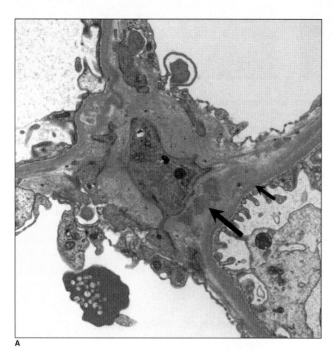

A

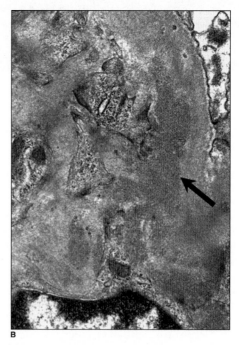

B

FIGURE 5.15: Sparse mesangial immune dense deposits in IgAN. (A,B) Mesangial dense deposits (larger arrows) may be sparse and in such cases, are almost always localized to the periphery of the mesangium, just underneath the GBM (smaller arrow). There is only mild increase in mesangial matrix [UA-LC stain, original magnifications: × 17,800 (A) and × 35,100 (B)].

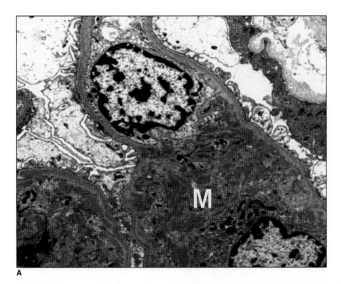
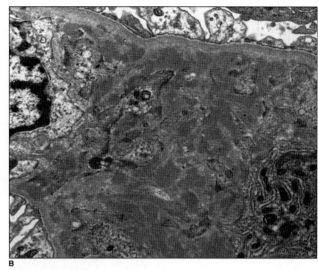

FIGURE 5.16: Abundant mesangial immune dense deposits in IgAN. (A,B) Immune dense deposits fill and expand the mesangium (M), and are embedded within increased matrix [UA-LC stain, original magnifications: × 3,500 (A) and × 8,900 (B)].

and little to no progression to ESRD over decades, to patients with active proliferative glomerulonephritis and a rapid descent to ESRD within 1–2 years. Long-term follow-up shows a wide spectrum of renal survival rates with ten-year renal survival ranging from 5 to 25 percent and twenty-year rates ranging from 25 to 50 percent. Remission rates vary between 5 and 30 percent. Like adult disease, pediatric IgAN was thought for many years to be a benign disease. Long-term studies, however, found renal survival in the 70–80 percent range after 20 years in children.

Investigations into the rate of disease progression are fraught with bias. The natural history of IgAN shares similarities worldwide but clinical outcomes are biased by regional differences in management and diagnostic approaches such as screening practices, the role or timing of renal biopsies, and referral tactics (so-called lead-time bias) [66]. In addition, regional diets, geographic differences in treatment, failure to adjust for treatment, and variability in follow-up and other selection biases conspire to produce divergent views on the clinical course of IgAN. Furthermore, evidence is accruing suggesting that IgAN progresses in an accelerated rather than linear fashion. This seems to be the case when serum creatinine reaches 3.0 mg/dL, which appears to be the point where renal function declines at a rapidly accelerated pace [67].

Thus, the highly variable clinical course of IgAN makes it difficult to encapsulate its natural history. Suffice it to say that perhaps the two largest cohorts of IgAN patients are (1) those who present with macroscopic hematuria with or without prodromal infection, and (2) those who present with persistent microhematuria with or without mild proteinuria. Many patients in the first group will see their hematuria resolve completely, only to return later as recurrent bouts of gross hematuria. Long-term follow-up studies found that patients who present with intermittent gross hematuria but do not develop proteinuria or persistent microscopic hematuria have an excellent prognosis [68]. Unfortunately, majority of these patients eventually develop persistent microhematuria with increasing proteinuria and are at risk for ESRD. Arguably, the second group comprises the largest segment of the IgAN population. Most patients in this group

present with persistent microhematuria and mild proteinuria and tend to exhibit a slow insidious march to ESRD, which is hastened by the development of hypertension. The more aggressive forms with rapid progression to ESRD represent a small minority of patients. Acute renal failure is sometimes observed with episodes of gross hematuria but is usually transient and has no impact on overall clinical progression [11].

Prognosis and Clinicopathologic Correlation

Genetic Prognostic Factors

The search for susceptibility genes in IgAN (Table 5.5) is often coupled with attempts to identify genetic polymorphisms that might also predict disease outcome [69]. Table 5.6 contains a partial list of candidate genes whose polymorphic variants are linked to disease progression. Many of them have inflammatory or immunologic functions (MCP-1, TCR Cα, TCR Cβ, IL-1Ra, selectin, TNF-α, TGF-β, CD14, and CCCR-5). Similar to the susceptibility genes in IgAN, prognostic polymorphisms linked to certain kindreds or specific racial/ethnic groups may not extend to others.

Some polymorphic genotypes within the renin-angiotensin-aldosterone system (RAAS) result in its partial activation and are associated with cardiovascular, neurologic, and renal disease, including IgAN. The kidney is affected since increased levels of angiotensin II and decreased levels of bradykinin are thought to alter glomerular hemodynamics and produce tuft hypertrophy and sclerosis, as well as exert proliferative effects upon mesangial and smooth muscle cells. The three major polymorphisms of the human angiotensin-converting enzyme (ACE) gene, termed I/I, I/D, and D/D, arise because of insertion or deletion of DNA sequence containing a putative silencer motif within intron 16, and are the best characterized polymorphisms in the RAAS. The D/D genotype is associated with higher serum and tissue levels of ACE when compared to the wild-type allele. A potential relationship between genetic polymorphisms of the RAAS and IgAN is evidenced by ACE inhibitors and angiotensin II type 1 receptor (ATR) antagonists (or so-called

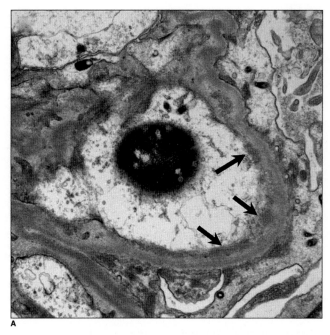

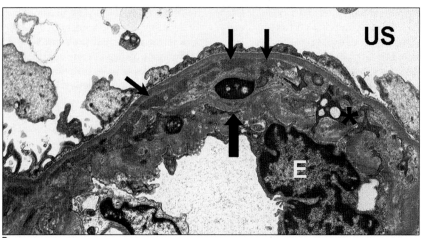

FIGURE 5.17: Subendothelial immune dense deposits in IgAN. (A) When present, subendothelial immune deposits (arrows) are usually small and sparsely distributed along occasional capillary walls (UA-LC stain, original magnification: × 8,900). (B) Subendothelial immune deposits are more abundant in membranoproliferative forms of IgAN and are typically sandwiched between the original and reduplicated glomerular basement membranes (larger arrow). The asterisk (*) denotes mesangial interposition (E, glomerular endothelial cell; US, urinary space. UA-LC stain, original magnification: × 17,800).

"ARBs") slowing progression of IgAN in some patients. Subsequent investigations claimed a link between expression of the ACE D/D genotype and progression to ESRD in IgAN [70,71]. Linkage has been reported in Scottish, North American, and Italian patients, as well as in some but not all Japanese cohorts, but absent in patients from France, Germany, and China. Many of the studies claiming prognostic significance of the D allele in IgAN are heavily biased [72] and therefore, better designed studies are still needed before the ACE D/D genotype can be exploited for prognostic or therapeutic purposes.

Other genetic polymorphisms of the RAAS have been implicated in disease progression in IgAN (Table 5.6). They include a second polymorphic variant (A2350G) present within exon 17 of the ACE gene and a polymorphic variant (M235T) in the gene encoding angiotensinogen.

Clinical Prognostic Factors

Innumerable studies document clinical risk factors for disease progression in IgAN. The data are often inconsistent. In an attempt to clarify the confusion, D'Amico [73] critically analyzed the most statistically reliable of these studies and found that the strongest independent predictors of progression in adult and pediatric IgAN included: (1) severe proteinuria at presentation and during follow-up, (2) arterial hypertension at presentation and during follow-up, and (3) increased serum creatinine at presentation. Weaker predictors included: (1) absence of recurrent gross hematuria, (2) male sex, (3) older age at presentation, and (4) marked erythocyturia in the early stages of disease.

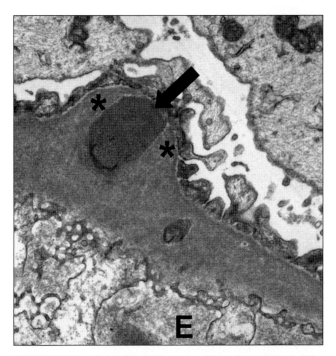

FIGURE 5.18: *Subepithelial immune dense deposits in IgAN. Subepithelial deposits are small and sparsely distributed (arrow). Isolated deposits maybe surrounded by basement membrane neosynthesis or so-called spike formations (asterisks) (E, glomerular endothelial cell. UA-LC stain, original magnification: × 27,500).*

Meanwhile, the European IgA Nephropathy Consortium [74] investigated the long-term follow-up of 437 patients and found that poor prognosis was associated with: (1) 1.0 g/24 hours incremental rises in proteinuria, (2) 1.0 mg/dL incremental rises in serum creatinine, and (3) microscopic hematuria at onset.

Of note, no risk for ESRD was found with arterial hypertension, although two-thirds of the patients were on ACE inhibitor or angiotensin receptor blocker (ARB) therapy. In a study that investigated the natural history of IgAN across three continents (Europe, North America, and Australia), Geddes et al. [66] found that the following were independent predictors of poor outcome in multivariate analysis: (1) Increased urinary protein, (2) decreased CrCl at presentation, and (3) younger-aged adults. In addition, there were no gender differences in the outcome. Furthermore, hypertension failed multivariate analysis as an independent risk factor for ESRD.

Morphologic Prognostic Factors

A large number of studies have assessed histologic risk factors for disease progression in IgAN. Summation of these studies [21,73] reveals that, in general, the strongest independent predictors of poor outcome in adult and pediatric IgAN include: (1) extensive interstitial fibrosis and tubular atrophy, (2) high index scores for glomerular and/or tubulointerstitial damage (based on semiquantitative scales), and (3) higher class designations, as per the Lee and Haas classification systems.

Of these, extensive tubulointerstitial scarring consistently carries the worst prognosis. Correlation of high index scores and poor prognosis is derived from semiquantitative scales that are the culmination of both active and chronic lesions. Weaker predictors of poor outcome in adult and pediatric IgAN include: (1) extensive segmental to global glomerulosclerosis, (2) cellular crescents, (3) prominent hyaline arteriolosclerosis, and (4) immune deposits extending into glomerular capillary loops.

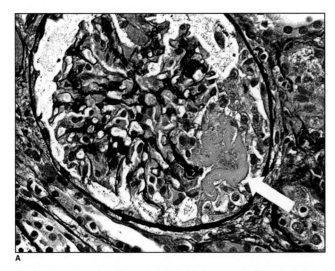
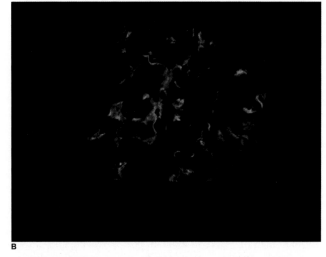

A

B

FIGURE 5.19: *Acute necrotizing GN in a case of IgAN with antineutrophil cytoplasmic antigen (ANCA). (A) A glomerulus shows segmental fibrinoid necrosis (arrow) consistent with acute necrotizing GN (JMS stain). (B) Immunofluorescence microscopy reveals dominant IgA in mesangium (original magnification: × 400). Underlying ANCA should be ruled out in cases of IgAN where acute necrotizing GN is the predominant lesion.*

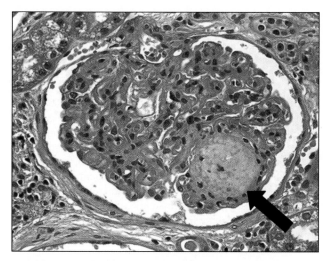

FIGURE 5.20: *IgAN in the setting of cirrhosis. A large mesangial nodule (arrow) resembling a Kimmelstiel-Wilson lesion is superimposed upon a background of mild mesangial proliferation (PAS stain, original magnification: × 400).*

Table 5.4 Putative Etiologic Agents in IgAN

Viral	Cytomegalovirus
	Adenovirus
	Herpes simplex
	Epstein-Barr virus
	Hepatitis B
Bacterial	Staphylococcus aureus
	Haemophilus parainfluenzae
	Group A β-hemolytic streptococcus
Dietary	Gluten proteins
	Milk proteins
	Soy proteins
	Rice proteins
	Bovine serum albumin
Endogenous	Fibronectin
	Aberrantly glycosylated IgA

The weaker predictors are statistically relevant by univariate analysis in most studies, but defined as independent risk factors in only a minority of studies [21,73].

Endocapillary proliferation, diffuse/florid mesangial hypercellularity, crescents, karyorrhexis, and acute necrotizing lesions (i.e., fibrinoid necrosis) of the glomerular tuft are traditional indicators of histologic activity in IgAN. Most studies imply through univariate analysis that IgAN patients harboring these indices tend to progress to ESRD faster than patients do without them (reviewed in Refs. 13,73,75). Active lesions, however, are not as reliable as chronic lesions in predicting clinical outcome. Multivariate analyses do not identify florid mesangial proliferation as an independent prognostic factor, with exception of one notable study [76]. Endocapillary proliferation by

Table 5.5 A Partial List of Candidate Susceptibility Genes Associated with IgAN

Gene Product	Locus	Population
E- and L-selectins	1q24-25	Japanese
Polymeric immunoglobulin receptor	1q31-41	Japanese
HLA-DRA	6p21.3	Japanese
Immunoglobulin μ-binding protein	11q13.2-13.4	Japanese
T-cell receptor Cα	14q11	Chinese
Gal-NAc-α-R β1,3-galactosyltransferase (C1GALT1)	17p13-14	Chinese
Interleukin-1 receptor antagonist	2q12-21	Chinese/Finnish
Interleukin-1β	2q12-21	Finnish
Transient receptor potential channel 3	4q26-31	Italian
Interleukins-2 and –21	4q26-31	Italian
IGNA1[a]	6q22-23	Italian/US
Ser/Thr protein kinase	6q23	Italian
Vanin 3	6q23	Italian
Histone deacetylase 5	17q12-22	Italian
Granulin	17q12-22	Italian

[a] The gene product of IGAN1 has not yet been established.

itself is a poor predictor of outcome. Although the clinical course of IgAN patients with acute necrotizing and crescentic glomerulonephritis is characterized by frequent acute flare-ups and progression to ESRD, actuarial renal survival is not significantly worse than control patients without these lesions [73]. Thus, multivariate analysis often renders active lesions impotent as independent risk factors.

Most statistical analyses, however, do not account for the fact that active and chronic lesions in IgAN commonly occur as an amalgam. For example, the combination of mesangial hypercellularity, endocapillary proliferation, and cellular crescents is a precursor to glomerular sclerosis, which is an independent risk factor for progression of IgAN [77]. Furthermore, the mere presence of a lesion is not as important prognostically as its extent within the biopsy. These variables are overcome in large part by the classification systems popularized by Lee and Haas, which segregate the amalgamated lesions and their extent of involvement into higher class designations. Higher designations carry incremental risks. For instance, 45 percent of patients in Haas class IV (diffuse proliferative IgAN) developed ESRD within five years, whereas progressive renal disease was far less common in classes I and II [20]. The prognosis of Haas class III (focal proliferative IgAN) is intermediate between classes II and IV. These results are consistent with several clinical studies that find a worse prognosis in those patients presenting with more proliferative (histologically active) forms of IgAN [23,78,79]. These studies also correlate histologically active forms of IgAN with clinical risk factors, such as nephrotic range proteinuria, hypertension or both. Not surprisingly, patients with Haas class V (≥40 percent global glomerulosclerosis and/or ≥40 percent tubular atrophy) progress faster to ESRD than any other class [20]. In a

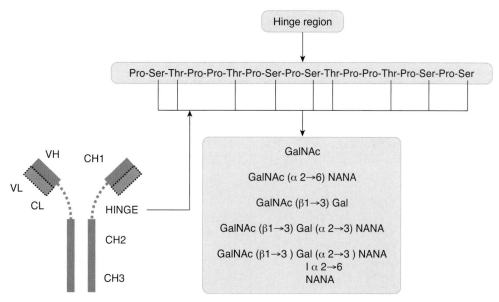

FIGURE 5.21: *Basic structure of IgA1. IgA1 also has a unique 18-amino acid hinge region between the CH1 and CH2 portions of the molecule that is rich in serine (Ser) and threonine (Thr) residues. These amino acids serve as putative sites for O-glycosylation and differentiate IgA1 from IgA2. Under normal circumstances, O-glycosylation of IgA1 involves binding of N-acetylgalactosamine (GalNAc) to any of the nine Ser/Thr residues occurring along the hinge region of the molecule. Galactose (Gal) may subsequently bind to GalNAc via a β1-3 linkage, depending on the expression and activity of galactosyl transferases. Sialic acid (N-acetylneuraminic acid, NANA) may also bind to either the GalNAc or penultimate Gal moieties, or to both via α2-6 or α2-3 linkages, respectively. Thus, any number of combinations can result in various permutations of IgA1 O-glycoforms.*

seeming paradox, Haas class II (FSGS-like IgAN) is also characterized by a sclerosing process but carries a good prognosis regardless of its association.

The prognostic implications of ultrastructural changes in IgAN remain uncertain. Subendothelial or subepithelial immune deposits, GBM abnormalities, mesangial cell interposition, and mesangiolysis correlate with histologically active disease by light microscopy but a statistical association with prognosis remains unproven. Haas [20] found no correlation between subendothelial/subepithelial dense deposits and prognosis, whereas extension of immune complex deposition into peripheral capillary loops is ranked as a weak predictor of disease progression by D'Amico [73].

Treatment

Nonimmunosuppressive Therapy

In general, most patients with IgAN appear to benefit from control of hypertension, particularly via blockade of the RAAS. Numerous reports show the effectiveness of ACE inhibitors or ARBs in the treatment of IgAN. Although most of these studies are limited to patients with favorable prognoses, some demonstrate efficacy of ACE inhibitors against proteinuria and disease progression in patients with hypertension and high-grade proteinuria [80]. Others advocate a role for a combined regimen of ACE inhibitor and ARBs [81]. In summary, the evidence generally supports use of RAAS blockade in all hypertensive and probably all proteinuric patients with IgAN [82]. This approach also helps to reduce risk of cardiovascular disease in IgAN patients.

Omega-3 fatty acid–containing fish oil supplements are widely used as adjunctive therapy for reducing proteinuria and slowing the progression of IgAN, although the data are extremely variable. Although some studies document that omega-3 fatty acids lower urinary protein beyond the effects of ACE inhibitors, others show no beneficial effects [83]. Nevertheless, several prospective studies have demonstrated that, for patients with higher grades of proteinuria, omega-3 fatty supplements can slow progression of renal disease and impart a survival advantage.

Immunosuppressive Therapy

The therapeutic decision to treat IgAN patients with ACE inhibitors alone or to add steroids or fish oil supplements largely depends on the presence of clinical signs associated with a poor prognosis. For example, patients with minimal proteinuria may be limited to ACE inhibitor therapy, whereas patients with high-grade or nephrotic-range proteinuria may have steroid hormones added to their treatment. Like fish oils, the efficacy of steroid hormones in the treatment of IgAN is controversial. Consensus is impeded by differences in trial design, limited sample size, heterogeneous patient populations, and the slow progression of IgAN. Nevertheless, it appears that steroids decrease proteinuria in IgAN, even in studies where they have no effect on renal survival [84]. Meta-analyses and prospective randomized studies tend to favor steroid usage in IgAN, especially in cases with significant proteinuria or more aggressive forms of the disease [85–88]. On the other hand, when and how to implement steroid hormones is equivocal. To quote Samuels and colleagues, "At present, steroids are the most promising intervention in terms of

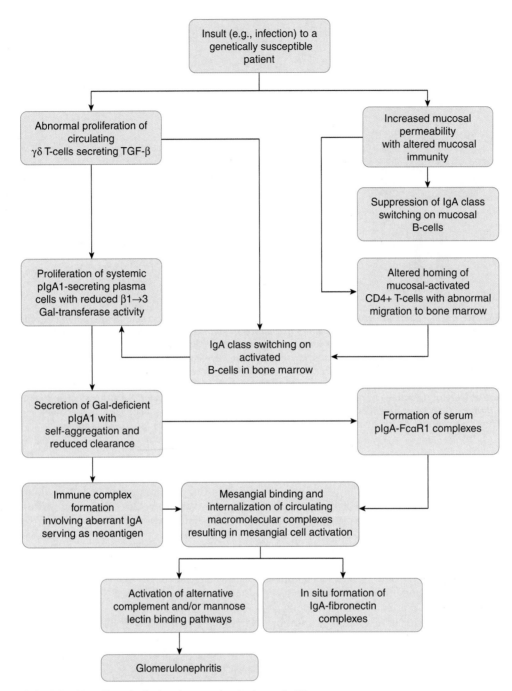

FIGURE 5.22: *Hypothetical pathogenesis of primary IgAN.*

both renal function and proteinuria, but there is not enough information to provide strong recommendations" [87].

There is a growing recognition that more aggressive forms of IgAN require more aggressive therapeutic interventions. Taking cues from lupus nephritis, certain studies advocate corticosteroids and cyclophosphamide to abrogate clinical and histologic activity in progressive IgAN [23,76,90,91]. In these studies, all patients had biopsy-proven IgAN and the vast majority exhibited clinical activity in the form of increased serum creatinine, proteinuria ≥ 1.0 g/24h, hypertension, and

hematuria with combinations of two or more clinical parameters. Trial-entry biopsies evidenced histologic activity to various degrees but required at least focal proliferative IgAN with extra- and/or endocapillary proliferation (Haas subclass III) as the least common denominator for initiation of cytotoxic immunosuppression. Treatment with steroids and cyclophosphamide halted clinical activity except hypertension and sent nearly all patients into remission. Furthermore, combination therapy virtually eradicated histologic activity in studies where follow-up biopsies were performed (Figure 5.23). Thus, subsets

Table 5.6 A Partial List of Genetic Polymorphisms Associated with Progression Of IgAN

Gene Product	Polymorphism	Population
Monocyte chemoattractant protein-1	A-2518G	Japanese
T-cell receptor Cα	RFLP(Taq I)	Japanese
T-cell receptor Cβ	RFLP(Bgl II)	Japanese
Interleukin-1 receptor antagonist	VNTR	Japanese
E-selectin	C1402T	Japanese
L-selectin	C712T	Japanese
Plasminogen activator inhibitor-1	G994T	Japanese
eNOS	ecNOS4 b/a	Japanese
Neuropeptide-Y Y1 receptor	Y/y genotype	Japanese
Aldosterone synthase	C344T	Japanese females[a]
Megsin	A23167G	Chinese
MUC20	SL/LL genotype	Chinese
Tumor necrosis factor-α	−308A/G	Chinese/Korean
TGF-β	C-509T/T869C	Korean
CC-chemokine receptor 5	d32	French
CD14	−159	Korean
Angiotensin-converting enzyme	Insertion/ deletion	Scottish
	Intron 16	Japanese[b] North American Italian
	A2350G/ exon 17	Japanese
Angiotensinogen	M235T	Canadian

[a] Prognosis in Japanese males is not affected.

[b] Some Japanese cohorts but not others showed linkage.

of IgAN patients with clinically and histologically active disease benefit significantly from cytotoxic immunosuppressive therapy.

Transplantation

In the United States, IgAN accounts for about 10 percent of kidney transplants among patients with primary GN. On average, about one-third of patients will develop recurrence, although it usually takes years to evolve. Regardless of the seemingly high recurrence rate, several studies report a higher five- and ten-year graft survival in patients receiving allografts for IgAN than other diseases [92]. The reasons for higher allograft survival are unclear. Some argue that elevated anti-HLA IgA, which is unique to the majority of transplanted IgAN patients, is somehow protective [93]. Others argue that the slow evolution of recurrent IgAN plays little role in allograft dysfunction until five or more years posttransplantation. Indeed, the only established predictor of graft loss is the time elapsed following transplantation. No indicators can reliably predict recurrence. The rate of recurrence is similar between cadaveric and living-related donors. In summary, end-stage IgAN is highly amenable to

kidney transplantation, since afflicted patients tend to be young healthy adults and graft survival is excellent.

HENOCH-SCHONLEIN PURPURA

Introduction

The earliest descriptions of Henoch-Schonlein purpura extend back to the turn of the nineteenth century when London physician William Heberden described a five-year-old boy who presented with skin rash ("bloody points"), joint pain and swelling, gross hematuria, and colic associated with bloody stools [94]. This constellation of symptomatology was initially referred to as Heberden-Willan disease. Several decades later, German physician Johann Schonlein recapitulated some of Heberden's findings in his descriptions of "peliosis rheumatica" (a.k.a., Schonlein's purpura), a disease characterized by arthritis associated with petechial skin rash [95]. After his death in 1864, Schonlein's pupil, German pediatrician Eduard Henoch extended the criteria of "Schonlein-Henoch purpura" to include abdominal pain and subsequently renal disease [96]. Eventually, the disease manifesting as a hemorrhagic skin rash, colic (often with bloody diarrhea), joint pain, and gross hematuria evolved into what is now termed "Henoch-Schonlein purpura" (HSP).

The International Consensus Conference on Nomenclature of Systemic Vasculitis (the Chapel Hill Consensus Conference) characterizes HSP as a leukocytoclastic vasculitis related to deposition of "IgA-dominant immune deposits" along small vessels and causing insult to the skin, intestine, kidney, and joints [97]. Thus, much of the damage in HSP is attributed to vascular IgA deposition. Kidney involvement ranges from 20 to 85 percent and includes additional deposition of IgA in glomeruli, identical to IgAN. This similarity, as well as commonalities in pathogenesis, led to the speculation that primary IgAN may represent a limited form of HSP. Although HSP is a systemic disease, this chapter will focus predominantly on the renal manifestations.

Epidemiology and Clinical Presentation

HSP is primarily a disease of children and young adults and is the most common vasculitis of childhood. Little is known about the epidemiology of HSP worldwide, since most of the studies are limited to Europe and the Middle East. The incidence approximates 10–14 cases per 100,000, although this figure is tenuous at best due to geographic variations in diagnostic approach [98]. It typically strikes children with a mean age of about 6 years [99]. The vast majority of patients are under 10 years of age. Presentation prior to 3 years of age is rare. Afflicted boys outnumber girls by about 3:2. A prodromal respiratory infection occurs in about one-third of children but rarely in adults, similar to IgAN. There appears to be seasonal skewing with increased incidence during fall and winter. The incidence of HSP in adults is about 10 percent or fewer than that of children with a range of 1–14 cases per 1,000,000 adults per year [100]. The mean age of onset in adults is about 50 years with a 1.7:1 male:female ratio [101]. Although the incidence of HSP is significantly less in adults than in children, the frequency of renal involvement is higher in adults. The disease also tends to be more aggressive in adults with a significantly higher incidence of ESRD than in children [102].

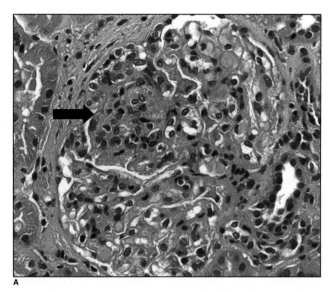
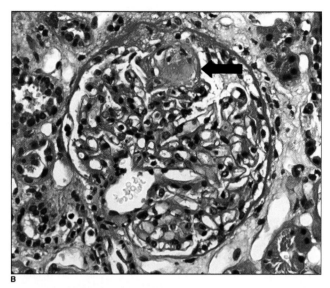

FIGURE 5.23: *Histological response to oral prednisone and intravenous cyclophosphamide in proliferative IgAN. (A) A representative glomerulus from a case of focal proliferative IgAN (Haas class III) shows segmental endocapillary proliferation (arrow) on a background of mesangial proliferation (H&E stain, original magnification: × 400). (B) A representative glomerulus six months after treatment shows abrogation of histologic activity and regression to FSGS-like IgAN (Haas class II). The arrow denotes a healed segmental lesion adhered to Bowman's capsule. Proteinuria and serum creatinine also normalized in response to treatment (PAS stain, original magnification: × 400).*

Although the presence of renal or cutaneous deposition of IgA is helpful, the diagnosis of HSP is made primarily on clinical criteria. For example, the American College of Rheumatology utilizes four criteria for the diagnosis of HSP: (1) presentation before 20 years of age, (2) palpable cutaneous purpura (not attributable to thrombocytopenia), (3) acute abdominal pain (including ischemic bowel disease) with or without bloody diarrhea, or (4) biopsy-proven leukocytoclastic vasculitis [103]. Although the Chapel Hill Consensus Conference states that the presence of small-vessel vasculitis with IgA deposition is sufficient for the diagnosis of HSP, the classification of Helander and colleagues require the documentation of vascular IgA deposition in conjunction with clinical symptoms including abdominal pain with or without gastrointestinal bleeding and the presence of renal involvement [104].

The protean features of HSP including gross hematuria and abdominal pain are not immediately life threatening but garner rapid medical attention. Most patients describe a recent viral infection that may include gastroenteritis or upper respiratory infection followed by the development of acute abdominal pain, diffuse myalgias, malaise, and low-grade fevers. The viral prodrome is typically short-lived (1–5 days) and is followed by the development of gross hematuria and a purpuric rash. In cases of HSP nephritis, renal involvement may be limited to a few days of gross hematuria followed by rapid progression to crescentic glomerulonephritis and renal failure. Pediatric patients with prolonged abdominal pain and hematochezia that are unresponsive to steroids or other forms of immunosuppressive therapy are at risk for volvulus. This severe complication can result in complete bowel obstruction and the potential for visceral perforation.

HSP has also been associated with CNS manifestations including small-vessel vasculitis. In children, CNS involvement is typically mild and characterized by persistent headache with associated photophobia; however, delirium and generalized seiz-

ure disorders have also been reported. The diagnosis of CNS vasculitis in the setting of HSP is challenging given that sensitivity of conventional angiography is insufficient to detect vascular inflammation. Magnetic resonance imaging (MRI), on the other hand, frequently detects small foci of hyperintensive signaling within the deep cortical white matter, although these lesions are not specific for HSP and are similar to those associated with hypertensive encephalopathy [105]. For children presenting with HSP following a typical viral prodrome, the clinician will need to establish whether the existing neurologic findings are a consequence of HSP or evolution into a viral meningoencephalitis.

The clinical presentation of adult HSP is similar to that found in pediatric populations, but is typically more refractory to therapy and associated with a worse prognosis.

Approach to Interpretation

Light Microscopy

The incidence of renal involvement in HSP varies from 20 to 100 percent. The wide range probably stems from the same selection and lead-time biases that plague IgAN. The renal histopathology of HSP is indistinguishable from that of primary IgAN (Figure 5.24). Like IgAN, the light microscopic patterns of glomerular injury are extremely variable, although there is a tendency for HSP nephritis to exhibit more histologic activity than IgAN, especially in children (Figure 5.25) [9]. Several histologic classification systems for HSP nephritis are in use. The classification of Meadow and colleagues is older and serves as the foundation for Lee's classification for IgAN (Table 5.3). A more recent classification system was published by the International Study of Kidney Disease in Childhood (ISKDC) in 1977 (Table 5.7) [106]. This system depends largely on the presence of cellular crescents and is in wider use than the older Meadow's classification. An estimated 40 percent of biopsied patients with

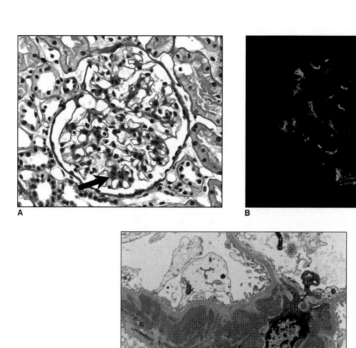

FIGURE 5.24: *HSP nephritis. (A) A glomerulus from a case of mesangioproliferative HSP nephritis (ISKDC grade II) shows mild segmental mesangial hypercellularity and matrix increase (arrow) (PAS stain, original magnification: × 400). (B) Immunofluorescence microscopy reveals mesangial deposition of IgA (Original magnification: × 400). (C) Electron microscopy demonstrates numerous granular "immune-type" dense deposits restricted to the mesangium (M) (UA-LC stain, original magnification: × 11,000). These morphologic findings are indistinguishable from IgAN.*

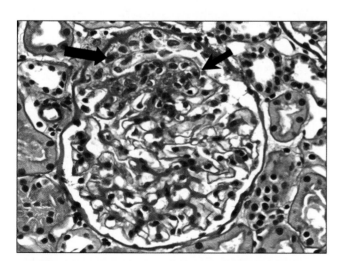

FIGURE 5.25: *Extra- and endocapillary proliferation in pediatric HSP nephritis. Mild segmental endocapillary proliferation (smaller arrow) is accompanied by an adjacent incipient cellular crescent (larger arrow) (PAS stain, original magnification: × 400).*

HSP exhibit crescents (Figure 5.26) [107]. The overwhelming majority of cases shows fewer than 50 percent crescentic involvement and is classified as grade III or lower. Membrano-proliferative forms of HSP occur in only about 2 percent of patients (Figure 5.27). An acute necrotizing component (i.e., segmental fibrinoid glomerular necrosis) is detected in as many as 50 percent of biopsied cases (Figure 5.28) [108]. Tubulointer-stitial scarring and inflammation tends to be commensurate with the degree of glomerular scarring and activity, respectively.

HSP is characterized as a small-vessel leukocytoclastic vascu-litis, which is frequently documented in skin biopsies of afflicted patients. Typically, arterioles, capillaries, and postcapillary venules evidence fibrinoid necrosis and karyorrhexis along the vascular wall (Figure 5.29A). Fibrinoid change is usually accom-panied by varying degrees of perivascular and/or transmural acute and chronic inflammation. Microthrombi may also be present. Immunofluorescence microscopy demonstrates IgA deposition along blood vessel walls, which is considered central to the patho-genesis of HSP (Figure 5.29B). Sometimes, the vasculitis may manifest in the biopsy solely as capillaritis, as in rare cases of lung involvement. In contrast to skin, leukocytoclastic vasculitis is seen in 1 percent or less of renal biopsies of HSP patients [102].

Table 5.7 The International Study of Kidney Disease in Childhood (ISKDC) Classification of HSP Nephritis

Grade	Histologic Findings
Grade I	Minimal histologic findings
Grade II	Pure mesangioproliferative lesions, focal or diffuse
Grade III	Mesangial proliferation, focal (IIIa) or diffuse (IIIb), associated with <50% cellular crescents
Grade IV	Mesangial proliferation, focal (IVa) or diffuse (IVb), associated with 50–75% cellular crescents
Grade V	Mesangial proliferation, focal (Va) or diffuse (Vb), associated with >75% cellular crescents
Grade VI	Membranoproliferative glomerulonephritis

Immunofluorescence Microscopy

The demonstration of IgA deposition in tissues is considered by some to be the gold standard for the diagnosis of HSP. The distribution and pattern of (co)dominant IgA immunofluorescence between HSP nephritis and primary IgAN are indistinguishable. Staining is invariably mesangial in location with extension of IgA into glomerular capillary loops in the more histologically active disease. IgA is accompanied by IgG deposition, and to a lesser extent IgM deposition, in the majority of cases. C3 is present in at least three-quarters of cases, whereas C4 and C1q are generally absent. Fibrinogen is present in cellular crescents and acute necrotizing lesions, as it is seen in other forms of acute necrotizing and crescentic GN. Fibrinogen is also commonly detected in the mesangium in HSP nephritis, as is κ/λ light chain deposition.

Electron Microscopy

Like light and immunofluorescence microscopy, the electron microscopic features of HSP nephritis are very similar to primary IgAN and will not be reiterated here. There are some subtle differences, however. Because HSP nephritis tends to be more histologically active than IgAN, the frequency of subendothelial immune deposits is increased in the former than the latter. In addition, the incidence of intramembranous and subepithelial immune deposits is also increased in HSP nephritis – indeed, in as many as half of the cases (Figure 5.30A) [109]. Subepithelial deposits are sometimes "hump-like" in appearance, similar to that seen in a postinfectious process (Figure 5.30B).

Differential Diagnosis

The differential diagnosis of HSP nephritis is derived from Table 5.1 and distinguished from IgAN by the presence of systemic disease (Figure 5.2). In short, HSP nephritis is part of a systemic disease and therefore needs to be differentiated from other systemic diseases manifesting as vasculitis and hematuric renal disease. These include: (1) ANCA-associated disease (namely, Wegener's granulomatosis and microscopic polyangiitis); (2) infectious GN related to deep-seated visceral or cutaneous abscesses, endocarditis, or osteomyelitis; (3) IgA-dominant postinfectious GN; (4) "shunt nephritis"; (5) lupus

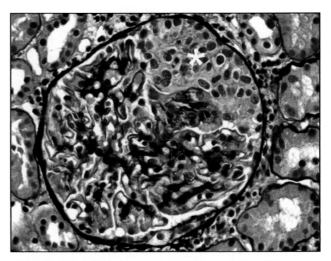

FIGURE 5.26: Cellular crescent (white asterisk) in HSP nephritis. Crescents occur more frequently in HSP than IgAN (JMS stain, original magnification: × 400).

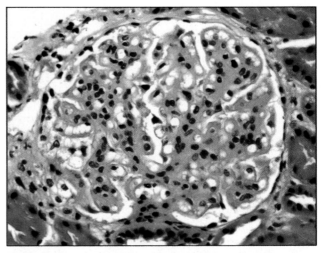

FIGURE 5.27: Membranoproliferative GN in HSP nephritis. Global mesangial proliferation and increased mesangial matrix are associated with variable thickening of glomerular capillary loops (H&E stain, original magnification: × 400).

nephritis; (6) cryoglobulinemic GN; and (7) acute thrombotic microangiopathies. Clinicopathologic features that distinguish each of these from primary IgAN are also applicable to HSP nephritis, as alluded to in the differential diagnosis section of IgAN. Some of these entities deserve further clarification, however.

A primary distinction between HSP and ANCA-associated disease includes serologic evidence of IgG ANCA with failure to demonstrate immune complex deposition in the latter. As with IgAN, a subset of patients with HSP nephritis exhibits positive ANCA serologies. However, most of the ANCA is of the IgA rather than IgG subclass and its role in the pathogenesis is controversial [110]. Serum IgA ANCA may simply represent a nonspecific interaction [111]. There is also a speculation that

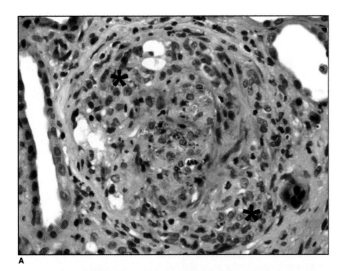

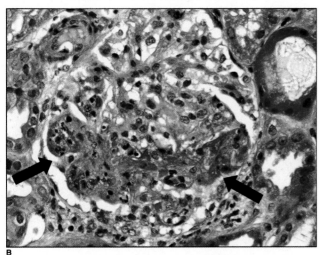

FIGURE 5.28: *Acute necrotizing and crescentic glomerulonephritis in HSP (ISKDC Class III). (A) The glomerular tuft is markedly compressed by a fulminant circumferential cellular crescent (asterisks) (H&E stain, original magnification: × 400). (B) Another glomerulus from the same case depicted in (A) shows segmental fibrinoid necrosis (arrows) (MAS stain, original magnification: × 400).*

number of clinical features with HSP including acute renal failure, hematuria, purpura, and arthralgias. However, these patients often appear septic and are hypocomplementemic. Furthermore, the kidney biopsy shows a preponderance of glomerular C3 deposition without immunoglobulin and especially not IgA. "Shunt nephritis" is a specialized form of infectious GN that can also present with hematuria, purpura, and arthralgias. Membranoproliferative GN is the most common histologic finding. It is one of the few infectious GNs where IgA deposits occur in a significant number of cases. IgA is rarely, if ever, the dominant or even codominant immunoglobulin, however. Moreover, a clinical history of ventriculovascular shunt placement would seem to exclude HSP.

Although most cases of mixed cryoglobulinemia occur as IgG-IgM, rare cases can present as IgA-IgG and involve the kidney in the form of cryoglobulinemic GN [112,113]. These patients can exhibit hematuria, mild proteinuria, and cutaneous vasculitis with IgA deposition in glomeruli and skin vasculature. The renal histology may or may not resemble cryoglobulinemic GN and in some cases, the only clue to its etiology is the serologic evidence of cryoglobulins containing IgG and IgA either in monoclonal form or as rheumatoid factor.

Although there are no established associations between HSP nephritis and the thrombotic microangiopathies, recent studies have demonstrated that the majority of adults and children with HSP, when tested, showed elevated serum levels of IgA antiphospholipid antibodies, particularly in the earlier phases of disease [114,115]. Although the role of antiphospholipid antibodies in thrombotic microangiopathies is well known, their action in HSP is unknown. Interestingly, correlation between elevated antibody and disease activity, and eventual onset of proteinuria has been reported.

Secondary Forms of HSP Nephritis

Many of the diseases associated with secondary forms of IgAN listed in Table 5.1 are also reported for secondary HSP nephritis, including hepatitis B, HIV, cirrhosis, Crohn's disease, polycythemia vera, IgA myeloma, lymphoma, lung cancer, ankylosing spondylitis, Behcet's disease, and alpha-1 antitrypsin deficiency. As shown in Table 5.8, a number of drugs are also associated with the development of HSP with nephritis.

Etiology and Pathogenesis

Etiology

Like primary IgAN, the cause of HSP is unknown. Numerous exogenous agents have been linked to the disease but have never been proven as causative (Table 5.8). Infection has always been suspected because of seasonal variations in HSP and the prodromal upper respiratory infections that occur in about one-third of patients [116]. Accordingly, a number of viruses have been implicated but none is proven. Most bacteria linked to HSP tend to infect the respiratory or GI tract and include *Helicobacter, Group A β-hemolytic streptococcus, Salmonella, Mycobacterium,* and *Mycoplasma* species. These infections are often related to overproduction of serum IgA, which might facilitate IgA deposition in predisposed patients. A few microbial antigens have been detected in mesangial immune deposits in HSP. For example,

the target antigens in IgA ANCA are different from those of IgG ANCA, and are not pathogenic. Regardless, IgA ANCA is detected more often in HSP than other vasculitidies and has been suggested as a useful adjunct in diagnosis, particularly in the early phase of the disease in children.

Certain infectious or postinfectious GN may exhibit systemic manifestations that can mimic HSP. For example, sepsis or endocarditis caused by methicillin-resistant forms of *Staph. aureus* and *epidermidis* may be associated with proliferative GN and (co)dominant deposition of IgA, thereby simulating HSP nephritis [35]. These cases are usually characterized by positive blood cultures, hypocomplementemia, or positive changes on echocardiogram in the case of endocarditis, which reveals their infectious nature and distinguishes them from HSP. Other infectious GNs, such as those associated with deep-seated visceral or cutaneous abscesses and osteomyelitis, may share a

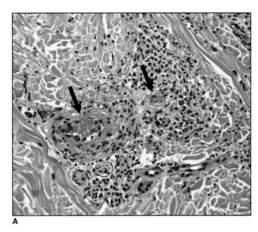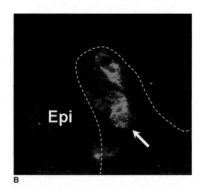

FIGURE 5.29: *Skin biopsy of purpuric lesion from an HSP patient. (A) Dermal blood vessels (arrows) exhibit severe leukocytoclastic vasculitis. (H&E stain, original magnification: × 400). (B) The walls of blood vessels in the papillary dermis immunofluoresce brightly for IgA (arrows). The dashed line approximates the epidermal basement membrane (Epi, epidermis) (original magnification: × 600).*

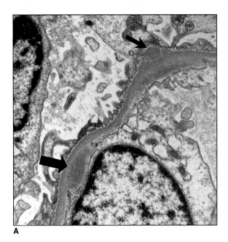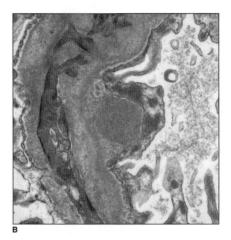

FIGURE 5.30: *Immune deposits along glomerular capillary walls in HSP nephritis. (A) Although the prevalence of subendothelial immune deposits (larger arrows) and subepithelial deposits (smaller arrow) are higher in HSP than IgAN, they tend to be sparsely distributed (UA-LC stain, original magnification: × 22,300). (B) Subepithelial immune deposits sometimes form "humps" reminiscent of postinfectious GN (UA-LC stain, original magnification: × 35,100).*

nephritis-associated plasmin receptor, a group A streptococcal antigen, has been identified in the glomeruli of about 30 percent of patients with HSP nephritis [117]. Likewise, an antigen derived from *H. parainfluenzae* was localized in the mesangium of about 35 percent of patients biopsied for HSP [118]. These studies are important for bolstering the infectious etiology of HSP, at least in a subset of patients.

Like IgAN, linkage between HSP and certain neoplasms has been reported in greater than 30 patients (Table 5.8) [119]. Since the vast majority is males with a mean age of 60 years, neoplasia should be ruled out in this demographic. In contrast to IgAN, HSP has a modest association with medicinal and illicit drugs (Table 5.8). This relationship attests to the hyper-

sensitivity component of HSP that is not typically encountered in IgAN. In fact, it is sometimes difficult to discern if HSP is related to the infection or its treatment [120].

Genetic Susceptibility

Little is known about the molecular pathogenesis of HSP. Familial clustering is reported but less frequently than in IgAN [121]. A partial list of candidate susceptibility genes are listed in Table 5.9. Of interest, polymorphisms of genes encoding components of the RAAS, which appear to play a role in progression of IgAN, may also serve as candidate susceptibility genes in HSP. The ACE I/D genotype and the ATG/M235T polymorphism are associated with development of HSP in

Table 5.8 Potential Etiologic Factors in HSP

Infections	*Helicobacter pylori*, methicillin-sensitive and -resistant *Staphylococcus aureus*, Group A *β*-hemolytic streptococcus, *Haemophilus parainfluenzae*, *Salmonella typhi*, *Bartonella henselae*, *Mycobacterium tuberculosis*, *Mycoplasma pneumoniae*, hepatitis A/B/C, HIV, *Parvovirus B19*, and *Varicella zoster*
Drugs	Vancomycin, ciprofloxacin, clarithromycin, propylthiouracil, cocaine, levodopa, carbidopa, carbamazepine, anastrozole, ACE inhibitors, acetylsalicylic acid, streptokinase, intravesicular bacilli Calmette-Guerin, and immunization for hepatitis B
Neoplasia	Lung, prostate, breast, kidney, GI tract, IgA myeloma, and Hodgkin's/non-Hodgkin's lymphoma
Environmental factors	Insect bites, food allergies, and cold exposure
Miscellaneous	Pregnancy

Table 5.9 A Partial List of Candidate Susceptibility Genes Associated with HSP Nephritis

Gene or Gene Product	Polymorphism	Population
HLA-B35	–	Great Britain
HLA-DRB1	–	Spain
Angiotensinogen	M235T	Turkish
Angiotensin-converting enzyme[a] [18]	D/D genotype	Japanese
IL-1*β*	−511 C/T	Spanish
IL-8	Allele A	Spanish
PAX2	1410CT/1521AC	Chinese
VEGF	−1154 G	Spanish
Inducible nitric oxide	(8−10)CCTTTn	Spanish
TGF-*β*	TT genotype	Taiwanese
Complement 4	C4B*Q0	Icelandic

Turkish children, but only the AGT polymorphism is related to increased risk of HSP nephritis [122]. Any relationship between the ACE homozygous D/D genotype and development of HSP nephritis is merely implied.

Genetic polymorphisms or defects of the complement system may also contribute to the pathogenesis of HSP. The *C4* gene is the most polymorphic gene in MHC III, which provides for diverse antigen–antibody interactions in infection, neoplasia and autoimmunity. It encodes for two polymorphic proteins (called isotypes): complement 4A (C4A) and complement 4B

(C4B). Each isotype is different in its antigen-binding affinity, rate of activation, and half-life, and has different functions. C4 deficiencies have been linked to IgAN, HSP, and systemic lupus erythematosus, with C4B deficiencies carrying a higher risk for HSP nephritis than C4A deficiencies [123,124]. Different alleles have been characterized for the two isotypes, including nonexpressed or "null" alleles termed *C4A*Q0* and *C4B*Q0*. These "null" alleles can produce partial C4 deficiencies. The *C4B*Q0* allele was identified in as many as 43 percent of Icelandic children with HSP [125]. In contrast to partial C4 deficiencies, complete C4 deficiency is extremely rare with fewer than 30 known cases worldwide. These patients are also at risk for the development of HSP nephritis [126]. C2 deficiency, which is also rare, has also been cited as a possible risk factor for HSP.

Role of Aberrantly Glycosylated Forms of Polymeric IgA

In all likelihood, HSP nephritis and IgAN share many of the same pathogenic mechanisms, although far less is known about the former than the latter (reviewed in Refs. 21,107). Total serum IgA (monomeric and polymeric IgA) is elevated in 40–50 percent of both patients. Both diseases are characterized by glomerular deposition of pIgA1 [127]. Aberrant *O*-linked glycosylation of the hinge region of the pIgA1 molecule, which appears to be a key element in the pathogenesis of IgAN, may also play a role in HSP [128]. Preliminary data suggest that aggregation of NeuNAc- and Gal-deficient *O*-glycoforms of pIgA1, which are major components of both circulating and deposited IgA complexes in IgAN, also occur in HSP [61,129]. It is not yet known if the source of this pIgA1 in HSP results from a translocation of immune response from gut to bone marrow, as speculated for primary IgAN. Nevertheless, there is limited data implying that aggregated Gal-deficient pIgA1 from the sera of HSP patients activate cultured mesangial cells (i.e., proliferation and secretion of matrix material) [130]. In all likelihood, mechanisms of mesangial cell activation in HSP are common to other forms of immune complex–mediated GN.

Role of Complement

Complement seems to participate in the disease process but just like in IgAN, its exact role is unclear. Complement consumption is marginal at best in HSP, such that hypocomplementemia is an atypical but not an unheard finding in afflicted patients. Certain observations hint at activation and include the deposition of C3, properdin, and membrane attack complex (MAC) C3b-5 in glomeruli; depressed CH_{50} and serum properdin; and elevated serum C3d and MAC. These findings are inconsistent among patient cohorts, however, as some studies report activation of the classical pathway, others report activation of the alternative pathway, and a few report no evidence of complement activation [131]. The vast majority of HSP patients with nephritis evidence activation of the alternative pathway, with about one-half of all patients exhibiting additional activation of the MBL pathway [132,133]. Complement activation through the MBL pathway correlates with codeposition of IgA1 and IgA2 in the mesangium, similar to IgAN discussed earlier.

Role of Immunomodulatory Factors

The role of cytokines, chemokines, and other immunomodulatory factors in HSP is poorly understood. Observations about cytokines are sporadic and sometimes conflicting. TNF-α is not only a proinflammatory cytokine but also promotes activation of mesangial cells by stimulating cellular proliferation and secretion of mesangial matrix. Its role in pathogenesis is suggested by increased levels in both urine and sera of HSP patients in the acute but not remitting phase [134,135]. Some reports describe higher levels of serum TNF-α correlating with renal involvement, whereas others fail to detect raised levels of TNF-α or its soluble receptors in the sera of HSP patients [136,137]. In some but not all studies, elevated levels of urinary TNF-α are matched by increased urinary excretion of IL-1β, another proinflammatory cytokine and activator of mesangial cells [134,138]. Concomitant increases in serum IL-1 have not been identified yet, however.

Cytokines IL-4, IL-5, and IL-6 derived from Th2 lymphocytes have also been found to be significantly elevated in HSP. IL-5 has been linked to eosinophilia and raised levels of eosinophilic cationic protein (ECP) in HSP [139,140] All three parameters are closely associated with HSP nephritis but not the severity of kidney disease. IL-4 is elevated in patients with HSP but not HSP nephritis, even though IL-4 is more closely tied to class switching to IgE production. Like most other cytokines in HSP, remission of disease correlates with a significant reduction of IL-4 and IL-5.

Prognosis, Natural History, and Clinicopathologic Correlation

A few studies attempt to correlate genetic polymorphisms of genes encoding components of the RAAS with clinical outcomes in HSP nephritis. In Japanese patients, the expression of the ACE D allele is related to the severity and persistence of proteinuria, especially the homozygous D/D genotype that can predict proteinuria as far out as eight years [141]. A cohort of Italian patients with HSP nephritis followed for 20 years showed no such correlation between ACE polymorphic expression (I/I, ID, or D/D) and renal outcomes [142]. Moreover, a study of British subjects with HSP nephritis found no relationship between the D/D genotype and severity of proteinuria or disease progression [143].

Of the primary components of HSP, nephritis has the greatest chance of becoming chronic and therefore has the greatest impact on patient prognosis. The incidence of renal involvement in HSP ranges from about 20 to 58 percent in children and about 30 to 85 percent in adults [144–146]. The severity of renal and extrarenal disease tends to increase with age. In adult patients, the incidence of chronic kidney disease ranges from 10 to 75 percent and ESRD, 8–16 percent [101]. HSP in children exhibits a relatively benign course. The incidence of ESRD is generally lower in pediatric HSP and ranges from 1 to 8 percent, although long-term follow-up studies of U.S. children with HSP nephritis show a significantly higher rate of ESRD hovering around 20 percent [147]. Prior univariate and multivariate analyses identify factors that predict renal disease in pediatric HSP [148,149]. Independent risk factors for renal involvement include: (1) recurrent or persistent purpura,

(2) older age of onset (>4 years of age), (3) severe abdominal involvement (colic with melena), and (4) diminished factor XIII activity (<80 percent).

In addition, there was a strong correlation between persistent purpura and decreased factor XIII activity with moderate to heavy proteinuria.

The vast majority of studies investigating prognostic features in adult HSP are predominantly European in origin. Examples of previously reported risk factors associated with progression of HSP include (1) the presence of cellular crescents as per renal biopsy, (2) evidence of kidney failure at presentation, (3) proteinuria exceeding 1.0 g/24h, (4) hypertension, (5) hematuria and anemia at presentation, (6) summertime onset of disease, and (7) disease relapse [101]. However, multivariate analysis of 250 adult patients with a fifteen-year follow-up identified the following as independent risk factors for renal failure in HSP: (1) serum Cr >1.4 mg/dL, (2) greater than 10 percent interstitial fibrosis, (3) poteinuria >1 g/24 hours, (4) greater than 20 percent glomerulosclerosis, and (5) fibrinoid necrosis affecting >10 percent of glomeruli [102].

Endocapillary proliferation and cellular crescents increase the relative risk for severe renal failure by univariate analysis. These trends did not survive multivariate analysis, however. Overall renal prognosis in this series was poor with nearly 40 percent of patients exhibiting various degrees of renal insufficiency, including an ESRD prevalence of 11 percent. The rate of renal insufficiency and ESRD was higher than that seen in other studies, probably because of a longer term of follow-up.

In childhood HSP nephritis, hematuria and mild proteinuria (<500 mg/24 hours) carry a good prognosis with <5 percent of patients progressing to ESRD in 10–25 years [150]. In contrast, acute nephritic syndrome, increasing proteinuria, nephrotic syndrome, or combined nephritic–nephrotic features impart a poorer prognosis and occurs in 5–20 percent of pediatric HSP. Most of these children (>50 percent) will development hypertension and chronic renal failure with about 20 percent progressing to end-stage [145], although hypertension by itself is not an independent predictor of poor prognosis [146]. Despite the aforementioned indicators of risk, pediatric HSP is basically a self-limited disease with greater than 90–95 percent of patients enjoying complete or nearly complete recovery [151].

The Italian Group of Renal Immunopathology conducted collaborative studies that investigated the prognosis of biopsy-proven HSP nephritis in adults and children as a contiguous group [152,153]. The first report found that proteinuria was the only independent risk factor for progression. Although proteinuria exceeding 1.5 gm/24h was unfavorable for adults, no such cutoff could be established for children. There was no difference in outcome if children displayed mild or heavy proteinuria. Hypertension was also identified as a risk factor, but not as an independent variable. Moreover, hypertension had greater impact upon progression in adults than children. Impaired renal function at onset was another poor prognostic indicator but only in adults. Hence, outcomes in children were harder to predict than adults, a finding echoed by other long-term studies of pediatric HSP spanning more than 20 years after onset [150,154]. Despite occasional differences in prognostic factors, there was surprisingly little statistical difference in clinical presentation, clinical outcomes, and renal morphology between children and adults. Extended follow-up from the second report helped to clarify the role of proteinuria in prognosis of HSP nephritis [153]. Multivariate analysis showed that increasing proteinuria established during follow-up was an independent risk factor for progression, whereas baseline proteinuria at onset was not. Thus, relative risk increases significantly with every 1g/24h increase recorded during follow-up. The predictive value of follow-up proteinuria is applicable to both children and adults. In terms of age at onset, prognosis was poorer for adult than pediatric HSP nephritis. Almost twice as many adult patients progressed to dialysis as children (7.2 vs. 13.2 percent, respectively). Accordingly, ten-year renal survival for adult patients was 76 percent, as opposed to 90 percent for children. Multivariate analysis identified female gender as an independent risk factor.

Several studies have implicated cellular crescents as a poor prognostic indicator in HSP [150,155]. However, recent reports utilizing multivariate analysis conclude that cellular crescents have limited prognostic significance in HSP nephritis [102,152,153]. On the other hand, acute necrotizing GN, glomerular sclerosis, and interstitial fibrosis withstand multivariate analysis and are independent risk factors for progression in adult HSP nephritis.

Treatment

As previously noted the clinical presentation of HSP is broad and can range from a limited course of cutaneous vasculitis to rapidly progressive glomerulonephritis with life threatening pulmonary hemorrhage. There are few prospective controlled trials to guide management. Consequently, treatment options are often determined by the patient's individual clinical presentation. Steroid therapy, whether oral or intravenous, is often used in the treatment of HSP. In a study of 171 children with HSP, patients were randomized either to placebo or a one-month course of prednisone to determine its effect on both renal and nonrenal manifestations of the disease. Of note, non-renal symptoms including abdominal pain, hematochezia, and joint stiffness were significantly improved following steroids, but they were unable to prevent the development of hematuria and proteinuria. However, long-term follow-up at six months demonstrated that patients randomized to the steroid group had reduced hematuria and proteinuria [156].

Guidelines for treatment of more aggressive forms of pediatric HSP nephritis are tentative at best. Although a number of uncontrolled studies document improved outcomes with corticosteroids, azathioprine, alkylating agents, or plasmapheresis [157], no single modality proves superior for the treatment of severe HSP nephritis. A full recovery is expected in about 40 percent of these patients regardless of the treatment being supportive or aggressive with alkylating agents [157,158]. Children with proteinuria and whose kidney biopsies are beyond ISKDC grade IIIa (Table 5.7) are at ~20 percent risk for developing complications of persistent renal disease over the long term, despite treatment with cyclophosphamide, long-term steroids and/or azathioprine. About one in ten of these patients resist all forms of treatment and progress to ESRD, especially if they are older, exhibit nephrotic-range proteinuria or nephrotic syndrome, and have ≥50 percent crescents on biopsy. However, the degree of proteinuria at presentation does not correlate with long-term outcome. Thus, patients presenting with suspected

HSP and demonstrating hematuria and proteinuria should undergo a renal biopsy as a part of the initial workup. The rationale is that previous studies in IgAN and other related GNs have shown that the amount of hematuria or the level of urinary protein does not correlate with the severity of the underlying histopathology. Assessing the extent of histologic activity may help the clinician determine the type and duration of therapy. Early intervention is deemed essential by some but inconsequential by others [157,159,160]. It is noteworthy that the addition of pulse urokinase to methylprednisolone and cyclophosphamide increases the efficacy of combination therapy against more aggressive forms of HSP nephritis [161].

For patients with more extensive and systemic manifestations of HSP, alternative therapies including high-dose γ globulin therapy or plasmapheresis might be considered. High-dose gamma globulin has been shown to be effective in reversing severe nephritis, abdominal pain and other visceral manifestations of HSP [162–164]. Aberrant deposition of IgA in blood vessels and development of target organ vasculitis has led many clinicians to utilize plasmapheresis as treatment for life-threatening manifestations of HSP. It has been used to stabilize highly aggressive HSP nephritis in a small number of cases [165]. Plasmapheresis has also been used to treat potentially life-threatening extrarenal manifestations of HSP including pulmonary hemorrhage and cerebral vasculitis. The rarity of these manifestations complicates the design and implementation of controlled studies and thus the use of plasmaphoresis should only be considered as adjunction therapy for severe complications of HSP [166].

ALPORT SYNDROME (HERIDITARY NEPHRTITIS) AND THIN BASEMENT MEMBRANE NEPHROPATHY

Introduction

In 1902, L.B. Guthrie reported clustering of recurrent hematuria in a London family [167]. The family was followed by Kendall and Hertz, who later described progression of the disease, which they termed "nephritis," and discovered female carrier status [168]. In 1923, Arthur Frederick Hurst found that certain members of that same family eventually progressed to ESRD [169]. Arthur Cecil Alport researched and expanded the pedigree to several generations and discovered the following: (1) deafness accompanied renal failure, (2) males were more severely affected than females, (3) affected males died of their kidney disease, and (4) females lived to old age [170]. Ocular abnormalities in the form of macular lesions and deformation of the lens (anterior lenticonus) were eventually recognized as an important association, and "Alport's disease" came to be defined as a progressive hereditary nephritis (hematuria and proteinuria) associated with sensorineural high-tone deafness and ocular abnormalities affecting the lens and fundus. The genetic component of Alport's disease remained a mystery for half a century until the late 1970s when the X-linked form was discovered [171]. Subsequent genetic benchmarks in Alport's disease included: (1) mapping of the primary locus to the X-chromosome by linkage analysis; (2) the first association of mutations in *COL4A5*, the X-chromosome gene that encodes the α5 chain of collagen type IV; and (3) identification of autosomal recessive and autosomal dominant forms, both attributable to mutations along *COL4A3* and *COL4A4*, the genes that encode the α3 and α4 chains of collagen type IV, respectively [172–175].

Another form of familial hematuria evolved alongside Alport's disease. In 1926, George Baehr reported a "benign and curable form of hemorrhagic nephritis" in fourteen young adults [176]. These patients exhibited painless microscopic hematuria without hypertension or edema. The hematuria was often incidental and follow-up revealed an excellent prognosis. Subsequently, McConville and McAdams discovered kindreds with benign hematuria who demonstrated an autosomal dominant pattern of inheritance [177]. In 1973, Rogers and colleagues reported a correlation between the so-called benign familial hematuria and extensive thinning of GBMs [178]. Eventually, the terms "thin basement membrane disease" and "thin basement membrane nephropathy" (TBMN) became the pathologic correlate to the clinical diagnosis of benign familial hematuria.

Clinicopathologic similarities between TBMN and Alport syndrome sparked investigations into common genetic events [179]. Consequently, in 1996, Lemmink and colleagues discovered a mutation in *COL4A4*, the same gene affected in autosomal forms of Alport syndrome in a kindred of familial benign hematuria [180]. Despite the exponential leaps in our understanding of the etiology and pathogenesis of Alport syndrome and TBMN, a cloud of uncertainty still lingers over the differential between the two diseases.

Of note, the reader should understand that much of the discussion here focuses on the renal aspects of Alport syndrome. The intent is to stay true to the book's intended scope and purpose and not meant to diminish the importance of the extrarenal manifestations. Furthermore, the terms hereditary nephritis, Alport's disease, and Alport syndrome will be used interchangeably. Finally, we will depart from the normal format of the book to discuss the etiology and pathogenesis of hereditary nephritis and TBMN prior to the pathology section. This is intended to enhance the reader's understanding about the pathology.

Epidemiology

Very little is known about the epidemiology of Alport syndrome and TBMN. There is no geographic clustering, and all ethnic groups are affected. The gene frequency in Alport syndrome is estimated in the United States at about 1:5,000 to 1:10,000. Alport's disease comprises about 1–2 percent of the dialysis patients in Europe and about 2 percent of renal transplant patients in the United States and India. It accounts for about 3 percent of cases of chronic renal failure in childhood. In parts of Sweden, the frequency of X-linked disease in males is about 1:17,000 births with a prevalence of about 1:40,000. In Finland, the prevalence is about 1:53,000 live births. Mass screening of schoolchildren for hematuria in Korea detected Alport's disease in about 0.4 percent of children. Thus, statistics are sporadic and the incidence worldwide is unknown.

The prevalence of TBMN is unknown but can be estimated from the (1) frequency of persistent glomerular hematuria within given populations, (2) prevalence of biopsy-proven diagnoses within large-scale surveys, and (3) frequency of the carrier state within kindreds, harboring autosomal recessive Alport syndrome [181]. Using these parameters, the prevalence extrap-

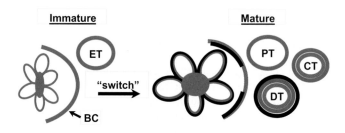

Type IV Collagen Networks

α1, α1, α2 (IV)- α1, α1, α2 (IV)

α3, α4, α5 (IV)- α3, α4, α5 (IV)

α1, α1, α2 (IV)- α5, α5, α6 (IV)

FIGURE 5.31:   Redistribution of α(IV) collagen networks in the developing kidney. See text for details (ET, embryonal tubules; BC, Bowman's capsule; PT, proximal tubules; DT, distal tubules; CT, collecting tubules).

olates broadly to >1 percent but <10 percent of the population. If these figures are accurate, then they suggest that TBMN is the most frequently encountered inherited kidney disease, is the most common cause of persistent hematuria, and is more common than IgAN or Alport's disease.

Etiology, Pathogenesis, and Clinical Presentation

Background

Both Alport syndrome and TBMN are hereditary in nature and arise from mutations of the genes encoding type IV collagen. Six different chains of collagen type IV are produced in mammals – α1 (IV) through α6 (IV) – and are encoded by genes *COL4A1* through *COL4A6*, respectively [182]. *COL4A1* and *COL4A2* are located on chromosome 13, *COL4A3* and *COL4A4* on chromosome 2, and *COL4A5* and *COL4A6* on the X chromosome. Each gene pair is oriented head-to-head along the three chromosomes. Each collagen chain is composed of three domains. The N-terminus is capped by the 7S domain that consists of about 25 residues including asparagine with N-linked oligosaccharides. The helical or collagenous domain is an extended single helical structure consisting of about 1,400 residues with numerous glycine (Gly)-XY repeats, where X is commonly a proline (Pro) residue and Y is often a hydroxyproline (Hpr) residue. Both Pro and Hpr allow for folding and provide stability for the helical structure of collagens. The C-terminus is capped by the noncollagenous (NC1) domain, which contains about 230 residues. The NC1 domain is largely responsible for combining the single helices into protomers, or triple helices. Although the six collagen chains could theoretically form fifty-six different combinations, hypervariable regions within the NC1 domain limit the number of protomers to three: α1, α1, α2 (IV); α3, α4, α5 (IV); and α5, α5, α6 (IV). The substructure of GBM begins with a collagenous network that is formed when protomers bind to one another. The NC1 domains of two protomers bind end-to-end to form dimers, whereas the 7S domains of four protomers overlap and bind through disulfide linkages to form tetramers. Dimers and tetramers intertwine to form network complexes. Three different network complexes are reported: α1, α1, α2 (IV)-α1, α1, α2 (IV); α3, α4, α5 (IV)-α3, α4, α5 (IV); and α1, α1, α2 (IV)-α5, α5, α6 (IV). These networks bind together to form the scaffolding for glomerular and tubular basement membranes in kidney.

The α1, α1, α2 (IV) complexes are ubiquitous to all mammalian basement membranes, whereas expression of α3, α4, α5, and α6 (IV) collagen chains is tissue-dependent. In the developing human kidney, immature basement membranes consist mainly of the α1, α1, α2 (IV) complexes. By three months postnatally, however, a molecular "switch" occurs whereby most but not all of the α1, α1, α2 (IV) complexes in GBM are replaced by α3, α4, α5 (IV)-α3, α4, α5 (IV) network (Figure 5.30). Podocytes appear to be the source of this new collagen. Residual deposition of α1 (IV) and α2 (IV) continues along the subendothelial aspect of mature GBM and is derived from endothelial and possibly mesangial cells [183]. Mesangial matrix of mature glomeruli remains rich in α1 (IV) and α2 (IV) collagen, as do all tubular basement membranes. Basement membranes surrounding distal tubules contain additional amounts of α3, α4, α5 (IV) complexes and probably α1, α1, α2 (IV)-α5, α5, α6 (IV) networks, whereas collecting ducts contain additional content of α1, α1, α2 (IV)-α5, α5, α6 (IV) networks [184]. Mature basement membranes surrounding Bowman's capsule are revamped to consist predominantly of the α1, α1, α2 (IV)-α5, α5, α6 (IV) networks with segmental distribution of α3, α4, α5 (IV) complexes (Figure 5.31).

Etiology

Three genetic forms of Alport syndrome are recognized: X-linked dominant (or semidominant), autosomal recessive, and autosomal dominant. The X-linked form accounts for about 80–85 percent of cases and arises when *COL4A5* is mutated on chromosome Xq26-48. Mutations of the *COL4A3* or *COL4A4* genes on chromosome 2q35-37 result in autosomal forms of the disease. About 15 percent of all cases are autosomal recessive and are associated with identical mutations of both alleles (homozygous mutations) or different mutations of both alleles (compound heterozygotes) of *COL4A3* or *COL4A4*. Autosomal dominant Alport syndrome, which accounts for about 5 percent of all cases, results from mutation(s) of a single allele (heterozygous mutations) of *COL4A3* or *COL4A4*.

Greater than 300 mutations are associated with hereditary nephritis (reviewed in Ref. 185). The vast majority of these is reported for X-linked Alport syndrome and is detected along the entire length of the *COL4A5* gene with no obvious hot spots. In general, each kindred harbors a unique mutation. About 10–15 percent of mutations in the X-linked disease are de novo. Virtually every type of mutation has been described, including missense, in-frame, frameshift, nonsense (including small deletions and insertions), and large rearrangements (typically large deletions). Large rearrangements (gross deletions) account for about 20 percent of mutations and small mutations (missense, deletional, insertional, nonsense, and splice site), account for about 80 percent of mutations in X-linked Alport syndrome [186]. Missense mutations associated with Gly substitutions along the collagenous domain of α5 (IV) are the most frequently encountered. Because they involve the Gly-XY repeats, Gly substitutions usually disrupt the tertiary structure of the α5 (IV) protein and therefore, can dramatically affect the

quaternary structure of type IV collagen. Missense mutations may completely inhibit protomer formation if it involves the NC1 domain. They may also affect posttranslational modification of the α5 (IV) protein. In general, protein truncation is not a feature of missense mutations. Major rearrangements of *COL4A5* are detected in about 5–15 percent of families harboring X-linked disease [187]. They are usually large deletions of varying length that can sometimes extend into the adjacent 5′ end of the *COL4A6* gene. The consequence of such an extended deletion is the additional development of diffuse leiomyomatosis (leiomyomas of the esophagus, trachea, bronchi, and genital tract) in the setting of X-linked Alport's disease. Large deletions may result in complete absence of the α5 (IV) protein or its truncation if the open reading frame is conserved. Truncation is frequent in X-linked Alport's disease and commonly associated with mutations producing premature stop codons (splice site mutations, nonsense mutations, and small deletions and insertions) [187]. More severe truncations are associated with frameshift mutations.

Autosomal recessive Alport syndrome is linked to homozygous and compound heterozygous mutations of *COL4A3* and *COL4A4*. More than thirty mutations have been described. Most are nonsense or missense mutations but frameshift, splice site, deep intronic, and large deletion mutations have also been reported [188–192]. Autosomal dominant Alport syndrome is linked to heterozygous mutations of *COL4A3* and *COL4A4*. At least nine mutations have been reported and are mainly missense and splice site mutations [175,193]. Similar to the X-linked form, mutations associated with autosomal Alport syndrome occur all along *COL4A3* and *COL4A4* without any obvious hot spots.

Investigations into the mutational events in hereditary nephritis have also enhanced our understanding about the etiology of TBMN. Hematuria in TBMN is transmitted as an autosomal dominant trait and is associated with mutations of *COL4A3* and *COL4A4*, analogous to autosomal Alport syndrome [180]. To date, about twenty-seven heterozygous mutations are documented in *COL4A3* and *COL4A4* for TBMN [194,195]. About 40 percent of TBMN patients segregate to the *COL4A3/COL4A4* locus [193]. Most are missense and nonsense mutations, whereas the rest are splice site, frameshift, small insertional, and small/large deletional mutations. Point mutations (substitutions) in the NC1 domains have also been described. Similar to autosomal Alport syndrome, TBMN mutations occur all along *COL4A3* and *COL4A4* without any obvious hot spots. It has been suggested that TBMN represents the carrier state for autosomal recessive Alport syndrome, since both share specific mutations and the latter manifests as diffuse GBM attenuation early on.

Also known as benign familial hematuria, TBMN is not always familial. In fact, about one-third of patients have no known relatives with hematuria. Furthermore, many families harboring TBMN do not show linkage to the *COL4A3/COL4A4* locus. The reasons are often attributed to de novo mutations, incomplete penetrance, coincidental hematuria in unaffected family members, or linkage to genes other than *COL4A3* or *COL4A4* [196]. Attempts to establish linkage with mutational events in other structural protein genes such as α1 (IV), α2 (IV), perlecan, fibronectin, and laminins were unsuccessful.

Pathogenesis

The pathogenesis of hereditary nephritis is not completely understood. It is generally assumed that mutations of the genes encoding $\alpha3$ (IV), $\alpha4$ (IV), or $\alpha5$ (IV) result in absent or altered monomers that are ultimately degraded or excluded from protomer assembly. In the example of X-linked Alport syndrome, mutation of $\alpha5$ (IV) will inhibit or interfere with self-assembly of $\alpha3$, $\alpha4$, $\alpha5$ (IV) complexes and $\alpha1$, $\alpha1$, $\alpha2$ (IV)-$\alpha5$, $\alpha5$, $\alpha6$ (IV) networks. Thus, vital accrual of the $\alpha3$, $\alpha4$, $\alpha5$ (IV) complexes in mature GBM is either completely inhibited or severely perturbed. Consequently, the GBM fails to mature properly and relies on the $\alpha1$, $\alpha1$, $\alpha2$ (IV) complexes for structural integrity. The GBM remains functional despite its structural deficiencies, at least for a few years or even decades. However, $\alpha1$ (IV) and $\alpha2$ (IV) apparently lack the stability inherent to $\alpha3$, $\alpha4$, $\alpha5$ (IV) complexes. The latter network contains more cysteine residues and therefore exhibits more disulfide bridging, which imparts greater resistance to protease degradation [197]. Over time, the physical integrity of the immature GBM is compromised. Podocyte injury leads to foot process effacement. The glomerular filtration barrier begins to falter, allowing for nonselective passage of protein (proteinuria) and RBCs (hematuria). In most instances, glomeruli undergo sclerosis leading to progressive renal insufficiency. Of note, data from animal models implicate a number of other noncollagenous proteins as either directly or indirectly involved in the pathogenesis of hereditary nephritis [198–202].

The pathogenesis of TBMN is seemingly simple. GBMs are poorly developed due to genetic mutation of type IV collagen, or perhaps some other gene(s). GBMs are diffusely attenuated and develop periodic breaks or small gaps that allow for passage of RBCs into the ultrafiltrate. The consequence is gross or microscopic hematuria. It is not clear, however, why some cases of benign familial hematuria lose their benignity and develop significant proteinuria and renal insufficiency. The controversial presumption is that certain patients are susceptible to a "gene dosage" effect where a more aggressive course is related to a more severe mutational defect of collagen.

Clinical Presentation

Male patients with X-linked Alport syndrome usually present, prior to seven years of age, with isolated gross or microscopic hematuria, and within the context of familial disease. At the very least, they exhibit persistent rather than intermittent microhematuria. Exercise or upper respiratory infections may provoke episodes of gross hematuria in children, adolescents, and teenagers. Proteinuria at presentation is uncommon in younger children and appears later in the disease. However, a child whose clinical course is characterized only by microhematuria may go undiagnosed for several years and can therefore present later with hematuria and mild proteinuria. Children rarely, if ever, present with the sensorineural hearing loss and ocular complications (anterior lenticonus, dot-and-fleck maculopathy, and posterior polymorphous dystrophy) that are characteristic of Alport syndrome, since these complications develop much later in the disease.

The vast majority of affected females exhibit only microscopic hematuria at presentation. Unlike males, microhematuria in females has a greater tendency to be intermittent and therefore, has a greater chance of evading detection. Thus, female patients may present at a later age than males. A minor subset of women with X-linked Alport syndrome and almost all women with autosomal recessive disease develop proteinuria and progress to ESRD. Hence, Alport disease can declare itself as microhematuria and proteinuria during the teen years in females.

Like Alport's disease, TBMN usually presents with isolated painless microhematuria. It presents in children at a median age of 7 years, and in adults at a median age of 37 years. The male:female ratio is not known. In contrast to Alport's disease, about 30 percent of patients do not have a family history of hematuria. Most patients present only with persistent microhematuria detected incidentally. Episodes of macrohematuria are less frequent than in Alport's disease and are usually exacerbated with exercise and infection. Children rarely present with proteinuria but it can evolve later in the disease in some patients. Hence, adults can sometimes present with TBMN complicated by mild to moderate proteinuria.

Approach to Interpretation

Light Microscopy

The light microscopic features of TBMN and hereditary nephritis are nonspecific. The glomerular changes of hereditary nephritis are ill-defined during the early phase of the disease and are often nil (Figures 5.32A,B). Other findings may include persistence of immature glomeruli, mesangial prominence without mesangial hypercellularity, prominent or mildly thickened glomerular capillary loops, and segmental glomerulosclerosis, among others. Progression of the disease is characterized by nonspecific patterns of segmental to global glomerulosclerosis (Figures 5.32C,D). Sclerotic lesions are sometimes accompanied by hyalinosis. These changes occur on a background of increased mesangial matrix with mild mesangial proliferation and thickening of capillary loops. Silver stains may reveal simple to complex reduplication of the capillary loops and segmental tuft collapse. Glomerulosclerosis tends to occur with greater frequency in autosomal recessive Alport syndrome [203]. Crescents are infrequent and thought to be reactive in nature. The extent of tubulointerstitial scarring is usually commensurate with the degree of glomerular sclerosis. Scattered RBC casts are typical. Both tubular and interstitial foam cells may also be present in abundance (Figure 5.33). The presence of foam cells in the absence of hyperlipidemia or nephrotic range proteinuria is strongly suggestive of hereditary nephritis. Vascular changes (medial wall thickening and intimal fibrosis) are essentially limited to older patients with hypertension. Kidney biopsies from heterozygous female carriers of X-linked disease and male/female carriers of autosomal recessive disease show the first signs of glomerular and tubulointerstitial scarring during late childhood, but X-linked carrier females show a higher rate of scarring with age.

Glomeruli in TBMN are essentially unremarkable by light microscopy (Figure 5.34A). Detection of diffuse GBM thinning is beyond the resolution of the light microscope. Markedly affected cases, however, may show reduced argyrophilia of glomerular capillary loops by virtue of reduced substrate available for silver impregnation. Mesangial hypercellularity and matrix increase are usually nominal but occasionally increased. Kidney biopsies from children with TBMN rarely show any chronic

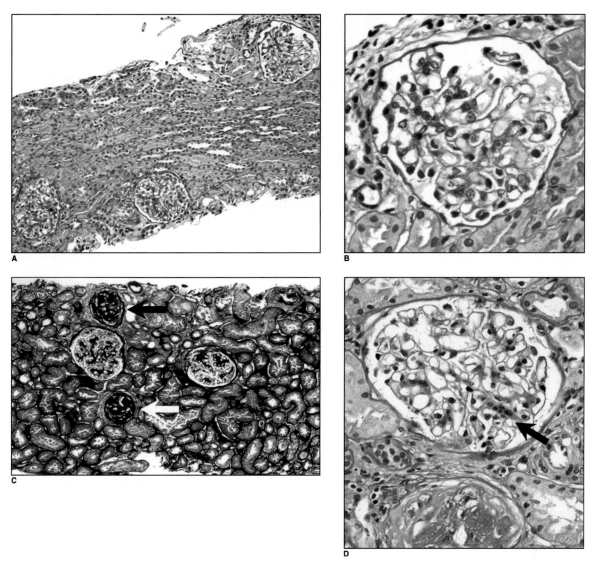

FIGURE 5.32: *Light microscopic findings in Alport's disease. (A,B) A biopsy from a four-year-old boy with early onset of hereditary nephritis shows virtually no glomerular or tubulointerstitial changes by light microscopy [PAS stain, original magnifications: × 100 (A) and × 400 (B)]. (C,D) In contrast to the case depicted in (A) and (B), a biopsy from a fifteen-year-old male with advanced hereditary nephritis exhibits a nonspecific pattern of glomerulosclerosis (white and black arrows) and tubulointerstitial scarring. Glomeruli evidence mild segmental mesangial hypercellularity and matrix increase (arrow) [(C) Combined MAS/JMS stain, original magnification: × 100; (D) PAS stain, original magnification: × 400].*

changes. Biopsies from some adult patients with TBMN may exhibit focal nonspecific glomerulosclerosis with varying degrees of tubulointerstitial and vascular scarring (Figure 5.34B). These changes are often attributed to secondary processes such as coincidental hypertension or age-related senescence. Yet, some nonelderly adult patients with TBMN exhibit focal glomerulosclerosis prior to onset of hypertension and proteinuria. This finding of "premature" glomerulosclerosis has been suggested as a risk factor for disease progression [204].

Immunofluorescence Microscopy

Since Alport's disease and TBMN are not immune complex–mediated, screening for deposition of immunoglobulin and complement has limited utility and only serves to rule out other glomerulopathies. Occasional glomerular deposits of IgG, IgM, or C3 are sometimes detected but are ambiguous. Instead, immunofluorescence microscopy is useful in cataloging the distribution of type IV collagens in glomeruli, tubular basement membranes, and skin. These data are extremely helpful in the diagnosis of Alport's disease.

Commercially available kits utilize monoclonal antibodies against selected collagen type IV α-chains to assist in the diagnosis of Alport syndrome. These kits usually contain monoclonal antibodies against α1 (IV), α3 (IV), and α5 (IV). Figure 5.34 compares the distribution of type IV collagen α-chains in normal adult kidney and X-linked Alport syndrome. In normal kidney, anti-α1 (IV) antibodies mark the α1, α1, α2 (IV)-α1,

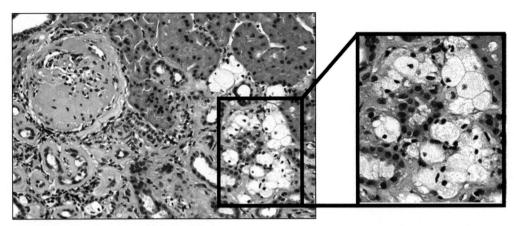

FIGURE 5.33: *Interstitial foam cells in a case of advanced Alport's disease (H&E stain, original magnification: × 100; inset: × 600).*

α1, α2 (IV) networks in mesangial matrix and tubular basement membranes, as well as the α1, α1, α2 (IV)-α5, α5, α6 (IV) networks along Bowman's capsule (Figure 5.35A, and Table 5.10). These antibodies also identify residual amounts of α1, α1, α2 (IV)-α1, α1, α2 (IV) networks in mature GBM (Figure 5.35A). Antibodies targeting α3 (IV) and α5 (IV) detect α3, α4, α5 (IV)-α3, α4, α5 (IV) networks along GBMs and basement membranes surrounding Bowman's capsule and distal tubules (Figures 5.35C,E, and Table 5.10). Anti-α5 (IV) antibodies also mark the α3, α4, α5 (IV) complexes and α1, α1, α2 (IV)-α5, α5, α6 (IV) networks in Bowman's capsule (Figure 5.35E).

In males, X-linked Alport syndrome results in the failure to assimilate the α5 (IV) molecule into collagen protomers, which subsequently inhibits assembly of the α3, α4, α5 (IV)-α3, α4, α5 (IV) and α1, α1, α2 (IV)-α5, α5, α6 (IV) networks. Consequently, antibodies against α3 (IV) and α5 (IV) do not react with affected kidney tissue (Figures 5.35D,F and Table 5.10). Since there is little or no affect on the assembly of the α1, α1, α2 (IV) complexes, immunofluorescence for α1 (IV) in the Alport kidney persists (Figure 5.35B and Table 5.10). The failure to detect α3 (IV) and α5 (IV) by immunofluorescence is not an ubiquitous finding among male patients with X-linked disease. Negative immunofluorescence for α3 (IV) and α5 (IV) occurs in only about two-thirds of male patients. The discrepant one-third who continue to show expression of α3 (IV) and/or α5 (IV) apparently harbor *COL4A5* mutations that may perturb the collagen molecule but may not be enough to inhibit protomer and network assembly. These cases maybe associated with mutations related to less aggressive forms of hereditary nephritis. In some X-linked male patients, α5 (IV) is not expressed but α3 (IV) is expressed to varying degrees [205].

X-linked heterozygous females, most of whom have very mild disease, tend to exhibit a mosaic pattern of α3 (IV) and/ or α5 (IV) expression. Here, immunofluorescence for α3 (IV) and α5 (IV) exhibits a segmental, irregular, or discontinuous linear pattern along glomerular capillary loops and tubular basement membranes. This mosaic expression of collagen along basement membranes is thought to be secondary to random or nonrandom X-inactivation resulting in production of wild-type collagen by one cell but a mutant form from an adjacent cell [206]. This mechanism is purely speculative at the moment.

Autosomal recessive Alport syndrome is characterized by the failure to assimilate the α3 (IV) or α4 (IV) chains into collagen protomers that inhibits assembly of the α3, α4, α5 (IV)-α3, α4, α5 (IV) networks. Thus, immunofluorescence for α3 (IV) and α5 (IV) is lost along glomerular capillary loops and α3 (IV) is no longer detected around Bowman's capsule or distal tubules (Table 5.10). Because the mutations have no effect on the α1, α1, α2 (IV)-α5, α5, α6 (IV) networks, linear immunofluorescence for α5 (IV) persists along Bowman's capsule and tubular basement membranes (Table 5.10). This pattern of persistence of α5 (IV) immunofluorescence in the absence of α3 (IV) is a key feature distinguishing X-linked from autosomal disease.

The sensitivity of collagen type IV detection using immunofluorescence microscopy for the diagnosis of hereditary nephritis is modest (about 65–75 percent). The reason is that the type of mutation and the gene dosing effect have a profound effect on the expression, or lack thereof, of collagens along basement membranes. Considering the hundreds of private mutations associated with Alport syndrome, it is amazing that a consistent phenotypic distribution of collagen is found two-thirds of the time. Nevertheless, there are variations in presence and absence of collagens in affected organs [205,207]. Accordingly, failure to identify any change in collagen expression in a patient with suspected Alport's disease does not rule it out.

The distribution of collagen type IV along the epidermal basement membrane (EBM) can also be exploited in the diagnosis of X-linked Alport's disease. EBM contains large amounts of α1 (IV), α2 (IV), α5 (IV), and α6 (IV). The linear immunofluorescence for α1 (IV) seen along the EBM in normal skin persists in patients with X-linked disease. In contrast, the normal linear pattern of immunofluorescence for α5 (IV) is absent from male patients and segmental (mosaic) in female patients with X-linked disease. Skin testing has no utility in diagnosing autosomal Alport syndrome, since the EBM is normally devoid of α3 (IV). The relative ease and lower cost of obtaining a skin versus kidney biopsy has caused many to advocate skin testing as the diagnostic procedure of choice in X-linked Alport syndrome [208].

To date, immunohistochemical localization of type IV collagen has been performed on only a handful of patients with autosomal dominant Alport syndrome [209]. They show no

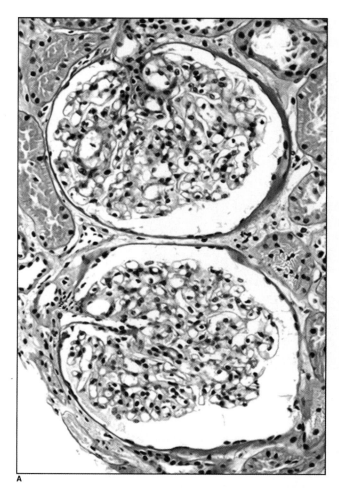 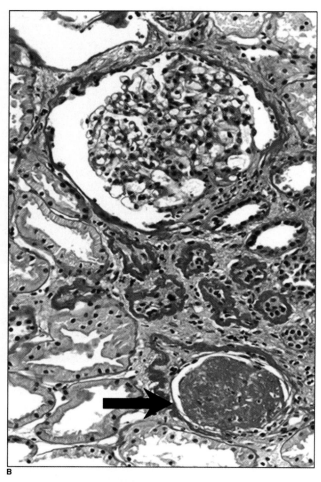

FIGURE 5.34: Light microscopic changes in TBMN. (A) In many instances, glomeruli are essentially unremarkable by light microscopy. (B) A biopsy from a thirty-three-year-old patient with thin basement membrane nephropathy but no history of hypertension shows evidence of "premature" glomerulosclerosis (arrow) and tubulointerstitial scarring. (PAS stain, original magnification: × 100).

difference between affected and control patients. Likewise, kidney biopsies from patients with TBMN typically show no change in the expression of collagen type IV, despite the presence of heterozygous mutations of *COL4A3* and *COL4A4*.

Electron Microscopy

Advances in the pathologic diagnosis of Alport's disease were at a standstill until the late 1960s when electron microscopy was applied [210,211]. The most important morphologic clues to the diagnosis of hereditary nephritis occur at the ultrastructural level and are manifested primarily as alterations in the fine structure of the GBM. Ultrastructural alterations of hereditary nephritis can be detected as early as one year of age. A key diagnostic feature is the presence of reduplication or splitting of the GBM lamina densa, a pattern that is often referred to as "basket weaving" (Figure 5.36). The typical appearance is that of intertwining electron-dense lamellae that represent the frayed or duplicated segments of lamina densa. Basket weaving within thickened GBMs increases the likelihood of hereditary nephritis, since GBM thickening is also considered a salient diagnostic feature (Figure 5.37). Another characteristic finding

is the presence of electron-lucent areas between the electron-dense strands. These spaces contain fine granular particles measuring up to 900 angstroms in diameter and are referred to affectionately as "crumbs" by Liapis and colleagues (Figure 5.38) [212]. Affected GBM often shows irregular contouring along both the subepithelial and subendothelial sides (Figure 5.36B). An accentuated bulge will periodically erupt on the subepithelial side. The extent of podocyte injury is variable; reactive changes include vacuolization and hypertrophy. Foot processes maybe mildly distorted or completely effaced over affected GBM segments (Figure 5.36). Reduplication of the GBM with mesangial interposition is occasionally observed (Figure 5.39).

It should be noted that thickened GBMs with evidence of basket weaving is hereditary nephritis until proven otherwise, but is only pathognomonic if diffuse and global. The lesion has also been reported in IgAN, poststreptococcal GN, focal sclerosis, and membranous glomerulopathy [213,214].

Although specific GBM changes tend to cluster in many but not all Alport kindreds, the degree and extent of GBM changes vary considerably among unrelated patients [184,215]. Some may show global GBM thickening where multiple lamellae span

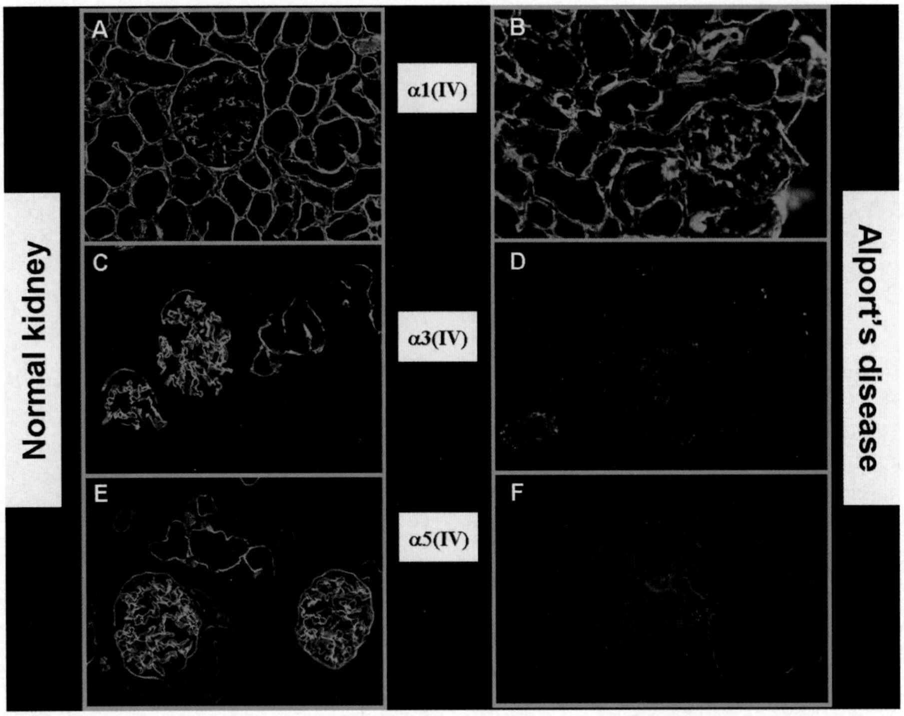

FIGURE 5.35: *Distribution of type IV collagen α-chains in normal adult kidney and X-linked Alport syndrome. See text for details (original magnification: × 100).*

Table 5.10 Basic Immunohistochemical Distribution of Type IV Collagens in Normal Human Kidney and Hereditary Nephritis

	Normal Kidney					
	α1(IV)	α3(IV)	α5(IV)			
Glomerulus	+	+	+			
Bowman's capsule	+	−/+	+			
Distal nephron (TBM)	+	+	+			

	Hereditary Nephritis					
	X-linked (males)			Autosomal recessive		
	α1(IV)	α3(IV)	α5(IV)	α1(IV)	α3(IV)	α5(IV)
Glomerulus	+	−	−	+	−	−
Bowman's capsule	+	−	−	+	−	+
Distal nephron (TBM)	+	−	−	+	−	+

−/+: Mosaic pattern of immunofluorescence.

TBM, Tubular basement membranes.

the full thickness of expanded membranes (Figure 5.40). These findings maybe seen in (1) older male children with juvenile onset X-linked hereditary nephritis, (2) older male adults with adult onset of X-linked hereditary nephritis, (3) male and female patients with advancing autosomal recessive Alport syndrome, and (4) rarely, in female X-linked carriers [216]. These changes tend to carry a poor prognosis and portend onset of ESRD. Other patients may exhibit segmental thickening and basket weaving of GBMs adjacent to long segments of normal or even attenuated GBMs (Figure 5.37). Attenuated GBMs may also show signs of mild basket weaving. This alternating pattern of thick and thin GBMs with segmental basket weaving has been reported in X-linked, autosomal recessive or autosomal dominant Alport's disease, including female carriers of X-linked disease [216]. These findings may represent an intermediate stage between early and late disease. Still other Alport patients may exhibit diffuse attenuation of GBMs with no thickening and little or no evidence of basket weaving. They therefore mimic

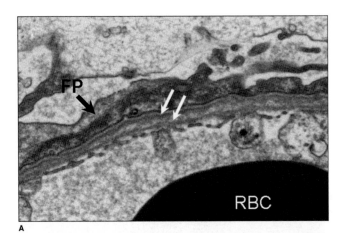

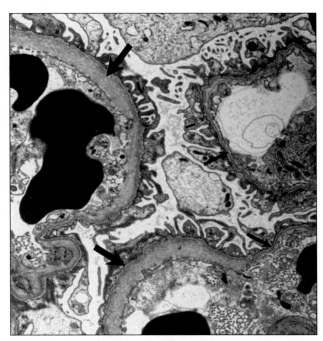

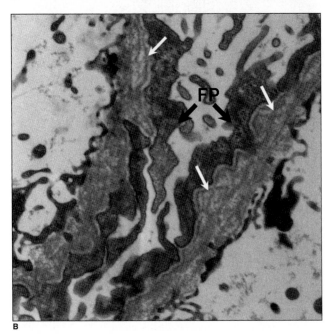

FIGURE 5.36: *Ultrastructural alterations of the GBM in Alport's disease. (A) An important diagnostic feature of hereditary nephritis is splitting or reduplication of the lamina densa, also referred to as a "basket weave" pattern. The GBM depicted here is attenuated and shows simple splitting of the lamina densa (arrows). The foot processes (FP) are also effaced (RBC, red blood cell, UA-LC stain, original magnification: × 22,300). (B) Another example shows more extensive splitting and reduplication of the lamina densa (arrows), resulting in irregular thickening and contouring of the GBM along the subendothelial and subepithelial sides. Foot processes (FP) are effaced (UA-LC stain, original magnification: × 27,500).*

FIGURE 5.37: *Ultrastructural alterations of the GBM in Alport's disease. The diagnosis of hereditary nephritis is bolstered by exuberant splitting and reduplication of lamina densa resulting in abnormally thickened GBMs (larger arrows). Segmental attenuation of membranes may also be seen (smaller arrows), even in advanced disease. Indeed, alternating thick and thin GBMs are common in hereditary nephritis. In the lower right hand corner, an attenuated portion of GBM (smaller arrow) gives rise to a much thicker one (bigger arrow) (UA-LC stain, original magnification: × 11,000).*

TBMN histologically. These kinds of changes may represent the earliest stages of hereditary nephritis and are commonly seen in female carriers of X-linked disease. Indeed, serial biopsies in humans have mapped progression from a TBMN-like histology in childhood to advanced hereditary nephritis in adulthood and are recapitulated in a number of experimental models [202,217]. However, some patients with progressive hereditary nephritis continue to show diffuse attenuation of GBMs [212]. Consequently, the presence of TBMN-like changes does not necessarily carry a good prognosis. Since the earliest stages of hereditary nephritis and female carriers of the Alport gene may manifest as TBMN, immunofluorescence testing of a current or previous biopsy for type IV collagens should be considered under the following circumstances: (1) evidence of clinical progression of disease, such as new-onset proteinuria (>500 mg/24h), increasing proteinuria, new-onset hypertension, and/or renal insufficiency; (2) a family history of Alport's disease or chronic renal failure; and (3) minor Alport-like changes by electron microscopy. Finally, a small subset of patients with hereditary nephritis show completely normal GBMs [179].

Thus, changes in the fine structure of the glomerulus vary widely among patients with hereditary nephritis. There are loose associations between certain changes and mode of transmission. For example, female carriers of X-linked disease tend to show greater variation in GBM thickness and a higher frequency of basket weaving than carriers of autosomal disease. Some ultrastructural features also correlate with genotype in hereditary nephritis. For instance, Mazzuccio et al. attribute more severe ultrastructural changes to null mutations (major rearrangements, mutations involving the start codon, and frameshift mutations), and less severe lesions to missense mutations involving Gly-XY sequences and small in-frame deletions/insertions [205]. Attempts to correlate ultrastructural findings with collagen type IV expression have been mixed.

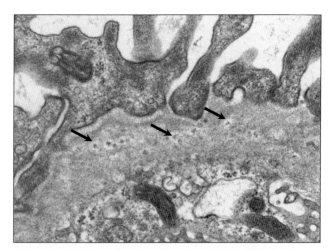

FIGURE 5.38: "Crumbs" in Alport's disease. Fine dense-core granular particles (arrows) reside between reduplicated lamina densa (UA-LC stain, original magnification: × 45,100).

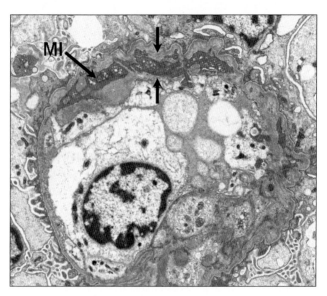

FIGURE 5.39: Mesangial interposition in Alport's disease. The arrows depict splitting and reduplication of GBM around mesangial interposition (MI) (UA-LC stain, original magnification: × 3,500).

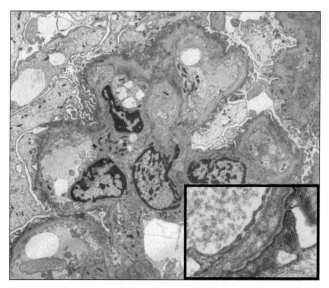

FIGURE 5.40: Global thickening of GBMs in Alport's disease (UA-LC stain, original magnification: × 5,510; inset: × 35,100).

Light and immunofluorescence microscopic findings in TBMN are nonspecific and therefore provide few clues to the diagnosis. Electron microscopy is required since the key diagnostic feature is the diffuse thinning of GBMs (Figure 5.41). The diagnosis is seemingly simple but inherently flawed [218]. For example, there are no established criteria for normal GBM thickness, although estimates can be gleaned from the literature. The mean GBM width is estimated at 150 nm at birth; 200 nm by 1 year of age; 208–245 nm between 1 and 6 years of age; 244–307 nm between 6 and 11 years of age; 320 ± 50 nm in female adults; and 370 ± 50 nm in male adults (reviewed in Ref. 194). A number of other factors confound standardization of the diagnosis. Age, gender, and technical artifacts such as fixation and embedding media effect GBM width. There is lack of consensus

about the best approach to measure GBM thickness. Finally, there is no consensus on the morphologic criteria for TBMN. Most laboratories develop their own criteria based on the literature or on studies of their local patient population. In general, the literature estimates that the lower limits of normal GBM thickness in adults range between 200 and 265 nm. WHO criteria sets the lower limits at 250 nm for adults and 180 nm for children between 2 and 11 years of age, but does not account for gender [219]. Some pathologists confide that they do not measure GBMs and simply make a subjective judgment based on overall appearance (unpublished data). Although different laboratories employ different diagnostic protocols, most agree that their data are derived from multiple measurements taken from the periphery of multiple capillary loops (Figure 5.42). GBMs are usually measured between cell membranes of podocyte and endothelium where they contact with the membrane. Some, on the other hand, advocate measuring the width of the lamina densa [214].

Optimal diagnostic criteria for TBMN include: (1) a clinical history of hematuria without significant proteinuria or renal impairment; (2) a family history of hematuria but not chronic renal failure or hearing loss; (3) nonspecific findings by light and immunofluorescence microscopy; and (4) diffuse or global (>50 percent) thinning of GBMs without any other significant glomerular pathology. The trilaminar structure of the GBM is preserved, although attenuated (Figures 5.41 and 5.42). The lamina densa shows little or no evidence of splitting, fraying, or reduplication (Figure 5.42). Even minor evidence of basket weaving should alert the pathologist to the possibility of Alport's disease. Irregular contouring of the GBM maybe present but is usually mild. Foot processes are well preserved or show evidence of patchy mild effacement. Interestingly, a significant percentage of patients with isolated hematuria show only segmental (<50 percent) rather than global GBM thinning [220]. Segmental versus diffuse attenuation is simply one of many confounding issues that hinder standardization of the diagnosis of TBMN.

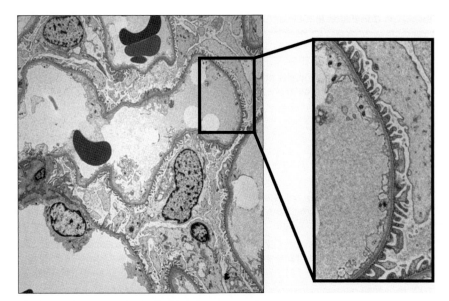

FIGURE 5.41: Global attenuation of GBMs in TBMN. GBMs are abnormally thin (UA-LC stain, original magnification: × 4,510; inset: × 14,000).

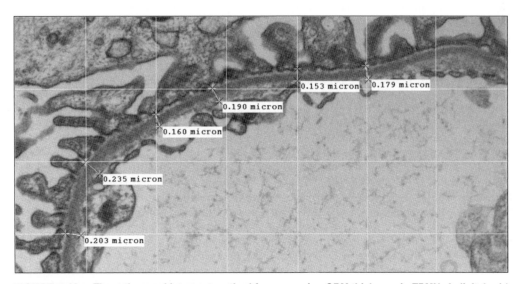

FIGURE 5.42: The orthogonal intercept method for measuring GBM thickness in TBMN. A digital grid is superimposed over peripheral GBM. To ensure random sampling, measurements of GBM thickness are taken where the grid intersects with membrane. Measurements span between cell membranes of podocyte and endothelial cells where they contact with basement membrane. In the field shown, the average GBM width is 187 nm, and is well below the normal value for this adult male patient. (Courtesy of Dr. Vanesa Bijol, Emory University Hospital, Atlanta, Georgia.)

Differential Diagnosis

The differential diagnosis of Alport's disease includes other inherited forms of glomerular disease that result in hematuria and proteinuria (Table 5.1). They include familial IgAN, nail-patella syndrome, and TBMN. Familial IgAN may mimic hereditary nephritis clinically but does not have the extrarenal manifestations and is differentiated further from Alport's disease by the presence of IgA deposits on renal biopsy. Nail-patella syndrome is distin-

guished from Alport syndrome by a completely different set of extrarenal manifestations, and by a renal biopsy showing the large distinctive collagen fibrils located along thickened GBMs.

An important and potentially difficult task is differentiating early X-linked or autosomal recessive Alport syndrome from TBMN, since the prognosis between the two diseases is so disparate. There are some obvious differences. TBMN has no extrarenal manifestations, in either the patient or the patient's

Table 5.11 Genotype–Phenotype Correlation in X-Linked Alport Syndrome

Reference	COL4A5 Mutations	Clinical Outcome
Jias et al. [186]	Large rearrangements and smaller mutations (nonsense, small insertions/deletions) leading to a premature stop codon	Highest risk: 90% probability of ESRD in males before 30 years of age (50% renal survival rate at 20 years)
	Splice site mutations	Higher risk: 70% probability of ESRD in males before 30 years of age (50% renal survival rate at 25 years)
	Missense mutations	High risk: 50% probability of ESRD in males before 30 years of age (50% renal survival rate at 32 years)
Gross et al. [185]	Large rearrangements, donor splice site mutations, and mutations leading to a premature stop codon or involving the NC1 domain	Type S (Severe): Males reach ESRD at ~20 years of age with an 80% chance of hearing loss and 40% chance of ocular lesions
	Non-Gly-XY missense mutations, Gly-XY missense mutations in exons 21–47, in-frame and acceptor splice site mutations	Type MS (Moderate-severe): Males reach ESRD at ~26 years of age with a 65% chance of hearing loss and 30% chance of ocular lesions
	Gly-XY missense mutations in exons 1–20	Type M (Moderate): Males reach ESRD at ~30 years of age with a 70% chance of hearing loss and 30% chance of ocular lesions

family history. The mode of transmission is autosomal dominant. Disease progression in TBMN should increase suspicion of early Alport's disease and either a skin or kidney biopsy, or both are warranted. Workup of the biopsy should include immunofluorescence for the type IV collagens. The skin biopsy has utility in diagnosing X-linked Alport syndrome but not autosomal recessive disease. The kidney biopsy yields data for both but the false- negative rate [positive staining for α3 (IV) and/or α5 (IV) is 20–30 percent. The utility of electron microscopy is limited in differentiating the two diseases, but evidence of basket weaving even in the absence of GBM thickening supports early Alport's disease. If the examination of pedigree and pathologic analysis of tissue fail to differentiate TBMN from Alport's syndrome, then the only viable option is wait for the disease to declare itself. Genetic testing is an option but is not cost-effective. The test only has meaning if a mutation is somehow detected in *COL4A5*, since TBMN and autosomal recessive Alport syndrome are associated with mutations of *COL4A3* and *COL4A4*.

Prognosis, Natural History, and Clinicopathologic Correlation

The general premise is that males who develop mutation(s) of the X-linked *COL4A5* gene invariably progress to ESRD before 30 years of age. The rate of progression varies between families and appears to be dependent on the type of mutation. In fact, some investigators produced constructs of genotype–phenotype relationships that attempt to classify and predict disease outcomes in X-linked disease based on the type of mutation. These schemata are listed in Table 5.11. Although each has caveats, these schemata will serve as the framework for future molecular prognostication, when genetic testing becomes broader based.

Females who are heterozygous for a mutated X-linked *COL4A5* gene are carriers of Alport syndrome. Phenotypic expression of these carriers is variable but most exhibit clinicopathologic features of TBMD. About 12 percent progress to ESRD prior to 40 years of age [216]. The probability of ESRD increases to 30 percent by 60 years of age, however. Onset of hearing loss, and onset and incremental rises of proteinuria are the best predictors for progression to ESRD, although no significant genotype–phenotype relationships have yet been established in females with X-linked Alport syndrome. In contrast to males with X-linked disease, clinical presentation and clinical course show tremendous variability among affected females within a given family. Inactivation of the X chromosome is thought to account for this variability but has not yet been proven.

Patients who exhibit homozygous or compound heterozygous mutations of *COL4A3* or *COL4A4* develop autosomal recessive Alport syndrome. Male and female patients with autosomal recessive Alport syndrome invariably progress to ESRD before 30 years of age. On the other hand, males or females who are heterozygous for *COL4A3* or *COL4A4* mutations have variable outcomes. Some are completely asymptomatic, whereas others exhibit clinical and pathologic features of TBMD. A few progress to proteinuria and renal insufficiency. Preliminary data suggest that missense mutations tend to impart a more aggressive clinical course than null mutations in these patients [191]. A rare subset of patients heterozygous for *COL4A3* or *COL4A4* mutations develop autosomal dominant Alport syndrome, which is usually defined by male-to-male transmission and associated with consanguinity. Clinical outcomes are unpredictable with inconsistent progression to ESRD, usually after 50 years of age [175]. No genotype–phenotype correlations have been defined.

Certain ultrastructural features are touted as prognosticators in hereditary nephritis [215]. Extensive basket weaving along GBMs is considered more ominous than extensive thinning. Indeed, the latter seems to impart a more favorable prognosis in males. These findings have not yet withstood the rigors of statistical analysis, however.

Table 5.12 Findings Associated with Loin Pain Hematuria Syndrome

GBM thickening and attenuation
Mild cortical infarction
Renal microaneurysms
Renal vasospasm
Renocalyceal fistulas
Renal arteriovenous malformations
Renovascular disease
Abnormal ureteral peristalsis
"Occult" nephrolithiasis
Hypersensitivity
Altered coagulability
Psychological factors

In general, TBMD carries an excellent prognosis. The only acknowledged risk factors for progression are proteinuria and hypertension. These complications are extremely rare in children. In adults with biopsy-proven TBMD, the incidence of proteinuria (>500 mg/24 hours) is about 20 percent and hypertension, about 35 percent [221]. Renal impairment develops in about 7 percent of these patients and usually has a late onset (>50 years of age). Progression to ESRD is generally a rare event, although the incidence of ESRD may reach as high as 20 percent in some cohorts carrying *COL4A3/COL4A4* mutations. Finally, association of TBMN with other glomerulopathies increases risk for progression; the most common is IgAN [29].

Treatment

To date, therapy for Alport's disease or TBMN is merely supportive. ACE inhibitors or cyclosporine reduce urinary protein excretion in some Alport patients, but the data are too preliminary to draw reasonable conclusions for the long term [222,223]. A number of other therapeutic approaches are being tested in experimental animals, including gene therapy, but it is not clear if these modalities will extrapolate to the human condition.

Alport's disease is not a contraindication for renal transplantation. In general, renal allograft survival is no different in Alport patients than the general population of recipients. A small minority of Alport patients, however, run the risk of developing rapidly progressive GN within the first year post transplant. Apparently, these patients are sensitized to idiotypic mutations of collagen type IV. Implantation of the renal allograft exposes them to the unfamiliar wild type collagens that their immune systems recognize as foreign. The result is the production of anti-GBM autoantibodies, crescentic GN, and acute renal failure. Prognosis is generally poor, unless plasmaphoresis is employed earlier in the course of the disease.

LOIN PAIN HEMATURIA SYNDROME

Loin pain hematuria syndrome (LPHS) was first defined in 1967 in a small cadre of young women who suffered from chronic recurrent pain in the lower flanks and intermittent hematuria [224]. Extensive workups failed to reveal any overt cause for their symptomatologies, although arteriograms suggested slight alterations in renal cortical perfusion and renal biopsies demonstrated mild nonspecific scarring of the interstitium and vasculature. Today, the clinical criteria first described by Little et al. still apply but with some permutations. The typical patient remains a white female in her late twenties who presents with recurrent loin pain and microscopic or gross hematuria that may be intermittent [225]. Hematuria and loin pain do not always synchronize, however. Onset of back pain can precede hematuria and is usually severe, debilitating, and may radiate to the abdomen, thigh, or groin. It often presents unilaterally but eventually progresses to both sides of the back. Fever, dysuria, and mild proteinuria are atypical features that are sometimes observed. As many as one-half of patients diagnosed with LPHS also have a history of nephrolithiasis.

There are a number of negative findings in LPHS, since it is a diagnosis of exclusion. The physical exam is essentially unremarkable, except for occasional tenderness along the costovertebral angle. Hypertension is infrequent. There is no evidence for infection. Urologic and laboratory workups tend to be unremarkable, although various abnormalities along the coagulation cascade are observed in some patients. The subtle abnormalities in renal cortical perfusion and blood vessel integrity seen in earlier arteriography studies were not observed in later studies. Consequently, radiographic studies are nonspecific and inconsistent in LPHS. Of note, we have seen at least two cases of arteriovenous (AV) malformations of the renal pelvis mimicking LPHS. A urologic, nephrologic, and pathologic workup was unrevealing, until renal arteriograms detected the highly elusive AV malformations in the calyses.

The pathology of LPHS is nonspecific. Light microscopy is usually unremarkable but may occasionally show mild glomerular, tubulointerstitial, and vascular scarring, which is not attributable to hypertension or senescence in younger patients. RBCs are frequently seen within tubules. Immunofluorescence and electron microscopy are also nonspecific and rule out an immune-mediated process, such as IgAN. Electron microscopy, however, may reveal varying degrees of GBM thickening and attenuation. In one series, about 15 percent of patients met the diagnostic criteria for TBMN [226].

LPHS is a diagnosis of exclusion and therefore prone to ambiguity. A full diagnostic workup can involve expensive procedures such as ultrasound, MRI, cystoscopy, ureteroscopy, renal isotope scintigraphy, renal angiography, and renal biopsy. For many patients, a complete workup may be cost-prohibitive and thereby leave the cause of LPHS undiscovered. Strong associations with nephrolithiasis, TBMN, and psychological factors also lend an air of uncertainty to the concept that LPHS is a distinct clinical entity [227]. Moreover, the etiology of LPHS is linked to a number of inconsistent findings (Table 5.12), which adds to the equivocation. One of the more unifying theories of pathogenesis supposes that structural alterations of the GBM (manifested ultrastructurally as thickening or thinning) lead to hematuria, obstruction of the tubules by RBC casts, backleak of glomerular filtrate, acute tubular injury, interstitial edema, capsular distention, and flank pain [226]. The theory includes hypercalciuria or hyperuricosuria with microcrystalline formation in tubules ("occult" nephrolithiasis) as a mechanism to further exacerbate hematuria, tubular injury, and back pain [228].

Despite dozens of studies attempting to validate the disease (for review, see Ref. 225), there is only partial agreement on diagnostic criteria, management, and treatment. Pain is managed by a variety of modalities including nonsteroidal antiinflammatory drugs, opioid analgesics, tricyclic antidepressants, transcutaneous electrical nerve stimulation (TENS), and anesthetic nerve blocks. Opioids can be deployed by implantable intrathecal devices. High-dose opioids may be required to combat persistently severe pain. The success of these treatments is extremely variable; overall, only about 30 percent of patients experience remission after several years of conservative therapy. Surgical procedures aimed at denervating the kidney are also available but have limited success; they include renal nerve excision, surgical sympathectomy, and capsulectomy. Whereas renal nerve excision provides temporary pain relief, it has a higher incidence of recurrence than autotransplantation. Autotransplantation, the relocation of a native kidney to the iliac fossa, is touted as a safe and effective surgical approach to treating LPHS. It can be performed laproscopically. Pain remission rates are variable and range from 25 to 75 percent, whereas hematuria tends to persist in most cases. In an extreme example, LPHS was treated successfully by bilateral nephrectomy followed by cadaveric transplantation [229]. Interestingly, hematuria recurred even though the pain associated with it did not.

Despite all the difficulties encountered with diagnosis, treatment, and management, patients with LPHS have an excellent prognosis and do not develop significant impairment of renal function.

REFERENCES

1. Berger J, Hinglas N. (1968). Les depots intercapillaires IgA–IgG. *J Urol Nephrol (Paris)* 74:694–5.
2. Berger J, Hinglas N, Striker L. (2000). Intercapillary deposits of IgA-IgG. *J Am Soc Nephrol* 11:1957–9.
3. Berger J. (1969). IgA glomerular deposits in renal disease. *Transplant Proc* 1:939–944.
4. D'Amico G. (1987). The commonest glomerulonephritis in the world: IgA nephropathy. *Quart J Med* 64:709–27.
5. Levy M, Berger J. (1988). Worldwide perspective of IgA nephropathy. *Am J Kidney Dis* 12:340–7.
6. Donadio JV, Grande JP. (2002). IgA nephropathy. *N Engl J Med* 347:738–48.
7. Galla J. (1995). IgA nephropathy. *Kidney Int* 47:377–87.
8. Emancipator S.N. "IgA Nephropathy and Henoch-Scholein Syndrome." In J.C. Jennette, J.L. Olson, M.M. Schwartz, and F.G. Silva, eds., *Heptinstall's Pathology of the Kidney*, 5th ed., vol. 1 (Philadelphia: Lippincott-Raven, 1998), pp. 479–539.
9. Davin J-C, Ten Berge IJ, Weening JJ. (2001). What is the difference between IgA nephropathy and Henoch-Schönlein purpura nephritis? *Kidney Int* 59:823–34.
10. Frimat L, Hestin D, Aymard B, Mayeux D, Renoult E, Kessler, M. (1996). IgA nephropathy in patients over 50 years of age: a multicentre, prospective study. *Nephrol Dial Transplant* 11:1043–7.
11. Praga M, Guitirrez-Millet V, Navas J, Ruilope L, Morales J, Alcazar J, Bello I, Rodicio J. (1985). Acute worsening of renal function during episodes of macroscopic hematuria in IgA nephropathy. *Kidney Int* 28:69–74.
12. Hogg RJ, Silva FG, Wyatt RJ, Reisch JS, Argyle JC, Savino DA. (1994). Prognostic indicators in children with IgA nephropathy–report of the Southwest Pediatric Nephrology Study Group. *Pediatr Nephrol* 8:15–20.
13. Ibels LS, Gyory AZ. (1994). IgA nephropathy: analysis of the natural history, important factors in the progression of renal disease, and a review of the literature. *Medicine* 73:79–102.
14. Tang Z, Wu Y, Wang QW, Yu YS, Hu WX, Yao XD, Chen HP, Liu ZH, Li LS. (2002). Idiopathic IgA nephropathy with diffuse crescent formation. *Am J Nephrol* 22:480–6.
15. Tumlin JA, Hennigar RA. (2004). Clinical presentation, natural history, and treatment of crescentic proliferative IgA nephropathy. *Sem Nephrol* 24:256–68.
16. D'Amico G, Napodano P, Ferrario F, Rastaldi MP, Arrigo G. (2001). Idiopathic IgA nephropathy with segmental necrotizing lesions of the capillary wall. *Kidney Int* 59:682–92.
17. Haas M, Jafri J, Bartosh SM, Karp SL, Adler SG, Meehan SM. (2000). ANCA-associated crescentic glomerulonephritis with mesangial IgA deposits. *Am J Kidney Dis* 36:709–18.
18. Lee SM, Rao VM, Franklin WA, Schiffer MS, Aronson AJ, Spargo BH, Katz AI. (1982). IgA nephropathy: morphologic predictors of progressive renal disease. *Hum Pathol* 13:314–22.
19. Meadow SR, Glasgow EF, White RH, Moncrieff MW, Cameron JS, Ogg CS. (1972). Schonlein-Henoch nephritis. *Quart J Med* 41:241–58.
20. Haas M. (1997). Histological subclassification of IgA Nephropathy: a clinicopathologic study of 244 cases. *Am J Kidney Dis* 29:829–42.
21. Haas, M, . "IgA Nephropathy and Henoch-Schonlein Purpura Nephritis." In J.C. Jennette, J.L. Olson, M.M. Schwartz, and F.G. Silva, eds., *Heptinstall's Pathology of the Kidney*, 6th ed., vol. 1 (Philadelphia: Lipincott, Williams and Wilkins, 2006), pp. 423–486.
22. Haas M. (1996). IgA nephropathy histologically resembling focal-segmental glomerulosclerosis: a clinicopathologic study of 18 cases. *Am J Kidney Dis* 28:365–71.
23. Tumlin JA, Lohavichan V, Hennigar R. (2003). Crescentic proliferative IgA nephropathy: clinical and histologic response to methyl prednisolone and intravenous cyclophosphamide. *Nephrol Dial Transplant* 18:1321–92.
24. Tolkoff-Rubin NE, Cosimi AB, Fuller T, Rublin RH, Colvin RB. (1978). IgA nephropathy in HLA-identical siblings. *Transplantation* 26:430–3.
25. Gu X, Herrera GA. (2003). The value of electron microscopy in the diagnosis of IgA nephropathy. *Ultrastruct Pathol* 26:203–10.
26. Lee HS, Choi Y, Lee JS, Yu BH, Koh HI. (1989). Ultrastructural changes in IgA nephropathy in relation to histologic and clinical data. *Kidney Int* 35:880–6.
27. Morita M, Sakaguchi H. (1988). A quantitative study of glomerular basement membrane changes in IgA nephropathy. *J Pathol* 154:7–18.
28. Vogler C, Eliason SC, Wood EG. (1999). Glomerular membranopathy in children with IgA nephropathy and Henoch Schonlein purpura. *Pediatr Dev Pathol* 2:227–35.

29. Norby SM, Cosio FG. (2005). Thin basement membrane nephropathy associated with other glomerular diseases. *Sem Nephrol* 25:176–9.

30. Clive DM, Galvanek EG, Silva FG. (1990). Mesangial immunoglobulin A deposits in minimal change nephrotic syndrome: a report of an older patient and review of the literature. *Am J Nephrol* 10:31–6.

31. Tsukada M, Honda K, Nitta K, Yumura W, Nihei H. (2003). Incidental mesangial IgA deposition in minimal change nephrotic syndrome (MCNS). *Jap J Nephrol* 45:681–8.

32. Westhoff TH, Waldherr R, Loddenkemper C, Ries W, Zidek W, van der Giet M. (2006). Mesangial IgA deposition in minimal change nephrotic syndrome: coincidence of different entities or variant of minimal change disease? *Clin Nephrol* 65:203–7.

33. Nasr SH, Markowitz GS, Whelan JD, Albanese JJ, Rosen RM, Fein DA, Kim SS, D'Agati VD. (2003). IgA-dominant acute poststaphylococcal glomerulonephritis complicating diabetic nephropathy. *Hum Pathol* 34:1235–41.

34. Long JA, Cook WJ. (2006). IgA deposits and acute glomerulonephritis in a patient with staphylococcal infection. *Am J Kidney Dis* 48:851–5.

35. Satoskar AA, Nadasdy G, Plaza JA, Sedmak D, Shidham G, Hebert L, Nadasdy T. (2006). Staphylococcus infection-associated glomerulonephritis mimicking IgA nephropathy. *Clin J Am Soc Nephrol* 1:1179–86.

36. Newell G. (1987). Cirrhotic glomerulonephritis: incidence, morphology, clinical features and pathogenesis. *Am J Kidney Dis* 9:183–90.

37. Koyama A, Sharmin S, Sakurai H, Shimizu Y, Hirayama K, Usui J, Nagata M, Yoh K, Yamagata K, Muro K, Kobayashi M, Ohtani K, Shimizu T, Shimizu T. (2004). Staphylococcus aureus cell envelope antigen is a new candidate for the induction of IgA nephropathy. *Kidney Int* 66:121–32.

38. Scolari F. (1999). Familial IgA nephropathy. *J Nephrol* 12:213–19.

39. Izzi C, Ravani P, Torres D, Prati E, Viola BF, Guerini S, Foramitti M, Frasca G, Amoroso A, Ghiggeri GM, Schena FP, Scolari F. (2006). IgA nephropathy: the presence of familial disease does not confer an increased risk for progression. *Am J Kidney Dis* 47:761–9.

40. Gharavi AG, Yan Y, Scolari F, Schena FP, Frasca GM, Ghiggeri GM, Cooper K, Amoroso A, Viola BF, Battini G, Caridi G, Canova C, Farhi A, Subramanian V, Nelson-Williams C, Woodford S, Julian BA, Wyatt RJ, Lifton RP. (2000). IgA nephropathy, the most common cause of glomerulonephritis, is linked to 6q22-23. *Nat Genet* 26:354–7.

41. Bisceglia L, Cerullo G, Forabosco P, Torres DD, Scolari F, Di Perna M, Foramitti M, Amoroso A, Bertok S, Floege J, Mertens PR, Zerres K, Alexopoulos E, Kirmizis D, Ermelinda M, Zelante L, Schena FP; European IgAN Consortium. (2006). Genetic heterogeneity in Italian families with IgA nephropathy: suggestive linkage for two novel IgA nephropathy loci. *Am J Hum Genet* 79: 1130–4.

42. Barrett J, Feehally J, Smith AC. (2006). Pathogenesis of IgA nephropathy. *Sem Nephrol* 24:197–217.

43. Rifai A, Millard K. (1985). Glomerular deposition of immune complexes prepared with monomeric or polymeric IgA. *Clin Exp Immunol* 60:363–8.

44. Suzuki S, Kobayashi H, Sato H, Arakawa M. (1990). Immunohistochemical characterization of glomerular IgA deposits in IgA nephropathy. *Clin Nephrol* 33:66–71.

45. Novak J, Vu HL, Novak L, Julian B. (2002). Interactions of human mesangial cells with IgA and IgA-containing immune complexes. *Kidney Int* 62:465–75.

46. Monteiro RC, Halbwachs-Mecarelli L, Roque-Barreira MC, Noel LH, Berger J, Lesavre P. (1985). Charge and size of mesangial IgA in IgA nephropathy. *Kidney Int* 28:666–71.

47. Silva FG, Chander P, Pirani CL, Hardy MA. (1982). Disappearance of glomerular mesangial IgA deposits after renal allograft transplantation. *Transplantation* 33:241–6.

48. Harper SJ, Allen AC, Pringle JH, Feehally J. (1996). Increased dimeric IgA producing B cells in the bone marrow in IgA nephropathy determined by in situ hybridisation for J chain mRNA. *J Clin Pathol* 49:38–42.

49. Buck KS, Foster EM, Watson D, Barratt J, Pawluczyk IZ, Knight JF, Feehally J, Allen AC. (2002). Expression of T cell receptor variable region families by bone marrow $\gamma\delta$ T cells in patients with IgA nephropathy. *Clin Exp Immunol* 127:527–32.

50. Batra A, Smith AC, Feehally J, Barratt J. (2007). T-cell homing receptor expression in IgA nephropathy. *Nephrol Dial Transplant* 22:2540–8.

51. Toyabe S, Harada W, Uchiyama M. (2001). Oligoclonally expanding $\gamma\delta$ T lymphocytes induce IgA switching in IgA nephropathy. *Clin Exp Immunol* 124:110–17.

52. Allen AC, Bailey EM, Brenchley PE, Buck KS, Barratt J, Feehally J. (2001). Mesangial IgA1 in IgA nephropathy exhibits aberrant O-glycosylation: observations in three patients. *Kidney Int* 60:969–73.

53. Smith AC, Feehally J. (2003). New insights into the pathogenesis of IgA nephropathy. *Springer Sem Immunopathol* 24:477–93.

54. Allen AC, Topham PS, Harper SJ, Feehally J. (1997). Leucocyte ß1,3 galactosyltransferase activity in IgA nephropathy. *Nephrol Dial Transplant* 12:701–6.

55. Sano T, Hiki Y, Kokubo H, Iwase H, Shigematsu H, Kaboyashi Y. (2002). Enzymatically deglycosylated human IgA1 molecules accumulate and induce inflammatory cell reaction in rat glomeruli. *Nephrol Dial Transplant* 17: 50–6.

56. Haddad E, Moura IC, Arcos-Fajardo M, Macher MA, Baudouin V, Alberti C, Loirat C, Monteiro RC, Peuchmaur M. (2003). Enhanced expression of the CD71 mesangial IgA1 receptor in Berger disease and Henoch-Schonlein nephritis: association between CD71 expression and IgA deposits. *J Am Soc Nephrol* 14:327–37.

57. Moura IC, Arcos-Fajardo M, Gdoura A, Leroy V, Sadaka C, Mahlaoui N, Lepelletier Y, Vrtovsnik F, Haddad E, Benhamou M, Monteiro RC. (2005). Engagement of transferrin receptor by polymeric IgA1: evidence for a positive feedback loop involving increased receptor expression and mesangial cell proliferation in IgA nephropathy. *J Am Soc Nephrol* 16:2667–76.

58. Hisano S, Matsushita M, Fujita T, Endo Y, Takebayashi S. (2001). Mesangial IgA2 deposits and lectin pathway-mediated complement activation in IgA glomerulonephritis. *Am J Kidney Dis* 38:1082–8.

59. Roos A, Rastaldi MP, Calvaresi N, Oortwijn BD, Schlagwein N, van Gijlswijk-Janssen DJ, Stahl GL, Matsushita M, Fujita T, van Kooten C, Daha MR. (2006). Glomerular activation of the lectin pathway of complement in IgA nephropathy is associated with more severe renal disease. *J Am Soc Nephrol* 17:1724–34.

60. Lasseur C, Allen AC, Deminiere C, Aparicio M, Feehally J, Combe C. (1997). Henoch-Schonlein purpura with immunoglobulin A nephropathy and abnormalities of immunoglobulin A in a Wiskott-Aldrich syndrome carrier. *Am J Kidney Dis* 29:285–7.

61. Zickerman AM, Allen AC, Talwar V, Olczak SA, Brownlee A, Holland M, Furness PN, Brunskill NJ, Feehally J. (2000). IgA myeloma presenting as Henoch-Schonlein purpura with nephritis. *Am J Kidney Dis* 36:E19.

62. Roccatello D, Picciotto G, Torchio M, Ropolo R, Ferro M, Franceschini R, Quattrocchio G, Cacace G, Coppo R, Sena LM, et al. (1993). Removal systems of immunoglobulin A and immunoglobulin A containing complexes in IgA nephropathy and cirrhosis patients. The role of asialoglycoprotein receptors. *Lab Invest* 69:714–23.

63. Pouria S, Feehally J. (1999). Glomerular IgA deposition in liver disease. *Nephrol Dial Transplant* 14:2279–82.

64. Feehally J, Beattie TJ, Brenchley PE, Coupes BM, Mallick NP, Postlethwaite RJ. (1987). Response of circulating immune complexes to food challenge in relapsing IgA nephropathy. *Pediatr Nephrol* 1:581–6.

65. Nagura H. (1989). IgA nephropathy and mucosal immune system. *Tokai J Exp Clin Med* 14:1–4.

66. Geddes CC, Rauta V, Gronhagen-Riska C, Bartosik LP, Jardine AG, Ibels LS, Pei Y, Cattran DC. (2003). A tricontinental view of IgA nephropathy. *Nephrol Dial Transplant* 18:1541–8.

67. Coppo R, D'Amico G. (2005). Factors predicting progression of IgA nephropathies. *J Nephrol* 18:503–12.

68. Donadio J, Grande J. (1997). Immunoglobulin A nephropathy: a clinical perspective. *J Am Soc Nephrol* 1324–32.

69. Hsu SI. (2001). The molecular pathogenesis and experimental therapy of IgA nephropathy: recent advances and future directions. *Curr Mol Med* 1:183–96.

70. Harden PN, Geddes C, Rowe PA, McIlroy JH, Boulton-Jones M, Rodger RS, Junor BJ, Briggs JD, Connell JM, Jardine AG. (1995). Polymorphisms in angiotensin-converting-enzyme gene and progression of IgA nephropathy. *Lancet* 345:1540–2.

71. Hunley TE, Julian BA, Phillips JA, Summar ML, Yoshida H, Horn RG, Brown NJ, Fogo A, Ichikawa I, Kon V. (1996). Angiotensin converting enzyme gene polymorphism: potential silencer motif and impact on progression in IgA nephropathy. *Kidney Int* 49:571–7.

72. Hsu SI, Ramirez SB, Winn MP, Bonventre JV, Owen WF. (2000). Evidence for genetic factors in the development and progression of IgA nephropathy. *Kidney Int* 57:1818–35.

73. D'Amico G. (2004). Natural history of idiopathic IgA nephropathy and factors predictive of disease outcome. *Semin Nephrol* 24:179–96.

74. Manno C, Strippoli GF, D'Altri C, Torres D, Rossini M, Schena FP. (2007). A novel simpler histological classification for renal survival in IgA nephropathy: a retrospective study. *Am J Kidney Dis* 49:763–75.

75. D'Amico G. (2000). Natural history of idiopathic IgA nephropathy: role of clinical and histological prognostic factors. Am.. *J Kidney Dis* 36:227–37.

76. Ballardie FW, Roberts IS. (2002). Controlled prospective trial of prednisolone and cytotoxics in progressive IgA nephropathy. *J Am Soc Nephrol* 13:142–8.

77. Hisano S, Kiyoshi Y, Tanaka I, Tokieda K, Niimi K, Tsuru N, Takebayashii S, Iwasaki H. (2004). Clinicopathological correlation of childhood IgA glomerulonephritis presenting diffuse endocapillary proliferation. *Pathol Int* 54:174–80.

78. Boyce NW, Holdsworth SR, Thomson NM, Atkins RC. (1986). Clinicopathological associations in mesangial IgA nephropathy. *Am J Nephrol* 6:246–52.

79. Welch TR, McAdams AJ, Berry A. (1988). Rapidly progressing IgA nephropathy. *Am J Dis Child* 142:789–93.

80. Praga M, Gutierrez E, Gonzalez E, Morales E, Hernandez E. (2003). Treatment of IgA nephropathy with ACE inhibitors: a randomized and controlled trial. *J Am Soc Nephrol* 14:1578–83.

81. Nakao N, Yoshimura A, Morita H, Takada M. Kayano T. Ideura T. (2003). Combination treatment of angiotensin-II receptor blocker and angiotensin-converting-enzyme inhibitor in non-diabetic renal disease (COOPERATE): a randomized controlled trial. *Lancet* 361:117–24.

82. Appel GB, Waldman M (2006). The IgA nephropathy treatment dilemma. *Kidney Int* 69:1939–44.

83. Hogg RJ, Lee J, Nardelli N, Julian BA, Cattran D, Waldo B, Wyatt R, Jennette JC, Sibley R, Hyland K, Fitzgibbons L, Hirschman G, Donadio JV Jr, Holub BJ. (2006). Southwest Pediatric Nephrology Study Group. Clinical trial to evaluate omega-3 fatty acids and alternate day prednisone in patients with IgA nephropathy: report from the Southwest Pediatric Nephrology Study Group. *Clin J Am Soc of Nephrol* 1:467–74.

84. Katafuchi R, Ikeda K, Mizumasa T. (2003). Controlled, prospective trial of steroid treatment in IgA nephropathy: a limitation of low dose prednisolone therapy. *Am J Kidney Dis* 41:972–83.

85. Schena FP, Montenegro M, Scivittaro V. (1990). Meta-analysis of randomised controlled trials in patients with primary IgA nephropathy (Berger's disease). *Nephrol Dial Transplant* [5, Suppl 1]:47–52.

86. Pozzi C, Andrulli S, Del Vecchio L. (2004). Corticosteroid effectiveness in IgA nephropathy: long-term results of a randomized, controlled trial. *J Am Soc Nephrol* 15:157–63.

87. Samuels JA, Strippoli GF, Craig JC, Schena FP, Molony DA, (2004). Immunosuppressive treatments for immunoglobulin A nephropathy: a meta-analysis of randomized controlled trials. *Nephrology* 9:177–85.

88. Tumlin JA, Madaio MP, Hennigar R. (2007). Idiopathic IgA nephropathy: pathogenesis, histopathology, and therapeutic options. *Clin J Am Soc Nephrol* 2:1054–61.

89. Ballardie FW, Roberts ISD. (2002). Controlled prospective trial of prednisolone and cytotoxics in progressive IgA nephropathy. *J Am Soc Nephrol* 13:142–8.

90. Roccatello D, Ferro M, Cesano G. (2000). Steroid and cyclophosphamide in IgA nephropathy. *Nephrol Dial Transplant* 15:833–5.

91. McIntyre CW, Fluck RJ, Lambie SH. (2001). Steroid and cyclophosphamide therapy for IgA nephropathy associated with crescenteric change: an effective treatment. *Clin Nephrol* 56:193–8.

92. Ponticelli C, Traversi L, Banfi G. (2004). Renal transplantation in patients with IgA mesangial glomerulonephritis. *Pediatr Transplant* 8:334–8.

93. Lim EC, Chia D, Gjertson DW, Koka P, Terasaki PI. (1993). In vitro studies to explain high renal allograft survival in IgA nephropathy patients. *Transplantation* 55:996–9.

94. Heberden W. *Commentaries on the History and Cure of Diseases.* Chapter 78: De purpureis maculis. London, 1802.

95. *Dr. J.L. Schönleins allgemeine und specielle Pathologie und Therapie. Nach seinen Vorlesungen niedergeschrieben von einigen seiner Zuhörer und nicht autorisiert herausgegeben.* Würzburg, Etlinger, 1832.

96. *Über eine eigentümliche Form von Purpura.* Berliner klinische Wochenschrift, 1874; 11:641

97. Jennette JC, Falk RJ, Andrassy K, Bacon PA, Churg J, Gross WL, Hagen EC, Hoffman GS, Hunder GG, Kallenberg CG, et al. (1997). Nomenclature of systemic vasculitides. Proposal of an international consensus conference. *Arthritis Rheum* 37:187–92.

98. Saulsbury FT. (2007). Clinical update: Henoch-Schonlein purpura. *Lancet* 369:976–8.

99. Garcia-Porrua C, Calvino MC, Llorca J, Couselo JM, Gonzalez-Gay MA. (2002). Henoch-Schonlein purpura in children and adults: clinical differences in a defined population. *Sem Arthritis Rheum* 32:149–56.

100. Saulsbury FT. (2002). Epidemiology of Henoch-Schonlein purpura. *Clev Clin J Med* [69, Suppl 2]:SII87–9.

101. Kellerman PS. (2006). Henoch-Schonlein purpura in adults. *Am J Kidney Dis* 48:1009–16.

102. Pillebout E, Thervet E, Hill G, Alberti C, Vanhille P, Nochy D. (2002). Henoch-Schonlein Purpura in adults: outcome and prognostic factors. *J Am Soc Nephrol* 13:1271–8.

103. Mills JA, Michel BA, Bloch DA, Calabrese LH, Hunder GG, Arend WP, Edworthy SM, Fauci AS, Leavitt RY, Lie JT, et al. (1990). The American College of Rheumatology 1990 criteria for the classification of Henoch-Schonlein purpura. *Arthritis Rheum* 33:1114–21.

104. Helander SD, De Castro FR, Gibson LE. (1995). Henoch-Schönlein purpura: clinicopathologic correlation of cutaneous vascular IgA deposits and the relationship to leukocytoclastic vasculitis. *Acta Derm Venereol* 75:125–32.

105. Perez C, Maravi E, Olier J, Guarch R. (2000). MR imaging of encephalopathy in adult Henoch-Shönlein purpura. *AJR Am J Roentgenol* 175:922–3.

106. Heaton JM, Turner DR, Cameron JS. (1977). Localization of glomerular "deposits" in Henoch–Schonlein nephritis. *Histopathology* 1:93–104.

107. Rai A, Nast C, Adler S. (1999). Henoch-Schonlein purpura nephritis. *J Am Soc Nephrol* 10:2637–44.

108. Szeto CC, Choi PC, To KF, Li PK, Hui J, Chow KM, Leung CB, Lui SF, Mac-Moune Lai F. (2001). Grading of acute and chronic renal lesions in Henoch-Schonlein purpura. *Mod Pathol* 14:635–40.

109. Zollinger HU, Mihatsch MJ, Gaboardi F, Banfi G, Edefonti A, Bardare M, Gudat F. (1980). Schonlein-Henoch glomerulonephritis. Characteristic ultrastructural changes in the glomerular basement membrane and localisation of osmiophilic deposits. Virchows Archiv. A, *Pathol Anat Histol* 388:155–65.

110. Ozaltin F, Bakkaloglu A, Ozen S, Topaloglu R, Kavak U, Kalyoncu M, Besbas N. (2004). The significance of IgA class of antineutrophil cytoplasmic antibodies (ANCA) in childhood Henoch-Schonlein purpura. *Clin Rheumatol* 23:426–9.

111. Coppo R, Cirina P, Amore A, Sinico RA, Radice A, Rollino C. (1997). Properties of circulating IgA molecules in Henoch-Schonlein purpura nephritis with focus on neutrophil cytoplasmic antigen IgA binding (IgA-ANCA): new insight into a debated issue. Italian Group of Renal Immunopathology Collaborative Study on Henoch-Schonlein purpura in adults and in children. *Nephrol Dial Transplant* 12:2269–76.

112. Mookerjee BK, Maddison PJ, Reichlin M. (1978). Case report: mesangial IgA-IgG deposition in mixed cryoglobulinemia. *Am J Med Sci* 276:221–5.

113. Rollino C, Dieny A, Le Marc'hadour F, Renversez JC, Pinel N, Cordonnier D. (1992). Double monoclonal cryoglobulinemia, glomerulonephritis and lymphoma. *Nephron* 62:459–64.

114. Yang YH, Huang MT, Lin SC, Lin YT, Tsai MJ, Chiang BL. (2000). Increased transforming growth factor-beta (TGF-beta)-secreting T cells and IgA anti-cardiolipin antibody levels during acute stage of childhood Henoch-Schonlein purpura. *Clin Exp Immunol* 122:285–90.

115. Kawakami T, Watabe H, Mizoguchi M, Soma Y. (2006). Elevated serum IgA anticardiolipin antibody levels in adult Henoch-Schonlein purpura. *Br J Dermatol* 155:983–7.

116. Coppo R, Amore A, Gianoglio B. (1999). Clinical features of Henoch-Schonlein purpura. Italian Group of Renal Immunopathology. *Annal Med Intern* 150:143–50.

117. Masuda M, Nakanishi K, Yoshizawa N, Iijima K, Yoshikawa N. (2003). Group A streptococcal antigen in the glomeruli of children with Henoch-Schonlein nephritis. *Am J Kidney Dis* 41:366–70.

118. Ogura Y, Suzuki S, Shirakawa T, Masuda M, Nakamura H, Iijima K, Yoshikawa N. (2000). Haemophilus parainfluenzae antigen and antibody in children with IgA nephropathy and Henoch-Schönlein nephritis. *Am J Kidney Dis* 36:47–52.

119. Zurada JM, Ward KM, Grossman ME. (2006). Henoch-Schonlein purpura associated with malignancy in adults. *J Am Acad Dermatol* [55, Suppl 5]:S65–70.

120. Gonzalez-Gay MA, Calvino MC, Vazquez-Lopez ME, Garcia-Porrua C, Fernandez-Iglesias JL, Dierssen T, Llorca J. (2004). Implications of upper respiratory tract infections and drugs in the clinical spectrum of Henoch-Schonlein purpura in children. *Clin Exp Rheumatol* 22: 781–4.

121. Levy M. (2001). Familial cases of Berger's disease and anaphylactoid purpura. *Kidney Int* 60:1611–12.

122. Ozkaya O, Soylemezolu O, Gonen S, Misirliolu M, Tuncer S, Kalman S, Buyan N, Hasanolu E. (2006). Renin-angiotensin system gene polymorphisms: association with

susceptibility to Henoch-Schonlein purpura and renal involvement. *Clin Rheumatol* 25:861–5.

123. Jin DK, Kohsaka T, Koo JW, Ha IS, Cheong HI, Choi Y. (1996). Complement 4 locus II gene deletion and DQA1*0301 gene: genetic risk factors for IgA nephropathy and Henoch-Schonlein nephritis. *Nephron* 73:390–5.

124. Ault BH, Stapleton FB, Rivas ML, Waldo FB, Roy S, 3rd, McLean RH, Bin JA, Wyatt RJ. (1990). Association of Henoch-Schonlein purpura glomerulonephritis with C4B deficiency. *J Pediatr* 117:753–5.

125. Stefansson Thors V, Kolka R, Sigurdardottir SL, Edvardsson VO, Arason G, Haraldsson A. (2005). Increased frequency of C4B*Q0 alleles in patients with Henoch-Schonlein purpura. *Scand J Immunol* 61:274–8.

126. Yang Y, Lhotta K, Chung EK, Eder P, Neumair F, Yu CY. (2004). Complete complement components C4A and C4B deficiencies in human kidney diseases and systemic lupus erythematosus. *J Immunol* 173:2803–14.

127. Tomino Y, Endoh M, Suga T, Miura M, Kaneshige H, Nomoto Y, Sakai H. (1982). Prevalence of IgA1 deposits in Henoch-Schoenlein purpura (HSP) nephritis. *Tokai J Exp Clin Med* 7:527–32.

128. Saulsbury FT. (1997). Alterations in the O-linked glycosylation of IgA1 in children with Henoch-Schonlein purpura. *J Rheumatol* 24:2246–9.

129. Allen AC, Willis FR, Beattie TJ, Feehally J. (1998). Abnormal IgA glycosylation in Henoch-Schonlein purpura restricted to patients with clinical nephritis. *Nephrol Dial Transplant* 13:930–4.

130. Novak J, Moldoveanu Z, Renfrow MB, Yanagihara T, Suzuki H, Raska M, Hall S, Brown R, Huang WQ, Goepfert A, Kilian M, Poulsen K, Tomana M, Wyatt RJ, Julian BA, Mestecky J. (2007). IgA nephropathy and Henoch-Schoenlein purpura nephritis: aberrant glycosylation of IgA1, formation of IgA1-containing immune complexes, and activation of mesangial cells. *Contr Nephrol* 157:134–8.

131. Smith GC, Davidson JE, Hughes DA, Holme E, Beattie TJ. (1997). Complement activation in Henoch-Schonlein purpura. *Pediatr Nephrol* 11:477–80.

132. Endo M, Ohi H, Ohsawa I, Fujita T, Matsushita M. (2000). Complement activation through the lectin pathway in patients with Henoch-Schonlein purpura nephritis. *Am J Kidney Dis* 35:401–7.

133. Hisano S, Matsushita M, Fujita T, Iwasaki H. (2005). Activation of the lectin complement pathway in Henoch-Schonlein purpura nephritis. *Am J Kidney Dis* 45:295–302.

134. Wu TH, Wu SC, Huang TP, Yu CL, Tsai CY. (1996). Increased excretion of tumor necrosis factor alpha and interleukin 1 beta in urine from patients with IgA nephropathy and Schonlein-Henoch purpura. *Nephron* 74:79–88.

135. Besbas N, Saatci U, Ruacan S, Ozen S, Sungur A, Bakkaloglu A, Elnahas AM. (1997). The role of cytokines in Henoch Schonlein purpura. *Scand J Rheumatol* 26:456–60.

136. Ha TS. (2005). The role of tumor necrosis factor-alpha in Henoch-Schonlein purpura. *Pediatr Nephrol* 20:149–53.

137. Gattorno M, Vignola S, Barbano G, Sormani MP, Sabatini F, Buoncompagni A, Picco P, Pistoia V. (2000). Tumor necrosis factor induced adhesion molecule serum concen-

trations in Henoch-Schonlein purpura and pediatric systemic lupus erythematosus. *J Rheumatol* 27:2251–5.

138. Rauta V, Teppo AM, Tornroth T, Honkanen E, Gronhagen-Riska C. (2003). Lower urinary-interleukin-1 receptor-antagonist excretion in IgA nephropathy than in Henoch-Schonlein nephritis. *Nephrol Dial Transplant* 18:1785–91.

139. Namgoong MK, Lim BK, Kim JS. (1997). Eosinophil cationic protein in Henoch-Schonlein purpura and in IgA nephropathy. *Pediatr Nephrol* 11:703–6.

140. Kawasaki Y, Hosoya M, Suzuki H. (2005). Possible pathologenic role of interleukin-5 and eosino cationic protein in Henoch-Schonlein purpura nephritis. *Pediatr Int* 47:512–17.

141. Yoshioka T, Xu YX, Yoshida H, Shiraga H, Muraki T, Ito K. (1998). Deletion polymorphism of the angiotensin converting enzyme gene predicts persistent proteinuria in Henoch-Schonlein purpura nephritis. *Arch Dis Child* 79:394–9.

142. Amoroso A, Danek G, Vatta S, Crovella S, Berrino M, Guarrera S, Fasano ME, Mazzola G, Amore A, Gianoglio B, Peruzzi L, Coppo R. (1998). Polymorphisms in angiotensin-converting enzyme gene and severity of renal disease in Henoch-Schoenlein patients. Italian Group of Renal Immunopathology. *Nephrol Dial Transplant* 13:3184–8.

143. Dudley J, Afifi E, Gardner A, Tizard EJ, McGraw ME. (2000). Polymorphism of the ACE gene in Henoch-Schonlein purpura nephritis. *Pediatr Nephrol* 14:218–20.

144. Saulsbury FT. (1999). Henoch-Schonlein purpura in children. Report of 100 patients and review of the literature. *Medicine* 78:395–409.

145. Fervenza FC. (2003). Henoch-Schonlein purpura nephritis. *Int J Dermatol* 42:170–7

146. Mir S, Yavascan O, Mutlubas F, Yeniay B, Sonmez F. (2007). Clinical outcome in children with Henoch-Schonlein nephritis. *Pediatr Nephrol* 22:64–70.

147. Butani L. (2001). Long-term outcome of children with Henoch-Schonlein purpura (HSP) nephritis. *J Am Soc Nephrol* 12:194A

148. Kaku Y, Nohara K, Honda S. (1998). Renal involvement in Henoch-Schonlein purpura: a multivariate analysis of prognostic factors. *Kidney Int* 53:1755–9.

149. Sano H, Izumida M, Shimizu H, Ogawa Y. (2002). Risk factors of renal involvement and significant proteinuria in Henoch-Schonlein purpura. *Eur J Pediatr* 161:196–201.

150. Goldstein AR, White RH, Akuse R, Chantler C. (1992). Long-term follow-up of childhood Henoch-Schonlein nephritis. *Lancet* 339:280–2.

151. Stewart M, Savage JM, Bell B, McCord B. (1998). Long term renal prognosis of Henoch-Schonlein purpura in an unselected childhood population. *Eur J Pediatr* 147:113–15.

152. Coppo R, Mazzucco G, Cagnoli L, Lupo A, Schena FP. (1997). Long-term prognosis of Henoch-Schonlein nephritis in adults and children. Italian Group of Renal Immunopathology Collaborative Study on Henoch-Schonlein purpura. *Nephrol Dial Transplant* 12:2277–83.

153. Coppo R, Andrulli S, Amore A, Gianoglio B, Conti G, Peruzzi L, Locatelli F, Cagnoli L. (2006). Predictors of outcome in Henoch-Schonlein nephritis in children and adults. *Am J Kidney Dis* 47:993–1003.

154. Ronkainen J, Nuutinen M, Koskimies O. (2002). The adult kidney 24 years after childhood Henoch-Schonlein purpura: a retrospective cohort study. *Lancet* 360:666–70.

155. Yoshikawa N, White RH, Cameron AH. (1981). Prognostic significance of the glomerular changes in Henoch-Schoenlein nephritis. *Clin Nephrol* 16:223–9.

156. Ronkainen J, Koskimies O, Ala-Houhala M, Antikainen M, Merenmies J, Rajantie J, Ormälä T, Turtinen J, Nuutinen M. (2006). Early prednisone therapy in Henoch-Schönlein purpura: a randomized, double-blind, placebo-controlled trial. *J Pediatr* 149:241–7.

157. Shenoy M, Bradbury MG, Lewis MA, Webb NJ. (2007). Outcome of Henoch-Schönlein purpura nephritis treated with long-term immunosuppression. *Pediatr Nephrol* 22:1717–22.

158. Tarshish P, Bernstein J, Edelmann CM Jr. (2007). Henoch-Schönlein purpura nephritis: course of disease and efficacy of cyclophosphamide. *Pediatr Nephrol* 22: 1717–22.

159. Niaudet P, Habib R. (1998). Methylprednisolone pulse therapy in the treatment of severe forms of Schönlein-Henoch purpura nephritis. *Pediatr Nephrol* 12:238–43.

160. Foster BJ, Bernard C, Drummond KN, Sharma AK. (2000). Effective therapy for severe Henoch-Schonlein purpura nephritis with prednisone and azathioprine: a clinical and histopathologic study. *J Pediatr* 136:370–5.

161. Kawasaki Y, Suzuki J, Suzuki H. (2004). Efficacy of methylprednisolone and urokinase pulse therapy combined with or without cyclophosphamide in severe Henoch-Schonlein nephritis: a clinical and histopathological study. *Nephrol Dial Transplant* 19:858–64.

162. Heldrich FJ, Minkin S, Gatdula CL. (1993). Intravenous immunoglobulin in Henoch-Schonlein purpura: a case study. *Md Med J* 42:577–9.

163. Rostoker G, Desvaux-Belghiti D, Pilatte Y, Petit-Phar M, Philippon C, Deforges L, Terzidis H, Intrator L, André C, Adnot S, Bonin P, Bierling P, Remy P, Lagrue G, Lang P, Weil B. (1994). High-dose immunoglobulin therapy for severe IgA nephropathy and Henoch-Schönlein purpura. *Ann Intern Med* 120:476–84.

164. Hamidou MA, Pottier MA, Dupas B. (1996). *Intravenous immunoglobulin in Henoch-Schonlein purpura Ann Intern Med* 125:1013–14.

165. Hattori M, Ito K, Konomoto T, Kawaguchi H, Yoshioka T, Khono M. (1999). Plasmapheresis as the sole therapy for rapidly progressive Henoch-Schönlein purpura nephritis in children. *Am J Kidney Dis* 33:427–33.

166. Eun SH, Kim SJ, Cho DS, Chung GH, Lee DY, Hwang PH. (1999). Cerebral vasculitis in Henoch-Schönlein purpura: MRI and MRA findings, treated with plasmapheresis alone. *Am J Kidney Dis* 33:427–33.

167. Guthrie LB. (1902). "Idiopathic," or congenital, hereditary and familial haematuria. *Lancet* 1:1243–6.

168. Kendall G, Hertz AF. (1912). Hereditary familial congenital haemorrhagic nephritis. *Guy's Hosp Rep* 66:137–44.

169. Hurst AF. (1923). Hereditary familial congenital haemorrhagic nephritis occurring in sixteen individuals in three generations. *Guy's Hosp Rep* 3:368–70.

170. Alport AC. (1927). Hereditary familial congenital haemorragic nephritis. *Br Med J* 1:504–6.

171. O'Neill WM Jr, Atkin CL, Bloomer HA. (1978). Hereditary nephritis: a re-examination of its clinical and genetic features. *Ann Intern Med* 88:176–82.

172. Atkin CL, Hasstedt SJ, Menlove L, Cannon L, Kirschner N, Schwartz C, Nguyen K, Skolnick M. (1988). Mapping of Alport syndrome to the long arm of the X chromosome. *Am J Hum Genet* 42:249–55.

173. Barker DF, Hostikka SL, Zhou J, Chow LT, Oliphant AR, Gerken SC, Gregory MC, Skolnick MH, Atkin CL, Tryggvason K. (1990). Identification of mutations in the COL4A5 collagen gene in Alport syndrome. *Science* 248:1224–7.

174. Mochizuki T, Lemmink HH, Mariyama M, Antignac C, Gubler MC, Pirson Y, Verellen-Dumoulin C, Chan B, Schroder CH, Smeets HJ. et al. (1994). Identification of mutations in the alpha 3(IV) and alpha 4(IV) collagen genes in autosomal recessive Alport syndrome. *Nat Genet* 8: 77–81.

175. Pescucci C, Mari F, Longo I, Vogiatzi P, Caselli R, Scala E, Abaterusso C, Gusmano R, Seri M, Miglietti N, Bresin E, Renieri A. (2004). Autosomal-dominant Alport syndrome: natural history of a disease due to COL4A3 or COL4A4 gene. *Kidney Int* 65:1598–1603.

176. Baehr G. (1926). Benign and curable form of hemorrhagic nephritis. *JAMA* 86:1001–4.

177. McConville JM, McAdams AJ. (1966). Familial and nonfamilal benign hematuria. *J Pediatr* 69:207–14.

178. Rogers PW, Kurtzman NA, Bunn SM, White MG. (1973). Famalial benign essential hematuria. *Arch Intern Med* 131:237–62.

179. Habib R, Gubler MC, Hinglais N, Noel LH, Droz D, Levy M, Mahieu P, Foidart JM, Perrin D, Bois E, Grunfeld JP. (1982). Alport's syndrome: experience at Hopital Necker. *Kidney Int* [Suppl 11]:S20–8.

180. Lemmink HH, Nillesen WN, Mochizuki T, Schroder CH, Brunner HG, van Oost BA, Monnens LA, Smeets HJ. (1996). Benign familial hematuria due to mutation of the type IV 4 gene.acollagen *J Clin Invest* 98:1114–18.

181. Wang YY, Savige J. (2004). The epidemiology of thin basement membrane nephropathy. *Sem Nephrol* 25:136–9.

182. Hudson BG, Tryggvason K, Sundaramoorthy M, Neilson EG. (2003). Alport's syndrome, Goodpasture's syndrome, and type IV collagen. *N Eng J Med* 348:2543–56.

183. Heidet L, Cai Y, Guicharnaud L, Antignac C, Gubler MC. (2000). Glomerular expression of type IV collagen chains in normal and X-linked Alport syndrome kidneys. *Am J Pathol* 156:1901–10.

184. Grubler M-C, Heidet L, Antignac C. "Alport's Syndrome, Thin Basement Membrane Nephropathy, Nail-Patella Syndrome, and Type III Collagen Glomerulopathy." In J.C. Jennette, J.L. Olson, M.M. Schwartz, and F.G. Silva, eds., *Heptinstall's Pathology of the Kidney*, 6th ed., vol. 1 (Philadelphia: Lipincott, Williams and Wilkins, 2006), pp. 487–515.

185. Gross O, Netzer KO, Lambrecht R, Seibold S, Weber M. (2002). Meta-analysis of genotype-phenotype correlation in X-linked Alport syndrome: impact on clinical counselling. *Nephrol Dial Transplant* 17:1218–27.

186. Jais JP, Knebelmann B, Giatras I, De Marchi M, Rizzoni G, Renieri A, Weber M, Gross O, Netzer KO, Flinter F, Pirson Y, Verellen C, Wieslander J, Persson U, Tryggvason K,

Martin P, Hertz JM, Schroder C, Sanak M, Krejcova S, Carvalho MF, Saus J, Antignac C, Smeets H, Gubler MC. (2000). X-linked Alport syndrome: natural history in 195 families and genotype- phenotype correlations in males. *J Am Soc Nephrol* 11:649–57.

187. Kashtan CE. (2000). Alport syndrome: abnormalities of type IV collagen genes and proteins. *Renal Failure* 22:737–49.

188. Heidet L, Arrondel C, Forestier L, Cohen-Solal L, Mollet G, Gutierrez B, Stavrou C, Gubler MC, Antignac C. (2001). Structure of the human type IV collagen gene COL4A3 and mutations in autosomal Alport syndrome. *J Am Soc Nephrol* 12:97–106.

189. Longo I, Porcedda P, Mari F, Giachino D, Meloni I, Deplano C, Brusco A, Bosio M, Massella L, Lavoratti G, Roccatello D, Frasca G, Mazzucco G, Muda AO, Conti M, Fasciolo F, Arrondel C, Heidet L, Renieri A, De Marchi M. (2002). COL4A3/COL4A4 mutations: from familial hematuria to autosomal-dominant or recessive Alport syndrome. *Kidney Int* 61:1947–56.

190. Nagel M, Nagorka S, Gross O. (2005). Novel COL4A5, COL4A4, and COL4A3 mutations in Alport syndrome. *Hum Mutat* 26:60.

191. Longo I, Scala E, Mari F, Caselli R, Pescucci C, Mencarelli MA, Speciale C, Giani M, Bresin E, Caringella DA, Borochowitz ZU, Siriwardena K, Winship I, Renieri A, Meloni I. (2006). Autosomal recessive Alport syndrome: an in-depth clinical and molecular analysis of five families. *Nephrol Dial Transplant* 21:665–71.

192. Rana K, Tonna S, Wang YY, Sin L, Lin T, Shaw E, Mookerjee I, Savige J. (2007). Nine novel COL4A3 and COL4A4 mutations and polymorphisms identified in inherited membrane diseases. *Pediatr Nephrol* 22:652–7.

193. Rana K, Wang YY, Buzza M, Tonna S, Zhang KW, Lin T, Sin L, Padavarat S, Savige J. (2005). The genetics of thin basement membrane nephropathy. *Semin Nephrol* 25: 163–70.

194. Tryggvason K, Patrakka J. (2006). Thin basement membrane nephropathy. *J Am Soc Nephrol* 17:813–22.

195. Slajpah M, Gorinsek B, Berginc G, Vizjak A, Ferluga D, Hvala A, Meglic A, Jaksa I, Furlan P, Gregoric A, Kaplan-Pavlovcic S, Ravnik-Glavac M, Glavac D. (2007). Sixteen novel mutations identified in COL4A3, COL4A4, and COL4A5 genes in Slovenian families with Alport syndrome and benign familial hematuria. *Kidney Int* 71: 1287–95.

196. Rana K, Wang YY, Powell H, Jones C, McCredie D, Buzza M, Udawela M, Savige J. (2005). Persistent familial hematuria in children and the locus for thin basement membrane nephropathy. *Pediatr Nephrol* 20:1729–37.

197. Kalluri R, Shield CF, Todd P, Hudson BG, Neilson EG. (1997). Isoform switching of type IV collagen is developmentally arrested in X-linked Alport syndrome leading to increased susceptibility of renal basement membranes to endoproteolysis. *J Clin Invest* 99:2470–8.

198. Miner JH, Sanes JR. (1996). Molecular and functional defects in kidneys of mice lacking collagen alpha 3(IV): implications for Alport syndrome. *J Cell Biol* 135:1403–13.

199. Miner JH. (2003). Of laminins and delamination in Alport syndrome. *Kidney Int* 63:1158–9.

200. Kashtan CE. (2005). Familial hematurias: what we know and what we don't. *Pediatr Nephrol* 20:1027–35.

201. Greer KA, Higgins MA, Cox ML, Ryan TP, Berridge BR, Kashtan CE, Lees GE, Murphy KE. (2006). Gene expression analysis in a canine model of X-linked Alport syndrome. *Mammalian Genome* 17:976–90.

202. Cosgrove D, Kalluri R, Miner JH, Segal Y, Borza DB. (2007). Choosing a mouse model to study the molecular pathobiology of Alport glomerulonephritis. *Kidney Int* 71:615–18.

203. Dagher H, Buzza M, Colville D, Jones C, Powell H, Fassett R, Wilson D, Agar J, Savige J. (2001). A comparison of the clinical, histopathologic, and ultrastructural phenotypes in carriers of X-linked and autosomal recessive Alport's syndrome. *Am J Kidney Dis* 38:1217–28.

204. Nieuwhof CM, de Heer F, de Leeuw P, van Breda Vriesman PJ. (1997). Thin GBM nephropathy: premature glomerular obsolescence is associated with hypertension and late onset renal failure. *Kidney Int* 51:1596–601.

205. Mazzucco G, Barsotti P, Muda AO, Fortunato M, Mihatsch M, Torri-Tarelli L, Renieri A, Faraggiana T, De Marchi M, Monga G. (1998). Ultrastructural and immunohistochemical findings in Alport's syndrome: a study of 108 patients from 97 Italian families with particular emphasis on COL4A5 gene mutation correlations. *J Am Soc Nephrol* 9:1023–31.

206. Kashtan CE. (2007). Alport syndrome and the X chromosome: implications of a diagnosis of Alport syndrome in females. *Nephrol Dial Transplant* 22:1499–505.

207. Wei G, Zhihong L, Huiping C, Caihong Z, Zhaohong C, Leishi L. (2006). Spectrum of clinical features and type IV collagen alpha-chain distribution in Chinese patients with Alport syndrome. *Nephrol Dial Transplant* 21:3146–54.

208. Rizzoni G, Massella L. (2004). Differential diagnosis between X-linked Alport syndrome and thin basement membrane nephropathy. *Kidney Int* 66:1289–90.

209. van der Loop FT, Heidet L, Timmer ED, van den Bosch BJ, Leinonen A, Antignac C, Jefferson JA, Maxwell AP, Monnens LA, Schroder CH, Smeets HJ. (2000). Autosomal dominant Alport syndrome caused by a COL4A3 splice site mutation. *Kidney Int* 58:1870–5.

210. Antonovych TT, Deasy PF, Tina LU, D'Albora JB, Hollerman CE, Calcagno PL. (1969). Hereditary nephritis: early clinical, functional, and morphological studies. *Pediatr Res* 3:545–56.

211. Spear GS, Slusser RJ. (1972). Alport's syndrome. Emphasizing electron microscopic studies of the glomerulus. *Am J Pathol* 69:213–24.

212. Liapis H, Gokden N, Hmiel P, Miner JH. (2002). Histopathology, ultrastructure, and clinical phenotypes in thin glomerular basement membrane disease variants. *Hum Pathol* 33:836–45.

213. Hill GS, Jenis EH, Goodloe S Jr. (1974). The nonspecificity of the ultrastructural alterations in hereditary nephritis with additional observations on benign familial hematuria. *Lab Invest* 31:516–32.

214. Meleg-Smith S. (2001). Alport disease: a review of the diagnostic difficulties. *Ultrastruct Pathol* 25:193–200.

215. Mazzucco G, De Marchi M, Monga G. (2002). Renal biopsy interpretation in Alport Syndrome. *Sem Diag Pathol* 19: 133–45.

216. Jais JP, Knebelmann B, Giatras I, De Marchi M, Rizzoni G, Renieri A, Weber M, Gross O, Netzer KO, Flinter F, Pirson Y, Dahan K, Wieslander J, Persson U, Tryggvason K, Martin P, Hertz JM, Schroder C, Sanak M, Carvalho MF, Saus J, Antignac C, Smeets H, Gubler MC. (2003). X-linked Alport syndrome: natural history and genotype-phenotype correlations in girls and women belonging to 195 families: a "European Community Alport Syndrome Concerted Action" study. *J Am Soc Nephrol* 14:2603–10.

217. Cangiotti AM, Sessa A, Meroni M, Montironi R, Ragaiolo M, Mambelli V, Cinti S. (1996). Evolution of glomerular basement membrane lesions in a male patient with Alport syndrome: ultrastructural and morphometric study. *Nephrol Dial Transplant* 11:1829–34.

218. Foster K, Markowitz GS, D'Agati VD. (2005). Pathology of thin basement membrane nephropathy. *Sem Nephrol* 25:149–58.

219. Churg J, Bernstein J, Glassock RJ (eds). *Renal Disease: Classification and Atlas of Glomerular Diseases*, 2nd ed. New York: Igaku-Shoin, 1995.

220. Ivanyi B, Pap R, Ondrik Z. (2006). Thin basement membrane nephropathy: diffuse and segmental types. *Arch Pathol Lab Med* 130:1533–7.

221. Tonna S, Wang YY, MacGregor D, Sinclair R, Martinello P, Power D, Savige J. (2005). The risks of thin basement membrane nephropathy. *Sem Nephrol* 25:171–5.

222. Proesmans W, Van Dyck M. (2004). Enalapril in children with Alport syndrome. *Pediatr Nephrol* 19:271–5.

223. Charbit M, Gubler MC, Dechaux M, Gagnadoux MF, Grünfeld JP, Niaudet P. (2007). Cyclosporine therapy in patients with Alport syndrome. *Pediatr Nephrol* 22:57–63.

224. Little PJ, Sloper JS and de Wardener H.E. (1967). A syndrome of loin pain and haematuria associated with disease of peripheral renal arteries. *Quart J Med* 36:253–9.

225. Dube GK, Hamilton SE, Ratner LE, Nasr SH, Radhakrishnan J. (2006). Loin pain hematuria syndrome. *Kidney Int* 70:2152–5.

226. Spetie DN, Nadasdy T, Nadasdy G, Agarwal G, Mauer M, Agarwal AK, Khabiri H, Nagaraja HN, Nahman NS Jr, Hartman JA, Hebert LA. (2006). Proposed pathogenesis of idiopathic loin pain-hematuria syndrome. *Am J Kidney Dis* 47:419–27.

227. Lall R, Mailis A, Rapoport A. (1997). Hematuria-loin pain syndrome: its existence as a discrete clinicopathological entity cannot be supported. *Clin J Pain* 13:171–7.

228. Praga M, Martinez MA, Andres A, Alegre R, Vara J, Morales E, Herrero JC, Novo O, Rodicio JL. (1998). Association of thin basement membrane nephropathy with hypercalciuria, hyperuricosuria and nephrolithiasis. *Kidney Int* 54:915–20.

229. Diwakar R, Andrews PA. (2006). Renal transplantation in a patient with loin pain hematuria syndrome. *Clin Nephrol* 66:144–6.

CHAPTER 6

Glomerular Diseases Associated with Nephritic Syndrome and/or Rapidly Progressive Glomerulonephritis

Thomas E. Rogers, MD, Dinesh Rakheja, MD, and Xin J. Zhou, MD

INTRODUCTION

Acute nephritic syndrome is a clinical symptom complex characterized by hematuria (often accompanied by red cell casts in the urine), mild to moderate proteinuria, hypertension, and renal insufficiency, the latter manifested by increased serum creatinine. The clinical onset of nephritic syndrome is typically abrupt and the clinical course may be self-limited or evolve into a chronic nephritis. The histomorphologic correlates of nephritic syndrome are protean and include acute diffuse proliferative glomerulonephritis, membranoproliferative glomerulonephritis, dense deposit disease, focal glomerulonephritis, and crescentic glomerulonephritides. The last category is usually defined by the presence of crescents in at least 50 percent of the sampled glomeruli in a biopsy. This strict definition is important because it may predict a poor clinical outcome. Crescentic glomerulonephritides often lead to a greater than 50 percent decline in glomerular filtration rate (GFR) within three months of clinical presentation, a clinical course that is christened "rapidly progressive glomerulonephritis (RPGN)" or rapidly progressive renal failure [1]. Nephritic syndrome and RPGN are etiologically heterogeneous and an accurate etiologic diagnosis often requires the combination of clinical history, laboratory tests, and renal biopsy examination by light microscopy, immunofluorescence, and electron microscopy. A simplified, algorithmic approach to the interpretation of these conditions is shown in Figure 6.1.

ACUTE DIFFUSE INTRACAPILLARY PROLIFERATIVE GLOMERULONEPHRITIS

Acute diffuse intracapillary proliferative glomerulonephritis describes a pattern of glomerular injury characterized by an enlargement of the majority of glomeruli (i.e., diffuse) because of a global increase in endocapillary cellularity (i.e., proliferative), usually with numerous neutrophils (i.e., acute). It is an immune complex-mediated injury seen most commonly following transient infections (postinfectious acute diffuse proliferative glomerulonephritis or simply acute postinfectious glomerulonephritis). In the past, the most common infections associated with postinfectious acute diffuse proliferative glomerulonephritis were pharyngitis and skin infection caused by group A β-hemolytic streptococci (*Streptococcus pyogenes*), giving rise to the term poststreptococcal acute diffuse proliferative glomerulonephritis or simply acute poststreptococcal glomer-

ulonephritis. In addition to transient infections, persistent infections can also cause acute diffuse proliferative glomerulonephritis, in which case the term infectious acute diffuse proliferative glomerulonephritis is used. The latter has been associated with infectious endocarditis, bacterial infections of cerebrospinal fluid shunts, osteomyelitis, and deep-seated abscesses. Occasionally, postinfectious and infectious glomerulonephritides may have other histologic patterns such as crescentic, membranoproliferative, and mesangioproliferative. The mesangioproliferative pattern, though nonspecific, is usually seen during the resolving phase of postinfectious or infectious glomerulonephritis. Other immune complex mediated diseases such as lupus nephritis and IgA nephropathy can also give rise to acute diffuse proliferative glomerulonephritic histomorphology. In this section, we will limit ourselves to the discussion of postinfectious and infectious acute proliferative glomerulonephritides. The other entities are discussed elsewhere in this book.

Acute Postinfectious Glomerulonephritis

Acute postinfectious glomerulonephritis (APIGN) was first described in 1812, when Wells noted anasarca and bloody urine in patients with scarlet fever [2]. In 1836, Bright noted the association of scarlet fever with self-limited hematuria and facial swelling [3], which led to the eponym "Bright disease" [4].

Epidemiology and Clinical Presentation

In colder regions of the world, acute poststreptococcal glomerulonephritis (APSGN) usually follows streptococcal infections of the upper respiratory tract, pharynx, or tonsils [5], while in the warmer regions, streptococcal skin infections are the more common prequels to renal disease [6]. Only infections with certain "nephritogenic" strains of group A streptococci, *S. pyogenes*, are associated with renal disease: M-types 1, 4, 12, and 25 are the most frequently implicated in upper respiratory infection-associated APSGN, while M-types 2, 42, 49, 56, 57, and 60 are the frequent suspects in cases of skin infection-associated APSGN [7]. The overall risk of developing APSGN after an infection with a nephritogenic streptococcal strain is estimated to be 15 percent, but risk varies with the M-type as well as the site of the infection [8]. APSGN usually occurs in children and young adults, although no age is immune to the occurrence of

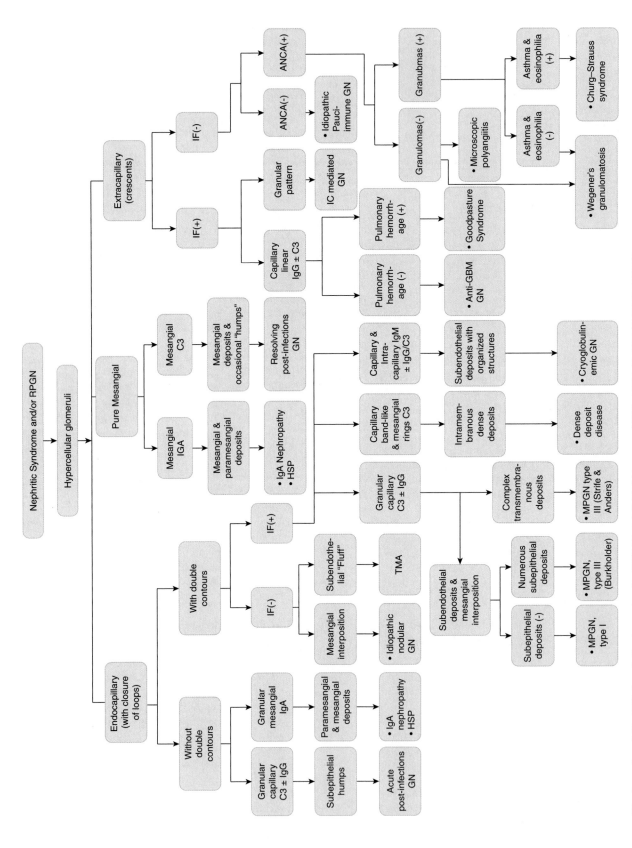

GN: glomerulonephritis; **TMA:** thrombotic microangiopathy; **ANCA:** antineutrophil cytoplasmic antibody; **HSP:** Henoch-Schönlein purpura; **ANCA:** antineutrophil cytoplasmic antibody
MPGN: membranoproliferative glomerulonephritis; **RPGN:** rapidly progressive glomerulonephritis; **IF:** immunofluorescence; **IC:** immune complex

FIGURE 6.1: Algorithmic approach to the interpretation of nephritic syndrome and rapidly progressive glomerulonephritis.

the disease. Males are affected twice as often as females. The incidence of APSGN has steadily declined in the United States and Europe over the last several decades, but remains high in the developing countries [1,7,9]. In recent years, staphylococci and gram-negative bacilli have become more prevalent as the causes of APIGN. APIGN because of nonstreptococcal bacteria is more often seen in adults, where it is associated with predispositions such as alcohol abuse, diabetes mellitus, and intravenous drug use. The prognosis tends to be worse than APSGN, with development of chronic renal failure in up to 50 percent of the patients [10,11].

The latent interval between streptococcal infection and the onset of renal symptoms is 1–2 weeks in cases of upper respiratory infections and 3–6 weeks in cases of skin infections. The usual patient with APSGN presents with the classic signs and symptoms of nephritic syndrome that include gross hematuria (dark, "smoky," "cola or coffee-colored" urine due to hemolysis of red cells in the renal tubular system), microscopic hematuria, and proteinuria that may be in the nephrotic range in 5 to 10 percent of patients. Hematuria tends to persist longer than proteinuria. The urine sediment contains red blood cells, red cell casts, granular casts, and sometimes leukocyte casts [1], and the urine usually has a high specific gravity. There may be oliguria, particularly in older patients and with more severe disease, but it is usually transient with diuresis occurring in one to two weeks [12]. Anuria is uncommon. There may be facial and peripheral edema [1]. Hypertension is not uncommon, especially in the older patients, but it usually resolves with resolution of the renal disease [1]. Blood urea nitrogen and serum creatinine are elevated during the acute stages of the illness. Serum complement levels, especially C3 and occasionally C4 are low, but return to normal with resolution of the disease. Harbingers of a poor prognosis include persistent hypertension, persistent and especially nephrotic range proteinuria, and persistent hematuria [13].

In the majority of the patients, a history of a recent infection is easily established. In addition to the clinical symptoms, the patients may have undergone rapid streptococcal carbohydrate antigen tests in throat swabs, or routine throat swab cultures may have isolated the streptococcus [14]. The patients usually show elevated and rising titers of antistreptococcal antibodies, most commonly antistreptolysin O (ASO) in cases of pharyngitis and antideoxyribonuclease B (anti-DNase B) in cases of skin infections [1].

The classical clinical picture and laboratory tests are diagnostic in the majority of the cases of APSGN and thus, most patients do not undergo renal biopsy, which is reserved for patients with an atypical presentation or with persistent or progressive disease (Table 6.1).

Approach to Interpretation

Gross Pathology. The kidney is enlarged and may have many pinpoint red dots on the surface, giving rise to a "flea-bitten" appearance. The red dots represent red blood cells within the Bowman's spaces and tubular lumens.

Light Microscopy. Acute diffuse proliferative glomerulonephritis is the classical histomorphologic pattern of glomerular injury seen with APSGN and nonstreptococcal APIGN. All or nearly all glomeruli are enlarged. Glomerular tufts are hyper-

Table 6.1 Indications for Renal Biopsy in Children with Suspected Postinfectious Glomerulonephritis

Lack of clinical or serologic evidence of streptococcal infection or immune complex disease
    Lack of rise in anti-streptococcal antibody titers
    Normal serum complement levels
Atypical clinical features at onset of disease
No latency period following infection
Anuria
Persistence of hypertension
Nephrotic syndrome
Atypical recovery
    Failure of recovery of renal function
    Continued decline in renal function
    Continued low complement levels
    Persistence of proteinuria
    Persistence of hematuria

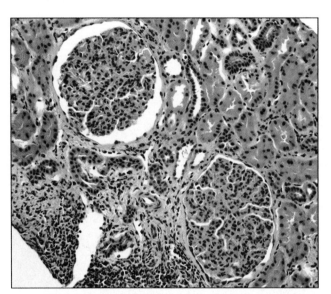

FIGURE 6.2: *Acute postinfectious glomerulonephritis. There is diffuse global intracapillary hypercellularity with an accentuated lobularity caused by mesangial hypercellularity and infiltration of monocytes and neutrophils. Glomerular capillary loops are obscured. There is also prominent interstitial inflammation (H&E, 200×).*

cellular and capillary lumens are obscured (Figure 6.2). The hypercellularity is due to increased numbers of mesangial cells, swelling and proliferation of the capillary endothelial cells, and filling of the capillary lumens by leukocytes such as monocytes and neutrophils, occasionally eosinophils, and rarely lymphocytes [15–18]. The "endocapillary" nature of this glomerular hypercellularity is best appreciated with periodic acid Schiff (PAS) or methenamine silver stains (Figure 6.3). The term "exudative" glomerulonephritis, used when neutrophils are prominent, is erroneous because neutrophils are present within the glomerular capillary lumens and not extravasated

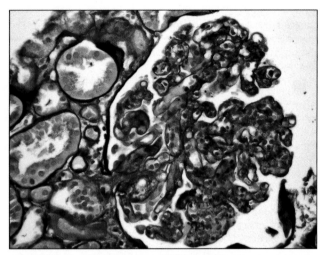

FIGURE 6.3:   Acute postinfectious glomerulonephritis. The methenamine silver stained section highlights the "endocapillary" nature of the hypercellularity with obliterated capillary lumens by the cellular proliferation (Methenamine silver, 400×).

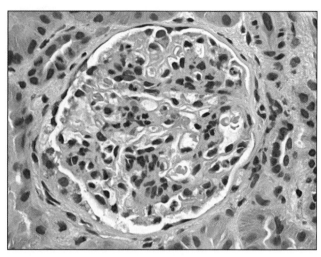

FIGURE 6.5:   Resolving postinfectious glomerulonephritis. The H&E-stained section displays mesangial hypercellularity and expansion of the mesangial matrix (400×).

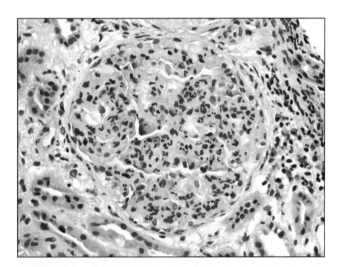

FIGURE 6.4:   Acute postinfectious glomerulonephritis. There is global endocapillary hypercellularity caused mainly by an infiltration of neutrophils warranting a diagnosis of "exudative" glomerulonephritis (H&E, 400×).

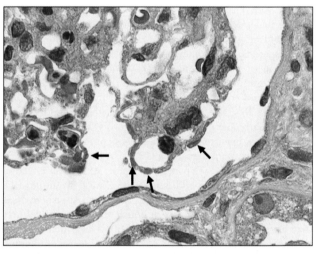

FIGURE 6.6:   Acute postinfectious glomerulonephritis. The trichrome-stained section discloses a segment of glomerular tufts with subepithelial fuchsinophilic (red) deposits (arrows) (1,000×, courtesy of Dr. Tibor Nadasdy).

(Figure 6.4). The relative proportion of neutrophils as well as the overall cellularity decline over time [19]. In a study of thirty-six patients over nearly four years, mesangial hypercellularity and some degree of mesangial matrix expansion (mesangioproliferative glomerulonephritis) was the only late light microscopic finding (Figure 6.5) [19,20]. Under oil immersion objective, Masson trichrome stain may demonstrate fuchsinophilic deposits along the outer aspect of glomerular capillary loops (Figure 6.6) corresponding to the large "hump-like" subepithelial immune deposits seen by electron microscopy. Foci of necrosis and crescents are rare (Figure 6.7). The latter, especially if numerous, may portend a severe form of the disease warranting prompt and aggressive treatment with corticoste-

roids and antihypertensive agents [18,21]. However, a recent study showed that on multivariate analysis, the presence of cellular crescents did not significantly correlate with serum creatinine >2 mg/dl or with the risk of end-stage renal disease [22]. Proximal renal tubules may contain protein resorption droplets, and there may be red cells or red cell casts as well as hyaline casts in tubular lumens. Neutrophils may also be present in tubular lumens (Figure 6.8). Florid cases have been described with acute tubulitis and tubular damage [23,24]. Interstitial changes, usually minor, include edema and mild infiltrates of mononuclear cells and occasionally neutrophils. Vascular changes are not common, although cases of necrotizing arteritis in association with APIGN have been described. In such cases, a

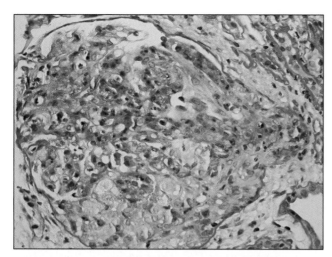

FIGURE 6.7: *Acute postinfectious diffuse proliferative glomerulonephritis. The glomerulus contains a cellular crescent with compressed capillary tufts. The glomerulus shows global endocapillary hypercellularity as well (PAS, 400×).*

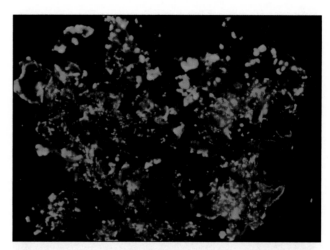

FIGURE 6.9: *Acute postinfectious glomerulonephritis. There is coarse ("lumpy-bumpy") staining of glomerular capillary loops for C3. Significant mesangial deposits are also present (FITC conjugated anti-C3, 400×, courtesy of Dr. Zoltan Laszik).*

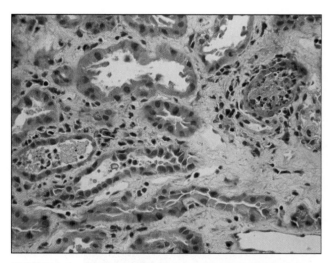

FIGURE 6.8: *Acute postinfectious glomerulonephritis. A few tubular lumens contain clusters of neutrophils and apoptotic cells. There is also interstitial edema with patchy inflammatory infiltration composed of lymphocytes, plasma cells, and neutrophils (H&E, 400×).*

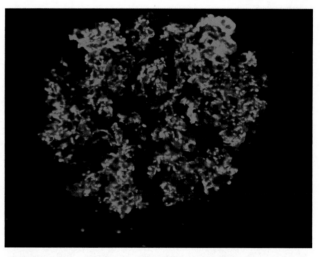

FIGURE 6.10: *Acute postinfectious glomerulonephritis. There is extensive granular staining along the capillary walls and in the mesangial regions for C3, giving rise to a "starry sky" appearance (FITC conjugated anti-C3, 400×, courtesy of Dr. Tibor Nadasdy).*

primary or systemic vasculitic process should also be considered [25].

Immunofluorescence Microscopy. Immunofluorescence reveals coarse granular, "lumpy-bumpy" staining of glomerular capillary loops with IgG and C3 (Figures 6.9 and 6.10). Less frequently, IgM, IgA, light chains, and the early complement components such as C1q and C4 may be present. In cases where the subepithelial deposits are numerous, immunofluorescent staining may have a band-like quality. Some cases may show staining only with C3. The localization of the deposits in the glomeruli changes over time. Late in the course, the pattern of immunofluorescence staining is predominantly or even exclusively mesangial (Figure 6.11).

Sorger et al. described three immunofluorescent staining patterns: the "garland-type" pattern of densely packed, sometimes confluent, staining of peripheral capillary loops with IgG and C3, is seen in all stages of the disease and frequently in patients with more severe disease; the "starry sky" pattern with irregular, fine staining with IgG and C3 is most commonly seen early on in the disease process; and the "mesangial" pattern of staining with IgG and C3 or predominantly C3, usually corresponds to a mesangioproliferative pattern by light microscopy and mesangial/paramesangial deposits by electron microscopy [20]. However, it should be noted that mixed staining patterns, which do not readily fit any one category, are common.

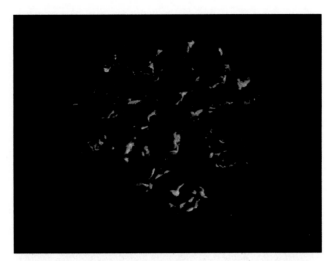

FIGURE 6.11: *Resolving postinfectious glomerulonephritis. There is mainly mesangial staining and less peripheral capillary loop staining for FITC conjugated anti-C3 (400×). However, this staining pattern is non-specific and the integration of the light and electron microscopic findings as well as clinical information is needed to reach an accurate diagnosis.*

Electron Microscopy. Ultrastructural examination confirms the increased numbers of mesangial cells, endothelial cells, and infiltrative leukocytes that obscure glomerular capillary lumens (Figure 6.12). The lamina densa of the glomerular basement membranes (GBM) usually remains unaltered. There may rarely be patchy areas of thickening of the lamina densa, focal areas of widening of the lamina rara interna, or scalloping of the outer aspect of the lamina densa or lucencies within the lamina densa possibly due to resorbed deposits. Areas of endothelial disruption are frequently present with white cells directly abutting the lamina densa of the capillary wall. The classic alteration is the presence of subepithelial, variably electron-dense, "hump-like" deposits present along the peripheral and paramesangial regions of glomerular capillary loops (Figure 6.13). These are most abundant early in the course of the disease and gradually decline in number with time, usually completely disappearing by six weeks [26]. The subepithelial deposits along the paramesnagial regions of the glomerular capillary loops persist the longest. Intramembranous, subendothelial, and mesangial deposits may be present, but are usually fewer and

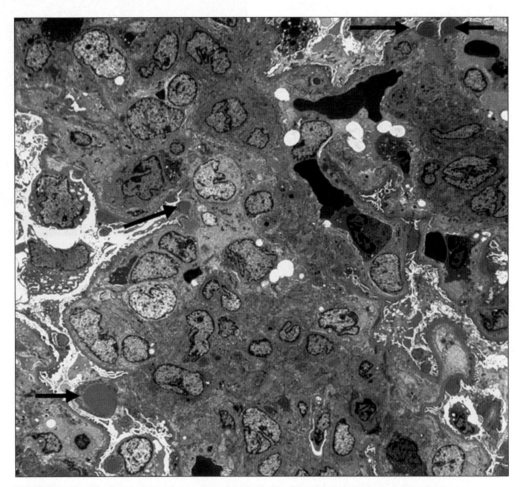

FIGURE 6.12: *Acute postinfectious glomerulonephritis. Electron microphotograph shows endocapillary hypercellularity with increased numbers of mesangial cells, infiltrative leukocytes, and endothelial cells. Capillary lumens are obscured by the cellular proliferation. Large, "hump-like" subepithelial electron-dense deposits are present (arrows).*

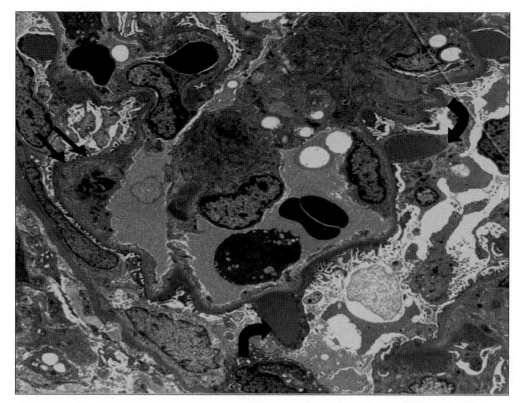

FIGURE 6.13: *Acute postinfectious glomerulonephritis. This electron photomicrograph shows a capillary lumen containing neutrophils. One neutrophil is directly abutting the denuded GBM (straight arrows). A number of large, discrete electron-dense subepithelial humps (occasional flame shaped) are seen (curved arrows).*

are not as prominent as the subepithelial deposits (Figure 6.14). The visceral epithelial cells overlying the subepithelial deposits show effaced foot processes.

Differential Diagnosis

The morphologic differential diagnostic considerations for APIGN are numerous and include various infection-related nephritides (Table 6.2), membranoproliferative glomerulonephritis (MPGN), dense deposit disease (DDD), cryoglobulinemic glomerulonephritis, lupus nephritis, and IgA nephropathy. In various nonstreptococcal postinfectious or infection-associated glomerulonephritides, diffuse proliferative glomerulonephritis as well as other morphologic patterns including crescentic glomerulonephritis, focal proliferative glomerulonephritis or glomerulosclerosis, mesangial proliferative glomerulonephritis, cryoglobulinemic glomerulonephritis, and type I MPGN can be seen. In many of these cases, electron-dense deposits are smaller and not limited to the subepithelial location but are present anywhere within the glomerular capillary wall or mesangium. In some cases of histologically classic diffuse proliferative glomerulonephritis, an underlying etiology is never found.

In some cases of type I MPGN and DDD, the glomeruli may be very cellular and may contain neutrophils. Both APSGN and MPGN are positive for C3 and IgG by immunofluorescence and may contain electron-dense deposits of similar appearance

and location. Thus, it may be difficult to classify accurately, rare cases of acute glomerulonephritis as APSGN or type I MPGN if the clinical history of a recent streptococcal infection is lacking and there are no medical conditions that might be associated with type I MPGN. Patient follow-up is often required to determine the exact nature of the disease as APSGN usually resolves while MPGN type I is usually progressive, especially if untreated. DDD can be distinguished from APSGN by the pathognomonic electron-dense transformation of GBM and mesangial matrix on electron microscopy. It should be noted that DDD occasionally has hump-like deposits similar to those seen in APIGN.

Some cases of cryoglobulinemic glomerulonephritis lacking characteristic glomerular capillary thrombi and organized electron-dense deposits may be difficult to distinguish from APSGN. Diffuse proliferative lupus nephritis (Class IV) may appear similar to APSGN on routine light microscopy. However, it is easy to make a diagnosis of Class IV lupus nephritis on immunofluorescence (a "full house" pattern) and electron microscopic (numerous electron-dense deposits, predominantly in the subendothelial and mesangial regions) examinations. IgA nephropathy can rarely present with a pattern of acute diffuse proliferative glomerulonephritis. In addition, the resolving phase of APIGN can have a mesangioproliferative pattern resembling typical IgA nephropathy. Immunofluorescence microscopy is most helpful in these situations, since IgA

Table 6.2 Infectious Agents Associated with Glomerulonephritis

Bacteria
Staphylococci
Gram negative bacilli
Group A Streptococci
Streptococcus pneumoniae
Treponema pallidum
Salmonella species
Brucella species
Mycobacteria
Campylobacter species
Meningococci
Nocardia species
Actinobacillus species
Borrelia species
Bartonella species
Propionibacterium species
Coxiella burnetii
Legionella species
Mycoplasma species

Viruses
Varicella
Coxsackie
Rubeola (measles)
Mumps
Epstein-Barr
Influenza
Hepatitis B and C
Enteric Cytopathic Human Orphan (ECHO)
Adenovirus
Parvovirus B19
Vaccinia
Herpes

Fungi
Aspergillus fumigatus
Histoplasma
Candida albicans

Parasites
Schistosoma species
Plasmodium species

nephropathy has dominant/codominant mesangial IgA staining, while APIGN does not.

Etiology and Pathogenesis

APSGN and nonstreptococcal APIGN are immunologically mediated disorders. The development of antibodies against intracellular and extracellular streptococcal or other bacterial antigens explains the latency between onset of the infection and development of the renal disease. These antibodies are not only useful in establishing the diagnostic link between the infection and the renal disease, but also are involved in the formation of in situ and circulating immune complexes that initiate the development of renal disease through a variety of effector mechanisms [7,8,27–29].

Rodriquez-Iturbe and Batsford [27] noted that glomerular immune complex formation is the initiating event. Numerous mechanisms have been proposed to explain the formation of immune complexes in APSGN. These mechanisms have included molecular mimicry, autoimmune reactivity, and streptococcal-related glomerular plasmin-binding activity. For many years, the concept of molecular mimicry was the favored explanation. It was hypothesized that antigenic similarity between streptococcal antigens and human antigens explained the formation of autoantibodies against human antigens. However, nonnephritogenic streptococci also have the same antigens and yet do not cause kidney disease [30]. The autoimmune phenomena seen in APSGN likely represent epiphenomena. Streptococcal-related glomerular plasmin-binding activity has gained prominence in recent years as the likely pathogenesis of APSGN. A recently described streptococcal antigen, nephritis-associated plasmin receptor (NAPlr) or streptococcal glyceraldehyde-3-phosphate dehydrogenase (GAPDH), binds plasmin maintaining its proteolytic activity, activates the alternate complement pathway, incites an inflammatory response, and damages GBM and mesangial matrix leading to formation and penetration of immune complexes [8,16,27,29,31]. Several proteins have been postulated to be "nephritogenic." However, streptococcal pyrogenic exotoxin B (SPEB) and its zymogen precursor (zSPEB) are currently felt to be the most important "nephritogenic" antigens. These streptococcal proteinases are highly antigenic and stimulate the formation of antibodies that can then form circulating immune complexes and in situ immune complexes [8,27,28,32]. Both GAPDH and SPEB have been identified in renal biopsy specimens of APSGN. Rising antibody titers to SPEB/zSPEB and GAPDH are now considered to be the best evidence of nephritogenic streptococcal infection and may replace the current serologic methods used for diagnosis of APSGN [27].

Clinical Course, Prognosis, Treatment, and Clinical Correlation

APSGN occurring in children and adolescents has an excellent prognosis, with complete recovery of renal function in over 90 percent of patients. The presence of another underlying renal disease, persistent proteinuria, persistent renal insufficiency, oliguria/anuria, hypertension, and numerous crescents in the renal biopsy may portend a poor prognosis [1,13,18,33,34]. A recent study showed that, on multivariate analysis, the correlates of seum creatinine >2 mg/dl included only hypoalbuminemia, interstitial inflammation, endocapilalry proliferation, and acute tubular injury [22]. In children, there is a very high rate of complete glomerular healing (97 percent) although it may take a considerable amount of time (2 to 12 years) [35]. The outcome in adults may be less favorable especially at older ages, with underlying medical illnesses, and with interstitial inflammation on biopsy. [11,36]. The reported proportions of complete recovery in adults are in the range of 53 to 76 percent [1]. In a recent study of adult patients with APIGN, 56.1 percent of the patients without underlying diabetic glomerulosclerosis and none with underlying diabetic glomerulosclerosis achieved complete remission; 26.8 percent of the former and 18.2 percent of the latter had persistent renal dysfunction; and the remainder of the patients in both groups progressed to end stage renal disease. By multivariate analysis, age, and serum creatinine at the time of the renal biopsy correlated inversely with complete remission [22].

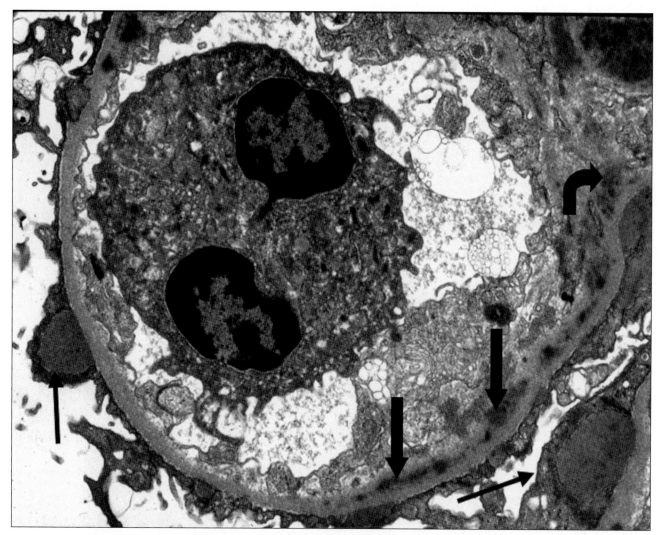

FIGURE 6.14: *Acute postinfectious glomerulonephritis. Electron micrograph shows a neutrophil in the capillary lumen. There is a large subepithelial electron-dense deposit (hump, thin arrows) with scattered subendothelial (thick arrows) and mesangial (curved arrow) electron-dense deposits. Significant foot process effacement is present. Another large hump is noted at the right lower corner of the field (courtesy of Dr. Zoltan Laszik).*

Treatment is directed towards appropriate medical therapy for the infection and supportive care for the patients and their renal disease. Corticosteroids have been used effectively in cases with features suggesting a poorer outcome [21].

Infectious Endocarditis-Associated Glomerulonephritis

Infectious endocarditis-associated glomerulonephritis can be caused by either acute or subacute infectious endocarditis. In addition, renal infarcts and abscesses, and interstitial nephritis are other renal complications of endocarditis [37,38].

Epidemiology and Clinical Presentation

The most common infectious organisms in endocarditis-associated glomerulonephritis are *Staphylococcus aureus* and the viridans streptococci. However, a number of other bacteria and fungi have been reported as causative agents. Patients usually present with features of endocarditis including fever, heart mur-

murs, anemia, Roth spots, purpura, and hepatosplenomegaly. In some cases, renal involvement may be the first sign of disease. The signs and symptoms of renal disease include hematuria, proteinuria, depressed serum complement levels, and renal insufficiency and failure. Renal complications, including glomerulonephritis, renal infarcts, renal abscesses, and interstitial nephritis affect up to 40 to 50 percent of patients with infectious endocarditis [37,39].

Approach to Interpretation

Gross Pathology. Renal infarcts may be caused by emboli arising from heart vegetations. Other gross findings include petechial hemorrhages in cases of severe glomerulonephritis such as those associated with crescents.

Light Microscopy. The histologic appearance of infectious endocarditis-associated glomerulonephritis varies from acute

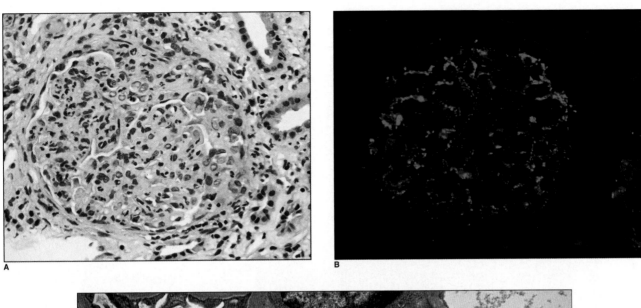

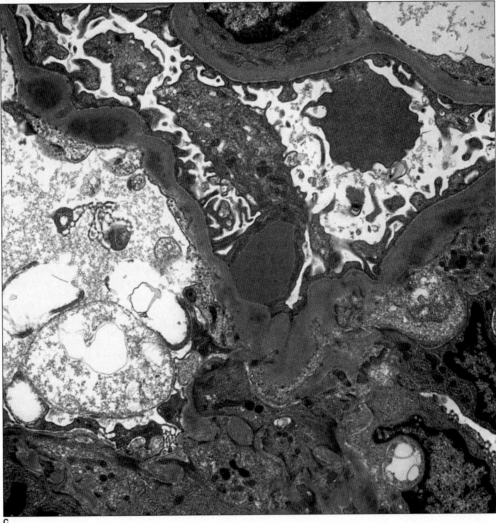

FIGURE 6.15: *Infectious endocarditis-associated glomerulonephritis. (A). Light microscopy reveals glomerular intracapillary hypercellularity with a significant influx of neutrophils. A small cellular crescent is also observed (H&E, 400x). (B). Immunofluorescence microscopy displays coarse granular staining along the capillary walls and segmentally in the mesangial regions for C3 (400x, courtesy of Dr. Tibor Nadasdy). (C). Electron micrograph shows a large subepithelial hump-like electron-dense deposit. Scattered subendothelial deposits are also noted.*

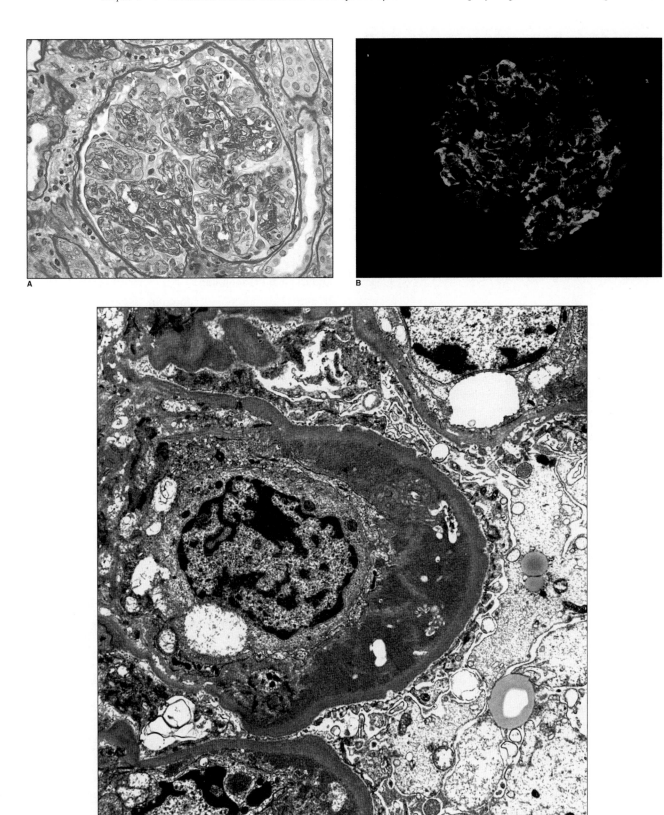

FIGURE 6.16: *Infectious endocarditis-associated glomerulonephritis. (A). Light microscopy reveals a membranoproliferative pattern of glomerular injury characterized by global intracapillary hypercellularity with frequent double-contoured capillary walls (PAS, 400x). (B): Immunofluorescence microscopy displays intense granular staining along the capillary walls and segmentally in the mesangial regions for IgG (400x). (C:. Electron micrograph shows capillary loops with numerous large subendothelial electron-dense deposits.*

diffuse proliferative glomerulonephritis indistinguishable from APSGN (Figure 6.15A), to focal proliferative, necrotizing, or sclerosing glomerulonephritis with or without immune complex deposition, crescentic glomerulonephritis, and type I MPGN (Figures 6.16A and 6.17). Focal glomerulonephritis (focal necrotizing glomerulonephritis, in particular) is the most common pattern. In those with proliferative glomerulonephritis, there are varying degrees of focal or global hypercellularity, and some have changes of MPGN type I, which is more likely associated with subacute rather than acute infectious endocarditis. With treatment of the endocarditis, the renal disease may resolve with complete healing, but more commonly, the renal glomerular lesions evolve into segmental or global sclerosis. Tubulointerstitial disease usually parallels the degree of renal glomerular injury. It may include acute tubular necrosis in severe cases, or drug-related or immune-mediated tubulointerstitial nephritis with numerous eosinophils [38].

Immunofluorescence Microscopy. Staining for immunoglobulins and complement may or may not be present and is usually lacking in cases of necrotizing glomerulonephritis. When present, the staining may be band-like or granular along the capillary wall as well in the mesangium (Figures 6.15B, 6.16B). A patient with diffuse proliferative glomerulonephritis associated with subacute infectious endocarditis due to viridans streptococci showed a "full-house" immunofluorescence pattern with reactivity for C3, C4, C1q, IgG, IgA, and IgM [40]. Another patient with enterococcal endocarditis-associated focal and segmental glomerular endocapillary proliferation, glomerular fibrinoid necrosis, and prominent crescents showed diffuse and global mesangial and capillary wall staining for IgG, IgM, and C3 [41].

Electron Microscopy. Cases with light microscopic features of acute diffuse proliferative glomerulonephritis may have "hump-like" subepithelial electron-dense deposits (Figure 6.15C). In addition, subendothelial, subepithelial, and mesangial deposits may be present with both diffuse proliferative and focal proliferative glomerular morphology. In patients with MPGN, there are subendothelial deposits and areas of mesangial cellular interposition in glomerular capillary basement membranes (Figure 6.16C). Cases of necrotizing glomerulonephritis frequently lack deposits [38].

Differential Diagnosis

Given the broad range of histologic manifestations of endocarditis-associated glomerulonephritis, the differential diagnostic considerations are wide-ranging. Immune complex-mediated focal or diffuse proliferative glomerulonephritis may be due to a variety of immune complex-mediated diseases including systemic lupus erythematosus. In particular, the rare patient with diffuse proliferative glomerulonephritis and a "full-house" immunofluorescent study may be confused with lupus nephritis [40]. The MPGN pattern is indistinguishable from the MPGN pattern seen with other infections such as hepatitis B and C. Pauci-immune, focal, necrotizing glomerulonephritis needs to be distinguished from an ANCA-associated vasculitic process.

Etiology and Pathogenesis

S. aureus and the viridans streptococci are currently the most common causes of infectious endocarditis, although numerous other bacteria and fungi may be responsible. Intravenous drug users, patients with diseased native cardiac valves, and prosthetic valve recipients are at the highest risk for infection [37]. Circulating immune complexes, in situ immune complex formation, in situ localization of nephritogenic bacterial molecules, and cell-mediated mechanisms are postulated to be responsible for the development of the renal disease [42]. Immune complex deposition certainly plays a role in membranoproliferative cases, while pauci-immune cases may be due to cell-mediated immune mechanisms or associated with ANCA [38, 43].

Clinical Course, Prognosis, Treatment, and Clinical Presentation

If untreated, infectious endocarditis-associated glomerulonephritis has a worse prognosis than APIGN. Prompt treatment of the infection may lead to a resolution or healing of the glomerulonephritis. Treatment includes antibiotics and possibly steroids, and surgery for replacement or repair of severely diseased cardiac valves, drainage of abscesses, and removal of infectious vegetations. Plasmapheresis, corticosteroids, and immunosuppression in combination with antibiotics have been effective in cases of rapidly progressive renal failure and those refractory to antibiotic therapy alone [44–46]. Prophylaxis with antibiotics has reduced the incidence of endocarditis in patients known to be at risk.

Infected Ventriculoatrial Shunt Related Glomerulonephritis (Shunt Nephritis)

Shunt nephritis refers to glomerulonephritis associated with infections in shunts used to treat hydrocephalus, occurring more commonly with ventriculoatrial than with

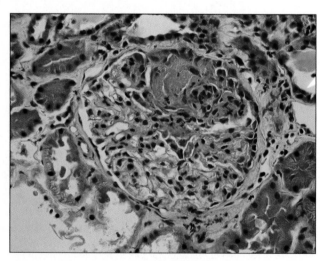

FIGURE 6.17: *Infectious endocarditis-associated glomerulonephritis. The glomerulus reveals small segmental fibrinoid necrosis with an early small cellular crescent. The non-necrotic segments are essentially unremarkable (H&E, 400x).*

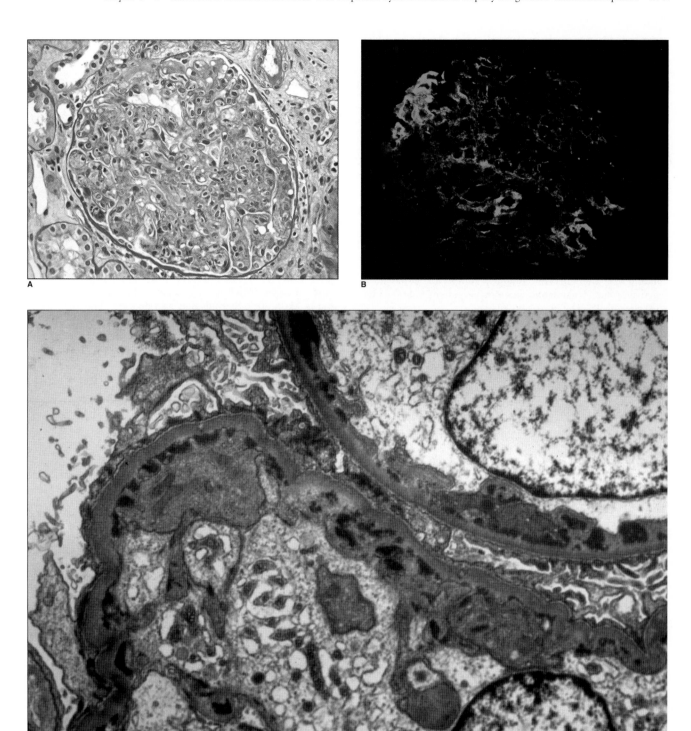

FIGURE 6.18: Shunt nephritis. (A). The glomerulus reveals significant intracapillary hypercellularity with an exaggerated lobular configuration and segmental basement membrane reduplication (PAS; 400x). (B). Immunofluorescence microscopy shows granular staining along the capillary walls and in the mesangial regions for IgG (400x). (C). The electron micrograph reveals glomerular capillary loops with many subendothelial electron-dense deposits.

ventriculoperitoneal shunts. Fortunately, ventriculoperitoneal shunts are replacing ventriculoatrial and ventriculojugular shunts as the surgical treatment of choice for hydrocephalus. Therefore, shunt nephritis is rarely seen nowadays. Patients

with infections of portosystemic shunts for problems associated with chronic liver disease may develop an IgA predominant form of MPGN-like glomerulonephritis and should not be referred to as "shunt nephritis." The offending organisms in shunt nephritis are usually low virulence bacteria like *Staphylococcus epidermidis*, although other infectious agents have also been reported [47–49].

Epidemiology and Clinical Presentation

Patients with shunt nephritis may present with symptoms related to infection of the shunt such as fever, malaise, and nausea and vomiting due to increased intracranial pressure. Shunt infections typically occur 4 to 5 years after shunt placement (with a range of 1 month to more than 20 years). The renal manifestations are those of acute nephritic syndrome and include hematuria and proteinuria that may be in the nephrotic range. Varying degrees of renal insufficiency may be present as well. Consistent with an immunologically mediated renal injury, the patients frequently have hypocomplementemia, circulating cryoglobulins and immune complexes, elevated C-reactive protein, rheumatoid factor, hypergammaglobulinemia, and occasionally ANCA [47,48,50].

Approach to Interpretation

Light Microscopy. An MPGN-pattern is seen in nearly half of all patients (Figure 6.18A), while a third have focal or diffuse proliferative glomerulonephritis. Rarely, the renal biopsies show mesangioproliferative glomerulonephritis. A few crescents may develop, but rarely do they involve greater than half of all glomeruli to warrant a diagnosis of crescentic glomerulonephritis [1,48–50].

Immunofluorescence Microscopy. IgG, IgM, and IgA as well as complement components including the early components are positive in most cases of shunt nephritis. Some patients have positivity for complement components alone. The pattern of immunofluorescence is compatible with the histologic form of the disease. Thus, granular to band-like staining of the glomerular capillary loops and mesangial regions occurs in cases with MPGN pattern (Figure 6.18B), coarse granular staining of the glomerular capillary loops in focal and diffuse proliferative glomerulonephritis, and mesangial staining in mesangioproliferative glomerulonephritis. Immunoglobulin and complement staining of peritubular capillaries has also been noted.

Electron Microscopy. Most cases of shunt nephritis have electron-dense deposits in the mesangium and in subendothelial location along the glomerular capillary walls (Figure 6.18C). The latter are more common than subepithelial deposits, which may be "hump-like." In cases with the morphology of MPGN, mesangial cell interposition in glomerular capillary basement membranes is also present.

Differential Diagnosis, Etiology, and Pathogenesis

Shunt-related glomerulonephritis develops in 0.7–2.3 percent of patients with ventriculoatrial shunts even though shunt infections occur more frequently in these patients [47]. Analogous forms of glomerulonephritis also develop in patients with other implanted vascular devices such as permanent indwelling catheters and medication injection reservoirs. The most common offending organisms are staphylococci such as *S. epidermidis*, although a variety of other bacterial and fungal infections have been reported. Low complement levels, circulating cryoglobulins and immune complexes, rheumatoid factor, and ANCA suggest underlying immune-mediated mechanisms [47–50]. Glomerular localization of bacterial antigens, antibodies, and immune complexes are thought to be etiopathogenetically related to the development of the renal disease.

Clinical Course, Prognosis, Treatment, and Clinical Correlation

Shunt nephritis typically resolves with treatment of the underlying infection, which usually requires shunt removal in addition to antibiotics. Steroids may also be used. The majority of the treated patients recover completely while some go on to develop persistent renal insufficiency and progress to end stage renal disease [47–51].

Deep-Seated Abscess and Osteomyelitis Related Glomerulonephritis

Epidemiology and Clinical Presentation

Deep-seated visceral and soft tissue abscesses and osteomyelitis are occasionally associated with development of glomerulonephritis. The patients present with signs and symptoms referable to their infections. Skin purpura may be present if there is a concomitant small vessel vasculitis. The signs and symptoms of renal disease include hematuria and proteinuria, with varying degrees of renal insufficiency and hypertension that depend on the severity of the renal disease. Hypocomplementemia and cryoglobulinemia are common [1,52–54].

Approach to Interpretation

Light Microscopy. Like other infection-related glomerulonephritides, these patients may have focal or diffuse proliferative glomerulonephritis, MPGN, crescentic glomerulonephritis, and mesangioproliferative glomerulonephritis (Figure 6.19A). Some degree of crescent formation is common; occasionally the crescents affect more than 50 percent of the glomeruli, qualifying for a diagnosis of crescentic glomerulonephritis. Medical and surgical treatment of the underlying infection usually leads to a restoration of normal renal function and glomerular architecture, although renal biopsies in some patients may show segmental or global glomerulosclerotic lesions [52,53].

Immunofluorescence Microscopy. The glomeruli stain for immunoglobulin and complement in the glomerular capillary loops and mesangium, consistent with the light microscopic pattern of the disease (Figure 6.19B).

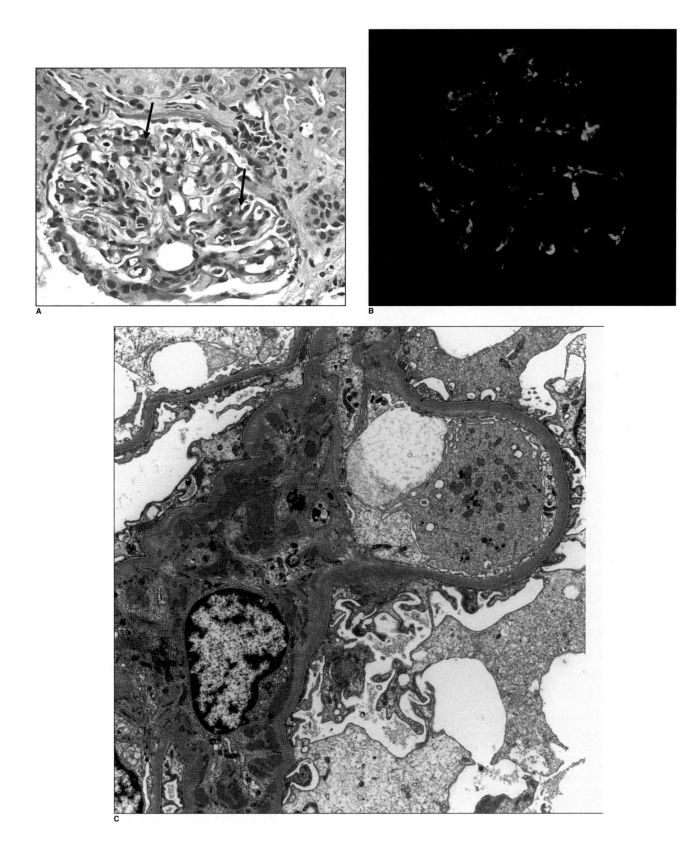

FIGURE 6.19: *Glomerulonephritis associated with deep-seated abscess. (A). There is mild segmental mesangial hypercellularity (i.e., three or more mesangial and/or inflammatory cells per mesangial area away from the vascular pole in a 2-3 μm thick section; arrows) (PAS, 400x). (B). Immunofluorescence microscopy reveals granular staining in the mesangial regions for C3 (400x). (C). Electron micrograph reveals mesangial electron-dense deposits.*

Electron Microscopy. The location and morphology of the electron-dense deposits correspond to the light and immunofluorescence patterns of the disease (Figure 6.19C).

Differential Diagnosis, Etiology, Pathogenesis, Clinical Course, Prognosis, Treatment, and Clinical Correlation

The sites of abscess formation most often associated with glomerulonephritis are the lungs and the most common pathogen is *S. aureus*. However, abscesses at any site and osteomyelitis may be associated with glomerulonephritis. Immune mechanisms similar to those described for other infection-related renal disease are thought to be involved in the pathogenesis of glomerulonephritis associated with deep-seated abscesses and osteomyelitis. Effective medical and surgical treatment with eradication of the infection usually results in a complete recovery of the renal function whereas delays in therapy or failure to clear the infection may result in persistent or progressive renal failure [52–54].

MEMBRANOPROLIFERATIVE GLOMERULONEPHRITIS (MESANGIOCAPILLARY GLOMERULONEPHRITIS)

Idiopathic Membranoproliferative Glomerulonephritis

Membranoproliferative glomerulonephritis (MPGN) defines a histopathologic pattern of glomerular injury that has also been called mesangiocapillary glomerulonephritis [55]. MPGN is characterized by thickening of the glomerular capillary walls (membrano-), and hypercellularity in the glomerular capillary tufts (proliferative). In addition, the glomeruli often have a lobular configuration because of the prominent mesangial hypercellularity and matrix expansion. In addition to occurring as a primary (idiopathic) disease, an MPGN-pattern may be seen with a variety of underlying diseases (Table 6.3). Indeed, most cases of MPGN-pattern in adults are secondary to an identifiable cause (most often chronic hepatitis C infection), while most cases in children are primary [56,57]. Some of the glomerulonephritides with MPGN-pattern are discussed elsewhere in the text. Later in this chapter, we will focus on the glomerulonephritides associated with chronic hepatitis B and hepatitis C infections.

Historically, primary MPGN has been subclassified into three types based on the histomorphologic patterns. MPGN type I is characterized by the typical light microscopic features described above, along with the presence of immune deposits in the subendothelial and mesangial regions. A few small immune deposits may also be present in subepithelial location. Burkholder, in 1970, described a case of MPGN with double contouring of the GBM as well as a "spiked" appearance with subepithelial electron-dense deposits reminiscent of membranous glomerulopathy [58]. While this form of renal disease has been called MPGN type III of Burkholder, many consider it an example of type I MPGN with unusually prominent subepithelial deposits or undiagnosed lupus or postinfectious glomerulo-

Table 6.3 Diseases That May Be Associated With a Membranoproliferative Glomerulonephritis Pattern

Infections
Chronic hepatitis C infection
Chronic hepatitis B infection
Infectious endocarditis
Visceral and deep seated infections
Infected ventriculoatrial shunts
Brucellosis
Plasmodial infections (malaria)
Schistosomiasis
Mycoplasma infection

Immunologic diseases
Systemic lupus erythematosus
Anti-phospholipid antibody syndrome
Mixed connective tissue disease
Rheumatoid arthritis

Dysproteinemias
Light chain deposition disease
Heavy chain deposition disease
Waldenstrom macroglobulinemia
Fibrillary glomerulonephritis
Immunotactoid glomerulonephritis
Cryoglobulinemia

Malignancies
Leukemias and lymphomas

Chronic liver disease/Cirrhosis
Chronic infectious hepatitis (C and B)
Alpha1-antitrypsin deficiency

Thrombotic microangiopathies
Radiation nephritis
Sickle cell anemia
Transplant glomerulopathy

nephritis. MPGN type III described by Strife and Anders has complex GBM formation and electron-dense deposits at both subendothelial and subepithelial areas that are bridged by intramembranous deposits blending into the GBM [57,59,60]. The histopathologic pattern of glomerular injury designated MPGN type II is more appropriately referred to as dense deposit disease (DDD). It is now recognized as a disorder distinct from MPGN types I and III [61], and is discussed separately in this chapter.

Epidemiology and Clinical Presentation

Primary or idiopathic MPGN comprises <5 percent of all primary glomerulonephritides and accounts for 4–10 percent of the cases of primary nephrotic syndrome in children. While the prevalence of primary MPGN appears to be declining in North America and Europe, MPGN remains one of the most common causes of nephrotic syndrome in the Middle East, South America, and Africa, accounting for 30–40 percent of the cases [57].

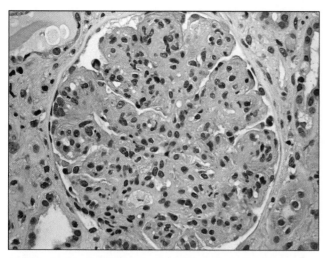

FIGURE 6.20: *MPGN type I. The glomerulus is hypercellular with obliterated capillary lumens caused by proliferation of mesangial and endothelial cells as well as infiltrating leukocytes (H&E, 400×).*

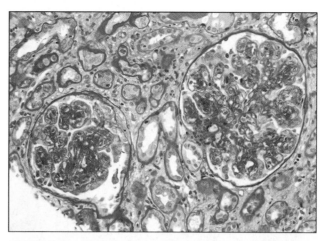

FIGURE 6.21: *MPGN type I. Both glomeruli disclose global intracapillary hypercellularity and expansion of mesangial matrix with accentuated lobularity of glomerular tufts. The glomerular capillary lumens are narrowed. There is also focal tubular atrophy and interstitial fibrosis (PAS, 200×).*

MPGN may occur at any age, but is most common in older children and young adults between 7 and 30 years. The clinical picture may be one of nephrotic syndrome (in approximately 50 percent of the cases) with or without hematuria and red cell casts [62–67]. Ten to 20 percent of the patients may present with nephritic syndrome [68]. Approximately one third of the patients develop hypertension at the onset of disease. An upper respiratory tract infection frequently precedes the first clinical recognition of the renal disease. Serum complement levels are low at some point in a majority of the patients. Thus, low levels of C3 may be seen in up to 80 percent of patients with MPGN type I and 50 percent of patients with MPGN type III. In MPGN type I, the serum levels of the components of both the classical complement pathway (C1, C2, and C4) and the alternative pathway (properdin and factor B) are decreased. Blood urea nitrogen and creatinine levels are elevated in a quarter of the patients. In patients with MPGN type III, asymptomatic hematuria and proteinuria may remain subclinical for a long time before diagnosis [59,69]. Patients with MPGN type III have low serum levels of C3, C5, and properdin but normal serum levels of C1q and C4, suggesting activation of the alternative complement pathway alone without activation of the classical pathway.

Approach to Interpretation of MPGN Type I

Gross Pathology. With advancing disease and nephron loss, there is progressive renal cortical atrophy resulting in progressively smaller kidneys with a finely granular surface. Both kidneys are similarly affected. The most important determinant of gross morphology appears to be the degree of glomerulosclerosis. The gross features of MPGN types I and III are similar.

Light Microscopy. Glomeruli are enlarged with global hypercellularity and frequently, an accentuated lobular configuration where it is much easier to see individual tufts as separate from one

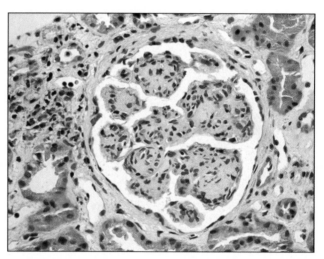

FIGURE 6.22: *MPGN type I. The glomerulus reveals moderate mesangial hypercellularity with nodular mesangial sclerosis (H&E, 400×).*

another (Figures 6.20 and 6.21). There is an increase in the number of mesangial cells and a variable increase in mesangial matrix. In some case, the increase in the amount of mesangial matrix may be pronounced, giving a nodular appearance to the glomeruli (Figure 6.22). A variable number of monocytes and neutrophils may also contribute to the increased cellularity. When prominent, the increased neutrophils may create the appearance of an "exudative glomerulonephritis," not unlike that seen in APSGN. The increased glomerular cellularity tends to obscure the glomerular capillary lumens. In addition, variable thickening of the glomerular capillary walls compromises the glomerular capillary lumens. Often, the glomerular capillary basement membranes show double contours or a "tram track" appearance, best appreciated in the peripheral portions of the capillary loops on PAS and methenamine silver stains (Figures 6.21 and 6.23). In some instances, the glomerular capillary basement membranes may

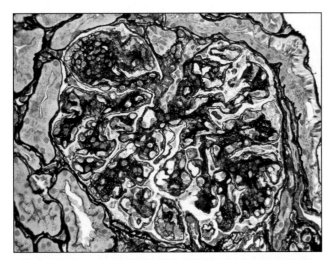

FIGURE 6.23: *MPGN type I. The methenamine silver stained glomerulus shows modest intracapillary hypercellularity with expanded mesangial matrix, narrowed capillary lumens, and diffuse double contours (400×).*

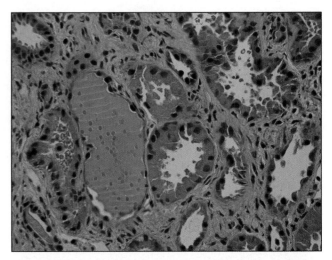

FIGURE 6.25: *MPGN type I. There are red blood cells (RBC) and RBC casts in the tubular lumens. Scattered tubules display numerous intracytoplasmic protein resorption droplets. Mild interstitial fibrosis and inflammation are also noted (H&E, 400x).*

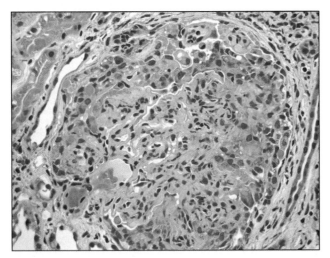

FIGURE 6.24: *MPGN type I. The H&E stained section reveals a cellular crescent with compressed hypercellular capillary tufts (H&E, 400x).*

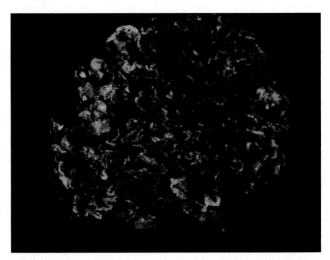

FIGURE 6.26: *MPGI type I. Immunofluorescence microscopy reveals intense granular peripheral and mesangial staining for C3 (400x).*

have a complex laminated appearance. The double contours of the glomerular capillary basement membranes are due to mesangial cell interposition or mononuclear cell infiltration into the subendothelial regions at the periphery of the glomerular capillary loops, and deposition of immune complexes in the same region with formation of new basement membrane matrix material by mesangial and endothelial cells on the inside of the interposed cells and immune deposits. Fuchsinophilic deposits may be seen on trichrome staining on the subendothelial aspect of the glomerular capillary loops [55,62,64,68,70,71]. While usually diffuse and global, a small percentage of cases show only focal and segmental involvement by the disease process. The latter cases may represent an early stage of the disease and have a better prognosis compared to cases showing more uniform, global glomerular pathology [65,66,72]. Cellular crescents may be present in a small percentage of cases (Figure 6.24) and often indicative of a poorer prognosis

[63,64,68,73,74]. Over time, the glomerular hypercellularity decreases and glomeruli assume a more globally sclerotic appearance. This is often accompanied by tubular atrophy and interstitial fibrosis and inflammation. In cases with heavy proteinuria, there are protein and lipid resorption droplets in proximal tubular epithelial cells (Figure 6.25). Tubules may contain red cells in their lumens. With progression and the development of chronic renal disease and hypertension, secondary arterial and arteriolar sclerosis may be seen. The presence of vasculitis should prompt a search for cryoglobulinemia.

Immunofluorescence Microscopy. There is consistent, usually intense, staining for C3 in a fine to coarse or broad, granular staining pattern along the periphery of the glomerular capillary

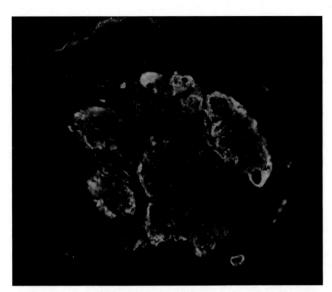

FIGURE 6.27: *MPGN type I. Immunofluorescence microscopy discloses predominantly peripheral capillary wall staining with a band-like pattern for IgG (FITC conjugated anti-IgG, 400×).*

loops as well as in the mesangium (Figure 6.26 and 6.27). Similar staining patterns are often seen for IgG and IgM, and occasionally IgA, and for early complement components, C1q and C4. In some cases, the dominant staining is along the capillary walls, whereas in other cases it is mainly in the mesangial regions. The peripheral capillary wall deposits have a smooth outer contour, highlighting their subendothelial location confined by the outer normal GBM. The degree of staining of different capillary loops may be quite variable. The staining is gradually lost as the disease progresses, the deposits are resorbed, and glomerulosclerosis ensues.

Electron Microscopy. Ultrastructural examination confirms an increase in the mesangial cells and mesangial matrix with an influx of inflammatory cells in some cases (Figure 6.28). The periphery of the glomerular capillary loops is variably thickened with interposition of mesangial and inflammatory cells into the subendothelial space as well as deposition of homogeneous, electron-dense deposits in the same regions with formation of new basement membrane-like material by mesangial and endothelial cells "sandwiching" the deposits and interposed cells between an outer normal GBM and an inner basement membrane-like material (Figures 6.29 and 6.30). The electron-dense deposits may be numerous and large, but in some cases are fewer and smaller and may be quite inconspicuous. Scattered, subepithelial and mesangial deposits may be present as well [55,62,65,66,68,71,72,74]. The degree to which the cellular interposition and/or electron-dense deposit formation contribute to the thickening of glomerular capillary walls is variable. There is usually widespread visceral epithelial foot process effacement associated with podocyte hypertrophy and focal microvillous transformation. Changes of tubular atrophy, interstitial fibrosis and inflammation, and arteriolar sclerosis parallel the degree of glomerulosclerosis and hypertension.

Approach to Interpretation of MPGN Type III

Light Microscopy. The glomeruli show varying degrees of mesangial matrix expansion, often resulting in a "lobular glomerulonephritis" appearance. While the mesangial hypercellularity is of a lesser degree than seen in type I MPGN, the glomerular capillary wall thickening is more diffuse and pronounced with prominent "splitting" or "tram tracking." On methenamine silver staining, spikes of basement membrane may be seen in the peripheral glomerular capillary loops (Figure 6.31) in MPGN type III of Burkholder [58,69,71,75]. In MPGN type III of Strife and Anders, the glomerular capillary walls may appear disrupted and frayed because of the presence of complex deposits in the subendothelial, intramembranous, and subepithelial locations (Figure 6.32 and 6.33). The glomerular changes are usually global and diffuse, but may sometimes be focal and segmental.

Immunofluorescence Microscopy. In 50 percent of the cases, there is coarse granular staining of the glomerular capillary loops and mesangial regions for C3. The remaining 50 percent of cases show combined staining for C3 and immunoglobulins, mainly IgG, with less intense and more variable staining for IgM and/or IgA (Figures 6.34, 6.35).

Electron Microscopy. In MPGN type III of Burkholder, electron-dense deposits are located in a pattern similar to that seen in MPGN type I [58], with the addition of prominent subepithelial deposits and deposition of basement membrane material in between the subepithelial deposits (Figure 6.36). The latter are responsible for the appearance of spikes on light microscopy. In MPGN type III of Strife and Anders, there are prominent deposits in the subendothelial and intramembranous locations. The deposits appear to extend from the subendothelial location across the lamina densa to the subepithelial location and are associated with disruption and lamination of the lamina densa (Figure 6.37) [59,60,69]. The deposits blend into the lamina densa (because the deposits are less electron-dense) and may be easier to appreciate in silver-impregnated semithin sections. This complex laminated appearance is believed to be due to multiple generations of deposits associated with repetitive disruption and generation of new lamina densa.

Differential Diagnosis

The diagnosis of primary MPGN is one of exclusion [56]. There are numerous diseases associated with secondary MPGN (Table 6.3). In addition to clinical history, the microscopic examination of the kidney allows one to suggest an underlying etiology. For instance, in immune complex-mediated diseases with an MPGN pattern, such as cryoglobulinemia and systemic lupus erythematosus, the renal biopsy shows features characteristic of these diseases detailed elsewhere in this text. In monoclonal immunoglobulin deposition disease, there may be glomerular deposition of a variety of paraproteins in different patients. In fibrillary or immunotactoid glomerulonephritis, ultrastructural features are pathognomonic. In nonimmune complex-mediated diseases such as subacute and chronic thrombotic microangiopathies with an MPGN pattern, subendothelial electron-lucent material (fluff) on electron microscopy can help with the differential diagnosis. In addition to MPGN, a "nodular" appearance to the glomeruli may be produced by

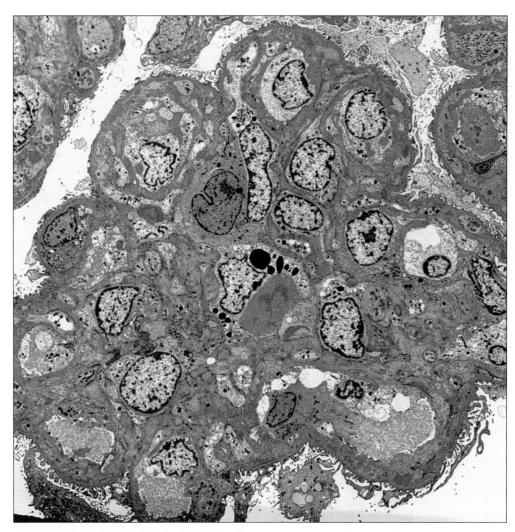

FIGURE 6.28: *MGN type I. Electron micrograph discloses a hypercellular capillary tuft with increased numbers of mesangial cells, endothelial cells, and leukocytes obscuring many of the glomerular capillary lumens. There is extensive circumferential mesangial interposition with numerous subendothelial electron-dense deposits and an irregular subendothelial layer of the neomembrane.*

diabetic glomerulosclerosis, amyloidosis, light chain deposition disease, as well as idiopathic lobular glomerulonephritis. Therefore, knowledge of the clinical history and laboratory tests coupled with a careful analysis of the light microscopic, immunofluorescent, and ultrastructural findings are required to accurately diagnose MPGN.

Etiology and Pathogenesis

MPGN was initially described in association with hypocomplementemia. In fact, West called the disease "membranoproliferative hypocomplementemic glomerulonephritis" [76]. Depressed serum levels of C3 are present in all subtypes of MPGN. Type I MPGN is an immune complex-mediated disease [57]. The circulating immune complexes are deposited in the subendothelial space and mesangium. The deposited immune complexes activate the complement cascade via the classical pathway, leading to the generation of chemoattractants

(C3a, C5a) for leukocytes and the membrane attack complex (C5b-9) that directly mediates cell injury. In some patients, complement is activated by the C4 nephritic factor (C4NeF), an autoantibody directed against the classic pathway C3 convertase (C4b2a). Activation of complement may also occur via the mannose-binding lectin (a lectin which binds IgG and activates the complement cascade) pathway since mannose-binding lectin has been identified in the immune deposits of patients with MPGN type I. In addition, activation of innate immune responses via toll-like receptor (TLR) binding of foreign and endogenous proteins has also been shown to occur. The activation of TLRs leads to the release of inflammatory mediators and activation of the classical complement pathway [57]. Complement activation via these various mechanisms leads to the release of chemotactic factors causing platelet and leukocyte accumulation, which in turn, release reactive oxygen species and proteases that mediate renal injury. Both infiltrating and native glomerular cells can release cytokines and growth factors

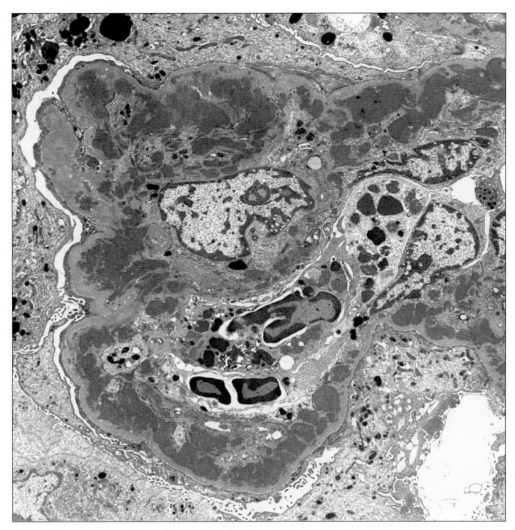

FIGURE 6.29: *MPGN type I. Numerous, subendothelial, electron-dense deposits are "sandwiched" between the original basement membrane of the glomerular capillary loops on the outside and the newly formed basement membrane-like material on the inside. Glomerular tufts also contain infiltrating leukocytes and there is effacement of visceral epithelial foot processes.*

leading to mesangial proliferation and matrix expansion. Other postulated pathogenetic mechanisms include complement deficiency states, cellular and humoral immune activation, platelet activation, and inheritable genetic predisposition [57].

The pathogenesis of MPGN type III is probably similar to MPGN type I. However, nephritic factor of the terminal pathway (NeFt) has been found in 78 percent of patients with MPGN type III. NeFt is a properdin-dependent factor that slowly activates C3 and terminal complement components. In addition, genetic factors may also play a role in MPGN type III [57].

Clinical Course, Prognosis, Treatment, and Clinical Correlation

Idiopathic MPGN Types I and III are usually progressive renal disorders, although the course of disease progression may be quite variable [62,63,65–68,70,72,77–79]. The 10-year renal survival rate is approximately 50 percent. The signs and symp-

toms of the renal disease may persist continuously or appear episodically. Only an occasional patient becomes completely asymptomatic. Clinical features and histomorphologic findings that may predict a worse outcome with rapid disease progression include nephrotic syndrome, renal insufficiency, and/or hypertension at the time of initial diagnosis, and the presence of cellular crescents or tubulointerstitial disease on biopsy [65,73,74,77–79]. Patients with focal glomerular involvement on biopsy tend to have a better prognosis [65,72]. Many therapeutic agents, such as steroids, immunosuppressive and cytotoxic agents, and antiplatelet drugs, have been used in patients with MPGN, with variable outcomes in slowing progression of the renal disease. [66,67,69,72,74,77–79]. The most promising is the alternate day use of high dose prednisone (40 mg/m^2 body surface area every other day for 1–2 years, tapered gradually to 20 mg on alternate days for 3–10 years) [66]. These drugs are used in conjunction with the management of hypertension, proteinuria, and hyperlipidemia. In patients who receive a renal transplant, MPGN type I recurs in 40–48 percent of the

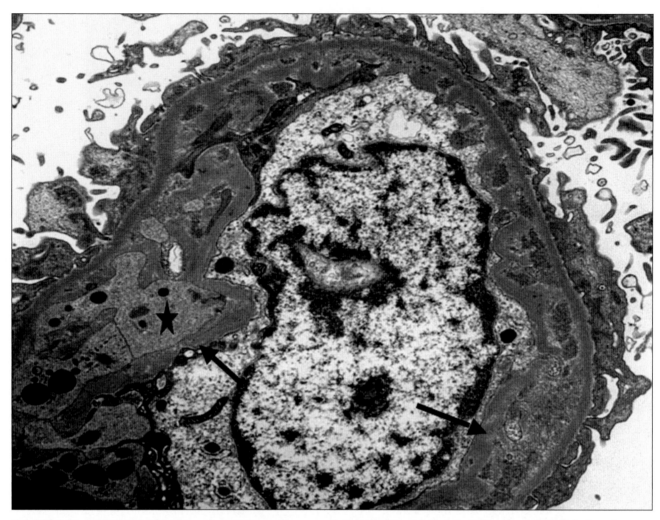

FIGURE 6.30: *MPGN type I. Electron micrograph reveals mesangial interposition (star) along with subendothelial electron-dense deposits between the original glomerular basement membrane on the outside and the newly formed basement membrane-like material on the inside (arrows). Visceral epithelial foot process effacement is also present.*

allografts, with graft failure in up to 40 percent of the recurrences. A few cases of recurrent MPGN type III with detrimental effect on graft survival have also been reported [80].

Conditions Associated With Membranoproliferative Glomerulonephritis Pattern

Glomerular injury characterized by the histomorphologic pattern of MPGN may be seen in association with a variety of underlying conditions such as infections, autoimmune disorders, dysproteinemias, and chronic liver diseases (Table 6.3). Some of these disorders are discussed elsewhere in this book. Here, we will focus on the glomerulonephritides associated with chronic hepatitis B and hepatitis C infections.

(Hepatitis C-Associated Glomerulonephritis)

Epidemiology and Clinical Presentation

Hepatitis C-associated glomerulonephritis is an immune complex-mediated disease that usually occurs many years after initial infection, with or without cryoglobulinemia. When asso-

ciated with cryoglobulins in the serum and cryoglobulin deposition in the glomeruli, the term cryoglobulinemic, hepatitis C-associated glomerulonephritis is more appropriate [81–85]. These patients often have advanced chronic liver disease with cirrhosis present in up to half of the cases. The patients often present with proteinuria, frequently in the nephrotic range, and varying degrees of renal insufficiency. A nephritic picture is seen in 25 percent of the patients and hypocomplementemia is frequent [84, 86]. Given the high prevalence of chronic hepatitis C infection (affecting about 3 percent of the world's population) and the proclivity to develop renal disease in this form of liver disease, it is not surprising that hepatitis C-associated glomerulonephritis is currently the most common cause of secondary MPGN. Hepatitis C-associated glomerulonephritis accounts for up to 60 percent of MPGN cases in Japan and 10–20 percent of MPGN cases in the United States [81].

Light Microscopy. Hepatitis C-associated glomerulonephritis manifests most commonly (in 80 percent of the cases) as type I MPGN, followed by type III MPGN [81,84,86,87]. Membranous glomerulopathy nephropathy, IgA nephropathy, acute

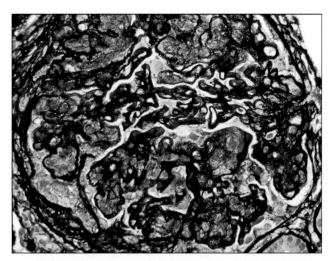

FIGURE 6.31: *MPGN type III of Burkholder. The methenamine silver stained section reveals a glomerulus with endocapillary hypercellularity, narrowed or obliterated capillary lumens, and double contoured capillary walls coupled with numerous "spikes" (400×).*

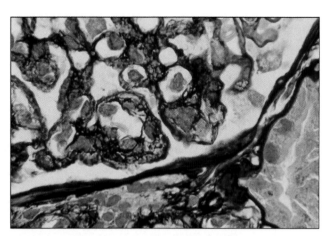

FIGURE 6.33: *MPGN type III of Strife and Anders. The methenamine silver stained section reveals the glomerular capillary walls with a frayed, disrupted, and moth-eaten appearance (1,000x, courtesy of Dr. William Kern).*

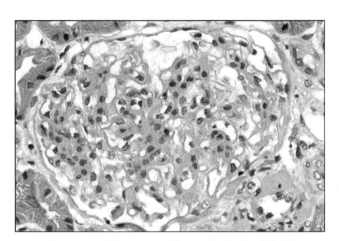

FIGURE 6.32: *MPGN type III of Strife and Anders. There is mild to moderate mesangial hypercellularity with increased mesangial matrix and thickened capillary walls (H&E, 400x, courtesy of Dr. William Kern).*

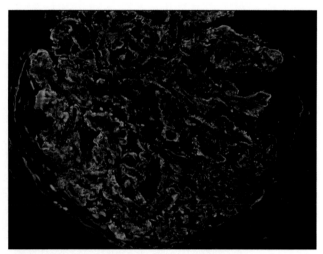

FIGURE 6.34: *MPGN type III of Burkholder. Immunofluorescence microscopy shows strong granular staining along the capillary walls, in the mesangium, and along the Bowman's capsule for IgG (400x).*

diffuse and exudative proliferative glomerulonephritis, focal segmental glomerulosclerosis, thrombotic microangiopathy, fibrillary, and immunotactoid glomerulopathies (Figure 6.38A) have also been reported in patients with chronic hepatitis C infection [81,83–85].

Immunofluorescence and Electron Microscopy. In MPGN, there is granular staining of glomerular capillary walls and mesangium for IgG, IgM, and C3. There may also be staining for IgA and other complement components. The histologic form of renal injury dictates the staining pattern on immunofluorescence microscopy (Figure 6.38B). Likewise, the immunofluorescent staining corresponds to the electron-dense deposits in the same locations. In cryoglobulinemic, hepatitis C-associated glomerulonephritis, the ultrastructural

appearance is characteristic and is described in detail in Chapter 10.

Etiology and Pathogenesis

Hepatitis C-associated glomerulonephritis is believed to be caused by glomerular deposition of circulating immune complexes associated with chronic viral antigenemia. [81,83,84,88]. Chronic hepatitis C infection stimulates the production of antiviral antibodies and rheumatoid factor. Indeed, the binding of immunoglobulins to rheumatoid factor is the cause of mixed cryoglobulinemia. Studies have also shown that hepatitis C proteins bind to TLRs and trigger inflammatory pathways and the complement cascade.[89]. Hepatitis C virus is a single-stranded RNA virus, whose genome may be a ligand for TLR7 and

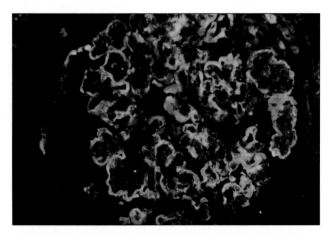

FIGURE 6.35:   MPGN type III of Strife and Anders. There is confluent granular staining of the peripheral capillary walls and mesangium for C3. (FITC conjugated anti-C3, 400×)

TLR8 [88]. It has been postulated that immune complexes containing hepatitis C RNA activate the mesangial TLR3, effecting proliferation and apoptosis and inducing the production of chemokines such as CCL5 (chemokine, CC motif, ligand 5) and CCL2 (chemokine, CC motif, ligand 2) [90]. Reverse transcriptase PCR-based methods have demonstrated hepatitis C viral RNA in the renal tissue affected by hepatitis C-associated glomerulonephritis [83].

Clinical Course, Prognosis, Treatment, and Clinical Correlation

The natural history of hepatitis C-associated glomerulonephritis is similar to other forms of MPGN. Once developed, the renal disease is progressive, leading usually to renal failure. Antiviral therapy with interferon and ribavirin has proven beneficial in reducing circulating cryoglobulins, decreasing proteinuria, and stabilizing renal function. [81,84,86,88]. However, the renal disease returns once the treatment is discontinued. In

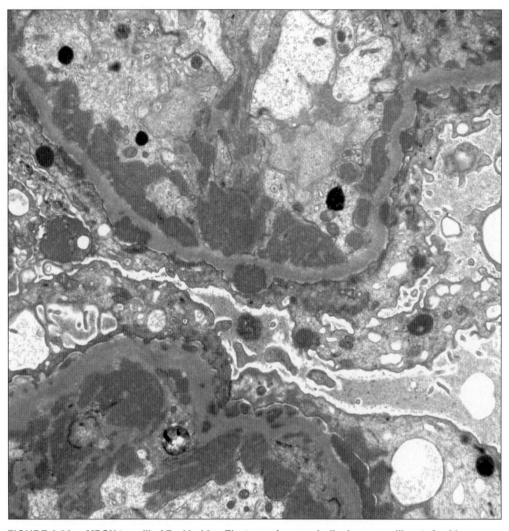

FIGURE 6 36:   MPGN type III of Burkholder. Electron micrograph displays a capillary tuft with numerous subendothelial and subepithelial electron-dense deposits as well as mesangial interpositions.

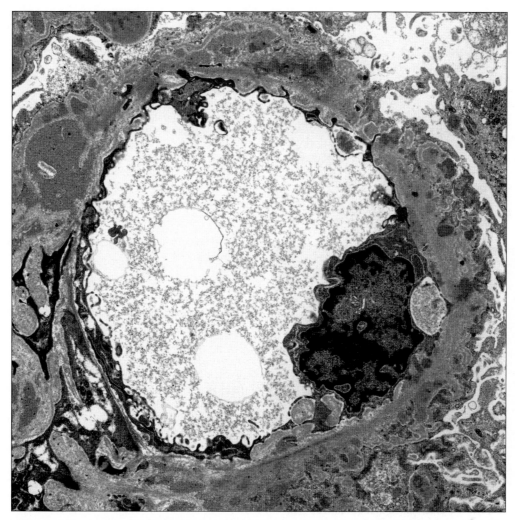

FIGURE 6.37: *MPGN type III of Strife and Anders. Ultrastructurally, the subepithelial and subendothelial electron-dense deposits appear to interconnect throughout the basement membranes of glomerular capillary loops. The complex deposits give a laminated appearance to the lamina densa of the glomerular capillary loops. Visceral epithelial foot processes are effaced (courtesy of Dr. Zoltan Laszik).*

severe cases, treatment with steroids, immunosuppressive agents, rituximab (anti-CD20 that targets B-lymphocytes), and plasmapheresis has been employed for short-term success either before or concurrent with the antiviral therapy [82,86,87].

(Hepatitis B-Associated Glomerulonephritis)

Epidemiology and Clinical Presentation

Unlike hepatitis C virus, hepatitis B virus is a DNA virus. Chronic infection with hepatitis B virus continues to be an endemic problem in parts of Africa and Asia. Similar to hepatitis C, glomerulonephritis associated with chronic hepatitis B infections is believed to be an immune complex-mediated process that is most often associated with membranous glomerulopathy

and MPGN types I and III [91–95]. Patients with renal disease develop proteinuria that may be in the nephrotic range, hematuria, and often, renal insufficiency. Hypocomplementemia is present in the majority of the patients. Multisystem vasculitis may develop within weeks to months after the development of the renal disease. These patients manifest fever, rash, arthralgia, and abdominal pain.

Light, Immunofluorescence, and Electron Microscopies. In addition to membranous glomerulopathy and MPGN types I and III (Figure 6.39A) patients may develop IgA nephropathy, mesangial proliferative glomerulonephritis, focal segmental sclerosis, minimal change disease (minimal change nephrotic syndrome), and polyarteritis nodosa [84,91–95]. The pattern of immunofluorescence staining for immunoglobulins and complement components, and the localization of electron-dense deposits

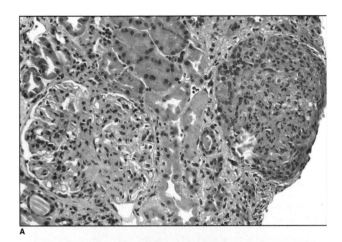

A

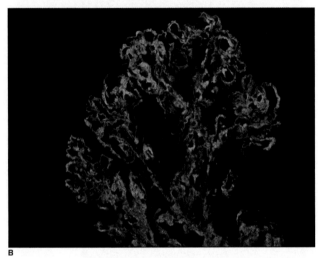

B

FIGURE 6.38: Fibrillary glomerulonephritis associated with hepatitis C. (A). One glomerulus reveals mesangial hypercellularity with significant global mesangial matrix expansion and focal thickening of capillary walls by acidophilic amorphous material. The second glomerulus discloses a large circumferential cellular crescent with compressed capillary tufts (H&E, 200x). (B). Immunofluorescence microscopy displays band-like staining of capillary walls and confluent mesangial staining for IgG (400x).

correspond to the pattern of the glomerular disease (Figures 6.39B and 6.39C).

Etiology and Pathogenesis

Mechanisms, postulated to explain the development of renal injury in patients with chronic hepatitis B infection, include deposition of immune complexes composed of viral antigens and host antibodies; direct cytopathic effects of hepatitis B virus that is known to infect glomerular mesangial cells; induction of T- and B-lymphocyte mediated immunomodulatory processes; and injury mediated by hepatitis B virus-induced cytokines [91,93–95]. Hepatitis B virus antigens, antiviral antibodies, and hepatitis B DNA have all been detected in the kidneys of affected patients. It has been suggested that genetic factors may

Table 6.4 Diseases Associated with Histomorphologic Appearance of Lobular Glomerulonephritis or Nodular Glomerulosclerosis

Diabetic glomerulosclerosis
Monoclonal immunoglobulin deposition disease
Amyloidosis
Chronic thrombotic microangiopathies
Membranoproliferative glomerulonephritis, types I and III
Dense deposit disease
Fibronectin glomerulopathy
Fibrillary glomerulopathy
Immunotactoid glomerulopathy
Idiopathic nodular glomerulosclerosis

predispose certain chronic hepatitis B patients to develop renal disease [91, 95].

Clinical Course, Prognosis, and Clinical Correlation

Hepatitis B-associated glomerulonephritis has a more favorable prognosis in children than in adults. [91,93,95]. Sixty-seven to ninety-five percent of the children with hepatitis B-associated glomerulonephritis undergo remission either spontaneously or in response to therapy [95]. Treatment strategies include antiviral regimens such as interferon and ribavirin. The antiviral drugs are much more effective at inducing remission of active viral infection in cases of hepatitis B than in hepatitis C, and the renal disease subsides with the clearance of the virus [84,91, 94–96]. Prospectively, the most effective means of eliminating hepatitis B-associated glomerulonephritis is the effective use of the hepatitis B vaccine in high-risk populations [91].

IDIOPATHIC NODULAR GLOMERULOSCLEROSIS

Epidemiology and Clinical Presentation

Nodular glomerulosclerosis or lobular glomerulonephritis describes a histomorphologic pattern of glomerular injury in which there is exaggerated mesangial sclerosis and glomerular lobularity. This form of renal disease may be idiopathic or seen in cases of MPGN, diabetic glomerulosclerosis, dysproteinemias, and organized glomerular deposition diseases (Table 6.4) [97]. Patients with idiopathic nodular glomerulosclerosis are typically older (mean age of approximately 68 years) Caucasians with long histories of hypertension and cigarette smoking, and often present with renal insufficiency and nephrotic range proteinuria. The term "smoking-associated nodular glomerulosclerosis" has been proposed to highlight the strong association with cigarette smoking [98]. This entity is discussed here because of its morphologic similarity to MPGN.

Approach to Interpretation

Light, Immunofluorescence, and Electron Microscopy. Glomeruli show accentuated lobularity and "nodular," acellular

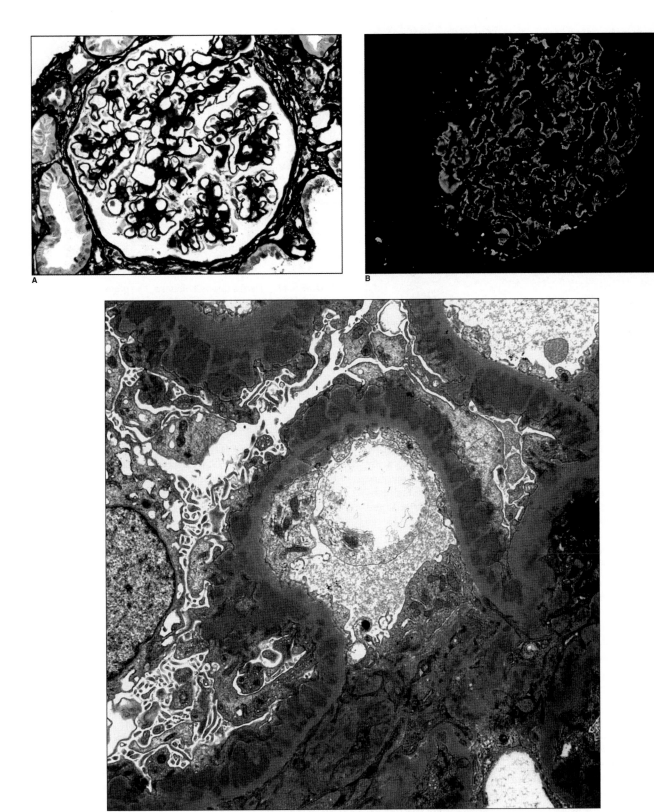

FIGURE 6.39: *Membranous nephropathy (glomerulopathy) associated with hepatitis B. (A). The glomerulus is normocellular with patent capillary lumens. The glomerular capillary walls are thickened with numerous spikes (Methenamine silver, 400x). (B). Immunofluorescence microscopy reveals strong granular staining along the capillary walls for IgG (400x). (C). Electron micrograph reveals numerous subepithelial electron-dense deposits with diffuse foot process effacement. Scattered mesangial electron-dense deposits are also noted, suggesting the possibility of a secondary membranous glomerulopathy.*

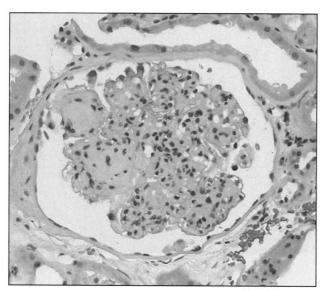

FIGURE 6.40:   Idiopathic nodular glomerulosclerosis. There is mild mesangial hypercellularity with nodular expansion of the mesangial matrix (H&E, 400×, courtesy of Dr. Tibor Nadasdy)

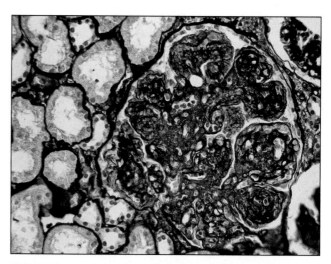

FIGURE 6.41:   Dense deposit disease. The glomerulus displays global endocapillary hypercellularity with mesangial matrix expansion and double contoured capillary walls reminiscent of MPGN type I. The "split" appearance is due to the presence of intramembranous deposits that are non-argyrophilic (Methenamine silver, 400×).

expansion of the mesangial matrix with compression of the capillary loops (Figure 6.40). The histomorphologic features are often best appreciated with PAS and trichrome stains. By definition, the stains for amyloid are negative and no immune complex or organized deposits are demonstrated by immunofluorescent or electron microscopic examinations. Arterial and arteriolar sclerosis is almost always present [97].

Differential Diagnosis

Table 6.4 lists the conditions that may give rise to the morphologic appearance of lobular/nodular glomerulosclerosis.

Etiology, Pathogenesis, Clinical Course, Prognosis, Treatment, and Clinical Correlation

The typical patient with idiopathic lobular/nodular glomerulosclerosis is a hypertensive elderly chronic smoker. Presumably, the age, smoking, and hypertension all play a role in the pathogenesis of this disorder resulting in excess deposition of extracellular matrix in the mesangium. Age and hypertension-associated arterial and arteriolar sclerosis may be worsened by the intrarenal hemodynamic effects of cigarette smoking. This may occur via sympathetic activation either directly by nicotine or secondary to chronic hypoxia due to the smoking-related chronic obstructive airway disease. Advanced glycosylation end products may also play a role in the pathogenesis of the disease. Continued smoking, lack of angiotensin II receptor blockade when treating these patients' hypertension, advanced glomerulosclerosis with associated tubular atrophy, and severe arteriosclerosis are predictors of progressive renal disease [97,98].

DENSE DEPOSIT DISEASE

Epidemiology and Clinical Presentation

Dense deposit disease (DDD) was originally characterized by Habib as type II MPGN [99]. However, it has become clear that DDD is epidemiologically, morphologically, and etiopathogenetically distinct from MPGN and therefore merits a separate designation [61, 100–102]. DDD is characterized by an electron-dense transformation of the GBM and mesangium as well as the basement membranes of the tubules and Bowman's capsules. Dense deposits have been reported in renal interstitial capillary and arteriolar walls. DDD is very rare, affecting 2–3 people/million, and occurring primarily in children and young adults. It has a strong association with upper respiratory tract infections that precede the onset of renal signs and symptoms in 50 percent of the patients. [99,100] The patients may present with acute nephritic syndrome, hematuria, proteinuria that may be in the nephrotic range, and usually some degree of renal insufficiency. Serum complement levels, especially C3, are low. Unlike MPGN type I, the early components of the classical complement pathway, C1q and C4, are frequently normal [55,61–63,70,99–101,103]. C3 nephritic factor (C3NeF; a circulating IgG or IgM autoantibody) is found in 70–80 percent of the cases and plays a major role in the pathogenesis of this disease. Twenty to twenty-five percent of patients with DDD have partial lipodystrophy, which may precede the renal disease by many years. Interestingly, dense deposits may also be found in the spleen and in Bruch membrane in the eye. The latter, called drusen, may lead to decreased visual acuity in nearly 20 percent of the patients with DDD [100].

Approach to Interpretation

Light Microscopy. Dense deposit disease (DDD) has a varied morphologic appearance with only 25 percent of cases showing

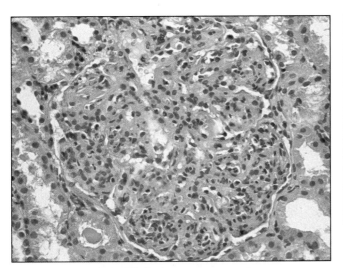

FIGURE 6.42: *Dense deposit disease. There is global intracapillary hypercellularity with significant infiltration of neutrophils reminiscent of acute "exudative" intracapillary proliferative glomerulonephritis (H&E, 400×).*

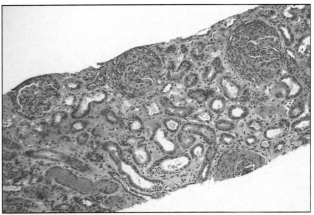

FIGURE 6.44: *Dense deposit disease. The H&E-stained section reveals numerous crescents. There is interstitial edema with mild inflammatory infiltration and significant tubular injury (100x).*

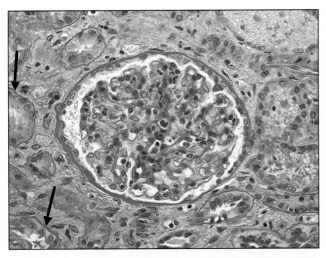

FIGURE 6.43: *Dense deposit disease. The glomerulus reveals mild mesangial hypercellularity with scattered leukocytes within the capillary lumens. There are prominent ribbon-like deposits in the Bowman's capsule and a few tubular basement membranes (arrows) (PAS, 400x).*

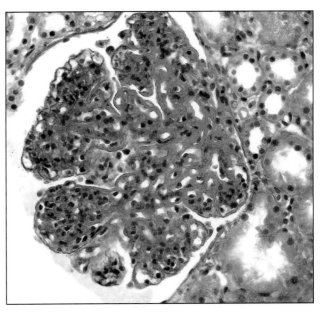

FIGURE 6.45: *Dense deposit disease. There is global intracapillary hypercellularity with accentuated lobularity of glomerular tufts and large, "ribbon-like", fuchsinophilic (red) deposits along the periphery capillary walls. Significant mesangial deposits (red) are also observed (Trichrome, 400×).*

MPGN pattern by light microscopy (Figure 6.41). [57,70 71,73,99–101,103]. In some cases, the glomeruli appear relatively normal with only capillary wall thickening. Other cases feature hypercellular and occasionally "exudative" glomerular tufts reminiscent of APIGN (Figure 6.42). There may be variable expansion of the mesangial matrix, which in occasional cases has a nodular appearance ("lobular glomerulonephritis"). Other patterns of glomerular injury that have been reported in DDD include mesangioproliferative glomerulonephritis (Figure 6.43), focal and segmental necrotizing glomerulonephritis, and membranous glomerulopathy. Crescents may occur as well (Figure 6.44). As the renal disease progresses, the glomeruli

become more sclerotic. The thickening of the glomerular capillary walls reflects the presence of elongate, often "ribbon-like," intramembranous deposits that vary greatly in size and number. The deposits are PAS positive and often fuchsinophilic on trichrome stain (Figure 6.45) and stain negatively with methenamine silver giving a "double contour" appearance in some cases. Similar deposits may be present within the basement membranes of proximal and distal tubules. The tubular epithelial cells may contain protein resorption droplets or may appear vacuolated. The degree of tubular atrophy, interstitial fibrosis, and interstitial chronic inflammation parallels the degree of

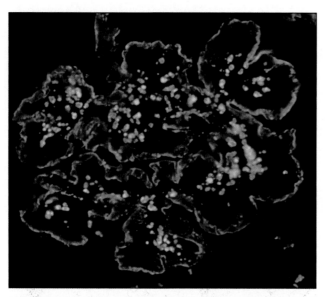

FIGURE 6.46:   Dense deposit disease. Immunofluorescence microscopy reveals band-like staining of glomerular capillary walls and granular staining in the mesangium (with ring-shaped forms in some areas) with FITC conjugated anti-C3 (400×, courtesy of Dr. Stephen Bonsib).

glomerulosclerosis. Arterial sclerosis accompanies the development of hypertension with progressive renal disease.

Immunofluorescence Microscopy.   Immunofluorescence microscopy shows intense staining of the glomerular capillary walls for C3 (Figure 6.46). The capillary wall staining has been variously described as linear, "double linear", "pseudo-linear," smooth, "ribbon-like", granular, or nodular. Mesangial staining may be granular or form a ring around a central nonstaining region (Figure 6.46) [61,102]. There may be C3 staining of the Bowman's capsules and tubular basement membranes. Early complement components such as C1q and C4 are usually absent. Staining for immunoglobulin IgM, IgG, and rarely IgA, is usually absent or seen only focally and segmentally and with lower intensity than the staining for C3 [55,62,70, 71,99,101,103,104].

Electron Microscopy.   The ultrastructural features of the glomerular changes in DDD are highly distinctive and their identification is required for a definitive diagnosis. There are very dense, homogeneous deposits within the basement membranes of the glomerular capillary walls. The deposits may replace the entire lamina densa or only a portion (Figures 6.47 and 6.48). The deposits may be widespread within the glomerular capillary loops or discontinuous with stretches of basement membrane

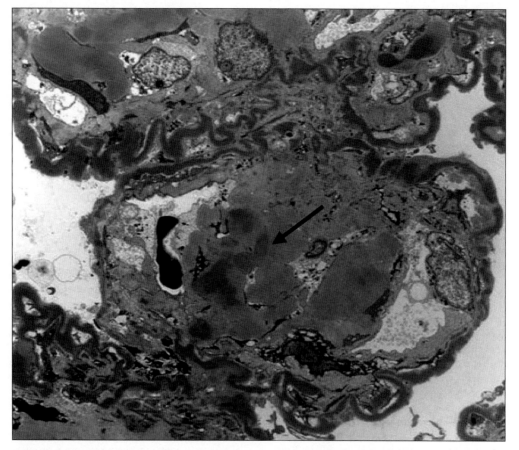

FIGURE 6.47:   Dense deposit disease. Electron micrograph reveals linear band-like (occasionally interrupted) electron densities within the lamina densa and ring-shaped electron-dense deposits within the mesangium (arrows).

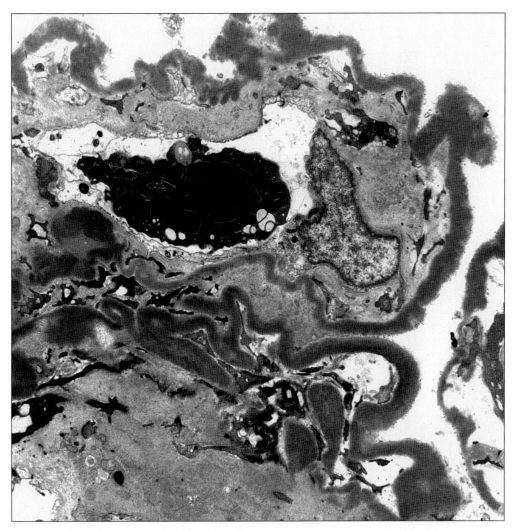

FIGURE 6.48: Dense deposit disease. Electron microphotograph reveals irregular electron-dense thickening of the lamina densa with alternating thinner segments.

without any deposits. Paramesangial deposits may also occur. Later in the course of the disease, the deposits may show areas of lucency that indicate dissolution. In cases with the light microscopic features of acute proliferative glomerulonephritis or membranous glomerulopathy, deposits may also be present in the subendothelial and subepithelial locations, respectively. In addition, deposits may also be present within the glomerular mesangium, along the Bowman's capsule, and within the blood vessel walls and tubular basement membranes [55,61,70,71,99–101,103,104]. The mesangial electron-dense deposits may reveal a distinct ring shape corresponding to the "mesangial rings" observed on immunofluorescence microscopy. The mesangial electron-dense deposits may be associated with a poor clinical outcome [105]. In addition to the deposits, the glomerular mesangium may also show an increase in the number of mesangial cells, an influx of inflammatory cells, and an increase in matrix. Mesangial cell interposition may occur between the glomerular capillary endothelial cells and their basement membranes.

Etiology and Pathogenesis

The characteristic feature of DDD is the intramembranous deposition of peculiar electron-dense material. While the precise composition of these dense deposits remains unknown, they differ from the normal GBM in their amino acid and carbohydrate compositions and contain large amounts of N-acetyl glucosamine. Since immunoglobulins are either absent or not a significant constituent of the dense deposits, it is clear that immune complexes do not play a major role in the pathogenesis of this disease. On the other hand, the presence of C3 but not of C1q or C4 (early components of the classical pathway of complement activation) in the glomeruli, along with the reduced serum levels of C3 and normal serum levels of C1q and C4, indicates that an uncontrolled activation of the alternative complement pathway plays a central role in the pathogenesis of DDD. High levels of activation of the alternative complement pathway are achieved by stabilization of C3bBb, the alternative pathway C3 convertase. C3bBb is normally stabilized by properdin and inhibited by factor H. In more than 80 percent of

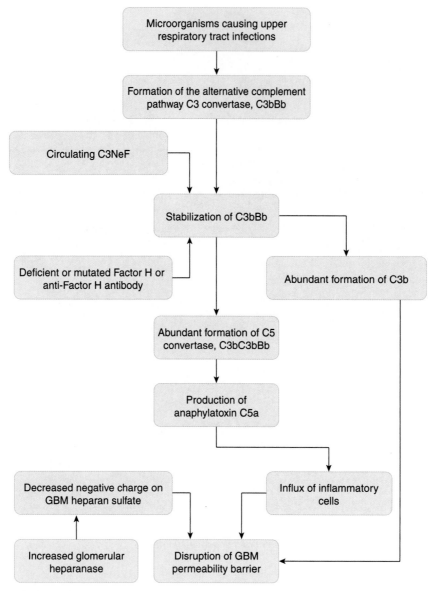

FIGURE 6.49: Pathogenesis of dense deposit disease (see text for detail). C3NeF: C3 nephritic factor; GBM: glomerular basement membrane.

patients with DDD, a circulating IgG or IgM autoantibody, known as the C3 nephritic factor (C3NeF or the nephritic factor of amplification loop) binds to and stabilizes C3bBb by preventing its inactivation by factor H [106]. An inherited deficiency of factor H has been associated with the development of familial DDD [107]. Further illustrating the importance of the uncontrolled activation of the alternative pathway of complement are the reports of DDD in patients with a mutation in the regulatory domain of factor H [108] or with an inhibitory autoantibody to factor H [109]. The unregulated cleavage of C3 by C3bBb leads to the formation of abundant C3bC3bBb, the C5 convertase. While the chronic deposition of C3b along the GBM, by itself, may be sufficient to disrupt the GBM permeability barrier and lead to proteinuria, the formation of C3b-

C3b dimers on the GBM effectively promotes the local formation of the C5 convertase with the formation of the anaphylatoxin C5a that attracts neutrophils and produces GBM damage leading to proteinuria [110,111]. The expression of glomerular heparanase is increased in DDD and contributes to its pathogenesis by degrading the negatively charged glycosaminoglycan side chains of heparan sulfate in the GBM and at podocyte and endothelial surfaces, leading to altered permeability, local release of cytokines, and weakening of interactions with factor H [112,113]. Podocytes are also affected, with interferences in podocyte-GBM interactions resulting in detachment of the podocytes and associated physiologic alterations. Figure 6.49 illustrates the current understanding of the pathogenesis of DDD.

Clinical Course, Prognosis, Treatment, and Clinical Correlation

The overall prognosis of DDD is poor with end stage renal disease developing in the majority of patients over a year to several decades, with a median renal survival of 5–12 years. DDD tends to have a worse prognosis and more aggressive course to renal failure compared to MPGN types I and III [63,70,73,78,99,102,104,114,115]. The disease recurs in many transplant recipients (67–100 percent) and is progressive, with recurrence directly accounting for 15 percent or more of failed grafts [116]. Clinical and histologic features predictive of rapid disease progression include hypertension, hematuria, and the presence of nephrotic syndrome or renal insufficiency at the time of diagnosis, and crescents, focal glomerulonephritis, tubulointerstitial disease, mesangial deposits, mesangial hypercellularity, and glomerulosclerosis in the diagnostic biopsy [55,63,68,70,99,101]. Nonspecific treatment modalities such as steroids, immunosuppression, anticoagulation, antiplatelet therapy, ACE inhibitors, and angiotensin type I receptor blockers have been used with variable success in slowing the progression of the renal disease [66,79,99,100,104]. In the presence of circulating C3NeF, as in most patients with DDD, plasmapheresis may be a therapeutic option to remove C3NeF. Plasmaphereis may also be useful in removing inactivating autoantibodies to factor H. The anti-CD20 antibody, rituximab, has also been suggested for use in patients with positive C3NeF, evidence of C3 consumption, and functionally normal factor H. In patients with factor H deficiency, plasma infusion or exchange may be used to correct the deficiency. More recently, the use of anti-C5 antibody to block the release of C5a and the use of sulodexide, an effective heparanase inhibitor, have been proposed to target downstream effector pathways involved in the pathogenesis of DDD, but their effectiveness requires further study [117].

CRESCENTIC GLOMERULONEPHRITIS

Crescentic glomerulonephritis is characterized by the presence of glomerular crescents, an extracapillary proliferative lesion partially or completely filling the glomerular Bowman's space. While an occasional crescent may be seen in other glomerulonephritides, the presence of crescents in more than 50 percent of the glomeruli defines "crescentic glomerulonephritis" [118,119]. Yet, the presence of any crescent in a kidney biopsy should be noted because of the potential for a rapid progression of the renal disease. "Rapidly progressive glomerulonephritis (RPGN)" is a clinical term that describes a progressive renal disease that results in 50 percent or greater loss of renal function within three months. While the clinical syndrome of RPGN may be associated with tubulointerstitial diseases (i.e., acute tubular necrosis and acute interstitial nephritis) and vascular diseases (i.e., malignant hypertension and thrombotic microangiopathy), the most common pattern of glomerular injury associated with RPGN is crescentic glomerulonephritis. Crescentic glomerulonephritis is a morphologically and etiologically diverse entity. Morphologically, it is subclassified into three categories: pauci-immune crescentic glomerulonephritis, immune complex-associated

Table 6.5 Frequency (%) of the Types of Crescentic Glomerulonephritis

Age (years)	Pauci-immune	Immune Complex-Mediated	Anti-GBM
All ages	60	24	15
1–20	42	45	12
21–60	48	35	15
61–100	79	6	15

Adapted from Jennette JC. *Kidney Int*, 2003; 63(3): 1164–77.

crescentic glomerulonephritis, and anti-GBM antibody-associated crescentic glomerulonephritis (Table 6.5). Most, but not all, patients of crescentic glomerulonephritis with a pauci-immune immunofluorescence pattern have a positive serum antineutrophil cytoplasmic antibody (ANCA) [119].

The initial event in crescent formation is damage to the glomerular capillary endothelium and GBM mediated by anti-GBM antibodies, immune complexes, and/or ANCA [119]. The injured glomerular capillary endothelium and GBM allow fibrin and other plasma proteins to enter the Bowman's space and stimulate the proliferation of visceral as well as parietal epithelial cells, and the recruitment of inflammatory cells especially T-lymphocytes and macrophages [120]. This cellular process is accompanied by a release of inflammatory cytokines and activation of the coagulation cascade. Over time, the cellular crescents either resolve completely or develop into fibrocellular and fibrous crescents. The formation of the latter involves processes such as the fibronectin-mediated chemotaxis of fibroblasts, transforming growth factor-β-induced synthesis of collagen, matrix production by crescent cells, and removal of cellular constituents by apoptosis [119,121].

Pauci-Immune or Antineutrophil Cytoplasmic Antibody-Associated Crescentic Glomerulonephritis

In 1979, Stilmant showed that sixteen (35 percent) of his forty-six patients with crescentic glomerulonephritis had no evidence of immune deposits by immunofluorescence and ultrastructural examination [122]. This, pauci-immune crescentic glomerulonephritis, may occur as a component of systemic small vessel vasculitides such as Wegener's granulomatosis, microscopic polyangiitis, and Churg–Strauss syndrome, or may occur as a primary renal small vessel vasculitis. Pauci-immune crescentic glomerulonephritis is the most common form of crescentic glomerulonephritis and therefore is the pathologic correlate of the majority of the glomerular causes of RPGN. Pauci-immune crescentic glomerulonephritis also accounts for many cases of pulmonary–renal vasculitic syndromes. Antineutrophil cytoplasmic antibodies (ANCA) are detected in 80–90 percent of patients with pauci-immune crescentic glomerulonephritis [123,124]. Conversely, 80–90 percent of the cases of crescentic glomerulonephritis that occur in ANCA-positive patients belong to the pauci-immune category [119]. Hence, pauci-immune crescentic glomerulonephritis is also known as

ANCA-associated glomerulonephritis or simply ANCA glomerulonephritis.

Epidemiology and Clinical Presentation

Pauci-immune crescentic glomerulonephritis is the most common cause of crescentic glomerulonephritis, accounting for 50 to 60 percent of the cases [119]. It is especially common in older patients, being responsible for 79 percent of the cases of crescentic glomerulonephritis in patients older than 60 years of age but only 42–48 percent of crescentic glomerulonephritis in those younger than 60 years (Table 6.5) [119]. Patients present with rapidly progressive renal failure, hematuria, and proteinuria, which is usually in the nonnephrotic range. Occasional patients with a more indolent course have glomerular sclerosis and only focally active disease manifested histologically as necrosis and crescents. [125,126]. About 75 percent of patients have synchronous or metachronous manifestations of systemic small vessel vasculitis [127]. These include "flu-like" illness, fever, arthralgias, myalgias, purpura, cutaneous nodules or ulcers, abdominal pain, gastrointestinal bleeding, upper and lower respiratory tract complaints, pulmonary nodules or cavitary lesions, pulmonary hemorrhage with hemoptysis, optic involvement, and peripheral neuropathy [126]. Churg–Strauss syndrome is distinguished from other forms of small vessel vasculitis by the presence of asthma or severe allergic rhinitis and peripheral blood eosinophilia [126]. Patients with Wegener's granulomatosis have necrotizing, granulomatous inflammation in the upper and/or lower respiratory tracts [126]. Patients with microscopic polyangiitis lack the granulomatous inflammation seen in Wegener's granulomatosis and the history of asthma and peripheral eosinophilia seen in Churg–Strauss syndrome [126].

Serologic testing for ANCA is extremely useful in the evaluation of crescentic glomerulonephritis [124]. They are detected in 80–90 percent of cases of Wegener's granulomatosis and microscopic polyangiitis, and 60 percent of cases of Churg–Strauss syndrome [124,126]. In patients with RPGN, a positive ANCA test predicts the presence of Wegner's granulomatosis or microscopic polyangiitis with 95 percent certainty (positive predictive value), while a negative ANCA test rules out these disorders with 85 percent certainty (negative predicitive value) [124,128]. The antigens against which the ANCA are directed are proteins in the cytoplasm of neutrophils and lysosomes of monocytes. Indirect immunofluorescence microscopy, on alcohol fixed neutrophils, shows two distinct staining patterns: diffuse cytoplasmic staining (C-ANCA) or perinuclear staining (P-ANCA). The determination of the actual protein antigen is performed by enzyme-linked immunosorbent assay (ELISA). C-ANCA is most commonly directed against proteinase 3 (PR3), while the most common antigenic specificity for P-ANCA is myeloperoxidase (MPO) [124]. PR3 is a serine protease involved in tissue breakdown during neutrophil migration into inflammatory foci. MPO is involved in the generation of bactericidal hypochlorite molecules and reactive oxygen species [124]. ANCA, both C-ANCA and P-ANCA, may be directed against other neutrophil proteins as well. ANCA may be associated with other diseases such as inflammatory bowel disease, autoimmune liver disease, systemic lupus erythematosus, primary sclerosing cholangitis, rheumatoid arthritis, cystic fibro-

sis, and a few parasitic diseases, and it may also be induced by drugs [124,128]. While there is a higher prevalence of C-ANCA with anti-PR3 activity in Wegener's granulomatosis and microscopic polyangiitis, and a higher prevalence of P-ANCA with anti-MPO specificity in Churg–Strauss syndrome, there is sufficient overlap to preclude the use of these antibodies as the sole means of diagnosing these diseases [124].

Of note, circulating ANCA and a corresponding association with systemic small vessel vasculitis is seen in a quarter of patients with anti-GBM antibody disease and in a few patients with immune complex-mediated crescentic glomerulonephritis [119, 124].

Approach to Interpretation

Gross Pathology. Kidneys are of normal size or slightly enlarged with red spots visible on the surface due to blood within the Bowman's space and tubular lumens or periglomerular hemorrhage due to rupture of the Bowman's capsule. Larger, irregular areas of hemorrhage correlate with the presence of associated small vessel vasculitis. Infarcts and arterial aneurysms are also evidence of vasculitis.

Light Microscopy. Numerous morphologic patterns of injury have been described in pauci-immune glomerulonephritis [119,125,129]. Renal biopsies from nine out of ten patients with ANCA-associated glomerulonephritis show some degree of crescent formation, while crescentic glomerulonephritis (defined by the presence of crescents involving at least 50 percent of the glomeruli in a biopsy) is present in about half of the cases. The glomerular capillary tufts are compressed by the extracapillary cellular crescents surrounding them (Figures 6.50 and 6.51). The endocapillary hypercellularity, typical of immune complex-mediated glomerulonephritides, is lacking. Frequently, there is segmental, and sometimes global, fibrinoid necrosis with lysis of the mesangial matrix and capillary basement membranes, most easily seen with PAS and methenamine

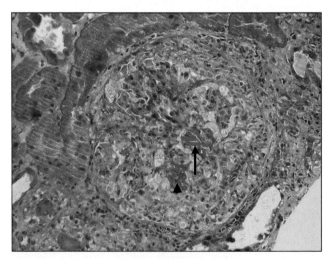

FIGURE 6.50: *Pauci-immune (ANCA) crescentic glomerulonephritis. The glomerulus reveals segmental fibrinoid necrosis (red, arrows) and areas of sclerosis (blue). The Bowman's space is completely filled by a cellular crescent admixed with fibrin tactoids (arrowheads) (Trichrome, 400x).*

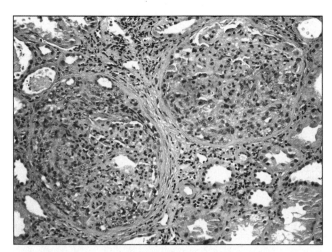

FIGURE 6.51: *Pauci-immune (ANCA) crescentic glomerulonephritis. The H&E-stained section reveals two glomeruli compressed by large circumferential cellular crescents. There is significant inflammation in the adjacent interstitium and tubules (200×).*

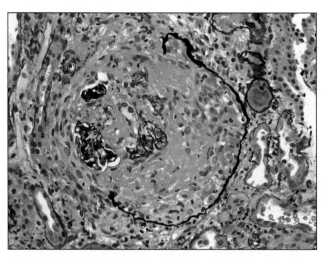

FIGURE 6.52: *Pauci-immune (ANCA) crescentic glomerulonephritis. There is extensive destruction of the glomerular tufts and Bowman's capsule coupled with extensive periglomerular inflammation (Methenamine silver, 400×).*

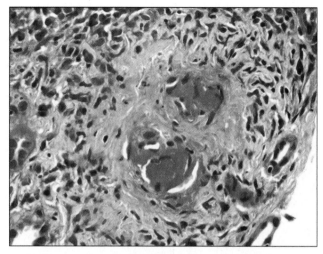

FIGURE 6.53: *Global sclerosing pauci-immune (ANCA) crescentic glomerulonephritis. The PAS-stained section reveals a glomerulus with complete destruction of the Bowman's capsule and fragmented sclerotic capillary tufts suggesting earlier destructive necrotizing injury (400x).*

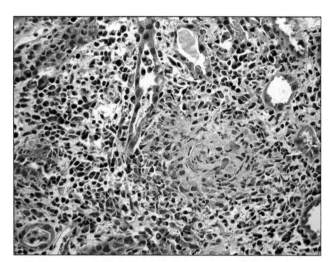

FIGURE 6.54: *Churg-Strauss syndrome. The H&E-stained section reveals interstitial granulomatous inflammation with numerous eosinophils. The patient had a history of asthma and peripheral eosinophilia (400x).*

silver stains. Intact neutrophils as well as karyorrhectic debris and fibrin thrombi are frequently seen within the affected glomerular capillary lumens. As the lesions progress, macrophages become a part of the inflammatory infiltrate. Marginated neutrophils and glomerular capillary luminal thrombi may also be present in intact glomerular tufts adjacent to the areas of glomerular capillary wall necrosis. Breaks along the Bowman's capsule, best seen on silver methenamine stain, are often associated with intense, sometimes granulomatous, interstitial inflammatory reaction (Figure 6.52). As with other forms of crescentic glomerulonephritis, the crescents may be cellular, fibrocellular, or fibrous, reflecting the stage of evolution and chronicity of the disease. All stages of crescents may be present in the same biopsy. The fibrous crescents are often associated with sclerosis of the involved glomeruli (Figure 6.53). Tubular epithelial simplification resembling acute tubular necrosis,

tubulitis, and tubular atrophy with interstitial fibrosis are often seen. Areas of tubular epithelial cell coagulative necrosis should alert the pathologist to look for associated vasculitis and infarction. The interstitium shows variable inflammation, predominantly composed of lymphocytes, histiocytes, plasma cells, and sometimes a brisk number of eosinophils. The presence of discrete interstitial granulomas suggests the possibility of underlying Wegener's granulomatosis or Churg–Strauss syndrome (Figure 6.54). However, as a note of caution, an apparent interstitial granuloma may turn out to be adjacent to a disrupted Bowman's capsule on deeper levels of the biopsy. The granulomatous interstitial inflammation adjacent to a disrupted Bowman's capsule does not carry the same connotation, and may be observed in any form of crescentic glomerulonephritis. Vasculitis, with or without fibrinoid necrosis, is seen in 10–20 percent

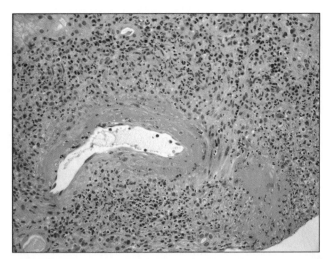

FIGURE 6.55: ANCA small vessel vasculitis. The interlobular artery shows extensive fibrinoid necrosis of the wall with heavy neutrophilic inflammation in the adventitia (H&E 400x).

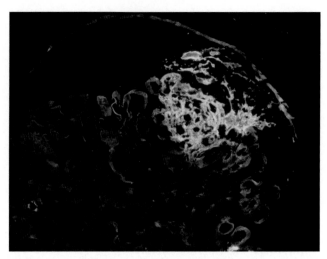

FIGURE 6.56: Pauci-immune (ANCA) crescentic glomerulonephritis. Immunofluorescence microscopy reveals a segmental strong staining with FITC conjugated anti-fibrinogen corresponding to segmental fibrinoid necrosis. The non-necrotic segments are negative (400×).

of the biopsies from patients with associated systemic vasculitides [119,125]. The vasculitis may involve arterioles, arteries, or medullary vessels, with a preference for the interlobular arteries (Figure 6.55). Vascular injury eventually results in irregular parenchymal and perivascular scarring. Necrotizing, leukocytoclastic angiitis of the medullary vasa recta has been seen in all forms of pauci-immune glomerulonephritis, and appears to be a specific characteristic of this disease. In addition to leukocytoclasia of neutrophils, the medullary leukocytoclastic angiitis is frequently associated with interstitial hemorrhage and the presence of neutrophilic tubulitis and neutrophils within tubular lumens. Severe medullary angiitis may result in papillary necrosis.

Immunofluorescence Microscopy. Pauci-immune glomerulonephritis, by definition, is characterized by an entirely negative or a very weakly positive immunofluorescence study. Nonspecific staining for immunoglobulins especially IgM, complement components, and plasma proteins may be noted in areas of glomerular necrosis. Cellular crescents, foci of glomerular necrosis, and fibrinoid vascular necrosis stain with antibodies to fibrin and fibrinogen (Figure 6.56), with loss of this staining as these lesions progress to fibrous crescents, glomerulosclerosis, and healed vascular scars, respectively. Areas of glomerular necrosis also stain for antibodies to neutrophil granule contents such as MPO, PR3, elastase, and lactoferrin, although these antibodies are not routinely used for diagnosis. It is important to note that some cases of crescentic glomerulonephritis, with positive circulating ANCA, do show strong linear or granular immunofluorescent staining of the glomeruli. These cases represent concurrent anti-GBM antibody disease and immune complex-associated glomerulonephritis, respectively.

Electron Microscopy. The absence of prominent glomerular electron-dense deposits is a defining characteristic of pauci-immune glomerulonephritis. However, as noted above, there are cases of ANCA-positive immune complex-mediated glomerulonephritis that do show glomerular electron-dense deposits. With vascular injury, endothelial swelling and necrosis occur with expansion of the subendothelial lucent zone and accumulation of electron-dense fibrin in these regions. Glomeruli contain areas of necrosis with breaks in the GBM and along the Bowman's capsule, mesangial matrix lysis, and associated accumulation of electron-dense fibrin and fibrin tactoids (Figure 6.57). The adjacent intact glomerular capillary tufts may contain marginated neutrophils and luminal thrombi with fibrin tactoids and platelets. Fibrin tactoids have more irregular and angular contours and are more electron-dense than immune complex deposits.

Differential Diagnosis

Pauci-immune glomerulonephritis and anti-GBM antibody glomerulonephritis are indistinguishable by light and electron microscopy. The presence of vasculitis in vessels other than the glomerular capillaries is suggestive of ANCA-associated disease. Immunofluorescence microscopy and serologic testing for ANCA and anti-GBM antibodies are required to distinguish the two entities or to establish the concurrent presence of both diseases. Immune complex-mediated crescentic glomerulonephritis may show more intracapillary hypercellularity and thickened glomerular capillary walls in nonnecrotic and nonsclerotic glomerular capillary tufts. However, distinguishing pauci-immune glomerulonephritis from immune complex disease is often difficult by light microscopic examination alone. The diagnosis of immune complex-mediated crescentic glomerulonephritis requires the demonstration of the immune complexes by immunofluorescence and/or ultrastructural examinations. In cases of immune complex-mediated crescentic glomerulonephritis with disproportionate glomerular necrosis

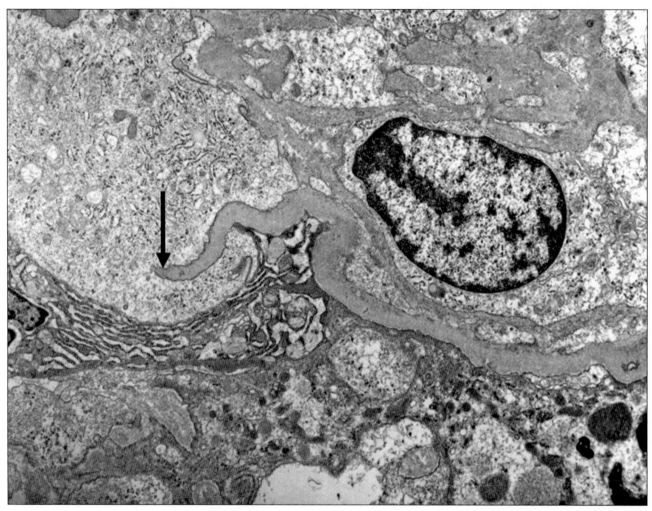

FIGURE 6.57: *Pauci-immune (ANCA) crescentic glomerulonephritis. Electron micrograph reveals a ruptured segment of glomerular basement membrane (arrow) (courtesy of Dr. Zoltan Laszik).*

or crescent formation and/or with vasculitis, the presence of coexisting ANCA-associated disease should be considered.

Pauci-immune glomerulonephritis may be induced by drugs and may need to be distinguished from drug-induced lupus nephritis. Serologic testing for ANCA and antinuclear, and antidouble stranded DNA antibodies can help distinguish the two entities. Cases with both ANCA and antinuclear antibodies usually have a severe glomerulonephritis similar to the typical pauci-immune glomerulonephritis and a clinical picture of RPGN, requiring aggressive medical intervention.

Pauci-immune glomerulonephritis must also be distinguished from medium size vasculitides, classic polyarteritis nodosa, and Kawasaki disease, all of which can cause necrotizing arteritis. Classic polyarteritis nodosa and Kawasaki disease do not cause glomerulonephritis or vasculitis in arterioles, capillaries, or venules [130]. Atheroembolic disease and thrombotic microangiopathies may appear similar to vasculitis. Careful histologic examination should detect atheroemboli containing cholesterol clefts in the former disease and fibrinoid necrosis of the arterioles in the latter. Correlation with the clinical history and other laboratory data should also help in distinguishing these entities.

Etiology and Pathogenesis

In vitro studies show that ANCA activate cytokine-primed neutrophils via direct F(ab)$_2$ ligation and Fc receptor engagement and cause their degranulation and respiratory bursts with release of toxic oxygen metabolites. Cytokine priming of neutrophils causes significant surface expression of neutrophil granule contents such as MPO and PR3, to which ANCA bind. The resultant activation of neutrophils also results in their adherence to endothelial cells via expression of adhesion molecules such as β2-integrins and via in situ formation of ANCA-MPO or ANCA-PR3 immune complexes that bind to endothelial surfaces by charge-dependent mechanisms and produce endothelial cell injury. MPO and PR3 are also internalized by the endothelial cells inducing intracellular oxidant release and endothelial cell apoptosis. ANCA also bind to monocytes causing their activation and release of toxic oxygen metabolites, chemoattractant proteins, and other inflammatory mediators. The activated monocytes migrate to the affected tissues such as the renal glomeruli, where they become macrophages seen in ANCA-associated glomerulonephritis [128,131–133]. Furthermore, recent studies have suggested that activation of

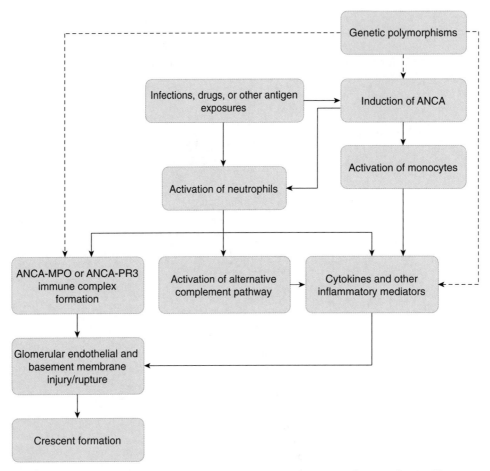

FIGURE 6.58: *Pathogenesis of ANCA-associated glomerulonephritis (see text for detail). ANCA: antineutrophil cytoplasmic antibody; MPO: myeloperoxidase; PR3: proteinase 3.*

neutrophils by ANCA may generate yet unknown factor(s), which activate the alternative complement pathway that, in turn, amplifies the inflammation likely mediated by the production of C5a [134]. A synergistic, proinflammatory event, such as exposure to cytokines like tumor necrosis factor-α, is very likely required in the development of ANCA-mediated endothelial injury. Indeed, 90 percent of the patients with ANCA-associated crescentic glomerulonephritis have "flu-like" symptoms preceding the development of specific renal or systemic vasculitis-associated symptomatology. The production of ANCA is a subject of current research. It has been suggested that the development of ANCA is initiated by immune responses to endogenously derived antisense peptides or complementary peptide mimics introduced by infectious pathogens (such as *S. aureus, Entamoeba histolytica*, and Ross River virus) that are known to have such peptides, or by drugs, or other exposures (such as solvents, farm pollens, silica, propylthiouracil, penicillamine, minocycline, and hydralazine) that are known to be associated with pauci-immune glomerulonephritis and small vessel vasculitis [128,131,132]. The antibody response to the complementary peptides induces antiidiotypic antibodies that cross-react with the sense peptides of the autoantigen. Circulating and tissue T-lymphocytes show persistent activation during active disease. The activated T-lymphocytes are predominantly of the Th-1 phenotype and are responsible for the production of a variety of proinflammatory substances, including interferon-γ and tumor necrosis factor-α [132]. The etiopathogenesis of pauci-immune glomerulonephritis and small vessel vasculitis appears to be a multifactorial process involving, in addition to the above environmental factors, the genetic make-up of the subjects that influences the expression level of ANCA antigens in neutrophils, polymorphisms in genes encoding antiproteinase, and polymorphisms in genes that produce mediators of adaptive and innate immune responses [131,132,134,135]. Figure 6.58 illustrates the current etiopathogenetic concepts of pauci-immune glomerulonephritis.

Clinical Course, Prognosis, and Clinical Correlation

Pauci-immune crescentic glomerulonephritis and ANCA-associated small vessel vasculitis are aggressive diseases with 1-year mortality rates of approximately 80 percent. With treatment, 5-year patient and renal survival rates are about 75 percent [119,132,136]. Patients, who respond to therapy or go into remission, frequently relapse [119,137,138]. Patients with antibodies to PR3 have threefold higher relapse rates (>50 percent) compared to those with antibodies to MPO [119,138]. Other predictors of poor outcome and advanced disease include high serum creatinine levels at presentation, older age, pulmonary hemorrhage, and more severe tubulointerstitial disease with tubular atrophy and interstitial fibrosis, and higher degrees of glomerulosclerosis on initial biopsy. Cellular crescents, necrotizing glomerulonephritis, and active tubulointerstitial inflammation likely represent early active disease and correlate with better treatment response [119,139]. Patients with ANCA-negative pauci-immune glomerulonephritis are younger and have lower prevalence rates of extrarenal disease, higher levels of proteinuria with a higher incidence of nephrotic syndrome, and lower rates of renal survival as compared to ANCA-positive patients. Nephrotic syndrome at presentation is seen in 46 percent of ANCA-negative patients compared to 9 percent of ANCA-positive patients [139,140]. ANCA have been reported in up to a third of the patients with anti-GBM glomerulonephritis. These patients tend to be older, frequently have other manifestations of systemic small vessel vasculitis, and have better outcome and survival rates with treatment than patients with ANCA-negative anti-GBM disease.

The clinical management of pauci-immune glomerulonephritis involves three stages: remission induction, remission maintenance, and relapse treatment. Cyclophosphamide and corticosteroids have been the mainstays of therapy, with improvement in renal function noted in 90 percent of the patients and complete remission in 75 percent [119,132,136]. Relapses typically respond to re-treatment with similar regimens. With a better understanding of the pathobiology of pauci-immune glomerulonephritis and in an effort to reduce toxicity associated with the use of aggressive immunosuppression, other treatment modalities are being tried, especially directed at maintenance of remission. A recent study showed that, compared to intravenous methylprednisolone, the addition of plasma exchange to a regimen of oral cyclophosphamide and oral prednisolone increased the rate of renal recovery in ANCA-associated systemic vasculitis that presented with severe acute renal failure. However, patient survival and severely adverse event rates were similar in both groups [141]. Presumably, the plasma exchange helps by removing or diluting the pathogenic circulating ANCA. In another recent study, the addition of plasma exchange as adjuvant therapy increased the likelihood of renal recovery even in severely affected, dialysis-dependent patients with ANCA-associated glomerulonephritis [142].

Antiglomerular Basement Membrane Disease

Antiglomerular basement membrane (GBM) glomerulonephritis is one manifestation of a disease process that can involve the lung as well as the kidney and is secondary to vascular injury mediated by antibodies directed against the GBM. Ernest Goodpasture described a patient with glomerulonephritis who also had hemoptysis and dyspnea due to pulmonary hemorrhage [143]. The name, Goodpasture syndrome, was later applied to patients presenting with this constellation of clinical signs and symptoms. While ANCA-associated vasculitides such as microscopic polyangiitis, Wegener's granulomatosis, and Churg–Strauss syndrome, can result in a similar clinical presentation,

the term Goodpasture syndrome is reserved for those patients known to have anti-GBM antibodies [144]. The term "anti-GBM disease" is sometimes used as an umbrella term that includes Goodpasture syndrome, isolated anti-GBM glomerulonephritis, and isolated anti-GBM antibody-mediated pulmonary hemorrhage.

Epidemiology and Clinical Presentation

Anti-GBM disease has a bimodal age distribution, with one peak occurring in adolescents and young adults and another after the sixth decade of life. Among younger patients, males are more commonly affected, while females predominate at the older age. The disease affects Caucasians nine times more commonly than African-Americans [119,145]. Nearly half of the patients with anti-GBM disease present with glomerulonephritis alone, while less than 5 percent present with pulmonary capillaritis and hemorrhage alone and 45 percent have Goodpasture syndrome at presentation [119,145–147]. Young men are more likely to have pulmonary involvement than older women [119,145]. Patients with renal disease most often present with rapidly progressive glomerulonephritis, hematuria, and proteinuria that is usually in the non-nephrotic range. Anti-GBM glomerulonephritis is pathologically and clinically the most severe form of glomerulonephritis [119,147]. Only rare patients have a mild nephritic presentation or present with nephrotic syndrome [148,149]. The patients with pulmonary involvement present with hemoptysis and dyspnea, which may be life-threatening.

Approach to Interpretation

Gross Pathology. The kidneys of patients with anti-GBM glomerulonephritis have numerous petechial spots corresponding to blood within Bowman's spaces and tubular lumens. The lungs of patients with pulmonary involvement have focal or diffuse areas of dark red discoloration corresponding to intra-alveolar hemorrhages.

Light Microscopy. Nearly all cases of anti-GBM glomerulonephritis have glomerular crescents at the time of diagnosis, with 50 percent or more crescents present in the biopsies of the majority (>80 percent) of the patients (Figure 6.59). The earliest identifiable glomerular lesion is focal and segmental, necrotizing glomerulonephritis (Figure 6.60), which is usually accompanied by variable neutrophilic infiltrate at the sites of necrosis. PAS and methenamine silver stains highlight the areas of segmental necrosis and the breaks in the GBM and Bowman's capsule that sometimes accompany these segmental lesions (Figure 6.60). By staining the GBM, these stains also highlight the glomerular tufts as separate from the overlying cellular crescents. The glomerular capillaries and mesangium are most often normocellular, similar to ANCA-associated glomerulonephritis but differing from immune complex-mediated crescentic glomerulonephritis, which typically has both endocapillary and extracapillary proliferative appearance. The glomerular crescents may be small and only partial, or large and circumferential with compression of the underlying glomerular

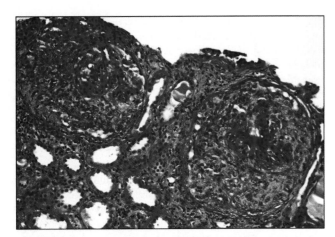

FIGURE 6.59: *Anti-glomerular basement membrane glomerulonephritis. Both glomeruli are compressed by large circumferential cellular crescents (PAS, 200×).*

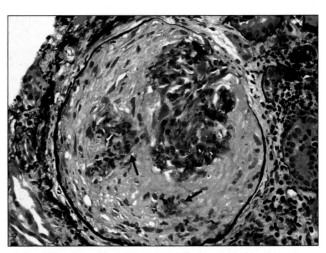

FIGURE 6.61: *Anti-glomerular basement membrane glomerulonephritis. The glomerulus has a large fibrocellular crescent with fragmented and sclerotic glomerular tufts (arrows) (Methenamine silver, 400×).*

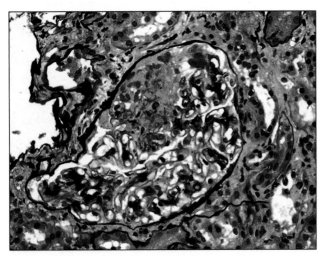

FIGURE 6.60: *Anti-glomerular basement membrane glomerulonephritis. The glomerulus shows segmental necrosis highlighted by dissolution of the methenamine silver positive glomerular capillary basement membranes. The nonnecrotic segments are histologically unremarkable (Methenamine silver, 400×).*

capillary tufts. The crescents may be associated with disruption of the Bowman's capsule and extension into the surrounding, periglomerular interstitium. This may incite a granulomatous inflammatory reaction. Giant cells may be seen in the crescents and sometimes along the tubular basement membranes. With time, the cellular crescents evolve from fibrocellular into fibrous crescents (Figure 6.61). Tubularization of the Bowman's space may also occur. The segmentally necrotic areas within glomeruli gradually undergo sclerosis, which is better appreciated by special stains such as trichrome and methenamine silver. Early in the active stages of the disease, there are red cells, red cell casts, and pigment casts formed from breakdown of red cells in the tubular lumens. These tubular changes are accompanied by varying degrees of interstitial edema and interstitial inflamma-

tory infiltrates that consist predominantly of mononuclear cells. Scattered neutrophils and eosinophils may be present as well. Tubular epithelial simplification may accompany severe renal failure. As the disease evolves, these changes progress to tubular atrophy and interstitial fibrosis. Arteritis rarely accompanies anti-GBM glomerulonephritis [150] and, when present, may represent concurrent ANCA-associated disease. All patients with RPGN or crescentic glomerulonephritis should be tested for the presence of both ANCA and anti-GBM antibodies in their serum. Patients who have both diseases simultaneously tend to be older and show a better response to treatment than patients with anti-GBM glomerulonephritis alone.

Immunofluorescence Microscopy. The diagnostic feature of anti-GBM glomerulonephritis is marked diffuse, global, linear staining of GBM for immunoglobulins, usually IgG (Figure 6.62). Distal tubular basement membrane staining may be present as well. Lesser degrees of staining for IgM and IgA are often present. There are a few reports of IgA-dominant anti-GBM glomerulonephritis. The immunoglobulin staining pattern may be discontinuous in areas with destruction of the GBM due to necrotizing glomerulonephritis. Granular or discontinuous linear staining for C3 and other complement components may be present as well. The linear staining of the GBM may be confused with the nonspecific, linear staining of basement membranes seen in diabetics, older individuals, and autopsy material. A careful study of the staining pattern of albumin is very useful because the intensity of albumin staining is generally equal to or stronger than IgG staining in these conditions. However, in anti-GBM disease, the intensity of albumin staining is far weaker than IgG staining. If in doubt, a diagnosis of anti-GBM glomerulonephritis should be correlated with positive serum antibody test results and the clinical picture. Anti-GBM glomerulonephritis may rarely coexist with membranous glomerulopathy [151–153]. In these instances, it may be difficult to tease out the granular staining pattern from the coexisting linear staining pattern and the diagnosis requires the ultrastructural

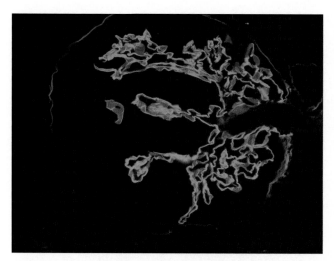

FIGURE 6.62: *Anti-glomerular basement membrane glomerulonephritis. Intense linear staining along the glomerular capillary walls for IgG, with GBM breaks (400×).*

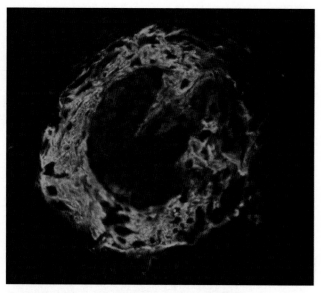

FIGURE 6.63: *Anti-glomerular basement membrane glomerulonephritis. Immunofluorescence microscopy reveals a strong, irregular staining for fibrin in a crescent surrounding the compressed glomerulus tuft (400×).*

presence of subepithelial electron-dense deposits. Staining for fibrin is positive in areas of glomerular necrosis, in crescents (Figure 6.63), and in the periglomerular interstitium in areas where the Bowman's capsule is disrupted. In the lungs of patients with pulmonary disease, there is linear staining of the alveolar capillary basement membranes for IgG and C3; however, the inetrpretation of immunofluorescent staining in the lung may be difficult and requires experience. The alveolar spaces stain for fibrin in the presence of pulmonary capillaritis.

Electron Microscopy. There are no ultrastructural diagnostic features of anti-GBM glomerulonephritis. The findings are those common to all necrotizing and crescentic glomerulonephritides and include breaks in the GBM, margination of leukocytes within capillary lumens, areas of segmental necrosis with fibrin deposits in the necrotic tufts and in capillary lumens, and areas of endothelial disruption within glomerular capillaries (Figure 6.64). Fibrin deposition in areas of necrosis is typically electron-dense and may be amorphous or organized into curvilinear or angular fibrillary material. It should not be confused with electron-dense immune complex deposits. The glomerular crescents contain epithelial cells, macrophages, occasional neutrophils, and fibrinous material. As crescents evolve and undergo sclerosis, they accumulate more collagen and lose cells.

Differential Diagnosis

The light microscopic differential diagnosis of anti-GBM glomerulonephritis includes all forms of glomerulonephritis that are associated with crescents including pauci-immune or ANCA-associated glomerulonephritis and immune complex-mediated glomerulonephritides. [119,154] The majority of patients presenting with combined pulmonary and renal vasculitic syndromes have pauci-immune or ANCA-associated vasculitis (55 percent), while a minority have anti-GBM disease (7 percent), or concurrent anti-GBM disease and ANCA-associated vasculitis (8 percent). Immune complex-mediated pulmonary

and renal vasculitic disease is rare [154]. Anti-GBM glomerulonephritis, like pauci-immune glomerulonephritis, tends to have more necrosis and less endocapillary cellularity than immune complex-mediated glomerulonephritis. Immunofluorescence studies distinguish the three types of crescentic glomerulonephritides. Patients with anti-GBM glomerulonephritis may have concurrent ANCA-associated or immune complex-mediated disease [119,151,152]. Therefore, it is prudent to perform serologic testing for anti-GBM antibodies in patients with ANCA-associated or immune complex-mediated glomerulonephritis. Linear staining with immunoglobulins may be noted in patients with diabetic glomerulosclerosis and monoclonal immunoglobulin deposition disease. These diseases have distinctly different light microscopic appearances and clinical presentations.

Etiology and Pathogenesis

In 1967, Lerner, Glassock, and Dixon found antibodies to GBM antigens in patients with linear IgG-positive glomerulonephritis [155]. They showed that injection of these antibodies into animals resulted in a similar form of glomerulonephritis, establishing the antibodies to be the causative agents of this disease. The major epitopes for anti-GBM antibodies are in the α_3 chain of the noncollagenous domain of type IV collagen and include the immunodominant target epitope EA (encompassed by α_3-NC$_1$ residues 17–31) and a homologous region EB (encompassed by α_3-NC$_1$ residues 121–141). The latter is recognized by only a small number of patients. Although the target epitopes are known, the mechanisms whereby the normally hidden target epitopes become accessible to circulating autoantibodies remain unknown. In addition, the stimuli and mechanisms leading to autoantibody formation are still unclear [156,157]. The specificity of antibodies is the same in patients with glomerulonephritis and pulmonary disease. Agents in

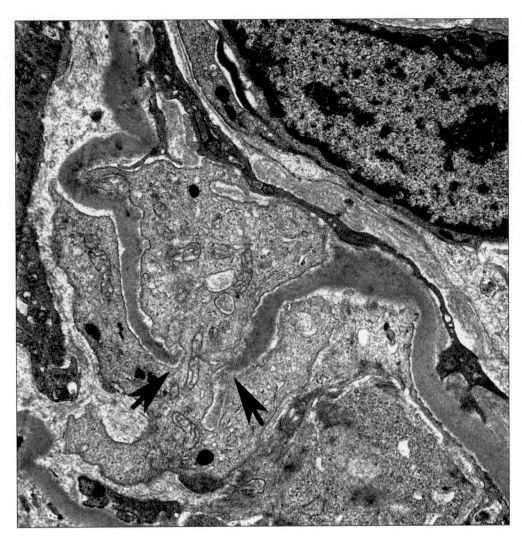

FIGURE 6.64: *Anti-glomerular basement membrane glomerulonephritis. Electron micrograph reveals disruption of the glomerular basement membrane (arrows). No immune-type electron-dense deposits are seen.*

Table 6.6 Frequency of Crescent Formation in Various Diseases

	Any Crescent Formation	>50% Crescents
Anti-GBM disease	97.1	84.8
Pauci-immune GN	89.5	50.3
Lupus nephritis, class III/IV	56.5	12.9
Henoch-Schönlein purpura	61.3	9.7
IgA nephropathy	32.5	4.0
Acute postinfectious GN	33.3	3.3
MPGN Type I	23.8	4.6
Dense deposit disease	43.8	18.8
Fibrillary glomerulopathy	22.8	5.0
Monoclonal Ig deposition disease	5.6	0
Thrombotic microangiopathies	5.6	0.9
Diabetic nephropathy	3.2	0.3
Membranous glomerulopathy	3.2	0.1

Adapted from Jennette JC *Kidney Int*, 2003; 63(3): 1164–77.

cigarette smoke, other hydrocarbons, or respiratory tract infections may be required as cofactors for the development of the pulmonary disease. Such environmental irritants and toxins likely injure the glomerular and pulmonary basement membranes, thereby exposing cryptic epitopes to preexisting antibodies that then incite an immune-mediated injury [157]. The vascular injury is likely mediated by T-lymphocytes and macrophages. [158,159]. The strong association between HLA DR and DQ antigens and anti-GBM disease suggests that the development of anti-GBM antibodies and disease is likely influenced by genetic factors [160].

Clinical Course, Prognosis, Treatment, and Clinical Correlation

Anti-GBM glomerulonephritis, either alone, or associated with pulmonary disease in patients with Goodpasture syndrome, is an aggressive disease [119]. Rapid institution of immunosuppressive therapy, which usually consists of high-dose

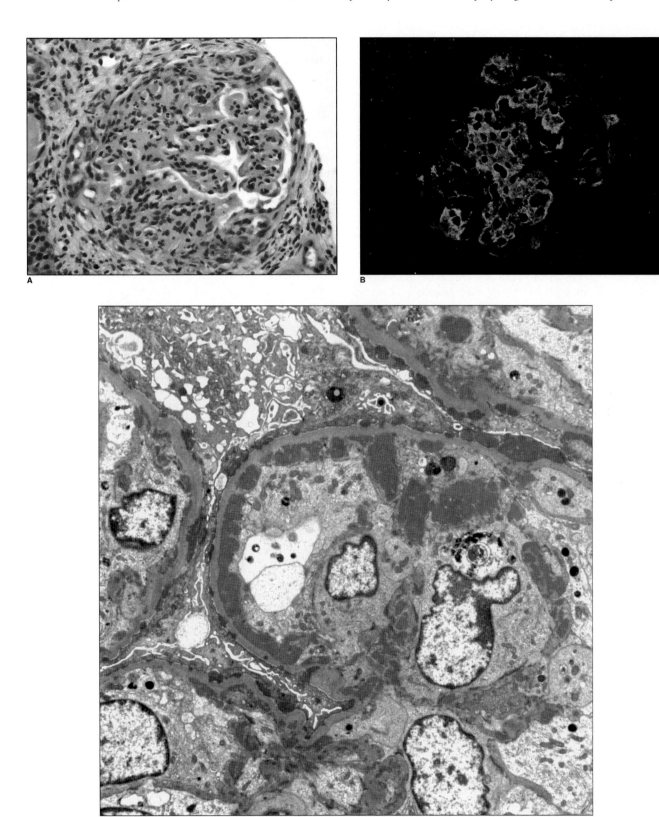

FIGURE 6.65: *Diffuse lupus nephritis with crescent formation. (A) The glomerulus displays global intracapillary hypercellularity with obliterated capillary lumens and thickened capillary walls. A small cellular crescent is present (H&E 400×). (B) Immunofluorescence microscopy reveals intense granular staining along the capillary walls and in the mesangium for IgG (400×). (C). Electron micrograph reveals numerous subendothelial, subepithelial, and mesangial electron-dense deposits. Many subepithelial electron-dense deposits are also noted.*

corticosteroids and cytotoxic drugs such as cyclophosphamide are the mainstays of therapy [161,162]. Plasmapheresis plays a major role in treatment. In patients with serum creatinine values of less than 5.7 mg/dl, plasmapheresis in addition to immuno-suppression resulted in 100 percent patient survival and 95 percent renal survival rates at one year. In patients on dialysis, patient survival was 68 percent with a renal survival rate of only 8 percent [161]. Thus, rapid diagnosis and institution of therapy can have a dramatic impact on patient survival and retention of renal function. As the pathobiologic mechanisms leading to the development of crescentic glomerulo-nephritides are being better understood, newer therapies such as leflunomide (a pyrimidine synthesis inhibitor), deoxysper-gualin (an immunosuppressant), infliximab (antitumor necrosis factor α antibody), calcineurin inhibitors, and antibodies directed against T-lymphocytes are finding their way into experimental treatment protocols for crescentic glomerulo-nephritides of all types [119,163]. The prognosis of anti-GBM disease is worse than pauci-immune crescentic glomerulonephritis and immune complex-mediated crescentic glomerulonephritis [119]. In patients who do respond to ther-apy, disease recurrences are uncommon, but may occur years after the initial presentation. The disease may recur in renal transplants, but this is uncommon in patients who are nega-tive for serum anti-GBM antibodies at the time of their transplant.

Immune Complex-Mediated Crescentic Glomerulonephritis

Epidemiology and Clinical Presentation

Crescents have been noted in virtually every type of immune complex-mediated glomerulonephritis (Table 6.6). Detailed descriptions of these forms of disease are given elsewhere in this book. In addition, there are cases that are best classified as idiopathic immune complex-mediated glomerulonephritis. These are the cases where no definitive underlying diganotic pattern is present. The relative percentage of crescents varies considerably and in general, when crescents occur in immune complex-mediated glomerulonephritis, they affect a smaller percentage of glomeruli than in cases of anti-GBM disease or ANCA-associated glomerulonephritis. Immune complex-asso-ciated crescentic glomerulonephritis also shows lesser degrees of glomerular necrosis compared to the other forms of cres-centic glomerulonephritis [119].

Approach to Interpretation

Gross Pathology. Kidneys are normal or slightly enlarged. Petechial hemorrhage may be seen.

Light Microscopy. The specific type of immune complex-medi-ated disease determines the light microscopic appearance of the glomeruli. Examination of the glomeruli that are not severely affected by crescents or necrosis (i.e. the most preserved glomer-uli) may allow the identification of disease-specific histomorpho-logic patterns such as the tram-track appearance of GBM in MPGN, GBM spikes in membranous glomerulopathy, and endocapillary hypercellularity with "wireloop" lesions in diffuse proliferative lupus nephritis (Figure 6.65A).

Immunofluorescence Microscopy. Immunofluorescence microscopy reflects the underlying immune complex disease. Examples include the IgA predominant or codominant staining in IgA nephropathy, the "full house" staining in proliferative lupus glomerulonephritis (Figure 6.65B), and the uniformly gran-ular staining of glomerular capillary loops with IgG in membra-nous glomerulopathy.

Electron Microscopy. Electron microscopic examination con-firms the presence of electron-dense immune complex deposits. The location of the deposits reflects the underlying disease. Thus, IgA nephropathy shows predominantly mesangial deposits, APSGN shows the characteristic large subepithelial "humps," membranous glomerulopathy shows diffuse regularly distributed subepithelial deposits, while lupus glomerulonephritis shows widely distributed deposits in the mesangial, subendothelial, and subepithelial locations (Figure 6.65C). The endothelial cells in the latter disease may contain tubuloreticular inclusions.

Clinical Course, Prognosis, Treatment, and Clinical Correlation

The underlying diseases dictate the management of immune-complex mediated crescentic glomerulonephritis and are dis-cussed elsewhere in this book. In general, crescent formation portends a worse prognosis and requires aggressive treatment [119,164,165]. Crescent formation occurs because of unusually severe endothelial injury with breaks in the GBM. Crescent formation may also reflect coexistent ANCA-associated disease such as has been reported with cases of membranous glomer-ulopathy. Therefore, such patients should undergo serologic testing to detect ANCA.

REFERENCES

1. Nadasdy T, and Silva FG, . Acute postinfectious glomer-ulonephritis and glomerulonephritis caused by persistent bacterial infection. *Heptinstall's Pathology of the Kidney*. J.C. Jennette, et al., Eds. 2007, Lippincott Williams and Wil-kins: Philadelphia, PA, pp. 322–395.
2. Wells CD. Observations on the dropsy which succeeds scarlet fever. *Trans Soc Imp Med Chir Knowledge* 1812; 3: 167–186.
3. Bright R. Cases and observations illustrative of renal disease accompanied with the secretion of albuminous urine. *Guy's Hosp Rev* 1836; 1: 338.
4. Volhard F and Fahr T. Die Brightsche Nierenkrankheit. 1914; Berlin: Springer.
5. Rammelkamp CH. Microbiologic aspects of glomerulo-nephritis. *J Chronic Dis* 1957; 5(1): 28–33.
6. Dillon HC, Reeves MS, and Maxted WR. Acute glomeru-lonephritis following skin infection due to streptococci of M-type 2. *Lancet* 1968; 1(7542): 543–5.
7. Cunningham MW. Pathogenesis of group A streptococcal infections. *Clin Microbiol Rev* 2000; 13(3): 470–511.
8. Yoshizawa N. Acute glomerulonephritis. *Intern Med* 2000; 39(9): 687–94.

9. Markowitz M. Changing epidemiology of group A streptococcal infections. *Pediatr Infect Dis J* 1994; 13(6): 557–560.

10. Mazzucco G, Bertani T, Fortunato M, Bernardi M, Leutner M, Boldorini R, and Monga G. Different patterns of renal damage in type 2 diabetes mellitus: a multicentric study on 393 biopsies. *Am J Kidney Dis* 2002; 39(4): 713–720.

11. Montseny JJ, Meyrier A, Kleinknecht D, and Callard P. The current spectrum of infectious glomerulonephritis. Experience with 76 patients and review of the literature. *Medicine (Baltimore)* 1995; 74(2): 63–73.

12. Haas M, Spargo BH, Wit EJ, and Meehan SM. Etiologies and outcome of acute renal insufficiency in older adults: a renal biopsy study of 259 cases. *Am J Kidney Dis* 2000; 35(3): 433–47.

13. El-Husseini AA, Sheashaa HA, Sabry AA, Moustafa FE, and Sobh MA. Acute postinfectious crescentic glomerulonephritis: clinicopathologic presentation and risk factors. *Int Urol Nephrol* 2005; 37(3): 603–9.

14. Nadler H. Group A strep detection. *Diagn Clin Test* 1989; 27: 34.

15. Parra G, Platt JL, Falk RJ, Rodriguez-Iturbe B, and Michael AF. Cell populations and membrane attack complex in glomeruli of patients with poststreptococcal glomerulonephritis: identification using monoclonal antibodies by indirect immunofluorescence. *Clin Immunol Immunopathol* 1984; 33(3): 324–32.

16. Rastaldi MP, Ferrario F, Yang L, Tunesi S, Indaco A, Zou H, and D'Amico G. Adhesion molecules expression in non-crescentic acute poststreptococcal glomerulonephritis. *J Am Soc Nephrol* 1996; 7(11): 2419–27.

17. Fish AJ, Herdman RC, Michael AF, Pickering RJ, and Good RA. Epidemic acute glomerulonephritis associated with type 49 streptococcal pyoderma. II. Correlative study of light, immunofluorescent and electron microscopic findings. *Am J Med* 1970; 48(1): 28–39.

18. Lewy JE, Salinas-Madrigal L, Herdson PB, Pirani CL, and Metcoff J. Clinico-pathologic correlations in acute poststreptococcal glomerulonephritis. A correlation between renal functions, morphologic damage, and clinical course of 46 children with acute poststreptococcal glomerulonephritis. *Medicine (Baltimore)* 1971; 50(6): 453–501.

19. Jennings RB and Earle DP. Poststreptococcal glomerulonephritis: histopathologic and clinical studies of the acute, subsiding acute and early chronic latent phases. *J Clin Invest* 1961; 40: 1525–95.

20. Sorger K. Postinfectious glomerulonephritis. Subtypes, clinico-pathological correlations, and follow-up studies. *Veroff Pathol* 1986; 125: 1–105.

21. Raff A, Hebert T, Pullman J, and Coco M. Crescentic poststreptococcal glomerulonephritis with nephrotic syndrome in the adult: is aggressive therapy warranted? *Clin Nephrol* 2005; 63(5): 375–80.

22. Nasr SH, Markowitz GS, Stokes MB, Said SM, Valeri AM, and D'Agati VD. Acute postinfectious glomerulonephritis in the modern era: experience with 86 adults and review of the literature. *Medicine (Baltimore)* 2008; 87(1): 21–32.

23. Morel-Maroger L, Kourilsky O, Mignon F, and Richet G. Antitubular basement membrane antibodies in rapidly progressive poststreptococcal glomerulonephritis: report of a case. *Clin Immunol Immunopathol* 1974; 2(2): 185–94.

24. Watt MF, Howe JS, and Parrish AE. Renal tubular changes in acute glomerulonephritis. *AMA Arch Intern Med* 1959; 103(5): 690–5.

25. Bodaghi E, Kheradpir KM, and Maddah M. Vasculitis in acute streptococcal glomerulonephritis. *Int J Pediatr Nephrol* 1987; 8(2): 69–74.

26. Herdson PB, Jennings RB, and Earle DP. Glomerular fine structure in poststreptococcal acute glomerulonephritis. *Arch Pathol* 1966; 81(2): 117–28.

27. Rodriguez-Iturbe B and Batsford S. Pathogenesis of poststreptococcal glomerulonephritis a century after Clemens von Pirquet. *Kidney Int* 2007; 71(11): 1094–104.

28. Batsford SR, Mezzano S, Mihatsch M, Schiltz E, and Rodriguez-Iturbe B. Is the nephritogenic antigen in poststreptococcal glomerulonephritis pyrogenic exotoxin B (SPE B) or GAPDH? *Kidney Int* 2005; 68(3): 1120–9.

29. Oda T, Yamakami K, Omasu F, Suzuki S, Miura S, Sugisaki T, and Yoshizawa N. Glomerular plasmin-like activity in relation to nephritis-associated plasmin receptor in acute poststreptococcal glomerulonephritis. *J Am Soc Nephrol* 2005; 16(1): 247–54.

30. Robinson JH and Kehoe MA. Group A streptococcal M proteins: virulence factors and protective antigens. *Immunol Today* 1992; 13(9): 362–7.

31. Yoshizawa N, Yamakami K, Fujino M, Oda T, Tamura K, Matsumoto K, Sugisaki T, and Boyle MD. Nephritis-associated plasmin receptor and acute poststreptococcal glomerulonephritis: characterization of the antigen and associated immune response. *J Am Soc Nephrol* 2004; 15(7): 1785–93.

32. Parra G, Rodriguez-Iturbe B, Batsford S, Vogt A, Mezzano S, Olavarria F, Exeni R, Laso M, and Orta N. Antibody to streptococcal zymogen in the serum of patients with acute glomerulonephritis: a multicentric study. *Kidney Int* 1998; 54(2): 509–17.

33. Buzio C, Allegri L, Mutti A, Perazzoli F, and Bergamaschi E. Significance of albuminuria in the follow-up of acute poststreptococcal glomerulonephritis. *Clin Nephrol* 1994; 41(5): 259–64.

34. Rodriguez-Iturbe B. Postinfectious glomerulonephritis. *Am J Kidney Dis 2000*; 35(1): XLVI–XLVIII.

35. Roy S, 3rd, Pitcock JA, and Etteldorf JN. Prognosis of acute poststreptococcal glomerulonephritis in childhood: prospective study and review of the literature. *Adv Pediatr* 1976; 23: 35–69.

36. Moroni G, Pozzi C, Quaglini S, Segagni S, Banfi G, Baroli A, Picardi L, Colzani S, Simonini P, Mihatsch MJ, and Ponticelli C. Long-term prognosis of diffuse proliferative glomerulonephritis associated with infection in adults. *Nephrol Dial Transplant* 2002; 17(7): 1204–1211.

37. Sexton DJ and Spelman D. Current best practices and guidelines. Assessment and management of complications in infective endocarditis. *Cardiol Clin* 2003; 21(2): 273–82, vii–viii.

38. Majumdar A, Chowdhary S, Ferreira MA, Hammond LA, Howie AJ, Lipkin GW, and Littler WA. Renal pathological

findings in infective endocarditis. *Nephrol Dial Transplant* 2000; 15(11): 1782–7.

39. Eknoyan G, Lister BJ, Kim HS, and Greenberg SD. Renal complications of bacterial endocarditis. *Am J Nephrol* 1985; 5(6): 457–69.

40. Lee LC, Lam KK, Lee CT, Chen JB, Tsai TH, and Huang SC. "Full house" proliferative glomerulonephritis: an unreported presentation of subacute infective endocarditis. *J Nephrol* 2007; 20(6): 745–9.

41. Kirkpantur A, Altinbas A, Arici M, Baydar DE, Altun B, and Arslan S. Enterococcal endocarditis associated with crescentic glomerulonephritis. *Clin Exp Nephrol* 2007; 11(4): 321–5.

42. Bayer AS and Theofilopoulos AN. Immunopathogenetic aspects of infective endocarditis. *Chest* 1990; 97(1): 204–12.

43. Fukuda M, Motokawa M, Usami T, Oikawa T, Morozumi K, Yoshida A, and Kimura G. PR3-ANCA-positive crescentic necrotizing glomerulonephritis accompanied by isolated pulmonic valve infective endocarditis, with reference to previous reports of renal pathology. *Clin Nephrol* 2006; 66(3): 202–9.

44. Daimon S, Mizuno Y, Fujii S, Mukai K, Hanakawa H, Otsuki N, Yasuhara S, Saga T, and Koni I. Infective endocarditis-induced crescentic glomerulonephritis dramatically improved by plasmapheresis. *Am J Kidney Dis* 1998; 32(2): 309–13.

45. Koya D, Shibuya K, Kikkawa R, and Haneda M. Successful recovery of infective endocarditis-induced rapidly progressive glomerulonephritis by steroid therapy combined with antibiotics: a case report. *BMC Nephrol* 2004; 5(1): 18.

46. Le Moing V, Lacassin F, Delahousse M, Duval X, Longuet P, Leport C, and Vilde JL. Use of corticosteroids in glomerulonephritis related to infective endocarditis: three cases and review. *Clin Infect Dis* 1999; 28(5): 1057–61.

47. Legoupil N, Ronco P, and Berenbaum F. Arthritis-related shunt nephritis in an adult. *Rheumatology (Oxford)* 2003; 42(5): 698–9.

48. Haffner D, Schindera F, Aschoff A, Matthias S, Waldherr R, and Scharer K. The clinical spectrum of shunt nephritis. *Nephrol Dial Transplant* 1997; 12(6): 1143–8.

49. Vella J, Carmody M, Campbell E, Browne O, Doyle G, and Donohoe J. Glomerulonephritis after ventriculo-atrial shunt. *Qjm* 1995; 88(12): 911–8.

50. Iwata Y, Ohta S, Kawai K, Yamahana J, Sugimori H, Ishida Y, Saito K, Miyamori T, Futami K, Arakawa Y, Hirota Y, Wada T, Yokoyama H, and Yoshida K. Shunt nephritis with positive titers for ANCA specific for proteinase 3. *Am J Kidney Dis* 2004; 43(5): e11–6.

51. Fukuda Y, Ohtomo Y, Kaneko K, and Yabuta K. Pathologic and laboratory dynamics following the removal of the shunt in shunt nephritis. *Am J Nephrol* 1993; 13(1): 78–82.

52. Beaufils M. Glomerular disease complicating abdominal sepsis. *Kidney Int* 1981; 19(4): 609–18.

53. Beaufils M, Morel-Maroger L, Sraer JD, Kanfer A, Kourilsky O, and Richet G. Acute renal failure of glomerular origin during visceral abscesses. *N Engl J Med* 1976; 295(4): 185–9.

54. Kilincer C, Hamamcioglu MK, Simsek O, Hicdonmez T, Aydoslu B, Tansel O, Tiryaki M, Soy M, Tatman-Otkun M, and Cobanoglu S. Nocardial brain abscess: review of clinical management. *J Clin Neurosci* 2006; 13(4): 481–5.

55. Chung J, Habib R, and White RH. Pathology of the nephrotic syndrome in children: A report for the International Study of Kidney Disease in Children. *Lancet* 1970; 1: 1299.

56. Rennke HG. Secondary membranoproliferative glomerulonephritis. *Kidney Int* 1995; 47(2): 643–56.

57. Zhou XJ, and Silva FG. Membranoproliferative glomerulonephritis, in *Heptinstall's Pathology of the Kidney*. J.C. Jennette, et al., Eds. 2006, Lippincott Williams and Wilkins: Philadelphia, PA, pp. 253–319.

58. Burkholder PM, Marchand A, and Krueger RP. Mixed membranous and proliferative glomerulonephritis. A correlative light, immunofluorescence, and electron microscopic study. *Lab Invest* 1970; 23(5): 459–79.

59. Strife CF, McEnery PT, McAdams AJ, and West CD. Membranoproliferative glomerulonephritis with disruption of the glomerular basement membrane. *Clin Nephrol* 1977; 7(2): 65–72.

60. Anders D, Agricola B, Sippel M, and Thoenes W. Basement membrane changes in membranoproliferative glomerulonephritis. II. Characterization of a third type by silver impregnation of ultra thin sections. *Virchows Arch A Pathol Anat Histol* 1977; 376(1): 1–19.

61. Walker PD, Ferrario F, Joh K, and Bonsib SM. Dense deposit disease is not a membranoproliferative glomerulonephritis. *Mod Pathol* 2007; 20(6): 605–16.

62. Nakopoulou L. Membranoproliferative glomerulonephritis. *Nephrol Dial Transplant* 2001; 16 Suppl. 6: 71–3.

63. Cameron JS, Turner DR, Heaton J, Williams DG, Ogg CS, Chantler C, Haycock GB, and Hicks J. Idiopathic mesangiocapillary glomerulonephritis. Comparison of types I and II in children and adults and long-term prognosis. *Am J Med* 1983; 74(2): 175–92.

64. Kim Y and Michael AF. Idiopathic membranoproliferative glomerulonephritis. *Annu Rev Med* 1980; 31: 273–88.

65. Watson AR, Poucell S, Thorner P, Arbus GS, Rance CP, and Baumal R. Membranoproliferative glomerulonephritis type I in children: correlation of clinical features with pathologic subtypes. *Am J Kidney Dis* 1984; 4(2): 141–6.

66. West CD. Idiopathic membranoproliferative glomerulonephritis in childhood. *Pediatr Nephrol* 1992; 6(1): 96–103.

67. Yalcinkaya F, Ince E, Tumer N, and Ekim M. The correlation between the clinical, laboratory and histopathological features of childhood membranoproliferative glomerulonephritis and response to treatment. *Turk J Pediatr* 1992; 34(3): 135–44.

68. Levy M, Gubler MC, and Habib R. New concepts in membranoproliferative glomerulonephritis, in *Progress in Glomerulonephritis*. P. Kincaid-Smith, A.J.F. d'Apice, and R.C. Atkins, Eds. 1979, Wiley: New York.

69. Strife CF, Jackson EC, and McAdams AJ. Type III membranoproliferative glomerulonephritis: long-term clinical and morphologic evaluation. *Clin Nephrol* 1984; 21(6): 323–34.

70. Davis AE, Schneeberger EE, Grupe WE, and McCluskey RT. Membranoproliferative glomerulonephritis (MPGN type I) and dense deposit disease (DDD) in children. *Clin Nephrol* 1978; 9(5): 184–93.

71. Ferrario F and Rastaldi MP. Histopathological atlas of renal diseases. Membranoproliferative glomerulonephritis. *J Nephrol* 2004; 17(4): 483–6.

72. Strife CF, McAdams AJ, and West CD. Membranoproliferative glomerulonephritis characterized by focal, segmental proliferative lesions. *Clin Nephrol* 1982; 18(1): 9–16.

73. Miller MN, Baumal R, Poucell S, and Steele BT. Incidence and prognostic importance of glomerular crescents in renal diseases of childhood. *Am J Nephrol* 1984; 4(4): 244–7.

74. Swainson CP, Robson JS, Thomson D, and MacDonald MK. Mesangiocapillary glomerulonephritis: a long-term study of 40 cases. *J Pathol* 1983; 141(4): 449–68.

75. Meyers KE, Finn L, and Kaplan BS. Membranoproliferative glomerulonephritis type III. *Pediatr Nephrol* 1998; 12(6): 512–22.

76. West CD. Membranoproliferative hypocomplementemic glomerulonephritis. *Nephron* 1973; 11(2): 134–46.

77. Levin A. Management of membranoproliferative glomerulonephritis: evidence-based recommendations. *Kidney Int Suppl* 1999; 70: S41–6.

78. Schwertz R, de Jong R, Gretz N, Kirschfink M, Anders D, and Scharer K. Outcome of idiopathic membranoproliferative glomerulonephritis in children. Arbeitsgemeinschaft Padiatrische Nephrologie. *Acta Paediatr* 1996; 85(3): 308–12.

79. Uszycka-Karcz M, Stolarczyk J, Wrzolkowa T, Kaminska H, Zurowska A, Marczak E, Schramm K, and Mierzewski P. Mesangial proliferative glomerulonephritis in children. *Int J Pediatr Nephrol* 1982; 3(4): 251–6.

80. Noris M and Remuzzi G. Translational mini-review series on complement factor H: therapies of renal diseases associated with complement factor H abnormalities: atypical haemolytic uraemic syndrome and membranoproliferative glomerulonephritis. *Clin Exp Immunol* 2008; 151(2): 199–209.

81. Ali A and Zein NN. Hepatitis C infection: a systemic disease with extrahepatic manifestations. *Cleve Clin J Med* 2005; 72(11): 1005–8, 1010–4, 1016 passim.

82. Canada R, Chaudry S, Gaber L, Waters B, Martinez A, and Wall B. Polyarteritis nodosa and cryoglobulinemic glomerulonephritis related to chronic hepatitis C. *Am J Med Sci* 2006; 331(6): 329–33.

83. Hoch B, Juknevicius I, and Liapis H. Glomerular injury associated with hepatitis C infection: a correlation with blood and tissue HCV-PCR. *Semin Diagn Pathol* 2002; 19(3): 175–87.

84. Lai AS and Lai KN. Viral nephropathy. *Nat Clin Pract Nephrol* 2006; 2(5): 254–62.

85. Uchiyama-Tanaka Y, Mori Y, Kishimoto N, Nose A, Kijima Y, Nagata T, Umeda Y, Masaki H, Matsubara H, and Iwasaka T. Membranous glomerulonephritis associated with hepatitis C virus infection: case report and literature review. *Clin Nephrol* 2004; 61(2): 144–50.

86. Kamar N, Rostaing L, and Alric L. Treatment of hepatitis C-virus-related glomerulonephritis. *Kidney Int* 2006; 69(3): 436–9.

87. Kamar N, Izopet J, Alric L, Guilbeaud-Frugier C, and Rostaing L. Hepatitis C virus-related kidney disease: an overview. *Clin Nephrol* 2008; 69(3): 149–60.

88. Alpers CE and Smith KD. Cryoglobulinemia and renal disease. *Curr Opin Nephrol Hypertens* 2008; 17(3): 243–9.

89. Dolganiuc A, Oak S, Kodys K, Golenbock DT, Finberg RW, Kurt-Jones E, and Szabo G. Hepatitis C core and nonstructural 3 proteins trigger toll-like receptor 2-mediated pathways and inflammatory activation. *Gastroenterology* 2004; 127(5): 1513–24.

90. Wornle M, Schmid H, Banas B, Merkle M, Henger A, Roeder M, Blattner S, Bock E, Kretzler M, Grone HJ, and Schlondorff D. Novel role of toll-like receptor 3 in hepatitis C-associated glomerulonephritis. *Am J Pathol* 2006; 168(2): 370–85.

91. Bhimma R and Coovadia HM. Hepatitis B virus-associated nephropathy. *Am J Nephrol* 2004; 24(2): 198–211.

92. Fabrizi F, Dixit V, and Martin P. Meta-analysis: anti-viral therapy of hepatitis B virus-associated glomerulonephritis. *Aliment Pharmacol Ther* 2006; 24(5): 781–8.

93. Han SH. Extrahepatic manifestations of chronic hepatitis B. *Clin Liver Dis* 2004; 8(2): 403–18.

94. Mason A. Role of viral replication in extrahepatic syndromes related to hepatitis B virus infection. *Minerva Gastroenterol Dietol* 2006; 52(1): 53–66.

95. Ozdamar SO, Gucer S, and Tinaztepe K. Hepatitis-B virus associated nephropathies: a clinicopathological study in 14 children. *Pediatr Nephrol* 2003; 18(1): 23–8.

96. Farrell GC and Teoh NC. Management of chronic hepatitis B virus infection: a new era of disease control. *Intern Med J* 2006; 36(2): 100–13.

97. Markowitz GS, Lin J, Valeri AM, Avila C, Nasr SH, and D'Agati VD. Idiopathic nodular glomerulosclerosis is a distinct clinicopathologic entity linked to hypertension and smoking. *Hum Pathol* 2002; 33(8): 826–35.

98. Nasr SH and D'Agati VD. Nodular glomerulosclerosis in the nondiabetic smoker. *J Am Soc Nephrol* 2007; 18(7): 2032–6.

99. Habib R, Gubler MC, Loirat C, Maiz HB, and Levy M. Dense deposit disease: a variant of membranoproliferative glomerulonephritis. *Kidney Int* 1975; 7(4): 204–15.

100. Appel GB, Cook HT, Hageman G, Jennette JC, Kashgarian M, Kirschfink M, Lambris JD, Lanning L, Lutz HU, Meri S, Rose NR, Salant DJ, Sethi S, Smith RJ, Smoyer W, Tully HF, Tully SP, Walker P, Welsh M, Wurzner R, and Zipfel PF. Membranoproliferative glomerulonephritis type II (dense deposit disease): an update. *J Am Soc Nephrol* 2005; 16(5): 1392–403.

101. Sibley RK and Kim Y. Dense intramembranous deposit disease: new pathologic features. *Kidney Int* 1984; 25(4): 660–70.

102. Antoine B and Faye C. The clinical course associated with dense deposits in the kidney basement membranes. *Kidney Int* 1972; 1(6): 420–7.

103. Mampaso F, Leyva-Cobian F, Martinez-Montero JC, Gonzalo A, Bellas C, Moneo I, and Junquera E. Mesangial proliferative glomerulonephritis with unusual intramembranous granular dense deposits. *Clin Nephrol* 1983; 19(2): 92–8.

104. Klein M, Poucell S, Arbus GS, McGraw M, Rance CP, Yoon SJ, and Baumal R. Characteristics of a benign subtype of dense deposit disease: comparison with the progressive form of this disease. *Clin Nephrol* 1983; 20(4): 163–71.

105. SPNSG. Dense deposit disease in children: prognostic value of clinical and pathologic indicators. The Southwest

Pediatric Nephrology Study Group. *Am J Kidney Dis* 1985; 6(3): 161–9.

106. Schwertz R, Rother U, Anders D, Gretz N, Scharer K, and Kirschfink M. Complement analysis in children with idiopathic membranoproliferative glomerulonephritis: a long-term follow-up. *Pediatr Allergy Immunol* 2001; 12(3): 166–72.

107. Levy M, Halbwachs-Mecarelli L, Gubler MC, Kohout G, Bensenouci A, Niaudet P, Hauptmann G, and Lesavre P. H deficiency in two brothers with atypical dense intramembranous deposit disease. *Kidney Int* 1986; 30(6): 949–56.

108. Licht C, Heinen S, Jozsi M, Loschmann I, Saunders RE, Perkins SJ, Waldherr R, Skerka C, Kirschfink M, Hoppe B, and Zipfel PF. Deletion of Lys224 in regulatory domain 4 of Factor H reveals a novel pathomechanism for dense deposit disease (MPGN II). *Kidney Int* 2006; 70(1): 42–50.

109. Meri S, Koistinen V, Miettinen A, Tornroth T, and Seppala IJ. Activation of the alternative pathway of complement by monoclonal lambda light chains in membranoproliferative glomerulonephritis. *J Exp Med* 1992; 175(4): 939–50.

110. Rawal N and Pangburn M. Formation of high-affinity C5 convertases of the alternative pathway of complement. *J Immunol* 2001; 166(4): 2635–42.

111. Pickering MC, Warren J, Rose KL, Carlucci F, Wang Y, Walport MJ, Cook HT, and Botto M. Prevention of C5 activation ameliorates spontaneous and experimental glomerulonephritis in factor H-deficient mice. *Proc Natl Acad Sci U S A* 2006; 103(25): 9649–54.

112. Levidiotis V, Freeman C, Tikellis C, Cooper ME, and Power DA. Heparanase is involved in the pathogenesis of proteinuria as a result of glomerulonephritis. *J Am Soc Nephrol* 2004; 15(1): 68–78.

113. Levidiotis V, Freeman C, Tikellis C, Cooper ME, and Power DA. Heparanase inhibition reduces proteinuria in a model of accelerated anti-glomerular basement membrane antibody disease. *Nephrology (Carlton)* 2005; 10(2): 167–73.

114. Kleinknecht D, Kourilsky O, Morel-Maroger L, Adhemar JP, Droz D, Masselot JP, and Adam C. Dense deposit disease with rapidly progressive renal failure in a narcotic addict. *Clin Nephrol* 1980; 14(6): 309–12.

115. Schena FP, Pertosa G, Stanziale P, Vox E, Pecoraro C, and Andreucci VE. Biological significance of the C3 nephritic factor in membranoproliferative glomerulonephritis. *Clin Nephrol* 1982; 18(5): 240–6.

116. Braun MC, Stablein DM, Hamiwka LA, Bell L, Bartosh SM, and Strife CF. Recurrence of membranoproliferative glomerulonephritis type II in renal allografts: The North American Pediatric Renal Transplant Cooperative Study experience. *J Am Soc Nephrol* 2005; 16(7): 2225–33.

117. Smith RJ, Alexander J, Barlow PN, Botto M, Cassavant TL, Cook HT, de Cordoba SR, Hageman GS, Jokiranta TS, Kimberling WJ, Lambris JD, Lanning LD, Levidiotis V, Licht C, Lutz HU, Meri S, Pickering MC, Quigg RJ, Rops AL, Salant DJ, Sethi S, Thurman JM, Tully HF, Tully SP, van der Vlag J, Walker PD, Wurzner R, and Zipfel PF. New approaches to the treatment of dense deposit disease. *J Am Soc Nephrol* 2007; 18(9): 2447–56.

118. Churg J, and Sobin L, . Classification of glomerulonephritis, in *Renal Disease Classification and Atlas of Glomerular Diseases*. J. Churg, J. Bernstein, and R. Glassock, Eds. 1995, Igaku-Shoin: Tokyo. p. 3–19.

119. Jennette JC. Rapidly progressive crescentic glomerulonephritis. *Kidney Int* 2003; 63(3): 1164–77.

120. Thorner PS, Ho M, Eremina V, Sado Y, and Quaggin S. Podocytes contribute to the formation of glomerular crescents. *J Am Soc Nephrol* 2008; 19(3): 495–502.

121. Tipping PG and Kitching AR. Glomerulonephritis, Th1 and Th2: what's new? *Clin Exp Immunol* 2005; 142(2): 207–15.

122. Stilmant MM, Bolton WK, Sturgill BC, Schmitt GW, and Couser WG. Crescentic glomerulonephritis without immune deposits: clinicopathologic features. *Kidney Int* 1979; 15(2): 184–95.

123. Falk RJ and Jennette JC. Anti-neutrophil cytoplasmic autoantibodies with specificity for myeloperoxidase in patients with systemic vasculitis and idiopathic necrotizing and crescentic glomerulonephritis. *N Engl J Med* 1988; 318(25): 1651–7.

124. Savige J, Davies D, Falk RJ, Jennette JC, and Wiik A. Antineutrophil cytoplasmic antibodies and associated diseases: a review of the clinical and laboratory features. *Kidney Int* 2000; 57(3): 846–62.

125. Hauer HA, Bajema IM, van Houwelingen HC, Ferrario F, Noel LH, Waldherr R, Jayne DR, Rasmussen N, Bruijn JA, and Hagen EC. Renal histology in ANCA-associated vasculitis: differences between diagnostic and serologic subgroups. *Kidney Int* 2002; 61(1): 80–9.

126. Samarkos M, Loizou S, Vaiopoulos G, and Davies KA. The clinical spectrum of primary renal vasculitis. *Semin Arthritis Rheum* 2005; 35(2): 95–111.

127. Woodworth TG, Abuelo JG, Austin HA, 3rd, and Esparza A. Severe glomerulonephritis with late emergence of classic Wegener's granulomatosis. Report of 4 cases and review of the literature. *Medicine (Baltimore)* 1987; 66(3): 181–91.

128. Malenica B, Rudolf M, and Kozmar A. Antineutrophil cytoplasmic antibodies (ANCA): diagnostic utility and potential role in the pathogenesis of vasculitis. *Acta Dermatovenerol Croat* 2004; 12(4): 294–313.

129. Ferrario F and Rastaldi MP. Histopathological atlas of renal diseases: ANCA-associated vasculitis (first part). *J Nephrol* 2005; 18(2): 113–6.

130. Jennette JC and Falk RJ. Nosology of primary vasculitis. *Curr Opin Rheumatol* 2007; 19(1): 10–6.

131. Jennette JC, Xiao H, and Falk RJ. Pathogenesis of vascular inflammation by anti-neutrophil cytoplasmic antibodies. *J Am Soc Nephrol* 2006; 17(5): 1235–42.

132. Morgan MD, Harper L, Williams J, and Savage C. Antineutrophil cytoplasm-associated glomerulonephritis. *J Am Soc Nephrol* 2006; 17(5): 1224–34.

133. Langford CA and Balow JE. New insights into the immunopathogenesis and treatment of small vessel vasculitis of the kidney. *Curr Opin Nephrol Hypertens* 2003; 12(3): 267–72.

134. Jennette JC and Falk RJ. New insight into the pathogenesis of vasculitis associated with antineutrophil cytoplasmic autoantibodies. *Curr Opin Rheumatol* 2008; 20(1): 55–60.

135. Lionaki S, Jennette JC, and Falk RJ. Anti-neutrophil cytoplasmic (ANCA) and anti-glomerular basement membrane (GBM) autoantibodies in necrotizing and crescentic glomerulonephritis. *Semin Immunopathol* 2007; 29(4): 459–74.

136. Little MA and Pusey CD. Glomerulonephritis due to anti-neutrophil cytoplasmic antibody-associated vasculitis: an update on approaches to management. *Nephrology (Carlton)* 2005; 10(4): 368–76.

137. Feldmann M and Pusey CD. Is there a role for TNF-alpha in anti-neutrophil cytoplasmic antibody-associated vasculitis? Lessons from other chronic inflammatory diseases. *J Am Soc Nephrol* 2006; 17(5): 1243–52.

138. Sanders JS, Stassen PM, van Rossum AP, Kallenberg CG, and Stegeman CA. Risk factors for relapse in anti-neutrophil cytoplasmic antibody (ANCA)-associated vasculitis: tools for treatment decisions? *Clin Exp Rheumatol* 2004; 22(6 Suppl. 36): S94-101.

139. Alexopoulos E, Gionanlis L, Papayianni E, Kokolina E, Leontsini M, and Memmos D. Predictors of outcome in idiopathic rapidly progressive glomerulonephritis (IRPGN). *BMC Nephrol* 2006; 7: 16.

140. Chen M, Yu F, Wang SX, Zou WZ, Zhao MH, and Wang HY. Antineutrophil cytoplasmic autoantibody-negative Pauci-immune crescentic glomerulonephritis. *J Am Soc Nephrol* 2007; 18(2): 599–605.

141. Jayne DR, Gaskin G, Rasmussen N, Abramowicz D, Ferrario F, Guillevin L, Mirapeix E, Savage CO, Sinico RA, Stegeman CA, Westman KW, van der Woude FJ, de Lind van Wijngaarden RA, and Pusey CD. Randomized trial of plasma exchange or high-dosage methylprednisolone as adjunctive therapy for severe renal vasculitis. *J Am Soc Nephrol* 2007; 18(7): 2180–8.

142. de Lind van Wijngaarden RA, Hauer HA, Wolterbeek R, Jayne DR, Gaskin G, Rasmussen N, Noel LH, Ferrario F, Waldherr R, Bruijn JA, Bajema IM, Hagen EC, and Pusey CD. Chances of renal recovery for dialysis-dependent ANCA-associated glomerulonephritis. *J Am Soc Nephrol* 2007; 18(7): 2189–97.

143. Goodpasture WE. The significance of certain pulmonary lesions in relation to the etiology of influenzae. *Am J Med Sci* 1919; 158: 863–70.

144. Martinez JS and Kohler PF. Variant "Goodpasture's syndrome"? The need for immunologic criteria in rapidly progressive glomerulonephritis and hemorrhagic pneumonitis. *Ann Intern Med* 1971; 75(1): 67–76.

145. Savage CO, Pusey CD, Bowman C, Rees AJ, and Lockwood CM. Antiglomerular basement membrane antibody mediated disease in the British Isles 1980-4. *Br Med J (Clin Res Ed)* 1986; 292(6516): 301–4.

146. Saraf P, Berger HW, and Thung SN. Goodpasture's syndrome with no overt renal disease. *Mt Sinai J Med* 1978; 45(4): 451–4.

147. Daly C, Conlon PJ, Medwar W, and Walshe JJ. Characteristics and outcome of anti-glomerular basement membrane disease: a single-center experience. *Ren Fail* 1996; 18(1): 105–12.

148. Qunibi WY, Taylor K, Knight TF, Senekjian HO, Gyorkey F, and Weinman EJ. Nephrotic syndrome in antiGBM antibody mediated glomerulonephritis. *South Med J* 1979; 72(11): 1396–8.

149. Knoll G, Rabin E, and Burns BF. Antiglomerular basement membrane antibody-mediated nephritis with normal pulmonary and renal function. A case report and review of the literature. *Am J Nephrol* 1993; 13(6): 494–6.

150. Wu MJ, Rajaram R, Shelp WD, Beirne GJ, and Burkholder PM. Vasculitis in Goodpasture's syndrome. *Arch Pathol Lab Med* 1980; 104(6): 300–2.

151. Kurki P, Helve T, von Bonsdorff M, Tornroth T, Pettersson E, Riska H, and Miettinen A. Transformation of membranous glomerulonephritis into crescentic glomerulonephritis with glomerular basement membrane antibodies. Serial determinations of antiGBM before the transformation. *Nephron* 1984; 38(2): 134–7.

152. Pettersson E, Tornroth T, and Miettinen A. Simultaneous anti-glomerular basement membrane and membranous glomerulonephritis: case report and literature review. *Clin Immunol Immunopathol* 1984; 31(2): 171–80.

153. Jennette JC, Lamanna RW, Burnette JP, Wilkman AS, and Iskander SS. Concurrent antiglomerular basement membrane antibody and immune complex mediated glomerulonephritis. *Am J Clin Pathol* 1982; 78(3): 381–6.

154. Leatherman JW, Sibley RK, and Davies SF. Diffuse intrapulmonary hemorrhage and glomerulonephritis unrelated to anti-glomerular basement membrane antibody. *Am J Med* 1982; 72(3): 401–10.

155. Lerner RA, Glassock RJ, and Dixon FJ. The role of antiglomerular basement membrane antibody in the pathogenesis of human glomerulonephritis. *J Exp Med* 1967; 126(6): 989–1004.

156. Borza DB. Autoepitopes and alloepitopes of type IV collagen: role in the molecular pathogenesis of antiGBM antibody glomerulonephritis. *Nephron Exp Nephrol* 2007; 106(2): e37–43.

157. Borza DB, Bondar O, Colon S, Todd P, Sado Y, Neilson EG, and Hudson BG. Goodpasture autoantibodies unmask cryptic epitopes by selectively dissociating autoantigen complexes lacking structural reinforcement: novel mechanisms for immune privilege and autoimmune pathogenesis. *J Biol Chem* 2005; 280(29): 27147–54.

158. Bolton WK, Innes DJ, Jr., Sturgill BC, and Kaiser DL. T-cells and macrophages in rapidly progressive glomerulonephritis: clinicopathologic correlations. *Kidney Int* 1987; 32(6): 869–76.

159. Reynolds J, Tam FW, Chandraker A, Smith J, Karkar AM, Cross J, Peach R, Sayegh MH, and Pusey CD. CD28-B7 blockade prevents the development of experimental autoimmune glomerulonephritis. *J Clin Invest* 2000; 105(5): 643–51.

160. Huey B, McCormick K, Capper J, Ratliff C, Colombe BW, Garovoy MR, and Wilson CB. Associations of HLA-DR and HLA-DQ types with antiGBM nephritis by sequence-specific oligonucleotide probe hybridization. *Kidney Int* 1993; 44(2): 307–12.

161. Levy JB, Turner AN, Rees AJ, and Pusey CD. Long-term outcome of antiglomerular basement membrane antibody disease treated with plasma exchange and immunosuppression. *Ann Intern Med* 2001; 134(11): 1033–42.

162. Jones DA, Jennette JC, and Falk RJ. Goodpasture's syndrome revisited. A new perspective on glomerulonephritis and alveolar hemorrhage. *N C Med J* 1990; 51(8): 411–5.

163. Lee RW and D'Cruz DP. Novel Therapies for anti-neutrophil cytoplasmic antibody-associated vasculitis. *Drugs* 2008; 68(6): 747–770.

164. Srivastava RN, Moudgil A, Bagga A, Vasudev AS, Bhuyan UN, and Sundraem KR. Crescentic glomerulonephritis in children: a review of 43 cases. *Am J Nephrol* 1992; 12(3): 155–61.

165. Jindal KK. Management of idiopathic crescentic and diffuse proliferative glomerulonephritis: evidence-based recommendations. *Kidney Int Suppl* 1999; 70: S33–40.

CHAPTER 7

Systemic Lupus Erythematosus and Other Autoimmune Diseases (Mixed Connective Tissue Disease, Rheumatoid Arthritis, and Sjogren's Syndrome)

Michael B. Stokes MD, Samih H. Nasr MD, and Vivette D. D'Agati MD

SYSTEMIC LUPUS ERYTHEMATOSUS

Introduction

Systemic lupus erythematosus (SLE) is an autoimmune disease of unknown etiology characterized by inflammation of multiple organ systems including joints, skin, serosal membranes, central nervous system, and kidney. The American College of Rheumatology has identified eleven cardinal features of SLE: malar rash, discoid rash, photosensitivity, oral ulcers, nondeforming arthritis, serositis, renal disease (defined as persistent proteinuria ≥500 mg/day or 3+ by dipstick, or cellular casts of any kind), neurologic disease, hematologic disorders (including hemolytic anemia, leukopenia, lymphopenia, or thrombocytopenia), immunologic disorders [including antidouble-stranded DNA (dsDNA) antibody, anti-Smith antibody test, antiphospholipid antibody, lupus anticoagulant, or false-positive Venereal Disease Research Laboratories (VDRL)] and positive antinuclear antibody (ANA) test [1]. Development of any four of these features, either simultaneously or sequentially, is highly sensitive and specific for a diagnosis of SLE

Clinically apparent renal disease (lupus nephritis) occurs in up to 50 percent of SLE patients, usually within the first year of disease onset, and is a major cause of morbidity and mortality [2]. Renal disease also occurs, albeit less frequently, in other autoimmune diseases, including mixed connective tissue disease (MCTD), rheumatoid arthritis (RA), and Sjogren's syndrome.

Epidemiology and Clinical Presentation

The reported prevalence of SLE ranges from 4 to 250 cases per 100,000, reflecting the impact of geographic and demographic variables and different criteria for defining SLE in different studies. SLE is more common among women of reproductive age (female to male ratio approximately 10:1) with less pronounced female predominance in childhood and older age. In the United States, SLE is more common among women of African and Asian descent compared to Caucasians. Lupus nephritis may affect SLE patients at any age but tends to be more prevalent and more severe in children, in males and in individuals of African descent.

The clinical manifestations of SLE-associated renal disease are extremely diverse, ranging from asymptomatic hematuria and proteinuria to full nephrotic syndrome and rapidly progressive renal failure. Renal disease usually develops within the first year of SLE onset but may occur at any time. The pathologic manifestations of renal disease in SLE patients are similarly heterogeneous (Table 7.1). However, most patients have immune complex-mediated glomerular disease (lupus nephritis), with variable tubulointerstitial and vascular lesions. An algorithm for classification of glomerular disease in lupus patients based on pathologic findings is provided in Table 7.2.

A minority of lupus patients present with tubulointerstitial or vascular disease (usually associated with immune complex deposits), without glomerular lesions. Renal disease without immune deposits in SLE patients is termed nonlupus nephritis. Silent lupus nephritis refers to the presence of glomerular immune deposits and pathologic abnormalities in patients who lack clinical evidence of renal disease.

Table 7.1 Spectrum of Renal Disease in SLE

Glomerular immune deposits (lupus nephritis)
Minimal mesangial lupus nephritis
Mesangial proliferative lupus nephritis
Focal lupus nephritis
Diffuse lupus nephritis (diffuse segmental or diffuse global)
Membranous lupus nephritis
Advanced sclerosing lupus nephritis
Tubulointerstitial immune deposits[a]
Tubulointerstitial nephritis
Vascular lesions[a]
Uncomplicated vascular immune deposits
Lupus vasculopathy
Necrotizing arteritis
Thrombotic microangiopathy
Non-lupus nephritis (no immune deposits)
Minimal change disease
Focal segmental glomerulosclerosis (FSGS)
Thin basement membrane disease
Hypertensive arterionephrosclerosis
Amyloidosis
Acute allergic interstitial nephritis

[a] Tubulointerstitial and vascular immune deposits usually coexist with glomerular immune deposits.

In most patients with lupus nephritis, the diagnosis of SLE will already have been established by clinical and laboratory criteria prior to the renal biopsy. Thus, the primary purpose of the renal biopsy is to determine the class and activity of renal disease and to guide the choice of therapy. Transformations between different clinical and pathologic forms of lupus nephritis are not uncommon, both spontaneously and following therapy and repeat renal biopsy plays an important role in monitoring the course of lupus nephritis.

Spectrum of Renal Pathologic Findings

Lupus nephritis may involve all renal compartments, including glomeruli, tubules, interstitium, and blood vessels. Many types of lesions may occur in lupus nephritis and some apply to more than one class. Therefore, a general description of the spectrum of glomerular findings is presented here, with more specific description of the individual classes to follow in the next section.

Light Microscopy

For each glomerulus, the presence of increased cellularity and its location within the glomerular tuft, that is, whether mesangial, endocapillary or extracapillary, is determined. Mesangial hypercellularity, defined as three or more cells per mesangial stalk region in 3 μm sections in areas away from the vascular pole, is a common finding in classes II through V. Mesangial hypercellularity, often accompanied by mesangial immune deposits, can be considered the substratum on which the higher classes are built.

Endocapillary hypercellularity is characterized by luminal attenuation by infiltrating leukocytes (including neutrophils, monocytes, and/or lymphocytes) and proliferation of indigenous endothelial and mesangial cells. Extracapillary hypercellularity

Table 7.2 Algorithm for Classification of Glomerular Disease in SLE

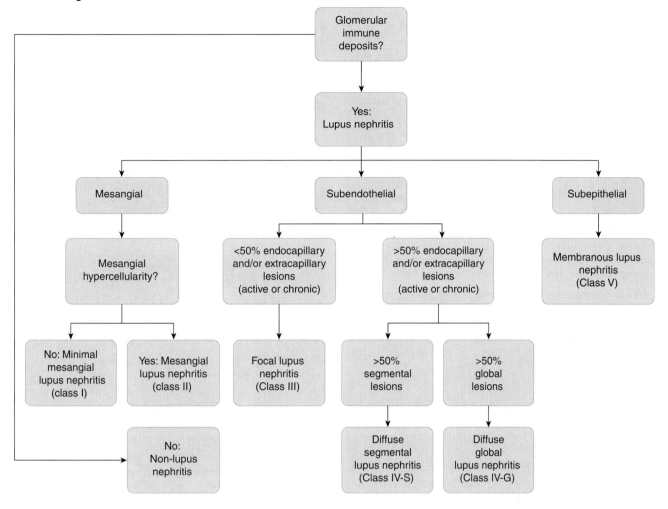

(crescent formation) is defined as a proliferation of two or more cell layers occupying at least 25 percent of Bowman's space. The distribution of endocapillary and extracapillary hypercellularity within the biopsy may be either focal (<50 percent glomeruli affected) or diffuse (>50 percent glomeruli affected). The extent of endocapillary hypercellularity within each affected glomerulus may be segmental (involving <50 percent of the glomerular tuft) or global (involving >50 percent of the glomerular tuft).

In active class III and IV lupus nephritis, a common finding is the necrotizing glomerular lesion. Histologic characteristics of the necrotizing lesion, which may be present in varying combinations, include endocapillary fibrin (termed fibrinoid necrosis), rupture of glomerular basement membrane, and apoptosis of the infiltrating leukocytes producing pyknotic or karyorrhectic nuclear debris. Immune deposits may be visible by light microscopy in mesangial, subendothelial, or subepithelial sites and characteristically stain fuchsinophilic (red) with the trichrome stain and eosinophilic with H&E and Jones methenamine silver stains. Large subendothelial deposits that extend along broad segments of glomerular capillary wall impart a thickened glassy

appearance to the glomerular basement membrane forming "wire loops" (Figures 7.1 to 7.3). In some areas, the large subendothelial deposits may be incorporated into the glomerular capillary wall by a subendothelial layer of neomembrane, producing a double contour. Large subendothelial deposits that bulge into the capillary lumen may form intraluminal immune aggregates termed "hyaline thrombi" (Figures 7.2 and 7.3). This term is a misnomer because the intraluminal material does not represent true fibrin thrombi, but rather immune deposits with similar composition by immunofluorescence and electron microscopy as the adjacent subendothelial deposits. In areas of active proliferation, true fibrin also may accumulate; it stains more darkly eosinophilic and exhibits a more granular/fibrillar texture than the more homogeneous immune deposits.

Hematoxylin bodies are a rare but distinctive feature of lupus nephritis (Figure 7.4). These smudgy, lilac-colored structures represent naked nuclei (probably derived from infiltrating leukocytes) that have been extruded following cell death. The binding of antinuclear antibodies to these nuclei results in coarse chromatin clumping and increased basophilia, producing a

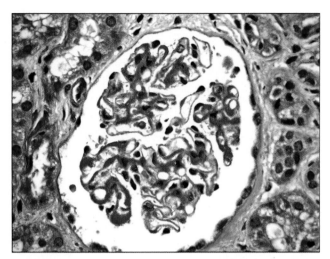

FIGURE 7.1: *Lupus nephritis class IV. Trichrome stain reveals global, wire-loop, red subendothelial immune deposits. There is no mesangial or endocapillary hypercellularity (×400).*

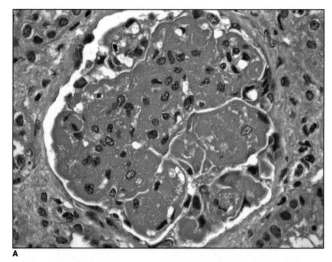

A

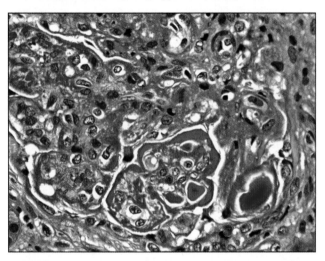

FIGURE 7.2: *Lupus nephritis class IV. The glomerular capillary walls are segmentally thickened by large, wire-loop subendothelial red deposits. Multiple, large intraluminal red immune deposits "hyaline thrombi" are also present. The glomerular capillary lumina are narrowed by moderate endocapillary and mesangial hypercellularity. (Trichrome stain, ×600).*

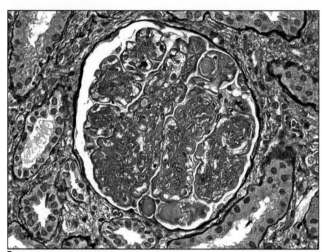

B

FIGURE 7.3: *Lupus nephritis class IV. Glomeruli are obliterated by massive mesangial, wire-loop subendothelial, and intraluminal immune deposits that stain hypereosinophilic on H&E stain (A, ×400) and red on JMS stain (B, ×400).*

hematoxylin (or "LE") body. Hematoxylin bodies are usually seen in the setting of active endocapillary proliferative (class III or IV) disease, but are rarely encountered in modern biopsy material.

In membranous forms of lupus nephritis, glomerular basement membranes may be thickened due to the presence of subepithelial immune deposits accompanied by intervening basement membrane "spikes." Jones methenamine silver stain best demonstrates the argyrophilic spikes and intervening eosinophilic subepithelial deposits.

As lupus nephritis evolves to chronicity in class III, IV, and V, glomeruli typically develop segmental or global glomerulosclerosis. These lesions should be examined closely for evidence of old inflammatory injury, such as fibrous crescents, disruption of Bowman's capsule, residual hypercellularity, or leukocyte infiltration. The International Society of Nephrology (ISN)

and Renal Pathology Society (RPS) classification requires that both proliferative and sclerosing glomerular lesions (attributed to postinflammatory scarring) be taken into account when determining the overall percentage of glomeruli affected by lupus nephritis. Wherever possible, globally sclerotic glomeruli attributed to ischemic sclerosis (such as due to aging or arteriosclerosis), which are more common in the subcapsular region, should be excluded from consideration.

Tubulointerstitial and vascular findings include interstitial inflammation, tubular atrophy, interstitial fibrosis, arteriosclerosis, vascular immune deposits, thrombosis and arteritis. These lesions should be graded semiquantitatively (absent, mild, moderate, or severe), based on the extent of tissue involvement.

Immunofluorescence Microscopy

Immunofluorescence microscopy (IF) staining should include a panel of antibodies to detect immunoglobulin (Ig) classes IgG,

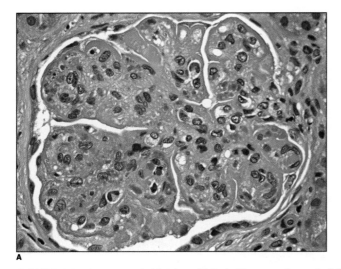
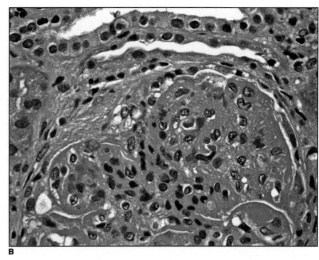

A   B

FIGURE 7.4:   Lupus nephritis class IV-G. A. Clusters of rounded, lilac-staining hematoxylin bodies are present in multiple glomerular capillaries. There is a background of global endocapillary hypercellularity and abundant hypereosinophilic mesangial and wire-loop subendothelial deposits (H&E, x400). B. The rounded, smudgy, basophilic hematoxylin bodies contrast with the massive, hypereosinophilic mesangial, subendothelial, and intraluminal immune deposits that obliterate the glomerular capillaries (H&E, × 600).

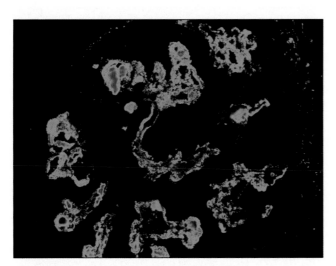

FIGURE 7.5:   Lupus nephritis class IV. The immunofluorescence micrograph shows heavy, global C1q deposits in glomerular capillary walls and lumina (× 400).

IgM, and IgA, kappa and lambda light chains, and complement C3 and C1q components. In addition, staining for fibrinogen may identify necrotizing lesions and fibrin thrombi. Immune deposits typically stain strongest for IgG, with frequent codeposition of other immunoglobulin classes (IgM and IgA), C3 and C1q. "Full-house" staining of immune deposits for all three immunoglobulin classes (IgG, IgM, and IgA) and both C3 and C1q is highly characteristic of lupus nephritis (Figure 7.5). Subendothelial peripheral capillary wall deposits may be comma-shaped and display a smooth outer contour, whereas subepithelial deposits are more punctate and granular.

Wire-loop deposits and intraluminal hyaline thrombi typically appear ring-shaped and globular, respectively. Immune deposits are also commonly identified in the tubulointerstitial and vascular compartments, where they may involve tubular basement membranes (TBM), interstitial capillary walls, inter-

stitial collagen, arterial intima, and media. Rarely, extraglomerular immune deposits are present without glomerular deposits.

Nuclei may show staining for IgG ("tissue ANA"), reflecting binding of ambient ANA to nuclei that have been exposed during the course of cryosectioning (Figure 7.6). Of note, tissue ANA does not correlate with disease activity and may be found in any class of lupus nephritis. Importantly, strong tissue ANA (particularly speckled patterns) may obscure or mimic the presence of immune deposits, emphasizing the importance of correlation with electron microscopy findings.

Electron Microscopy

Discrete electron-dense deposits are seen at sites in electron microscopy (EM) corresponding to IF findings. Virtually all cases of lupus nephritis demonstrate mesangial deposits. The deposits in lupus nephritis are usually uniformly granular but may display an organized substructure consisting of "finger print," lattice-like, microtubular (Figure 7.7), or fibrillar arrays. Finger print substructure consists of parallel arrays of band-like structures measuring 10 to 15 nm in diameter (Figure 7.8). These arrays are usually curved, resembling human fingerprints, but may be straight or tubular. Organized deposits may be associated with a circulating type III mixed cryoglobulin.

A common ultrastructural finding in lupus biopsies is the presence of intracellular tubuloreticular inclusions (TRI), usually in endothelial cells and rarely in glomerular epithelial and mesangial cells. TRI consist of interanastamosing tubular structures that measure 23 nm in external diameter and are located in the dilated cisternae of endoplasmic reticulum (Figure 7.9). TRI are also encountered following interferon therapy and in the setting of human immunosufficiency virus (HIV) infection and other retroviral infections and may represent a response to elevated interferon levels in the circulation ("interferon footprints"). Podocyte foot process effacement generally

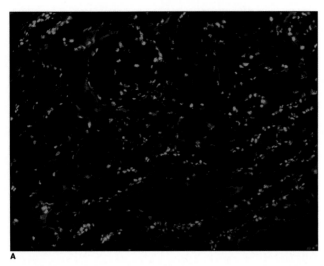
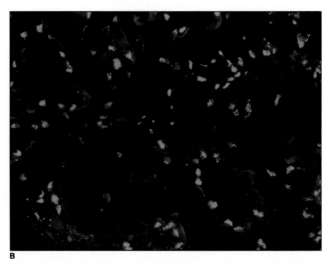

A   B

FIGURE 7.6:   Lupus nephritis class III. There is diffuse speckled staining of tubular epithelial cell nuclei for IgG. This phenomenon referred to as "tissue ANA" may also be seen in other autoimmune diseases associated with high-titer ANA. (Immunofluorescence micrographs; A, ×200; B, ×400).

reflects the extent of peripheral capillary wall injury and immune deposition and correlates roughly with the severity of proteinuria.

Classification of Lupus Nephritis and Clinical-pathologic Correlates

The ISN/RPS classification was introduced in 2003 (Table 7.3) [3]. This classification is based on the original 1974 World Health Organization (WHO) Classification of lupus nephritis, and incorporates some refinements of the two subsequent modifications [4,5]. The classification is based on an integrated evaluation of the glomerular pathologic alterations by light microscopy and IF findings (Table 7.4). Although EM is not required for this classification (so that it can be used in parts of the world where EM is not available), it is highly recommended. Because lesions may be focal and/or segmental, it is important to examine multiple tissue sections with standard histologic stains (H&E, periodic acid Schiff (PAS), trichrome, and silver stain). It is also preferable that the same pathologist evaluate the biopsy by the three modalities. Proper classification requires assessment of the presence of glomerular hypercellularity in mesangial, endocapillary and extracapillary zones and the percentage of glomeruli affected in the context of the distribution (mesangial, subendothelial, and/or subepithelial) of immune deposits by IF and/or EM. Details of the ISN/RPS Classification are provided in Table 7.3 and an abbreviated version is presented in Table 7.5.

Class I (Minimal Mesangial Lupus Nephritis)

Definition. Class I is defined as normal glomeruli by LM with mesangial immune deposits by IF and EM.

Clinical Features. There is usually no clinical evidence of hematuria or proteinuria and renal function is typically normal. However, systemic manifestations of lupus and lupus serologies may be active.

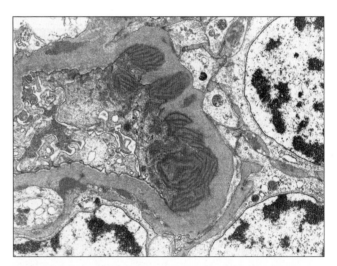

FIGURE 7.7:   Lupus nephritis class III and V. A subepithelial electron-dense deposit exhibits an organized substructure composed of parallel arrays of straight or slightly curved microtubules. Several small, non-organized electron dense subendothelial deposits are also present. (Electron micrograph, ×8,000).

Renal Biopsy Findings. Light microscopy reveals normal appearing glomeruli, with no significant hypercellularity (Figure 7.10) but IF microscopy shows mesangial immune deposits (Figure 7.11). EM usually reveals small immune type, electron-dense deposits confined to the mesangial regions. Podocyte foot process effacement is generally minimal. ISN/RPS Class I lupus nephritis corresponds to class IIa in the original WHO classification and class Ib lupus nephritis in the 1982 modified WHO classification [4].

Class II (Mesangial Proliferative Lupus Nephritis)

Definition. Class II is defined as pure mesangial hypercellularity of any degree and/or mesangial matrix expansion by light microscopy with mesangial immune deposits detectable by IF and EM.

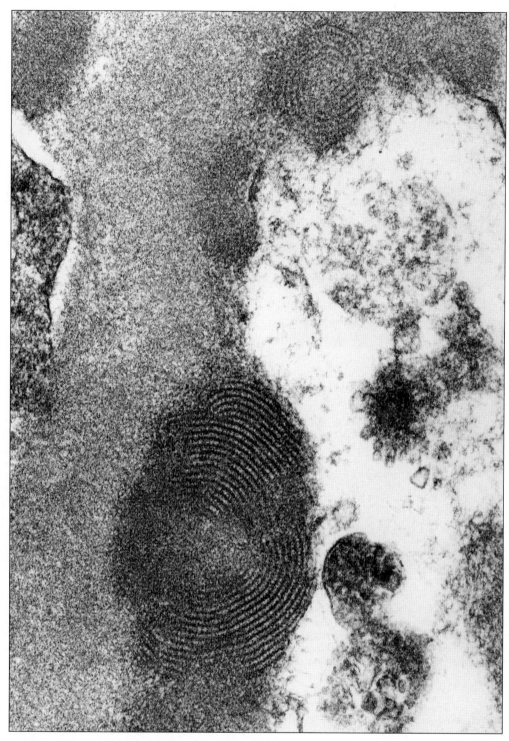

FIGURE 7.8: *A subendothelial electron-dense deposit with a fingerprint substructure. (Electron micrograph, × 40,000).*

Clinical Features. Most patients have no or only mild clinical renal abnormalities. Fewer than 50 percent of patients have mild hematuria or proteinuria, which generally does not exceed 1 gram per day. Renal function tests are usually normal although up to 15 percent of patients may have mildly reduced creatinine clearance. The presence of heavy proteinuria, active urinary sediment, or renal insufficiency may indicate superimposed non-lupus related glomerular disease. The nephrotic syndrome is virtually never observed unless there is a superimposed podocytopathy (vide infra).

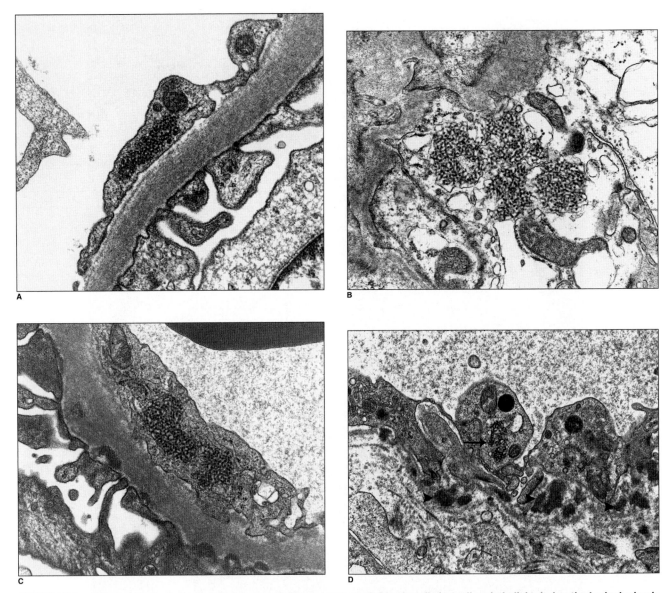

FIGURE 7.9: *Tubuloreticular inclusions in lupus nephritis. A. lupus nephritis class II. A small endothelial tubuloreticular inclusion is present in this glomerular endothelial cell. B. Lupus nephritis class IV. A large endothelial tubuloreticular inclusion in a glomerular endothelial cell is seen. C. Lupus nephritis class V. Glomerular endothelial tubuloreticular inclusions as well as several small electron-dense subepithelial immune deposits are shown. D. Lupus nephritis class IV. The micrograph depicts a portion of peritubular capillary. The arrow highlights a small endothelial tubuloreticular inclusion. Several electron-dense immune deposits involving the interstitial capillary basement membrane are present (arrowheads). (Electron micrographs; A–C, ×20,000; D, ×15,000).*

Despite the relatively mild and inactive glomerulonephritis, serologic tests for SLE may be strongly positive in up to 25 percent of cases.

Renal Biopsy Findings. Light microscopy shows mesangial hypercellularity, defined as ≥3 cells in a mesangial region in 3-μm thick sections, in areas away from the vascular pole (Figures 7.12 and 7.13). Mesangial hypercellularity is generally mild to moderate but occasionally may be severe. Immune deposits are seen by IF and/or EM microscopy, and rarely by light microscopy, in the mesangium (Figures 7.14 to 7.17). Rare minute subendothelial immune deposits extending out from the mesangium or paramesangial region may be seen by IF or EM. However, the presence of subendothelial peripheral capillary wall deposits that are visible by light microscopy is incompatible with class II and warrants classification as focal or diffuse lupus nephritis (class III or class IV), depending on the percentage of glomeruli affected.

Differential Diagnosis. This includes IgA nephropathy, Henoch-Schonlein purpura nephritis, mild membranoproliferative glomerulonephritis, and early or resolving acute postinfectious glomerulonephritis. By definition, IgA nephropathy

Table 7.3 ISN/RPS Classification of Lupus Nephritis (LN)

Class I	*Minimal mesangial LN* Normal glomeruli by LM, but mesangial immune deposits by IF
Class II	*Mesangial proliferative LN* Purely mesangial hypercellularity of any degree or mesangial matrix expansion by LM, with mesangial immune deposits. There may be a few isolated subepithelial or subendothelial deposits visible by IF or EM, but not by LM.
Class III	*Focal LN[a]* Active or inactive focal, segmental and/or global endo- and/or extracapillary GN involving <50% of all glomeruli, typically with focal subendothelial immune deposits, with or without mesangial alterations. *III (A):* Purely active lesions: focal proliferative LN *III (A/C):* Active and chronic lesions: focal proliferative and sclerosing LN *III (C):* Chronic inactive with glomerular scars: focal sclerosing LN
Class IV	*Diffuse LN[a]* Active or inactive diffuse, segmental and/or global endo- and/or extracapillary GN involving ≥50% of all glomeruli, typically with diffuse subendothelial immune deposits, with or without mesangial alterations. This class is divided into diffuse segmental (IV-S) when > 50% of the involved glomeruli have segmental lesions, and diffuse global (IV-G) when >50% of the involved glomeruli have global lesions. Segmental is defined as a glomerular lesion that involves less than half of the glomerular tuft. *IV-S (A) or IV-G (A):* Purely active lesions: diffuse segmental or global proliferative LN *IV-S (A/C) or IV-G (A/C):* Active and chronic lesions: diffuse segmental or global proliferative and sclerosing LN *IV-S (C) or IV-G (C):* inactive with glomerular scars: diffuse segmental or global sclerosing LN
Class V	*Membranous LN* Global or segmental subepithelial immune deposits or their morphologic sequelae by LM and by IF or EM, with or without mesangial alterations *May occur in combination with III or IV in which case both will be diagnosed; may show advanced sclerosis*
Class VI	*Advanced sclerosing LN* ≥ 90% of glomeruli globally sclerosed without residual activity

[a] Indicate the proportion of glomeruli with active and with sclerotic lesions.

[a] Indicate the proportion of glomeruli with fibrinoid necrosis and with cellular crescents.

[a] Indicate and grade (mild, moderate, severe) tubular atrophy, interstitial inflammation and fibrosis, severity of arteriosclerosis or other vascular lesions.
LM: light microscopy; IF: immunofluorescence microscopy; EM: electron microscopy.

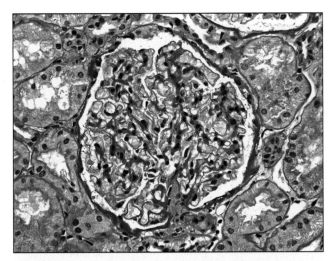

FIGURE 7.10:   *Lupus nephritis class I. The glomerulus is normocellular. There is no mesangial hypercellularity or matrix expansion, and the peripheral capillaries are fully patent. (PAS, ×400).*

FIGURE 7.11:   *Lupus nephritis class I. By immunofluorescence, there is global, granular to semilinear staining for IgG limited to the mesangium (×400).*

Table 7.4 Classification of Lupus Nephritis: Integration of LM, IF, and EM Findings

CLASS	LM		IF		EM		
	MES	PCW	MES	PCW	MES	SENDO	SEPI
I	0	0	+	0	+	0	0
II	+	0	+	0	+	0	0
III	+	+	++	+	++	+	+/-
IV	++	++	++	++	++	++	+/-
V	+	++	+	++	+	+/-	++

MES, mesangial; PCW, peripheral capillary wall; SENDO, subendothelial;

SEPI, subepithelial; LM, light microscopic abnormalities; IF, immunofluorescence location of deposits; EM, electron microscopic location of deposits.

Table 7.5 Abbreviated ISN/RPS Classification of Lupus Nephritis

Class I	Minimal mesangial lupus nephritis
Class II	Mesangial proliferative lupus nephritis
Class III	Focal lupus nephritis[a]
Class IV	Diffuse segmental (IV-S)[b] or diffuse global (IV-G) lupus nephritis[b]
Class V	Membranous lupus nephritis[c]
Class VI	Advanced sclerosing lupus nephritis

[a] Indicate the proportion of glomeruli with active or sclerosing lesions.

[b] Indicate the proportion of glomeruli with cellular crescents and/or fibrinoid necrosis.

[c] May coexist with either class III or class IV, in which case both classes are reported.

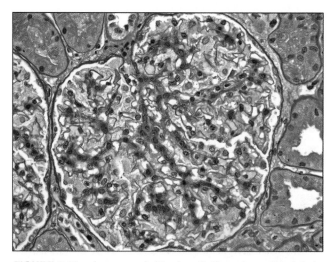

FIGURE 7.13: Lupus nephritis class II. There is a mild global increase in mesangial cell number. The glomerular capillary walls are thin and the peripheral capillaries are patent. (PAS, ×400).

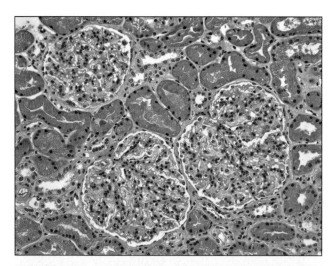

FIGURE 7.12: Lupus nephritis class II. Three glomeruli showing moderate global mesangial hypercellularity. (H&E, ×200).

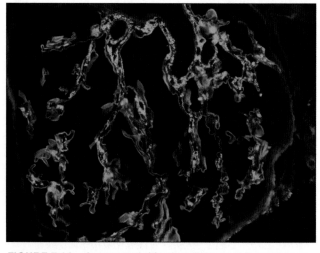

FIGURE 7.14: Lupus nephritis class II. Immunofluorescence microscopy reveals small granular, global mesangial deposits of IgG (×400).

displays dominant or codominant staining for IgA, whereas most cases of lupus nephritis have dominant staining for IgG. Other IF findings in favor of IgA nephropathy are the presence of weak or absent C1q and lambda dominance [6].

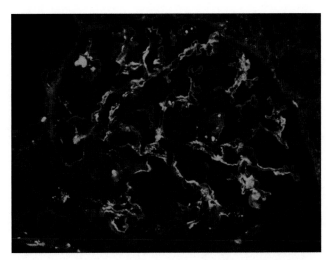

FIGURE 7.15: *Lupus nephritis class II. Another example of LN II showing semilinear, global mesangial deposits of IgG by immunofluorescence (×400).*

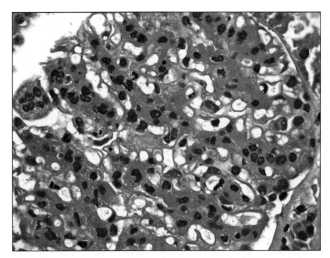

FIGURE 7.17: *Lupus nephritis class III. Rarely, the mesangial deposits are so large that they are visible by light microscopy. The glomerulus pictured here shows global mesangial expansion by glassy, hypereosinophilic immune deposits with less prominent mesangial hypercellularity, and segmental subendothelial deposits. (H&E, ×600).*

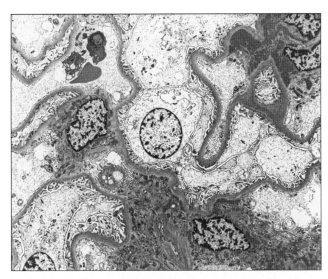

FIGURE 7.16: *Lupus nephritis class II. Abundant electron-dense deposits are present within the expanded mesangium. No deposits involving the peripheral capillary walls are identified. (Electron micrograph, ×2,000).*

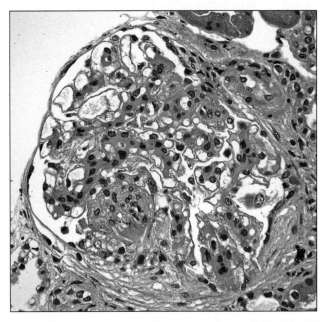

FIGURE 7.18: *Lupus nephritis class III. Lupus nephritis class III with moderate global mesangial hypercellularity, mild segmental endocapillary hypercellularity, and a small fibrocellular crescent. (H&E, ×400).*

Class III (Focal Lupus Nephritis)

Definition. Class III lupus nephritis is defined as active and/or chronic endocapillary and/or extracapillary glomerulonephritis affecting <50 percent of the total glomeruli sampled, with or without mesangial alterations.

Clinical Features. Class III lupus nephritis has a variable clinical picture. Over 50 percent of class III patients demonstrate serologic evidence of active disease, that is, high titer ANA, anti-dsDNA, and hypocomplementemia. However, these serologic findings do not always correlate with the severity of histologic abnormalities. About 50 percent of the patients have active urinary sediment and 25 to 50 percent of the patients

have proteinuria, which may be accompanied by nephrotic syndrome in up to one-third of the patients. Renal insufficiency, however, is uncommon, affecting only 10 to 25 percent of the patients. Hypertension may develop in up to one-third of cases. Patients with more scarred, inactive glomerular lesions have more chronic disease, with more frequent associated hypertension and reduced renal function. Class III with more extensive glomerular involvement (approaching 50 percent), particularly

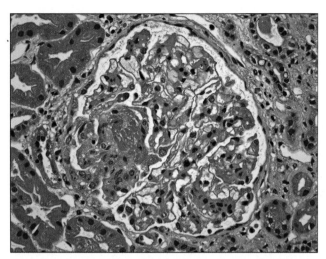

FIGURE 7.19: Lupus nephritis class III. There is segmental fibrinoid necrosis and small crescent formation. A background of global mesangial hypercellularity is present. (H&E, × 400).

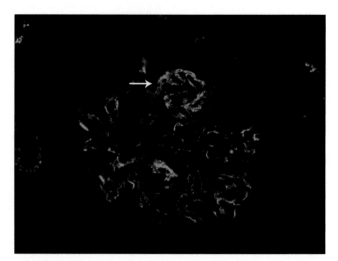

FIGURE 7.21: Lupus nephritis class III. The immunofluorescence micrograph shows IgG deposits segmentally in glomerular capillary walls (arrow) and globally in the mesangium (× 400).

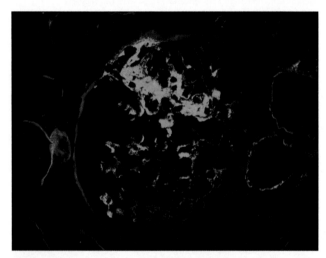

FIGURE 7.20: Lupus nephritis class III. By immunofluorescence, there is heavy segmental deposition of IgG in glomerular capillary walls and lumina. Less heavy deposits are seen in the mesangium of the remaining glomerular segments and focally in tubular basement membranes (× 400).

when accompanied by necrotizing lesions, may behave more like active Class IV lupus nephritis.

Renal Biopsy Findings. Most cases demonstrate segmental endocapillary hypercellularity with or without crescents and necrotizing lesions (Figures 7.18 and 7.19); global lesions are less frequently encountered. Hyaline thrombi and hematoxylin bodies may be present. In some cases, the segmental proliferative component has membranoproliferative features, including mesangial interposition and duplication of glomerular basement membrane. Glomeruli without endocapillary lesions often display background mesangial hypercellularity (Figures 7.18 and 7.19). Chronic lesions of segmental or global glomerulosclerosis may occur. Class III lupus nephritis with exclusively active (A) lesions is designated class III (A), whereas cases with

exclusively chronic (C) lesions are designated class III (C). Those with mixed active and chronic features in any proportion are designated class III (A/C). The degree of acute and chronic tubulointerstitial injury generally correlates with the severity of acute and chronic glomerular changes.

IF and EM display subendothelial peripheral capillary wall immune deposits, usually in a segmental distribution, and virtually always accompanied by mesangial deposits (Figures 7.20 to 7.23). Small subepithelial deposits may be seen. Only if the subepithelial deposits affect >50 percent of the glomerular surface area in at least 50 percent of glomeruli is an additional diagnosis of membranous lupus nephritis (class V) warranted.

Tubulointerstitial and vascular immune deposits may be present. Occasional cases of focal lupus nephritis display relatively sparse immune deposits relative to the degree of necrotizing lesions seen by light microscopy. These cases resemble pauci-immune segmental and necrotizing glomerulonephritis and a subset may be related pathogenetically to antineutrophil cytoplasmic autoantibodies (ANCA) (Figure 7.24) [7].

Differential Diagnosis. This includes IgA nephropathy, Henoch-Schonlein purpura nephritis, pauci-immune focal segmental necrotizing and crescentic glomerulonephritis, endocarditis-associated glomerulonephritis, and other forms of acute postinfectious glomerulonephritis. In pauci-immune focal segmental necrotizing and crescentic glomerulonephritis, the uninvolved glomeruli are usually normocellular whereas most cases of focal lupus nephritis show a background of mesangial hypercellularity.

Class IV (Diffuse Lupus Nephritis)

Definition. Class IV is defined as active and/or chronic endocapillary and/or extracapillary glomerulonephritis involving ≥50 percent of all glomeruli-sampled, typically with subendothelial immune deposits, and usually with mesangial alterations. In determining the overall percentage of glomeruli

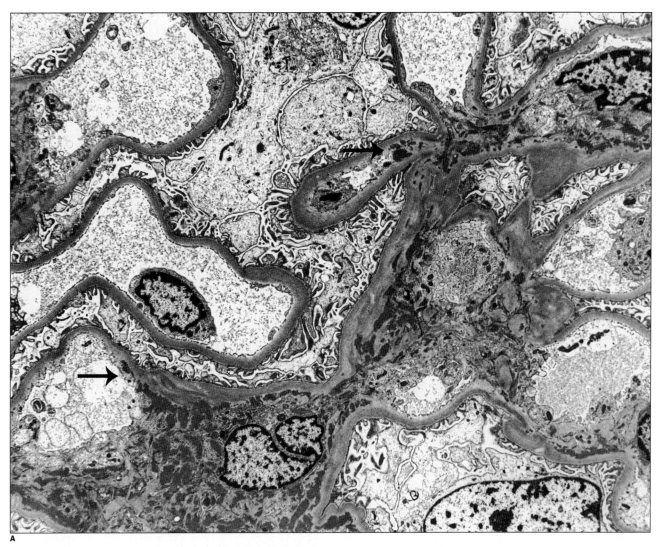

A

FIGURE 7.22: *Lupus nephritis class III. Electron micrographs A and B show abundant electron dense mesangial deposits that focally extend to the subendothelial zone (arrows). (A, ×2,000; B, ×8,000).*

affected, both proliferative and scarred glomeruli should be taken into account. In active forms, the endocapillary lesions are typically proliferative, but may also consist of wire loop type subendothelial deposits without endocapillary proliferation.

Clinical Features. Class IV is associated with the most severe renal presentation. Patients typically have active serologic markers including elevated anti-dsDNA titer and low complements. Nearly 75 percent have active urinary sediment. Hypertension is common and proteinuria is almost universal, in the nephrotic range in up to 50 percent of individuals. Renal insufficiency, however, is detectable in just over half of cases using measurements of GFR, although serum creatinine levels may be in the normal range.

Renal Biopsy Findings. Active diffuse proliferative lupus nephritis may demonstrate leukocyte infiltration, wire loops, and hyaline thrombi, hematoxylin bodies, and necrotizing lesions and crescents in varying combinations (Figures 7.2,

7.3 and 7.25 to 7.27). In some cases, there are membranoproliferative features with mesangial interposition and duplication of glomerular basement membranes (Figure 7.28). The term "diffuse lupus nephritis" was used rather than diffuse proliferative lupus nephritis to allow for endocapillary lesions such as extensive wire loops that may not be accompanied by endocapillary proliferation.

Class IV is subclassified as diffuse segmental lupus nephritis (class IV-S) if >50 percent of affected glomeruli show segmental lesions (Figure 7.29) or diffuse global lupus nephritis (class IV-G) if >50 percent of affected glomeruli show global lesions (Figure 7.30). This more controversial aspect of the classification was introduced to allow multicenter studies with standardized terminology addressing potential differences in outcome between these subgroups.

Cases with chronic proliferative lesions typically progress to segmental or global glomerulosclerosis. Residual features of underlying proliferation (hypercellularity, membranoproliferative changes, or fibrous crescents) may still be identified in these

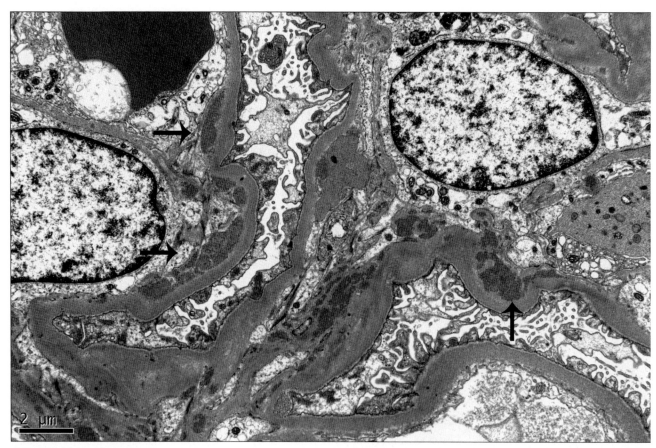

FIGURE 7.22: (continued)

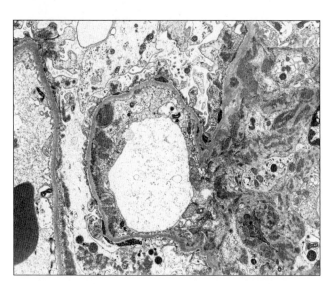

FIGURE 7.23: Lupus nephritis class III. There are electron dense subendothelial and mesangial deposits. The glomerular capillaries are patent. (Electron micrograph, ×5,000).

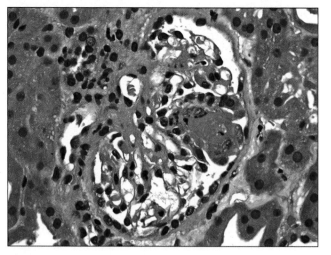

FIGURE 7.24: Lupus nephritis class III with ANCA seropositivity. The biopsy is from a patient with SLE and P-ANCA seropositivity. Light microscopy revealed a glomerular pattern similar to pauci-immune crescentic and necrotizing glomerulonephritis. The glomerulus pictured shows segmental fibrinoid necrosis without associated hypercellularity (H&E, x600). There was "full house" mesangial staining on immunofluorescence. Ultrastructurally, abundant endothelial tubuloreticular inclusions and mesangial deposits, but not subendothelial deposits, were seen. This case likely represents an overlap between lupus nephritis and ANCA necrotizing glomerulonephritis.

scarring glomeruli. Chronic proliferative lesions should be distinguished wherever possible from nonspecific glomerular scarring due to noninflammatory mechanisms of disease progression, age-related glomerular obsolescence, or hypertensive

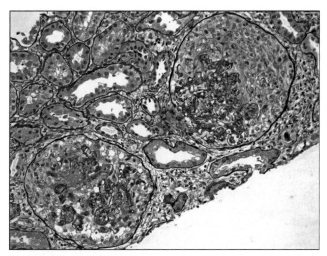

FIGURE 7.25: *Lupus nephritis class IV-G. Two glomeruli exhibit global endocapillary hypercellularity and circumferential cellular crescents. Fibrinoid necrosis is present in the glomerulus at left (JMS, ×200).*

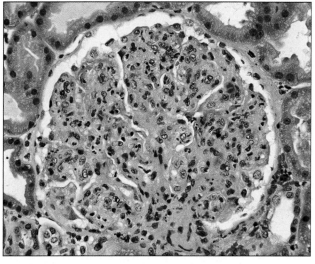

FIGURE 7.27: *Lupus nephritis class IV-G. There is global mesangial and endocapillary hypercellularity including numerous infiltrating neutrophils (H&E, ×500).*

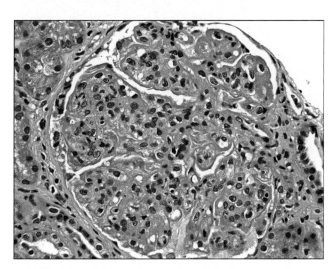

FIGURE 7.26: *Lupus nephritis class IV-G. There is global narrowing of glomerular capillaries by mesangial and endocapillary proliferation. Segmental wire-loop deposits are also present (H&E, ×400).*

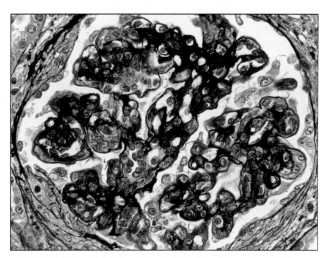

FIGURE 7.28: *Lupus nephritis class IV. Membranoproliferative variant with lobular accentuation, mesangial expansion, and global duplication of the glomerular basement membrane (JMS; ×500).*

arterionephrosclerosis, all of which lack evidence of underlying proliferation.

The percentage of glomeruli with active and chronic proliferative lesions is determined, and the proportion of glomeruli with fibrinoid necrosis and/or cellular crescents is assessed. Class IV with purely active lesions is designated class IV(A), cases with exclusively chronic lesions are designated class IV(C), and those with mixed features are designated class IV (A/C).

The degree of acute and chronic tubulointerstitial injury generally correlates with the severity of acute and chronic glomerular changes. Nonspecific arteriosclerosis is common in patients with hypertension or chronic features. Lupus-related vascular disease is more common in class IV than in the other classes (see "Lupus-Related Vascular Disease").

IF and EM usually reveal diffuse segmental or global subendothelial peripheral capillary wall immune deposits and mesangial deposits (Figures 7.31 to 7.35). As in class III, scattered subepithelial deposits are not uncommon in class IV disease. If the subepithelial deposits affect >50 percent of the glomerular surface area in at least 50 percent of glomeruli, an additional diagnosis of membranous (class V) lupus nephritis is warranted (Figure 7.34).

Tubulointerstitial and vascular immune deposits are not uncommon in class IV. Rare cases of diffuse lupus nephritis display relatively sparse immune deposits relative to the degree of necrotizing lesions seen by light microscopy. These cases resemble pauci-immune segmental and necrotizing glomerulonephritis and some examples may be related pathogenetically to ANCA [7].

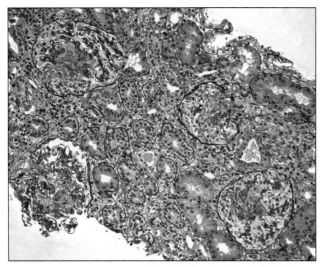

FIGURE 7.29: Lupus nephritis class IV-S. A low-power microscopic view shows diffuse and segmental distribution of cellular crescents. Crescents affected more than 50% of the total glomeruli in this biopsy. (JMS, ×100).

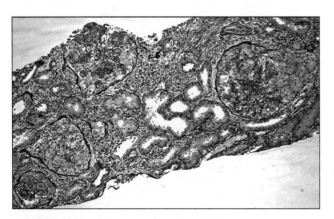

FIGURE 7.30: Lupus nephritis class IV-G. A low-power microscopic view shows diffuse and global distribution of cellular crescents. Crescents affected more than 50% of the total glomeruli in this biopsy. (JMS, ×100).

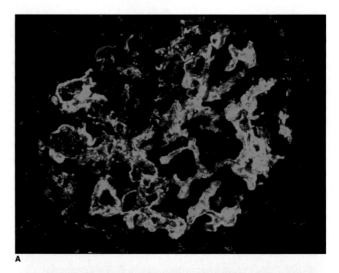

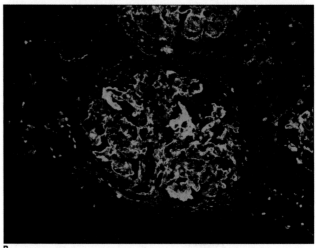

FIGURE 7.31: Lupus nephritis class IV-G. By immunofluorescence, there is intense, global staining for IgG (A) and C1q (B) in the glomerular mesangium and peripheral capillary loops (A, ×400; B, ×200).

Differential Diagnosis. This includes IgA nephropathy, Henoch-Schonlein purpura nephritis, membranoproliferative glomerulonephritis, cryoglobulinemic nephritis, acute postinfectious glomerulonephritis, and pauci-immune focal segmental necrotizing and crescentic glomerulonephritis. "Full-house" IF staining, intense C1q staining, extraglomerular deposits, and abundant endothelial TRI are all features that favor a diagnosis of diffuse lupus nephritis.

Class V (Membranous Lupus Nephritis)

Definition. Class V is defined as global or segmental continuous subepithelial immune deposits or their morphologic sequelae by light microscopy and by IF or EM, with or without mesangial alterations.

Clinical Features. Class V typically presents with heavy proteinuria and nephrotic syndrome. However, up to 40 percent

have subnephrotic proteinuria (<3 g/day) and up to 20 percent have < 1 g/day proteinuria at time of biopsy. Hematuria is detectable in about half of the patients. Active serologies, hypertension, and renal insufficiency are less common than in class III or class IV lupus nephritis. Approximately 50 percent have hypocomplementemia. Renal insufficiency and active urine sediment are more common in combined endocapillary proliferative and membranous (modified WHO class Vc or Vd) lupus nephritis than in pure membranous forms (modified WHO class Va or Vb). Patients may lack extrarenal manifestations and the onset of renal disease may precede the diagnosis of SLE by months or years. Patients with membranous lupus nephritis are at risk of developing renal vein thrombosis and pulmonary emboli [8].

It has long been recognized that patients with membranous lupus nephritis differ significantly from the proliferative classes III and IV with respect to presenting serologic findings and multisystem disease. Up to one-third of patients with Class V

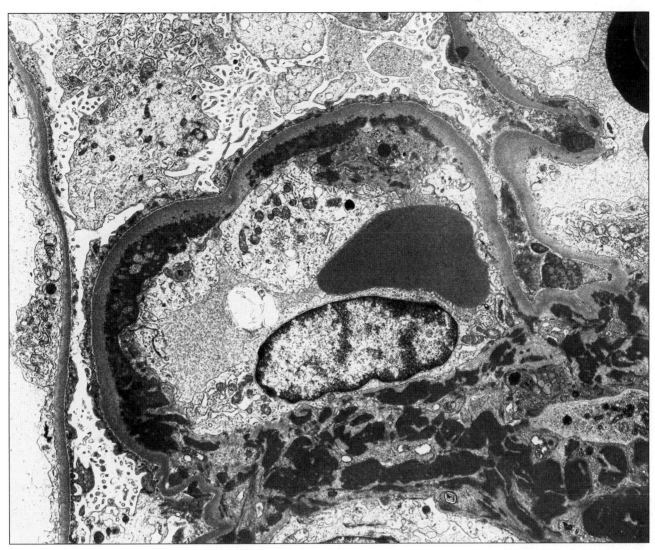

FIGURE 7.32: *Lupus nephritis class IV-G. The electron micrograph shows large circumferential subendothelial electron-dense deposits together with numerous mesangial deposits. Few subepithelial deposits are also present (×3,000).*

lupus nephritis present with isolated renal disease before other systemic manifestations are manifest, and some may be initially ANA negative [9]. Careful attention to pathologic features may help distinguish membranous lupus nephritis form idiopathic membranous glomerulonephritis.

Renal Biopsy Findings. Global or segmental continuous subepithelial capillary wall immune deposits are seen (Figures 7.36 to 7.39). In early stages, there may be no visible thickening of glomerular capillary walls by light microscopy. As the lesions evolve, glomerular basement membrane thickening owing to spike formation is seen. Later lesions may display vacuolation of basement membranes due to incorporation of immune deposits by overlying neomembrane formation. Most, but not all, cases of class V display underlying mesangial alterations (hypercellularity and/or immune deposits) (Figure 7.40). By IF and EM, class V may have sparse small subendothelial immune deposits. However, if subendothelial deposits are sizeable or visible by light microscopy, an additional diagnosis of

class III or class IV lupus nephritis is warranted depending on the percentage of glomeruli affected. As membranous lupus nephritis evolves to chronicity, segmental, or global glomerulosclerosis lesions may develop, without the superimposition of a more proliferative class.

The coexistence of proliferative lesions (either focal or diffuse) in membranous lupus nephritis is designated class III + V or class IV + V (Figures 7.41 and 7.42). In the prior modified WHO classification, these mixed classes had been classified under membranous lupus nephritis as subclasses Vc and Vd, respectively [4,5] . Because these mixed lesions behave aggressively as predicted by their proliferative component, the ISN/RPS classification eliminated these subclassifications.

As in primary membranous glomerulonephritis, the ultrastructural appearance of the deposits evolves over time, with the earliest findings of subepithelial deposits followed by basement membrane spike formation (Figures 7.43 to 7.45), incorporation of deposits within a new layer of basement membrane,

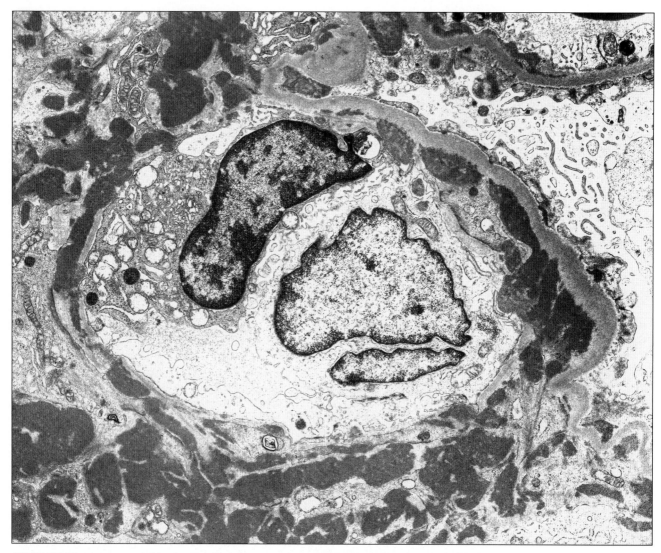

FIGURE 7.33: *Lupus nephritis class IV. The electron micrograph shows abundant mesangial and large subendothelial electron-dense deposits (×4,000).*

and increased electron lucency and resorption of deposits. In late stages, it may be difficult to identify the deposits by IF and EM; only their morphologic sequelae in the form of basement membrane remodeling, spiking, and internal vacuolizations at sites of deposit resorption provide evidence of an old membranous lesion.

Renal biopsy features of renal vein thrombosis include red blood cell and neutrophil congestion within glomerular capillaries, focal glomerular fibrin thrombus, and diffuse interstitial edema. Chronic renal vein thrombosis may lead to disproportionately severe diffuse tubular atrophy and interstitial fibrosis relative to the degree of glomerulosclerosis.

Differential Diagnosis. This includes idiopathic membranous glomerulonephritis and other secondary causes of membranous glomerulonephritis, including drug reaction, infection (e.g., hepatitis B and C) and neoplasia. Because membranous lupus nephritis may present prior to the development of other clinical and serologic evidence of SLE, differentiation from

idiopathic membranous glomerulonephritis is a particularly common problem. Pathologic features that favor lupus membranous nephritis, either alone or in combination, include mesangial hypercellularity, mesangial immune deposits, full-house IF staining, C1q staining, small subendothelial deposits, extraglomerular deposits, tissue ANA, and endothelial tubuloreticular inclusions [9].

Class VI (Advanced Sclerosing Lupus Nephritis)

Definition. Class VI is defined as extensive glomerular scarring with ≥ 90 percent global glomerulosclerosis and no residual activity.

Clinical Features. Renal insufficiency and hypertension are common. Many patients have inactive serologies but they may have persistent microhematuria and low-grade proteinuria. Most cases of class VI lupus nephritis represent "burnt out" class III or class IV proliferative lupus nephritis. There may have been a single episode of overwhelmingly proliferative nephritis, or more commonly, repeated bouts of proliferative nephritis that did not respond to therapy. Progression of class V lupus nephritis may also evolve into class VI.

Renal Biopsy Findings. By definition at least 90 percent of glomeruli are sclerotic. Most of the glomerulosclerosis is global, although some segmental scars may occur (Figures 7.46 and 7.47). There may be residual mesangial hypercellularity, thickening of glomerular basement membranes, or old fibrous crescents with disruption of Bowman's capsule. There is usually concomitant severe tubular atrophy, interstitial fibrosis, and arteriosclerosis. IF and EM may reveal residual immune deposits in sclerosing glomeruli, in the tubulointerstitial compartment, and in vessel walls.

Differential Diagnosis. This includes any cause of end-stage kidney disease associated with advanced glomerulosclerosis. Pathologic findings of residual immune deposits, tissue ANA, and endothelial tubuloreticular inclusions support a diagnosis of advanced sclerosing lupus nephritis. When these features are absent, a clinical history of SLE and previous renal biopsies documenting active lupus nephritis support this diagnosis.

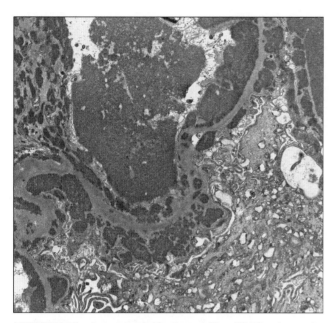

FIGURE 7.34: *Lupus nephritis classes IV and V. The glomerular capillary lumina are segmentally occluded by large intraluminal electron-dense deposits "hyaline thrombi". Large subendothelial, subepithelial and mesangial deposits are also present. (Electron micrograph, ×4,000).*

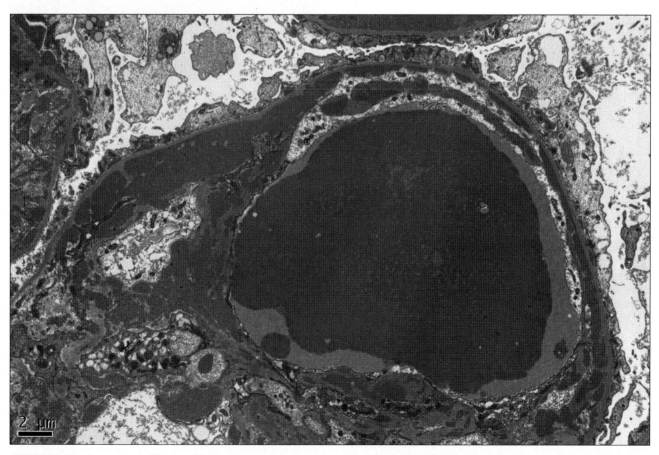

FIGURE 7.35: *Lupus nephritis class IV. The electron micrograph reveals a large "hyaline thrombus" that appears less electron dense at the periphery. There are also numerous mesangial and subendothelial immune deposits (×5,000).*

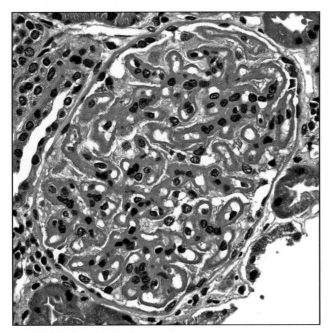

FIGUE 7.36:   Lupus nephritis class V. There is marked global thickening of the glomerular capillary walls with mild mesangial proliferation and swelling of podocytes. (H&E, ×400).

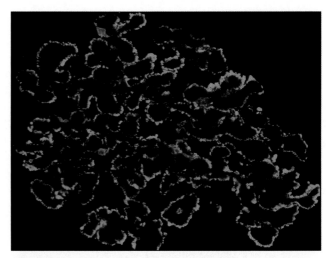

FIGURE 7.38:   Lupus nephritis class V. This immunofluorescence micrograph shows intense, granular subepithelial staining for C1q. No mesangial staining is noted (×400).

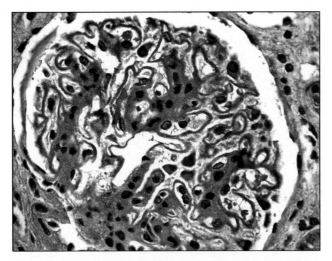

FIGURE 7.37:   Lupus nephritis class V. On trichrome stain, there are global, red subepithelial deposits contrasting with blue-staining glomerular basement membrane (×600).

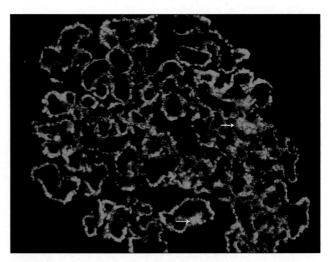

FIGURE 7.39:   Lupus nephritis class V. There are global, granular subepithelial deposits of lambda with segmental mesangial deposits (arrows). (Immunofluorescence micrograph, ×400).

Activity and Chronicity Indices in Lupus Nephritis

Semiquantitative grading of pathologic features of active and chronic injury may provide useful information in monitoring response to treatment and disease progression in individual patients [1,10]. These findings should be included in the renal biopsy report. The NIH [10] and ISN-RPS [3] definitions of pathologic activity and chronicity are listed in Table 7.6 and 7.7, respectively.

The NIH activity index is calculated by semiquantitatively scoring six pathologic features (including endocapillary proliferation, glomerular neutrophil infiltration, wire loop deposits, fibrinoid necrosis and karyorrhexis, cellular crescents, and interstitial inflammation) on a scale of 0 to 3+ (Table 7.6). Crescents and fibrinoid necrosis are assigned double weight because these are considered markers of more severe disease. The sum of the individual components yields a total histologic activity index score from 0 to 24. The NIH chronicity index (ranging from 0 to 12) is derived from the sum of four features, each graded on a scale of 0 to 3+, including glomerulosclerosis, fibrous crescents, tubular atrophy, and interstitial fibrosis.

Although there is debate about the reproducibility and predictive value of these indices [11,12], a combination of

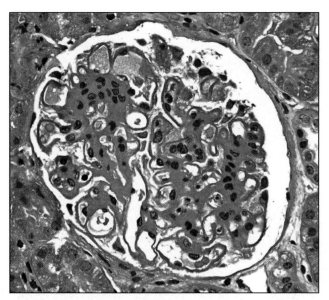

FIGURE 7.40: *Lupus nephritis class V. There is marked mesangial hypercellularity accompanied by thickening of the glomerular capillary walls. (H&E, ×400).*

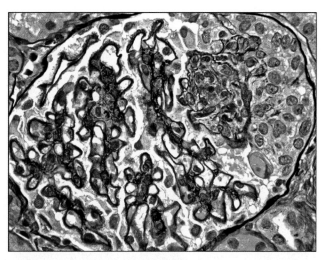

FIGURE 7.42: *Lupus nephritis class III and V. The glomerulus exhibits segmental endocapillary proliferation with an overlying cellular crescent. The glomerular capillary walls are thickened with numerous eosinophilic subepithelial deposits (JMS, ×400).*

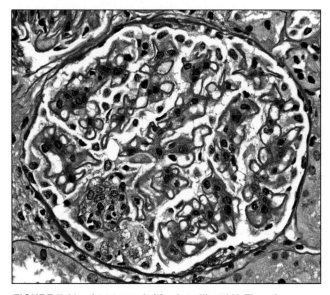

FIGURE 7.41: *Lupus nephritis class III and V. There is segmental endocapillary hypercellularity with an overlying small cellular crescent. The glomerular capillary walls appear thickened with a rigid aspect. (PAS, ×400).*

high activity (activity index >7) and increased chronicity (chronicity index >3) correlates with worse outcomes [13]. Interestingly, pathologic features of activity and chronicity in repeat renal biopsy performed six months after initiation of maximal treatment for lupus nephritis show greater correlation with renal outcome at five years than findings in the initial biopsy [14].

The ISN/RPS classification recommends semiquantitative grading and reporting of several glomerular markers of disease activity and chronicity. Markers of activity include cellular or fibrocellular crescents, fibrinoid necrosis, karyorrhexis, glomerular leukocyte infiltration, endocapillary hypercellularity, rupture of glomerular basement membranes, subendothelial immune deposits visible by light microscopy (wire-loop lesions), and intraluminal immune aggregates ("hyaline thrombi") (Table 7.7). Markers of chronicity include segmental or global glomerulosclerosis, fibrous crescents, and fibrous adhesions. Other pathologic features that may correlate with prognosis include intensity of IF staining, tubulointerstitial inflammation, macrophage infiltrates, tubular atrophy, interstitial fibrosis, and arteriosclerosis [15].

Other Pathologic Findings in SLE Biopsies

Tubulointerstitial Lesions

Tubulointerstitial injury is common in lupus nephritis and usually correlates with the degree of glomerular injury. In the setting of nephrotic range proteinuria, proximal tubules may show cytoplasmic lipid vacuoles and protein resorption droplets (Figure 7.48). Acute proximal tubular injury, characterized by loss of apical brush border, nuclear enlargement, prominent nucleoli, mitotic figures, and cytoplasmic simplification or sloughing, is common in cases of active class III and class IV lupus nephritis (Figure 7.49) [15]. Red blood cell casts can be seen, especially in active proliferative lupus nephritis (Figure 7.50). Interstitial edema and interstitial inflammation are frequent findings in severe proliferative lupus nephritis and may be accompanied by tubulointerstitial immune deposits (usually of IgG and complement) in up to 50 percent of cases (Figures 7.51

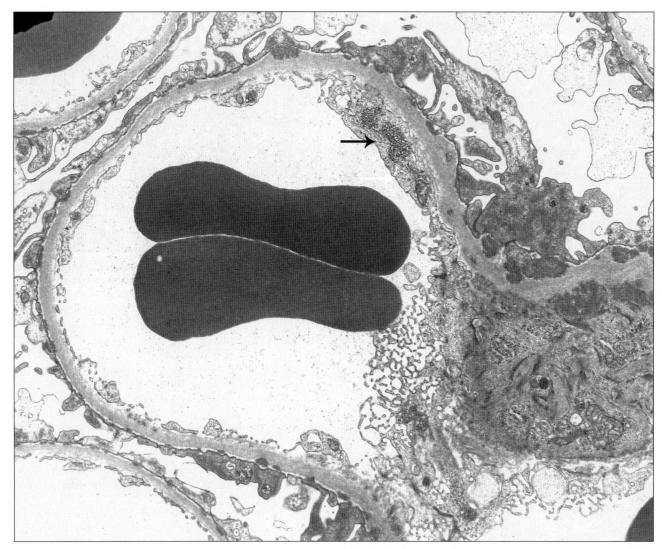

FIGURE 7.43: *Early lupus nephritis class V. The electron micrograph shows small sparse electron dense subepithelial deposits present predominantly along the glomerular basement membrane covering the mesangium. There are medium-sized paramesangial deposits and endothelial tubuloreticular inclusions (arrow) (×5,000).*

to 7.57) [16]. Deposits may involve TBM, interstitial capillary walls, and/or interstitial collagen.

Occasional cases of immune complex-associated tubulointerstitial nephritis without evidence of glomerular disease have been reported [17], as have rare cases associated with linear anti-TBM staining for IgG [18]. Tubular atrophy and interstitial fibrosis are markers of chronic renal injury that are more common in longstanding lupus nephritis. The severity of interstitial inflammation correlates well with degree of renal insufficiency and the extent of tubular atrophy is a good predictor of renal prognosis [19,20].

Vascular Lesions

It is easy to overlook vascular lesions in lupus nephritis because they are not considered when determining the class of nephritis and are not factored into assessments of activity and chronicity. However, some of these lesions have important clinical and prognostic implications. Therefore, attention should be directed to the vessels, not only by light microscopy, but when evaluating IF and EM, as well.

The commonest vascular lesions in lupus biopsies consist of ordinary arteriosclerosis and arteriolosclerosis. These may be related to aging and/or hypertension, and likely contribute to disease severity and prognosis.

Uncomplicated vascular immune deposits are highly characteristic of lupus nephritis. These are most commonly associated with class III and class IV but may be encountered in any class. IF typically reveals granular IgG, with or without IgM, IgA, C3, and C1q in the intima or media of arteries and arterioles (Figure 7.58). Corresponding granular electron-dense deposits are seen at these sites by EM (Figure 7.59). There is no associated

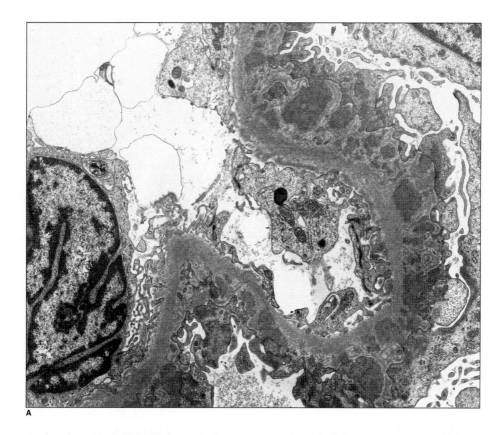

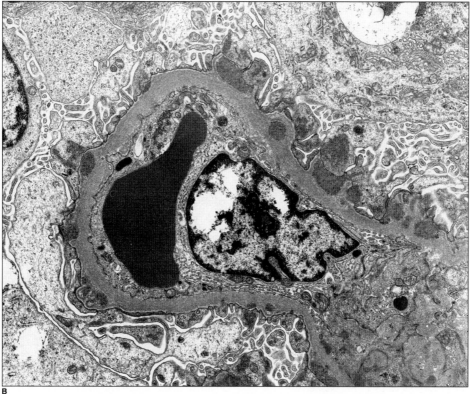

FIGURE 7.44: *Severe lupus nephritis class V. Electron micrographs (A-C) from 3 different patients show medium-sized electron-dense subepithelial deposits, many of which are separated by glomerular basement membrane spikes. Podocytes display marked foot process effacement (×5,000).*

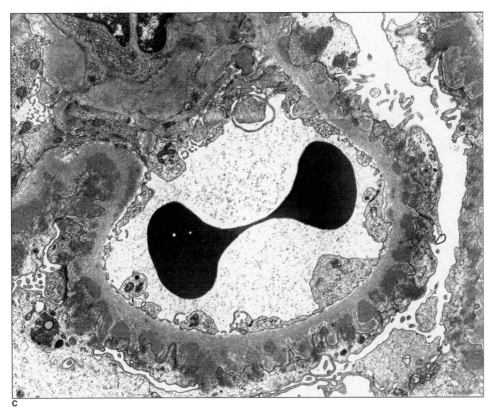

c

FIGURE 7.44: (continued)

inflammation of the vessel wall and the vessel lumen typically is not compromised. This form of vascular disease has not been shown to have a significant effect on prognosis.

Lupus vasculopathy is defined by LM findings of smudgy, eosinophilic, fibrinoid material, most commonly in arterioles,

that frequently narrows or occludes the vascular lumen and may be accompanied by necrosis of medial myocytes and endothelial cells (Figure 7.60) [21]. Importantly, there is no evidence of inflammation in the vessel wall hence the designation vasculopathy is preferable to vasculitis. These deposits stain for IgG,

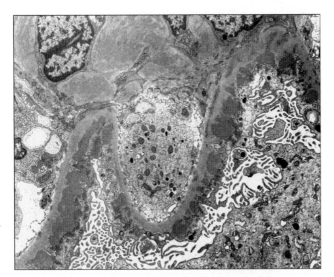

FIGURE 7.45: *Lupus nephritis class V. The glomerular basement membranes are thickened by the presence of numerous electron-dense subepithelial deposits. There are also abundant mesangial electron-dense deposits. Podocytes exhibit cytoplasmic microvillous transformation and marked foot process effacement. (Electron micrograph, ×4,000).*

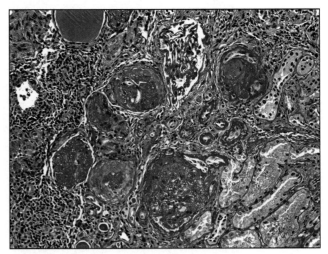

FIGURE 7.46: *Lupus nephritis class VI. Diffuse glomerulosclerosis with old fibrous crescents. The non-sclerotic glomerulus does not show residual activity. In this biopsy, 13 of the 15 glomeruli sampled were globally sclerotic. The patient had a previous biopsy 2 years prior that showed lupus nephritis class IV. (PAS, ×200).*

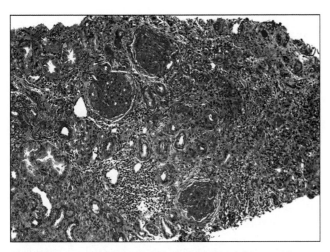

FIGURE 7.47: *Lupus nephritis class VI. There is extensive glomerulosclerosis, severe tubular atrophy and interstitial fibrosis, and moderate interstitial inflammation. (PAS, × 100).*

Table 7.7 ISN/RPS Active and Chronic Glomerular Lesions

Active lesions
- Endocapillary hypercellularity with or without leukocyte infiltration and with substantial luminal reduction
- Karyorrhexis
- Fibrinoid necrosis
- Rupture of glomerular basement membrane
- Crescents, cellular or fibrocellular
- Subendothelial deposits identifiable by light microscopy (wire loops)
- Intraluminal immune aggregates (hyaline thrombi)

Chronic lesions
- Glomerular sclerosis (segmental, global)
- Fibrous adhesions
- Fibrous crescents

Table 7.6 NIH Markers of Activity and Chronicity

Index of Activity (0–24)	Score
Endocapillary hypercellularity	(0–3+)
Neutrophil infiltration	(0–3+)
Subendothelial hyaline deposits	(0–3+)
Fibrinoid necrosis/karyorrhexis	(0–3+) × 2
Cellular crescents	(0–3+) × 2
Interstitial inflammation	(0–3+)

Index of Chronicity (0–12)	Score
Glomerular sclerosis	(0–3+)
Fibrous crescents	(0–3+)
Tubular atrophy	(0–3+)
Interstitial fibrosis	(0–3+)

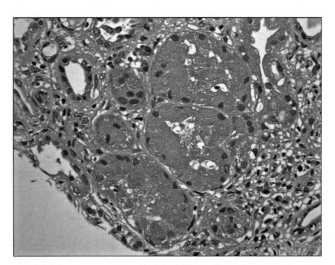

FIGURE 7.48: *Lupus nephritis class V. Several proximal tubules contain numerous intracytoplasmic hypereosinophilic protein resorption droplets (H&E, × 600).*

complement and fibrin, indicating a combination of immune deposition and intravascular coagulation (Figures 7.61 and 7.62). This lesion is most commonly encountered in cases of severe active class IV lupus nephritis and carries a poor prognosis. Patients are frequently severely hypertensive and develop rapidly progressive renal failure.

Necrotizing arteritis is rare in SLE. This may be renal-limited or associated with systemic vasculitis. Vessel walls demonstrate fibrinoid necrosis and inflammatory cell infiltration resembling microscopic polyangiitis (Figure 7.63). Immune deposits may or not be identified by IF and EM (Figure 7.64). This lesion may complicate any class of lupus nephritis.

Thrombotic microangiopathy in lupus patients occurs in variety of clinical settings including antiphospholipid antibody nephropathy/lupus anticoagulant syndrome (see the following discussion), overlap with systemic sclerosis, hemolytic uremic syndrome and thrombotic thrombocytopenic purpura. Laboratory findings may include positive lupus anticoagulant, antiphospholipid antibody, or autoantibody to von Willebrand

factor cleaving protease. Thrombotic microangiopathy is characterized by fibrin thrombi involving small arteries, arterioles, and/or glomerular capillaries (Figures 7.65 and 7.66). In addition, glomeruli may show capillary necrosis, widening of the subendothelial zone and mesangiolysis (Figure 7.67), and arterial vessels may show mucoid intimal edema (Figure 7.68), entrapped fragmented red blood cells, and fibrinoid necrosis. Thrombotic microangiopathy may coexist with any class of lupus nephritis, or may be the sole renal biopsy finding.

Antiphospholipid Antibody Syndrome

Definition

The antiphospholipid antibody (APL) syndrome (or lupus anticoagulant syndrome) is defined by the occurrence of thrombosis or pregnancy morbidity in patients who have serologic evidence of antiphospholipid antibodies on two or more occasions, at least twelve weeks apart [22]. APL syndrome may be primary, but more commonly develops in patients who have either SLE or a lupus-like illness that does not fulfill ARA criteria for SLE.

Antiphospholipid antibodies are detected by lupus anticoagulant (LA) test or enzyme linked immunosorbent assay (ELISA) for anticardiolipin (ACL) antibodies and/or anti-β2-glycoprotein antibodies [22]. The LA test consists of prolongation of the activated partial thromboplastin time that is not reversed by addition of normal platelet-free plasma to the patient's plasma. ACL antibodies are directed to naturally occurring phospholipids and/or β2-glycoprotein. Antiphospholipid antibodies may be detected in up to 50 percent of SLE patients but only a minority develops signs of APL syndrome.

The clinical manifestations of APL syndrome are highly variable and include vascular thromboses (arterial and deep venous), recurrent spontaneous abortion, premature births before the 34th week of gestation due to preeclampsia or placental insufficiency, pulmonary hypertension, Budd-Chiari syndrome, livedo reticularis, transient ischemic attacks, stroke, migraine, cardiac valvular disease, adrenal hemorrhage, thrombocytopenia, and renal disease (APL nephropathy) [22]. APL nephropathy is an important complication of SLE and related autoimmune connective tissue diseases.

Clinical Features of APL Nephropathy

The major clinical characteristics of APL nephropathy are hypertension (mild to malignant range) and chronic renal insufficiency, with variable proteinuria (ranging from mild to nephrotic range) and hematuria [22,23]. Rarely, patients present with rapidly progressive renal failure associated with severe hypertension [22]. However, features of microangiopathic hemolytic anemia are typically absent. In one study, APL nephropathy was detected in 32 percent of lupus biopsies, both with and without coexistent lupus nephritis [24]. APL nephropathy was associated with extrarenal arterial thromboses, but not venous thrombosis, and with LAC but not with ACL antibodies [23,24]. In addition, the presence of APL nephropathy in lupus patients was associated with hypertension, renal insufficiency, and increased interstitial fibrosis, suggesting that it may impact negatively on prognosis.

Renal Biopsy Findings in APL Nephropathy

The characteristic pathologic findings in APL nephropathy are vaso-occlusive lesions that may involve any level of the renal vasculature including main renal artery, intrarenal arteries and arterioles, glomerular capillaries and veins. The spectrum of lesions includes acute thromboses within glomeruli (Figure 7.69), arterioles and arteries (thrombotic microangiopathy), fibrous or mucoid intimal hyperplasia, and organizing thromboses with fibrous or fibrocellular luminal obliteration. The resulting ischemic injury to the tubular compartment produces focal cortical atrophy, particularly involving the subcapsular region. Zones of tubular thyroidization (atrophic tubules containing regular eosinophilic casts) may be found [23]. Such

lesions may occur in APL patients regardless of whether they have underlying SLE [23,24]. In those APL patients with SLE, the findings of thrombotic microangiopathy may coexist with any class of lupus nephritis [24].

Etiology and Pathogenesis of Lupus Nephritis

The etiology of SLE and the pathogenesis of lupus nephritis are poorly understood. A role for genetic factors is supported by the increased incidence of SLE and other autoimmune diseases in family members and by the high concordance of SLE in identical twins. There are weak associations of SLE with HLA-DR3, HLA-DR2, and heritable deficiencies of the early complement components, C2 and C4. Roles for genetic polymorphisms in T cell receptors, increased cytokine production, impaired scavenger mechanisms, and abnormal tolerance have also been described. The predominance of SLE in women of childbearing age may reflect the effect of sex hormones and possibly a role for pregnancy-induced chimerism in some individuals [25]. Pregnancy, drugs, and ultraviolet light all may trigger flares of SLE, providing evidence for hormonal and environmental factors.

Myriad immunological abnormalities have been described in SLE patients and in experimental models of lupus but their precise role in the initiation and maintenance of lupus nephritis remain poorly understood. SLE is characterized by loss of self-tolerance, leading to development of autoantibodies to a wide variety of nuclear antigens, including DNA, Smith, Ro, and La [26]. Dysregulation of T cell function, polyclonal B cell activation, and defective B cell tolerance all may predispose to autoantibody formation. IgM autoantibodies to single-stranded and double-stranded DNA occur naturally and display weak reactivity to self-antigens. Isotype switching (from IgM to IgG) may increase autoantibody pathogenicity. Toll-like receptor (TLR) signaling on B cells may play a role in such isotype switching [27]. Activation of the innate immune system via TLR also suggests a possible pathomechanism whereby exogenous triggers, such as infectious agents, could initiate SLE [28]. However, to date no specific etiologic pathogen has been identified in human SLE.

Autoantibodies with multiple specificities have been eluted from lupus kidneys but anti-dsDNA antibodies predominate [29]. Localization of anti-dsDNA autoantibodies within glomerular immune deposits may result from three mechanisms: (1) autoantibody-binding to planted autoantigens such as nucleosomes that have bound to the anionic glomerular basement membrane via electrostatic interactions [30]; (2) crossreactivity of anti-DNA antibodies with normal glomerular constituents, such as heparan sulfate proteoglycans, laminin, type IV collagen, and alpha actinin-4, leading to in situ immune complex formation [31]; and (3) deposition of preformed immune complexes from the circulation. These three mechanisms are not mutually exclusive and each may contribute in varying degrees to the pathogenesis of lupus nephritis.

Localization of immune deposits within glomeruli may also be influenced by the class and subclass of immunoglobulins, their electric charge, and antigen specificity, and the circulating immune complex load. Mesangial deposition is favored by

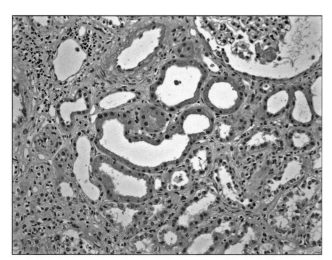

FIGURE 7.49: Lupus nephritis class III. Tubules exhibit degenerative and regenerative changes with luminal ectasia, epithelial simplification, and nuclear enlargement with hyperchromasia. There is also mild interstitial inflammation and segmental glomerular fibrinoid necrosis (H&E, ×200).

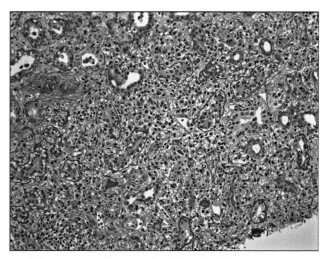

FIGURE 7.51: Lupus nephritis class IV. There is marked interstitial inflammation and focal tubulitis (PAS, ×400).

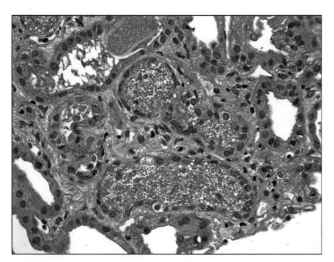

FIGURE 7.50: Lupus nephritis class IV. There are several degenerated erythrocyte casts accompanied by tubular dilatation and simplification. The interstitium is expanded by edema and mononuclear inflammatory cells. (H&E, ×400).

penetration exerts direct cellular effects, including enhanced proliferation or apoptosis, all of which may contribute to glomerular pathology. Dysregulation of apoptosis may promote increased release of autoantigens, accumulation of autoreactive lymphocytes, and increased autoantibody production. These effects may be aggravated by deficiencies in complement components, leading to impaired autoantigen clearance.

Activation of complement by immune deposits promotes leukocyte infiltration and the ensuing release of inflammatory mediators stimulates glomerular cell proliferation and progressive sclerosis. Microarray analysis of peripheral blood mononuclear cells and glomeruli from SLE patients reveal dysregulation of inflammatory cytokines, chemokines, and immune response-related genes, as well as genes involved in apoptosis, signal transduction, and the cell cycle [32]. Interferon (IFN)-regulated genes are highly overexpressed in the peripheral blood and glomeruli of SLE patients, supporting a central role for IFN in SLE [33,34].

Clinical Course, Prognosis, Treatment, and Clinical Correlations in Lupus Nephritis

Major determinants of poor renal outcome include African-American race, low socioeconomic status, higher initial serum creatinine, lower hematocrit levels and flares (recurrence) and pathologic severity [35–38]. Racial differences may reflect socioeconomic variables and/or increased incidence of more severe forms of lupus nephritis [36, 38]. Children and males also typically display more severe forms of lupus nephritis and tend to have worse renal outcomes.

Pathologic correlates of outcome include class of lupus nephritis, activity and chronicity indices, and transition from milder to more severe form of lupus nephritis.

One study of 85 lupus nephritis patients found a worse renal prognosis for "severe" focal proliferative Class III patients (ISN/RPS class IV-S) than for patients with diffuse proliferative Class IV lesions (ISN/RPS class IV-G) [37]. This

relatively small amounts of intermediate-sized, high-avidity complexes. When present in larger quantities, these may extend into the subendothelial areas. Subepithelial deposits may be favored by smaller, low-avidity, relatively cationic immune complexes formed in relative antigen excess. Such deposits may dissociate and reform in situ, allowing electrostatic interactions with the glomerular capillary wall's polyanionic constituents. The clearing ability of the mesangium and local hemodynamic factors also may play a role.

Binding of anti-dsDNA antibodies to the surface of endothelial, mesangial, and visceral epithelial cells and intracellular

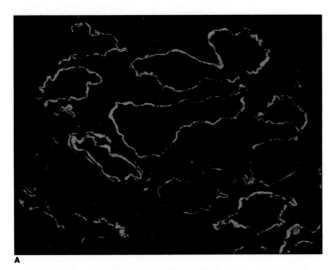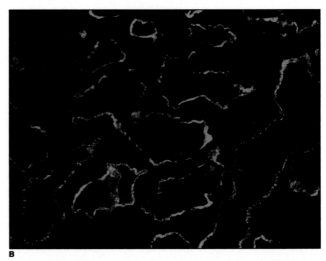

A B

FIGURE 7.52: *Lupus nephritis class IV and V. The immunofluorescence micrographs show abundant granular deposits of IgG (A) and C3 (B) in tubular basement membranes (× 400).*

study stresses the bad outcome for patients with segmental necrotizing lesions. A Japanese study of 60 lupus nephritis patients found that those patients with lupus nephritis class IV-S had worse renal survival than those with IV-G (95 months survival vs. 214 months), although this did not reach statistical significance [39]. By contrast, two studies from Boston [40] and Paris [41] have failed to find outcome differences between these subgroups. Moreover, the observation of transition between IV-S and IV-G in repeat biopsies in some patients argues against the hypothesis that these patterns reflect distinct pathomechanisms of disease. Patients with combined membranous and proliferative lupus nephritis (i.e., class V + III or class V + IV) have shown particularly poor renal outcomes, reflecting the complexity of the glomerular capillary wall lesions [42].

The optimum choice of drug and duration of therapy to achieve remission, prevent relapses of lupus nephritis, and minimize side-effects in lupus nephritis are the subject of ongoing investigation. Patients with class I or class II lupus nephritis require no specific treatment for their renal disease [43]. For cases of class III with mild focal glomerular involvement and without evidence of necrotizing lesions or large subendothelial immune deposits, treatment with steroids alone may suffice. Class III with more extensive glomerular involvement and/or high activity, and active class IV lupus nephritis have the worst renal outcomes. These are usually treated aggressively with a combination of prednisone, cyclophosphamide, azathioprine (AZA), and/or mycophenolate mofetil (MMF) [43].

The choice of treatment of class V lupus nephritis is influenced by the severity of renal disease. Individuals with subnephrotic proteinuria and normal renal function generally have a good prognosis and may be treated with short course of cyclosporine and low-dose steroids. Those with full nephrotic syndrome or reduced renal function may require treatment with steroids, cytotoxic agents, cyclosporine, and/or MMF [43].

Non-lupus Nephritis

Definition. Nonlupus nephritis is defined by renal biopsy findings other than lupus nephritis in SLE patients with clinically significant renal disease.

Clinical Features. These are variable and may include asymptomatic proteinuria, nephrotic syndrome, hematuria, active renal sediment, and renal failure.

Renal Biopsy Findings. Pathologic findings include minimal change disease, focal segmental glomerulosclerosis (FSGS), IgM nephropathy, thin basement membrane disease, hypertensive arterionephrosclerosis, amyloidosis, and acute allergic interstitial nephritis [44].

A primary podocytopathy (e.g., minimal change disease or idiopathic FSGS) may be suspected in patients who present with abrupt onset of full nephrotic syndrome and renal biopsy findings of little or no mesangial hypercellularity with extensive foot process effacement in the absence of peripheral capillary wall immune deposits [45–47] (Figure 7.70). Interestingly, these cases often show prompt remission response to immunosuppressive therapy, akin to idiopathic minimal change disease. It has been debated whether these cases represent the coincidental superimposition of minimal change disease on mild mesangial lupus nephritis. The close temporal relationship of renal symptoms to onset of clinical signs of SLE has suggested to some investigators that these cases may represent a lupus-related podocytopathy, favored by the heightened systemic cytokine activity of SLE [47].

Renal amyloidosis of the secondary type has been described in SLE patients, reflecting elevated serum amyloid A protein levels in the setting of chronic inflammatory disorders. However, secondary amyloidosis is rare in the modern era, presumably reflecting better therapy for the inflammatory manifestations of SLE. In cases where LM demonstrates prominent necrotizing lesions and IF and EM reveal only sparse subendothelial immune deposits [7] or features of membranous nephropathy [48], the possibility

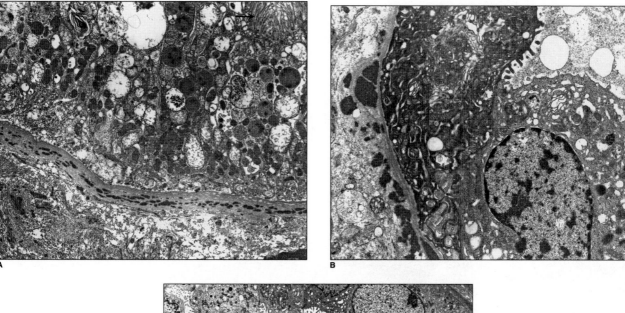

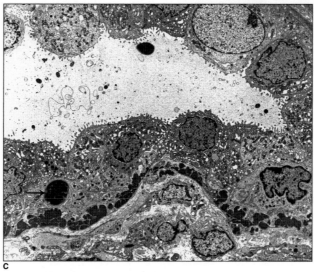

FIGURE 7.53: *Tubular basement membrane deposits. A. Lupus nephritis class V. There are numerous electron-dense deposits within a proximal tubular basement membrane. The arrow highlights a portion of tubular brush border. B. Lupus nephritis class V. The micrograph reveals several granular electron-dense deposits abutting a distal tubular basement membrane along the interstitial aspect. C. Lupus nephritis class IV. Numerous electron-dense deposits are seen within a distal tubular basement membrane. The arrow shows rounded electron dense material within an epithelial cell, suggesting invaginated immune deposits. (Electron micrographs; A, ×4,000; B, ×5,000; C, ×3,000).*

of superimposed ANCA vasculitis should be evaluated by serologic testing for ANCA.

Silent Lupus Nephritis

Definition. Silent lupus nephritis is defined by the presence of renal pathologic abnormalities in SLE patients who lack clinical signs of renal disease. Renal pathologic abnormalities have been detected in up to 80 percent of SLE patients without overt renal disease [49].

Clinical Features. Patients have normal urine sediment, normal creatinine clearance, and proteinuria <300 mg/day, but may have active serologies (elevated anti-dsDNA and hypocomple-

mentemia). Compared to overt lupus nephritis, duration of lupus was shorter in the silent lupus nephritis patients, and patients had less overall disease activity, less neurologic disease, hypertension, and ecchymosis. Interestingly, Raynaud's phenomenon was common in silent lupus nephritis in one series [49]. A variable number of silent lupus nephritis cases evolve into overt lupus nephritis [50, 51], suggesting that renal involvement may be underrecognized in SLE patients, particularly early in the course of their disease.

Renal Biopsy Findings. In silent diffuse proliferative lupus nephritis, the biopsy may show features of active class IV despite the absence of overt clinical manifestations.

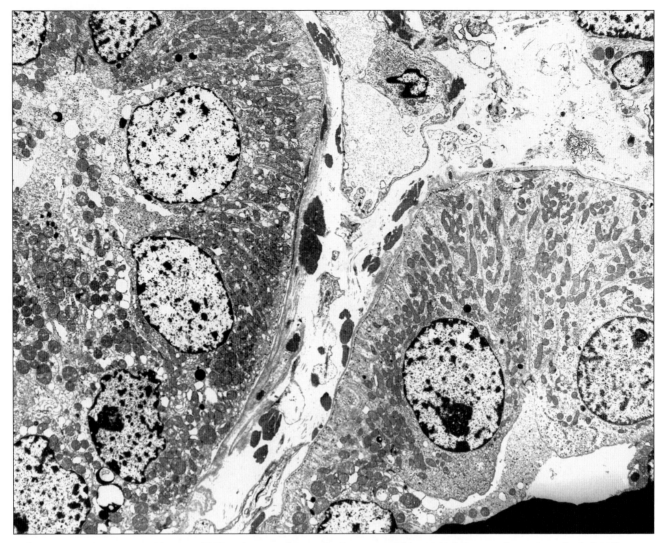

FIGURE 7.54: Lupus nephritis class IV. The electron micrograph shows several interstitial electron dense deposits (×3,000).

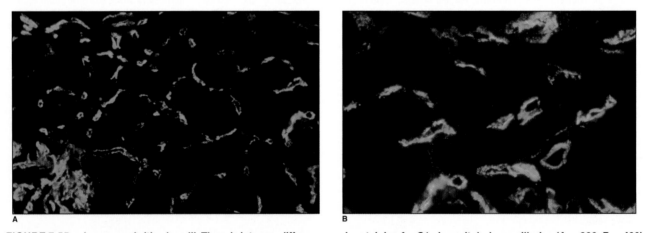

FIGURE 7.55: Lupus nephritis class III. There is intense, diffuse, granular staining for C1q in peritubular capillaries (A, ×200; B, ×400). Lupus nephritis is one of few immune-mediated renal diseases in which diffuse staining of peritubular capillaries for immunoglobulins and complements (C1, C3, and C4d) can be seen. In the renal allograft, this can be misinterpreted as evidence of antibody-mediated rejection. (Immunofluorescence micrographs; A, ×200; B, ×400).

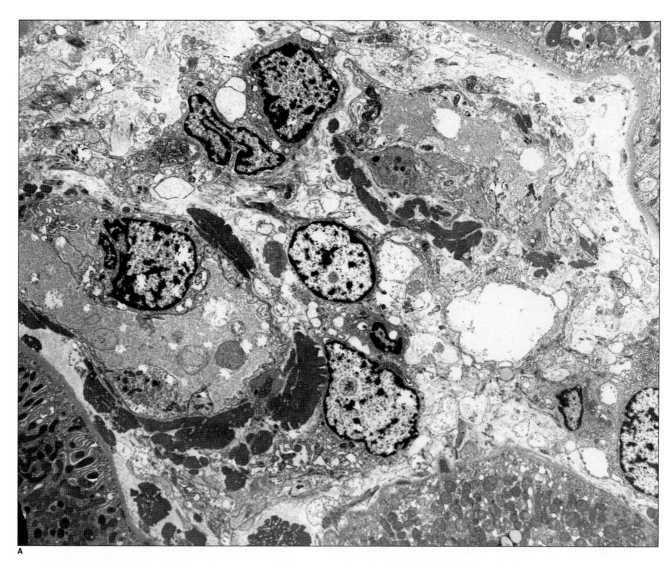

A

FIGURE 7.56: *Lupus nephritis class IV. Electron micrographs A–C reveal abundant electron immune deposits within the walls of interstitial capillaries (A,B, ×2,000; C, ×3,000).*

Drug-induced SLE

Definition. The diagnosis of drug-induced lupus is based on three criteria: absence of lupus prior to receiving the drug; development of ANA (usually with antihistone specificity) and at least one other clinical feature of SLE while receiving therapy; and serologic and clinical improvement following discontinuation of the drug.

More than 80 drugs have been reported to cause a lupus-like syndrome or exacerbate underlying lupus [52–54]. Drugs that have been definitely implicated in inducing SLE include hydralazine, procainamide, isoniazid, methyldopa, quinidine, minocycline, and chlorpromazine. Other agents that have a strong probable association include sulfasalazine, statins, penicillamine, hydrochlorothiazide, and fluorouracil. More recently, tumor necrosis factor (TNF) blockers for treatment of rheumatoid arthritis and other inflammatory diseases have been linked to induction of lupus-like syndrome, including some cases with nephritis [55,56].

Clinical Features. Compared to idiopathic SLE, drug-induced SLE patients are generally older and show an equal male to female ratio. Caucasians are affected more commonly than African-Americans and may have more severe manifestations [53]. The clinical spectrum varies from mild skin involvement to mild systemic disease. Clinical characteristics of drug-induced lupus include positive ANA (99 percent), positive antihistone antibodies (95 percent) arthralgia, myalgia, pleuritis, and fever. Anti-dsDNA and anti-Sm antibodies are usually absent and serum complements are usually normal. Malar rash, CNS disease, and renal involvement are rare. The onset is generally insidious and may develop from one month to several years after initiating drug therapy. Renal involvement in drug-induced lupus is rare (<5 percent of cases vs. 50 percent in idiopathic SLE), but may be clinically severe.

Importantly, drug-induced lupus usually resolves completely, with normalization of ANA following discontinuation of the offending drug. Treatment of drug-induced lupus includes

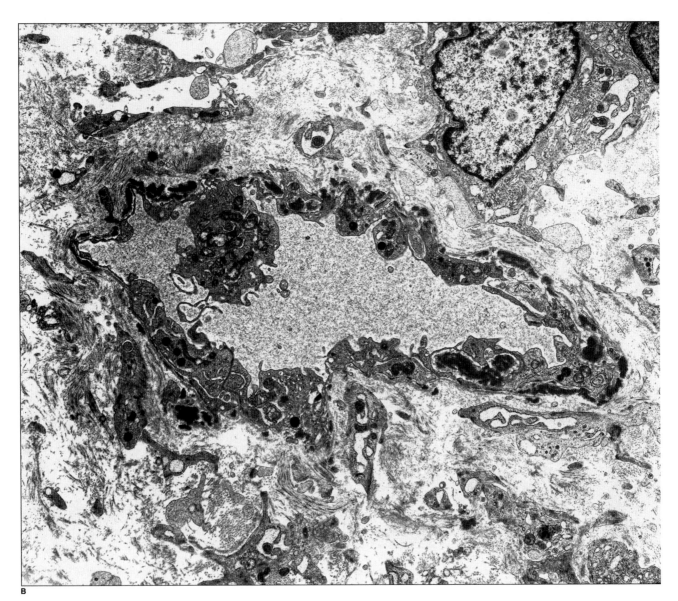

FIGURE 7.56: (continued)

discontinuing the offending agent. Immunosuppressive therapy may be indicated in cases that develop severe organ complications, such as class III, class IV, or class V lupus nephritis.

Renal Biopsy Findings. Any class of lupus nephritis may be seen, with particularly high incidence of focal proliferative and crescentic forms. Patients treated with hydralazine and propylthiouracil may also occasionally develop positive ANCA and features of systemic vasculitis with pauci-immune necrotizing and crescentic glomerulonephritis [57].

Lupus Nephritis Associated with HIV Infection

Some patients with HIV infection manifest clinical and pathologic signs of lupus nephritis. This phenomenon may be more prevalent in children with perinatal HIV infection who are African-American and male [58]. Presenting clinical features include hematuria, proteinuria, and renal insufficiency and renal biopsy examination may reveal any class of lupus nephritis (class II, Class III, class IV, class V, and combined class III+ V), with or without features of collapsing FSGS (HIV-associated nephropathy) [58].

MIXED CONNECTIVE TISSUE DISEASE

Definition

Mixed connective tissues disease (MCTD) is a group of disorders characterized by overlapping clinical features of SLE, scleroderma, and polymyositis, with high titer antibodies to ribonuclease-sensitive extractable nuclear antigens (ENA)

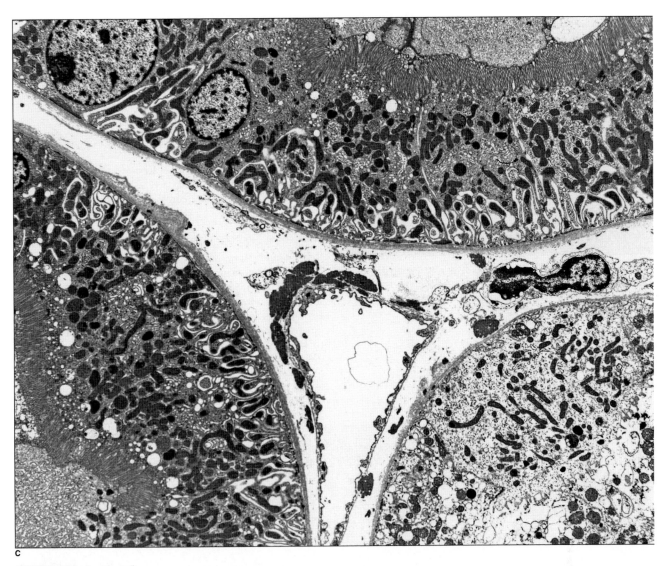

C

FIGURE 7.56: (continued)

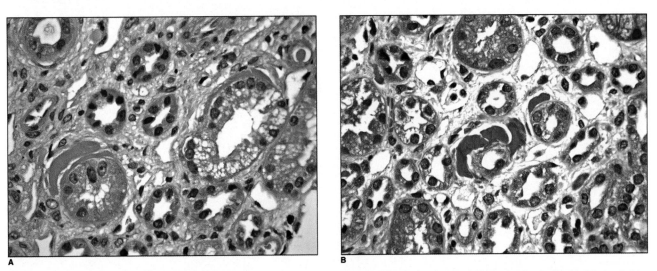

A

B

FIGURE 7.57: Lupus nephritis class IV and V. Rarely, the extraglomerular deposits are so large that they would be visible by light microscopy. A. This micrograph highlights focal hypereosinophilic immune deposits involving tubular basement membranes and interstitial capillaries (H&E, ×400). B. In another microscopic field from the same case, the tubular basement membranes and interstitial capillary wall deposits stain fuchsinophilic (red) with the trichrome stain (×400).

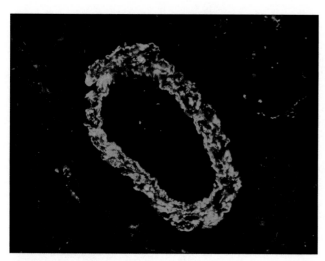

FIGURE 7.58: *Lupus nephritis class IV and V. Strong granular staining for IgG is seen in the wall of an interlobular artery. The vascular deposits are not seen on light microscopy. (Immunofluorescence micrograph, ×200).*

[59]. Some patients may have an undifferentiated autoimmune rheumatic and connective tissue disorder [60] that over time evolves into SLE, scleroderma or rheumatoid arthritis (RA) [61]. However, there may also be a distinct subset of MCTD characterized by high titers of IgG antibodies to U1 small ribonucleoprotein (U1RNP) and heterogeneous ribonucleoprotein (hnRNP)-A2 [62].

Clinical Features

Clinical features include arthritis, Raynaud's phenomenon, lymphadenopathy, alopecia. sclerodactyly, rash, and restrictive lung disease. Renal disease and neurological involvement are rare.

Pathologic Findings

Renal biopsy shows an immune complex glomerulonephritis resembling lupus nephritis and/or vascular lesions of thrombotic microangiopathy similar to scleroderma renal disease (see chapters on Thrombotic Microangiopathies [Chapter 9] and Vascular Diseases [Chapter 12]). Membranous nephropathy is the most common lupus-like glomerular disease, occurring in 35 to 40 percent of renal biopsies (Figure 7.71). Mesangial proliferative glomerulonephritis and focal or diffuse proliferative glomerulonephritides are less common. The vascular lesions include acute fibrinoid necrosis of arterioles and mucoid

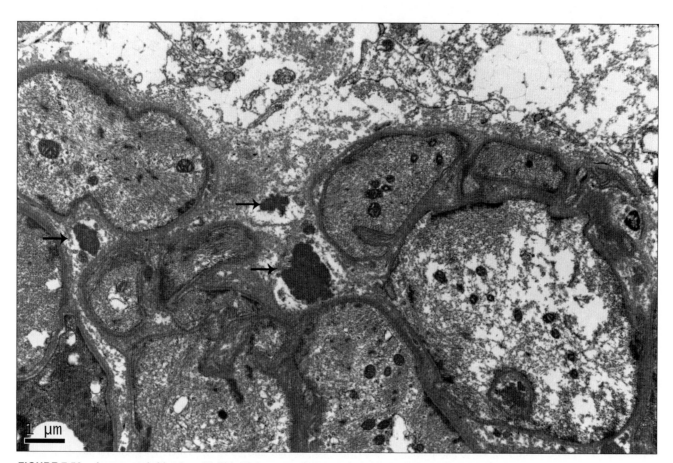

FIGURE 7.59: *Lupus nephritis class IV. This high-power electron micrograph of the wall of an interlobular artery shows several granular, electron-dense immune deposits (arrows) in the perimyocyte matrix (×12,000).*

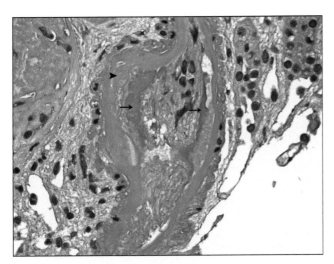

FIGURE 7.60: *Lupus vasculopathy. An arteriole is obliterated by endothelial cell swelling and intimal deposits of darkly eosinophilic material consistent with fibrin (arrows) together with paler eosinophilic material representing immune deposits (arrowhead). (H&E, ×600).*

edema of interlobular arteries, or more chronic concentric intimal fibroplasia affecting small or medium-sized arteries.

RHEUMATOID ARTHRITIS

Definition and Clinical Features

Rheumatoid arthritis (RA) is a chronic autoimmune disorder characterized by inflammatory joint disease, typically involving multiple joint areas (polyarthritis) with variable involvement of other organs and blood vessels. Extraarticular manifestations of RA include subcutaneous nodules on the extensor surface (rheumatoid nodules), vasculitis, mononeuritis multiplex, lung nodules, pericarditis, scleritis and serositis. The American Rheumatism Association (ARA) recognizes seven criteria for the diagnosis of RA, including morning stiffness in and around the joints, arthritis of three or more joint areas, arthritis of hand joints, symmetric arthritis, rheumatoid nodules, serum rheumatoid factor, and radiographic changes such as erosions or bony decalcification adjacent to involved joints (Table 7.8) [63]. The presence of any four of these criteria is diagnostic of RA.

The prevalence of renal abnormalities in autopsies of RA patients ranges from 8 to 90 percent, depending on the pathologic criteria and methodologies used. Renal disease is an important cause of morbidity and mortality in RA and falls into three major categories: amyloidosis; complications of drug therapy; and primary renal disease related to RA itself or overlap with other connective tissue diseases.

RA-Related Amyloidosis

Clinical Features. The prevalence of amyloidosis in RA ranges from 0 to 5 percent in cross-sectional renal biopsy studies but greater than 50 percent in renal biopsies performed for the evaluation of proteinuria [64]. It is more common in individuals with long-standing RA (mean duration 13.7 years) [65] and may involve multiple organ systems. However, renal involvement usually dominates the clinical presentation and course.

Most individuals present with heavy proteinuria or the nephrotic syndrome and 50 percent have renal insufficiency. Proteinuria generally correlates with the presence of peripheral capillary wall amyloid deposits. Occasional patients with predominantly vascular amyloid deposits may lack significant proteinuria. Tubular defects such as renal tubular acidosis and concentrating defects are seen in those with extensive tubulointerstitial deposits. Renal insufficiency is more common in those

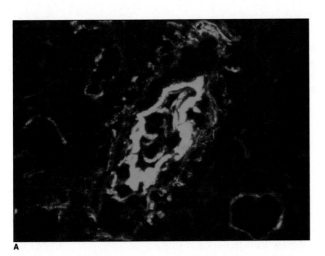

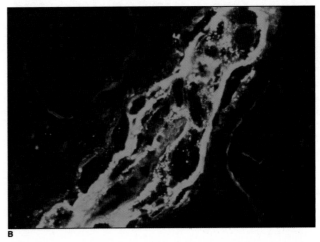

A   B

FIGURE 7.61: *Lupus vasculopathy. In this case of lupus nephritis class III and V, there was intense (3+) intraluminal and intimal positivity in small interlobular arteries for IgG (A) and C1q (B). Similar vascular positivity for IgM, IgA, C3, fibrin, kappa, and lambda was also present (not shown). (Immunofluorescence micrographs, ×400).*

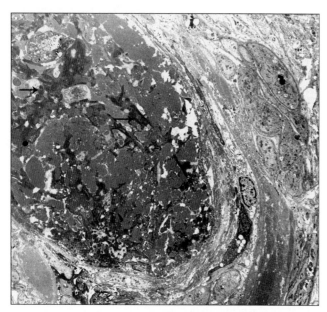

FIGURE 7.62: Lupus vasculopathy. An arteriole shows endothelial cell loss and numerous luminal and mural granular electron-dense immune deposits admixed with less abundant highly electron dense fibrin tactoids (arrows). (Electron micrograph, × 2,000).

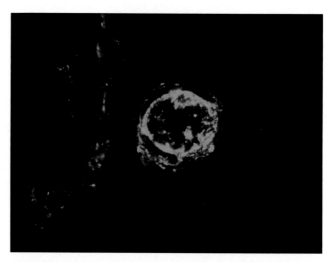

FIGURE 7.64: Lupus vasculitis. The biopsy is from a patient with lupus nephritis class IV and ANCA seropositivity. On immunofluorescence, there was a strong staining of arteriolar walls for IgG (shown) and fibrin (× 400). Focal transmural vasculitis was seen on light microscopy.

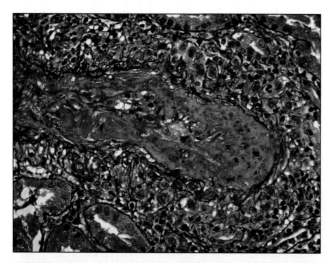

FIGURE 7.63: Lupus vasculitis. This biopsy is from a patient with systemic lupus erythematosus and negative ANCA. Renal biopsy showed lupus nephritis classes IV and V and necrotizing vasculitis. The small interlobular artery depicted exhibits intimal fibrinoid necrosis and circumferential, transmural inflammation. (JMS, × 400).

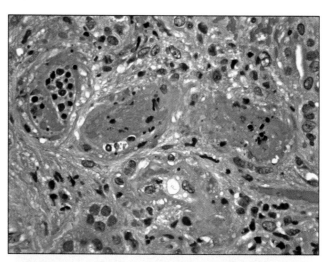

FIGURE 7.65: Thrombotic microangiopathy in SLE. Multiple arterioles are obliterated by intraluminal fibrin thrombi associated with endothelial cell necrosis and apoptosis, as well as entrapment of fragmented red blood cells. (H&E, × 400).

with more advanced disease. There is no specific therapy for RA-related amyloidosis and the prognosis is generally poor. Renal failure due to amyloidosis is an important cause of mortality in RA.

Renal Biopsy Findings. Amyloidosis may affect glomeruli, tubular basement membranes, interstitium, and blood ves-

sels in any combination. Amyloid deposits are palely eosinophilic (Figure 7.72A), weak PAS-positive, trichrome gray, and nonargyrophilic. Confirmation requires demonstration of red-green birefringent staining with Congo Red. The amyloid deposits demonstrate strong immunohistochemcal staining for serum amyloid A (AA) protein (Figure 7.72B) and may also display diffuse indistinct staining for immunoglobulins and albumin due to nonspecific trapping. Unlike primary (AL) amyloidosis, there is no dominant staining for kappa or lambda light chain. EM reveals randomly oriented, nonbranching fibrils measuring 8 to 12 nm in average thickness.

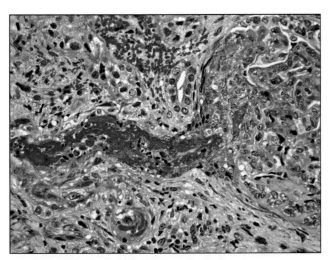

FIGURE 7.66: *Thrombotic microangiopathy in SLE. Two arterioles exhibit intraluminal and mural deposition of dark red fibrin with focal endothelial cell necrosis. (Trichrome stain, × 400).*

Renal Disease Due to Drug Therapy of RA

Analgesic Nephropathy

The frequency of analgesic nephropathy in RA patients has declined following the withdrawal of compound analgesics and phenacetin from the market. Pathologic features of analgesic nephropathy include papillary necrosis and chronic tubulointerstitial nephropathy [66].

Nonsteroidal Anti-inflammatory Agents (NSAID)

Renal complications of nonsteroidal anti-inflammatory agents (NSAID) include reversible acute renal failure due to inhibition of cyclooxygenase and reduction in prostaglandin synthesis. Predisposing factors include intrinsic renal disease, congestive heart failure, volume depletion, and ascites. The pathologic features of this complication are not well-described but these likely consist of acute tubular injury. Other described complications include acute interstitial nephritis, with or without minimal change nephrotic syndrome. Rare cases of membranous glomerulonephritis (usually early, stage 1 or 2) have been described [67]. Similar renal toxicities have been reported for selective cyclooxygenase 2 (COX-2) inhibitors. In all such cases, reversibility of symptoms may be achieved following discontinuation of therapy.

Cyclosporine

The renal complications of cyclosporine are similar to those seen in the transplant setting but tend to occur less frequently in RA, reflecting the lower doses employed [68]. These include reversible renal insufficiency without any morphologic alteration (due to vasomotor constriction) or with isometric cytoplasmic vacuolization of the proximal tubules; and chronic renal insufficiency associated with interstitial fibrosis (with either a diffuse or "striped" pattern) and/or nodular hyaline arteriolosclerosis [69]. Rare individuals may develop acute thrombotic microangiopathy accompanied by renal insufficiency and signs of hemolytic uremic syndrome.

Gold Salts and Penicillamine

The major renal complication of these agents is membranous glomerulonephritis [70]. Proteinuria may develop in up to 10 percent of patients treated with these agents and is not related to cumulative dose. In most cases, proteinuria disappears within one year of discontinuing the drug. The light microscopy and

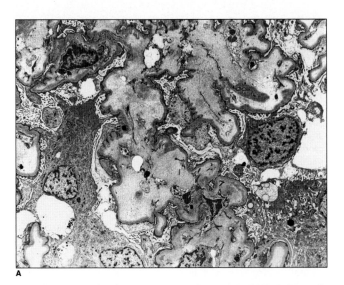

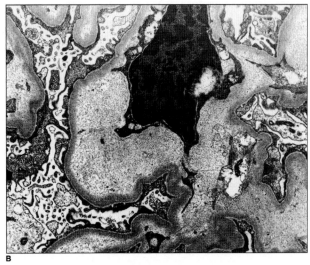

FIGURE 7.67: *Thrombotic microangiopathy in SLE. A. There is a global subendothelial accumulation of electron lucent, flocculent material ("fluff") as well as extensive loss of endothelial cells. The glomerular basement membrane is segmentaly wrinkled and thickened. B. The micrograph highlights prominent dissolution of the mesangial matrix consistent with mesangiolysis. (Electron micrographs; A, × 2,000; B, × 6,000).*

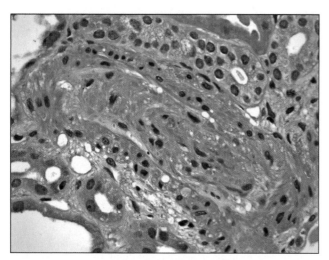

FIGURE 7.68: *Thrombotic microangiopathy in SLE. This small interlobular artery shows marked mucoid intimal expansion causing complete occlusion of the lumen. (H&E, × 400).*

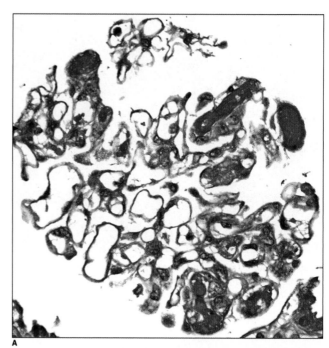

A

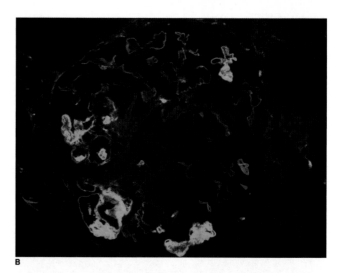

B

FIGURE 7.69: *Antiphospholipid antibody syndrome in SLE. The renal biopsy in this patient with SLE showed lupus nephritis class III and acute thrombotic microangiopathy associated with secondary antiphospholipid antibody syndrome. A. Trichrome stain highlights multiple intracapillary red thrombi (× 400). B. The glomerular thrombi stain strongly for fibrin by immunofluorescence. (× 400).*

IF findings are indistinguishable from idiopathic membranous glomerulonephritis. However, in gold-associated membranous glomerulonephritis, EM may reveal intralysosomal filamentous gold inclusions in proximal tubules, and rarely in glomerular epithelial cells and mesangial cells. Rare cases of pauci-immune focal segmental necrotizing and crescentic glomerulonephritis have been reported following penicillamine therapy, some in association with renal vasculitis and pulmonary hemorrhage [71]. Some of these cases demonstrate antimyeloperoxidase (anti-MPO) ANCA [72] but whether the development of ANCA in these patients represents a drug-related phenomenon or a manifestation of underlying RA is uncertain.

Tumor Necrosis Factor (TNA)-Alpha Antagonists

Treatment of RA with TNF-alpha antagonists, including etanercept, infliximab, and adalimumab, frequently leads to induction of autoantibodies (including ANA, anti-dsDNA, ANCA, and ACL antibodies) and some patients develop clinical signs of a lupus-like disease. Rare cases of renal disease have been reported including lupus-like nephritis (either focal or diffuse proliferative glomerulonephritis or membranous lupus nephritis [Figure 7.73], usually with new appearance of anti-dsDNA antibodies), new onset of pauci-immune necrotizing and crescentic glomerulonephritis (with or without ANCA), and renal vasculitis [55,56]. Some of these cases have shown resolution of serologic and renal abnormalities following discontinuation of the drug. The temporal relationship to drug use in these individuals suggests that the pathogenesis of renal disease is related to immune dysregulation associated with TNF-alpha blockade [55].

Glomerular Disease Related to RA

Rare cases of glomerular disease other than amyloidosis, or associated with a history of nephrotoxic drug use have been

described in RA patients. These include cases of mesangial proliferative glomerulonephritis (Figure 7.74) [73], membranous glomerulonephritis (Figure 7.75) [74], pauci-immune focal segmental necrotizing and crescentic glomerulonephritis (both with [75,76] or without [77] ANCA) (Figure 7.76), and thrombotic microangiopathy associated with antiphospholipid antibody [78]. Rare cases of large vessel vasculitis have also been described in RA patients [79].

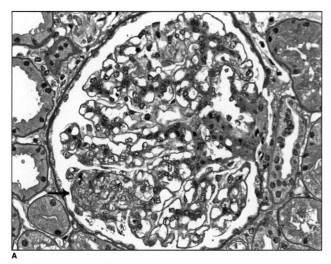
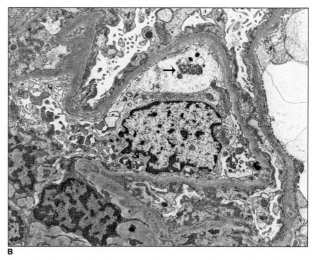

FIGURE 7.70: Podocytopathy in SLE. The biopsy is from a 28-year-old female with newly diagnosed systemic lupus erythematosus and new-onset nephrotic syndrome. On light microscopy, all fourteen glomeruli sampled showed global mesangial hypercellularity and two glomeruli revealed cellular lesions of focal segmental glomerulosclerosis (arrow). (PAS, × 400). B. Ultrastructurally, podocytes were swollen with complete foot process effacement (shown). There were many endothelial tubuloreticular inclusions (arrow) and only rare, minute mesangial and subepithelial deposits (not shown). (Electron micrograph, × 4,000). No subendothelial deposits were seen on electron microscopy or immunofluorescence. The biopsy was interpreted as lupus nephritis class II and podocytopathy with features of cellular focal segmental glomerulosclerosis. The patient was treated with steroids and had a full remission of nephrotic syndrome in several weeks.

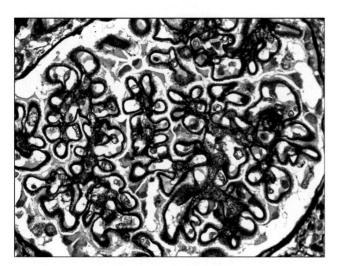

FIGURE 7.71: Membranous lupus nephritis in mixed connective tissue disease. Membranous glomerulonephritis in a patient with mixed connective tissue disease. JMS stain showed global, minute, eosinophilic subepithelial deposits separated by well-developed, black glomerular basement membrane spikes (× 600). On immunofluorescence, the deposits stained for IgG, IgA, IgM, C3, C1, kappa and lambda ("full house staining") resembling lupus nephritis class V.

Table 7.8 American Rheumatism Association Criteria for Diagnosis of Rheumatoid Arthritis

1. Morning stiffness of >1 hour
2. Arthritis and soft-tissue swelling of >3 of 14 joints/joint groups
3. Arthritis of hand joints
4. Symmetric arthritis
5. Subcutaneous nodules (rheumatoid nodules)
6. Rheumatoid factor (RF) titer above the 95th percentile
7. Radiological changes suggestive of joint erosion

The first four criteria must be present for at least 6 weeks to establish the diagnosis.

The clinical features of mesangial proliferative glomerulonephritis include hematuria and/or mild proteinuria [73]. IF most commonly reveals mesangial IgM, with variable weak staining for IgG, IgA, C3, and C1q. EM demonstrates small paramesangial electron-dense deposits [73]. Membranous glomerulonephritis typically presents with heavy proteinuria or the nephrotic syndrome [74]. The duration of RA prior to onset of renal disease ranges from three to thirteen years. The pathologic findings are usually indistinguishable from primary membranous glomerulonephritis (Figure 7.75), with glomerular capillary wall deposits of IgG and C3 [74]. Rare cases may demonstrate costaining for IgM, IgA and C1q, resembling membranous lupus nephritis [74].

Focal segmental necrotizing and crescentic glomerulonephritis may be accompanied by cutaneous or multisystem vasculitis. Although ANCA serologies were not tested in earlier reports, most cases in the modern era manifest are P-ANCA (anti-myeloperoxidase) positive [75,76]. In one study of 246 RA patients, 52 patients (21 percent) had positive P-ANCA and this was significantly associated with development of RA-related nephropathy [75]. These findings support the emerging view that ANCA-associated renal disease may be a form of primary RA-related glomerulonephritis.

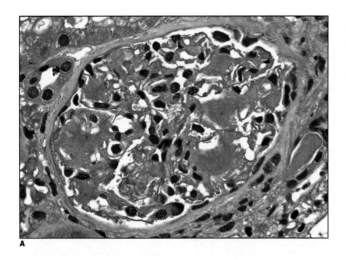

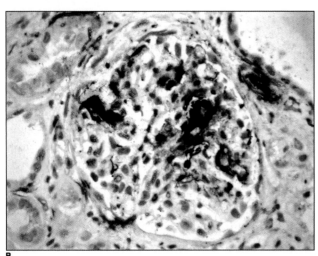

FIGURE 7.72: Secondary (AA) amyloidosis in rheumatoid arthritis. A. There is global glomerular mesangial expansion by eosinophilic amyloid deposits (H&E, ×600). B. The amyloid material stains strongly for serum amyloid A (SAA) protein by immunohistochemistry. Focal tubular basement membrane and interstitial amyloid positivity for SAA are also noted (×600).

SJOGREN'S SYNDROME

Definition

Sjogren's syndrome (SS) is a chronic, organ-specific autoimmune disease characterized by lymphocyte infiltration of the exocrine salivary glands and lacrimal glands giving rise to xerostomia and xerophthalmia (sicca complex) [80]. SS may be primary (40 percent of cases) or associated with a variety of other autoimmune disorders, including RA (50 percent), SLE (5 percent), and systemic sclerosis (5 percent) [81]. Multisystemic involvement occurs in a subset of patients with primary Sjogren's syndrome, with lymphocyte infiltrates affecting kidney, lungs, liver, bone marrow, thyroid, stomach, pancreas, and skin

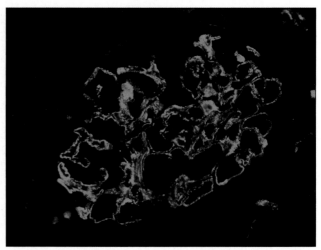

FIGURE 7.73: Membranous lupus nephritis in rheumatoid arthritis. The patient is a 64-year-old male with history of rheumatoid arthritis treated with the anti-TNF alpha agent: adalimumab. He developed nephritic-range proteinuria with positive ANA and anti-DNA antibody. The renal biopsy showed membranous lupus nephritis. The immunofluorescence micrograph shown reveals granular, global glomerular capillary wall and mesangial positivity for IgG (×400).

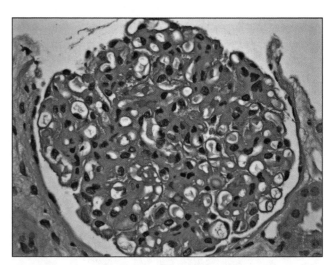

FIGURE 7.74: Mesangial proliferative glomerulonephritis in rheumatoid arthritis. The glomerulus shows mild global mesangial hypercellularity. The glomerular capillary lumina are patent (H&E, ×400).

Clinical Features

Serologic features include positive ANA (80 percent), hypergammaglobulinemia (80 percent), rheumatoid factor (75–95 percent), anti-Ro/SSA, and anti-La/SSB (60 percent). Hypocomplementemia is seen in lupus-associated SS but is uncommon in primary SS. Occasional patients develop mixed cryoglobulinemia. The reported prevalence of renal disease in primary SS ranges from 18 to 67 percent of cases, reflecting differences in diagnostic criteria [82]. The renal manifestations are variable and reflect the type of renal pathologic lesion. Most commonly, this consists of tubulointerstitial nephritis associated with distal renal tubular

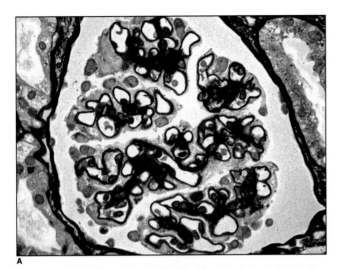

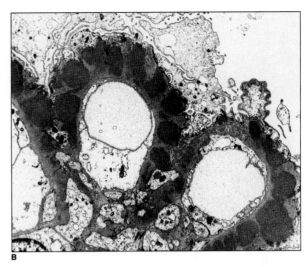

FIGURE 7.75:   Membranous glomerulonephritis in rheumatoid arthritis. Fifty-eight year-old male with history of rheumatoid arthritis for 17 years, not treated with penicillamine or gold. He developed sudden-onset nephrotic syndrome and the renal biopsy showed membranous glomerulonephritis. A. JMS stain delineates delicate, global glomerular basement membrane spikes (× 600). B. On electron microscopy, there are large, regularly- distributed, electron-dense subepithelial deposits with intervening glomerular basement membrane spikes (× 4,000).

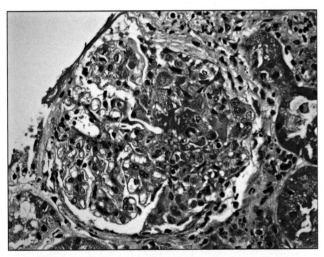

FIGURE 7.76:   ANCA-associated pauci-immune crescentic and necrotizing glomerulonephritis in rheumatoid arthritis. A glomerulus shows a cellular crescent with associated fibrin (red) extravasation into the urinary space. (Trichrome stain, × 400).

acidosis, impaired concentrating ability, with variable, generally mild renal insufficiency. Occasional patients may develop Fanconi syndrome, hypercalciuria, nephrocalcinosis, and osteomalacia. Glomerular disease and renal vasculitis are uncommon. Glomerulonephritis is characterized by proteinuria, active urinary sediment, and renal insufficiency [83,84]. Renal vasculitis is associated with hypertension and renal insufficiency and may be accompanied by signs of extrarenal vasculitis.

Renal Biopsy Findings

The commonest pattern of renal disease in SS is chronic tubulointerstitial nephritis, with patchy interstitial infiltrates of lymphocytes, monocytes, and occasional plasma cells (Figures

7.77A,B). There is frequently evidence of ongoing activity (tubulitis) (Figure 7.77C) with varying degrees of tubular atrophy and interstitial fibrosis. Granulomas are absent. IF and EM may reveal tubulointerstitial immune deposits but these are not uniformly present. Intratubular and interstitial calcifications may be seen in cases of nephrocalcinosis associated with hypercalcemia. Glomeruli may show nonspecific changes including pericapsular fibrosis.

Immune complex-mediated glomerulonephritis in SS is relatively rare and may include any class of lupus glomerulonephritis, including mesangial proliferative, focal and diffuse proliferative and membranous glomerulonephritis [83] or membranoproliferative glomerulonephritis related to cryoglobulinemia [84] (Figure 7.78). IF and EM reveal patterns of immune deposition, similar to lupus nephritis or cryoglobulinemic glomerulonephritis.

Differential Diagnosis

This includes sarcoidosis, drug-induced (allergic), and infectious tubulointersitital nephritis.

Etiology and Pathogenesis

These are largely unknown. The presence of lymphocytic infiltrates in the affected organs suggests a role for cell-mediated immunity. Some cases of primary SS may be related pathogenetically to Epstein-Barr virus infection of renal tubular epithelium [85]. The immune complex-associated glomerular lesions are likely related to autoantibody formation, analogous to lupus nephritis.

Treatment and Prognosis

Interstitial nephritis often responds to high-dose steroids. Treatment of immune complex glomerular disease should be directed to the particular class of lupus nephritis. Patients

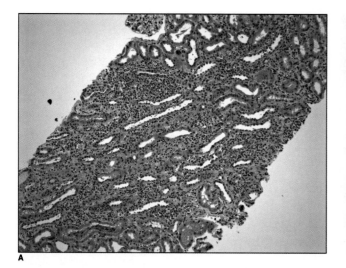

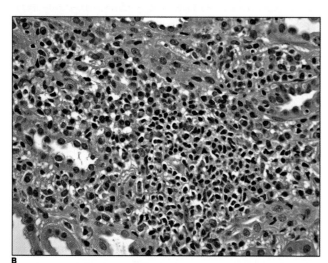

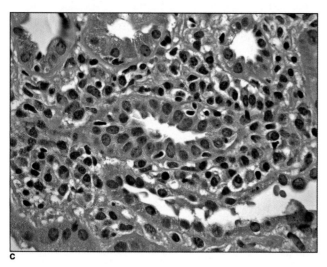

FIGURE 7.77: *Sjogren's syndrome. Low-power micrograph shows diffuse, dense interstitial inflammation. B. The interstitial infiltrate is composed of lymphocytes and abundant plasma cells. C. Multifocal mononuclear cell tubulitis is seen (H&E; A, ×100; B, ×400; C, ×600).*

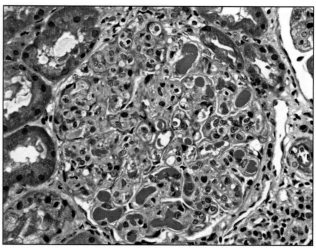

FIGURE 7.78: *Sjogren's syndrome. Cryoglobulinemic glomerulonephritis in Sjogren's syndrome. A glomerulus shows global monocyte infiltration and abundant intracapillary red deposits forming 'protein thrombi' (Trichrome stain, ×400).*

with necrotizing arteritis are treated similar to microscopic polyangiitis with a regimen including steroids and cyclophosphamide.

REFERENCES

1. Hochberg MC. Updating the American College of Rheumatology revised criteria for the classification of systemic lupus erythematosus. *Arthritis Rheum* 1997; 40: 1725.
2. Pollak VE, Pirani CL, Schwartz FD. The natural history of the renal manifestations of systemic lupus erythematosus. *J Lab Clin Med* 1964; 63: 537–550.
3. Weening JJ, D'Agati VD, Schwartz MM, et al. The classification of glomerulonephritis in systemic lupus erythematosus revisited. *J Am Soc Nephrol* 2004; 15: 241–250.
4. Churg J, Sobin LH. *Renal Disease: Classification and Atlas of Renal Disease.* Igaku-New Shoin; Tokyo, 1982.
5. Churg J, Bernstein J, Glassock R. Lupus nephritis, in *Renal Disease: Classification and Atlas of Renal Disease.* Igaku-New Shoin; New York, 1995, pp. 151–155.
6. Jennette JC. The immunohistology of IgA nephropathy. *Am J Kidney Dis* 1988; 12: 348–352.
7. Nasr SH, D'Agati VD, Park HR et al. Necrotizing and crescentic lupus nephritis with anti-neutrophil cytoplasmic antibody seropositivity. *Clinical JASN* 2008; 3: 682–90.
8. Appel GB, Williams GS, Meltzer JI et al. Renal vein thrombosis, nephrotic syndrome, and systemic lupus erythematosus: an association in four cases. *Ann Intern Med* 1976; 85:310–317.
9. Jennette JC, Iskandar SS, Dalldorf FG. Pathologic differentiation between lupus and nonlupus membranous glomerulopathy. *Kidney Int* 1983; 24: 377–385.
10. Austin HA, Muenz LR, Joyce KM, et al. Prognostic factors in lupus nephritis. Contribution of renal histologic data. *Am J Med* 1983; 75: 382–391.
11. Appel GB, Cohen DJ, Pirani CL, et al. Long-term follow-up of patients with lupus nephritis. a study based on the classification of the World Health Organization. *Am J Med* 1987; 83: 877–885.

12. Schwartz MM, Bernstein J, Hill GS, et al. Predictive value of renal pathology in diffuse proliferative lupus glomerulonephritis. Lupus Nephritis Collaborative Study Group. *Kidney Int* 1989; 36: 891–896

13. Austin HA, 3rd, Boumpas DT, Vaughan EM, et al. Predicting renal outcomes in severe lupus nephritis: contributions of clinical and histologic data. *Kidney Int* 1994; 45: 544–550.

14. Hill GS, Delahousse M, Nochy D, et al. Predictive power of the second renal biopsy in lupus nephritis: significance of macrophages. *Kidney Int* 2001; 59: 304–316.

15. Hill GS, Delahousse M, Nochy D, et al. A new morphologic index for the evaluation of renal biopsies in lupus nephritis. *Kidney Int* 2000; 58: 1160–1173.

16. Park MH, D'Agati V, Appel GB, et al. Tubulointerstitial disease in lupus nephritis: relationship to immune deposits, interstitial inflammation, glomerular changes, renal function, and prognosis. *Nephron* 1986; 44: 309–319.

17. Mori Y, Kishimoto N, Yamahara H, et al. Predominant tubulointerstitial nephritis in a patient with systemic lupus nephritis. *Clin Exp Nephrol* 2005; 9: 79–84.

18. Makker SP: Tubular basement membrane antibody-induced interstitial nephritis in systemic lupus erythematosus. *Am J Med* 1980; 69: 949–952.

19. Hunter MG, Hurwitz S, Bellamy CO, et al. Quantitative morphometry of lupus nephritis: the significance of collagen, tubular space, and inflammatory infiltrate. *Kidney Int* 2005; 67: 94–102.

20. Howie AJ, Turhan N, Adu D: Powerful morphometric indicator of prognosis in lupus nephritis. *Qjm* 2003; 96: 411–420.

21. Banfi G, Bertani T, Boeri V, et al. Renal vascular lesions as a marker of poor prognosis in patients with lupus nephritis. Gruppo Italiano per lo Studio della Nefrite Lupica (GISNEL). *Am J Kidney Dis* 1991; 18: 240–248.

22. Miyakis S, Lockshin MD, Atsumi T, et al. International consensus statement on an update of the classification criteria for definite antiphospholipid syndrome (APS). *J Thromb Haemost* 2006; 4: 295–306.

23. Nochy D, Daugas E, Droz D, et al. The intrarenal vascular lesions associated with primary antiphospholipid syndrome. *J Am Soc Nephrol* 1999; 10: 507–518.

24. Daugas E, Nochy D, Huong DL, et al. Antiphospholipid syndrome nephropathy in systemic lupus erythematosus. *J Am Soc Nephrol* 2002; 13: 42–52.

25. Kremer Hovinga IC, Koopmans M, Baelde HJ, et al. Chimerism occurs twice as often in lupus nephritis as in normal kidneys. *Arthritis Rheum* 2006; 54: 2944–2950.

26. Hahn BH: Antibodies to DNA. *N Engl J Med* 1998; 338: 1359–1368.

27. He B, Qiao X, Cerutti A: CpG DNA induces IgG class switch DNA recombination by activating human B cells through an innate pathway that requires TLR9 and cooperates with IL-10. *J Immunol* 2004; 173: 4479–4491.

28. Pawar RD, Patole PS, Ellwart A, et al. Ligands to nucleic acid-specific toll-like receptors and the onset of lupus nephritis. *J Am Soc Nephrol* 2006; 17: 3365–3373.

29. Mannik M, Merrill CE, Stamps LD, et al. Multiple autoantibodies form the glomerular immune deposits in patients with systemic lupus erythematosus. *J Rheumatol* 2003; 30: 1495–1504.

30. Kalaaji M, Fenton KA, Mortensen ES, et al. Glomerular apoptotic nucleosomes are central target structures for nephritogenic antibodies in human SLE nephritis. *Kidney Int* 2007; 71: 664–672.

31. Zhao Z, Weinstein E, Tuzova M, et al. Cross-reactivity of human lupus anti-DNA antibodies with alpha-actinin and nephritogenic potential. *Arthritis Rheum* 2005; 52: 522–530.

32. Peterson KS, Huang JF, Zhu J, et al. Characterization of heterogeneity in the molecular pathogenesis of lupus nephritis from transcriptional profiles of laser-captured glomeruli. *J Clin Invest* 2004; 113: 1722–1733.

33. Baechler EC, Batliwalla FM, Karypis G, et al. Interferon-inducible gene expression signature in peripheral blood cells of patients with severe lupus. *Proc Natl Acad Sci USA* 2003; 100: 2610–2615.

34. Qing X, Putterman C. Gene expression profiling in the study of the pathogenesis of systemic lupus erythematosus. *Autoimmun Rev* 2004; 3: 505–509

35. Lewis EJ, Kawala K, Schwartz MM. Histologic features that correlate with the prognosis of patients with lupus nephritis. *Am J Kidney Dis* 1987; 10:192–197.

36. Dooley MA, Hogan S, Jennette C, et al. Cyclophosphamide therapy for lupus nephritis: poor renal survival in black Americans. Glomerular Disease Collaborative Network. *Kidney Int* 1997; 51: 1188–1195.

37. Najafi CC, Korbet SM, Lewis EJ, et al. Significance of histologic patterns of glomerular injury upon long-term prognosis in severe lupus glomerulonephritis. *Kidney Int* 2001; 59: 2156–2163.

38. Korbet SM, Schwartz MM, Evans J, et al. Severe lupus nephritis: racial differences in presentation and outcome. *J Am Soc Nephrol* 2007; 18: 244–254.

39. Yokoyama H, Wada T, Hara A, et al. The outcome and a new ISN/RPS 2003 classification of lupus nephritis in Japanese. *Kidney Int* 2004; 66: 2382–2388.

40. Mittal B, Hurwitz S, Rennke H, et al. New subcategories of class IV lupus nephritis: are there clinical, histologic, and outcome differences? *Am J Kidney Dis* 2004; 44: 1050–1059.

41. Hill GS, Delahousse M, Nochy D, et al. Class IV-S versus class IV-G lupus nephritis: clinical and morphologic differences suggesting different pathogenesis. *Kidney Int* 2005; 68: 2288–2297.

42. Pasquali S, Banfi G, Zucchelli A, et al. Lupus membranous nephropathy: long-term outcome. *Clin Nephrol* 1993; 39: 175–182.

43. Waldman M, Appel GB: Update on the treatment of lupus nephritis. *Kidney Int* 2006; 70: 1403–1412.

44. Baranowska-Daca E, Choi YJ, Barrios R, et al. Nonlupus nephritides in patients with systemic lupus erythematosus: a comprehensive clinicopathologic study and review of the literature. *Hum Pathol* 2001; 32: 1125–1135.

45. Dube GK, Markowitz GS, Radhakrishnan J, et al. Minimal change disease in systemic lupus erythematosus. *Clin Nephrol* 2002; 57: 120–126.

46. Hertig A, Droz D, Lesavre P, et al. SLE and idiopathic nephrotic syndrome: coincidence or not? *Am J Kidney Dis* 2002; 40: 1179–1184.

47. Kraft SW, Schwartz MM, Korbet SM, et al. Glomerular podocytopathy in patients with systemic lupus erythematosus. *J Am Soc Nephrol* 2005; 16: 175–179.

48. Marshall S, Dressler R, D'Agati V: Membranous lupus nephritis with antineutrophil cytoplasmic antibody-associated

segmental necrotizing and crescentic glomerulonephritis. *Am J Kidney Dis* 1997; 29: 119–124.

49. Zabaleta-Lanz ME, Munoz LE, Tapanes FJ, et al. Further description of early clinically silent lupus nephritis. *Lupus* 2006; 15: 845–851.

50. Wada Y, Ito S, Ueno M, et al. Renal outcome and predictors of clinical renal involvement in patients with silent lupus nephritis. *Nephron Clin Pract* 2004; 98:c105–c111.

51. Bennett WM, Bardana EJ, Norman DJ, et al. Natural history of "silent" lupus nephritis. *Am J Kidney Dis* 1982; 1: 359–363.

52. Hess E: Drug-related lupus. *N Engl J Med* 1988; 318: 1460–1462.

53. Vasoo S: Drug-induced lupus: an update. *Lupus* 2006; 15: 757–761.

54. Sarzi-Puttini P, Atzeni F, Capsoni F, et al. Drug-induced lupus erythematosus. *Autoimmunity* 2005; 38: 507–518.

55. Stokes MB, Foster K, Markowitz GS, et al. Development of glomerulonephritis during anti-TNF-alpha therapy for rheumatoid arthritis. *Nephrol Dial Transplant* 2005; 20: 1400–1406.

56. Mor A, Bingham C, Barisoni L, et al. Proliferative lupus nephritis and leukocytoclastic vasculitis during treatment with etanercept. *J Rheumatol* 2005; 32: 740–743.

57. Vogt BA, Kim Y, Jennette JC, et al. Antineutrophil cytoplasmic autoantibody-positive crescentic glomerulonephritis as a complication of treatment with propylthiouracil in children. *J Pediatr* 1994; 124: 986–988.

58. Chang BG, Markowitz GS, Seshan SV, et al. Renal manifestations of concurrent systemic lupus erythematosus and HIV infection. *Am J Kidney Dis* 1999; 33: 441–449.

59. Sharp GC, Irvin WS, Tan EM, et al. Mixed connective tissue disease – an apparently distinct rheumatic disease syndrome associated with a specific antibody to an extractable nuclear antigen (ENA). *Am J Med* 1972; 52:148–159.

60. Kitridou RC, Akmal M, Turkel SB, et al. Renal involvement in mixed connective tissue disease: a longitudinal clinicopathologic study. *Semin Arthritis Rheum* 1986;16: 135–145.

61. Danieli MG, Fraticelli P, Salvi A, et al. Undifferentiated connective tissue disease: natural history and evolution into definite CTD assessed in 84 patients initially diagnosed as early UCTD. *Clin Rheumatol* 1998; 17: 195–201.

62. Aringer M, Steiner G, Smolen JS: Does mixed connective tissue disease exist? Yes. *Rheum Dis Clin North Am* 2005; 31: 411–420.

63. Arnett FC, Edworthy SM, Bloch DA, et al. The American Rheumatism Association 1987 revised criteria for the classification of rheumatoid arthritis. *Arthritis Rheum* 1988; 31: 315–324.

64. Boers M. Renal disorders in rheumatoid arthritis. *Semin Arthritis Rheum* 1990; 20: 57–68.

65. Couverchel L, Maugars Y, Prost A: Outcomes of thirty-four rheumatoid arthritis patients with renal amyloidosis, including twelve given alkylating agents. *Rev Rhum Engl Ed* 1995; 62: 79–85.

66. Nanra RS. Renal papillary necrosis in rheumatoid arthritis. *Med J Aust* 1975; 1: 194–197.

67. Radford MG, Holley KE, Grande JP, et al. Reversible membranous nephropathy associated with the use of nonsteroidal anti-inflammatory drugs *JAMA* 1996; 276: 466–469.

68. Cohen DJ, Appel GB: Cyclosporine: nephrotoxic effects and guidelines for safe use in patients with rheumatoid arthritis. *Semin Arthritis Rheum* 1992; 21: 43–48.

69. Rodriguez F, Krayenbuhl JC, Harrison WB, et al. Renal biopsy findings and followup of renal function in rheumatoid arthritis

patients treated with cyclosporin A. An update from the International Kidney Biopsy Registry. *Arthritis Rheum* 1996; 39: 1491–1498.

70. Hall CL: The natural course of gold and penicillamine nephropathy: a longterm study of 54 patients. *Adv Exp Med Biol* 1989; 252: 247–256.

71. Almirall J, Alcorta I, Botey A, et al. Penicillamine-induced rapidly progressive glomerulonephritis in a patient with rheumatoid arthritis. *Am J Nephrol* 1993; 13: 286–288.

72. Nanke Y, Akama H, Terai C, et al. Rapidly progressive glomerulonephritis with D-penicillamine. *Am J Med Sci* 2000; 320: 398–402.

73. Korpela M, Mustonen J, Pasternack A, et al. Mesangial glomerulopathy in rheumatoid arthritis patients. Clinical follow-up and relation to antirheumatic therapy. *Nephron* 1991; 59: 46–50.

74. Honkanen E, Tornroth T, Pettersson E, et al. Membranous glomerulonephritis in rheumatoid arthritis not related to gold or d-penicillamine therapy: a report of four cases and review of the literature. *Clin Nephrol* 1987; 27: 87–93.

75. Mustila A, Korpela M, Mustonen J, et al. Perinuclear anti-neutrophil cytoplasmic antibody in rheumatoid arthritis: a marker of severe disease with associated nephropathy. *Arthritis Rheum* 1997; 40: 710–717.

76. Goto A, Mukai M, Notoya A, Kohno M. Rheumatoid arthritis complicated with myeloperoxidase antineutrophil cytoplasmic antibody (MPO-ANCA)-associated vasculitis: a case report. *Mod Rheumatol* 2005; 15: 118–122.

77. Hsieh HS, Chang CF, Yang AH, et al. Antineutrophil cytoplasmic antibody-negative pauci-immune crescentic glomerulonephritis associated with rheumatoid arthritis: An unusual case report. *Nephrology (Carlton)* 2003; 8: 243–247.

78. Nomura M, Okada J, Tateno S, et al. Renal thrombotic microangiopathy in a patient with rheumatoid arthritis and antiphospholipid syndrome: successful treatment with cyclophosphamide pulse therapy and anticoagulant. *Intern Med* 1994; 33: 484–487.

79. Moreland L, DiBartolomeo A, Brick J. Rheumatoid vasculitis with intrarenal aneurysm formation. *J Rheumatol* 1988; 15: 845–849.

80. Sjogren H: Zur Kenntnis Der Keratoconjuctivitis Sicca (Kratitis Folliforms Bei Hypojunktion Der Tramemdrusen). *Acta Ophthalmol Copenh* 11:1–151, 1933.

81. Reveille JD, Wilson RW, Provost TT, et al. Primary Sjogren's syndrome and other autoimmune diseases in families. Prevalence and immunogenetic studies in six kindreds. *Ann Intern Med* 1984; 101: 748–756.

82. Aasarod K, Haga HJ, Berg KJ, et al. Renal involvement in primary Sjogren's syndrome. *Qjm* 2000; 93: 297–304.

83. Font J, Cervera R, Lopez-Soto A, et al. Mixed membranous and proliferative glomerulonephritis in primary Sjogren's syndrome. *Br J Rheumatol* 1989; 28: 548–550.

84. Kau CK, Hu JC, Lu LY, et al. Primary Sjogren's syndrome complicated with cryoglobulinemic glomerulonephritis, myocarditis, and multi-organ involvement. *J Formos Med Assoc* 2004; 103: 707–710.

85. Fox RI, Pearson G, Vaughan JH: Detection of Epstein-Barr virus-associated antigens and DNA in salivary gland biopsies from patients with Sjogren's syndrome. *J Immunol* 1986; 137: 3162–3168.

CHAPTER 8

Metabolic Diseases of the Kidney

Zoltan G. Laszik, MD, and Lukas Haragsim, MD

This chapter discusses a diverse group of metabolic diseases with significant renal manifestations. A few of these diseases, such as lipoprotein glomerulopathy (LPG), affect only the kidney while most of the diseases have systemic manifestations with renal involvement. Most of them are quite rare, however, some of them are common and diabetic nephropathy (DNP) represents the most common cause of end-stage renal disease (ESRD) in the western world. In addition to their diverse etiology, they also differ in clinical presentation, renal pathologic findings, pathogenesis, and outcome. The epidemiologic data, clinical presentation, morphologic findings, differential diagnosis, etiology and pathogenesis, clinical course, prognosis, and treatment will be discussed separately for each disease.

ALKAPTONURIA (ALKAPTONURIC OCHRONOSIS)

Introduction

Alkaptonuria is a rare mendelian autosomal recessive disorder of tyrosine catabolism and represents the first documented example of an autosomal recessive disease in humans [1].

Epidemiology and Clinical Presentation

The estimated incidence of alkaptonuria is 1 in 250,000 to 1 million live births [2]. Most patients are diagnosed in the third decade of life, however, a significant proportion of patients are diagnosed during infancy [2]. The diagnosis is often suggested by darkening of the urine upon standing. Discoloration of the skin and arthritic symptoms, both related to ochronotic pigment deposition, typically begin during the third or fourth decade of life. Cardiovascular manifestations include calcification of the coronary arteries, aortic dilatation, and aortic- and mitral-valve calcification. Renal involvement with renal insufficiency is a rare complication. Nephrolithiasis is relatively common; in a recent study 22.4 percent of fifty-eight patients with alkaptonuria had renal stones, however, only 1 of the fifty-eight patients, who also had DNP, had reduced creatinine clearance.

Approach to Interpretation

Gross Pathology. There are no characteristic gross findings in patients with ochronosis.

Light Microscopy. The light microscopic findings are mostly nonspecific, except for the presence of melanin-like (ochronotic) pigment deposited in various compartments of the kidney. The coarsely granular yellowish-brown pigment is found in the tubular epithelial cells, interstitium, interstitial histiocytes, tubular casts, and various constituents of the glomeruli. The pigment is well visualized on hematoxylin and eosin-stained sections; it also reacts with special stains for melanin. In advanced stages, often associated with renal failure, extensive tubular atrophy and interstitial fibrosis may be seen accompanied by slight to moderate chronic interstitial inflammatory cell infiltrates.

Immunofluorescence (IF) Microscopy. The IF findings are either nonspecific or negative.

Electron Microscopy. Ochronotic pigment can be seen in the glomeruli, tubules, and interstitium. Glomerular deposition involves visceral and parietal epithelial cells, mesangial cells, basement membranes, and extracellular spaces. It can also be found in the tubular epithelial cells, within tubular casts admixed with crystalline material, inside histiocytes, and free in the interstitium.

Differential Diagnosis

Deposition of a melanin-like (ochronotic) pigment in the kidney requires clinical-laboratory correlation to confirm the diagnosis of ochronosis. Melanin, which is histologically similar to the ochronotic pigment, can be seen in the kidney only in rare cases of pigmented primary or metastatic neoplasms. Lipofuscin, an irregular granular golden-brown pigment sometimes accumulated in the cytoplasm of the tubular epithelial cells, displays periodic acid Schiff (PAS) positivity and yellow-to-red autofluorescence.

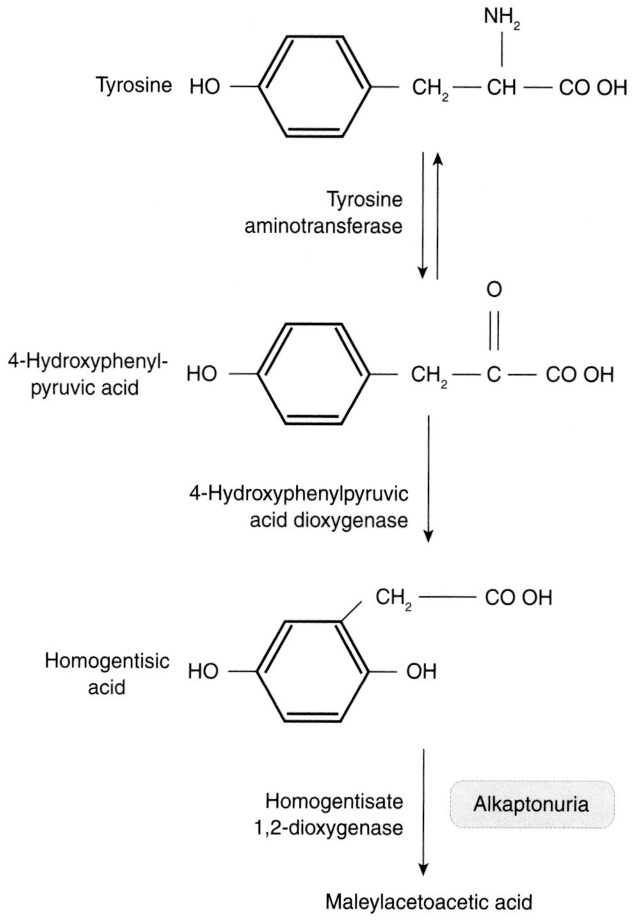

FIGURE 8.1: *The molecular pathogenesis of alkaptonuria.*
The basic defect of alkaptonuria is deficient homogentisate
1,2-dioxygenase (HGO) activity. Accumulation of homogentisic
acid leads to the formation of ochronotic pigment.

Etiology and Pathogenesis

Alkaptonuria is caused by deficient activity of homogentisate
1,2-dioxygenase (HGO) enzyme due to mutations of the
HGO gene [3] (Figure 8.1). Ensuing accumulation of homogentisic acid (HGA) leads to the formation of ochronotic pigment
that binds to connective tissue. The pigment causes ochronosis
with destruction of joints, spinal disks, and bones, and deterioration of cardiac valves. The black urine results from excretion
of large quantities of HGA through the kidney; HGA is color-
less in fresh urine but darkens on exposure to air. HGA is also
secreted by renal tubular epithelial cells, which may reduce the
burden of HGA on tissues; however, large quantities of HGA
excreted into the urine may also contribute to the increased rate
of kidney stone formation. Renal insufficiency may cause worsening of alkaptonuria by decreased excretion of HGA [4].

Clinical Course, Prognosis, Treatment, and Clinical Correlation

Although relatively rare, renal insufficiency may occur in alkaptonuria during the later stages of the disease with interstitial

fibrosis and tubular atrophy. There is no well-established effective therapy for alkaptonuria. Treatment with vitamin C to
enhance HGA degradation has not proved beneficial. Limited
experience with nitisinone (Orfadin), an inhibitor of the enzyme
that produces HGA, revealed dramatic reduction of urinary
excretion of HGA in individuals with alkaptonuria [5].

CYSTINOSIS

Introduction

Cystinosis is a rare inherited autosomal recessive lysosomal
transport disorder. Renal involvement is the major cause of
morbidity and mortality in the two most common forms (infantile and juvenile) of the disease.

Epidemiology and Clinical Presentation

The estimated incidence is 1 in 100,000 to 200,000 live births,
although higher incidences are reported from France and Que-
bec, Canada [6]. There are three clinical forms of the disease
based on age at onset and severity of symptoms: early-onset
nephropathic (infantile), late-onset nephropathic (juvenile),
and nonnephropathic (ocular). Among these various clinical
forms, the infantile form is the most severe with ESRD developing by 10 years of age [7]. The two other forms (juvenile and
ocular) are less frequent and somewhat less severe, with ESRD
developing at least in some patients with the juvenile form
[8]. The typical renal manifestations of the infantile and
juvenile forms are listed in Table 8.1. In the infantile form,
the onset of renal Fanconi syndrome is usually prior to 1 year
of age, followed by progressive renal functional deterioration. Cystinosis accounts for approximately 5 percent of
chronic renal failure in children [9]. The diagnosis of cystinosis is confirmed by measurement of the cystine levels in
mixed leukocyte preparations. Polymerase chain reaction-
based assays are also available for molecular diagnosis of the
more common mutations of the gene (see also "Etiology and
Pathogenesis") [8].

Approach to Interpretation

Gross Pathology. In advanced disease, the kidneys are grossly
contracted. In less advanced stages, no typical gross findings are
reported.

Light Microscopy. The characteristic light microscopic findings of the infantile form of cystinosis are summarized in Table
8.2. In the infantile form, the kidneys show progressive interstitial fibrosis, tubular atrophy, variable interstitial inflammation, and evolving glomerulosclerosis. During the early stages
of the disease, an increased number of immature glomeruli may
be present [10]. Multinucleated visceral and parietal epithelial
cells (polykaryocytosis) are also typical early findings, although
not unique to cystinosis [11]. Multinucleation of rare tubular
epithelial cells can be observed. Relatively large hexagonal, needle-shaped or rhomboid clefts corresponding to cystine crystals
can be seen in interstitial histiocytes, tubular epithelial cells, as
well as freely in the interstitium (Figure 8.2). Due to water

Table 8.1 Clinical Manifestations of Infantile and Juvenile Forms of Nephropathic Cystinosis

Early-Onset (Infantile)

Age	Presentation
Birth	Normal
Infancy	Renal tubular Fanconi syndrome – Dehydration, polyuria, polydipsia – Metabolic acidosis – Hypokalemia – Hypophosphatemic rickets – Hypocalcemic tetany Growth retardation Vomiting
Early childhood	Photophobia
Preadolescence	Renal failure Proteinuria Renal osteodystrophy Hypothyroidism

Late-Onset (Juvenile)

Average onset at 12–13 years of age	Progressive renal dysfunction Fanconi syndrome may not be present

Modified from Nesterova and Gahl [17].

Table 8.2 Light Microscopic Findings of the Infantile Form of Cystinosis

Multinucleated visceral and parietal epithelial cells (polykaryocytosis)
Increased number of immature glomeruli
Hexagonal/needle-shaped clefts (IH, IS)
Progressive interstitial fibrosis
Tubular atrophy
Interstitial inflammation
Glomerulosclerosis

Abbreviations: IH, interstitial histiocytes; IS, interstitium

solubility, the crystals are not retained in tissue sections of formalin-fixed material. However, they can be directly visualized under polarized light as birefringent cytoplasmic structures in frozen sections of fresh tissues or paraffin sections of alcohol-fixed material. A smaller number of crystalline structures may also be found in tubular and glomerular epithelial cells. Microdissection studies disclosed a characteristic "swan-neck" lesion of the first portion of the proximal tubule showing prominent atrophy of the epithelium with luminal narrowing [10]. This lesion seems to develop during the second six months of life and may be preceded by deposition of intracytoplasmic crystalline structures within tubular epithelial cells [10]. However, the "swan-neck" lesion is difficult to detect by light microscopy and may also occur in patients with other causes of Fanconi's syndrome posing significant limitations to its diagnostic utility. On Toluidine blue-stained thick sections, visceral epithelial cells, rare tubular epithelial cells, and occasional interstitial cells may have an opaque-dark appearance. This feature is likely due to

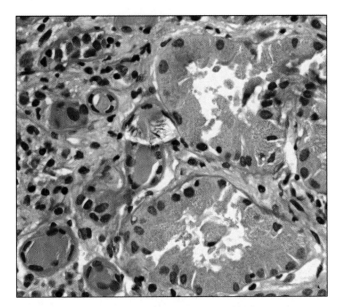

FIGURE 8.2: *Cystinosis with small intraepithelial needle-shaped clefts. Cystine crystals accumulate within interstitial histiocytes, freely in the interstitium, and also in tubular epithelial cells. Due to water solubility the crystals are dissolved during fixation with formalin leaving behind small needle-shaped clefts. (Hematoxylin and eosin, ×400).*

interaction of osmium with intracellular cystine. As the disease progresses, more and more glomerulosclerosis and interstitial fibrosis develop with ensuing ESRD usually before 10 years of age. Secondary FSGS can be seen especially in patients with significant proteinuria (Figure 8.3).

The juvenile form of the disease shows predominantly glomerular involvement with mesangial proliferative lesions and focal segmental and global glomerulosclerosis [8]. Tubulointerstitial changes may develop at advanced stages.

Immunofluorescence Microscopy. The IF is negative or shows only nonspecific staining.

Electron Microscopy. Typical early findings include membrane-bound intracytoplasmic rectangular-, needle-, or spindle-shaped clefts, corresponding to dissolved cystine crystals, within interstitial histiocytes and the neck region of the proximal tubules. Crystalline structures can also be found in the glomerular visceral and parietal epithelial cells [12]. Degenerative features of the proximal tubular epithelial cells with prominent vacuolization and increased number of lysosomes can be detected. In the more advanced stages the neck region of the proximal tubule exhibits thin simplified epithelium without lysosomes, crystalline spaces, and brush border [10]. Effacement of the foot processes of the visceral epithelial cells and thickening of the glomerular capillary basement membranes (GBM) is also noted.

Differential Diagnosis

In addition to cystinosis, crystalline deposits can also be seen in the kidney in primary and secondary forms of renal oxalosis, Fabry's disease, and dysproteinemias. In contrast with cystine deposits, the usually fan-shaped oxalate crystals are retained in

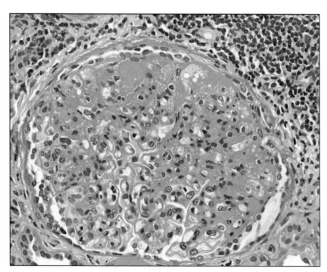

FIGURE 8.3: *Advanced cystinosis with focal segmental glomerulosclerosis. The glomerulus features hyperplastic and hypertrophic visceral epithelial cells, hyalinosis, and segmental sclerosis.(Periodic acid Schiff reaction, × 400).*

formalin-fixed paraffin embedded tissues. They do exhibit, just like cystine deposits, birefringence under polarized light. In Fabry's disease, frozen sections of fresh or formalin-fixed material show Maltese crosses under polarized light. The Maltese crosses correspond to glycolipid deposits that are most prominent in the glomeruli. In dysproteinemias, crystalline inclusions deposited within interstitial macrophages and tubular epithelial cells, are also retained in paraffin sections of formalin-fixed material. Monoclonality of the crystalline inclusions of dysproteinemias can be featured by immunofluorescence showing kappa or lambda light chain restriction. An algorithm for the differential diagnosis of crystal deposits in the kidney is provided (Figure 8.4). The presence of multinucleated visceral epithelial cells is highly characteristic, although not entirely specific for cystinosis, as these cells are also seen in rare cases of crescentic glomerulonephritis [13]. Cystinosis is not to be confused with cystinuria, a common inherited autosomal recessive disorder characterized by impaired reabsorption of cystin by the proximal tubules in the kidney [14]. The disease is caused by mutations of two genes (*SLC3A1* and *SLC7A9*) coding for transporter proteins responsible for tubular reabsorption of filtered positively charged amino acids. As a result of the reabsorption defect, increased urinary concentration of cystin may lead to the precipitation of cystin with formation of hexagonal crystals and renal stones.

Etiology and Pathogenesis

Cystinosis is an autosomal recessive disease caused by various mutations in the *CTNS* gene encoding cystinosin, a lysosomal cystine transporter [6,7]. More than 50 *CTNS* mutations have been described, the most common being a 57-kilobase deletion affecting nearly half of all North American and European patients [8,15]. Those patients with classical cystinosis have homozygous or compound heterozygous mutations associated

with the loss of a functional protein, whereas milder cases are heterozygous for a severe (e.g., nonsense) mutation and a milder (e.g., splice-site) mutation. Patients heterozygous for a severe mutation have no symptoms. The failure to transport cystine out of lysosomes results in intralysosomal cystine accumulation and crystallization, leading to cellular and organ dysfunction. In addition to the dominant renal manifestations, ocular, endocrinological, hepatic, muscular, and central nervous system complications can also occur. Although intrarenal cystine accumulation with crystalline deposits is a possible cause of renal structural and functional damage, the precise pathogenetic mechanisms that lead to progressive renal injury in cystinosis are not well understood. It has been postulated that the proximal tubular stricture at the "swan-neck" lesion may contribute to the progression of the disease [16].

Clinical Course, Prognosis, Treatment, and Clinical Correlation

Prior to the advent of renal transplantation most patients with nephropathic cystinosis died at a young age. Once kidney transplantation allowed longer survivals, the scope of the disease expanded with multisystemic involvement. Nonrenal complications include retinal blindness, vacuolar myopathy, swallowing dysfunction, diabetes mellitus, pancreatic exocrine insufficiency, central nervous system involvement, pulmonary dysfunction, male hypogonadism, benign intracranial hypertension, vascular calcifications, and nodular regenerating hyperplasia of the liver [17]. Without long-term treatment with the cystine-depleting cysteamine therapy, most transplant patients develop some of these major complications by the time they reach 30 years of age [18].

Early diagnosis is crucial to initiate preventive and therapeutic management. Prior to renal transplantation, therapy is primarily aimed at replacement of fluids and electrolytes due to losses from Fanconi syndrome. Targeted therapy involves oral administration of the free aminothiol cysteamine, which depletes leukocyte cystine content of up to 95 percent and reduces the cystine content of parenchymal tissues [19]. Long-term cysteamine oral administration in children with cystinosis helps maintain renal glomerular function and improves growth [20]. It has also been shown that children who are treated early and adequately with cysteamine have renal function that increases during the first five years of life and then declines at a normal rate [21]. Most recent data indicate that long-term oral cysteamine therapy can also retard or prevent serious late complications of cystinosis. Frequency of myopathy, diabetes, pulmonary insufficiency, hypothyroidism, hypercholesterolemia, and death decreased with time on cysteamine therapy and increased with time off cysteamine therapy [18].

DIABETIC NEPHROPATHY

Introduction

Diabetic nephropathy is a clinical syndrome characterized by persistent albuminuria (>300 mg/24 hours), a steady decline in glomerular filtration rate (GFR), and elevated blood pressure [22]. The clinical and morphologic features of DNP are similar, although not identical, in type 1 and type 2 diabetes. In

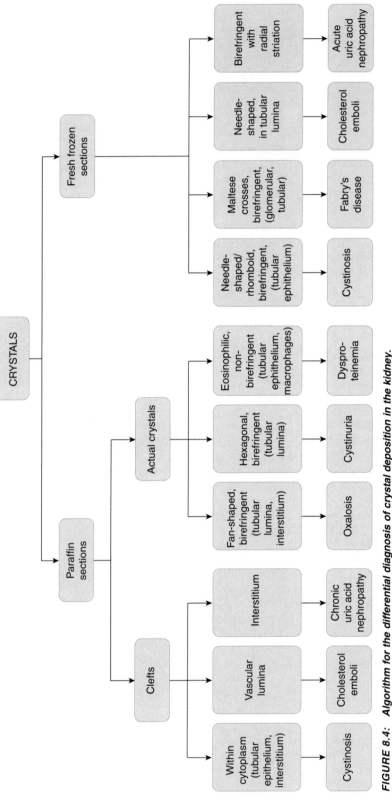

FIGURE 8.4: *Algorithm for the differential diagnosis of crystal deposition in the kidney.*

general, the renal lesions in patients with type 2 diabetes are more heterogenous [23].

Epidemiology and Clinical Presentation

Diabetic nephropathy is the most common cause of chronic renal failure in the United States and accounts for almost half of patients in long term dialysis programs [24]. Approximately one-third of patients with diabetes develop DNP with a high likelihood of progression to ESRD. Diabetic nephropathy is more common in the diabetic populations of certain ethnic and racial groups. The prevalence of DNP is highest in Native Americans, followed by African Americans, Hispanics, and Caucasians [25–27]. As a result of increasing prevalence of diabetes, predominantly of type 2, the incidences of DNP and ESRD due to diabetes continue to rise. The onset of overt DNP is preceded by a preclinical stage with microalbuminuria (30–299 mg/24 hours). Overt DNP presents with proteinuria (>300 mg/day) and declining GFR, which is usually associated with rising systemic blood pressure and the presence of other diabetic complications. Fully developed nephrotic syndrome is rare but microscopic hematuria is relatively common in patients with DNP [28].

Table 8.3 Key Morphologic Findings in Diabetic Nephropathy

Diabetic glomerulosclerosis
  Thickening of the basement membranes
  Mesangial matrix accumulation (diffuse form)
  Mesangial nodules (nodular form)
  Capsular drop
  Fibrin cap
Tubular atrophy and interstitial fibrosis
Afferent and efferent arteriolar hyalinosis
Arteriosclerosis

Approach to Interpretation

Gross Pathology. At early stages, the kidneys are enlarged. Although the size is becoming smaller as the disease progresses, kidneys with advanced DNP are often not grossly contracted. The finely granular surface resembles the surface seen in arterial and arteriolar nephrosclerosis; however, the granularity of DNP is usually slightly more coarse.

Light Microscopy. The most characteristic light microscopic features of DNP are summarized in Table 8.3. Diabetic nephropathy affects all four renal compartments. Glomerular enlargement (hypertrophy) represents the earliest diabetic change detectable by light microscopy (Figure 8.5). This change may eventually evolve into diffuse and nodular diabetic glomerulosclerosis. Out of these two main forms, the diffuse

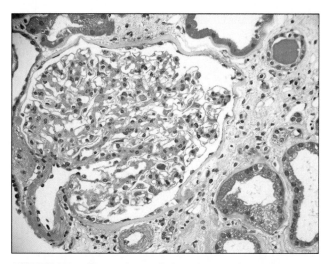

FIGURE 8.5: Glomerulomegaly is a characteristic feature of early diabetic renal disease. (Masson's trichrome, ×400).

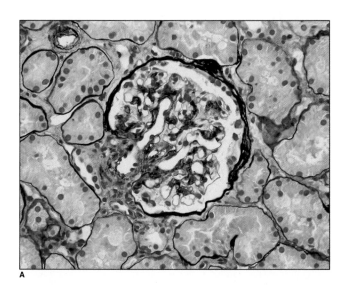

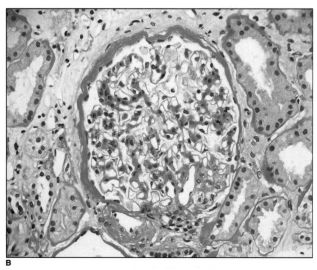

FIGURE 8.6: Incipient diabetic glomerulosclerosis. Light microscopic changes during the early stages of diabetic glomerular involvement can be very subtle. Mesangial matrix accumulation can be minimal or not apparent at all by light microscopy. However, thickening of the glomerular capillary basement membranes and/or mesangial matrix accumulation are readily detectable by electron microscopy at this early stage. A: minimal mesangial matrix accumulation (Jones' methenamine silver, ×400) B: slight mesangial matrix accumulation (Periodic acid Schiff, ×400).

A

B

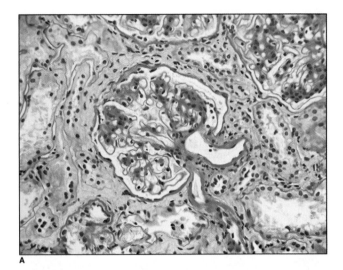

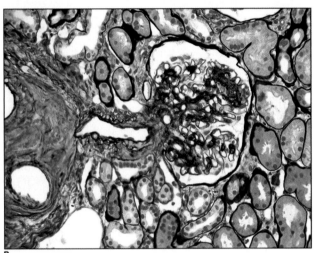

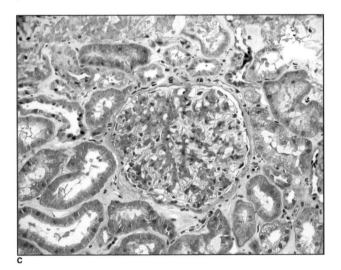

FIGURE 8.7: *Diffuse diabetic glomerulosclerosis. Mesangial matrix accumulation is seen without significant mesangial hypercellularity. The matrix is positive with periodic acid Schiff reaction, stains dark with Jones' methenamine silver and blue with Masson's trichrome. (A: Periodic acid Schiff, ×200; B: Jones' methenamine silver, ×200; C: Masson's trichrome, ×400).*

form represents the earlier and less severe manifestation of the disease. This form is characterized by an increase in mesangial matrix and uniform thickening of the glomerular capillary walls. Thickening of the capillary walls can be quite inconspicuous or may not be detectable at all by light microscopy (Figures 8.6 and 8.7). There is often slight mesangial hypercellularity present. As the disease progresses, capillary walls continue to thicken and mesangial volume continues to increase. Development of mesangial nodules (i.e., Kimmelstiel-Wilson type nodules) marks the onset of nodular diabetic glomerulosclerosis, considered to be the more severe and usually more advanced stage of diabetic glomerular involvement (Figures 8.8–8.10). Well-established nodular lesions are usually hypocellular or acellular. Prominent intra-, and interglomerular variation in the size of the nodules is typical. Also, the number of nodules may vary significantly from glomerulus to glomerulus. Nodular lesions often coexist with the diffuse form of the disease. The widened mesangial areas and nodules are eosinophilic, strongly PAS positive, and dark blue with Masson's trichrome. Fine lamellation can often be seen in well-developed nodular lesions especially with Jones' methenamine-silver (JMS) stain. At the periphery of the nodules, the patency of the capillary lumina is usually preserved until the very late stage(s) of the disease. Glomerular capillary microaneurysms may be present, especially in the nodular form (Figure 8.11). Mesangiolysis (i.e., loosening of the matrix) has been hypothesized as a possible pathogenetic event in the development of both the microaneurysms and the large lamellated nodules. The combination of mesangial expansion and thickened glomerular capillary walls will eventually result in decreasing patency of capillary lumina and decreased filtration surface area. As the glomeruli become obsolete, they usually do not shrink to the degree seen in other diseases resulting in global glomerulosclerosis. However, typical ischemic glomerular changes can sometimes be seen in at least some glomeruli secondary to arterial-, and arteriolosclerosis (Figure 8.12). Nodular glomerular lesions, reminiscent of those seen in DNP, can also occur in various other diseases in patients without diabetes. The morphologic features of various forms of nodular glomerulopathies are highlighted in Table 8.4 and Table 8.5.

The hyalinosis lesion (synonyms: exudative lesion or fibrin cap) is characterized by accumulation of homogenous eosinophilic hyaline material between the endothelial cells and the basement membranes of the glomerular capillaries (Figure 8.13). The lesion is considered to represent various plasma constituents and may contain lipid droplets and lipid laden macrophages. The hyaline material is pink with PAS but negative with methenamine silver stain. This lesion is identical to the hyalinosis lesion of focal and segmental glomerulosclerosis (FSGS) and may also be seen in other glomerular diseases including various forms of glomerulonephritides and reflux nephropathy. A lesion with similar staining properties, called the capsular drop, is found between the basement membrane and parietal epithelial cells of Bowman's capsule. Additional significant but less prominent glomerular changes include reduction in the number of podocytes [29] and the presence of atubular glomeruli (i.e., glomeruli that have open glomerular capillaries but have lost their connection to the proximal tubule).

Enlargement of the kidney during the early stages of the disease is, in part, linked to hypertrophy of the tubular compartment.

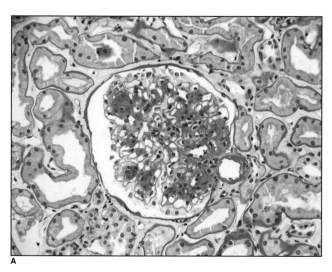
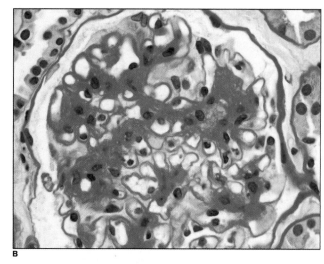

FIGURE 8.8: *Nodular diabetic glomerulosclerosis, early. The Kimmelstiel Wilson type mesangial nodules are relatively small and few (A: Periodic acid Schiff, × 400; B: Periodic acid Schiff, × 1000).*

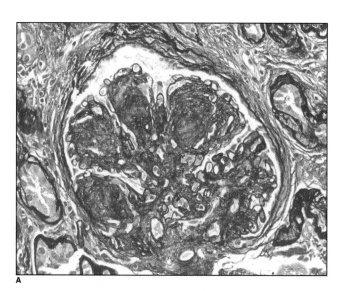
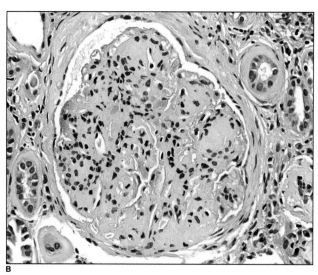

FIGURE 8.9: *Nodular diabetic glomerulosclerosis, well developed. The Kimmelstiel Wilson type mesangial nodules are large and numerous. Some of the nodules still contain cells, however, most of them are hypocellular or acellular (A: Jones' methenamine silver, × 400; B: Hematoxylin and eosin, × 400).*

As the disease progresses, chronic changes with tubular atrophy and interstitial fibrosis develop. The extent and severity of chronic tubulointerstitial injury usually correlates with the degree and severity of glomerular injury and chronic vascular disease. However, disparities in the severity of involvement between various compartments may occur. For such cases, glomerular disease often precedes the development of chronic tubulointerstitial injury. The thickened basement membranes of the atrophic tubules of diabetic kidneys are strongly PAS positive and may show lamellation and multiplication. Interstitial inflammatory cell infiltrates are often present, composed of mostly T lymphocytes and macrophages. Interstitial fibrosis, particularly when accompanied by inflammatory infiltrate, correlates with renal survival [30].

Arteriosclerosis and arteriolar hyalinization are integral parts of diabetic renal disease. Prominent hyaline arterioloscle-

rosis is a relatively early manifestation with frequent involvement of both afferent and efferent arterioles (Figure 8.14–8.17). Severe arteriolar hyalinosis without hypertension should raise suspicion for diabetes, especially in young people.

Immunofluorescence Microscopy. Linear positivity along the glomerular capillary walls and tubular basement membranes is common with IgG and albumin but may also be seen with IgM, the third component of complement (C3), and fibrinogen [31] (Figure 8.18). The positivities are considered to be nonspecific from entrapment of serum proteins secondary to structural changes in the basement membranes.

Electron Microscopy. Thickening of the GBM is considered to be the earliest ultrastructural change of diabetic renal

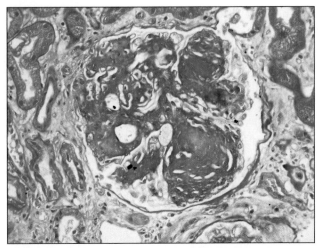

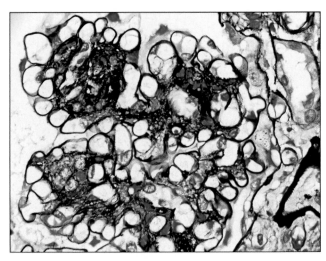

FIGURE 8.10: *Nodular diabetic glomerulosclerosis, advanced stage. The glomerulus exhibits severe expansion of the mesangium due to matrix accumulation with the formation of large Kimmelstiel-Wilson type nodules of various sizes. Note the paucity of nuclei within the nodules and the narrowing of the glomerular capillary lumina at the periphery of the nodules. (Masson's trichrome, × 400).*

FIGURE 8.11: *Small capillary microaneurysms at the periphery of the Kimmelstiel Wilson type nodules. (Jones' methenamine silver, × 1,000).*

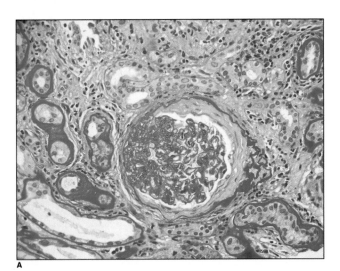

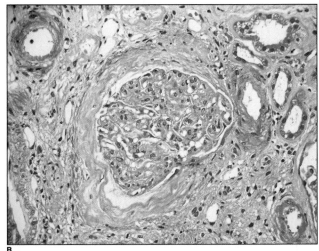

A

B

FIGURE 8.12: *Ischemic glomerular changes secondary to chronic vascular disease are often present especially during the advanced stages of diabetic nephropathy. A: Thickening and wrinkling of the glomerular capillary basement membranes with segmentally-accentuated glomerulosclerosis. Interstitial fibrosis and tubular atrophy are also present. (A: Periodic acid Schiff, × 400). B: Periglomerular fibrosis (Masson's trichrome, × 400).*

involvement [32], and if severe enough, is sufficient to make a diagnosis of early diabetic renal involvement in patients with diabetes even in the absence of any obvious light microscopic abnormalities. Although thickening of the GBMs remains one of the most characteristic features of DNP, focal prominent attenuations of the GBMs can also be seen in the more advanced stages of the disease, typically in association with capillary micro-aneurysms. Mesangial widening is due to increase in mesangial matrix and also in mesangial cells [33] (Figure 8.19). Mesangial matrix accumulation without thickening of the basement membranes can be observed occasionally during the early stages of the disease. Fibrin caps are characterized by accumulation of homo-

geneous electron-dense material between the endothelial cell and the GBM. The capsular drops, found between the Bowman's capsule and the parietal epithelium, reveal similar ultrastructural features. In well-developed DNP, there is an absolute loss in the number of visceral epithelial cells and widening of the foot processes; this latter feature shows a weak correlation with the degree of proteinuria.

Differential Diagnosis

The differential diagnoses of nodular diabetic glomerulosclerosis with characteristic light-, IF-, and electron microscopic findings are outlined in Table 8.4. Idiopathic nodular

Table 8.4 Morphologic Differential Diagnosis of Nodular Glomerulopathies: Light, Immunofluorescence, and Electron Microscopy

		DGS and INGS[a]	LCDD/LHCDD	AM	FI/IT	CFGP
LM	H&E	Eosinophilic	Eosinophilic	Pale/glassy	Pale/glassy	Pale
	PAS	Strongly (+++) positive	Positive (++)	Weakly (+) positive	Weakly (+) positive	Weakly (+) positive
	Silver	Argyrophilic	Usually non-A	Usually non-A	Usually non-A	Usually non-A
	Trichrome	Dark-blue	Red-blue	Gray-purple	Gray-purple	Pale-blue
	Congo-red	Negative	Negative	Positive	Negative	Negative
IF		IgG & albumin, linear; GBM/TBM	κ or λ, linear, with/without single HC; GBM/TBM	κ or λ, smudgy; mesangial, peripheral (AL type); negative (AA, other)	IgG, C3, κ & λ (FI); IgG, C3, κ or λ or κ & λ (IT); smudgy	Negative
EM		GBM thickening and mesangial matrix accumulation	Punctate deposits, GBM/TBM	Organized fibrillary (AM and FI) or non-amyloidotic microtubular glomerular fibrils/microtubules: 8—12 nm: AM; 12–30 nm: FI >30 nm: IT		Banding collagen fibers

[a]Distinction between DGS and INGS depends on the presence/absence of diabetes mellitus.

Table 8.5 Clinical Correlations, Immunohistochemical (IH) and Additional Morphologic Findings in Diabetic Glomerulosclerosis and Nodular Glomerulopathies

	DGS	INGS	LCDD/LHCDD	AM	FI/IT	CFGP
IH	–	–	–	AM AA (AA type)	–	Collagen (types 1, 3, or 5)
Common glomerular lesions other than nodular by LM	Diffuse mesangial widening	–	–	Mesangial widening	Proliferative or advanced sclerosing GN	–
Pertinent clinical correlations	History of DM	History of hypertension, smoking, and lack of DM	MM or MGUS	MM or MGUS	Lympho-proliferative diseases (IT)	–
Typical clinical presentation	Proteinuria, nephrotic range proteinuria					

Abbreviations (Tables 8.4 and 8.5) GBM, glomerular basement membrane; TBM, tubular basement membrane; DM, diabetes mellitus; DGS, diabetic glomerulosclerosis; INGS, idiopathic nodular glomerulosclerosis; LCDD, light chain deposition disease; HCD, heavy chain disease; LHCDD, light chain-heavy chain deposition disease; AM, amyloidosis/amyloid; AL, amyloid light chain; FI/IT, fibrillary-immunotactoid; CFGP, collagenofibrotic glomerulopathy; MM, multiple myeloma; MGUS, monoclonal gammopathy of uncertain significance; GN, glomerulonephritis; JMS, Jones' methenamine-silver; H&E, hematoxylin and eosin; M trichrome, Masson's Trichrome; non-A, non-argrophilic

glomerulosclerosis (INGS) [34] is morphologically almost identical to diabetic nodular glomerulosclerosis (Figure 8.20). The distinction between these diseases relies heavily upon clinical evidence for the presence or absence of diabetes in the affected individuals. Morphologically, the presence of fine capillary slits within the nodular lesions favors INGS [34].

The combination of characteristic IF and electron microscopic findings helps to differentiate light chain and light chain and heavy chain deposition diseases (LCD/LCHCD) [35] from other nodular glomerulosclerotic processes. Linear positivities highlighting glomerular and/or tubular basement membranes with a single light chain and/or heavy chain are diagnostic for

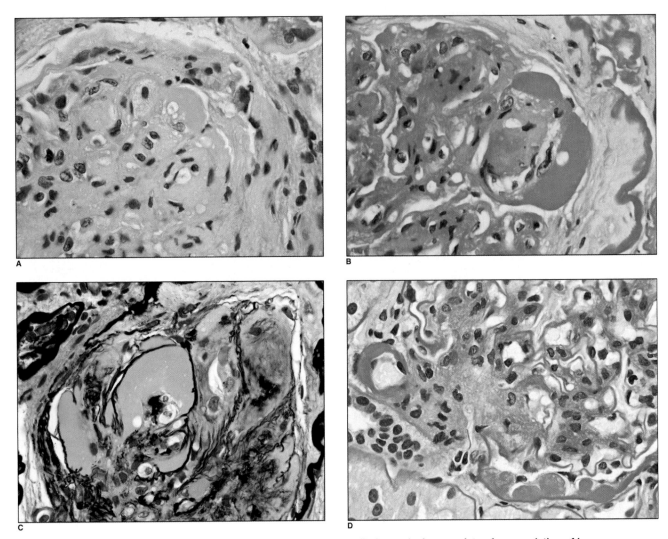

FIGURE 8.13: *Hyalinosis lesions of diabetic glomerulosclerosis. The fibrin cap lesion consists of accumulation of homogenous eosinophilic material between the glomerular capillary basement membrane and the endothelial cells. The material is positive with periodic acid Schiff and negative with Jones' methenamine silver. Note the presence of intracapillary foam cell (arrow). (A: hematoxylin and eosin, × 1,000; B: Periodic acid Schiff reaction, × 1,000; C: Jones' methenamine silver, × 1,000). Capsular drop, situated between the Bowman's capsule and the parietal epithelial cells, has similar staining characteristics. (D: Periodic acid Schiff, × 1,000).*

LCD/LCHCD by IF microscopy. Ultrastructurally, the finely granular ("punctate") deposits along the glomerular and tubular basement membranes are highly typical of LCD/LCHCD. Differentiation of amyloidosis from diabetic glomerulosclerosis is usually straightforward; amyloid deposits are typically pale with PAS, pale blue with trichrome, usually negative with Jones silver, and positive with Congo-red. In contrast, the widened mesangial areas of diabetic glomerulosclerosis are strongly PAS positive, stain dark blue with trichrome, black with Jones silver, and are negative with Congo-red stain. Smudgy glomerular staining by IF with IgG, C3, kappa, and/or lambda light chains helps to differentiate fibrillary and immunotactoid glomerulopathies (FI/IT) [36] from both diabetic and other forms of nodular glomerulosclerosis. Also, the light microscopic staining properties, Congo-red negativity, and the typical ultrastructural features with fibrillary or microtubular deposits secure the correct diagnosis of FI/IT. The diagnosis of collagenofibrotic glomerulopathy, a rare form of nodular glomerulosclerosis,

requires electron microscopic demonstration of banding collagen fibers in the glomeruli. Clinical and laboratory findings, as well as additional morphologic and immunohistochemical characteristics that aid differential diagnosis of nodular glomerulopathies are summarized in Tables 8.5. An algorithmic approach for the morphologic differentiation of various forms of nodular glomerulopathies is provided in Figure 8.21.

Glomerular diseases superimposed on diabetic glomerulosclerosis are relatively common (Figures 8.22–8.24). Some of the diseases, such as membranous nephropathy are easy to diagnose with the help of immunofluorescence and electron microscopy. However, a few of them may pose diagnostic challenges. For example, FSGS is difficult to diagnose in kidneys with nodular diabetic glomerulosclerosis showing advanced sclerotic features. In patients with a diffuse form of diabetic glomerulosclerosis the diagnosis of FSGS is more straightforward. Potential difficulties of recognizing amyloidosis or fibrillary glomerulonephritis superimposed on diabetic glomerulosclerosis may

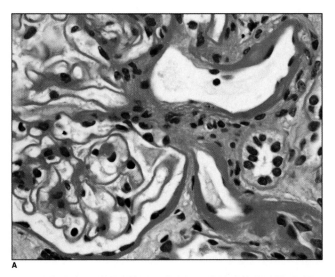
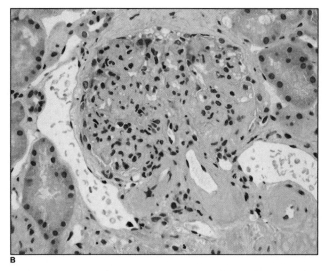

FIGURE 8.14: *Arteriolar hyalinization in diabetic nephropathy. Hyalinization of both afferent and efferent arterioles is a characteristic finding of diabetic renal disease. Subtle (A) and prominent (B) hyalinization affecting both the afferent and efferent arterioles is shown. (A: Periodic acid Schiff, ×1,000; B: hematoxylin and eosin, ×400).*

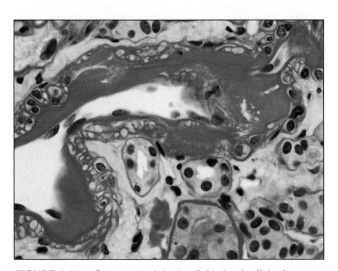

FIGURE 8.15: *Severe arteriolar hyalinization in diabetic nephropathy. (Periodic acid Schiff, ×1,000).*

stem from overlapping light microscopic features. In addition, fibrillary structures somewhat reminiscent of those seen in amyloidosis and fibrillary glomerulonephritis can also be present in diabetic glomerulosclerosis and the changes of amyloidosis can be focal or subtle. Shared morphologic features in DNP and membranoproliferative glomerulonephritis (MPGN), such as mesangial matrix accumulation and mesangial hypercellularity, may hamper recognition of MPGN superimposed on DNP. Large subepithelial humps might be the only morphologic feature of resolving postinfectious glomerulonephritis in diabetic glomerulosclerosis [37]. In diabetic patients who present with sudden-onset nephrotic syndrome the possibility of minimal change nephrotic syndrome superimposed on DNP should be considered in the differential diagnosis. In these cases, other causes of nephrotic syndrome should be excluded prior to ren-

dering a diagnosis of minimal change nephrotic syndrome. Collapsing variant of FSGS might be a particularly challenging diagnosis in patients with diabetic glomerulosclerosis. The presence of hyperplastic–hypertrophic visceral epithelial cells with heavy load of protein resorption droplets may be the only morphologic clue to the correct diagnosis.

Etiology and Pathogenesis

Susceptibility to the development of DNP and the risk of progression of DNP is determined by both genetic and environmental factors [38]. The risk of developing DNP is also increased by hypertension, glomerular hyperfiltration, poor glycemic and lipid control, and smoking [39] . Hyperglycemia plays a central role in the pathogenesis. Numerous molecular pathways and mediators participate in the pathogenetic process, among which the polyol pathway, advanced glycation end products (AGEs), protein kinase C activation, and various growth factors are the most significant [40]. Advanced glycation end products alter the structure and function of other intra- and extracellular molecules, modulate cell activation, signal transduction, the expression of cytokines, and growth factors through receptor-dependent and independent pathways [41].

Clinical Course, Prognosis, Treatment, and Clinical Correlation

In general, there is a good correlation between clinical stages of DNP, as described in patients with type I diabetes, and the renal morphologic changes [42]. Stage I is characterized by increased GFR and hypertrophy affecting both glomeruli and tubules. Insulin therapy is associated with decrease of both the hyperfunction and hypertrophy in this stage. Stage II develops silently over many years in some patients and is marked by the evolution of glomerular lesions in the absence of clinical

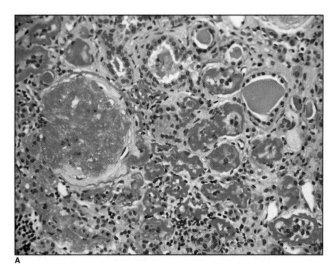
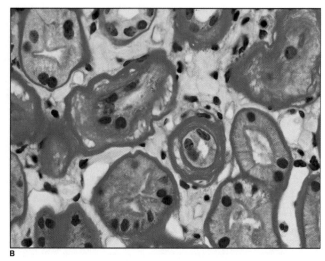

FIGURE 8.16:   Interstitial fibrosis, tubular atrophy, and global glomerulosclerosis in advanced diabetic nephropathy (A: Periodic acid Schiff, ×200). Atrophic tubules of diabetic nephropathy often show prominent multiplication of the basement membranes. (B: Periodic acid Schiff, ×1,000).

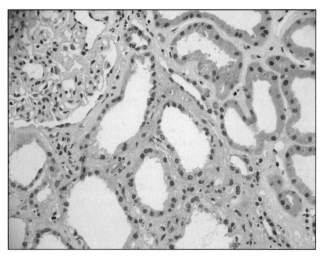
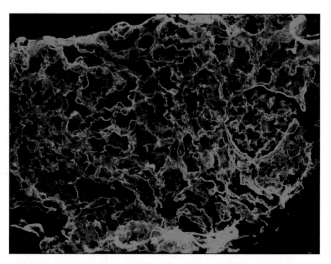

FIGURE 8.17:   Acute tubular epithelial injury ("acute tubular necrosis") in the background of diabetic nephrosclerosis. Flattening of the tubular epithelial cells in non-atrophic tubules is a characteristic feature of acute injury. (Hematoxylin and eosin, ×400).

FIGURE 8.18:   Linear staining along the tubular and glomerular capillary basement membranes with albumin. Albumin and IgG linear positivity is a typical, although nonspecific finding of diabetic nephropathy. (Direct immunofluorescence, albumin, × 400).

evidence of renal disease. Morphologically this stage is characterized by thickening of the GBM and mesangial matrix expansion [43]. There is also correlation between elevation of glycosylated hemoglobin and increased GFR at this stage [44]. Microalbuminuria (30 to 300 mg/day) marks the onset of incipient DNP (stage III) [28]. Renal function is preserved at this stage and proteinuria is typically intermittent with slowly increasing urinary albumin excretion over the years [45]. Clinical nephropathy is likely to occur once urinary albumin excretion attains levels of 0.075 to 0.1 g/day [43]. Hypertension may also be present, but it rarely occurs in patients with UAE < 100 mg/day [46]. Stage IV represents overt DNP as characterized by proteinuria of > 300 mg/day and steadily declining GFR rang-

ing from 1 to 24 ml/min/year (mean 12 ml/min/year) [22,47]. Nephrotic syndrome is relatively rare; however, microscopic hematuria has been reported in up to 48 percent of patients with DNP [28]. This stage is usually associated with rising systemic blood pressure and the presence of other diabetic complications. Stage V marks the development of ESRD as a direct result of DNP.

The clinical stages of DNP in patients with type 2 diabetes are less clearly elucidated, partly because of the difficulty of determination of the biological onset of the diabetes itself. It is especially difficult to establish the onset of stage III in a patient with type 2 diabetes. This is because microalbuminuria may be caused by frequent comorbidities in these patients,

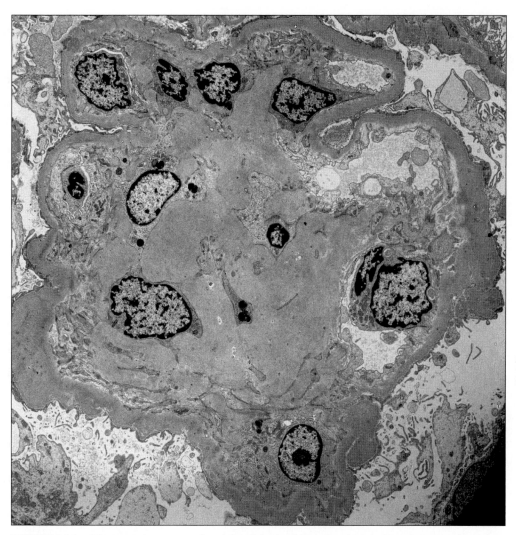

FIGURE 8.19: *Electron microscopy of nodular diabetic glomerulosclerosis. The picture shows severe widening of the mesangium due to matrix accumulation. The capillary loops are patent, although narrowed.*

such as hypertension, nephrosclerosis, or other related conditions.

ESRD usually develops 3 to 20 years after the onset of persistent proteinuria [48]. Once overt proteinuria occurs, progression to ESRD seems to be inevitable [45,49]. The cumulative incidence of ESRD is 50 percent in patients with type 1 diabetes 10 years after the onset of proteinuria [50], compared to 3 to 11 percent in proteinuric type 2 diabetic patients [51]. However, the course to ESRD is usually shorter in patients with type 2 diabetes [52]. Proteinuria and renal disease in patients with either type 1 or type 2 diabetes also decreases life expectancy, with cardiovascular disease being the leading cause of death [52].

Although a significant proportion of patients with stage IV disease progress to ESRD, patients with overt nephropathy may benefit from strict glycemic control, as documented in patients with type 1 diabetes [53,54]. Furthermore, antihypertensive treatment and strict blood glucose control may have beneficial effects on the progression and development of DNP in both type 1 and type 2 diabetic patients [55–57]. Antihypertensive treatment may not only slow down the rate of decline of GFR,

but in some patients, may lead to regression of the disease. [58]. Blockage of the renin-angiotensin system with angiotensin-converting enzyme (ACE) inhibitors or angiotensin receptor blockers (ARB) confers additional benefit on preserving renal function [59].

FABRY'S DISEASE

Introduction

Fabry's disease (angiokeratoma corporis diffusum) is an X-linked hereditary lysosomal storage disorder with systemic manifestations. Renal involvement is common and often severe.

Epidemiology and Clinical Presentation

The estimated incidence of the disease is 1:40,000 to 1:117,000 among Caucasian males [60]. Although it is the second most prevalent lysosomal storage disease after Gaucher's disease, it is still relatively rare and many of the symptoms and

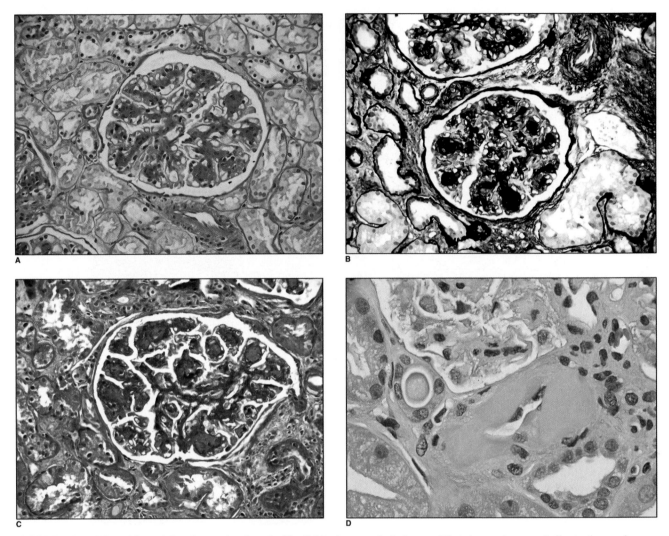

FIGURE 8.20: *Idiopathic nodular glomerulosclerosis. The light microscopic features of the glomerulus are similar to those of diabetic glomerulosclerosis; however, the patient did not have diabetes. (A: Hematoxylin and eosin, ×400; B: Jones' methenamine silver, ×400; C: Periodic acid Schiff, ×400). D: Severe arteriolar hyalinization can also be present. (Hematoxylin and eosin, ×1,000).*

manifestations are nonspecific, and therefore, the true incidence is uncertain. Symptoms usually develop in a predictable order which is more consistent in males than in females (Table 8.6). In heterozygous females, the clinical manifestations vary due to random X chromosome inactivation (Lyonization). Some female carriers may be asymptomatic and some may have only an attenuated form of the disease. [61] Atypical variants may have a milder phenotype with manifestations limited to the heart or the kidney [62–64].

The diagnosis of Fabry's disease is usually made on clinical grounds; however, the diagnosis is significantly delayed both in males and females (by 14 and 19 years, respectively) following the onset of the symptoms [65]. Absent or significantly decreased α-galactosidase A activity in the serum, white blood cells or cultured fibroblasts confirms the diagnosis. Mutational analysis of the α-galactosidase A gene may be needed for diagnosis in heterozygous females because of variable enzyme activity. Prenatal testing of carrier states is also readily available by molecular techniques. Renal biopsy is usually not needed for the

diagnosis; however, it is often performed in patients whose clinical presentation is not diagnostic.

Approach to Interpretation

Gross Pathology. The kidneys may be enlarged due to excessive glycolipid deposition. With various imaging modalities, cysts have been identified in up to 50 percent of patients studied with Fabry's disease [66].

Light Microscopy. In Fabry's disease, glycolipid [globotriaosylceramide (Gb3); see also "Etiology and Pathogenesis" in this section] is deposited in various tissues. However, Gb3 is dissolved during routine light microscopic processing, leaving behind only empty, foamy-appearing intracellular vacuoles (Figure 8.25). The typical light and electron microscopic findings in the kidney are summarized in Table 8.7. During the early stages of the disease, the kidney may be quite unremarkable with no or only minimal vacuolization present affecting

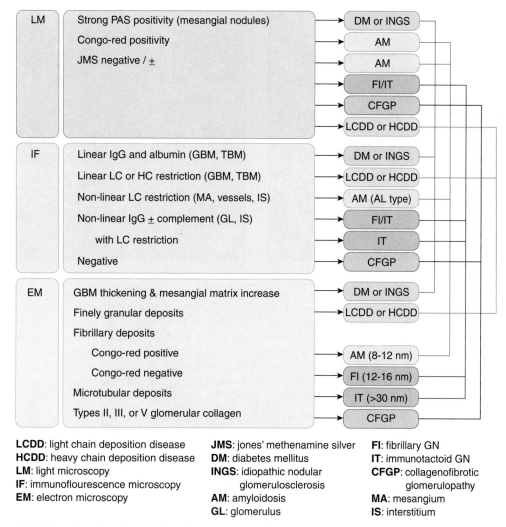

FIGURE 8.21: *Algorithm for the differential diagnosis of nodular glomerulopathies.*

mostly visceral epithelial cells. As the disease progresses, vacuolization becomes more prominent involving not only the podocytes, but also parietal epithelial cells, mesangial and glomerular endothelial cells, as well as distal and less frequently proximal tubular epithelial and interstitial cells. Fine vacuolization can also be seen in the endothelial cells of the peritubular capillaries; and endothelial and smooth muscle cells of the arteries and arterioles. At the more advanced stages, interstitial fibrosis, arterial and arteriolar sclerosis, mesangial sclerosis, and focal segmental and global glomerulosclerosis may develop. Under polarized light, frozen sections of fresh or formalin-fixed tissues show characteristic Maltese crosses, corresponding to glycolipid deposits (Figure 8.26). On frozen sections the glycolipid deposits are positive with Oil Red O and PAS stains. Because osmication preserves intracellular glycolipids, the deposits can also be visualized in Toluidine blue-stained semithin sections as lamellar intracytoplasmic structures (Figure 8.27).

Immunofluorescence Microscopy. No specific IF findings are present. Glomerular C3 deposits and IgM deposits in the areas of segmental sclerosis can sometimes be seen.

Electron Microscopy. Gb3 deposits appearing as whorled layers of alternating dense and pale material, often referred to as "myeloid or zebra bodies", are identified within enlarged secondary lysosomes virtually in every cell type in the kidney (Figure 8.28). The concentric layers have a periodicity of 3.5–5 nm. They are considered to be highly characteristic, although not entirely specific of Fabry's disease.

Differential Diagnosis

Prominent vacuolization of the visceral epithelial cells by light microscopy, similar to that seen in Fabry's disease, can also be seen in two additional lipid-storage diseases, I-cell disease and GM_1 gangliosidosis. Both I-cell disease and GM_1 gangliosidosis manifest during early childhood with a Hurler-like syndrome, however, neither disease has clinical renal manifestations. The vacuoles of the visceral epithelial cells in I-cell disease stain with colloidal iron, Sudan-black, and alcian-blue; in contrast, they are unstained in GM_1 gangliosidosis. Ultrastructurally, the vacuoles in I-cell disease and GM_1 gangliosidosis do not show the lamellation, characteristic of Fabry's disease. However,

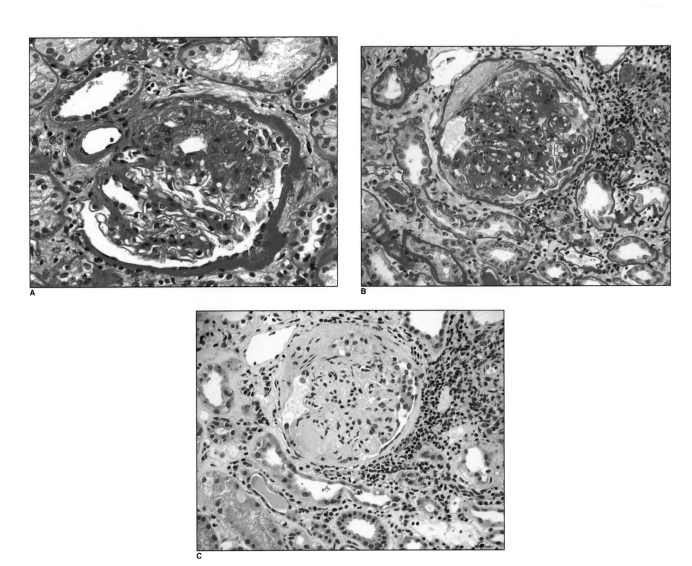

FIGURE 8.22: *Focal segmental glomerulosclerosis (FSGS) complicating diabetic nephrosclerosis. A: The glomerulus exhibits a large segmentally sclerotic lesion with hyperplastic visceral epithelial cells. The portion of the glomerulus without segmental sclerosis reveals mesangial widening with matrix accumulation, characteristic of diffuse type diabetic glomerulosclerosis (Periodic acid Schiff, ×400). In the advanced stages of diabetic glomerulosclerosis the diagnosis of superimposed FSGS can be challenging. The presence of prominent visceral epithelial cells hyperplasia may be a sign of FSGS, however, one should be careful not to overcall FSGS in this setting. (B: Periodic acid Schiff, ×400; C: Hematoxylin and eosin, ×400).*

lamellar inclusions, similar to those seen in Fabry's disease, have been described in gentamycin toxicity [67], silicone nephropathy [68], and chloroquine-induced lipidosis [69]. In contrast to Fabry's disease, lamellar inclusions of gentamycin toxicity are found primarily in the proximal tubular epithelial cells and not in the podocytes and distal tubular epithelial cells. In chloroquine toxicity, the tissue distribution of whorled lipid inclusions might be identical to those seen in Fabry's disease, however, glomerular intracapillary and mesangial histiocytes with clear lysosomes containing dense round and variably sized granules may also be present [69].

Etiology and Pathogenesis

The disease is caused by deficiency of α-galactosidase A, which catalyzes the lysosomal hydrolysis of Gb3. As a conse-

quence, Gb3 accumulates in the lysosomes in various organs leading to severe cellular and organ dysfunction and eventually death. The primary sites of Gb3 accumulation are glomerular and tubular epithelial cells, endothelial, perithelial and smooth muscle cells of the vasculature, myocardial cells, fibrocytes, and neurons of the dorsal root ganglion [70]. Over 300 mutations of the α-galactosidase A gene have been identified.

Proteinuria is likely related to Gb3 deposition in the podocytes and distal tubular dysfunction is the result of distal tubular epithelial deposition of Gb3. Chronic vascular changes seem to contribute to evolving renal chronicity through ischemia. Microvascular disease, podocyte injury, and interstitial fibrosis have all been proposed as potential mechanisms through which focal segmental and global glomerulosclerosis of Fabry's disease may develop [71].

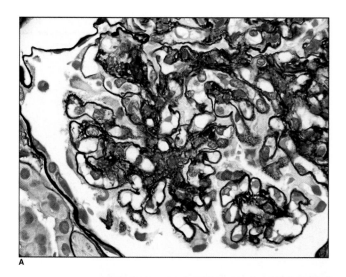

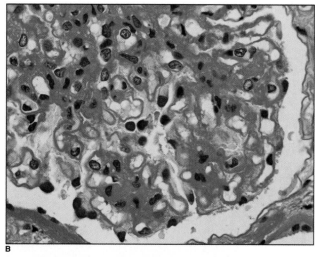

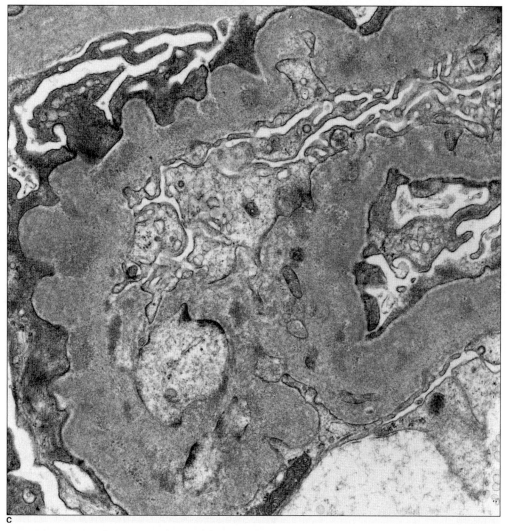

FIGURE 8.23: *Membranous nephropathy complicating diabetic glomerulosclerosis. The methenamine silver-stained section reveals spikes along the external aspects of the glomerular capillary basement membranes. Small silver-negative holes in the tangentially-cut thickened basement membranes are also seen. (A: Jones' methenamine silver, ×1,000). B: Periodic acid Schiff reaction highlights diffuse thickening of the glomerular capillary walls and mesangial widening (×1,000). C: Electron microscopy disclosed electron dense immunotype deposits embedded within the thickened glomerular capillary basement membranes. (Electron microphotograph, original magnification ×7,650).*

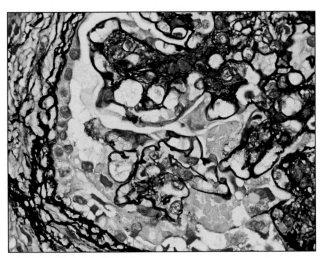

FIGURE 8.24: *Protein resorption droplets in hyperplastic visceral epithelial cells in a patient with nodular diabetic glomerulosclerosis and new-onset nephrotic range proteinuria. (Jones' methenamine silver, × 1,000).*

Clinical Course, Prognosis, Treatment, and Clinical Correlation

In hemizygous males, features of peripheral neuropathy with severe recurrent pain in the extremities often appear before the onset of skin lesions. Cardiac involvement (cardiomyopathy, coronary artery disease) is common, progressive with aging, and often severe. Cerebrovascular complications may also be present. The typical renal manifestations are listed in Table 8.8. The onset of proteinuria is usually in early adulthood; however, nephrotic range proteinuria was found only in 18 percent of patients with renal disease in a long-term study of natural history of Fabry's disease in male patients [60]. Chronic renal insufficiency (CRI) developed in 50 percent of patients at a median age of 42 years and ESRD in 23 percent of patients at a median age of 47 years [60]. Death usually results from renal failure or cardiac or cerebral complications before the age of 60 years [60]. Recombinant human α-galactosidase A replacement therapy – the only disease-specific therapy currently available for Fabry's disease – can reverse substrate storage in the lysosomes. It is recommended that enzyme replacement therapy in all males with Fabry's disease (including those with ESRD) and female carriers with disease manifestations should be initiated as early as possible [72]. The kidneys may show significant clearance of the deposits with the enzyme replacement therapy [73].

GAUCHER'S DISEASE

Introduction

Gaucher's disease is an inherited metabolic storage disorder in which abnormal accumulation of glucocerebrosidase in various organs, including spleen, liver, lungs, bone marrow, kidney, and sometimes brain may lead to severe functional impairment and death.

Epidemiology and Clinical Presentation

Although it is the most common lysosomal storage disorder, the prevalence is still relatively low occurring in about 1 in 40,000–

Table 8.6 Clinical Symptoms and Signs of Fabry's Disease

Childhood
Pain, numbness of fingers and toes
Telangiectasias on ears, conjunctiva
Blue-black angiomatous macules or papules
Edematous upper eyelids
Raynaud phenomenon
Ophthamological abnormalities

Early adulthood
Extensive telangectasias, angiokeratomas
Albuminuria, hematuria, oval fat bodies in urine
Edema
Fever, heat collapse, anhidrosis
Lymphadenopathy
Isothermia

30–40 years of age
Cardiac disease: coronary conduction defects,
   mitral insufficiency
Renal insufficiency
Cerebrovascular attacks
Neurological findings suggesting multiple sclerosis

Modified from Brady et al. [121]

60,000 in the general population [74,75]. It is, however, more common among Ashkenazi Jews with a prevalence of 1 in 500–800 and an estimated carrier frequency of 1 in 14 [74].

Among the three clinical types of the disease, type 1 is the most common comprising approximately 90–95 percent of the cases. The typical clinical manifestations of the three forms are summarized in Table 8.9. The clinical presentation of patients with type 1 disease is variable in presence and severity of symptoms as well as in the rate of progression. Patients can present with clinical symptoms as early as at 12 months of age but in many patients clinical signs develop in late adulthood. The most frequent mutation (N370S) is usually causing the development of symptoms at the age of approximately 30 years.

Hepatomegaly is almost universal but usually less clinically pronounced then splenomegaly. Hepatosplenomegaly might be asymptomatic or it can be associated with nonspecific signs like abdominal complains (distention, discomfort) and/or thrombocytopenia. Patients with Gaucher's disease type 1 do develop bone marrow disease but the anemia and thrombocytopenia seems to be more closely correlated with the degree of splenomegaly. Clinically the most debilitating effects are the skeletal manifestations that are associated with the highest degree of morbidity and impact on activities of daily living. Skeletal disease is characterized by osteopenia and patients may develop painful bone crisis similar to sickle cell disease as well as pathological fractures, vertebral compression, and osteonecrosis. In many affected children, Gaucher's disease type 1 is associated with delayed puberty and short stature.

Type 2 and type 3 diseases are rare. Type 2 disease occurs in infants with severe signs and symptoms including hepatomegaly, splenomegaly, and rapidly progressive brain damage. Type 3 occurs in children and adolescents; the disease progression is usually slower than in type 2 disease and the brain involvement is relative mild.

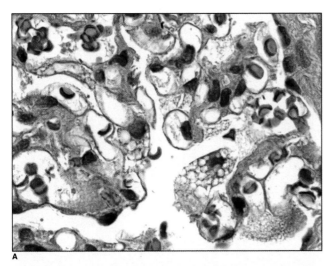 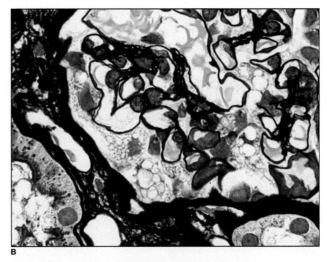

A **B**

FIGURE 8.25: *Fabry's disease. Visceral epithelial cells show prominent fine vacuolization. The accumulated glycolipid (globotriaosylceramide) is dissolved during routine light microscopic processing leaving behind fine cytoplasmic vacuolization. No other significant glomerular changes are noted. (A: Hematoxylin and eosin, × 1,000; B: Jones' methenamine silver, × 1,000).*

Renal involvement is rare in Gaucher's disease; in a study assessing renal functional abnormalities in 161 patients with Gaucher's disease, significant proteinuria was found only in patients with such comorbidities as diabetes mellitus or multiple myeloma [76]. Varying degrees of proteinuria and hematuria have been reported in a few patients [77].

Clinical differential diagnosis of Gaucher's disease is broad and includes differential diagnosis of splenomegaly, anemia, and thrombocytopenia as well as differential diagnosis of osteopenia, pathological fractures, and bone pain. In general, the diagnosis has to be confirmed by reduced glucocerebrosidase activity, which can be measured from peripheral leukocytes, cultured fibroblasts, or other nucleated cells. Subsequent DNA analysis to detect mutations can also be used. In patients with significant renal functional abnormalities, renal biopsy might be warranted.

Approach to Interpretation

Gross Pathology. A study assessing renal function and gross morphology in 161 patients with Gaucher's disease found no evidence of abnormal size, or alterations in sonographic images of the kidney [76].

Light Microscopy. The typical renal morphologic findings are summarized in Table 8.10. Accumulation of Gaucher's cells within glomerular capillary lumina is the most common finding in patients presenting with varying degrees of proteinuria and hematuria. Gaucher's cells are large cells of endothelial or macrophage origin showing characteristic wrinkled-paper "fluffy" appearance from intracytoplasmic accumulation of glucosylceramide. The cells display strong reactivity with PAS. Gaucher's cells have also been detected in the tubulointerstitial compartment [77,78], peritubular capillaries [77], and mesangial areas [78]. Accumulation of Gaucher's cells in the kidney typically follows splenectomy; this may, although rarely, lead to renal failure [79]. Rare cases of MPGN, FSGS, and amyloidosis have also been described in patients with Gaucher's disease.

Immunofluorescence Microscopy. There are no specific immunofluorescent findings.

Electron Microscopy. Gaucher's cells, located in glomeruli, peritubular capillaries and interstitial areas exhibit accumulation of membrane-bound tubular structures consisting of fibrils 60 to 80 nm in diameter. Some of the Gaucher's cells within the glomerular capillary lumina have been described as being directly apposed to basement membranes and also extending into the mesangium [77]. Mesangial cellular interposition and rare small mesangial electron dense deposits can also be seen [77]. Electron dense intracytoplasmic deposits (Gaucher's bodies) have been described in glomerular capillary endothelial, mesangial, and tubulointerstitial cells [78]. The foot processes of the visceral epithelial cells show effacement in patients with significant proteinuria.

Table 8.7 Renal Morphologic Findings of Fabry's Disease

Light Microcopy:
Cytoplasmic vacuolization
  Glomerular
    Visceral epithelial cells (most prominent)
    Parietal epithelial cells
    Mesangial cells
    Glomerular endothelial cells
  Tubulointerstitial/vascular
    Distal and proximal tubular epithelial cells
    Interstitial cells
    Peritubular capillaries
    Endothelial and smooth muscle cells of the arteries and
      arterioles
Interstitial fibrosis
Arterial and arteriolar sclerosis
Mesangial sclerosis
Focal segmental and global glomerulosclerosis

Electron Microscopy:
"Myeloid or zebra bodies" within secondary lysosomes

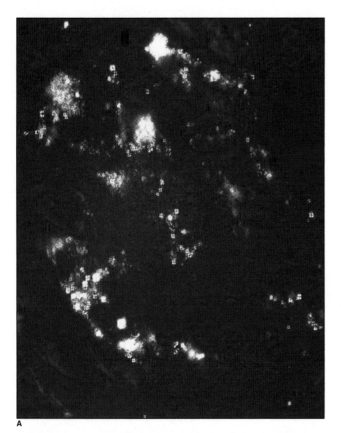
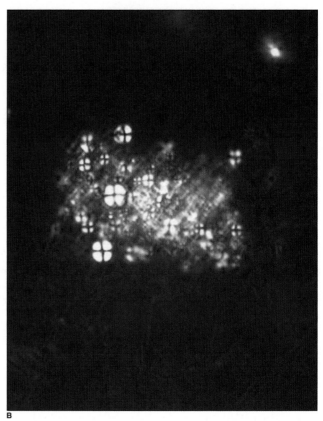

FIGURE 8.26: Fabry's disease. Glomerular visceral epithelial cells reveal Maltese crosses under polarized light, corresponding to glycolipid deposits. (Fresh frozen material, ×400 [A], ×400 [B]).

Differential Diagnosis

Glomerular intracapillary accumulation of large cells with fluffy PAS-positive cytoplasm is highly characteristic of Gaucher's disease. In context with the typical clinical history and ultrastructural findings of membrane-bound fibrils the diagnosis is usually straightforward. However, vacuolated intracapillary cells can also be seen in patients with Niemann-Pick disease and lecithin-cholesterol acyltransferase (LCAT) deficiency. In Niemann-Pick disease, large vacuolated cells known as "Niemann-Pick cells," stain with the Schultz method for cholesterol [80] and are only weakly positive by PAS stain. In addition to the glomerular intracapillary location, vacuolation in Niemann-Pick disease can also affect podocytes, tubular epithelial cells, and interstitial macrophages. LCAT deficiency can be distinguished from Gaucher's disease at the ultrastructural level. In LCAT deficiency, lipid deposits are mostly extracellular with partly electron dense and partly electron lucent appearance.

Etiology and Pathogenesis

Gaucher's disease is caused by deficient β-glucosidase enzyme activity, which leads to the accumulation of the substrate glucosylceramide. More than 200 mutations of the gene coding for β-glucosidase have been identified, however, there are only seven common mutations, six of which account for over 95 percent of genetic mutations of Gaucher's [74]. Most of the mutations are not associated with a specific phenotype and the clinical presentation varies widely. The inheritance is autosomal recessive. Progressive accumulation of glycolipid glucosylceramide in macrophages (Gaucher's cells) and to lesser extent in endothelial cells in various organs, including bone marrow, liver, spleen, lungs, and sometimes in kidneys may lead to severe organ dysfunction. Increased incidence of multiple myeloma in patients with Gaucher's [81] might be related to chronic stimulation of the immune system by abnormal macrophages. The precise mechanism of proteinuria is uncertain, however, cytokines produced by macrophages have been suggested as possible pathogenetic factors. Lending support to this hypothesis, amelioration of nephrotic range proteinuria has been observed in a patient following enzyme replacement therapy [77]; although the patient's renal biopsy, prior to initiation of therapy, did show glomerular accumulation of Gaucher's cells [77]. However, the presence of Gaucher's cells in the glomeruli may not always lead to proteinuria [82].

Clinical Course, Prognosis, Treatment, and Clinical Correlation

Gaucher's disease is one of the first of inherited metabolic disorders that can be treated with replacement of the deficient enzyme. The mainstay of the treatment is the use of recombinant glucocerebrosidase (imiglucerase), which is effective in patients with type 1 and type 3 diseases. The major goals of treatment are the elimination of symptoms and prevention of irreversible damage as well as improvement of overall health.

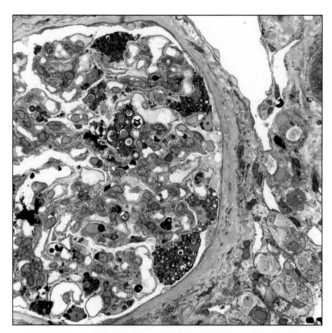

FIGURE 8.27: *Fabry's disease. Toluidine blue-stained semi-thin section shows lamellar intracytoplasmic structures in the visceral epithelial cells corresponding to glycolipid deposits. (×1,000).*

Enzyme replacement therapy should be continued as a life-long therapy. There is no effective treatment for brain damage that may occur in patients with type 2 and type 3 diseases. Enzyme replacement therapy has been shown to ameliorate nephrotic syndrome in a patient with Gaucher's disease and glomerular involvement [77].

TYPE I GLYCOGEN STORAGE DISEASES (VON GIERKE DISEASE)

Introduction

Glycogen storage diseases (GSD) (synonym: glycogenoses) comprise several types of inherited diseases caused by abnormalities of the enzymes that regulate the synthesis or degradation of glycogen. GSD type I (von Gierke Disease; GSD-I), the only form with significant renal manifestations, is caused by deficient catalytic activity of the glucose-6-phosphatase (G6Pase) enzyme (GSD-Ia), or deficiency of the glucose-6-phosphate (G6P) transporter (G6PT1) enzyme (GSD-Ib) (Table 8.11, Figure 8.29). Impaired production of glucose from glycogenolysis and gluconeogenesis results in severe hypoglycemia and increased production of lactic acid, triglyceride, and uric acid. Only GSD-I will be discussed in this chapter.

Epidemiology and Clinical Presentation

Glycogen storage disease I is relatively rare in the general population (1 in 100,000 to 1 in 400,000) but the frequency is increased in Ashkenazi Jewish population. GSD-Ia accounts for more than 80 percent of cases of GSD-I. Patients of both major subtypes, GSD-Ia and GSD-Ib, manifest phenotypic

G6Pase deficiency, characterized by hypoglycemia, hepatomegaly, nephromegaly, hyperlipidemia, hyperuricemia, lactic aciduria, and gross retardation [83]. GSD-Ib patients also suffer from chronic neutropenia and functional deficiencies of neutrophils and monocytes [83]. The common clinical features of GSD-I are listed in Table 8.12. A wide range of renal functional abnormalities may be present (Table 8.12).

Approach to Interpretation

Gross Pathology. The kidneys could be significantly enlarged, up to twice the normal weight.

Light Microscopy. Glycogen may be deposited in any or all portions of the nephron, including the glomerular tuft, Bowman's space, parietal epithelium, various tubular segments, and tubular lumina. Glomerular deposition of glycogen can cause two to three fold glomerular enlargements. Slight mesangial hypercellularity may be present. The tubular epithelial cells show extensive vacuolization due to intracytoplasmic glycogen accumulation. Progressive renal injury may lead to focal segmental and global glomerulosclerosis, interstitial fibrosis, tubular atrophy, and arteriolosclerosis. Renal morphologic abnormalities of GSD-I are summarized in Table 8.12.

Immunofluorescence Microscopy. Various immunoglobulins and complements are often deposited in the glomeruli. Also, glomerular deposition of apolipoprotein has been described [84].

Electron Microscopy. The GBM show extensive thickening with focal lamellations somewhat reminiscent of that seen in Alport's syndrome [85]. Fine glycogen granules can be observed in the thickened basement membranes, and also in mesangial, endothelial, and epithelial cells. Mesangial widening with matrix accumulation can be prominent, and along with the thickened basement membranes, may resemble changes seen in diabetic glomerulosclerosis [86]. Effacement of the visceral epithelial cell foot processes is seen in patients with proteinuria. Glycogen in the tubular epithelial cells is present freely and also in membrane-bound vesicles.

Differential Diagnosis

The diagnosis of GSD-I is usually made on the basis of characteristic clinical and biochemical features confirmed by mutation analysis. Renal biopsies may only be needed if renal abnormalities, such as significant degree of proteinuria are present. In context with the clinical presentation, interpretation of such biopsies is usually straightforward.

Etiology and Pathogenesis

Deficient catalytic activity of the G6Pase (type GSD-Ia), or G6PT1 (type GSD-Ib) (Table 8.10, Figure 29), caused by mutations in the corresponding genes, results in impaired production of glucose with severe hypoglycemia and multisystem glycogen deposition with functional impairment. A large number of mutations have been identified in both genes [83]. Hypercalciuria combined with low citrate excretion play a role in the pathogenesis of nephrocalcinosis and nephrolithiasis in these patients.

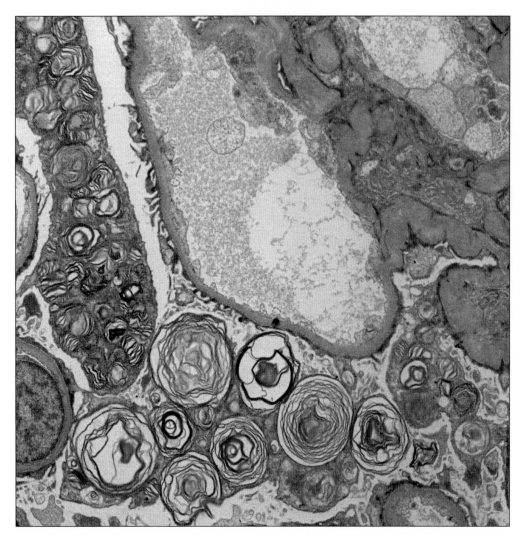

FIGURE 8.28: *Fabry's disease, electron microscopy. Visceral epithelial cells are loaded with "myeloid" bodies. (Electron microscopy, original magnification, ×6,800).*

Clinical Course, Prognosis, Treatment, and Clinical Correlation

Renal functional abnormalities are usually more prominent in those patients without treatment. Also, patients with persistently elevated concentrations of blood lactate, lipids, and uric acid are at increased risk of nephropathy. Children who are treated usually do not have any significant renal impairment except glomerular hyperfiltration. More severe renal involvement with proteinuria, hypertension, and decreased creatinine clearance may develop due to FSGS and interstitial fibrosis, which may, rarely, progress to renal failure in young adults [87] . Additional long-term complications include growth failure, gout, pulmonary hypertension, osteoporosis, and hepatic adenomas with the risk of the development of hepatocellular carcinoma (HCC) in type GSD-Ia and also recurrent infections and inflammatory bowel disease in type GSD-Ib. Current therapy is focused on maintaining normoglycemia through dietary therapy. ESRD and liver adenomas may be treated with kidney, and/or liver transplantation. Gene therapy might offer curative therapy in the future for GSD-Ia by expressing the missing enzyme in the liver [88]. Patients with the GSD-Ib type also suffer from chronic neutropenia and functional deficiencies of neutrophils and monocytes, which is treated with granulocyte colony stimulating factor to restore myeloid function.

Table 8.8 Typical Renal Manifestations of Fabry's Disease

Proteinuria (usually non-nephrotic, onset at age of 34 years)[a]
Decreased urinary concentrating ability
Polyuria, polydipsia
Fanconi syndrome (rare)
CRI (50% of patients at median age of 42 years)[a]
ESRD (23% of patients at median age of 47 years)[a]

Abbreviations: CRI, chronic renal insufficiency; ESRD, end-stage renal disease

[a] Data from Branton et al. (2002) [60]

Table 8.9 Clinical Features of Gaucher's Disease

	Type 1	Type 2	Type 3
Onset	>1 year	<1 year	2-20 years
Hepatospleno megaly	+	+/−	+
Bone disease	+	−	+/−
Cardiac value disease	−	−	+
Central nervous system disease	−	++	+/−
Age of death	60-90 years	<5 year	<30 years

Table 8.10 Typical Renal Morphologic Findings in Gaucher's Disease

Light Microscopy
   Gaucher cells with "fluffy" cytoplasm (GC, PTC, M, TI)
Electron Microscopy
   Gaucher cells with membrane bound tubular structures with fibrils (60-80 nm)
   Gaucher bodies (GCE, MC, TI)

Abbreviations: GC, glomerular capillaries; PTC, peritubular capillaries; M, mesangium; TI, tubulointerstitium; GCE, glomerular capillary endothelium; MC, mesangial cells.

LECITHIN CHOLESTEROL ACETYLTRANSFERASE DEFICIENCY

Introduction

Familial lecithin cholesterol acetyltransferase (LCAT) deficiency is a very rare autosomal recessive disorder of lipoprotein metabolism, resulting from loss of function of LCAT, a key enzyme in extracellular cholesterol metabolism and transport [89]. Approximately 50 families have been described in the literature so far.

Epidemiology and Clinical Presentation

The first cases were reported from Norway and in people of Northern European descent, but since then there have been several reports of patients from other parts of the world. Clinical manifestations include corneal opacities, anemia, and renal involvement with varying degrees of proteinuria and progressive renal insufficiency in some cases. Plasma LCAT activity is usually very low or completely absent. Plasma high-density lipopro-

tein (HDL) cholesterol levels are also very low and most plasma cholesterol is in a free form and triglycerides are elevated [89]. Proteinuria may begin in early childhood but most patients are diagnosed in early adulthood. Hypertension is common. Corneal opacities are frequently manifested during childhood.

Approach to Interpretation

Light Microscopy. The changes affect mostly glomeruli, however, vascular and tubulointerstitial disease may also be present [90,91]. The glomeruli show mesangial expansion usually without increased cellularity. There is irregular thickening of the GBM with focal vacuolization due to intramembranous lipid deposits. The GBM changes are best visualized on JMS and PAS stains and resemble those seen in advanced (stage 3) membranous nephropathy (Figure 8.30). Focal double contours of the GBM can be seen. The mesangial matrix may also have a finely vacuolated texture with a honeycomb appearance. Glomerular endocapillary foam cells can be seen occasionally. As the disease progresses, focal segmental and global glomerulosclerosis may develop with tubular atrophy, interstitial fibrosis, and arteriosclerosis.

Immunofluorescence Microscopy. The IF findings are typically negative or nonspecific.

Electron Microscopy. Lipid deposits are seen within the thickened GBM in epimembranous, intramembranous, and subendothelial locations [92,93] (Figure 8.31). The dense core of the lucent structures consists of curvilinear serpiginous fibrils and lamellar or granular densities located in the center or at the periphery. The lipid deposits correspond to the basement membrane vacuolization seen by light microscopy. Similar structures are also present within the increased mesangial matrix as irregularly distributed, rounded electron lucent inclusions with electron-dense cores. Mesangial deposits are usually large and granular. The mesangial extracellular lipid deposits resemble those seen in hepatic glomerulosclerosis. Similar lipid deposits can also be seen in the vascular endothelial cells and medial myocytes. Foam cells may be present mostly in mesangial location.

Differential Diagnosis

The differential diagnosis of LCAT deficiency includes advanced membranous nephropathy and hepatic glomerulosclerosis. Negative IF excludes membranous nephropathy. Clinical history of alcoholism and/or cirrhosis points to hepatic glomerulosclerosis.

Etiology and Pathogenesis

LCAT catalyzes the transfer of a preferentially unesterified fatty acid from phosphatidylcholine to cholesterol, and thereby produces lysophosphatidylcholine and a cholesteryl ester. Over fifty

Table 8.11 Glycogen Storage Disease-I: Molecular and Genetic Aspects and Incidence

Type	Enzyme Affected	Inheritance	Gene	Chromosome	Incidence
Type Ia	Glucose-6-phosphatase	AR	G6PC	17q21	1/100,000 to
Type Ib	Glucose-6-phosphate Transporter	AR	G6PT1	11q23	1/400,000 births

Abbreviations: AR, autosomal recessive.

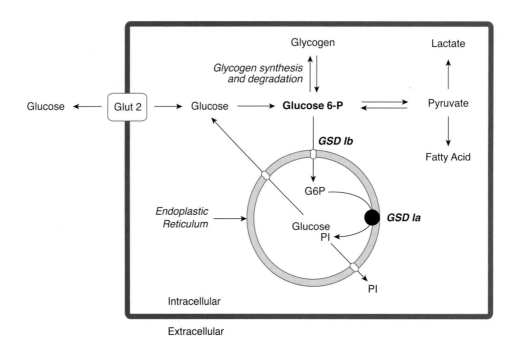

FIGURE 8.29: *Molecular pathogenesis of glycogen storage disease I (von Gierke Disease; GSD-I). GSD type I is caused by deficient catalytic activity of the glucose-6-phosphatase (G6Pase) enzyme (GSD-Ia), or deficiency of the glucose-6-phosphate (G6P) transporter (G6PT1) enzyme (GSD-Ib).*

mutations of the LCAT gene, localized to chromosome 16q21–q22, have been identified [89]. Patients with homozygous or compound heterozygous mutations may present with one of two clinical phenotypes, classical LCAT deficiency or fish-eye disease [89]. Altered or abolished LCAT enzyme

Table 8.12 Clinical Features, Renal Functional and Morphologic Changes in Glycogen Storage Disease-I

Clinical Features
Severe hypoglycemia
Lactic acidemia, hypertriglyceridemia, and hyperuricemia
Hepato,- and renomegaly
Failure to thrive
Delayed motor development
Bleeding tendency
Neutropenia, neutrophil dysfunction and recurrent infections[a]

Renal Functional Abnormalities
Proximal tubular dysfunction (glucosuria, phosphaturia, hypokalemia, and generalized aminoaciduria)
Glomerular hyperfiltration
Distal renal tubular acidification defect with hypercalciuria
Low citrate excretion
Albuminuria (adolescents)
Proteinuria (Hypertension)
Decreased creatinine clearance

Morphologic Changes
Glycogen accumulation in renal tubular epithelial cells
Glomerulomegaly
Focal segmental glomerulosclerosis
Interstitial fibrosis
Nephrocalcinosis and nephrolithiasis

a Typical in GSD-Ib but may also be present in GSD-Ia.

catalytic activity results in an abnormal lipid profile. Heterozygotes lack clinical symptoms, although they may have partial enzyme deficiency. Renal involvement results from abnormal glomerular deposition of various lipid constituents. However, the precise pathogenetic mechanisms of renal glomerular injury are uncertain. The role of inflammation as a result of glomerular lipid deposition has been postulated in a mouse model of LCAT deficiency displaying renal morphologic findings similar to those in humans with LCAT deficiency [94]. Also, mesangial deposition of lipoproteins can promote matrix production and glomerulosclerosis [95].

Clinical Course, Prognosis, Treatment, and Clinical Correlation

Renal involvement is the major cause of morbidity and mortality in patients with LCAT deficiency. Hypertension, nephrotic range proteinuria, and progressive renal insufficiency may lead to ESRD by the fourth to fifth decades of life. The disease may recur in allograft kidneys, however, graft function is usually preserved and long-term graft survival has been described [96]. The risk for atherosclerosis in patients with LCAT deficiency is uncertain. Some reports suggested increased atherosclerotic burden while others reported no atherosclerosis or endothelial dysfunction [89,97]. Currently, there is no well established therapy for the disease.

LIPOPROTEIN GLOMERULOPATHY

Introduction

Lipoprotein glomerulopathy is a rare hereditary renal disease with both familial and sporadic occurrence.

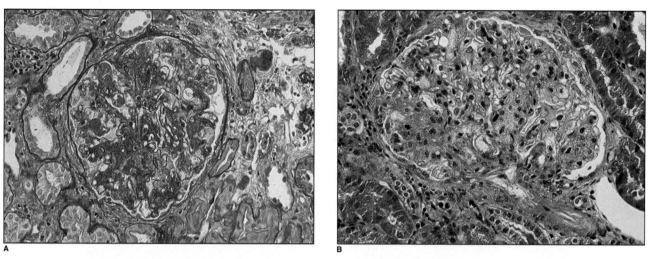

FIGURE 8.30: *LCAT deficiency. The glomerulus exhibits mesangial widening and thickening of the glomerular capillary walls. (A: Periodic acid Schiff, ×400; B: Masson's trichrome, ×400). Courtesy of Dr. Tibor Nadasdy.*

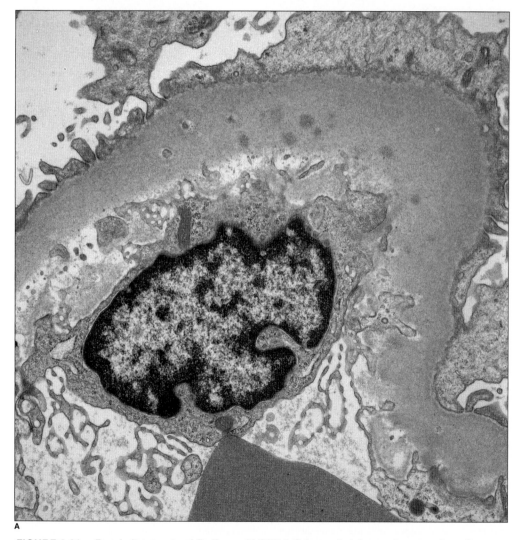

FIGURE 8.31: *Renal ultrastructural findings of LCAT deficiency. A: Intramembranous deposits are seen in the thickened glomerular capillary basement membranes. (Electron microphotograph, original magnification ×9,300).*

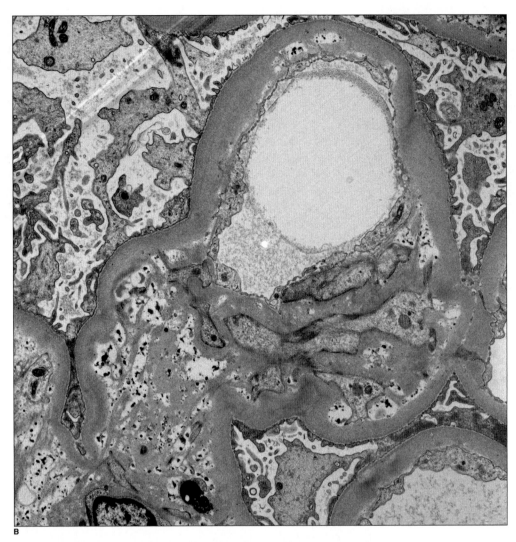

FIGURE 8.31: *B: Rounded electron lucent inclusions with electron dense cores are seen in the mesangial areas. (Electron microphotograph, original magnification ×6,800).*

Epidemiology and Clinical Presentation

Most of the cases are reported from Asia, particularly from Japan and China, and there is an apparent male predominance. Clinical renal manifestations include proteinuria, nephrotic range proteinuria, and microscopic or gross hematuria with or without impaired renal function [98,99] . Progression to ESRD may occur. Abnormal plasma lipoprotein profile resembling type III hyperlipoproteinemia and marked increase in serum apolipoprotein E (apo E) concentrations are characteristic laboratory findings. However, unlike type III hyperlipoproteinemia, LPG is not associated with arteriosclerosis and seems to be confined to the kidney.

Approach to Interpretation

Light Microscopy. The morphologic features of the disease were first reported by Faraggiana and Churg [100], however, Saito et al. [99] was the first to recognize it as a clinicopathologic entity. The most characteristic finding is the presence of pale eosinophilic lipoprotein "thrombi" within markedly dilated glo-

merular capillary lumina. The thrombi stain pale with PAS, pale blue with Masson's trichrome, and positive with Oil Red O on cryostat sections (Figure 8.32). Slight glomerulomegaly, focal reduplication of the GBMs with mesangial cell interposition, focal mesangial cellular proliferation, mesangiolysis, and small segmentally sclerotic lesions may occur [98,101,102]. No glomerular or tubulointerstitial accumulation of foamy macrophages is usually present. No "thrombi" in extrarenal locations have been described.

Immunofluorescence Microscopy. The glomerular capillary "thrombi" stain positive with antibodies against apoE and apoB. The conventional IF panel is either negative or show only nonspecific staining.

Electron Microscopy. Electron microscopy reveals glomeruli with dilated capillary lumina filled with osmiophilic finely vacuolated granular material showing a concentric lamellated appearance (Figure 8.32). Similar deposits can also be seen subendothelially as well as within the mesangial areas.

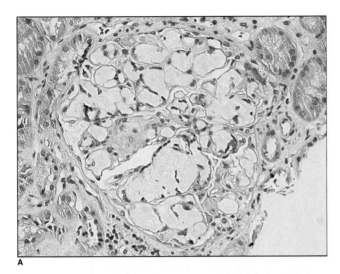

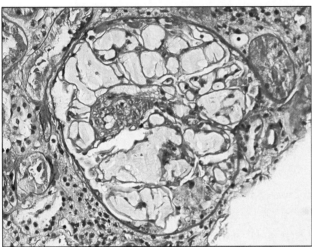

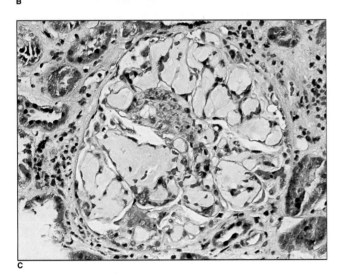

FIGURE 8.32: *Lipoprotein glomerulopathy. Dilated glomerular capillary lumina are filled with pale lipoprotein "thrombi".* (A: Hematoxylin and eosin, ×300; B: Periodic acid Schiff, ×200; C: Masson's trichrome, ×200). *Ultrastructurally, the "thrombi" are composed of finely vacuolated granular material with a concentric lamellate appearance. (Electron microscopy, original magnification, ×6,000). Courtesy of Dr. Tibor Nadasdy.*

Differential Diagnosis

The key to the correct morphologic diagnosis of LPG is the recognition of the glomerular lipoprotein "thrombi" within dilated capillary lumina. The diagnosis is usually straightforward because of the distinctly unique appearance of the glomerular lesions.

Etiology and Pathogenesis

Novel polymorphisms of the apoE gene, secondary to various genomic mutations, play a pivotal role in the development of LPG [103–105]. The most common apoE-Sendai variant (Arg145Pro) was found in eleven of fourteen Japanese patients in three unrelated kindreds [106]; all of the patients tested showed heterozygosity for the apoE variant, suggesting an autosomal recessive pattern of inheritance. In contrast, type III hyperlipoproteinemia, which has similar plasma lipoprotein profile but systemic manifestations of hyperlipidemia, is associated with homozygosity for the apoE2 isoform. The role of environmental and additional genetic factors has also been suggested as possible contributing factors in the pathogenesis of LPG [105]. A mouse model has been developed that reproduces the characteristic morphologic findings of LPG in apoE-deficient mice upon virus-mediated transduction of apoE-Sendai [107]. However, the precise mechanisms responsible for the development of lipoprotein "thrombi" remain unknown. It might be related to abnormal lipid trafficking due to structural alterations of the apoE molecule.

Clinical Course, Prognosis, Treatment, and Clinical Correlation

No effective treatment for LPG has been established yet. Therapeutic trials with immunosuppressants, hydroxymethyl/glutaryl-coenzyme A reductase inhibitors, and low density lipoprotein (LDL) apheresis revealed limited efficacy. However, with lipid lowering treatment disappearance of the glomerular capillary lipid thrombi has been reported [108,109]. Recurrence of the disease in transplants has also been reported in a few cases [102].

NEPHROCALCINOSIS

Introduction

Renal parenchymal deposition of calcium phosphate, termed nephrocalcinosis, is found in many different diseases and conditions (Table 8.13) [110]. Extensive deposition of calcium phosphate may lead to renal functional impairment.

Epidemiology and Clinical Presentation

Nephrocalcinosis is usually becoming clinically apparent only when significant parenchymal damage with renal functional compromise develops. This is in sharp contrast with nephrolithiasis, which usually produces symptoms early during the disease. The clinical presentation may also depend on the underlying conditions. If caused by hypercalcemia, either primary or secondary, nonspecific symptoms owing to hypercalcemia may include thirst, polyuria, and gastrointestinal symptoms, such as constipation. Hypercalcemia may also be

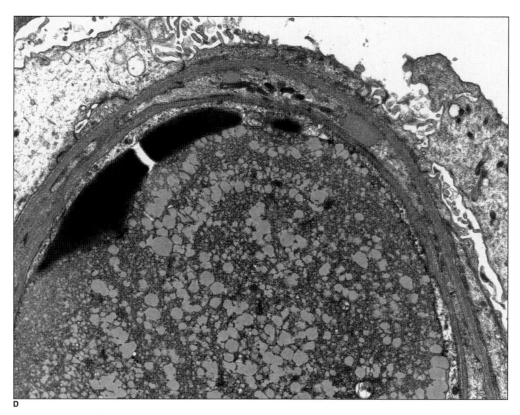

D

FIGURE 8.32: (continued).

the cause of aminoaciduria, salt and potassium wasting, and proximal and distal renal tubular acidosis [110]. However, most patients with primary hyperparathyroidism, the most common cause of hypercalcemia, are asymptomatic. Those who have renal manifestations with nephrocalcinosis, usually present with decreased GFR and tubular dysfunction.

Approach to Interpretation

Gross Pathology. The kidneys could be either normal size or smaller. Small wedge-shaped scars can be seen on the cut surface beneath the capsule.

Light Microscopy. The calcium phosphate deposits can be found within the tubular epithelial cells, inside the tubular lumina, along the tubular basement membranes, freely in the interstitium, and also in the arterial walls and Bowman's capsule (Figures 8.33 and 8.34). All tubular segments could be affected. On hematoxylin and eosin-stained sections, the deposits may appear as granular basophilic purplish concretions or as a purplish tinge or stippling along the tubular basement membranes. The deposits are nonpolarizable and stain positive with von Kossa. During the early stages of the disease, extensive acute tubular epithelial injury, slight interstitial edema, and inflammation may also be present. Interstitial fibrosis, tubular atrophy, and glomerulosclerosis may develop as the disease progresses. Wedge-shaped cortical scars may be formed alternating with better preserved areas, typically seen in patients with hypercalcemia. Arteries with medial calcifications usually do not show luminal compromise.

Immunofluorescent Microscopy. No specific immunofluorescent microscopic findings are present.

Electron Microscopy. Calcium phosphate deposits disclose a central nidus surrounded by electron dense radially oriented spicules with budding crystals. Severe tubular epithelial cell injury is secondary to calcium deposits.

Differential Diagnosis

A small number of renal parenchymal calcifications may be seen without any clinical significance. Only when the deposits are numerous, the diagnosis of nephrocalcinosis should be

Table 8.13 Causes of Nephrocalcinosis

Hypercalcemic/hypercalciuric states
Renal parenchymal injury
    Acute tubular necrosis
    Cortical necrosis
    Hemolytic uremic syndrome
Allograft rejection
Medications
    Oral sodium phosphate
    Acetazolamide
Intrarenal infections in patients with acquired immunodeficiency
    syndrome (mycobacterium avium, pneumocystis carinii)
Cystic fibrosis
Advanced/chronic renal disease (glomerulonephritis,
    pyelonephritis)
Renal tubular acidosis

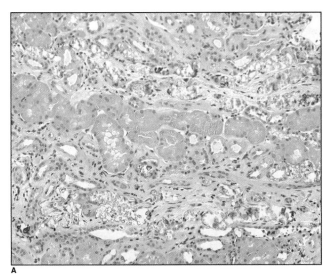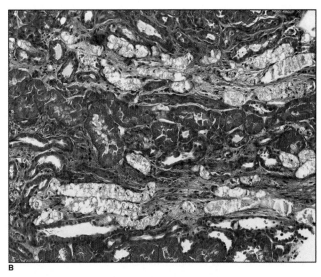

FIGURE 8.33: *Nephrocalcinosis. A: Calcium phosphate deposits are seen as basophilic purplish concretions in the interstitium. (Hematoxylin and eosin, ×200). B: On Masson's trichrome the deposits stain pale blue. (×200).*

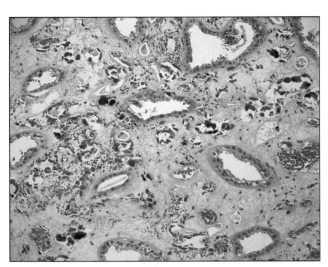

FIGURE 8.34: *Nephrocalcinosis, Randall's plaque. Calcification within the papilla (Randall's plaque) may serve as "nidus" for calcium-oxalate stones.*

considered. Calcium phosphate deposits should be distinguished from oxalate deposits that are birefringent and negative with the von Kossa stain. The distribution of calcifications within the kidney may help to determine the underlying etiology. For example, dystrophic calcification due to acute tubular necrosis develops at the site of tubular injury, most common in proximal tubules. Calcifications of distal tubules and collecting ducts in the renal cortex are typical of oral bowel-cleansing agents [111].

Etiology and Pathogenesis

Hypercalcemia, usually associated with hypercalciuria, is one of the common underlying conditions of nephrocalcinosis (Table 8.13). The cause of hypercalcemia is primary hyperparathyroidism or malignancy in over 90 percent of cases (Table 8.14). Less common causes include infantile and neonatal conditions, vitamin A and D excess, sarcoidosis, medications, milk-alkali syndrome, and rare genetic disorders. Among the many additional causes of nephrocalcinosis, unrelated to hypercalcemia, dystrophic parenchymal calcification may develop following ischemic or nephrotoxic acute tubular necrosis, cortical necrosis or hemolytic uremic syndrome. Nephrocalcinosis is also a well-known complication of oral sodium phosphate administration used for bowel-cleansing prior to colonoscopy [111]. Clinically, these patients present with acute renal failure although CRI may also develop. Increased incidence of nephrocalcinosis has been reported in association with distal renal tubular acidosis related to primary hereditary disorders, autoimmune diseases such as lupus and Sjögren's, and certain drugs [110]. Nephrocalcinosis is also relatively common in patients with nephropathic cystinosis [112]. Calcium phosphate deposits may cause tubular epithelial injury with interstitial fibrosis that leads to renal functional impairment. The scars seem to have more calcifications especially within the collecting ducts, raising the possibility of obstruction in the pathogenesis.

Clinical Course, Prognosis, Treatment, and Clinical Correlation

The clinical course, prognosis, and treatment depend primarily on the underlying conditions. If severe, nephrocalcinosis may have a significant impact on the progression of renal disease secondary to parenchymal damage, that is, interstitial fibrosis.

OXALOSIS

Introduction

Renal oxalosis is characterized by excessive deposition of calcium oxalate crystals in the kidney.

Table 8.14 Etiologic Factors of Hypercalcemia

Primary hyperparathyroidism
Malignancy
Genetic
Infantile neonatal conditions
Vitamin A and D excess
Sarcoidosis
Medications
Milk-alkali syndrome

Table 8.15 Causes of Hyperoxaluria

Primary
    Types 1, 2, and 3
Secondary
    Increased intestinal absorption
        Inflammatory small-bowel disease
        Status after partial small-bowel resection
        Status after small-bowel bypass surgery
    Massive oxalate load
        Excessive dietary intake of dark leafy vegetables, rhubarb,
            citrus fruits, or tea
    Ascorbate overdose
    Vitamin deficiency (Thiamine, Pyridoxine)
    Prolonged acute renal failure, chronic renal failure
    Ethylene glycol intoxication
    Methoxyfluorane

Epidemiology and Clinical Presentation

Renal oxalosis is common in patients with hyperoxaluria and may lead to acute or chronic renal failure. The common causes of hyperoxaluria are inborn errors of metabolism (i.e., primary hyperoxaluria [PH]) and increased oxalate intestinal absorption (Table 8.15) . Some patients with PH develop progressive renal parenchymal damage with CRI and ESRD typically before adulthood [113]. Other patients with PH may suffer only from recurrent urolithiasis or may have no symptoms at all. Increased intestinal absorption of oxalate due to small bowel resection, bypass surgery, or chronic inflammatory bowel disease may lead to progressive renal disease with CRI. Other, relatively rare causes of hyperoxaluria include massive oxalate overload, increased production of oxalate due to ethylene glycol intoxication, and excess intake of ascorbic acid, among others [110] (Table 8.18). These conditions may cause both acute and chronic renal insufficiency.

Approach to Interpretation

Light Microscopy. There are no specific gross renal findings associated with oxalosis. Microscopically, rhomboid or polyhedral birefringent oxalate crystals are seen mostly in the tubular lumina, and also in the tubular epithelial cells, and freely within the tubulointerstitium (Figure 8.35). The crystals are also readily visualized in hematoxylin and eosin-stained sections of formalin-fixed paraffin-embedded material without polarization. Tubular epithelial cell injury, secondary to crystal deposition, is usually present. As the disease progresses, chronicity develops with interstitial fibrosis, tubular atrophy, varying degree of chronic interstitial inflammation, and global glomerulosclerosis. Nephrocalcinosis may sometimes be present.

Immunofluorescence Microscopy. Immunofluorescence findings are typically negative or nonspecific.

Electron Microscopy. No specific ultrastructural findings are identified.

Differential Diagnosis

The shape and location of birefringent calcium oxalate crystals in sections of routinely fixed and processed paraffin-embedded tissues is highly characteristic. Needle-shaped crystalline deposits of dysproteinemias can also be seen in routinely processed paraffin embedded tissues in tubular epithelial cells and within interstitial macrophages. Crystals of cystinosis are only retained in alcohol-fixed material or fresh frozen sections.

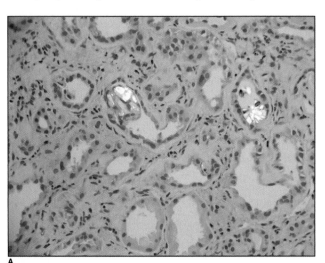
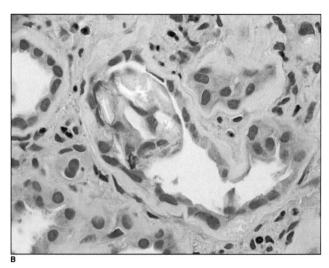

FIGURE 8.35: *Oxalosis. A: The birefringent calcium oxalate crystals are seen within tubular lumina and tubular epithelial cells. (Hematoxylin and eosin, under polarized light, ×200) B: The crystals within the epithelium exhibits polyhedral shape. (Hematoxylin and eosin, ×1,000).*

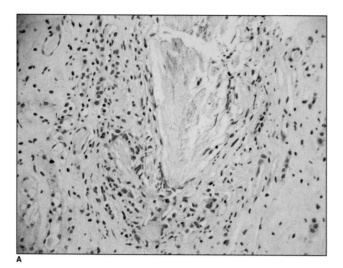
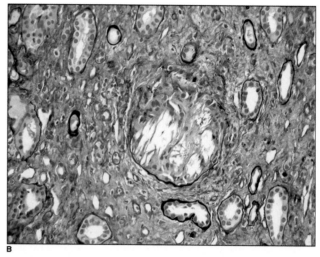

FIGURE 8.36: *Chronic uric acid nephropathy. A: Interstitial uric acid "tophus" reveals slightly basophilic matrix core surrounded by chronic inflammatory cell reaction. (Hematoxylin and eosin, × 400). B: Slit-like spaces corresponding to dissolved crystalline deposits of uric acid are surrounded by granulomatous inflammation. (Jones methenamine silver, × 400).*

Etiology and Pathogenesis

There are primary and secondary causes of hyperoxaluria (Table 8.18) . Primary hyperoxaluria type 1 (PH1) is an autosomal recessive disease caused by functional deficiency of a liver specific enzyme alanine-glyoxylate aminotransferase (AGT). AGT detoxifies the toxic metabolite of glyoxylate to glycine. Decreased activity of AGT results in excess production of oxalate and glycolate, leading to hyperoxaluria and hyperglycolic aciduria. Primary hyperoxaluria type 2 (PH2), which is the less common form, is caused by deficient glyoxylate reductase activity, leading to elevated levels of oxalate and L-glycerate in the urine. Several mutations have been identified for both genes [114]. The third type of primary hyperoxaluria (unclassified or atypical PH) has not been unraveled in terms of biochemical or molecular mechanism. In both the primary and the secondary forms of oxalosis, the marked excess of oxalate leads to the formation of insoluble calcium oxalate in the tubules, resulting in tubular epithelial damage, chronic tubulointerstitial injury, crystalluria, renal stone formation, and nephrocalcinosis.

Clinical Course, Prognosis, Treatment, and Clinical Correlation

PH1 is typically associated with more severe clinical manifestations. Approximately 50 percent of patients with PH1 reach ESRD by the age of 25 years [115]. Patients with ESRD require intensive dialysis to delay systemic oxalate deposition because the kidney is the only route of excretion of oxalate. Conservative treatment with hyperhydration, citrate, and pyridoxine can be successful in some patients. Combined liver–kidney transplantation has been used with some success.

URIC ACID NEPHROPATHY

Introduction

Precipitation of uric acid in the collecting ducts due to hyperuricemia is the underlying cause of uric acid nephropathy. Acute and chronic forms exist.

Epidemiology and Clinical Presentation

Acute uric acid nephropathy is the most frequent and clinically more important type of uric acid renal disease. It is characterized by acute oliguric or anuric renal failure due to precipitation of the uric acid crystals in the tubules. It is usually the result of the overproduction and overexcretion of uric acid in patients with malignancies especially lymphomas, leukemias, and less frequently myeloproliferative diseases including polycythemia vera. The acute uric acid nephropathy usually happens as a result of uric acid release from the tumor due to chemotherapy or radiation. But there have been cases of acute uric acid nephropathy in the setting of tissue catabolism due to seizures or primary overproduction of uric acid due to Lesch-Nyhan syndrome [116] . Usually there are no specific symptoms referable to the urinary tract except occasional flank pain. Tumor cell lysis results in rapid release of nucleotides followed by rapid rise in serum levels of uric acid. Rhabdomyolysis can also be the initiating factor.

Chronic uric acid nephropathy is a complication of gout. Gout is caused by hyperuricemia mainly due to decreased renal excretion of uric acid. Precipitated uric acid crystals, deposited in the kidney, induce tubular epithelial damage and interstitial granulomatous inflammation (Figure 8.36). Renal involvement, once common and often severe, now is typically mild and rare with only slight hypertension and slight reduction of renal function. It should be noted that epidemiological studies failed to demonstrate hyperuricemia

Table 8.16 Hereditary Disorders Associated With Hyperuricemia

Hypoxanthine–guanine phosphoribosyltransferase deficiency
5-Phophoribosyl pyrophosphate synthase superactivity
Glucose-6-phosphatase deficiency
Familial juvenile hyperuricemic nephropathy (familial nephropathy with gout)
Autosomal-dominant medullary cystic kidney disease (ADMCKD)

and gout as being independent risk factors for chronic kidney disease [117]. Patients with more significant renal impairment with gout may have comorbidities that contribute to the renal damage.

Patients who have hereditary disorders with various enzyme defects or tubular abnormalities (Table 8.16) that cause hyperuricemia may present with a range of renal manifestations including crystalluria, acute or chronic renal failure, and stones [118]. Crystalline deposits with interstitial microtophi (see section on "Light Microscopy" in this section) may be present in some, but not all of these hereditary disorders.

Approach to Interpretation

Gross Pathology. Linear yellow striations in the renal medulla and papillae, corresponding to precipitated uric acid in the collecting ducts, are the most typical findings of acute uric acid nephropathy. In the chronic form, yellow urate deposits may also be spotted in medulla. The size of the kidneys may be reduced accompanied by fine granularity of the surface and dilatation of the pelvis.

Light Microscopy. In the acute form, the collecting ducts contain large amounts of uric acid featuring amorphous masses in the paraffin sections and birefringent radially striated crystals in the frozen sections. Crystals may also be present penetrating the renal tubular epithelial cells. Secondary changes proximal to the obstruction include tubular dilatation and interstitial edema. In the chronic form, the collecting tubules in the renal medulla may contain monosodium urate crystals. The needle-shaped crystals are best seen in alcohol-fixed material; however, they may also be retained in formalin-fixed tissues. Some of the crystalline deposits may appear dark blue in the hematoxylin and eosin-stained sections possibly due to calcium content. When the typical birefringence of the crystals is lost, only faintly crystalline amorphous substance that stains blue on Masson's trichrome is seen. Due to deficiencies in the tubular walls crystalline deposits may appear interstitial and may evoke a mononuclear inflammatory cell reaction with granulomatous features showing foreign body giant cells, often referred to as "tophi" or "microtophi." During the early stages, the glomeruli may show slight enlargement with mesangial expansion, fibrillary thickening of the capillary walls and occasional reduplication of the basement membranes. Additional changes, usually regarded as secondary, include glomerulosclerosis, medullary scars with tubular atrophy, tubular dilatation (mostly in the medulla), and accumulation of intratubular polymorphonuclear leukocytes most common due to infections. Various degrees of interstitial fibrosis and tubular atrophy involving the renal cortex may also be present. In some of the hereditary disorders, such as hypoxanthine–guanine phosphoribosyltransferase deficiency, interstitial microtophi and crystalline tubular deposits may also be present. In others, microtophi are either absent or rare; focal segmental and global glomerulosclerosis with patchy tubular atrophy and interstitial fibrosis are the typical findings in familial juvenile hyperuricemic nephropathy [90].

Immunofluorescence Microscopy. No characteristic immunofluorescent findings are detected.

Electron Microscopy. During the early stages of the chronic form, prominent thickening of the GBMs with focal separation of the endothelial cells from the underlying membrane has been reported. Accumulation of finely granular material between the endothelial cells and the basement membranes may be seen.

Differential Diagnosis

Urate crystals with tophi have distinctive morphologic appearance. Although typically associated with gout, uric acid tophi are most commonly observed in biopsies from patients with advanced chronic renal disease. In acute uric acid nephropathy, calcium phosphate deposits may also form contributing to the renal failure. Also, the clinical presentation of unexplained severe renal failure particularly in young patients with hyperuricemia who have severe interstitial fibrosis and no specific glomerular or vascular disease in the biopsy should raise the possibility of autosomal dominant medullary cystic kidney disease.

Etiology and Pathogenesis

Hyperproduction of uric acid and/or diminished excretion through the kidney may lead to hyperuricemia and deposition of uric acid in various organs, including the kidneys. With higher plasma concentrations of uric acid, the filtered load surmounts the tubular capacity for reabsorption and a steep increase in uric acid excretion occurs. The excreted uric acid may exceed the limit of solubility resulting in crystal formation in the distal tubules. Acidic environment in the collecting ducts promotes the precipitation of uric acid.

Based upon the dynamics and severity of deposition, acute renal failure or CRI may develop. In addition to the hereditary disorders listed in Table 8.16, common causes of hyperuricemia include various drugs, ethanol, protein-rich diet, and obesity. Clinically significant renal disease due to impaired excretion through the kidney occurs mostly in gout; however, excretion is also hampered in lead toxicity, dehydration, renal insufficiency, and preeclampsia. Age, gender and race also affect the renal excretion of uric acid.

Clinical Course, Prognosis, Treatment, and Clinical Correlation

The treatment of fully developed acute uric acid nephropathy is not substantially different from treatment of acute oligo-anuric renal failure in general. The well-accepted mainstay of the prevention of acute uric acid nephropathy traditionally has been pretreatment with allopurinol as well volume expansion [116]. More questionable is the alkalinization of urine by sodium bicarbonate, with the aim of conversion of uric acid to more soluble urate salts. There seems to be very little added benefit and attempts to raise urine pH in the setting of fully developed acute renal failure are usually futile.

The relatively new approach to prevent and treat uric acid nephropathy relies on the increased degradation of uric acid. In humans and other primates uric acid is the final metabolite of the degradation of purines. In other mammals, uric acid can be converted into significantly more soluble allantoin. The reaction is catalyzed by uricase, which is missing in humans and other primates. Currently there is a recombinant uricase (rasburicase) available for replacement therapy and it has been shown to be effective in multiple clinical settings [119]. It can be used to treat hyperuricemia and also as a prophylactic measure in patients with tumor lysis syndrome [120].

REFERENCES

1. Idem. The Croonian lectures on inborn errors of metabolism. Lecture II. Alkaptonuria. *Lancet* 1908; 2:73–79.
2. Phornphutkul C, Introne WJ, Perry MB, Bernardini I, Murphey MD, Fitzpatrick DL, Anderson PD, Huizing M, Anikster Y, Gerber LH, Gahl WA. Natural history of alkaptonuria. *N Engl J Med* 2002;347:2111–21.
3. Held PK. Disorders of tyrosine catabolism. *Mol Genet Metab* 2006;88:103–6.
4. Introne WJ, Phornphutkul C, Bernardini I, McLaughlin K, Fitzpatrick D, Gahl WA. Exacerbation of the ochronosis of alkaptonuria due to renal insufficiency and improvement after renal transplantation. *Mol Genet Metab* 2002;77:136–42.
5. Suwannarat P, O'Brien K, Perry MB, Sebring N, Bernardini I, Kaiser-Kupfer MI, Rubin BI, Tsilou E, Gerber LH, Gahl WA. Use of nitisinone in patients with alkaptonuria. *Metabolism* 2005;54:719–28.
6. Gahl WA, Thoene JG, Schneider JA. Cystinosis. *N Engl J Med* 2002;347:111–21.
7. Kalatzis V, Antignac C. New aspects of the pathogenesis of cystinosis. *Pediatr Nephrol* 2003;18:207–15.
8. Servais A, Moriniere V, Grunfeld JP, Noel LH, Goujon JM, Chadefaux-Vekemans B, Antignac C. Late-onset nephropathic cystinosis: clinical presentation, outcome, and genotyping. *Clin J Am Soc Nephrol* 2008;3:27–35.
9. Middleton R, Bradbury M, Webb N, O'Donoghue D, Van't Hoff W. Cystinosis. A clinicopathological conference. "From toddlers to twenties and beyond" Adult-Paediatric Nephrology Interface Meeting, Manchester 2001. *Nephrol Dial Transplant* 2003;18:2492–5.
10. Mahoney CP, Striker GE. Early development of the renal lesions in infantile cystinosis. *Pediatr Nephrol* 2000;15:50–6.
11. Bonsib SM, Horvath F, Jr. Multinucleated podocytes in a child with nephrotic syndrome and Fanconi's syndrome: A unique clue to the diagnosis. *Am J Kidney Dis* 1999;34:966–71.
12. Jackson JD, Smith FG, Litman NN, Yuile CL, Latta H. The Fanconi syndrome with cystinossis. Electron microscopy of renal biopsy specimens from five patients. *Am J Med* 1962;33:893–910.
13. Nagata M, Yamaguchi Y, Komatsu Y, Ito K. Mitosis and the presence of binucleate cells among glomerular podocytes in diseased human kidneys. *Nephron* 1995;70:68–71.
14. Mattoo A, Goldfarb DS. *Cystinuria. Semin Nephrol* 2008;28:181–91.
15. Shotelersuk V, Larson D, Anikster Y, McDowell G, Lemons R, Bernardini I, Guo J, Thoene J, Gahl WA. CTNS mutations in an American-based population of cystinosis patients. *Am J Hum Genet* 1998;63:1352–62.
16. Chevalier RL, Forbes MS. Generation and Evolution of Atubular Glomeruli in the Progression of Renal Disorders. *J Am Soc Nephrol* 2008;19:197–206.
17. Nesterova G, Gahl W. Nephropathic cystinosis: late complications of a multisystemic disease. *Pediatr Nephrol* 2008;23:863–78.
18. Gahl WA, Balog JZ, Kleta R. Nephropathic cystinosis in adults: natural history and effects of oral cysteamine therapy. *Ann Intern Med* 2007;147:242–50.
19. Gahl WA. Early oral cysteamine therapy for nephropathic cystinosis. *Eur J Pediatr* 2003;162 Suppl. 1:S38–41.
20. Gahl WA, Reed GF, Thoene JG, Schulman JD, Rizzo WB, Jonas AJ, Denman DW, Schlesselman JJ, Corden BJ, Schneider JA. Cysteamine therapy for children with nephropathic cystinosis. *N Engl J Med* 1987;316:971–7.
21. Markello TC, Bernardini IM, Gahl WA. Improved renal function in children with cystinosis treated with cysteamine. *N Engl J Med* 1993;328:1157–62.
22. Parving HH, Smidt UM, Friisberg B, Bonnevie-Nielsen V, Andersen AR. A prospective study of glomerular filtration rate and arterial blood pressure in insulin-dependent diabetics with diabetic nephropathy. *Diabetologia* 1981;20:457–61.
23. Mazzucco G, Bertani T, Fortunato M, Bernardi M, Leutner M, Boldorini R, Monga G. Different patterns of renal damage in type 2 diabetes mellitus: a multicentric study on 393 biopsies. *Am J Kidney Dis* 2002;39:713–20.
24. United States Renal Data System. Annual data report. In USRDS Coordinating System, Minneapolis, MN, 2007.
25. Young BA, Maynard C, Boyko EJ. Racial differences in diabetic nephropathy, cardiovascular disease, and mortality in a national population of veterans. *Diabetes Care* 2003;26:2392–9.
26. Pugh JA. The epidemiology of diabetic nephropathy. *Diabetes Metab Rev* 1989;5:531–45.
27. Cowie CC, Port FK, Wolfe RA, Savage PJ, Moll PP, Hawthorne VM. Disparities in incidence of diabetic end-stage renal disease according to race and type of diabetes. *N Engl J Med* 1989;321:1074–9.
28. Mogensen CE, Schmitz O. The diabetic kidney: from hyperfiltration and microalbuminuria to end-stage renal failure. *Med Clin North Am* 1988;72:1465–92.
29. Li JJ, Kwak SJ, Jung DS, Kim JJ, Yoo TH, Ryu DR, Han SH, Choi HY, Lee JE, Moon SJ, Kim DK, Han DS, Kang SW. Podocyte biology in diabetic nephropathy. *Kidney Int Suppl* 2007;S36–42.
30. Bohle A, Wehrmann M, Bogenschutz O, Batz C, Muller CA, Muller GA. The pathogenesis of chronic renal failure in diabetic nephropathy. Investigation of 488 cases of diabetic glomerulosclerosis. *Pathol Res Pract* 1991;187:251–9.
31. Ainsworth SK, Hirsch HZ, Brackett NC, Jr., Brissie RM, Williams AV, Jr., Hennigar GR. Diabetic glomerulonephropathy: histopathologic, immunofluorescent, and ultrastructural studies of 16 cases. *Hum Pathol* 1982;13:470–8.
32. Drummond K, Mauer M. The early natural history of nephropathy in type 1 diabetes: II. Early renal structural changes in type 1 diabetes. *Diabetes* 2002;51:1580–7.
33. Steffes MW, Bilous RW, Sutherland DE, Mauer SM. Cell and matrix components of the glomerular mesangium in type I diabetes. *Diabetes* 1992;41:679–84.
34. Markowitz GS, Lin J, Valeri AM, Avila C, Nasr SH, D'Agati VD. Idiopathic nodular glomerulosclerosis is a distinct clinicopathologic entity linked to hypertension and smoking. *Hum Pathol* 2002;33:826–35.
35. Lin J, Markowitz GS, Valeri AM, Kambham N, Sherman WH, Appel GB, D'Agati VD. Renal monoclonal

immunoglobulin deposition disease: the disease spectrum. *J Am Soc Nephrol* 2001;12:1482–92.

36. Rosenstock JL, Markowitz GS, Valeri AM, Sacchi G, Appel GB, D'Agati VD. Fibrillary and immunotactoid glomerulonephritis: Distinct entities with different clinical and pathologic features. *Kidney Int* 2003;63:1450–61.

37. Haas M. Incidental healed postinfectious glomerulonephritis: a study of 1012 renal biopsy specimens examined by electron microscopy. *Hum Pathol* 2003;34:3–10.

38. Ng DP, Krolewski AS. Molecular genetic approaches for studying the etiology of diabetic nephropathy. *Curr Mol Med* 2005;5:509–25.

39. Olson JL, Laszik ZG, "Diabetic Nephropathy". in Jennette CJ, Olson JL, Schwartz MM, Silva FG (eds.), *Heptinstall's Pathology of the Kidney* (Philadelphia: Lippincott Williams & Wilkins, 2007), pp. 803–52.

40. Dronavalli S, Duka I, Bakris GL. The pathogenesis of diabetic nephropathy. *Nat Clin Pract Endocrinol Metab* 2008;4:444:52.

41. Tan AL, Forbes JM, Cooper ME. AGE, RAGE, and ROS in diabetic nephropathy. *Semin Nephrol* 2007;27:130–43.

42. Mogensen CE, Christensen CK, Vittinghus E. The stages in diabetic renal disease. With emphasis on the stage of incipient diabetic nephropathy. *Diabetes* 1983;32 Suppl. 2:64–78.

43. Selby JV, FitzSimmons SC, Newman JM, Katz PP, Sepe S, Showstack J. The natural history and epidemiology of diabetic nephropathy. Implications for prevention and control. *Jama* 1990;263:1954–60.

44. Mogensen CE, Christensen C, Christiansen J, Boye N, Pedersen MM, Schmitz A. Early hyperfiltration and late renal damage in insulin-dependent diabetes. *Pediatr Adolesc Endocrinol* 1988;17:197.

45. Viberti G, Keen H. The patterns of proteinuria in diabetes mellitus. Relevance to pathogenesis and prevention of diabetic nephropathy. *Diabetes* 1984;33:686–92.

46. Deckert T, Feldt-Rasmussen B, Borch-Johnsen K, Jensen T, Kofoed-Enevoldsen A. Albuminuria reflects widespread vascular damage. The Steno hypothesis. *Diabetologia* 1989;32:219–26.

47. Mogensen CE. Progression of nephropathy in long-term diabetics with proteinuria and effect of initial antihypertensive treatment. *Scand J Clin Lab Invest* 1976;36:383–8.

48. Krolewski AS, Canessa M, Warram JH, Laffel LM, Christlieb AR, Knowler WC, Rand LI. Predisposition to hypertension and susceptibility to renal disease in insulin-dependent diabetes mellitus. *N Engl J Med* 1988;318:140–5.

49. Grenfell A, Watkins PJ. Clinical diabetic nephropathy: natural history and complications. *Clin Endocrinol Metab* 1986;15:783–805.

50. Krolewski AS, Warram JH, Christlieb AR, Busick EJ, Kahn CR. The changing natural history of nephropathy in type I diabetes. *Am J Med* 1985;78:785–94.

51. Mogensen CE, Schmitz A, Christensen CK. Comparative renal pathophysiology relevant to IDDM and NIDDM patients. *Diabetes Metab Rev* 1988;4:453–83.

52. Pugh JA, Medina R, Ramirez M. Comparison of the course to end-stage renal disease of type 1 (insulin-dependent) and type 2 (non-insulin-dependent) diabetic nephropathy. *Diabetologia* 1993;36:1094–8.

53. Mulec H, Blohme G, Grande B, Bjorck S. The effect of metabolic control on rate of decline in renal function in insulin-dependent diabetes mellitus with overt diabetic nephropathy. *Nephrol Dial Transplant* 1998;13:651–5.

54. Bangstad HJ, Osterby R, Rudberg S, Hartmann A, Brabrand K, Hanssen KF. Kidney function and glomerulopathy over 8 years in young patients with Type I (insulin-dependent) diabetes mellitus and microalbuminuria. *Diabetologia* 2002;45:253–61.

55. Parving HH, Smidt UM, Hommel E, Mathiesen ER, Rossing P, Nielsen F, Gall MA. Effective antihypertensive treatment postpones renal insufficiency in diabetic nephropathy. *Am J Kidney Dis* 1993;22:188–95.

56. Hovind P, Rossing P, Tarnow L, Smidt UM, Parving HH. Progression of diabetic nephropathy. *Kidney Int* 2001;59:702–9.

57. Patel A, MacMahon S, Chalmers J, Neal B, Billot L, Woodward M, Marre M, Cooper M, Glasziou P, Grobbee D, Hamet P, Harrap S, Heller S, Liu L, Mancia G, Mogensen CE, Pan C, Poulter N, Rodgers A, Williams B, Bompoint S, de Galan BE, Joshi R, Travert F. Intensive blood glucose control and vascular outcomes in patients with type 2 diabetes. *N Engl J Med* 2008;358:2560–72.

58. Parving HH, Andersen AR, Smidt UM, Svendsen PA. Early aggressive antihypertensive treatment reduces rate of decline in kidney function in diabetic nephropathy. *Lancet* 1983;1:1175–79.

59. Lewis EJ, Hunsicker LG, Bain RP, Rohde RD. The effect of angiotensin-converting-enzyme inhibition on diabetic nephropathy. The Collaborative Study Group. *N Engl J Med* 1993;329:1456–62.

60. Branton MH, Schiffmann R, Sabnis SG, Murray GJ, Quirk JM, Altarescu G, Goldfarb L, Brady RO, Balow JE, Austin Iii HA, Kopp JB: Natural history of Fabry renal disease: influence of alpha-galactosidase A activity and genetic mutations on clinical course. *Medicine (Baltimore)* 2002;81:122–38.

61. Mehta A, Ricci R, Widmer U, Dehout F, Garcia de Lorenzo A, Kampmann C, Linhart A, Sunder-Plassmann G, Ries M, Beck M. Fabry disease defined: baseline clinical manifestations of 366 patients in the Fabry Outcome Survey. *Eur J Clin Invest* 2004;34:236–42.

62. Sawada K, Mizoguchi K, Hishida A, Kaneko E, Koide Y, Nishimura K, Kimura M. Point mutation in the alpha-galactosidase A gene of atypical Fabry disease with only nephropathy. *Clin Nephrol* 1996;45:289–94.

63. von Scheidt W, Eng CM, Fitzmaurice TF, Erdmann E, Hubner G, Olsen EG, Christomanou H, Kandolf R, Bishop DF, Desnick RJ. An atypical variant of Fabry's disease with manifestations confined to the myocardium. *N Engl J Med* 1991;324:395–9.

64. Meehan SM, Junsanto T, Rydel JJ, Desnick RJ. Fabry disease: renal involvement limited to podocyte pathology and proteinuria in a septuagenarian cardiac variant. Pathologic and therapeutic implications. *Am J Kidney Dis* 2004;43:164–71.

65. Eng CM, Fletcher J, Wilcox WR, Waldek S, Scott CR, Sillence DO, Breunig F, Charrow J, Germain DP,

Nicholls K, Banikazemi M. Fabry disease: baseline medical characteristics of a cohort of 1765 males and females in the Fabry Registry. *J Inherit Metab Dis* 2007;30:184–92.

66. Glass RB, Astrin KH, Norton KI, Parsons R, Eng CM, Banikazemi M, Desnick RJ. Fabry disease. renal sonographic and magnetic resonance imaging findings in affected males and carrier females with the classic and cardiac variant phenotypes. *J Comput Assist Tomogr* 2004;28:158–68.

67. Okuda S. Renal involvement in Fabry's disease. *Intern Med* 2000;39:601–2.

68. Banks DE, Milutinovic J, Desnick RJ, Grabowski GA, Lapp NL, Boehlecke BA. Silicon nephropathy mimicking Fabry's disease. *Am J Nephrol* 1983;3:279–84.

69. Albay D, Adler SG, Philipose J, Calescibetta CC, Romansky SG, Cohen AH.Chloroquine-induced lipidosis mimicking Fabry disease. *Mod Pathol* 2005;18:733–8.

70. Breunig F, Weidemann F, Beer M, Eggert A, Krane V, Spindler M, Sandstede J, Strotmann J, Wanner C. Fabry disease: diagnosis and treatment. *Kidney Int Suppl* 2003:S181–5.

71. Alroy J, Sabnis S, Kopp JB. Renal pathology in Fabry disease. *J Am Soc Nephrol* 2002;13 Suppl. 2:S134–8.

72. Desnick RJ, Brady R, Barranger J, Collins AJ, Germain DP, Goldman M, Grabowski G, Packman S, Wilcox WR. Fabry disease, an under-recognized multisystemic disorder: expert recommendations for diagnosis, management, and enzyme replacement therapy. *Ann Intern Med* 2003;138: 338–46.

73. Thurberg BL, Rennke H, Colvin RB, Dikman S, Gordon RE, Collins AB, Desnick RJ, O'Callaghan M. Globotriaosylceramide accumulation in the Fabry kidney is cleared from multiple cell types after enzyme replacement therapy. *Kidney Int* 2002;62:1933–46.

74. Mehta A. Epidemiology and natural history of Gaucher's disease. *Eur J Intern Med* 2006; Suppl.17:S2–5.

75. Meikle PJ, Hopwood JJ, Clague AE, Carey WF. Prevalence of lysosomal storage disorders. *JAMA* 1999;281:249–54.

76. Becker-Cohen R, Elstein D, Abrahamov A, Algur N, Rudensky B, Hadas-Halpern I, Zimran A, Frishberg Y.A comprehensive assessment of renal function in patients with Gaucher disease. *Am J Kidney Dis* 2005;46:837–44.

77. Santoro D, Rosenbloom BE, Cohen AH. Gaucher disease with nephrotic syndrome: response to enzyme replacement therapy. *Am J Kidney Dis* 2002;40:E4.

78. Chander PN, Nurse HM, Pirani CL. Renal involvement in adult Gaucher's disease after splenectomy. *Arch Pathol Lab Med* 1979;103:440–5.

79. Morimura Y, Hojo H, Abe M, Wakasa H. Gaucher's disease, type I (adult type), with massive involvement of the kidneys and lungs. *Virchows Arch* 1994;425:537–40.

80. Reiner CB. The Schultz histochemical reaction for cholesterol; observations on specificity and sensitivity. *Lab Invest* 1953;2:140–51.

81. Rosenbloom BE, Weinreb NJ, Zimran A, Kacena KA, Charrow J, Ward E. Gaucher disease and cancer incidence: a study from the Gaucher Registry. *Blood* 2005;105:4569–72.

82. Ross L.Gaucher's cells in kidney glomeruli. *Arch Pathol* 1969;87:164–7.

83. Chou JY, Matern D, Mansfield BC, Chen YT. Type I glycogen storage diseases: disorders of the glucose-6-phosphatase complex. *Curr Mol Med* 2002;2:121–43.

84. Yokoyama K, Hayashi H, Hinoshita F, Yamada A, Suzuki Y, Ogura Y, Kanbayashi H, Endo Y, Kawai T, Hara M.Renal lesion of type Ia glycogen storage disease: the glomerular size and renal localization of apolipoprotein. *Nephron* 1995;70:348–52.

85. Verani R, Bernstein J: Renal glomerular and tubular abnormalities in glycogen storage disease type I. *Arch Pathol Lab Med* 1988;112:271–4.

86. Obara K, Saito T, Sato H, Ogawa M, Igarashi Y, Yoshinaga K. Renal histology in two adult patients with type I glycogen storage disease. *Clin Nephrol* 1993;39:59–64.

87. Rake JP, Visser G, Labrune P, Leonard JV, Ullrich K, Smit GP. Glycogen storage disease type I: diagnosis, management, clinical course and outcome. Results of the European Study on Glycogen Storage Disease Type I (ESGSD I). *Eur J Pediatr* 2002;161 Suppl. 1:S20–34.

88. Koeberl DD, Kishnani PS, Chen YT: Glycogen storage disease types I and II: treatment updates. *J Inherit Metab Dis* 2007;30:159–64.

89. Calabresi L, Pisciotta L, Costantin A, Frigerio I, Eberini I, Alessandrini P, Arca M, Bon GB, Boscutti G, Busnach G, Frasca G, Gesualdo L, Gigante M, Lupattelli G, Montali A, Pizzolitto S, Rabbone I, Rolleri M, Ruotolo G, Sampietro T, Sessa A, Vaudo G, Cantafora A, Veglia F, Calandra S, Bertolini S, Franceschini G. The molecular basis of lecithin-cholesterol acyltransferase deficiency syndromes: a comprehensive study of molecular and biochemical findings in 13 unrelated Italian families. *Arterioscler Thromb Vasc Biol* 2005;25:1972–78.

90. Finn LS, Bernstein J, "Renal disease caused by familial metabolic and hematologic diseases" in Jennette CJ, , Olson JL, , Schwartz MM, , Silva FG (eds.), *Heptinstall's Pathology of the Kidney*. (Philadelphia: Lippincott Williams & Wilkins, 2007).

91. Gjone E. Familial lecithin-cholesterol acyltransferase deficiency – a new metabolic disease with renal involvement. *Adv Nephrol Necker Hosp* 1981;10:167–85.

92. Magil A, Chase W, Frohlich J. Unusual renal biopsy findings in a patient with familial lecithin:-cholesterol acyltransferase deficiency. *Hum Pathol* 1982;13:283–5.

93. Lager DJ, Rosenberg BF, Shapiro H, Bernstein J. Lecithin-cholesterol acyltransferase deficiency: ultrastructural examination of sequential renal biopsies. *Mod Pathol* 1991;4: 331–5.

94. Zhu X, Herzenberg AM, Eskandarian M, Maguire GF, Scholey JW, Connelly PW, Ng DS. A novel in vivo lecithin-cholesterol acyltransferase (LCAT)-deficient mouse expressing predominantly LpX is associated with spontaneous glomerulopathy. *Am J Pathol* 2004;165:1269–78.

95. Vaziri ND. Dyslipidemia of chronic renal failure: the nature, mechanisms, and potential consequences. *Am J Physiol Renal Physiol* 2006;290:F262–72.

96. Panescu V, Grignon Y, Hestin D, Rostoker G, Frimat L, Renoult E, Gamberoni J, Grignon G, Kessler M. Recurrence

of lecithin-cholesterol acyltransferase deficiency after kidney transplantation. *Nephrol Dial Transplant* 1997;12:2430–2.

97. Ayyobi AF, McGladdery SH, Chan S, John Mancini GB, Hill JS, Frohlich JJ. Lecithin- cholesterol acyltransferase (LCAT) deficiency and risk of vascular disease: 25 year follow-up. *Atherosclerosis* 2004;177:361–6.

98. Chen HP, Liu ZH, Gong RJ, Tang Z, Zeng CH, Zhu MY, Wang JP, Zhou H, Li LS. Lipoprotein glomerulopathy: clinical features and pathological characteristics in Chinese. *Chin Med J (Engl)* 2004;117:1513–7.

99. Saito T, Sato H, Kudo K, Oikawa S, Shibata T, Hara Y, Yoshinaga K, Sakaguchi H. Lipoprotein glomerulopathy: glomerular lipoprotein thrombi in a patient with hyperlipoproteinemia. *Am J Kidney Dis* 1989;13:148–53.

100. Faraggiana T, Churg J. Renal lipidoses: a review. *Hum Pathol* 1987;18:661–79.

101. Watanabe Y, Ozaki I, Yoshida F, Fukatsu A, Itoh Y, Matsuo S, Sakamoto N. A case of nephrotic syndrome with glomerular lipoprotein deposition with capillary ballooning and mesangiolysis. *Nephron* 1989;51:265–70.

102. Foster K, Matsunaga A, Matalon R, Saito T, Gallo G, D'Agati V, Stokes MB. A rare cause of posttransplantation nephrotic syndrome. *Am J Kidney Dis* 2005;45:1132–8.

103. Ogawa T, Maruyama K, Hattori H, Arai H, Kondoh I, Egashira T, Watanabe T, Kobayashi Y, Morikawa A. A new variant of apolipoprotein E (apo E Maebashi) in lipoprotein glomerulopathy. *Pediatr Nephrol* 2000;14:149–51.

104. Oikawa S, Matsunaga A, Saito T, Sato H, Seki T, Hoshi K, Hayasaka K, Kotake H, Midorikawa H, Sekikawa A, Hara S, Abe K, Toyota T, Jingami H, Nakamura H, Sasaki J. Apolipoprotein E Sendai (arginine 145–>proline): a new variant associated with lipoprotein glomerulopathy. *J Am Soc Nephrol* 1997;8:820–3.

105. Ando M, Sasaki J, Hua H, Matsunaga A, Uchida K, Jou K, Oikawa S, Saito T, Nihei H. A novel 18-amino acid deletion in apolipoprotein E associated with lipoprotein glomerulopathy. *Kidney Int* 1999;56:1317–23.

106. Saito T, Oikawa S, Sato H, Sasaki J. Lipoprotein glomerulopathy: renal lipidosis induced by novel apolipoprotein E variants. *Nephron* 1999;83:193–201.

107. Ishigaki Y, Oikawa S, Suzuki T, Usui S, Magoori K, Kim DH, Suzuki H, Sasaki J, Sasano H, Okazaki M, Toyota T, Saito T, Yamamoto TT. Virus-mediated transduction of apolipoprotein E (ApoE)-sendai develops lipoprotein glomerulopathy in ApoE-deficient mice. *J Biol Chem* 2000;275: 31269–73.

108. Ieiri N, Hotta O, Taguma Y. Resolution of typical lipoprotein glomerulopathy by intensive lipid-lowering therapy. *Am J Kidney Dis* 2003;41:244–9.

109. Arai T, Yamashita S, Yamane M, Manabe N, Matsuzaki T, Kiriyama K, Kanayama Y, Himeno S, Matsuzawa Y. Disappearance of intraglomerular lipoprotein thrombi and marked improvement of nephrotic syndrome by bezafibrate treatment in a patient with lipoprotein glomerulopathy. *Atherosclerosis* 2003;:293–9.

110. Weiss M, Liapis H, Tomaszewski JE, Arend LJ, "Pyelonephritis and other infections, reflux nephropathy, hydronephrosis, and nephrolithiasis", in Jennette CJ, Olson JL, Schwartz MM, Silva FG (eds.), *Heptinstall's Pathology of the Kidney*. Philadelphia, PA: Lippincott Williams & Wilkins, 2007, pp. 991–1081.

111. Markowitz GS, Nasr SH, Klein P, Anderson H, Stack JI, Alterman L, Price B, Radhakrishnan J, D'Agati VD. Renal failure due to acute nephrocalcinosis following oral sodiumphosphate bowel cleansing. *Hum Pathol* 2004;35: 675–84.

112. Theodoropoulos DS, Shawker TH, Heinrichs C, Gahl WA. Medullary nephrocalcinosis in nephropathic cystinosis. *Pediatr Nephrol* 1995;9:412–18.

113. van Woerden CS, Groothoff JW, Wanders RJ, Davin JC, Wijburg FA. Primary hyperoxaluria type 1 in The Netherlands: prevalence and outcome. *Nephrol Dial Transplant* 2003;18:273–9.

114. Danpure CJ. Primary hyperoxaluria: from gene defects to designer drugs? *Nephrol Dial Transplant* 2005;20: 1525–9.

115. Milliner DS, Wilson DM, Smith LH. Clinical expression and long-term outcomes of primary hyperoxaluria types 1 and 2. *J Nephrol* 1998;11 Suppl. 1:56–9.

116. Hochberg J, Cairo MS. Tumor lysis syndrome: current perspective. *Haematologica* 2008;93:9–13.

117. Becker MA, Jolly M. Hyperuricemia and associated diseases. *Rheum Dis Clin North Am* 2006;32:275–93, v–vi.

118. Zaka R, Williams CJ. New developments in the epidemiology and genetics of gout. *Curr Rheumatol Rep* 2006;8: 215–23.

119. Pui CH, Mahmoud HH, Wiley JM, Woods GM, Leverger G, Camitta B, Hastings C, Blaney SM, Relling MV, Reaman GH. Recombinant urate oxidase for the prophylaxis or treatment of hyperuricemia in patients With leukemia or lymphoma. *J Clin Oncol* 2001;19:697–704.

120. Hummel M, Reiter S, Adam K, Hehlmann R, Buchheidt D. Effective treatment and prophylaxis of hyperuricemia and impaired renal function in tumor lysis syndrome with low doses of rasburicase. *Eur J Haematol* 2008;80: 331–6.

121. Brady RO, Grabowski G, Thadhani R. *Fabry disease: review and new perspectives. SynerMed Commun* 2001:1–8.

CHAPTER 9

Thrombotic Microangiopathies

Zoltan G. Laszik, MD

INTRODUCTION

The term thrombotic microangiopathy (TMA) is applied to a cluster of various diseases featuring microvascular lesions; both thrombotic and nonthrombotic, secondary to endothelial injury (Table 9.1). According to the extent and severity of ensuing structural-organ damage, patients with TMA may show a wide variety of clinical manifestations. Also, because TMA is often associated with specific underlying diseases or conditions, the clinical presentation may be complex or nonspecific and recognition of TMA may require a high degree of clinical suspicion. Thrombocytopenia and microangiopathic hemolytic anemia are the primary diagnostic criteria of TMA; without an apparent alternative explanation for thrombocytopenia and microangiopathic hemolytic anemia, the presence of these laboratory find-

ings is sufficient to establish the clinical diagnosis of TMA (Table 9.2) [1]. In general, there are two major clinical forms of TMA: hemolytic uremic syndrome (HUS) and thrombotic thrombocytopenic purpura (TTP). HUS is characterized by predominant renal manifestations (i.e., acute renal failure). Multiorgan involvement with less prominent renal disease is typical of TTP. However, overlap in the clinical presentation between HUS and TTP may occur and precise clinical distinction between these two entities may occasionally be difficult, if not impossible. Additional forms of TMA include transplant rejection with microvascular thrombotic complications, malignant hypertension, preeclampsia–eclampsia, postpartum renal failure, scleroderma renal crisis, antiphospholipid antibody syndrome, and radiation nephritis (posttransplantation TMA).

Table 9.1 Classification of Thrombotic Microangiopathy

Hemolytic Uremic Syndrome
Typical (diarrhea-positive [D+], classic, "epidemic")
Atypical (diarrhea-negative [D−])
    Infections (bacterial and viral)
    Pregnancy
    Malignancy
    SLE
    Antiphospholipid antibodies
    Drugs (mitomycin C, cyclosporine, FK506, etc.)
    Other

Thrombotic Thrombocytopenic Purpura

Systemic sclerosis

Preeclampsia-eclampsia

Post-transplantation

Malignant hypertension

Renal allograft rejection

Other

Table 9.2 Presenting Signs and Symptoms of Patients With Thrombotic Microangiopathy

Primary diagnostic criteria
Thrombocytopenia
Microangiopathic hemolytic anemia (defined by negative
    findings on direct antiglobulin test, red blood cell
    fragmentation, and evidence of accelerated red cell
    production and destruction)
No clinically apparent alternative explanation
    for thrombocytopenia and anemia

Other common clinical features
Renal function abnormalities (proteinuria/hematuria common,
    acute renal failure and oliguria less common)
Neurologic abnormalities (mental status changes common, focal
    abnormalities less common)
Weakness
Abdominal symptoms (nausea, vomiting, diarrhea, pain)
Fever (high fever with chills is evidence against the
    diagnosis of TMA)

Modified from George 2000 [24].

HUS, TTP, systemic sclerosis, antiphospholipid antibody syndrome, preeclampsia–eclampsia, and posttransplantation TMA will be discussed in this chapter. Malignant hypertension is discussed in Chapter 12, while transplant rejection-associated TMA is presented in Chapter 16.

EPIDEMIOLOGY AND CLINICAL PRESENTATION

Thrombotic microangiopathy denotes various diseases (Table 9.1) that share a number of clinical, laboratory, and morphologic characteristics. There are, however, also significant differences in the clinical and laboratory features, pathogenesis, and morphology that set these diseases apart. Therefore, the epidemiological data and clinical presentations for the major groups of TMA, as well as those additional forms, will be individually discussed in this section.

Typical HUS (Synonyms: Classic, Diarrhea Positive [D+], or Epidemic HUS)

The classic form represents approximately 90 percent of HUS cases. It occurs mainly in young children and develops either in isolated (sporadic) cases or as outbreaks mostly in the summer. Most cases are caused by Shiga toxin-producing *Escherichia coli* (STEC) infection; however, in Southeast Asia infection with *Shigella dysenteriae* serotype 1 is the most common etiology. Among various serogroups and serotypes of STEC, O157:H7 is most frequently associated with the disease. However, regional differences do exist and an emerging role of non-O157 STEC serogroups has been reported from some countries in Europe [2]. The number of outbreaks caused by STEC O157:H7 has been steadily increasing in the United States between 1992 and 2002 [3]. During this time, there were a total of 350 reported outbreaks with 8,598 patients affected of whom 354 developed HUS (4.1 percent) [3]. Most of these outbreaks have resulted from undercooked ground beef or dairy products including raw milk; however, many additional routes and sources of infection also occurred including person to person transmission, animal contact, infected municipal water, and consumption of infected products such as lettuce, apple cider, apple juice, coleslaw, melons, and grapes [3]. Outbreaks due to contaminated drinking water tended to be the largest. Some data seem to indicate that most cases of HUS caused by STEC O157:H7 may be endemic, not related to outbreaks [4].

Shiga toxin-producing *E. coli* infection is associated with a spectrum of illnesses including asymptomatic infection, uncomplicated diarrhea, hemorrhagic colitis, and HUS [5]. Patients with the classic form of HUS, caused by STEC O157:H7, present with watery diarrhea, abdominal pain, fever and vomiting about three days following ingestion of the organisms. The diarrhea may progress to bloody diarrhea with hemorrhagic colitis one to three days thereafter. The second phase starts approximately ten days postinfection with the onset of various combinations of acute renal failure, anemia, bleeding abnormalities, central nervous system disorders, and cardiovascular changes. In rare instances, there is no prodromal diarrhea prior to the onset of renal failure. Laboratory abnormalities indicate thrombin generation and inhibition of fibrinolysis during the early stages of the disease with elevated serum levels of plasminogen activator inhibitor-1 (PAI-1), prothrombin fragment 1+2, and D-dimers [6]. These features of altered coagulation precede the development of renal injury [6]. Thrombocytopenia and microangiopathic hemolytic anemia, absent at the time when bloody diarrhea first develops, appear within a few days. Neutrophilia may be present. Additional laboratory findings include elevated serum lactic dehydrogenase level and a concomitant reduction in the serum haptoglobin level. Slight prolongation in prothrombin time is common. Laboratory confirmation of STEC infection requires positive polymerase chain reaction for Shiga toxin genes in stools and/or circulating antilipopolysaccharide antibodies; however, these tests are negative in approximately 15 percent of patients with D+ HUS [7].

Most of the clinical and laboratory features of Shigella dysenteriae type 1 infection-associated HUS resemble HUS caused by STEC infection. The median age at presentation is approximately three years and the median time from the onset of diarrhea to the development of HUS is seven days [8]. Signs of disseminated intravascular coagulation, a very rare event in patients with STEC-induced HUS, are more common in patients with HUS caused by Shigella dysenteriae type 1 infection. Also, neutrophilia at onset is typically greater than in HUS caused by STEC infection [9].

Atypical (Diarrhea-Negative [D-]) HUS

Patients with the atypical form of HUS comprise approximately 10 percent of all HUS cases [10]. Both children and adults might be affected. Most of the cases are sporadic, however, familial [11,12] and relapsing forms [12] do exist. In a significant proportion of patients with D– HUS, there will be associated conditions or diseases that may act as triggers or may be the cause of HUS. Such conditions and diseases include pregnancy, exposure to various drugs, malignancy, systemic lupus erythematosus (SLE), fever, certain bacterial and viral infections, upper respiratory tract infection, and gastroenteritis [12,13] (Table 9.1). Various genetic and acquired abnormalities of the complement regulatory proteins, as well as defective cobalamin metabolism have been identified as causative factors in approximately half of the patients with atypical HUS [11,14,15] (see also etiology and pathogenesis). The clinical onset of D– HUS is usually insidious; acute renal failure with or without proteinuria, micro-, or macrohematuria, and hypertension develop rapidly. Microangiopathic hemolytic anemia is present in most of the cases and thrombocytopenia in some. Serum levels of C3 may be normal or slightly decreased [12]. Extrarenal involvement is rare and prodromal diarrhea is usually absent; however, gastroenteritis was observed in up to 28 percent of pediatric patients with D- HUS with various mutations of the complement regulatory proteins [12].

In approximately one-third of women with atypical HUS, the first presentation is during pregnancy or following delivery [16]. TMA is most frequent in the second and third trimesters of pregnancy and approximately one-half of the cases occur during the postpartum period [17]. The typical features of postpartum HUS are sudden deterioration of renal function in association with microangiopathic hemolytic anemia and thrombocytopenia, usually within days, but ≤3 months after normal pregnancy and delivery. Blood pressure is usually normal at the onset of HUS, but severe hypertension frequently develops as the disease progresses.

Among various drugs, exposure to quinine, mitomycin-C, the antiplatelet agents ticlopidine and clopidogrel, and calcineurin inhibitors are most commonly associated with TMA [18]. The clinical presentation is usually, but not always, that of atypical HUS. Drug-induced TMA is a heterogeneous disorder as indicated by the number of drugs implicated as triggers, and by differences in clinical presentation, prognosis, and pathogenesis. Additional drugs and substances that have been reported in association with TMA include antibiotics, H-2 receptor antagonists, hormones, interferons, nonsteroidal antiinflammatory drugs, vaccines, and various other chemotherapeutic agents such as bleomycin, cisplatin, daunorubicin, cytosine arabinoside, cyclophosphamide, doxorubicin, gemcitabine, and vincristine. A list of drugs, vaccines, and agents implicated in TMA is provided in Table 9.3.

Patients with quinine-associated TMA are usually older and predominantly white women. The disease usually has an

Table 9.3 Drugs and Other Exogenous Substances Reported to Be Associated With Thrombotic Microangiopathy

Antineoplastic drugs
Mitomycin C (Mutamycin®) [Bristol-Myers Squibb; Princeton, NJ]
Bevacizumab (Avastin®) [Genentech; San Francisco, CA]
5-Fluorouracil (Adrucil®) [Pharmacia; North Peapack, NJ]
Cytarabine (Cytosar U®) [Pharmacia; North Peapack, NJ]
Chlorozotocin (DCNU)
Cisplatin (Platinol®) [Bristol-Myers Squibb; Princeton, NJ]
Daunorubicin [Bedford Laboratories; Bedford, OH]
Deoxycoformycin (Nipent®) [Super Gen; Dublin, CA]
Gemcitabine (Gemzar®) [Eli Lilly; Indianapolis, IN]
Hydroxyurea (Hydrea®) [Bristol-Myers Squibb; Princeton, NJ]

Immunosuppressants
Cyclosporin (Neoral, Sandimmune®) [Novartis; East Hanover, NJ]
OKT3 (Orthoclone®) [Ortho Biotech Products; Raritan, NJ]
Tacrolimus (Prograf®) [Fujisawa; Osaka, Japan]

Antiplatelet drugs
Ticlopidine (Ticlid®) [Hoffmann-La Roche; Nutley, NJ]
Clopidogrel (Plavix®) [Sanofi-Synthelabo; New York, NY]
Defibrotide (Dasovas®, others) [Pharmacia Upjohn; Milan, Italy]
Dipyridamole (Persantine®) [Boehringer Ingelheim; Ingelheim, Germany]

Antibiotics
Ampicillin (Omnipen®, others) [Wyeth-Ayerst Pharmaceuticals; St. David's, PA]
Clarithromycin (Biaxin®) [Abbott Laboratories; Abbott Park, IL]
d-Penicillamine (Cuprimine®, Merck; Whitehouse Station, New Jersey, USA), (Depen®, Wallace Laboratories; Cranbury, NJ)
Metronidazole (Flagyl®) [Searle Pharmaceuticals; Skokie, IL]
Oxytetracycline (Terramycin®) [Pfizer; New York, NY]
Penicillin (Pen Vee K®, others) [Wyeth-Ayerst Pharmaceuticals; St. David's, PA]
Rifampicin (Rifadin®, Aventis Pharmaceuticals; Bridgewater, NJ), (Rimactane®, Novartis; East Hanover, NJ)
Sulfisoxazole (Gantrisin®) [Hoffmann-La Roche; Nutley, NJ]

H-2 receptor antagonists
Cimetidine (Tagamet®) [GlaxoSmithKline; Research Triangle Park, NC]
Famotidine (Pepcid®) [Merck; Whitehouse Station, NJ]

Hormones
17-B Estradiol patch (Climara®, others) [Berlex Laboratories; Wayne, NJ]
Conjugated estrogens (Premarin®) [Wyeth-Ayerst Pharmaceuticals; St. David's, PA]
Danazol (Danocrine®) [Sanofi-Synthelabo; New York, NY]
Ethinyl estradiol (Estinyl®, various combination products) [Shering-Plough; Kenilworth, NJ]
Ethynodiol acetate (Various combination products)
Levonorgesterol (Norplant®) [Wyeth-Ayerst Pharmaceuticals; St. David's, PA]
Norethisterone (Aygestin®, various combination products) [ESI Lederle; St. David's, PA]

Interferons
Alpha interferon (Roferon®) [Hoffmann-La Roche; Nutley, NJ]
Alpha 2b interferon (Intron®) [Shering-Plough; Kenilworth, NJ]
Beta interferon (1a or 1b not specified)

Nonsteroidal antiinflammatory drugs
Diclofenac (Cataflam®, Voltaren®) [Novartis; East Hanover, NJ]

Table 9.3. *(continued)*

Ketorolac (Toradol®) [Hoffmann-La Roche; Nutley, NJ]
Nimesulide (Algimesil®, others) [Francia; Milan, Italy]
Piroxicam (Feldene®) [Pfizer; New York, NY]

Vaccines
Hepatitis-B (Engerix-B®, GlaxoSmithKline; Research Triangle
    Park, NC), (Recombivax HB®, Merck; Whitehouse Station, NJ)
Influenza (Fluarix®) [SmithKline Beecham;
    Hertfordshire, United Kingdom]
MMR (MMR II®) [Merck; Whitehouse Station, NJ]
Triple-antigen/t.a.b. (diphtheria, tetanus, pertussis vaccine,
    various brands)

Miscellaneous
Quinine (Formula Q®, various products available with some
    quinine content) [Major Pharmaceutical; Livonia, MI]
Simvastatin (Zocor®) [Merck; Whitehouse Station, NJ]
Albendazole (Albenza®) [GlaxoSmithKline; Research
    Triangle Park, NC]
Carbon tetrachloride (used as a hand washing agent in
    reported case)
Cocaine (used illicitly)
Heroin (used illicitly)
Hair dyes (unspecified brands)
Methapyrilene and salicylamide (Nytol®) [Block Drugs;
    Jersey City, NJ]
Valacyclovir (Valtrex®) [GlaxoSmithKline; Research
    Triangle Park, NC]

Modified from Medina et al. 2001. [18]

explosive-onset with acute renal failure; relapses after quinine reexposure are often seen. HUS develops in <10 percent of patients treated with mitomycin-C, and the onset is usually insidious and within four to eight weeks of the last dose of chemotherapy. Typical clinical presentation includes microangiopathic hemolytic anemia, thrombocytopenia, and renal failure. The course is potentially progressive even after discontinuation of the drug. The estimated incidence of ticlopidine-associated TMA range from 1 in 1,600 to 1 in 5,000 treated patients [19]. Onset of ticlopidine-associated TMA is relatively sudden, one to sixteen weeks after starting therapy. The clinical presentation is characterized by neurologic abnormalities, renal insufficiency, anemia, and thrombocytopenia. Calcineurin inhibitor-associated TMA is discussed in Chapter 16.

Although malignancies are often included among the etiologic factors of atypical HUS, in most patients with malignancy-associated TMA renal failure is not a common feature. Mucin-producing metastatic adenocarcinomas of stomach, breast, and lung are the most common underlying causes [20]. The patients present with hemolytic anemia of abrupt-onset and the clinical picture may resemble HUS or TTP. However, coagulation studies frequently indicate disseminated intravascular coagulation (DIC) with decreased number of platelets, elevated fibrin degradation products or D-dimers, prolonged bleeding time, and decreased levels of fibrinogen. These laboratory findings are suggestive of a different pathogenetic mechanism from classic TMA.

Among viral infections associated with TMA, infection with HIV is most common. Still, HIV-associated TMA is a relatively rare disease with a reported incidence of 0.3 percent from a large cohort of patients in the United States during the HAART (highly active antiretroviral therapy) era [21]. The incidence has declined significantly since the advent of HAART in the late 1990s. The disease has been reported in patients with both full-blown AIDS and asymptomatic HIV infection. The clinical and laboratory features appear to be similar but not necessarily identical to those of idiopathic HUS and TTP. The onset is usually gradual.

Thrombotic Thrombocytopenic Purpura

TTP is a relatively rare disease with a reported standardized incidence rate of 3.8/million/year in the United States for the years 1990 to 2000 [22]. A similar standardized incidence rate was reported for idiopathic TTP/HUS (i.e., TMA not associated with bloody diarrhea, drugs, pregnancy, and hematopoietic stem cell transplantation) from the Oklahoma TTP/HUS Registry database [13]. Incidence rates of idiopathic TTP/HUS are greater for women and patients with African-American heritage [13]; the peak incidence is during the third decade of life [23]. The classic clinical presentation includes fever, microangiopathic hemolytic anemia, thrombocytopenia, neurologic involvement, and renal manifestations (Table 9.2) [1]. However, clinical presentation with only limited features is more typical and most patients are lacking one or more of the classic signs and symptoms [1]. Also, due to the urgency for treatment, only microangiopathic hemolytic anemia and thrombocytopenia, without an apparent alternative etiology, are required to establish the clinical diagnosis and initiate plasma exchange treatment [1, 24]. Because of the limited clinical features at presentation, recognition of the disease during the early stages may be difficult. Most of the clinical manifestations are the consequence of widespread microvascular thrombotic lesions causing structural and functional organ damage. Renal involvement in TTP is less common and usually less severe than in HUS [23] and severe renal injury is quite rare.

Systemic Sclerosis

Systemic sclerosis is a relatively rare systemic connective tissue disorder. The prevalence and incidence in adults varies greatly among different surveys (7/million to 489/million and 0.6/million/year to 122/million/year, respectively) [25]. The estimated number of patients affected in the United States is 49,000 [26]. The disease is significantly more common in women and African-Americans have a higher age-specific incidence rate and more severe disease than whites [25]. The diagnosis of systemic sclerosis requires the presence of three clinicopathologic features: tissue fibrosis, unique vasculopathy, and the evidence of a systemic autoantibody response. Skin fibrosis is highly characteristic of systemic sclerosis and distinction between the two main forms of the disease, that is, diffuse or limited cutaneous forms, is based on the extent of skin involvement [27]. The diffuse cutaneous form is characterized by symmetrical skin involvement affecting both the distal and proximal parts of the extremities, and often the trunk and face. In the limited cutaneous form, there is a more confined symmetrical involvement of the skin affecting the fingers, hands, and the face. Visceral manifestations, including severe renal disease, develop earlier and considerably more often in the diffuse form of the disease. A third form, termed limited (early) systemic sclerosis may also exist with only subtle features of the disease [28]. The term "scleroderma renal crisis" denotes the most severe form of renal involvement in systemic sclerosis. This occurs in up to one-fifth of patients with the diffuse cutaneous form of the disease and in approximately 2 to 6 percent of patients with the limited cutaneous form. The disorder is characterized by rapidly developing acute renal failure that is often, but not always, accompanied by severe ("malignant") hypertension. Typical clinical and laboratory manifestations also include decreased glomerular filtration rate, oliguria/anuria, retinopathy, new-onset microscopic hematuria, and microangiopathic hemolytic anemia [29]. Other patients with systemic sclerosis but without scleroderma renal crisis may have various combinations of proteinuria, azotemia, and modest degrees of hypertension. Laboratory findings include anemia, hypergammaglobulinemia, positive rheumatoid factor, and antinuclear, anti-topoisomerase I, anticentromere, and anti-RNA polymerase antibodies. In spite of their common occurrence in systemic sclerosis, there is no compelling evidence that the antibodies play a direct role in the pathogenesis.

Preeclampsia–Eclampsia

Preeclampsia is a disease of pregnancy with clinical manifestations of new-onset hypertension (>140/90 mmHg) and subsequent proteinuria (>0.3 g/24 hours or >30 mg/dL in two random specimens) usually presenting after the 20th week of gestation [30]. It is encountered in 5 to 7 percent of all pregnancies and thus represents one of the most common renal-glomerular diseases worldwide [31]. Proteinuria is usually mild, however, it may reach nephrotic range and slight hematuria may also be present. Additional features include edema affecting mostly hands and face, decreased glomerular filtration rate, and hyperuricemia. Mild thrombocytopenia is common; however, microangiopathic hemolytic anemia is a rare feature in preeclampsia [16]. Preeclampsia is considered severe when blood pressure is higher (160–180/110 mmHg) and other signs of systemic involvement, including microangiopathic hemolytic anemia and thrombocytopenia are also present [16]. The occurrence of seizures in woman with preeclampsia defines eclampsia.

Preeclampsia is associated with increased fetal and maternal morbidity and mortality [32]. Maternal complications include renal failure, HELLP syndrome (hemolysis, elevated liver enzymes, and low platelet count), liver failure, and seizures (eclampsia). Preeclampsia is also responsible for approximately 15 percent of preterm births [33]. Prominent glomerular endothelial swelling ("endotheliosis"), the most characteristic morphologic abnormality of preeclampsia, represents a special form of TMA [34]. Clinical differential diagnosis of preeclampsia includes various glomerular diseases, such as chronic glomerulonephritis, minimal change nephrotic syndrome, focal segmental glomerulosclerosis, membranous nephropathy, postinfectious glomerulonephritis, diabetic nephropathy, and sickle cell nephropathy. In severe cases with significant microangiopathic hemolytic anemia and thrombocytopenia, HUS and TTP should also be considered in the clinical differential diagnosis [16].

Transplantation

Thrombotic microangiopathy can occur in patients with solid organ and bone marrow transplantation either as a de novo or recurrent disease. The term "posttransplantation thrombotic microangiopathy" (PTMA) is usually applied to cases with bone marrow transplantation (BMT) (synonyms: radiation nephropathy after total body irradiation, BMT nephropathy, thrombotic thrombocytopenic purpura or hemolytic uremic syndrome following BMT) [35]. The reported incidence of PTMA varies significantly with an average incidence of 8.2 percent [36]. Various comorbidities common in BMT patients, such as opportunistic infections, drug toxicity, radiation-related injury, and acute graft versus host disease (GVHD) can mimic the laboratory and clinical features of TMA, and therefore, clinical recognition of PTMA may be difficult. The disease may present with rapid or gradual decline in renal function along with hemolytic anemia and thrombocytopenia. The clinical course may be mild in some patients, and severe in others. The onset is usually >3 months, with the peak incidence of nine to twelve months, after BMT.

The reported incidence of de novo TMA in patients with kidney transplants also varies considerably. According to data from the U.S. Renal Data System (USRDS), the incidence is relatively low (0.8 percent) [37]. However, data from single centers indicate much higher incidences (3–14 percent) [38, 39]. The most important risk factors for de novo TMA in transplant kidneys are calcineurin inhibitors [38, 39], especially when used in combination with anti-mTOR (mammalian target of rapamycin) drugs [40, 41]. Additional risk factors include cytomegalovirus infection [42], parvovirus B 19 infection [43], BK polyoma virus nephropathy [44], malignancy [45], and marginal kidneys (i.e., kidneys from expanded criteria donors according to the United Network for Organ Sharing definition or non-heart beating donors) [46]. Rarely, valcyclovir [47], clopidogrel [48], and antiphospholipid or anticardiolipin antibodies [49, 50] can be the underlying cause. Thrombotic microangiopathy can also be seen in patients following renal transplantation as a recurrent disease [51] and rarely in association with acute antibody-mediated rejection [52] (see also Chapter 16). The risk of recurrence for D+ HUS is close to zero [53, 54], consistent with the infectious etiology of the disease. Recurrence rate in patients with atypical HUS is high and varies according to the etiology of the disease; data from three retrospective cohorts revealed recurrence rate of 76, 20, and 88 percent, for patients with complement factor H (CFH), membrane cofactor protein (MCP), and complement factor I (CFI) mutations, respectively [51]. Patients without demonstrable mutations in these three regulatory proteins exhibited a recurrence rate of 30 percent [51]. Data for disease recurrence in transplants for patients with less common mutations affecting factor B and C3, as well as those with anti-CFH antibodies, are limited.

Antiphospholipid Antibody Syndrome

The diagnosis of antiphospholipid antibody syndrome (APS) requires the combination of at least one clinical and one laboratory criterion such as vascular thrombosis or pregnancy morbidity and the presence of lupus anticoagulant, anticardiolipin, or anti-$\beta2$ glycoprotein-I antibody [55] (Table 9.4). The thrombotic complications of APS typically affect medium-sized and large arteries and veins, however, microvascular thromboses can also occur. The most common sites of large vessel thromboses are cerebral arteries and the deep veins of the legs. Typical

Table 9.4 Revised Classification Criteria for the Antiphospholipid Syndrome

Clinical criteria

Vascular thrombosis: One or more clinical episodes of arterial, venous, or small vessel thrombosis, in any tissue or organ.

Pregnancy morbidity

(a) One or more unexplained deaths of a morphologically normal fetus at or beyond the 10th week of gestation, with normal fetal morphology, or

(b) One or more premature births of a morphologically normal neonate before the 34th week of gestation because of eclampsia or severe preeclampsia, or recognized features of placental insufficiency, or

(c) Three or more unexplained consecutive spontaneous abortions before the 10th week of gestation, with maternal anatomic or hormonal abnormalities and paternal and maternal chromosomal causes excluded.

Laboratory criteria

Lupus anticoagulant (LA) present in plasma, on two or more occasions at least 12 weeks apart.

Anticardiolipin (aCL) antibody of IgG and/or IgM isotype in serum or plasma, present in medium or high titer (i.e. >40 GPL or MPL, or >the 99th percentile), on two or more occasions, at least 12 weeks apart.

Anti-b2 glycoprotein-I antibody of IgG and/or IgM isotype in serum or plasma (in titer >the 99th percentile), present on two or more occasions, at least 12 weeks apart.

Modified from Miyakis et al. [55].

clinical manifestations include cerebral infarctions, multiinfarct dementia, stroke, epilepsy, gangrene of the extremities, abdominal pain or intestinal infarction, pulmonary thromboembolism, Budd-Chiari syndrome, and livedo reticularis.

In addition to classic (primary) APS, microvascular thromboses can also be seen in association with antiphospholipid antibodies (aPL) (lupus anticoagulants and anticardiolipin antibodies) in a number of conditions, such as catastrophic APS, systemic lupus erythematosus (SLE), other rheumatic or autoimmune syndromes, HELLP syndrome, vasculitis, HIV infection, malignancy, drugs, trauma, and disseminated intravascular coagulation (DIC) [55–57]. Most patients with aPL-associated microthrombotic lesions suffer from primary APS or SLE ("secondary" APS) [58]. However, microvascular thromboses usually do not dominate the clinical picture in primary APS, and microangiopathic hemolytic anemia and thrombocytopenia, the classic laboratory features of TMA, are detected only in some of these cases. Furthermore, microvascular thrombotic complications are seen only in a small minority of patients with aPL-positivity. Therefore, the precise role of aPL in the development of microvascular thrombotic lesions is somewhat uncertain.

Characteristic small vessel lesions of primary APS in the kidney include intimal hyperplasia and recanalizing thrombi of the interlobular arteries and arterioles [59]. The term antiphospholipid syndrome nephropathy (APSN) refers to vasoocclusive lesions of the intrarenal vessels featuring acute thromboses and chronic arterial and arteriolar lesions in patients with primary or secondary APS [59, 60]. Antiphospho-

lipid syndrome nephropathy was reported in approximately one-third of patients with SLE [60]. In this study, APSN was statistically associated with lupus anticoagulant but not with anticardiolipin antibodies. In addition, APSN was shown to be an independent risk factor for more severely altered renal function and more severe interstitial fibrosis.

The term microangiopathic antiphospholipid-associated syndrome (MAPS) has been recently proposed for patients who have TMA with microangiopathic hemolytic anemia and often with thrombocytopenia in association with aPL-positivity but without large vessel thromboses [57]. These patients may have TTP, HELLP syndrome, or any form of TMA, with aPL-positivity being the distinguishing feature from "mainstream" TMA. In contrast, in patients with classic APS and coexistent small vessel thrombotic lesions but without microangiopathic hemolytic anemia, thrombocytopenia, or clinical presentation dominated by microvascular lesions, the term "microvascular manifestations of APS" is recommended [57].

Renal manifestations vary according to the type and extent of renal vascular involvement (i.e., capillary, arteriolar, arterial, or venous) and the presence or absence of associated diseases such as SLE. Arterial thrombotic obstruction may lead to parenchymal infarction, either focal or diffuse. In patients with APSN, hypertension is common and is likely related to vascular involvement. Renal insufficiency and subnephrotic range proteinuria are typical clinical–laboratory manifestations and hematuria is present in approximately half of the patients. Nephrotic syndrome is usually seen in those who have TMA with concurrent lupus nephritis.

APPROACH TO INTERPRETATION

Regardless of the clinical subgroup of TMA, the renal histologic findings are similar, although not necessarily identical in individual cases. The morphologic changes may vary according to the severity and the duration of the disease. The findings typical for all forms of TMA will be considered together in this chapter. Morphologic changes that are more characteristic or more prominent in certain forms of the disease will be emphasized. It should also be noted that distinction between various forms of TMA with different etiologies requires correlation of the morphologic changes with the clinical-laboratory and molecular genetic findings.

Gross Pathology

The size of the kidneys in TMA varies according to the severity and the stage of the disease and the presence or absence of preexisting renal diseases. The kidneys may be of normal size, enlarged, or contracted. Areas of necrosis, either patchy or large, are often present in patients who died during the acute stages of HUS or scleroderma renal crisis. Petechial hemorrhages are frequent findings in large swollen kidneys with mottled-yellowish appearance of the cortex during the acute stages in patients with severe disease. In patients with TTP, petechial hemorrhages involving both the renal parenchyma and the renal pelvis are the most typical gross findings. Nephrectomy specimens from patients who developed uncontrollable hypertension may show significant reduction in size, corresponding to chronicity with interstitial fibrosis. The subcapsular surface is usually smooth; however, fine granularity may also be present especially in older patients with arterial and arteriolar nephrosclerosis due to preexisting hypertension. In patients with pre-eclampsia–eclampsia, autopsy findings indicate no distinctive gross findings [61].

Light Microscopy

All four renal compartments can be affected. The characteristic light microscopic findings are listed in Table 9.5. The spectrum of the changes varies from subtle and focal affecting only a few glomeruli or a few glomerular capillary loops, to severe and widespread with concurrent glomerular, tubulointerstitial, and vascular involvement. Acute and chronic changes can also be present simultaneously. Multiple factors, such as the severity and the duration of the disease and the presence or absence of arterial changes, will alter the glomerular morphology. The early glomerular changes may involve the capillary walls, capillary lumina, and also the mesangium. Thickening of the capillary walls due to endothelial and subendothelial swelling represent early changes often accompanied by significant luminal narrowing. If severe, this may occlude the capillary lumina, often referred to as "acellular closure" with "bloodless" appearance of the glomeruli (Figure 9.1). Prominent swelling of the endothelial cells, coined by Spargo [34] as "endotheliosis," is

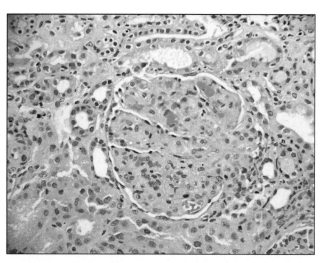

FIGURE 9.1: *Diarrhea-positive HUS in a 55-year-old patient. Most of the glomerular capillary lumina are closed ("acellular" closure) by thickened capillary walls and swollen endothelial cells. (Hematoxylin and eosin, ×400).*

particularly characteristic of preeclampsia–eclampsia. As a result, the glomeruli in preeclampsia–eclampsia are usually "bloodless" and enlarged. However, glomerulomegaly is typically not a feature in other forms of TMA. Additional changes in the glomerular capillary lumina may include the presence of fragmented red blood cells, fibrin, and platelet thrombi (Figures 9.2–9.8). Glomerular capillary thrombi, sparse or widespread, may be the only glomerular morphologic abnormality of TMA. This pattern of limited glomerular injury without significant arterial changes is often seen in patients with TTP. In contrast, glomerular capillary thrombi are virtually never seen in patients with preeclampsia–eclampsia. Sometimes, there will be glomeruli with dilated (ectatic) capillary loops filled with red blood cells, especially in cases with severe vascular involvement (Figure 9.9). Glomerular intracapillary accumulation of polymorphonuclear leukocytes can be seen in some cases, mostly in patients with D+ HUS [62].

As the disease progresses, some of the glomerular capillary walls may show reduplication (double contour appearance) of the basement membranes best seen with Jones methenamine-silver or periodic acid–Schiff (PAS) stains (Figures 9.2 and 9.5). Reduplication of the basement membranes is usually focal; however, it can also be widespread, especially in advanced disease (see below). Early mesangial changes, if present, reveal fibrillary appearance with or without fibrillar fibrin and fragmented red blood cells (Figure 9.2). Mesangial cells can often be swollen and hypertrophic. If mesangial cell proliferation occurs, it is usually slight (Figure 9.2). Mesangiolysis can also be seen, especially in some of the atypical forms of HUS following bone marrow transplantation or mitomycin therapy. However, in classic D+ HUS and TTP, mesangiolysis is a rare finding. The morphologic hallmark of well-established mesangiolysis is the presence of markedly dilated sometimes microcystic capillaries due to dissolution of the underlying mesangial matrix and cells and loss of mesangial anchoring of the capillary. However, during the early stages without dilated capillaries, mesangiolysis can be difficult to recognize. Mesangial edema and the

Table 9.5 Light Microscopic Features of Thrombotic Microangiopathy

Acute stage
Glomerular capillaries
  Luminal thrombi with or without fragmented RBCs
  Thickening of the walls (endothelial swelling;
    subendothelial widening)
  Narrowing/occlusion of the lumina ("acellular" closure)
  Reduplication of the GBMs
Glomerular mesangium
  Fibrillary appearance
  Mesangiolysis
  Fibrin deposition and fragmented RBCs
  Slight mesangial hypercellularity
Arteries and arterioles
  Endothelial swelling
  Subendothelial fibrin deposition
  Luminal thrombi
  Fibrinoid necrosis
  Edematous intimal thickening ("mucoid" intimal hyperplasia)
  Luminal narrowing/occlusion
  Myointimal cellular proliferation
  Organization and recanalization of luminal thrombi
  Intimal fibrosis
Chronic stage
Reduplication of the GBMs
Glomerulosclerosis
Organization and recanalization of luminal thrombi
Arterial intimal fibrosis
Interstitial fibrosis

Abbreviations: RBCs, red blood cells; GBM, glomerular basement membrane.

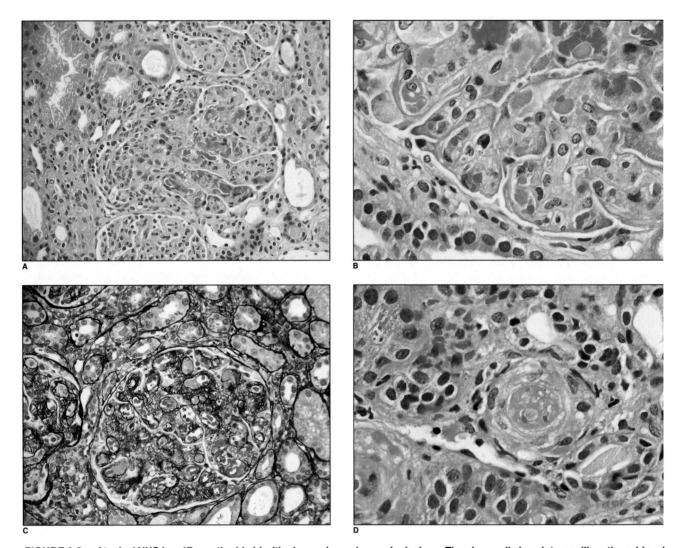

FIGURE 9.2: *Atypical HUS in a 17-month-old girl with glomerular and vascular lesions. The glomeruli show intracapillary thrombi and capillary congestion (A, B), reduplication of the basement membranes (C), mesangial fibrin deposits, mesangiolysis, and fibrillary appearance of the mesangium (B, C), and slight mesangial hypercellularity (A). (A: Hematoxylin and eosin, ×400. B: Hematoxylin and eosin, ×1,000. C: Jones' methenamine silver. ×400). D: A small artery is shown with thrombotic occlusion. (Hematoxylin and eosin, ×1,000).*

hazy appearance of the mesangium without well-delineated matrix are helpful signs to establish the diagnosis. During the healing stages of mesangiolysis, proliferating or sclerosing glomerular changes can develop and late stages are characterized by "bland" glomerular sclerosis with at least partial preservation of the lobular architecture. Ischemic glomerular changes during the acute stage of the disease may indicate severe vascular involvement by TMA or coexistent chronic hypertensive vascular disease. Focal necrotizing glomerular lesions are common in patients with malignant hypertension-associated TMA, but they are rarely seen in other forms of TMA. When present, the necrotizing glomerular lesions are usually small and may be associated with arteriolar thrombosis and/or fibrinoid necrosis of the arteriolar wall.

Chronic glomerular changes may develop as the disease progresses. This stage is characterized by mesangial matrix accumulation, thickening of the capillary walls with occasional double contours, segmentally sclerotic lesions, and chronic ischemic glomerular injury. Double contours result from mesangial cell interposition (i.e., mesangial cells interposed between the glomerular capillary endothelium and the lamina densa), and production of glomerular basement membrane-like material by glomerular capillary endothelial and interposed mesangial cells internal to the original basement membrane. Double contours with the mesangial sclerosis and occasional mild hypercellularity may mimic membranoproliferative glomerular injury. If the glomerular changes during the acute stage of the disease were relatively mild, such as capillary thrombi without significant capillary wall, mesangial and vascular changes, recovery may occur without any apparent residual chronic glomerular injury. Chronic ischemic-type glomerular changes are the result of long-standing or severe ischemia and can be seen during the late stages of TMA (Figures 9.3 and 9.9). These changes are similar to those seen in any other chronic

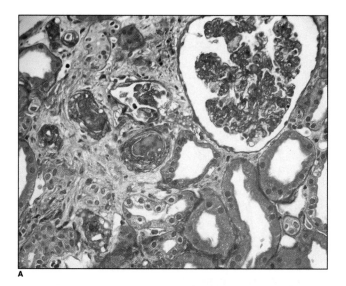
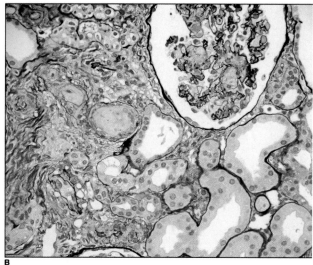

A   B

FIGURE 9.3: *Thrombotic microangiopathy with arteriolar thrombotic occlusion in a young child with atypical HUS. Note the presence of glomerular ischemia with thickening and wrinkling of the glomerular capillary basement membranes and simplification of the glomerular capillary tuft. (A: Masson's trichrome. ×400. B: Jones' methenamine silver. ×400).*

ischemic glomerular injury with thickening and wrinkling of the glomerular capillary basement membranes, simplification of the glomerular capillary tuft, and accumulation of PAS-negative collagen material internal to Bowman's capsule. The chronic ischemic changes may progress to complete glomerular ischemic obsolescence.

Thrombotic microangiopathy may also develop superimposed on other glomerular diseases, such as seen in patients with lupus nephritis, focal segmental glomerulosclerosis, IgA nephropathy, or in rare instances of crescentic glomerulonephritis or membranous nephropathy [63–67]. The morphologic findings in these cases will be the combination of underlying glomerular disease with features of TMA.

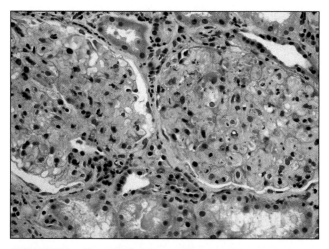

FIGURE 9.4: *Thrombotic microangiopathy with rare glomerular capillary thrombi and fragmented intraluminal red blood cells. The patient was a 70-year-old male with thrombotic thrombocytopenic purpura-like clinical presentation. ADAMTS 13 activity was normal. (Hematoxylin and eosin, ×400).*

Arteriolar involvement during early stages of TMA is characterized by swelling of the endothelial cells and subendothelial space often accompanied by severe luminal narrowing. Additional changes include fibrinoid necrosis and entrapment of red blood cells or fragmented red blood cells in the vessel wall (Figure 9.10). The lesion of fibrinoid necrosis results from non-specific trapping of plasma proteins and fibrin in the arteriolar wall secondary to increased vascular permeability. However, there is little evidence indicating that the lesion is associated with cellular necrosis. Typically, fibrinoid necrosis develops at the hilar region of the glomerulus and may affect the thickened intima or the entire thickness of the vessel wall. Sometimes, fibrin can only be seen underneath the intact-appearing or swollen endothelium. Often, there will be fibrin thrombi in the lumina in continuity with fibrinoid necrosis. In contrast to leukocytoclastic vasculitis, there is usually no inflammatory cellular infiltrates in association with fibrinoid necrosis in the setting of TMA. If healing takes place, hyalinization of the vessel wall may develop at the site of fibrinoid necrosis. Sometimes, arterioles with thrombotic occlusion reveal prominent dilatation. The organization and recanalization of the thrombotic lesions may show prominent cellular proliferation, somewhat reminiscent of small glomeruli, hence called "glomeruloid" structures. While this change is seldom seen in HUS, it is not uncommon in patients with TTP. Changes in the interlobular arteries are similar to those seen in the arterioles, although some differences do exist. In the larger vessels, edematous intimal thickening ("mucoid intimal hyperplasia") may become more prominent than in the smaller caliber arterioles (Figure 9.11). If severe, this change may lead to luminal occlusion. Fibrinoid necrosis, suffusion of the swollen edematous intima by red blood cells, and rare thrombotic lesions can also be seen during the early stages of the disease in patients with severe vascular involvement (Figures 9.12–9.18). In patients with Shigella dysenteriae infection, glomerular capillary thrombosis can be extensive and renal arterial thrombosis is often present [68].

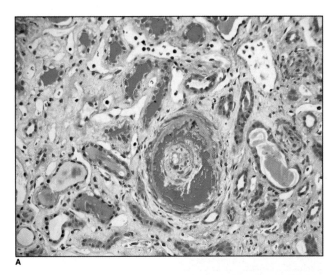

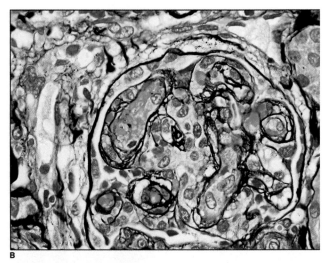

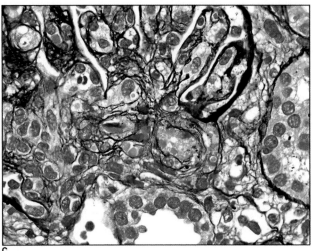

FIGURE 9.5: *Thrombotic microangiopathy in a 37-year-old African-American female who presented with a serum creatinine of 9.4 mg/dL, low platelet count, highly elevated LDH, and 4+ proteinuria. She also had new-onset joint pain but no significant prior medical history. She had no improvement in serum creatinine or platelet status after repeated plasma exchange treatments. ADAMTS-13 activity was below 5% of normal; all additional serologies were negative. A: Fibrinoid necrosis of a small artery. Note the red blood cells in the tubular lumina and the edematous widening of the interstitium. (Masson's trichrome, × 400). B: Glomerular capillary thrombosis and prominent new basement membrane formation ("reduplication" of the basement membrane). (Jones methenamine silver, × 1,000). C: The lumen of the arteriole is occluded by pale staining material admixed with fibrin and red blood cells. Similar material permeates the vessel wall. (Jones methenamine silver, × 1,000).*

During the healing stage, the edematous intima becomes cellular due to proliferating myointimal cells. With intimal deposition of delicate connective tissue fibrils, often in a concentric ring-like pattern (i.e., "onion-skinning"), severe arterial luminal narrowing or occlusion may develop. These changes will result in chronic ischemic damage affecting the glomeruli and the tubulointerstitium (Figures 9.19 and 9.20). Although interlobular arterial involvement is more common, arcuate and interlobar arteries can also be affected.

Among the various subtypes of TMA, arterial and arteriolar changes are more common and more severe in patients who have atypical HUS or scleroderma renal crisis [69, 70]. In contrast, patients with preeclampsia–eclampsia reveal only glomerular changes and vascular lesions are usually absent.

If there is a preexistent disease with vascular involvement, such as chronic hypertension, the acute vascular lesions of TMA may be seen side by side with arterial intimal fibroplasia, medial hypertrophy, and/or arterial/arteriolar hyalinosis. Patients with APSN often show acute lesions of TMA side by side with chronic vascular lesions [59, 60].

Acute tubular epithelial injury and acute tubular necrosis are common findings especially in patients with vascular involvement. Interstitial edema and mild mononuclear cell infiltrates may be present (Figure 9.9). Small patchy infarcts or larger necrotic areas can also be seen. The tubules may contain hyalin casts and red blood cells. Tubular atrophy and interstitial fibrosis may develop in the more advanced stages of the disease. Calcifications in the cortex may be the late sequel of cortical necrosis.

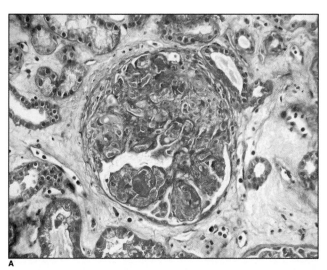
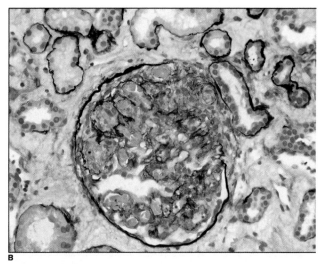

FIGURE 9.6: *Thrombotic microangiopathy with numerous glomerular intracapillary thrombi in a patient with recurrent mesangial lupus nephritis 2 years post-transplantation. The patient was on cyclosporine, mycofenolate mofetil, and prednisone at the time of the biopsy and had no prior history of TMA. Antiphospholipid antibodies were negative and microangiopathic hemolytic anemia was present without significant thrombocytopenia. No features of acute cellular or antibody-mediated rejection were seen. The thrombotic lesions resolved following cyclosporine withdrawal and plasma exchange therapy. (A: Masson's trichrome, × 400. B: Jones methenamine silver, × 400).*

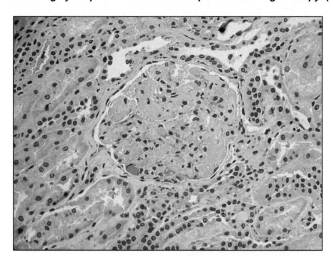

FIGURE 9.7: *Glomerular thrombotic microangiopathy in a transplant patient with C4d-positive acute antibody-mediated rejection. The glomerular capillary lumina are occluded by eosinophilic intracapillary thrombi. (Hematoxylin and eosin, × 400).*

Sometimes, the kidneys may lack distinctive pathologic features, especially in the advanced (chronic) stages of the disease. This is often seen in patients with history of longstanding systemic sclerosis and also in those patients who survived scleroderma renal crisis or malignant hypertension. Severe narrowing of the interlobular and arcuate arteries with intimal fibrosis and concentric reduplication of the elastic internal lamina may be present. The lesion is often referred to as "onionskin lesion," however, the same term is also applied for the earlier stages of arterial changes in TMA characterized by concentric intimal proliferation of myointimal cells embedded in loose mucoid material [71]. Some of these chronic vascular changes may probably develop without history of scleroderma renal crisis [72]. Nonspecific interstitial fibrosis or tubular atrophy may

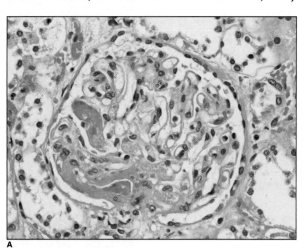
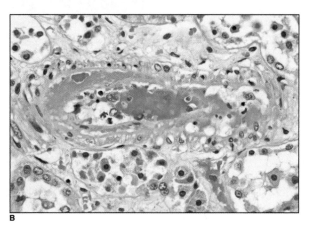

FIGURE 9.8: *Thrombotic microangiopathy following hematopoietic stem cell transplantation in an autopsy kidney. A: Glomerular TMA with intracapillary thrombi and mesangial fibrin deposits. (Hematoxylin and eosin. × 400). B: Fibrinoid necrosis of an arterial wall. There are no inflammatory cells in the vessel wall. (Hematoxylin and eosin. × 400).*

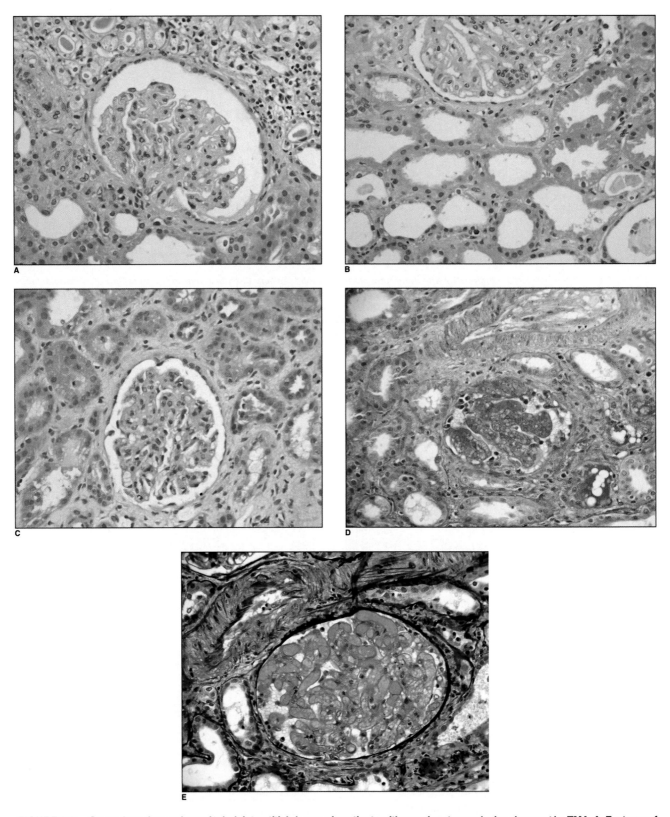

FIGURE 9.9: Secondary glomerular and tubulointerstitial changes in patients with prominent vascular involvement by TMA. A: Features of glomerular ischemia are seen with simplification and shrinkage of the glomerular capillary tufts. (Hematoxylin and eosin, × 400). B: Acute tubular epithelial injury with flattening of the tubular epithelial cells and dilatation of the tubular lumina. (Hematoxylin and eosin, × 400). C: Interstitial edema without glomerular changes. (Hematoxylin and eosin, × 400). D: Glomerular "paralysis" with dilatation of the glomerular capillary lumina filled with red blood cells. (Trichrome. × 400). E: Severe glomerular "paralysis" with capillary congestion. This lesion may progress into frank glomerular infarction. (Jones' methenamine silver. × 400). The secondary glomerular changes are usually focal; however, if the disease is severe, the glomerular and tubulointerstitial changes can progress into patchy or extensive cortical necrosis.

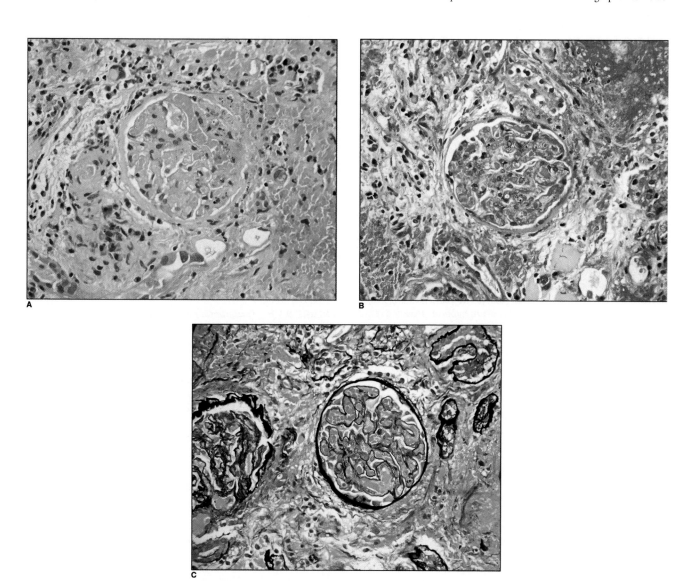

FIGURE 9.10: *Thrombotic microangiopathy with severe glomerular, vascular, and tubulointerstitial involvement in a transplant kidney with recurrent lupus membranous nephropathy. No features of acute cellular or antibody-mediated rejection were seen. Shown are glomerular capillary thrombi (A, B & C), arteriolar fibrinoid necrosis (A), mesangiolysis (C), and interstitial hemorrhage (B & C). (A: Hematoxylin and eosin, × 400. B: Masson's trichrome, × 400. C: Jones methenamine silver, × 400).*

also be present. Morphologic changes that are typical of specific subtypes of TMA are summarized in Table 9.6.

Immunofluorescence Microscopy

The immunofluorescence findings are not specific for any particular subtype of TMA. Fibrinogen positivity can be seen frequently during the acute stages of the disease in the glomeruli along the capillary walls, in the mesangial areas, and also within intracapillary thrombi [70, 71] (Figure 9.21). In TTP, the thrombi are considered to be platelet-rich and may show less prominent fibrinogen positivity [71]. The glomerular capillary walls can also exhibit granular IgM, C3, IgG, and rarely IgA staining [73-75]. Fibrinogen positivity is common in the wall of the arterioles and small arteries, often in a subendothelial position [70, 73, 74]. Vascular walls may also show IgM, C3, C1q, IgG, and IgA staining [70, 73, 74]. Fibrinogen is typically positive in the intravascular thrombi. In patients with pre-eclampsia–eclampsia, the characteristic findings include IgM and fibrinogen staining in the glomerular mesangial areas, capillary walls, and arterioles. The intensity of the fibrinogen staining seems to correlate with disease activity as fibrinogen positivity disappears within a few months postpartum [76].

Electron Microscopy

The ultrastructural findings are very similar in patients with TMA regardless of the etiology of the disease. However, the changes do vary according to the severity and the stage of the disease. Also, in patients who have immune complex-mediated glomerulonephritis, nephrosclerosis, or other renal disease in addition to TMA, the ultrastructural findings will show a combination of various features. A list of the common electron microscopic findings is provided in Table 9.7.

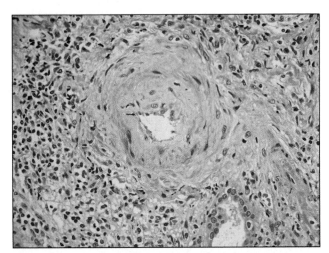

FIGURE 9.11: Edematous intimal thickening with luminal narrowing of a small interlobular artery. The patient had class IV lupus nephritis and presented with severe hypertension and renal failure. Edematous intimal thickening ("mucoid intimal hyperplasia") is a characteristic vascular change of acute TMA. (A: Hematoxylin and eosin, ×400).

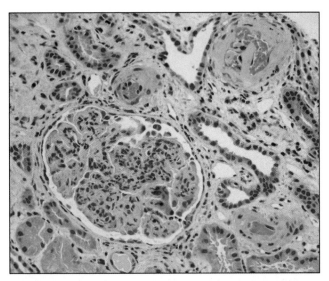

FIGURE 9.13: Thrombotic microangiopathy with vascular involvement in a patient with diffuse proliferative lupus nephritis in a 35-year-old female. One small artery shows fibrinoid necrosis of the vessel wall with re-canalization of the lumen. Endocapillary hypercellularity of the glomerulus with closure of the capillary lumina is present, however, no features of glomerular TMA are seen. The patient was negative for antiphospholipid antibodies. (Hematoxylin and eosin, ×400).

One of the most characteristic ultrastructural findings of TMA is focal or widespread thickening of the glomerular capillary walls. The thickening is due to widening of the subendothelial space, swelling of the endothelial cells, and occasional mesangial cell interposition (Figures 9.21–9.23). These changes seem to correlate with the severity and the stage of the disease. The widened subendothelial space in the lamina rara interna is pale and rarified with irregular collections of slightly electron-dense material usually without apparent fibrin. This material likely represents breakdown products of coagulation and cell debris. Features of endothelial cell activation and damage, most typical during the acute stages of the disease, include swelling

with loss of fenestration [75], localized areas of detachment from the basement membrane [77], and cytolysis [78]. Swelling of the endothelial cells, and to a lesser extent mesangial cells, is the most characteristic feature of preeclampsia–eclampsia (Figure 9.24) [34]. Intracapillary thrombi contain amorphous osmiophilic material admixed with fibrin, platelets, deformed red blood cells, and inflammatory cells (Figures 9.25 and 9.26). Platelets and remnants of platelets can be seen in the capillary lumina, between the endothelial cells, or within the glomerular

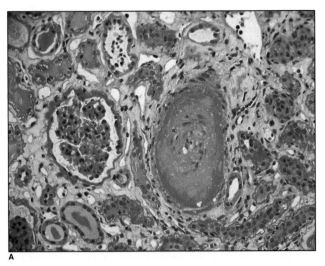

A

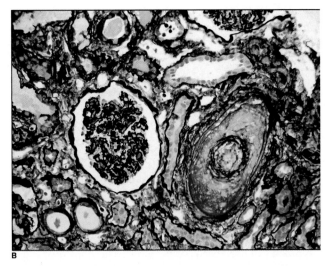

B

FIGURE 9.12: Thrombotic microangiopathy with small arterial involvement. The thickened vascular wall of a small artery with occluded lumen exhibits uneven pale staining on both the periodic acid-Schiff (A) and Jones methenamine silver (B)-stained sections. These staining characteristics correspond to fibrinoid necrosis with early organization in the vessel wall. Note prominent thickening and wrinkling of the glomerular capillary basement membranes and simplification of the glomerular capillary tufts typical of ischemia. Severe vascular involvement in TMA portends a poor renal prognosis. (×200).

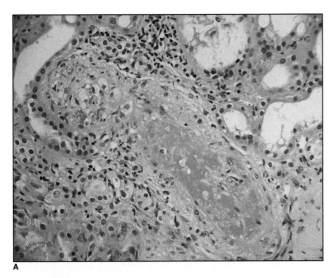
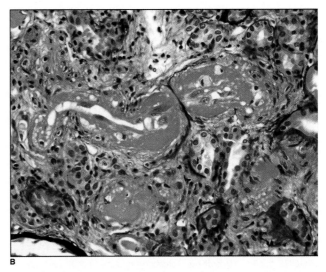

FIGURE 9.14: *Thrombotic microangiopathy in a young immunocompromised patient who presented with changes in mental status, fever, hemolysis, and acute renal failure. The patient did not respond to therapy and expired within 5 days of clinical presentation. Most of the arterioles and small interlobular arteries showed changes of acute TMA. A: Arteriolar thrombotic occlusion. (Hematoxylin and eosin, × 400). B: Fibrin is accumulated under the swollen endothelium in the arteriolar wall. (Hematoxylin and eosin, × 400).*

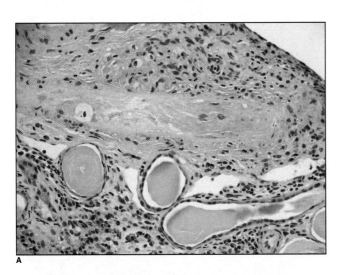
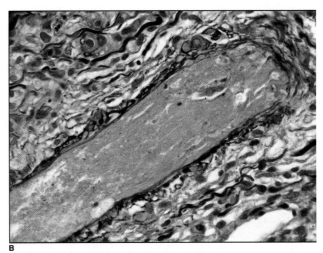

FIGURE 9.15: *Thrombotic occlusion of an interlobular artery in a 26-year-old patient with catastrophic antiphospholipid antibody syndrome. (A: Hematoxylin and eosin, × 400. B: Jones methenamine silver. × 1,000). A few endothelial cells and fragmented red blood cells are entrapped within the thrombus.*

capillary basement membrane. The mesangial matrix can also be swollen containing electron-dense, finely granular or fibrillar material similar to that seen in the widened subendothelial space [77]. Mesangiolysis and effacement of the foot processes of the visceral epithelial cells may be present.

In later stages, nonspecific wrinkling and thickening of the basement membranes may develop along with deposition of multiple basement membrane like layers in the capillary wall [74] with or without cellular (mesangial) interposition (Figure 9.27).

The endothelial cells of the arteries and arterioles show similar changes to those seen in the glomeruli. The thickened intima may have lucent appearance containing dense granules and fibrin (Figure 9.28). Luminal thrombi consist of platelets,

fibrin, and electron-dense granular material. In later stages, the thickened intima reveals myointimal cells and accumulated extracellular matrix.

DIFFERENTIAL DIAGNOSIS

The differential diagnosis of TMA includes both glomerular and vascular diseases. During the acute stages of TMA in patients with severe and extensive glomerular and vascular involvement, the light microscopic changes are highly characteristic and differentiation from other glomerular or vascular diseases is usually straightforward. The findings of acellular closure of the glomerular capillary lumina with thickened capillary walls, with or without capillary thrombotic lesions, in

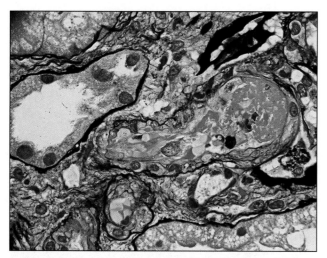

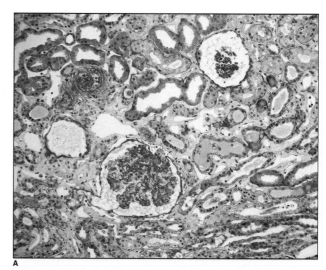

FIGURE 9.16: Thrombotic microangiopathy in a 57-year-old female following quinine ingestion. A large thrombus occludes the interlobular artery. Fibrin is also seen focally in the arterial wall. The patient did not recover renal function in spite of treatment with plasma exchange. (Jones methenamine silver. ×1,000).

combination with vascular changes such as mucoid intimal hyperplasia, intraluminal thrombosis, and/or fibrinoid necrosis of the vessel wall, are diagnostic of TMA. In patients who have less severe disease and the light microscopic findings are limited to rare glomerular intracapillary thrombi, TMA should not be overlooked. In biopsies that show only glomerular capillary thrombotic lesions, differential diagnosis includes disseminated intravascular coagulation (DIC); in these cases, DIC should be distinguished from TMA based on the clinical picture in combination with laboratory findings [79]. History of trauma, sepsis, obstetric emergency or malignancy is in favor of DIC. While individual laboratory tests may have high sensitivity, the specificity is usually low to diagnose DIC. Features of enhanced coagulation and fibrinolysis with elevated levels of soluble fibrin, fibrin degradation products (FDP), and D-dimers are characteristic laboratory findings of DIC. However, in spite of ongoing coagulation fibrinogen levels are usually not decreased in DIC. Global clotting times (aPTT and PT) are typically elevated in DIC and there is usually moderate to severe thrombocytopenia present. Furthermore, microangiopathic hemolytic anemia with schistocytes can also be seen in DIC making differentiation of DIC from TMA (i.e., HUS or TTP) difficult.

"Hyaline thrombi" within the glomerular capillary loops in patients with diffuse proliferative lupus nephritis (LN) or cryoglobulinemic glomerulonephritis (GN) may mimic the light microscopic appearance of glomerular capillary thrombi of TMA. In our experience, TMA can be easily missed by light microscopy or electron microscopy especially if another glomerular and/or vascular disease is present. In patients with LN or cryoglobulinemic GN with "hyaline thrombi," the immunofluorescent findings (positive glomerular staining with immunoglobulins and complements and negative staining with fibrinogen) are helpful to identify the nature of the thrombi. In addition, the presence of endocapillary cellular proliferation

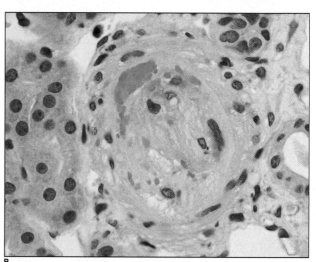

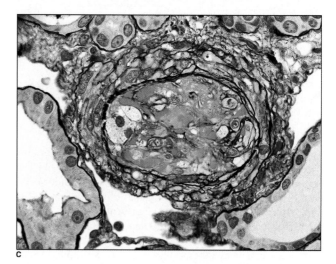

FIGURE 9.17: Scleroderma renal crisis in a 32-year-old patient. Arterial, glomerular and tubulointerstitial changes are shown. A: Ischemic glomerular changes, acute tubular injury and arterial thrombotic occlusion. (Masson's trichrome. ×200). B and C: Arterial occlusion with intimal edema and luminal thrombus admixed with red blood cells. (B: Hematoxylin and eosin, ×1,000. C: Jones methenamine silver. ×1,000).

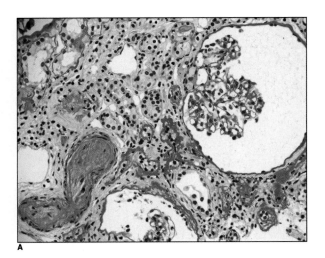

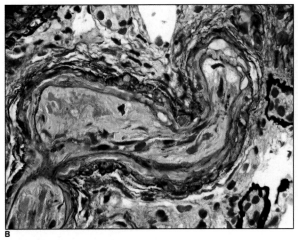

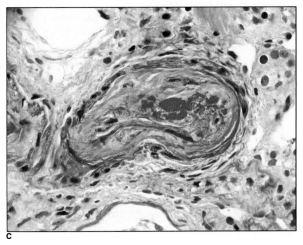

FIGURE 9.18: *Thrombotic microangiopathy in a 38-year-old patient with malignant hypertension. Serum creatinine was 5.6 mg/mL at presentation. A: A small artery is occluded by pale periodic acid-Schiff-positive matrix, corresponding to "mucoid intimal hyperplasia". Ischemic features in the glomerulus include thickening and wrinkling of the capillary basement membranes and simplification of the capillary tuft. Also note a few atrophic tubules with thickened tubular basement membranes. (Periodic acid-Schiff reaction. ×200). B: A small interlobular artery exhibits severe intimal thickening by subendothelial accumulation of fibrin and loose myxoid material. The endothelial cells are swollen and the lumen is almost occluded. (Jones methenamine silver. ×1,000). C: The same artery with Masson's trichrome stain. The subendothelial fibrin is highlighted in bright red. (×1,000).*

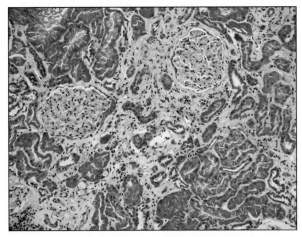

FIGURE 9.19: *Focally accentuated interstitial fibrosis in a patient with long-standing history of systemic sclerosis. No features of acute TMA were observed in this biopsy. (Masson's trichrome, ×200).*

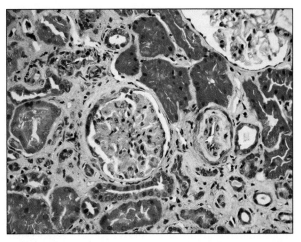

FIGURE 9.20: *Chronic vascular (arteriosclerotic) change from a patient with long-standing history of systemic sclerosis. Note the interstitial fibrosis and the ischemic glomerular changes. No features of acute TMA were present in the biopsy. Same patient as on Figure 19. (Masson's trichrome, ×200).*

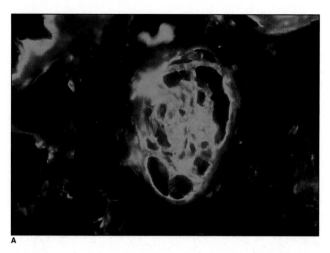

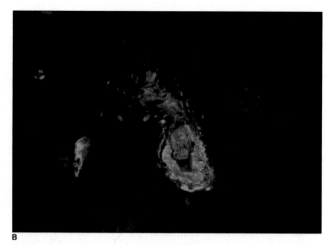

FIGURE 9.21: *Thrombotic microangiopathy. (Immunofluorescence microscopy). A: Strong global fibrinogen staining in a glomerulus. (Direct immunofluorescence. ×200). B: IgM positivity in an arteriole. (Direct immunofluorescence. ×400).*

Table 9.6 Characteristic Morphologic Changes in Specific Types of Thrombotic Microangiopathy

Preeclampsia-eclampsia
  Prominent endothelial swelling (endotheliosis)
Systemic lupus erythematosus and other immune complex-mediated glomerular diseases
  Glomerulonephritis in the background
Antiphospholipid antibody syndrome
  Organization and recanalization of luminal thrombi in arteries
Drugs
  Mesangiolysis may be prominent (mitomycin C)
Malignant hypertension
  Severe vascular changes with or without necrotizing
    glomerular lesions
Systemic sclerosis
  Ischemic changes (both glomerular and tubulointerstitial) are
    often prominent
  "Onion-skinning" of the arteries
Renal allograft rejection
  C4d-positivity of the tubulointerstitial capillaries may be present [a]
Hematopoietic stem cell transplantation
  Mesangiolysis may be severe

[a] C4d-positivity is a marker of acute antibody-mediated rejection.

Table 9.7 Electron Microscopic Features of Thrombotic Microangiopathy

Separation of the endothelial cells from the underlying basement
  membranes (lamina densa of the glomeruli, vessels)
Subendothelial accumulation of "fluffy" material
Endothelial swelling
Reduplication of the basement membranes
Fibrin and platelets (glomeruli, within vessel walls and their
  lumina)

with cellular closure of the glomerular capillary lumina, are in favor of GN. However, in rare instances patients who have GN with intracapillary hyaline thrombi in combination with mild TMA, recognition of TMA can be challenging. Differentiation of the various types of thrombi is aided by their special tinctorial properties. In contrast to "hyaline" thrombi, the thrombi of TMA have slightly granular texture on hematoxylin and eosin-stained sections and they are negative with PAS. In the more advanced stages of TMA, especially if reduplication of the glomerular capillary basement membranes is prominent, membranoproliferative glomerulonephritis (MPGN) enters the differential diagnosis. Morphologic differentiation should be aided by clinical history and laboratory features; in addition, glomerular cellular proliferation is usually absent or negligible in

patients with TMA. The lack of well-defined electron dense immunotype deposits on electron microscopy rules against an immune-mediated GN. In biopsies with arterial or arteriolar fibrinoid necrosis, especially if sampling is limited, necrotizing vasculitis should also be considered in the differential diagnosis. However, in contrast to necrotizing vasculitis, no significant number of acute inflammatory cells is present in association with fibrinoid necrosis of TMA (i.e., nonleukocytoclastic). In transplant biopsies, transplant glomerulopathy with extensive reduplication of the glomerular capillary basement membranes may mimic advanced TMA.

ETIOLOGY AND PATHOGENESIS

Over the past several years, there has been a major progress in our understanding of the specific causes and molecular pathways of various forms of TMA. However, regardless of the cause, the common pathogenetic pathway of TMA includes damage to the endothelial cells. This is supported by the pathologic findings of intimal swelling, coagulation both within the vessel wall and the vascular lumina, and the sequelae of vascular occlusion. Endothelial damage is seen in all forms of TMA affecting glomeruli, arteries, and arterioles. Features of coagulation include platelets and fibrin or fibrin thrombi in the glomeruli, small arteries, and arterioles. A particulate or fluffy,

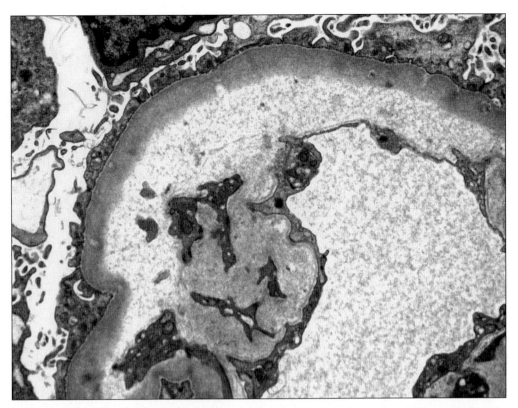

FIGURE 9.22: *Thrombotic microangiopathy. (Electron microscopy). Separation of the endothelial cells from the underlying glomerular capillary basement membrane. The appearance of the subendothelial "fluff" is similar to the luminal content. (×3,600).*

electron-dense material in the widened subendothelial region of the glomerular capillary wall likely represents fibrinogen (or fibrin) or other coagulation proteins admixed with matrix proteins, such as fibronectin. As new information emerges on specific etiologies and pathogenetic pathways in various forms of TMA, future classifications of TMA may incorporate this new information within the broad-based categories of the current classification system. Such "etiologic" classification of TMA will provide clinically useful information about specific underlying causes, including molecular pathways, prognosis and outcome, and may guide the decisions about specific therapies. A summary of various etiologies and an algorithmic approach to the etiologic classification is outlined in Table 9.8 and Figure 9.29.

Typical (D+) HUS

Most cases of typical HUS in the developed countries are caused by Shiga toxin-producing *E. coli* (STEC) infection. In Southeast Asia, infection with Shigella dysenteriae serotype 1 is the most common etiology. Shiga toxins produced by various strains of *E. coli* are two different bacteriophage-mediated protein exotoxins, composed of a single A subunit of 32-kD and five 7.7-kD B subunits [80]. Although the exotoxins produced by Shigella dysenteriae are closely related to Shiga toxin, they are not identical, and therefore, are generally referred to as Shiga-like toxins. The B subunits allow binding of the toxin to specific globotryaosyl ceramide (Gb3) cell surface receptors on the endothelial cells [81]. Binding to the receptor is followed by internalization of the toxin with subsequent retrograde transport from the Golgi-complex to the endoplasmic reticulum [82]. From there, the A subunit is translocated to the cytosol where it inhibits protein synthesis [82]. Oral infection with STEC results in bacterial adherence to the epithelial cells of colonic mucosa and local destruction of brush border microvilli ("attaching and effacing" lesion), a process mediated by outer membrane protein, intimin [83]. The toxins gain access to systemic circulation via translocation across polarized intestinal epithelial cells, a process facilitated by neutrophil transmigration [84]. Local cytokine production by intestinal epithelium may also contribute to the tissue damage. Transfer of Shiga toxin from the polymorphonuclear leukocytes, which serve as transporters in the circulation, to the endothelial cells is facilitated by the high affinity of the Gb3 endothelial cell receptor to the toxin [85]. Shiga toxin can also upregulate endothelial expression of various chemokines, cytokines, cell adhesion molecules, and transcription factors and stimulate the release of unusually large von Willebrand factor from the endothelial cells (ULvWF). High-level expression of Gb3 receptors by the renal microvasculature [86] may be responsible for preferential involvement of the kidney in HUS. Additional factors, such as lipopolysaccharide (endotoxin), tumor necrosis factor-alpha (TNFα), and interleukin-1 (IL-1) may also play a role in the pathogenesis [71]. Because

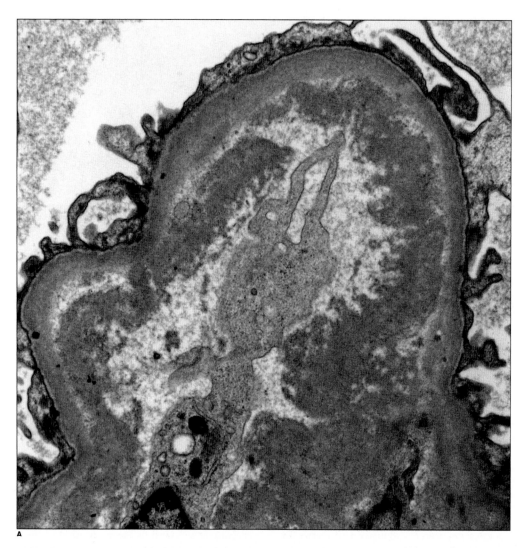

FIGURE 9.23: *Thrombotic microangiopathy. (Electron microscopy). A: Separation of the endothelial cells from the underlying glomerular capillary basement membrane. The subendothelial "fluff" is inhomogeneous with relatively dense areas. The foot processes of the visceral epithelial cells show prominent effacement (×3,600).*

Shigella dysenteriae bacteria can be entero-invasive, lipopolysaccharides may have a significant role in the pathogenesis of Shigella-induced HUS.

Atypical (D-) HUS (aHUS)

Complement Dysregulation

In more than half of the patients with aHUS, the disease is caused by complement dysregulation due to mutations in one of five proteins that regulate the complement alternative pathway and protect host cells from infections [11]. Complement activation generates C3 convertase (C3bBb), which sets the stage for an amplification cascade with further deposition of C3b onto target surfaces (opsonization). Ensuing formation of the membrane attack complex will lead to the lysis of microbes. With normal regulatory activity in place, complement activation is downregulated on intact host cells and tissue structures while efficient activation is permitted on foreign targets, such as microbial surfaces [87]. The mutations in aHUS may affect the plasma levels (Type I) or the function (Type II) of the regulatory proteins [15, 88]. Type II mutations of the negative regulators (complement factor H [CFH], complement factor I [CFI], and membrane cofactor protein [MCP]) are lack-of-function mutations while gain-of-function mutations affect the activation components (C3, and complement factor B [CFB]). As a result, there is impaired regulatory activity with accelerated complement activation and injury to the endogenous cells, including the endothelium. The majority of mutations affecting the regulatory proteins are heterozygous with dominant pattern of inheritance and variable (incomplete) penetrance. Rare cases with compound heterozygous or homozygous mutations affecting the CFH and MCP genes have been documented. Patients carrying the genetic mutation may develop the disease in infancy, later in life, or may remain disease free. A possible explanation for incomplete penetrance is

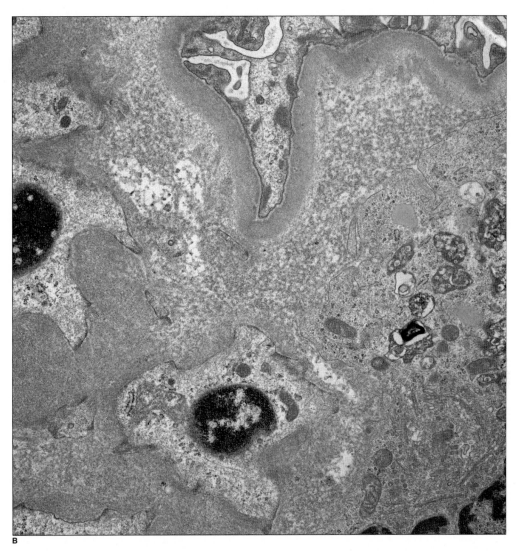

FIGURE 9.23: **B: Mesangial area with fibrillary appearance. This change often represents an early stage of mesangiolysis (×2,500).**

redundant capacity in the control of the alternative pathway that could, under normal circumstances, be sufficient to limit complement activation and protect endogenous cells even when activity of the negative regulators is decreased. Under special circumstances, such as systemic infections or pregnancy, protection of endogenous cells from increased complement activation may be insufficient if the alternative pathway regulatory activity is impaired, which may lead to the manifestation of TMA [13, 89]. The multiple hit theory implies that in addition to the "baseline" mutations, environmental factors, additional mutations, and/or genetic polymorphisms are necessary for the clinical disease to develop [90, 91].

Among the five complement regulatory proteins with mutations associated with aHUS, the prevalence is highest for complement factor H (CFH) (20–30 percent), followed by membrane cofactor protein (MCP) (5–10 percent), and complement factor I (CFI) (5 –13 percent) [51]. The rest of the mutations affecting complement factor B (CFB) and C3, are rare [92]. In addition, functional CFH deficiency due to anti-CFH antibodies is observed in approximately 10 percent of patients

with aHUS [93]. Some patients may have complex genetic abnormalities involving mutations of both ADAMTS13 (von Willebrand factor cleaving protease [a disintegrin and metalloproteinase with a thrombospondin type 1 motif, member 13]) and CFH genes (106). In pediatric population, the prognosis is most severe in patients with CFH mutations, with approximately 70 percent of patients reaching end-stage renal disease (ESRD) during childhood, frequently at the first episode [12, 94].

Neuraminidase

Neuraminidase can cleave sialic acid residues from cell surface glycoproteins exposing the hidden T-crypt antigens (Thomsen-Friedenreich antigen) on glomerular endothelial cells, platelets, and red blood cells. Naturally occurring (preformed) IgM antibodies in the circulation may react with the exposed T-crypt antigen which may lead to TMA [95, 96]. In addition to *Streptococcus pneumoniae* infection, other neuraminidase-producing organisms, such as Capnocytophaga canimorsus and possibly influenza A virus, are also reported as causes of HUS [96].

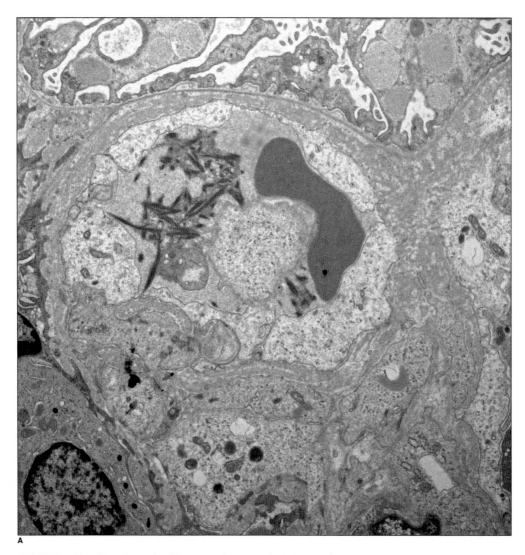

FIGURE 9.24: *Preeclampsia. (Electron microscopy). A: The endothelial cells are swollen causing narrowing of the glomerular capillary lumen. The patient had new-onset hypertension and severe proteinuria during pregnancy. The biopsy was taken 7 days post-partum. There were no features of focal segmental glomerulosclerosis in the biopsy. Although thrombotic lesions are very rare in preeclampsia, this biopsy shows a few fibrin wisps in the narrowed lumen. Both hypertension and proteinuria subsided eventually. (×3,000).*

Drugs

Drug-induced TMA is a heterogenous disorder and knowledge about the pathogenesis is limited. The pathogenesis of quinine-associated TMA is drug-dependent and antibody-mediated [18], and the same may be true for TMA associated with ticlopidine and clopidogrel. However, no antibodies have been identified so far in association with either ticlopidine or clopidogrel. The pathogenesis of mitomycin-C-associated TMA is not clear, however, the effects are dose-dependent pointing to direct toxicity. Also, dose-dependency with cyclosporine-associated TMA indicates direct toxicity.

Hematopoietic Stem Cell Transplantation

The etiology of posttransplantation TMA is likely multifactorial. Because of the close resemblance of the renal morphologic findings in posttransplantation TMA to radiation nephropathy, radiation has long been suspected to be the most significant factor in the pathogenesis. The cytotoxic effects of chemotherapy conditioning regimens [97] might further potentiate the effects of radiation. However, TMA can also develop without prior radiation [98]. A number of additional factors, such as cyclosporine and tacrolimus treatment, cytomegalovirus, fungal, and *Helicobacter pylori* infections, acute graft versus host disease (GVHD), and HLA-mismatched transplants may also contribute to the pathogenesis. [98] ADAMTS13 abnormalities do not seem to be a significant factor for TMA in this setting.

HIV Infection

The pathogenesis of HIV-associated TMA is not well understood. Direct injury of the endothelial cells by HIV, and factors

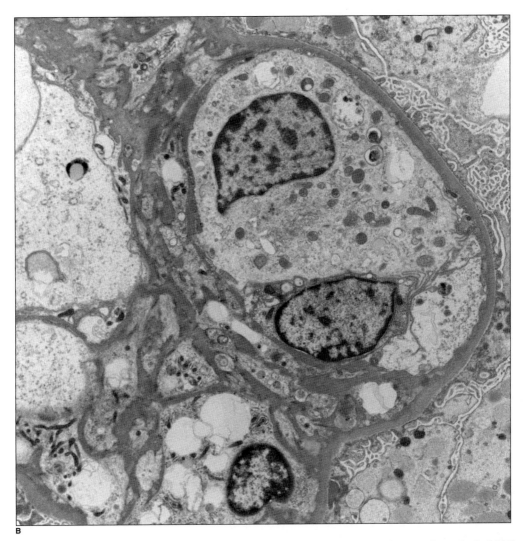

FIGURE 9.24: *B: Glomerular capillary loop with endotheliosis in a patient with preeclampsia. (×4,800).*

such as CMV infection, cryptosporidiosis, AIDS-related cancer, various drugs, and antiphospholipid antibodies have all been implicated in the pathogenesis [99].

von Willebrand Factor and ADAMTS13 Abnormalities

Endothelial cells are the primary source of circulating von Willebrand factor (vWF) multimers. vWF-cleaving metalloprotease (ADAMTS13) degrades the secreted multimers by cleaving vWF on the surface of the endothelial cells. Genetic or acquired deficiencies of ADAMTS13 activity result in deficient cleavage and persistence of unusually large (UL) vWF multimers (i.e., multimeric forms of vWF, larger than that in normal plasma) in circulation. Genetic deficiencies are linked to homozygous or compound heterozygous mutations of the ADAMTS13 gene while the more common acquired deficiencies are due to circulating inhibitory autoantibodies against ADAMTS13 [100, 101]. Thrombotic thrombocytopenic purpura in patients who have hereditary ADAMTS13 deficiency is often referred to as congenital

TTP [102] and the one associated with inhibitory antibodies against ADAMTS13 is referred to as acquired TTP [103]. Approximately half of the patients with genetic ADAMTS13 deficiency experience the first acute episode of TTP during childhood, and the other half during adulthood [104, 105]. Although some studies reported nearly perfect correlation between TTP and severe deficiency in ADAMTS13 activity, other studies showed that a significant proportion of patients with the clinical diagnosis of HUS (typical, atypical, and familial) can also have severe ADAMTS13 deficiency. Therefore, ADAMTS13 deficiency is not a reliable marker to distinguish TTP from HUS. However, severe deficiency of ADAMTS13 activity (i.e., lower than 5–10 percent of the activity of normal plasma) is highly specific for TMA, most often clinically diagnosed as TTP [103]. The interaction of large vWF multimers with platelet glycoprotein Ib-IX-V receptors might be mediated by high shear stress rates, followed by activation of platelets, platelet aggregation, and formation of platelet thrombi in the microcirculation [106]. The relative incidence rate for TMA associated with severe acquired ADAMTS13 deficiency is ninefold greater in

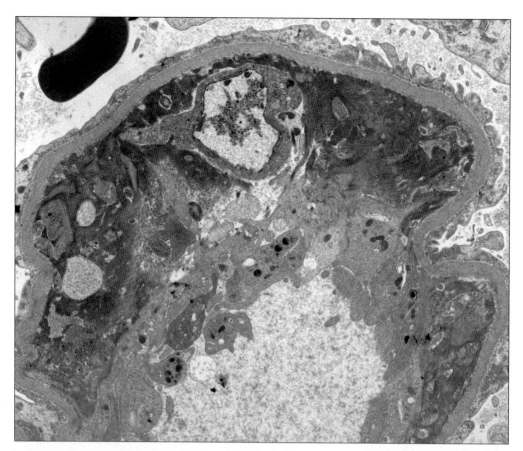

FIGURE 9.25: *Glomerular intracapillary fibrin deposition in a patient with TMA. (Electron microscopy). The endothelial cells are almost entirely destroyed and cellular debris is entrapped within the thrombus. A few platelets are also present along the luminal side of the clot. Effacement of the foot processes is present. (×3,200).*

African-Americans than in nonblacks [13], and among those with acquired ADAMTS13 deficiency, the frequency of obesity is also significantly increased [107]. Some data also indicate a possible role of functional impairment of ADAMTS13 in the pathogenesis of D+ (Shiga toxin-mediated) HUS [108].

Antiphospholipid Antibodies

Although there are data suggesting that antiphospholipid antibody positivity confers an increased risk of thrombotic microangiopathy, the role of antiphospholipid antibodies in this process is uncertain. Furthermore, the potential pathogenetic mechanisms that may link antiphospholipid antibodies to microvascular thrombosis, await identification [109, 110].

Preeclampsia–Eclampsia

Circulating antiangiogenic substances such as soluble fms-like tyrosine kinase (sF1t1) and endoglin are thought to play an important role in the pathogenesis of preeclampsia-eclampsia [111, 112]. sF1t1 is an endogenous inhibitor of vascular endothelial growth factor (VEGF) signaling. The serum levels of sF1t1, produced predominantly by the ischemic placenta, are highly elevated in patients with preeclampsia, even before the onset of hypertension [112]. Endothelial injury and swelling, the characteristic morphologic features of eclampsia, result from impaired VEGF signaling. Proteinuria might also be mediated by the endothelial injury; however, the role of diminished nephrin expression by the podocytes has also been raised as a possible mediator of proteinuria [113]. Thrombotic microangiopathy and proteinuria as a complication of anti-VEGF therapy lends support to the important role of diminished VEGF signaling in the pathogenesis of preeclampsia-eclampsia [114, 115].

Systemic Sclerosis

The pathogenesis of systemic sclerosis is complex. Altered collagen production, endothelial or vascular abnormalities, and immune factors are considered to be the major pathogenetic mechanisms. Cytokines, growth factors, autoantibodies, and additional mediators derived from various sources such as inflammatory cells, endothelial cells, platelets, and fibroblasts may have an important role in the pathophysiology of the disease. Although the role of genetic factors may be significant, environmental or acquired factors, such as viruses, chemical and physical agents, seem to play a more important role in the development of the disease.

The precise mediators and initiating events of scleroderma renal crisis are not well-delineated. Although renal pathologic

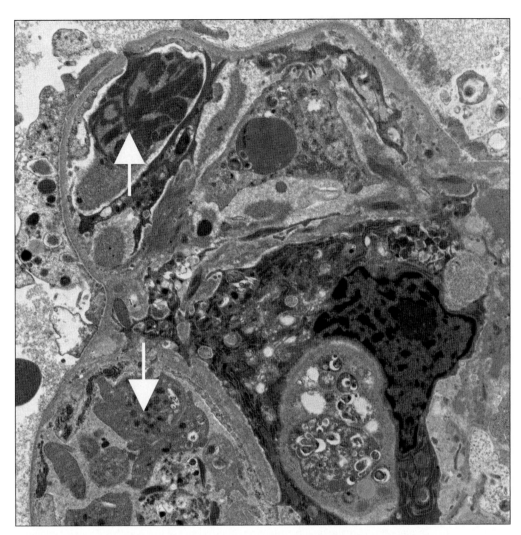

FIGURE 9.26: *Thrombotic microangiopathy in an HIV-infected patient showing glomerular intracapillary thrombotic lesion (arrows) and focal endothelial cell injury. (Electron microscopy. ×2,400).*

changes in scleroderma renal crisis indicate significant endothelial injury, similar to those seen in various other forms of TMA, it is unclear whether damage to the endothelial cells is the primary event or is it preceded by other changes such as activation of the immune system. The etiology of endothelial injury may be diverse; the role of a large number of cytokines and growth factors secreted by activated inflammatory cells, serum cytotoxic factors, downregulation of complement regulatory proteins, viruses, and antibody-dependent cell-mediated cytotoxicity have all been postulated [71]. Some data indicate that the renin–angiotensin system may play a significant role in the development of scleroderma renal crisis with malignant hypertension [116].

Polymorphonuclear Leukocyte Activation

Activated polymorphonuclear leukocytes may play a role in the endothelial injury in patients with D+ HUS. There are features of polymorphonuclear leukocyte activation in the setting of D+

HUS [117] and high polymorphonuclear leukocyte count at presentation in D+ HUS indicates a poor prognosis [118]. Endothelial injury can be mediated by superoxide anions generated by activated neutrophils in concert with endothelial-derived nitric oxide.

Platelet Activation or Aggregation

Thrombocytopenia is one of the defining features of TMA. Thrombocytopenia is caused by consumption of activated platelets in microthrombi, mechanical destruction in peripheral, damaged microvessels, or by antiplatelet antibodies, such as seen in quinine-associated TMA. Platelet activation is initiated by endothelial damage and thrombin generation, followed by platelet aggregation at the site of injury. Various factors, including cysteine proteinase (calpain), p37, large vWF multimers, and platelet-activating factor may promote platelet aggregation [119]. Activated or aggregated platelets may further contribute to vascular injury triggering intimal

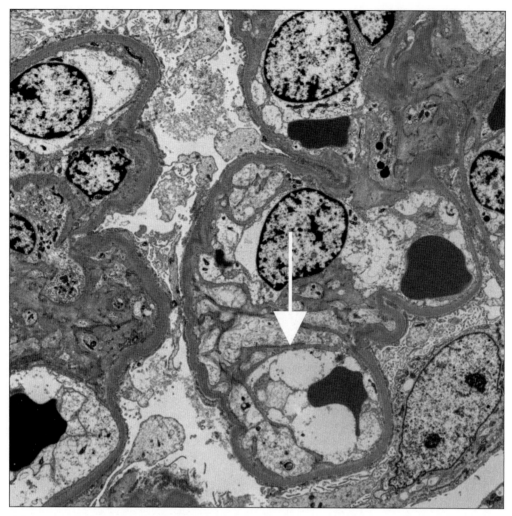

FIGURE 9.27: *Thrombotic microangiopathy. (Electron microscopy). A few capillary loops show thin newly-formed glomerular capillary basement membranes (arrow). (×2,800).*

proliferation and fibrosis through growth factors such as platelet-derived growth factor (PDGF) and transforming growth factor-β (TGF-β) [120].

Coagulation Disturbances

Many features of abnormal coagulation are seen in patients with TMA. In D+ HUS, thrombin generation and inhibition of fibrinolysis may precede or cause renal injury [6]. Laboratory features of altered coagulation include elevations in plasma concentrations of prothrombin fragment 1+2, tissue plasminogen activator (t-PA) antigen, t-PA-plasminogen-activator inhibitor type 1 (PAI-1) complex, and D-dimer levels [6]. Abnormal coagulation can be mediated by a number of factors, including PAI-1, t-PA, and urokinase-type plasminogen activator (uPA-R) [6, 71]. Decreased serum concentrations of tissue factor pathway inhibitor and increased concentrations of thrombomodulin were detected in patients with TTP [121].

Endothelial Damage

Injury to the endothelium plays a central role in the pathogenesis of TMA. Endothelial damage, initiated by multiple potential triggers, may lead to a switch of the endothelial anticoagulant properties to a procoagulant phenotype, decreased fibrinolytic activity, release of unusually large vWF multimers, activation with upregulation of adhesion molecules, chemokines, cytokines, transcription factors, platelet activation, and exposure of thrombogenic subendothelial surfaces. This may contribute to platelet aggregation, thrombus formation, and impaired removal of fibrin with subsequent severe vascular and organ damage.

CLINICAL COURSE, PROGNOSIS, TREATMENT AND CLINICAL CORRELATION

Correlation of the Pathologic Findings with Prognosis

In general, patients with only glomerular involvement are considered to have a better renal prognosis, and those with

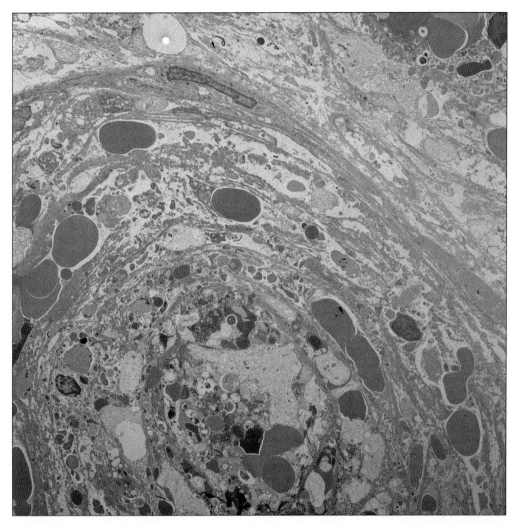

FIGURE 9.28: Vascular lesion of thrombotic microangiopathy. (Electron microscopy). Thickening of the arteriolar wall with edema, accumulation of fluffy material, cellular debris, fragmented red blood cells, and severe endothelial injury. (×2,000).

glomerular and vascular (i.e., arterial and arteriolar) involvement are associated with a less favorable outcome [69]. Accordingly, vascular changes seem to be more common and often more severe in patients with the atypical form of HUS versus those with typical HUS. However, the correlation is not absolute and the overall outcome may be affected by a number of extrarenal manifestations and there may also be overlaps between the glomerular and vascular lesions.

Typical (D+) HUS

D+ HUS caused by STEC infection is usually associated with a good prognosis. More than 80 percent of patients are reported to recover from renal failure with a case-fatality ratio of 5 percent [122]. Among pediatric patients, those with diarrhea-positive disease and evidence of STEC infection have significantly better prognosis than those: (1) without diarrhea and no evidence of STEC and (2) with diarrhea but no evidence of STEC [123]. However, approximately 12 percent of the

patients with D+ HUS who have recovered renal function after the initial episode will eventually progress to ESRD [124]. The higher severity of acute illness, particularly central nervous system symptoms and the need for initial dialysis, is strongly associated with worse long-term prognosis. The prognosis of HUS caused by Shigella dysenteriae infection is considered to be less favorable than HUS caused by STEC infection. However, Shigella dysenteriae infection with HUS is more common in developing countries where children may have significant comorbidities and poor access to health care. In epidemics in sub-Saharan Africa, mortality rates of up to 43 percent have been reported [125], while all five children recovered with normal renal function in an outbreak of HUS caused by Shigella dysenteriae type 1 infection reported from France [126].

Treatment of D+ HUS caused by STEC infection is nonspecific and mainly supportive. Antibiotics, antimotility agents, narcotics, and nonsteroidal anti-inflammatory drugs are not indicated. However, early antibiotic treatment is indicated in

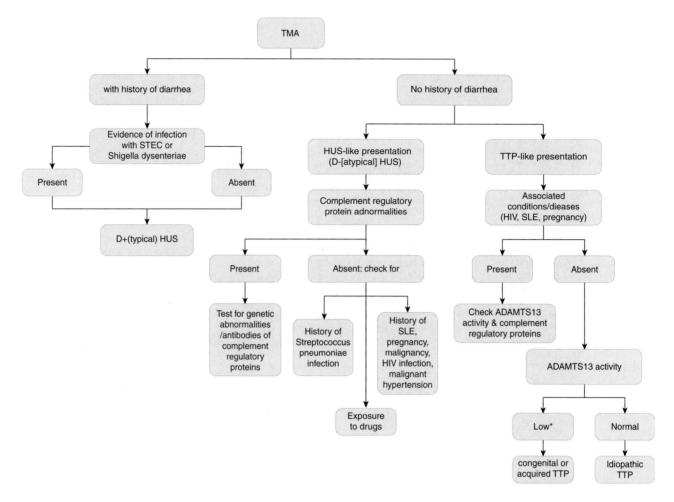

STEC: Shiga Toxin-producing Escherichia Coli
SLE : Systemic Lupus Erythematosus
HUS : Hemolytic Uremic Syndrome
TTP : Thrombotic Thrombocytopenic Purpura
* : < 5-10% of normal

FIGURE 9.29: *Algorithm for the etiologic classification of thrombotic microangiopathies.*

Shigella dysenteriae infection which may reduce bacterial enteroinvasion and the incidence of HUS [127].

Atypical (D-) HUS (aHUS)

The outcome of patients with aHUS is less favorable than with D+ HUS. The case-fatality ratio is approximately 20 percent and only 60 to 70 percent of patients recover renal function [128]. However, there are significant differences in outcome among patients with different etiologies of aHUS. Approximately 70 percent of patients with CFH mutations in the pediatric population reach ESRD during childhood, most frequently at the time of the first episode [94]. Approximately half of the patients with MCP mutations progress rapidly to ESRD or death and the other half recover [12]. The clinical course of patients with aHUS triggered by quinine or mitomycin toxicity is severe and the outcome is generally poor with high mortality. The mortality of HIV-associated TMA may

be as high as 100 percent [161]. Furthermore, patients without well-defined etiology of aHUS have a more variable outcome which may suggest various pathogenetic mechanisms.

Intensive plasmatherapy is the only therapeutic option for patients with aHUS, however, the benefits of the treatment are not clear and the success rate is low [12]. Results with liver or combined liver and kidney transplantation for those with genetic abnormalities of the complement regulatory proteins are disappointing.

Thrombotic Thrombocytopenic Purpura

Without plasma exchange treatment, TTP may follow a rapidly fatal course, with only approximately a 10 percent survival rate [1]. With the advent of plasma exchange therapy, prognosis has improved to between 75 and 92 percent [24]. Plasma exchange is the most important treatment and the value of additional treatment modalities is unknown [24]. However, the dramatic improvement in survival is not only related to treatment but also

Table 9.8 Etiologic Classification of Thrombotic Microangiopathy

Form		Etiology	Type	Associated diseases or conditions
HUS	Typical (D+)	Shiga-toxin-producing *E. coli* [3, 5] *Shigella dysenteriae* serotype 1 [135]		
	Atypical (D-)	*Streptococcus pneumoniae* [96]		
		Complement and regulatory protein abnormalities (CFH, MCP, CFI, CFB, C3, CFHR1, CFHR3)	Genetic [11, 51] Acquired (anti-CFH) (rare) [93]	
		Defective cobalamin metabolism [14]		
		Antiplatelet glycoprotein antibodies [18]		Exposure to quinine
		Uncertain		HIV infection SLE/APLAS Pregnancy Malignancy Drugs
		Multifactorial [98]		BMT
		Idiopathic		
TTP		ADAMTS13 deficiency	Genetic [101] Acquired [100]	
		Uncertain [17, 58, 99]		HIV infection SLE Pregnancy
		Idiopathic		
Renal allograft rejection		Multifactorial [52]		
Malignant hypertension		Uncertain		
Systemic sclerosis		Multifactorial		Severe hypertension

Abbreviations: CFH, complement factor H; CFI, complement factor I; CFB, complement factor B; MCP, membrane cofactor protein; C3, complement factor 3; ADAMTS13, von Willebrand factor cleaving protease; BMT, bone marrow transplantation; APLAS, antiphospholipid antibody syndrome; SLE, systemic lupus erythematosus.

to earlier detection and recognition of milder forms of the disease [1]. Relapses after initial response to treatment are relatively frequent (chronic or relapsing forms of TTP). For patients with the congenital forms of TTP, treatment with plasma infusions is sufficient for replacement of ADAMTS13 activity [129].

Bone marrow transplant-associated TMA has poor prognosis with a very high mortality rate. Most patients die from infection-related causes [98]. There is no consensus regarding the approach to treatment. The conventional treatment modalities of TMA, such as plasma exchange or plasma infusions are ineffective. However, plasma exchange or plasma infusion is the standard therapy for TTP in patients with HIV-infection [130, 131]. As a general rule, rapid diagnosis and institution of treatment is crucial for favorable outcome.

Systemic Sclerosis

Recent data indicate a ~11-year median survival for patients with systemic sclerosis [132]. Although, this represents a significant improvement in survival, systemic sclerosis still has the poorest prognosis among various connective tissue diseases. In general, the presence of major organ involvement (lung, kidney, heart) is associated with lower survival rates and patients with scleroderma renal crisis have the worse survival rates [133]. However, patients with scleroderma renal crisis who are treated with ACE inhibitors may have relatively good outcome (in up to 60 percent of patients) comparable to those without renal crisis [134].

Preeclampsia–Eclampsia

Quick resolution of both hypertension and proteinuria is the rule following delivery. In severe cases with significant microangiopathic hemolytic anemia, thrombocytopenia, renal failure, and neurological abnormalities, treatment with plasma exchange can be considered [16].

REFERENCES

1. George JN. Clinical practice. Thrombotic thrombocytopenic purpura. *N Engl J Med* 2006;354:1927–35.
2. Gerber A, Karch H, Allerberger F, Verweyen HM, Zimmerhackl LB. Clinical course and the role of shiga toxin-producing Escherichia coli infection in the hemolytic-uremic syndrome in pediatric patients, 1997-2000, in Germany and Austria: a prospective study. *J Infect Dis* 2002;186:493–500.
3. Rangel JM, Sparling PH, Crowe C, Griffin PM, Swerdlow DL. Epidemiology of Escherichia coli O157:H7 outbreaks, United States, 1982-2002. *Emerg Infect Dis* 2005;11:603–9.
4. Karpac CA, Lee A, Kunnel BS, Bamgbola OF, Vesely SK, George JN. Endemic Esherichia coil O157:H7 infections and hemolytic-uremic syndrome in Oklahoma, 2002–2005. *J Okla State Med Assoc* 2007;100:429–33.
5. Boyce TG, Swerdlow DL, Griffin PM. Escherichia coli O157:H7 and the hemolytic–uremic syndrome. *N Engl J Med* 1995;333:364–8.
6. Chandler WL, Jelacic S, Boster DR, Ciol MA, Williams GD, Watkins SL, Igarashi T, Tarr PI. Prothrombotic coagulation abnormalities preceding the hemolytic-uremic syndrome. *N Engl J Med* 2002;346:23–32.
7. Lynn RM, O'Brien SJ, Taylor CM, Adak GK, Chart H, Cheasty T, Coia JE, Gillespie IA, Locking ME, Reilly WJ, Smith HR, Waters A, Willshaw GA. Childhood hemolytic uremic syndrome, United Kingdom and Ireland. *Emerg Infect Dis* 2005;11:590–6.
8. Bhimma R, Rollins NC, Coovadia HM, Adhikari M. Postdysenteric hemolytic uremic syndrome in children during an epidemic of Shigella dysentery in Kwazulu/Natal. *Pediatr Nephrol* 1997;11:560–4.
9. Azim T, Islam LN, Halder RC, Hamadani J, Khanum N, Sarker MS, Salam MA, Albert MJ. Peripheral blood neutrophil responses in children with shigellosis. *Clin Diagn Lab Immunol* 1995;2:616–22.
10. Constantinescu AR, Bitzan M, Weiss LS, Christen E, Kaplan BS, Cnaan A, Trachtman H. Non-enteropathic hemolytic uremic syndrome: causes and short-term course. *Am J Kidney Dis* 2004;43:976–82.
11. Jokiranta TS, Zipfel PF, Fremeaux-Bacchi V, Taylor CM, Goodship TJ, Noris M. Where next with atypical hemolytic uremic syndrome? *Mol Immunol* 2007;44:3889–900.
12. Sellier-Leclerc AL, Fremeaux-Bacchi V, Dragon-Durey MA, Macher MA, Niaudet P, Guest G, Boudailliez B, Bouissou F, Deschenes G, Gie S, Tsimaratos M, Fischbach M, Morin D, Nivet H, Alberti C, Loirat C. Differential impact of complement mutations on clinical characteristics in atypical hemolytic uremic syndrome. *J Am Soc Nephrol* 2007;18:2392–400.
13. Terrell DR, Williams LA, Vesely SK, Lammle B, Hovinga JA, George JN. The incidence of thrombotic thrombocytopenic purpura-hemolytic uremic syndrome: all patients, idiopathic patients, and patients with severe ADAMTS-13 deficiency. *J Thromb Haemost* 2005;3:1432–6.
14. Sharma AP, Greenberg CR, Prasad AN, Prasad C. Hemolytic uremic syndrome (HUS) secondary to cobalamin C (cblC) disorder. *Pediatr Nephrol* 2007;22:2097–103.
15. Loirat C, Noris M, Fremeaux-Bacchi V. Complement and the atypical hemolytic uremic syndrome in children. *Pediatr Nephrol* 2008;23:1957–72.
16. McMinn JR, George JN. Evaluation of women with clinically suspected thrombotic thrombocytopenic purpura-hemolytic uremic syndrome during pregnancy. *J Clin Apher* 2001;16:202–9.
17. George JN. The association of pregnancy with thrombotic thrombocytopenic purpura-hemolytic uremic syndrome. *Curr Opin Hematol* 2003;10:339–44.
18. Medina PJ, Sipols JM, George JN. Drug-associated thrombotic thrombocytopenic purpura-hemolytic uremic syndrome. *Curr Opin Hematol* 2001;8:286–93.
19. Dlott JS, Danielson CF, Blue-Hnidy DE, McCarthy LJ. Drug-induced thrombotic thrombocytopenic purpura/hemolytic uremic syndrome: a concise review. *Ther Apher Dial* 2004;8:102–111.
20. Lesesne JB, Rothschild N, Erickson B, Korec S, Sisk R, Keller J, Arbus M, Woolley PV, Chiazze L, Schein PS, et al. Cancer-associated hemolytic-uremic syndrome: analysis of 85 cases from a national registry. *J Clin Oncol* 1989;7:781–9.
21. Becker S, Fusco G, Fusco J, Balu R, Gangjee S, Brennan C, Feinberg J. HIV-associated thrombotic microangiopathy in the era of highly active antiretroviral therapy: an observational study. *Clin Infect Dis* 2004;39 Suppl. 5:S267–75.
22. Miller DP, Kaye JA, Shea K, Ziyadeh N, Cali C, Black C, Walker AM. Incidence of thrombotic thrombocytopenic purpura/hemolytic uremic syndrome. *Epidemiology* 2004;15:208–15.
23. Ridolfi RL, Bell WR. Thrombotic thrombocytopenic purpura. Report of 25 cases and review of the literature. *Medicine (Baltimore)* 1981;60:413–28.
24. George JN: How I treat patients with thrombotic thrombocytopenic purpura-hemolytic uremic syndrome. *Blood* 2000;96:1223–9.
25. Chifflot H, Fautrel B, Sordet C, Chatelus E, Sibilia J. Incidence and prevalence of systemic sclerosis: a systematic literature review. *Semin Arthritis Rheum* 2008;37:223–35.
26. Helmick CG, Felson DT, Lawrence RC, Gabriel S, Hirsch R, Kwoh CK, Liang MH, Kremers HM, Mayes MD, Merkel PA, Pillemer SR, Reveille JD, Stone JH. Estimates of the prevalence of arthritis and other rheumatic conditions in the United States. Part I. *Arthritis Rheum* 2008;58:15–25.
27. LeRoy EC, Black C, Fleischmajer R, Jablonska S, Krieg T, Medsger TA, Jr., Rowell N, Wollheim F. Scleroderma (systemic sclerosis): classification, subsets and pathogenesis. *J Rheumatol* 1988;15:202–5.

28. LeRoy EC, Medsger TA, Jr. Criteria for the classification of early systemic sclerosis. *J Rheumatol* 2001;28:1573–6.

29. Penn H, Howie AJ, Kingdon EJ, Bunn CC, Stratton RJ, Black CM, Burns A, Denton CP. Scleroderma renal crisis: patient characteristics and long-term outcomes. *QJM* 2007;100:485–94.

30. Roberts JM, Gammill HS. Preeclampsia: recent insights. *Hypertension* 2005;46:1243–9.

31. Zhang J, Meikle S, Trumble A. Severe maternal morbidity associated with hypertensive disorders in pregnancy in the United States. *Hypertens Pregnancy* 2003;22:203–12.

32. Druzin ML, Charles B, Johnson AL. Editorial summary of symposium on hypertensive disorders of pregnancy. *Curr Opin Obstet Gynecol* 2008;20:91.

33. Goldenberg RL, Rouse DJ. Prevention of premature birth. *N Engl J Med* 1998;339:313–20.

34. Spargo B. "The renal lesions in preeclampsia" in Lindheimer M (ed.), *Hypertension in Pregnancy* (New York: Wiley Medical, 1976), pp. 129–37.

35. Ho VT, Cutler C, Carter S, Martin P, Adams R, Horowitz M, Ferrara J, Soiffer R, Giralt S. Blood and marrow transplant clinical trials network toxicity committee consensus summary: thrombotic microangiopathy after hematopoietic stem cell transplantation. *Biol Blood Marrow Transplant* 2005;11:571–5.

36. George JN, Li X, McMinn JR, Terrell DR, Vesely SK, Selby GB. Thrombotic thrombocytopenic purpura-hemolytic uremic syndrome following allogeneic HPC transplantation: a diagnostic dilemma. *Transfusion* 2004;44:294–304.

37. Reynolds JC, Agodoa LY, Yuan CM, Abbott KC. Thrombotic microangiopathy after renal transplantation in the United States. *Am J Kidney Dis* 2003;42:1058–68.

38. Zarifian A, Meleg-Smith S, O'Donovan R, Tesi RJ, Batuman V. Cyclosporine-associated thrombotic microangiopathy in renal allografts. *Kidney Int* 1999;55:2457–66.

39. Pham PT, Peng A, Wilkinson AH, Gritsch HA, Lassman C, Pham PC, Danovitch GM. Cyclosporine and tacrolimus-associated thrombotic microangiopathy. *Am J Kidney Dis* 2000;36:844–50.

40. Robson M, Cote I, Abbs I, Koffman G, Goldsmith D. Thrombotic micro-angiopathy with sirolimus-based immunosuppression: potentiation of calcineurin-inhibitor-induced endothelial damage? *Am J Transplant* 2003;3:324–7.

41. Saikali JA, Truong LD, Suki WN. Sirolimus may promote thrombotic microangiopathy. *Am J Transplant* 2003;3:229–30.

42. Waiser J, Budde K, Rudolph B, Ortner MA, Neumayer HH. De novo hemolytic uremic syndrome postrenal transplant after cytomegalovirus infection. *Am J Kidney Dis* 1999;34:556–9.

43. Murer L, Zacchello G, Bianchi D, Dall'Amico R, Montini G, Andreetta B, Perini M, Dossi EC, Zanon G, Zacchello F. Thrombotic microangiopathy associated with parvovirus B 19 infection after renal transplantation. *J Am Soc Nephrol* 2000;11:1132–7.

44. Petrogiannis-Haliotis T, Sakoulas G, Kirby J, Koralnik IJ, Dvorak AM, Monahan-Earley R, DEG PC, DEG U, Upton M, Major EO, Pfister LA, Joseph JT: BK-related polyomavirus vasculopathy in a renal-transplant recipient. *N Engl J Med* 2001;345:1250–5.

45. Gohh RY, Williams ME, Crosson AW, Federman M, Zambetti FX. Late renal allograft failure secondary to thrombotic microangiopathy associated with disseminated malignancy. *Am J Nephrol* 1997;17:176–80.

46. Pelle G, Xu Y, Khoury N, Mougenot B, Rondeau E. Thrombotic microangiopathy in marginal kidneys after sirolimus use. *Am J Kidney Dis* 2005;46:1124–8.

47. Balfour HH, Jr. Antiviral drugs. *N Engl J Med* 1999;340:1255–68.

48. Evens AM, Kwaan HC, Kaufman DB, Bennett CL. TTP/HUS occurring in a simultaneous pancreas/kidney transplant recipient after clopidogrel treatment: evidence of a nonimmunological etiology. *Transplantation* 2002;74:885–7.

49. Jumani A, Hala K, Tahir S, Al-Ghamdi G, Al-Flaiw A, Hejaili F, Qureshi J, Raza H, Ghalib M, Khader AA. Causes of acute thrombotic microangiopathy in patients receiving kidney transplantation. *Exp Clin Transplant* 2004;2:268–72.

50. Baid S, Pascual M, Williams WW, Jr., Tolkoff-Rubin N, Johnson SM, Collins B, Chung RT, Delmonico FL, Cosimi AB, Colvin RB. Renal thrombotic microangiopathy associated with anticardiolipin antibodies in hepatitis C-positive renal allograft recipients. *J Am Soc Nephrol* 1999;10:146–53.

51. Loirat C, Fremeaux-Bacchi V. Hemolytic uremic syndrome recurrence after renal transplantation. *Pediatr Transplant* 2008;12:619–29.

52. Haas M, Rahman MH, Racusen LC, Kraus ES, Bagnasco SM, Segev DL, Simpkins CE, Warren DS, King KE, Zachary AA, Montgomery RA. C4d and C3d staining in biopsies of ABO- and HLA-incompatible renal allografts: correlation with histologic findings. *Am J Transplant* 2006;6:1829–1840.

53. Loirat C, Niaudet P. The risk of recurrence of hemolytic uremic syndrome after renal transplantation in children. *Pediatr Nephrol* 2003;18:1095–101.

54. Ferraris JR, Ramirez JA, Ruiz S, Caletti MG, Vallejo G, Piantanida JJ, Araujo JL, Sojo ET. Shiga toxin-associated hemolytic uremic syndrome: absence of recurrence after renal transplantation. *Pediatr Nephrol* 2002;17:809–14.

55. Miyakis S, Lockshin MD, Atsumi T, Branch DW, Brey RL, Cervera R, Derksen RH, PG DEG, Koike T, Meroni PL, Reber G, Shoenfeld Y, Tincani A, Vlachoyiannopoulos PG, Krilis SA. International consensus statement on an update of the classification criteria for definite antiphospholipid syndrome (APS). *J Thromb Haemost* 2006;4:295–306.

56. Asherson RA, Cervera R, de Groot PG, Erkan D, Boffa MC, Piette JC, Khamashta MA, Shoenfeld Y. Catastrophic antiphospholipid syndrome: international consensus statement on classification criteria and treatment guidelines. *Lupus* 2003;12:530–534.

57. Asherson RA, Cervera R. Microvascular and microangiopathic antiphospholipid-associated syndromes ("MAPS"): semantic or antisemantic? *Autoimmun Rev* 2008;7:164–167.

58. Espinosa G, Bucciarelli S, Cervera R, Lozano M, Reverter JC, de la Red G, Gil V, Ingelmo M, Font J, Asherson RA. Thrombotic microangiopathic haemolytic anaemia and antiphospholipid antibodies. *Ann Rheum Dis* 2004;63:730–6.

59. Nochy D, Daugas E, Droz D, Beaufils H, Grunfeld JP, Piette JC, Bariety J, Hill G. The intrarenal vascular lesions associated with primary antiphospholipid syndrome. *J Am Soc Nephrol* 1999;10:507–18.

60. Daugas E, Nochy D, Huong DL, Duhaut P, Beaufils H, Caudwell V, Bariety J, Piette JC, Hill G. Antiphospholipid syndrome nephropathy in systemic lupus erythematosus. *J Am Soc Nephrol* 2002;13:42–52.

61. Sheehan H. *Pathology of Toxemia of Pregnancy*. (Edinburgh: Churchill Livingstone), 1973.

62. Inward CD, Howie AJ, Fitzpatrick MM, Rafaat F, Milford DV, Taylor CM. Renal histopathology in fatal cases of diarrhoea-associated haemolytic uraemic syndrome. British Association for Paediatric Nephrology. *Pediatr Nephrol* 1997;11:556–9.

63. George JN, Vesely SK, James JA. Overlapping features of thrombotic thrombocytopenic purpura and systemic lupus erythematosus. *South Med J* 2007;100:512–14.

64. Troxell ML, Pilapil M, Miklos DB, Higgins JP, Kambham N. Renal pathology in hematopoietic cell transplantation recipients. *Mod Pathol* 2008;21:396–406.

65. Abe H, Tsuboi N, Yukawa S, Tsuji S, Hayashi H, Yukawa N, Takanashi H, Tahara K, Tonozuka N, Hayashi T: Thrombotic thrombocytopenic purpura complicating Sjogren's syndrome with crescentic glomerulonephritis and membranous nephritis. *Mod Rheumatol* 2004;14:174–8.

66. Chang A, Kowalewska J, Smith KD, Nicosia RF, Alpers CE. A clinicopathologic study of thrombotic microangiopathy in the setting of IgA nephropathy. *Clin Nephrol* 2006;66:397–404.

67. Benz K, Amann K, Dittrich K, Dotsch J. Thrombotic microangiopathy as a complication in a patient with focal segmental glomerulosclerosis. *Pediatr Nephrol* 2007;22:2125–8.

68. Koster FT, Boonpucknavig V, Sujaho S, Gilman RH, Rahaman MM. Renal histopathology in the hemolytic-uremic syndrome following shigellosis. *Clin Nephrol* 1984;21:126–33.

69. Thoenes W, John HD. Endotheliotropic (hemolytic) nephroangiopathy and its various manifestation forms (thrombotic microangiopathy, primary malignant nephrosclerosis, hemolytic-uremic syndrome). *Klin Wochenschr* 1980;58:173–84.

70. Taylor CM, Chua C, Howie AJ, Risdon RA. Clinico-pathological findings in diarrhoea-negative haemolytic uraemic syndrome. *Pediatr Nephrol* 2004;19:419–425.

71. Laszik Z, Silva, FG, "Hemolytic Uremic Syndrome, Thrombotic Thrombocytopenic Purpura, and other Therombotic Microangiopathies"in Jennette J, Olson, JL., Schwartz, MM. , Silva, FG(ed.), *Heptinstall's Pathology of the Kidney* (Philadelphia, PA: Lippincott Williams & Wilkins, 2007), pp. 701–64.

72. Trostle DC, Bedetti CD, Steen VD, Al-Sabbagh MR, Zee B, Medsger TA, Jr.: Renal vascular histology and morph-ometry in systemic sclerosis. A case-control autopsy study. *Arthritis Rheum* 1988;31:393–400.

73. Gonzalo A, Mampaso F, Gallego N, Bellas C, Segui J, Ortuno J. Hemolytic uremic syndrome with hypocomple-mentemia and deposits of IgM and C3 in the involved renal tissue. *Clin Nephrol* 1981;16:193–9.

74. Bohle A, Helmchen U, Grund KE, Gartner HV, Meyer D, Bock KD, Bulla M, Bunger P, Diekmann L, Frotscher U, Hayduk K, Kosters W, Strauch M, Scheler F, Christ H. Malignant nephrosclerosis in patients with hemolytic ure-mic syndrome (primary malignant nephrosclerosis). *Curr Top Pathol* 1977;65:81–113.

75. Bohle A, Grabensee B, Fischer R, Berg H E, Klust. On four cases of hemolytic-uremic syndrome without microangiop-athy. *Clin Nephrol* 1985;24:88–92.

76. Petrucco OM, Thomson NM, Lawrence JR, Weldon MW: Immunofluorescent studies in renal biopsies in pre-eclamp-sia. *Br Med J* 1974;1:473–6.

77. Shigematsu H, Dikman SH, Churg J, Grishman E, Duffy JL. Mesangial involvement in hemolytic-uremic syndrome. A light and electron microscopic study. *Am J Pathol* 1976;85:349–62.

78. John HD, Thoenes W. The glomerular lesions in endothe-liotropic hemolytic nephroangiopathy (hemolytic uremic syndrome, malignant nephrosclerosis, post partum renal insufficiency). *Pathol Res Pract* 1982;173:236–59.

79. Taylor FB, Jr., Toh CH, Hoots WK, Wada H, Levi M. Towards definition, clinical and laboratory criteria, and a scoring system for disseminated intravascular coagulation. *Thromb Haemost* 2001;86:1327–30.

80. Fraser ME, Fujinaga M, Cherney MM, Melton-Celsa AR, Twiddy EM, O'Brien AD, James MN. Structure of shiga toxin type 2 (Stx2) from Escherichia coli O157:H7. *J Biol Chem* 2004;279:27511–17.

81. Lindberg AA, Brown JE, Stromberg N, Westling-Ryd M, Schultz JE, Karlsson KA. Identification of the carbohydrate receptor for Shiga toxin produced by Shigella dysenteriae type 1. *J Biol Chem* 1987;262:1779–85.

82. Paton JC, Paton AW. Shiga toxin 'goes retro' in human primary kidney cells. *Kidney Int* 2006;70:2049–51.

83. Xicohtencatl-Cortes J, Monteiro-Neto V, Ledesma MA, Jordan DM, Francetic O, Kaper JB, Puente JL, Giron JA. Intestinal adherence associated with type IV pili of enter-ohemorrhagic Escherichia coli O157:H7. *J Clin Invest* 2007;117:3519–29.

84. Hurley BP, Thorpe CM, Acheson DW. Shiga toxin trans-location across intestinal epithelial cells is enhanced by neu-trophil transmigration. *Infect Immun* 2001;69:6148–55.

85. te Loo DM, Monnens LA, van Der Velden TJ, Vermeer MA, Preyers F, Demacker PN, van Den Heuvel LP, van Hinsbergh VW. Binding and transfer of verocytotoxin by polymorphonuclear leukocytes in hemolytic uremic syn-drome. *Blood* 2000;95:3396–402.

86. Obrig TG, Louise CB, Lingwood CA, Boyd B, Barley-Maloney L, Daniel TO. Endothelial heterogeneity in Shiga toxin receptors and responses. *J Biol Chem* 1993;268:15484–8.

87. Atkinson JP, Goodship TH. Complement factor H and the hemolytic uremic syndrome. *J Exp Med* 2007;204:1245–8.

88. Saunders RE, Abarrategui-Garrido C, Fremeaux-Bacchi V, Goicoechea de Jorge E, Goodship TH, Lopez Trascasa M, Noris M, Ponce Castro IM, Remuzzi G, Rodriguez de Cor-doba S, Sanchez-Corral P, Skerka C, Zipfel PF, Perkins SJ. The interactive Factor H-atypical hemolytic uremic syn-drome mutation database and website: update and integra-tion of membrane cofactor protein and Factor I mutations with structural models. *Hum Mutat* 2007;28:222–34.

89. Olie KH, Goodship TH, Verlaak R, Florquin S, Groothoff JW, Strain L, Weening JJ, Davin JC. Posttransplantation cytomegalovirus-induced recurrence of atypical hemolytic uremic syndrome associated with a factor H mutation: successful treatment with intensive plasma exchanges and ganciclovir. *Am J Kidney Dis* 2005;45:e12–15.

90. Esparza-Gordillo J, Jorge EG, Garrido CA, Carreras L, Lopez-Trascasa M, Sanchez-Corral P, de Cordoba SR. Insights into hemolytic uremic syndrome: segregation of three independent predisposition factors in a large, multiple affected pedigree. *Mol Immunol* 2006;43:1769–75.

91. Fremeaux-Bacchi V, Kemp EJ, Goodship JA, Dragon-Durey MA, Strain L, Loirat C, Deng HW, Goodship TH. The development of atypical haemolytic-uraemic syndrome is influenced by susceptibility factors in factor H and membrane cofactor protein: evidence from two independent cohorts. *J Med Genet* 2005;42:852–6.

92. Goicoechea de Jorge E, Harris CL, Esparza-Gordillo J, Carreras L, Arranz EA, Garrido CA, Lopez-Trascasa M, Sanchez-Corral P, Morgan BP, Rodriguez de Cordoba S. Gain-of-function mutations in complement factor B are associated with atypical hemolytic uremic syndrome. *Proc Natl Acad Sci USA* 2007;104:240–5.

93. Dragon-Durey MA, Loirat C, Cloarec S, Macher MA, Blouin J, Nivet H, Weiss L, Fridman WH, Fremeaux-Bacchi V. Anti-Factor H autoantibodies associated with atypical hemolytic uremic syndrome. *J Am Soc Nephrol* 2005;16:555–63.

94. Caprioli J, Noris M, Brioschi S, Pianetti G, Castelletti F, Bettinaglio P, Mele C, Bresin E, Cassis L, Gamba S, Porrati F, Bucchioni S, Monteferrante G, Fang CJ, Liszewski MK, Kavanagh D, Atkinson JP, Remuzzi G. Genetics of HUS: the impact of MCP, CFH, and IF mutations on clinical presentation, response to treatment, and outcome. *Blood* 2006;108:1267–79.

95. Klein PJ, Bulla M, Newman RA, Muller P, Uhlenbruck G, Schaefer HE, Kruger G, Fisher R. Thomsen-Friedenreich antigen in haemolytic-uraemic syndrome. *Lancet* 1977;2:1024–5.

96. Copelovitch L, Kaplan BS. Streptococcus pneumoniae-associated hemolytic uremic syndrome. *Pediatr Nephrol* 2008;23:1951–6.

97. Antignac C, Gubler MC, Leverger G, Broyer M, Habib R. Delayed renal failure with extensive mesangiolysis following bone marrow transplantation. *Kidney Int* 1989;35:1336–44.

98. Siami K, Kojouri K, Swisher KK, Selby GB, George JN, Laszik ZG. Thrombotic microangiopathy after allogeneic hematopoietic stem cell transplantation: an autopsy study. *Transplantation* 2008;85:22–28.

99. Alpers CE. Light at the end of the TUNEL: HIV-associated thrombotic microangiopathy. *Kidney Int* 2003;63:385–396.

100. Rieger M, Mannucci PM, Kremer Hovinga JA, Herzog A, Gerstenbauer G, Konetschny C, Zimmermann K, Scharrer I, Peyvandi F, Galbusera M, Remuzzi G, Bohm M, Plaimauer B, Lammle B, Scheiflinger F. ADAMTS13 autoantibodies in patients with thrombotic microangiopathies and other immunomediated diseases. *Blood* 2005;106:1262–7.

101. Zheng XL, Sadler JE. Pathogenesis of thrombotic microangiopathies. *Annu Rev Pathol* 2008;3:249–77.

102. Loirat C, Veyradier A, Girma JP, Ribba AS, Meyer D. Thrombotic thrombocytopenic purpura associated with von Willebrand factor-cleaving protease (ADAMTS13) deficiency in children. *Semin Thromb Hemost* 2006;32:90–7.

103. Lammle B, Kremer Hovinga JA, George JN. Acquired thrombotic thrombocytopenic purpura: ADAMTS13 activity, anti-ADAMTS13 autoantibodies and risk of recurrent disease. *Haematologica* 2008;93:172–7.

104. Uchida T, Wada H, Mizutani M, Iwashita M, Ishihara H, Shibano T, Suzuki M, Matsubara Y, Soejima K, Matsumoto M, Fujimura Y, Ikeda Y, Murata M. Identification of novel mutations in ADAMTS13 in an adult patient with congenital thrombotic thrombocytopenic purpura. *Blood* 2004;104:2081–3.

105. Furlan M, Lammle B. Aetiology and pathogenesis of thrombotic thrombocytopenic purpura and haemolytic uraemic syndrome: the role of von Willebrand factor-cleaving protease. *Best Pract Res Clin Haematol* 2001;14:437–54.

106. Moake JL. Thrombotic microangiopathies. *N Engl J Med* 2002;347:589–600.

107. Vesely SK, George JN, Lammle B, Studt JD, Alberio L, El-Harake MA, Raskob GE. ADAMTS13 activity in thrombotic thrombocytopenic purpura-hemolytic uremic syndrome: relation to presenting features and clinical outcomes in a prospective cohort of 142 patients. *Blood* 2003;102:60–68.

108. Nolasco LH, Turner NA, Bernardo A, Tao Z, Cleary TG, Dong JF, Moake JL. Hemolytic uremic syndrome-associated Shiga toxins promote endothelial-cell secretion and impair ADAMTS13 cleavage of unusually large von Willebrand factor multimers. *Blood* 2005;106:4199–209.

109. Espinosa G, Bucciarelli S, Cervera R, Gomez-Puerta JA, Font J. Laboratory studies on pathophysiology of the catastrophic antiphospholipid syndrome. *Autoimmun Rev* 2006;6:68–71.

110. Safa O, Esmon CT, Esmon NL. Inhibition of APC anticoagulant activity on oxidized phospholipid by anti-{beta}2-glycoprotein I monoclonal antibodies. *Blood* 2005;106:1629–35.

111. Venkatesha S, Toporsian M, Lam C, Hanai J, Mammoto T, Kim YM, Bdolah Y, Lim KH, Yuan HT, Libermann TA, Stillman IE, Roberts D, D'Amore PA, Epstein FH, Sellke FW, Romero R, Sukhatme VP, Letarte M, Karumanchi SA. Soluble endoglin contributes to the pathogenesis of preeclampsia. *Nat Med* 2006;12:642–9.

112. Levine RJ, Maynard SE, Qian C, Lim KH, England LJ, Yu KF, Schisterman EF, Thadhani R, Sachs BP, Epstein FH, Sibai BM, Sukhatme VP, Karumanchi SA. Circulating angiogenic factors and the risk of preeclampsia. *N Engl J Med* 2004;350:672–83.

113. Garovic VD, Wagner SJ, Petrovic LM, Gray CE, Hall P, Sugimoto H, Kalluri R, Grande JP. Glomerular expression of nephrin and synaptopodin, but not podocin, is decreased in kidney sections from women with preeclampsia. *Nephrol Dial Transplant* 2007;22:1136–43.

114. Roncone D, Satoskar A, Nadasdy T, Monk JP, Rovin BH. Proteinuria in a patient receiving anti-VEGF therapy for

metastatic renal cell carcinoma. *Nat Clin Pract Nephrol* 2007;3:287–93.

115. Eremina V, Jefferson JA, Kowalewska J, Hochster H, Haas M, Weisstuch J, Richardson C, Kopp JB, Kabir MG, Backx PH, Gerber HP, Ferrara N, Barisoni L, Alpers CE, Quaggin SE: VEGF inhibition and renal thrombotic microangiopathy. *N Engl J Med* 2008;358:1129–36.

116. Lee S, Sharma K. The pathogenesis of fibrosis and renal disease in scleroderma: recent insights from glomerulosclerosis. *Curr Rheumatol Rep* 2004;6:141–8.

117. Fitzpatrick MM, Shah V, Filler G, Dillon MJ, Barratt TM. Neutrophil activation in the haemolytic uraemic syndrome: free and complexed elastase in plasma. *Pediatr Nephrol* 1992;6:50–3.

118. Walters MD, Matthei IU, Kay R, Dillon MJ, Barratt TM. The polymorphonuclear leucocyte count in childhood haemolytic uraemic syndrome. *Pediatr Nephrol* 1989;3:130–4.

119. Kelton JG, Moore JC, Warkentin TE, Hayward CP. Isolation and characterization of cysteine proteinase in thrombotic thrombocytopenic purpura. *Br J Haematol* 1996;93:421–6.

120. Levin M, Stroobant P, Walters MD, Cheng DJ, Waterfield MD, Barratt TM. Platelet-derived growth factors as possible mediators of vascular proliferation in the sporadic haemolytic uraemic syndrome. *Lancet* 1986;2:830–3.

121. Kobayashi M, Wada H, Wakita Y, Shimura M, Nakase T, Hiyoyama K, Nagaya S, Minami N, Nakano T, Shiku H. Decreased plasma tissue factor pathway inhibitor levels in patients with thrombotic thrombocytopenic purpura. *Thromb Haemost* 1995;73:10–14.

122. Remuzzi G, Ruggenenti P. The hemolytic uremic syndrome. *Kidney Int* 1995;48:2–19.

123. Gianviti A, Tozzi AE, De Petris L, Caprioli A, Rava L, Edefonti A, Ardissino G, Montini G, Zacchello G, Ferretti A, Pecoraro C, De Palo T, Caringella A, Gaido M, Coppo R, Perfumo F, Miglietti N, Ratsche I, Penza R, Capasso G, Maringhini S, Li Volti S, Setzu C, Pennesi M, Bettinelli A, Peratoner L, Pela I, Salvaggio E, Lama G, Maffei S, Rizzoni G. Risk factors for poor renal prognosis in children with hemolytic uremic syndrome. *Pediatr Nephrol* 2003;18:1229–35.

124. Garg AX, Suri RS, Barrowman N, Rehman F, Matsell D, Rosas-Arellano MP, Salvadori M, Haynes RB, Clark WF. Long-term renal prognosis of diarrhea-associated hemolytic uremic syndrome: a systematic review, meta-analysis, and meta-regression. *JAMA* 2003;290:1360–70.

125. Nathoo KJ, Porteous JE, Siziya S, Wellington M, Mason E. Predictors of mortality in children hospitalized with dysentery in Harare, Zimbabwe. *Cent Afr J Med* 1998;44:272–6.

126. Houdouin V, Doit C, Mariani P, Brahimi N, Loirat C, Bourrillon A, Bingen E. A pediatric cluster of Shigella dysenteriae serotype 1 diarrhea with hemolytic uremic syndrome in 2 families from France. *Clin Infect Dis* 2004;38:e96–9.

127. Bennish ML, Khan WA, Begum M, Bridges EA, Ahmed S, Saha D, Salam MA, Acheson D, Ryan ET. Low risk of hemolytic uremic syndrome after early effective antimicrobial therapy for Shigella dysenteriae type 1 infection in Bangladesh. *Clin Infect Dis* 2006;42:356–62.

128. Fitzpatrick MM, Walters MD, Trompeter RS, Dillon MJ, Barratt TM. Atypical (non-diarrhea-associated) hemolytic-uremic syndrome in childhood. *J Pediatr* 1993;122:532–7.

129. George JN. Congenital thrombotic thrombocytopenic purpura: Lessons for recognition and management of rare syndromes. *Pediatr Blood Cancer* 2008;50:947–8.

130. Ahmed S, Siddiqui RK, Siddiqui AK, Zaidi SA, Cervia J. HIV associated thrombotic microangiopathy. *Postgrad Med J* 2002;78:520–5.

131. Novitzky N, Thomson J, Abrahams L, du Toit C, McDonald A. Thrombotic thrombocytopenic purpura in patients with retroviral infection is highly responsive to plasma infusion therapy. *Br J Haematol* 2005;128:373–9.

132. Mayes MD, Lacey JV, Jr., Beebe-Dimmer J, Gillespie BW, Cooper B, Laing TJ, Schottenfeld D. Prevalence, incidence, survival, and disease characteristics of systemic sclerosis in a large US population. *Arthritis Rheum* 2003;48:2246–55.

133. Ferri C, Valentini G, Cozzi F, Sebastiani M, Michelassi C, La Montagna G, Bullo A, Cazzato M, Tirri E, Storino F, Giuggioli D, Cuomo G, Rosada M, Bombardieri S, Todesco S, Tirri G. Systemic sclerosis: demographic, clinical, and serologic features and survival in 1,012 Italian patients. *Medicine (Baltimore)* 2002;81:139–53.

134. Steen VD, Medsger TA, Jr. Long-term outcomes of scleroderma renal crisis. *Ann Intern Med* 2000;133:600–3.

135. Srivastava RN, Moudgil A, Bagga A, Vasudev AS. Hemolytic uremic syndrome in children in northern India. *Pediatr Nephrol* 1991;5:284–8.

CHAPTER 10

Renal Diseases Associated with Hematopoietic Disorders or Organized Deposits

Guillermo A. Herrera, MD

INTRODUCTION

A number of hematopoietic disorders are associated with renal manifestations. This chapter addresses those conditions associated with an underlying plasma cell dyscrasia and sickle cell disease. The pathologic spectrum of renal alterations seen in patients with underlying plasma cell dyscrasias (dysproteinemias) has been expanded considerably in the last two decades and exciting research advances have provided a much better understanding of the pathogenesis of these disorders. Waldenstrom macroglobulinemia is associated with a somewhat unique repertoire of pathological renal manifestations, and will be

discussed separately from the other plasma cell dyscrasia-associated renal disorders.

In addition, in the chapter, there are a number of other conditions that are associated with organized deposits or in their differential diagnosis. These conditions are quite heterogeneous as a group and the primary unifying aspect to consider them together in this chapter is that they present morphologically with so-called organized deposits or "unusual" ultrastructural findings. These include fibrillary, cryoglobulinemic, immunotactoid, fibronectin, collagenofibrotic, and nail-patella syndrome-associated glomerulopathies. Some of these conditions are rare. Although the ultrastructural findings are crucial in the diagnosis of many of these diseases, overall immunomorphologic findings and clinicopathologic correlates are essential to properly conceptualize and accurately diagnose these disorders, so that proper therapeutic interventions and adequate patients' management can follow. An algorithmic approach is useful to address the diagnosis of these conditions (see algorithm later). Finally, the renal pathology that occurs in patients with sickle cell-associated disorders will be discussed.

While renal pathologists may encounter patients with renal diseases associated with underlying plasma cell dyscrasias with some frequency in their practices, the great majority of the other conditions covered in this chapter are seen infrequently even in busy renal services. With newer therapies addressing molecular targets becoming available, recognition, pathologic assessment, and understanding of the pathogenesis of these disorders become extremely important.

RENAL PATHOLOGY IN PLASMA CELL DYSCRASIAS AND PARAPROTEINEMIA

Introduction

Patients with underlying plasma cell dyscrasias often develop renal manifestations. In the first large series of myeloma patients in 1975 by Kyle, 88 percent of 865 patients had proteinuria, and urinary Bence Jones proteins were noted in 49 percent of 631 patients in whom the search for the proteins was conducted. Amyloid was documented histologically in sixty-one patients with myeloma (7 percent), but it was only searched for in those patients with suggestive symptoms or findings [1]. More than thirty years later, those figures remain as today's reality.

The majority of the cases with renal manifestations are associated with alterations in the tubular interstitial compartment (70 percent) while only 30 percent develop glomerular pathology. In some instances, tubulopathic and glomerulopathic manifestations coexist [2–8]. Light and heavy chain components of the immunoglobulin molecule can be responsible and in a very small number of cases, both light and heavy chains can together be associated with the pathological manifestations. The physicochemical characteristics of the pathologic light or heavy chains are responsible for determining whether nephrotoxicity occurs and the specific pattern of damage in the kidney.

Monoclonal gammopathy of undetermined significance (MGUS) is relatively common occurring in approximately 0.15 percent of the population. MGUS is defined by a monoclonal immunoglobulin concentration in serum of 3 g/dl or less, associated with the absence of lytic bone lesions, anemia, hypercalcemia, and renal insufficiency related to the proliferation of monoclonal plasma cells that must be less than 10 percent of all cellular elements in the bone marrow aspirate/biopsy.

In large series from referral centers, it has been documented that 50 percent of the patients with a monoclonal gammopathy qualify for a diagnosis of MGUS while 15–20 percent had sufficient criteria for a diagnosis of myeloma [9]. Multiple myeloma eventually ensues in about 16 percent of patients with MGUS but it may occur many years (more than thirty years in some cases) after the initial diagnosis. MGUS is associated with progression to myeloma or a related lymphoplasmacytic condition of 1 percent per year [10,11]. It is because conversion to a full blown myeloma is not predictable that these patients must be followed in order to avoid any delays in diagnosis of overt disease.

Once any organ involvement is detected as a direct consequence of the monoclonal gammopathy, the diagnosis of MGUS is no longer tenable. A frequent indicator that transformation has taken place is the presence of renal manifestations, most often proteinuria. Renal biopsy can substantiate evidence of renal involvement, as a result of the effects of monoclonal paraproteins on any of the renal compartments. A high index of suspicion, however, is needed to detect subtle, early and unusual morphologic manifestations in the renal biopsies [12,13]; otherwise, the diagnosis may be completely missed.

Our understanding of light chain-associated diseases is far more advanced than that of heavy chain-associated disorders, primarily because the latter disorders were initially recognized less than twenty years ago when Eulitz recognized heavy chain-associated amyloidosis [14], whereas light chain deposition disease, the first light chain-associated disorder described, was first fully characterized in 1976 [15]. Some of the abnormal circulating proteins produced by the neoplastic plasma cells are highly nephrotoxic, and the amount of circulating monoclonal protein produced does not necessarily correlate with the degree of renal damage.

The pathology associated with underlying plasma cell dyscrasias will be discussed according to the main renal compartments affected in order to facilitate understanding and provide a platform to address pathogenesis. It should be clearly understood, however, that such approach is somewhat simplistic, as combinations of pathologic findings affecting more than one renal compartment occur in some cases [16–19]. The first three conditions listed below have only been documented in association with pathologic light chains, while the last two have been recognized in association with either abnormal circulating light or heavy chains. Diagnosis of heavy chain-associated glomerulopathies remains challenging, and they are likely under diagnosed at the present time. Therefore, renal manifestations are divided into the following categories:

(1) direct proximal tubular damage – acute tubulopathy (acute tubular necrosis-like), including proximal tubular lesion in Fanconi syndrome

(2) light chain cast nephropathy, also referred to as "myeloma" cast nephropathy

(3) acute tubular interstitial nephritis (inflammatory tubular interstitial nephritis) without casts

(4) light and heavy chain deposition diseases

(5) light and heavy chain-associated amyloidosis

Epidemiology and Clinical Presentation

Plasma cell dyscrasias are far more common in older individuals. Multiple myeloma can be conceptualized as the most blatant manifestation of a plasma cell dyscrasia with systemic manifestations that include punched-out bone lesions, a detectable paraprotein in the serum and/or urine and a significant population of monoclonal plasma cells in the bone marrow. Multiple myeloma represents approximately 1 percent of all malignant neoplasms, and almost 10 percent of all hematologic malignancies. Although the usual patients with a clinically detectable plasma cell dyscrasia are older than 60 years of age, due to advances in technology and increased awareness, younger patients are now being diagnosed. Overall the great majority of the patients are older than 40 years, and males are more commonly affected than females by a small percentage. Fewer than 2 percent of the patients diagnosed with myeloma are younger than 40. The incidence ranges from 1 per 100,000 individuals who are 40 to 49 years of age to 49 per 100,000 for those 80 years and older, highlighting a marked increase in incidence in older patients [20]. Typical signs and symptoms at presentation include anemia, increased serum calcium with associated thirst, fatigue and constipation, back pain, and an increase in serum creatinine (i.e., renal dysfunction).

Renal disease associated with plasma cell dyscrasias may present with various clinical manifestations including renal insufficiency or failure, proteinuria up to nephrotic range, tubular dysfunction with defects of urine acidification and concentration, and in a small number of patients, Fanconi syndrome with aminoaciduria, glucosuria, and phosphaturia occurs. Acute or chronic renal failure is commonly seen in patients with multiple myeloma, and the incidence of renal insufficiency reported in the two largest series has been 55 and 56 percent respectively [1,21]. Many of these patients have proteinuria (88 percent), mostly composed of light chains, but less than 15–25 percent of these patients develop nephrotic syndrome. In many instances, Bence Jones proteinuria can be massive. From a clinical standpoint, the determination of the presence of a circulating abnormal light or heavy chain is important, but not always possible. Approximately 80 percent of myeloma patients have a detectable monoclonal spike, and 97 percent exhibit monoclonal proteins in either serum or urine. A small number of myelomas (approximately 3 percent) are "nonsecretory"; those generally do not exhibit renal manifestations [22]. The most common causes of death in these patients are infection and complications associated with the renal damage and subsequent failure.

In a significant number of instances, detailed clinical information is not available to the pathologist examining the renal biopsy because of one of the following reasons: the clinical workup has not been performed or is incomplete; the results of the workup are pending; or the pertinent data is not communicated. Interestingly, the typical clinical presentation of plasma cell dyscrasias has shifted from overt symptoms to indolent or localized disease, making the role of the pathologist more critical. Renal pathologists are often the ones who diagnose the underlying plasma cell disorder by identifying evidence of renal damage as a consequence of the pathologic manifestations of light or heavy chains. It is because the findings in the bone marrow biopsy/aspirate may be subtle in some of these cases that immunohistochemical stains or flow cytometric determinations for kappa and lambda light chains may be indicated to identify a clone of plasma cells, even when the overall number of plasma cells is within the acceptable normal range and no atypical plasma cells or sheets are present.

The range of renal pathological alterations associated with an underlying plasma cell dyscrasia is varied and the circulating plasma cell products may affect any, or all of the renal compartments. Not all patients with plasma cell dyscrasias develop renal manifestations. Approximately 85 percent of patients with plasma cell dyscrasias have renal involvement as a direct consequence of the pathologic effect of light or heavy chains produced by the neoplastic plasma cells. In these patients, renal damage occurs in the tubular interstitial compartment in approximately 70 percent of the patients, and the remaining 30 percent develop glomerular manifestations [5]. The corresponding pathologic light chains are referred to as tubulopathic and glomerulopathic, respectively (Figure 10.1). In some cases, more than one renal compartment is involved.

Only glomerular manifestations have been associated with nephrotoxic heavy chains. Although little basic research has been conducted, it is believed that their pathogenic mechanisms may be quite similar to those of the corresponding light chain-associated disorders, as the final results are morphologically virtually identical. The schematic representation shown in Figure 10.1 highlights the main pathogenetic mechanisms involved in the various disease processes associated with light chain-associated nephropathies which will be discussed later in the chapter.

In the autopsy series of patients dying with myeloma, the most commonly found renal lesion is light chain cast nephropathy [23–25]. In the biopsy series, AL-amyloidosis and light chain cast nephropathy represent the two most common lesions, but this may be a selection bias reflecting the group of patients that are more frequently biopsied. Presently, the diagnosis of an underlying plasma cell dyscrasia often follows the evaluation of a renal biopsy from a patient who presents with renal dysfunction, failure or proteinuria, and monotypical deposition of light or heavy chains are identified in the renal parenchyma, and are responsible for the renal pathology.

Infiltration of the renal parenchyma by neoplastic plasma cells occurs uncommonly. It is quite unusual that in a renal biopsy such plasmacytic infiltration is determined to be the reason for the renal dysfunction. It is most often seen in autopsy specimens where small aggregates of such plasma cells can be seen in focal interstitial areas forming small nodules and replacing normal renal parenchyma [25]. In the great majority of the cases, most of the renal parenchyma is uninvolved, so that clinical renal manifestations are generally lacking in association with this type of pathology.

Approach to Interpretation of Pathologic Findings

Acute Tubulopathy (Acute Tubular Necrosis)

Clinical Presentation. These patients classically present with renal insufficiency, or renal failure. Interestingly, some cases with tubular changes noted on microscopic evaluation, fail to reveal significant clinical manifestations [5]. A group of these patients present with aminoaciduria, glucosuria, and phosphaturia (Fanconi syndrome) [26–28]. Patients with Fanconi syndrome are typically adults who exhibit low-grade proteinuria, renal insufficiency, and osteomalacia. Abnormal heavy chains have not been linked to proximal tubular damage. Only approximately half of these patients have a diagnosis of plasma cell dyscrasia established prior to the renal biopsy.

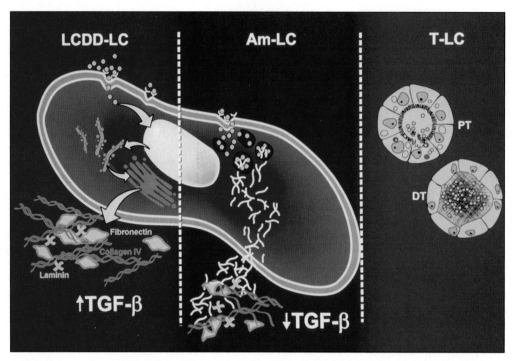

FIGURE 10.1: *Schematic representation of the various manifestations of light chain-associated renal disease. The panel on the left illustrates LCDD, emphasizing the increase in mesangial matrix that is characteristic of this disorder. The extracellular matrix accumulation is produced by the mesangial cells due to increased TGF-β secretion. In contrast, the middle panel illustrates the replacement of the normal mesangial matrix by amyloid fibrils produced intracellularly in mesangial cells and extruded into the matrix. TGF-β is decreased in amyloidosis, impairing the repair of the damaged mesangium. The right panel shows the two typical tubulopathic manifestations of light chains with proximal tubular damage shown on top, and light chain cast nephropathy at the bottom. The schematic drawing of the cell in the left and middle panels represents a mesangial cell. LCDD-LC, light chain deposition disease; Am-LC, light chain amylodosis; T-LC, light chain tubulopathy; PT, proximal tubule; DT, distal tubule.*

Gross Pathology. The gross appearance of the kidneys of patients with this condition is similar to that seen in acute tubular necrosis. Typically, the kidneys are enlarged and swollen and cortical areas appear pale. The corticomedullary junction becomes less distinct. The kidney weight in these cases is increased.

Light Microscopy. The main finding in these patients is characterized by variable degrees of proximal tubular damage, some associated with minor alterations in the proximal tubules (subtle vacuolization), and other cases with severe overt manifestations of proximal tubular damage, including apical blebing, desquamation, fragmentation, and frank necrosis (Figure 10.2) [5,13]. In some instances, mitotic figures are present, indicating ongoing regeneration. In some cases with clinical Fanconi syndrome, the cytoplasm of the damaged proximal tubular cells in the hematoxylin and eosin shows irregularly shaped empty spaces with sharp angles (Figure 10.3), with the spaces corresponding to cytoplasmic inclusions [26]. In rare instances, the crystals are readily apparent in the hematoxylin and eosin-stained sections [19]. Interstitial edema may be seen. Interstitial fibrosis is not part of this lesion initially, but repeated damage to the tubules may result in irreversible interstitial damage characterized by the presence of variably pronounced fibrosis. Interstitial inflammation is generally absent, or minimal, if present. Glomeruli and vasculature are normal.

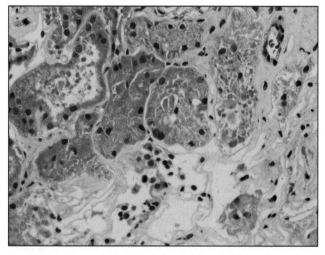

FIGURE 10.2: *Acute tubulopathy, monotypical λ light chain-associated. Hematoxylin and eosin. ×500. Marked alterations in proximal tubules, including apical cytoplasmic blebbing, desquamation, and fragmentation in proximal tubular cells.*

Immunofluorescene Microscopy. Granular to needle shaped fluorescence staining for monoclonal light chains may be detected in the cytoplasm of proximal tubular cells [12,13].

Staining for immunoglobulins, complement components, albumin, and fibrinogen are all negative. Likewise, staining for the other nonpertinent light chain is generally entirely negative. However, there may be some staining for the non-

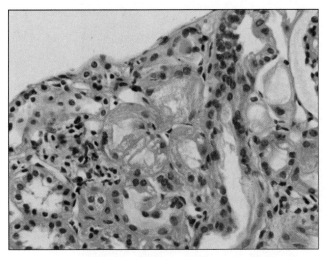

FIGURE 10.3: *Proximal tubular alterations in Fanconi syndrome. Hematoxylin and eosin. × 500. The cytoplasm of some proximal tubular cells exhibits empty spaces with angulated, sharp edges.*

pertinent light chain in the cytoplasm of the proximal tubular cells, although the intensity is generally much less. In a subset of these patients, those with Fanconi syndrome, κ positive needle-shaped structures may be primarily found in the cytoplasm of the proximal tubular cells [7]. It should be noted that in the majority of the cases with proximal tubulopathy, this finding is absent or subtle at the light microscopic level, requiring a high index of suspicion. Crystalline inclusions have also been found in visceral epithelial, endothelial and mesangial cells, and histiocytic cells in the interstitium, but much less frequently than in proximal tubular cells in these cases [29]. Lymphoplasmacytic cells may also exhibit similar cytoplasmic crystals in the bone marrow, or other locations where they may be present. However, crystallization is not a constant feature of Fanconi's syndrome [29].

Electron Microscopy. The most striking changes are seen by electron microscopy. The proximal tubules show prominent cytoplasmic alterations including apical blebbing, desquamation, fragmentation, vacuolization, and segmental loss of microvillous borders (Figures 10.4 and 10.5). The proximal tubular cells are filled with lysosomes containing monoclonal light chains (Figures 10.4 to 10.6). This can be confirmed by using immunogold labeling techniques (Figures 10.5 and 10.6) [12,13]. Some of the lysosomes are quite large and irregularly shaped (Figure 10.5) [13]. In some instances, the lysosomes are

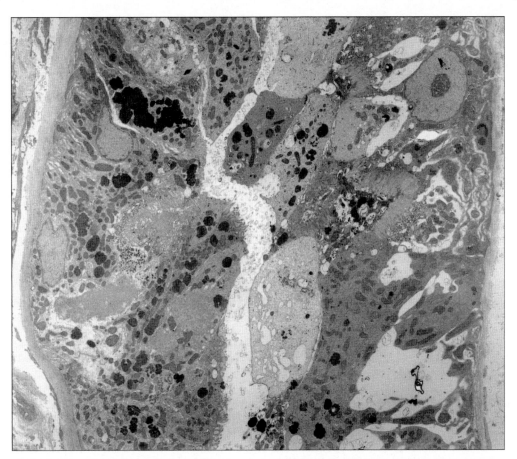

FIGURE 10.4: *Proximal tubular alterations in acute tubulopathy. Transmission electron microscopy. Uranyl acetate and lead citrate. × 7,500. Ultrastructural correlates to Figure 10.2. Markedly enlarged lysosomes with atypical shapes are noted in damaged proximal tubular cells. The lysosomal system appears quite prominent.*

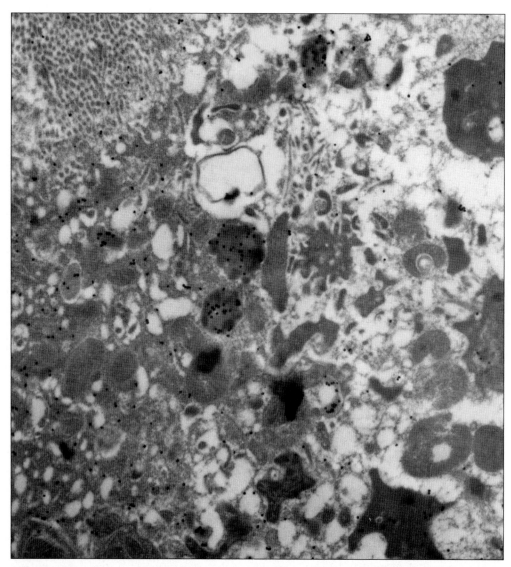

FIGURE 10.5: *Acute tubulopathy. Transmission electron microscopy. Immunogold labeling for κ light chains. Gold particles: 10 nm. Uranyl acetate and lead citrate. × 17 500. Gold particles label the lysosomes, including an atypical form noted at the bottom of the figure indicating the presence of monotypical kappa light chains in the lysosomes. Also, note the cytoplasmic alterations in the proximal tubular cell.*

so prominent that the other few organelles present are displaced toward the basolateral side (Figure 10.6) [5,13]. The patients with Fanconi syndrome typically display crystalline to fibrillary tubular geometric and angulated structures in the cytoplasm of proximal tubular cells, the morphologic hallmark of this condition (Figure 10.7). The crystals are generally rod-shaped or rectangular in shape with sharp angles. The crystalline inclusions have a lattice configuration with a periodicity of 8 to 11 nm. Most cases are first identified when the ultrastructural evaluation takes place. Ultrastructural labeling can be used to confirm monoclonality (κ almost exclusively) in the cytoplasmic inclusions (Figure 10.8) [5,13].

Differential Diagnosis. Other causes of acute tubular necrosis, especially as a result of nephrotoxins, which selectively affect the proximal tubules, need to be excluded. The lysosomal

prominence in the proximal tubular cells is not specific for light chain-induced tubular damage. Ultrastructural immunolabeling can provide definitive evidence of the causative role of the tubulopathic light chains in this lesion by demonstrating the monoclonal light chains within the crystalline inclusions. Unfortunately, this technique is not usually used for diagnostic purposes, and has been only mastered in selected electron microscopy laboratories. The hematological workup will often suffice to provide the clinical support required for establishing the suspected diagnosis. Demonstration of light chain restriction by immunofluorescence, in the proper clinicopathologic setting, is also diagnostic, and if crystalline structures can be discerned, a diagnosis of Fanconi syndrome can be strongly suspected. Negative staining for light chains does not exclude this lesion, as the commercially available antibodies may not be able to detect the abnormal light

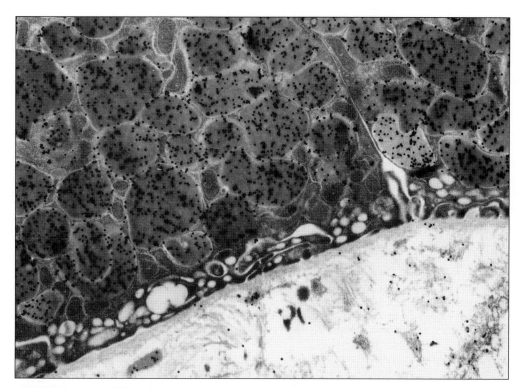

FIGURE 10.6: *Acute tubulopathy. Transmission electron microscopy. Immunogold labeling for λ light chains. Gold particles: 10 nm. Uranyl acetate and lead citrate. ×18,500. Proximal tubular cell filled with lysosomes which are intensely labeled for λ light chains. The few organelles that remain in the tubular cell are displaced toward the basolateral side.*

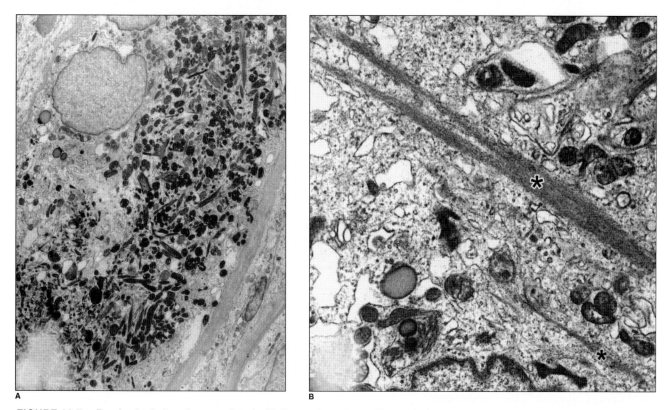

FIGURE 10.7: *Proximal tubulopathy associated with Fanconi syndrome. Transmission electron microscopy. Uranyl acetate and lead citrate. A: ×3,500; B: ×8,500. A: Fibrillary inclusions in the cytoplasm of proximal tubular cells; B: Note fibrillary appearance of the inclusions (*.)*

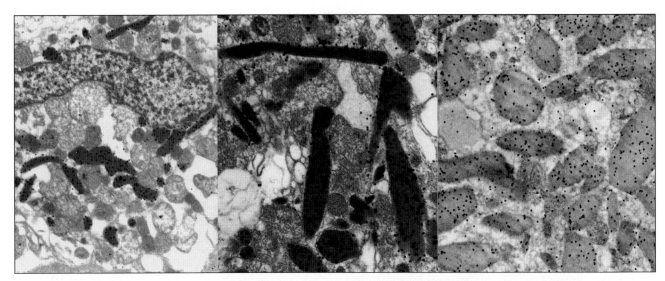

FIGURE 10.8: *Different types of cytoplasmic inclusions in Fanconi syndrome. Transmission electron microscopy. Immunogold labeling for k light chains. Left: ×6,500; middle: ×17,500; right: ×15,000. Two different ultrastructural appearances for inclusions (same in left and middle panels) that may be found in patients with acute tubulopathy associated with Fanconi syndrome. All inclusions are labeled intensely for κ light chains (gold particles on top of cytoplasmic inclusions.)*

chains present in the proximal tubules or other cellular elements, giving a false-negative result. The finding of intracytoplasmic crystals with light chain restriction (virtually exclusively κ) is diagnostic of Fanconi syndrome-associated nephropathy.

Clinical Course, Prognosis, Treatment, and Clinical Correlation. If the delivery of abnormal light chains to the tubules can be stopped, proximal tubular regeneration would occur, and renal function can be reestablished [5]. Unfortunately, it is generally not easy to effectively treat these patients' plasma cell dyscrasias to control the disease process. Treatment of the plasma cell disorder will however in most cases ameliorate the damage by reducing the overall concentration of light chains delivered to the kidneys. Therefore, chemotherapy to control the underlying plasma cell disorder is of paramount importance in the management of these cases. It is important to realize that this lesion is entirely reversible [5,13]. In some cases, proximal tubular damage is combined with other plasma cell dyscrasia-associated tubular interstitial or glomerular manifestations, creating additional difficulties in treatment. In cases of Fanconi syndrome, the process is usually indolent, and it may take years after the diagnostic finding in the renal biopsy for the patient to manifest definitive evidence of an underlying plasma cell dyscrasia. In one reported case, it took sixteen years for the plasma cell disorder to become evident [30]. While approximately 50 percent of patients with proximal tubulopathy without crystals are found to have underlying myeloma, a minority of those with Fanconi syndrome meet minimal criteria for a diagnosis of myeloma at the time of diagnosis. Information regarding long-term treatment and follow-up of these patients is not available, except that those with Fanconi syndrome generally exhibit a slow, smoldering clinical course, but eventually develop overt myeloma [30].

Light Chain ("Myeloma") Cast Nephropathy

Clinical Presentation. This is the most common renal manifestation associated with an underlying plasma cell dyscrasia in

autopsy series [24,25]. It is because these patients generally present with significant renal insufficiency or renal failure that they become excellent candidates for renal biopsy. In a study of renal biopsies from patients older than 60 years with unexpected acute renal failure, 5.9 percent had light chain cast nephropathy. Forty percent of these patients had undiagnosed myeloma at the time the renal biopsy was performed [31]. This pattern of nephron injury has not been described in association with heavy chain disorders.

Gross Pathology. No specific macroscopic findings have been described in the kidneys of patients with light chain (myeloma) cast nephropathy. In one autopsy series, the mean kidney weight was 166 g , but in one-third of the cases the kidneys were enlarged (more than 180 g) [23]. Subcapsular granularity and petechiae were noted in some of the kidneys [23], but these findings are likely vascular in origin rather than related to the obstructive nephron process. In another autopsy study, the average weight of the kidneys was 120 g and they showed findings most consistent with vascular disease [25].

Light Microscopy. The distal nephron is obstructed with casts, which contain the abnormal circulating light chains (Figures 10.9 and 10.10). The light chain interacts with Tamm-Horsfall protein which is secreted by the distal convoluted tubules [5,7,12]. The casts are generally variably eosinophilic on H&E stain, lamellated or fractured making them appear "brittle" and often contain neutrophils (Figure 10.9). Frequently surrounding the casts, there are reactive tubular cells. Multinucleated giant cells, of macrophage/histiocytic origin [32], are sometimes seen surrounding the distal tubular casts (Figure 10.10). The large casts may break through the nearby TBM with intense inflammatory reaction, with or without multinucleated cells [5]. Some casts may be Congo red positive. Variable degrees of interstitial inflammation, often including polymorphonuclear cells and at times eosinophiles, can be seen in association with the tubules, mostly distal containing the casts and tubules in

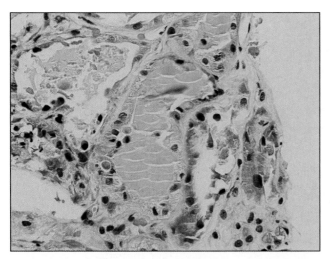

FIGURE 10.9: *Light chain cast nephropathy. Hematoxylin and eosin. ×500. Prominent fracture planes are shown in the distal nephron casts. The tubular cells show mild reactive changes. Also, note inflammatory cells associated with and surrounding casts.*

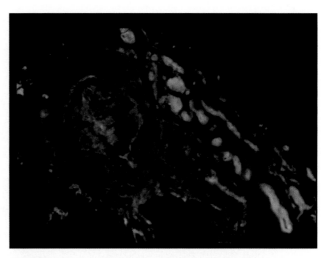

FIGURE 10.11: *Light chain cast nephropathy. Direct immunofluorescence stain for K light chain. Fluorescein isothiocyanate. ×500. Distal nephrons are full of kappa containing casts. Stain for λ light chains was negative.*

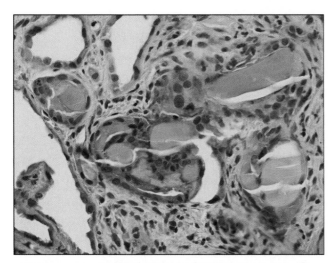

FIGURE 10.10: *Light chain cast nephropathy. Hematoxylin and eosin. ×500. Reactive tubular epithelial cells admixed with multinucleated giant cells are apparent. Fracture planes only noticeable in some of the casts.*

the immediate vicinity. Focal tubulitis may be present as well. The inflammatory cells include lymphocytes, eosinophiles, polymorphonuclear, and plasma cells [33]. In some cases, the casts contain crystals [5]. The degree of interstitial fibrosis does not correlate well with the extent of cast formation. Glomeruli and vasculature are normal in this condition.

Immunofluorescence Microscopy. The distal tubular obstruction by casts can be either acute or chronic. If acute, there is a great chance that the pertinent light chain can be detected as the sole light chain in association with the casts (Figure 10.11) [5,7]. If the casts have remained in place for prolonged periods of time, trapping of the other light chain is often noted, making it impossible at times to demonstrate monoclonality in the casts. It is because tubular casts in general

trap both kappa and lambda light chains that there may be difficulties in making a determination that the casts are monoclonal. In some of these cases, although staining for both light chains is present, one type of light chain exceeds the other in intensity, and this finding is also most compatible with the diagnosis [5,7]. Staining for IgM and IgA may be noted in the casts as most casts generally stain for these immunoreactants. Staining for the other immunoglobulins, complement, fibrinogen, and albumin is generally negative in all renal compartments.

Electron Microscopy. Glomeruli and vasculature are unremarkable. The tubular casts generally identified in distal nephrons can vary in ultrastructural appearance. Some of the casts are markedly electron-dense and appear fragmented with electron-dense material corresponding to light chains tightly apposed exhibiting a jig-zag puzzle-like type of arrangement (Figure 10.12). Other casts contain granular to grainy or flocculent material (Figure 10.13) [34]. Some myeloma casts contain abundant fibrillary material, in some instances arranged in a random fashion, mimicking amyloid. Ultrastructural labeling can definitely label the cast contents for the pertinent light chain [5], providing crucial evidence for a definitive diagnosis, especially if the immunofluorescence findings are equivocal. However, ultrastructural labeling is not needed for diagnosis in the great majority of the cases. When needle-shaped crystals are present in the casts, the ultrastructural appearance is rather unique and specific, also permitting an unequivocal diagnosis (Figure 10.14) [5]. Enlarged tubular epithelial cells, often showing evidence of damage, are frequently present surrounding the casts, especially if the casts have extended to proximal tubules as a result of their size. Cellular debris from proximal tubular cell damage may be found in the distal nephron casts.

Differential Diagnosis. At times, the morphology of the tubular casts is not classical, and it may be a challenge to differentiate them from other casts. A careful correlation with immunofluorescence findings is then indicated. If either light chain monotypicality

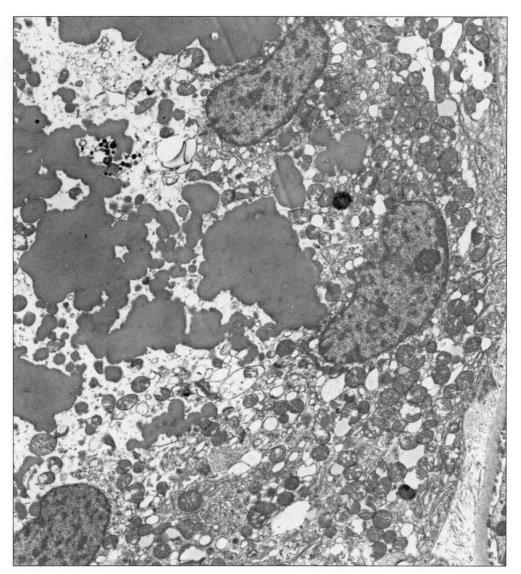

FIGURE 10.12: *Light chain cast nephropathy. Transmission electron microscopy. Uranyl acetate and lead citrate. ×8,500. Markedly electron-dense cast in collecting duct. Note the fragmented appearance of the cast and the jig-zag puzzle arrangement of its fragments. This is characteristic of "myeloma" casts.*

or preponderance of one type of light chain is demonstrated, the diagnosis is strengthened, and clinical correlation may provide confirmation of the diagnosis. In a subset of patients taking Rifampin, there is light chain proteinuria and when casts are found, the histological picture may resemble myeloma cast nephropathy [35]. The presence of crystals within tubular casts should strongly suggest a diagnosis of light chain cast nephropathy, but drugs like Indinavir (an antiretrovirus therapeutic agent) rarely results in a crystalline cast formation [36]. If light chain restriction can be demonstrated in association with the crystals, then the diagnosis of light chain cast nephropathy can be made unequivocally. Unfortunately, this is only possible in some cases.

Clinical Course, Prognosis, Treatment, and Clinical Correlations. Many of these patients require dialysis when they present acute renal failure. The purpose of the treatment is twofold: to disrupt and dissolve existing casts, and to prevent the formation of additional casts. Cysteamine, a reducing agent, and Dimethyl sulfoxide may be used to dissolve existing casts, and Colchicine, promoted as an agent to prevent new cast formation by removing carbohydrate moieties from the Tamm-Horsfall protein, but in the clinical arena, this has proven to be ineffective. Treating the underlying plasma cell dyscrasia by using an aggressive chemotherapeutic protocol to decrease the amount of circulating tubulopathic light chains represents the most fundamental component of the therapy for light chain cast nephropathy [37]. Hydration is also key to the treatment of this disorder. Other measures include alkalinization of the urine which aims at facilitating the solubility of the light chains, and in a select group of cases, generally the younger patients, plasmapheresis [38], although the data originating from three clinical trials have shown that plasmapheresis has no proven role to treat this condition [39]. Renal function improves in about 54 percent of the patients with the above measures; however,

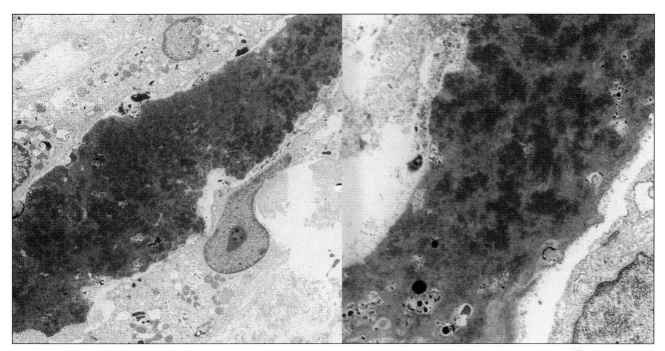

FIGURE 10.13: *Light chain cast nephropathy. Transmission electron microscopy. Uranyl acetate and lead citrate. Left: ×3,500; right: ×9,500. Cast with different appearance than the one illustrated in Figure 12. Granular material with different electron densities and cell fragments are present within the cast. These findings are present in some "myeloma" casts, but are not specific.*

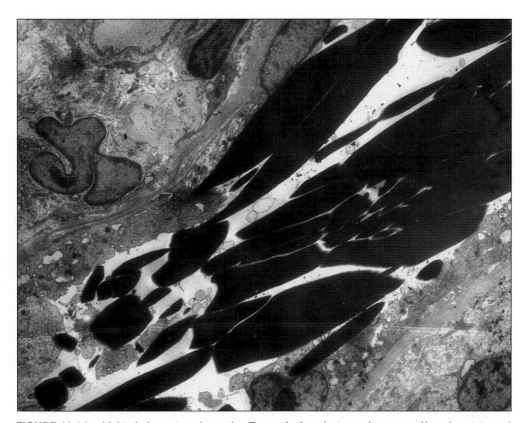

FIGURE 10.14: *Light chain cast nephropathy. Transmission electron microscopy. Uranyl acetate and lead citrate. ×8,500. Needle-shaped electron-dense crystals in a cast present in a collecting duct.*

progressive loss of renal function eventually occurs in most patients. The overall median survival for patients with this condition, and renal failure has been reported to be from 13 months to 20–30 months with a five-year survival rate of 18–27 percent [1,20,21]. Renal transplantation has not been considered a viable treatment modality for most patients with light chain cast nephropathy due to their poor prognosis. It has only been used selectively in a few patients with stable disease who were without extrarenal manifestations for more than one year.

Acute Tubular Interstitial Nephritis

Clinical Presentation. This is a rather newly recognized morphologic manifestation of renal involvement in plasma cell dyscrasias [40]. Therefore, the details regarding natural history of this condition are not well documented. This lesion has not been described in association with abnormal heavy chains. Conceptually speaking, this pattern may be considered a manifestation of light chain deposition disease restricted to the tubular interstitial compartment [41].

Gross Pathology. In an autopsy series, the kidneys of two patients with this condition showed normal weight, and no specific gross findings that could be linked to this disorder [25].

Light Microscopy. The findings in this condition are restricted to the tubular interstitial compartment. The glomeruli and vasculature are normal. In the interstitium, there is a variably prominent inflammatory infiltrate composed of lymphocytes, plasma cells, and occasionally, eosinophiles [40]. Acute inflammatory cells are rare in this condition, but a few may be seen as well. Tubulitis is seen generally in multifocal areas, (Figure 10.15) but in some cases may be localized to small interstitial areas. No casts of the type seen in light chain cast nephropathy are present and no multinucleated giant cells noted.

Immunofluorescence Microscopy/Immunohistochemistry. Demonstration of deposition of monoclonal light chains in the interstitial side of the tubular basement membranes is needed to make this diagnosis; therefore, immunofluorescence / immunohistochemistry and/or electron microscopy are essential to confirm the diagnosis [40]. The intensity and pattern of staining can be quite striking and may involve large areas of the interstitium, or very small foci [40]. Monotypic staining along tubular basement membranes with a linear pattern may be demonstrated using either immunofluorescence (usually more sensitive and easier to interpret) (Figure 10.16), or immunohistochemistry. Kappa light chains are more often involved in this pattern of renal injury than λ light chains [40]. The areas with the most inflammatory activity are the ones most commonly associated with the typical staining pattern for the pertinent light chain [40]. Staining for the other light chain is entirely negative or with much less intensity than the pertinent light chain, representing nonspecific background staining. Staining for other immunoglobulins, complement components, fibrinogen, and albumin are also negative.

Electron Microscopy. The glomeruli and vasculature are unremarkable in these cases. Specifically, no light chain deposits are present and nor is there any evidence of amyloid deposition. In some instances, deposition of light chains represented by punctuate to powdery deposits can be found alongside the tubular basement membranes, predominantly in association with tubules surrounded by the most inflammatory activity [40,41]. The lysosomal system may be prominent in proximal tubules. Using ultrastructural immunolabeling, the pertinent light chain can be labeled along tubular basement membranes even in the absence of typical deposits identifiable by electron microscopy (Figure 10.17). These light chain deposits are sometimes detected in focal interstitial areas and in proteinaceous material not forming solid casts that may be present in tubular lumina [40].

Differential Diagnosis. The main differential diagnosis is acute tubular interstitial nephritis, either related to a systemic

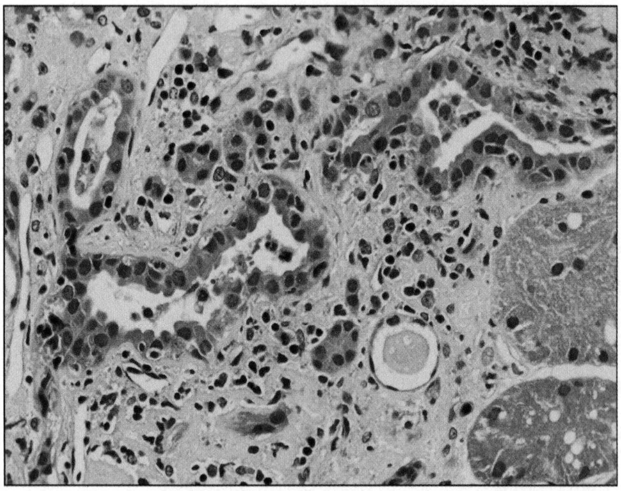

FIGURE 10.15: *Tubular interstitial nephritis. Hematoxylin and eosin. ×350. Interstitial inflammatory infiltrate composed primarily of lymphocytes associated with focal tubulitis.*

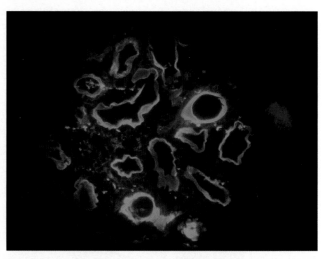

FIGURE 10.16: *Tubular interstitial nephritis. Direct immunofluorescence stain for κ light chain. Fluorescein isothiocyanate. ×350. Linear fluorescence along tubular basement membranes, which may be focal, represents a characteristic finding in this lesion.*

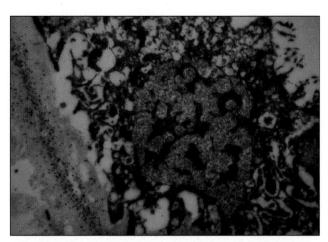

FIGURE 10.17:   Tubular interstitial nephritis. Immunogold labeling for κ light chains. Transmission electron microscopy. Uranyl acetate and lead citrate. Distinct labeling of tubular basement membrane for K light chain.

infection, or a hypersensitivity reaction (i.e., drug reaction). The only way to differentiate them from this entity is by using techniques to demonstrate the association of the interstitial inflammatory findings with monoclonal light chain deposition. There are no light microscopic findings that allow distinction of these entities. In some cases, punctuate to powdery electron-dense material may be seen ultrastructurally along the tubular basement membranes of tubules associated with the inflammatory process facilitating or confirming the diagnosis [40].

Clinical Course, Prognosis, Treatment, and Correlation. There has not been a study to analyze critically the clinical course or prognosis in this condition. It appears that treatment of the underlying plasma cell dyscrasia should be the primary approach to the treatment at this time. The use of steroids, as is the case in acute tubular interstitial nephritis, is also likely to be beneficial to these patients. Interestingly, in approximately 50 percent of these cases, the renal biopsy findings provide the first indication that the patient has an underlying plasma cell dyscrasia, and therefore, recognition of this unusual pattern of injury is important to uncover the underlying pathologic process [40].

Monoclonal Immunoglobulin Deposition Diseases

Clinical Presentation. Light chain deposition disease (LCDD) was coined as a specific entity in 1976 [15], and heavy chain deposition disease (HCDD) in 1993 [42]. Extremely rarely do these two diseases have been found to coexist [7]. They are both characterized by light and/or heavy chain deposits that may be identified in any or all renal compartments. The incidence of LCDD in autopsy series of patients with myeloma has been reported to be 3 to 5 percent [24,25]. Light chain deposits can frequently be seen in other organs (in up to 75 percent of the cases), most notably liver, heart, and lungs [43]. Cardiac (21 percent) and liver (19 percent) involvement are the most commonly recognized in LCDD [8]. The clinical and morphologic findings in both the diseases are identical [42, 44–46]. It is because of the

similarities that they will be discussed together. Monoclonal κ light chains (κIV preferentially) are more often involved in LCDD and the λ light chains (λVI most commonly) and γ heavy chains (mostly γ3) are most often associated with HCDD.

These diseases predominantly affect patients older than 50 years. The mean age in a study compiling twenty-three cases of renal monoclonal immunoglobulin deposition disease performed at a large institution was 57.4 years [7]. In the recently compiled author's ten- years experience (1996–2006), the mean age for LCDD patients at presentation was virtually the same (thirteen cases), and that of HCDD, 32.5 years, but with only two patients represented [47]. Overall, HCDD appears to occur more often in the younger patients [47] but as more cases are reported, this age difference may disappear.

The most common clinical presentation is proteinuria, not uncommonly in the nephrotic range, hypertension and renal insufficiency. Initial interactions of glomerulopathic light chains with peripheral glomerular capillary walls result in alterations of the glomerular permeability leading to proteinuria. In cases of HCDD, hypocomplementemia may also be present [6–8,42,44–46,48]. Monoclonal immunoglobulin deposition disease may coexist with light chain cast nephropathy in up to 21 percent of the affected patients [6], depending on the criteria used for diagnosis of cast nephropathy, and may also be associated, but much less commonly, with AL-amyloidosis [3,6].

Gross Pathology. There are two autopsy studies demonstrating no specific alterations in the kidneys of LCDD patients [24,25]. In one study, the mean weight of the kidneys of these patients was 271 g, and in the other study, there were two kidneys with an average weight of 130 g with coexistent vascular disease, which was attributed to the gross alterations [24,25]. There is no recorded data regarding gross pathological findings in kidneys from patients with HCDD.

Light Microscopy. The glomerulopathies associated with this disorder can present a variety of morphological patterns which result from a combination of glomerular proliferative activity and mesangial matrix expansion [2,4–8]. When the glomerulopathic light/heavy chains reach the mesangium and interact with mesangial cells, mesangial cell proliferation, and later,

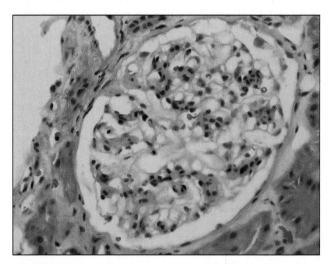

FIGURE 10.18:   LCDD. Hematoxylin and eosin. × 500. Mesangial proliferative pattern in LCDD.

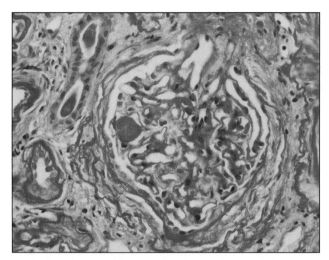

FIGURE 10.19: *LCDD, early nodular glomerulosclerosis. Periodic acid Schiff stain. ×500. Note focal mesangial nodule formation in an early nodular glomerulosclerosis as a manifestation of k LCDD.*

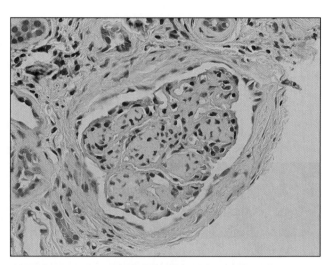

FIGURE 10.21: *γ HCDD. Hematoxylin and eosin. ×500. Mesangial nodularity with mild mesangial proliferation.*

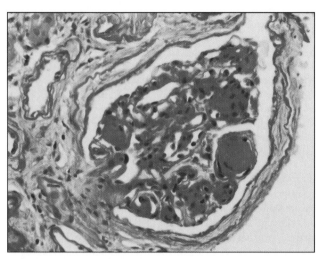

FIGURE 10.20: *LCDD, nodular glomerulosclerosis. Periodic acid Schiff. ×500. Well-defined nodular glomerulosclerosis as a manifestation of KLCDD.*

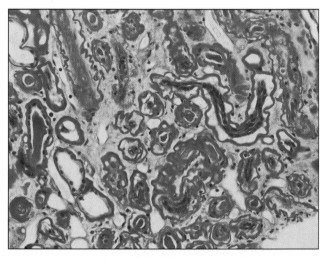

FIGURE 10.22: *LCDD. Periodic acid Schiff. ×350. Thickened and tortuous tubular basement membranes, as a result of light chain deposits on the outer aspect of the tubular basement membranes.*

matrix production and deposition occurs. As a result, there is much variability in the glomerular morphology that can be associated with these disorders. In early cases, glomeruli may appear essentially unremarkable and mimic minimal change glomerulopathy [2,12]. Mesangial proliferation (Figure 10.18) represents the earliest appreciable manifestation by light microscopy evolving into a membranoproliferative pattern with time. In the advanced stages, mesangial nodule formation occurs as a result of the excess extracellular matrix deposited in the mesangium, and the overall appearance is that of nodular glomerulosclerosis, the characteristic light microscopic pattern associated with these disorders. In the early phases of the process, mesangial nodules may be very focal and segmental (Figure 10.19), but as the disease process progresses striking mesangial nodularity and variable thickening of peripheral capillary walls develops; the overall light microscopic appearance becomes reminiscent

of diabetic nephropathy (Figure 10.20). The mesangial nodules typically stain with PAS (Figures 10.19 and 10.20) but show variable loss of argyrophilia. The nodules in LCDD and HCDD tend to be uniform in size, whereas in diabetic nephropathy, they are generally irregular in distribution, and vary in size and shape within a given glomeruli and among glomeruli. Significant mesangial proliferative activity can be present (Figure 10.21). Varying degrees of capillary wall thickening is also detected. Crescentic glomerulonephritis may be associated with LCDD and HCDD [6–8,49,50]. Interestingly, when LCDD is seen in combination with cast nephropathy, mesangial nodule formation is rarely seen. Only 18 percent of the cases in the series by Lin et al. demonstrated a pattern of nodular glomerulosclerosis [6]. Thickened and tortuous tubular basement membranes are often noted; these are highlighted on the PAS stain (Figure 10.22). Vessel walls of all sizes, both arterial and

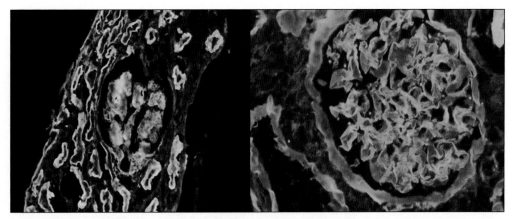

FIGURE 10.23: *LCDD. Direct immunofluorescence stain for κ light chains; fluorescein isothiocyanate. Left: ×250; right: ×500. Left panel: Linear staining pattern along peripheral capillary walls, a characteristic glomerular pattern in LCDD. Right panel: Linear staining along some peripheral capillary walls and granular mesangial fluorescence in a glomerulus with linear staining along tubular basement membranes, a distinct fluorescence pattern associated with LCDD, is shown.*

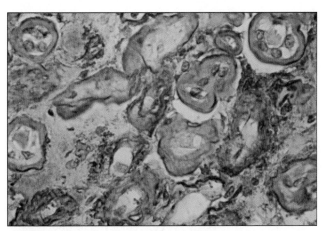

FIGURE 10.24: *LCDD. Immunohistochemical stain for κ light chains. Peroxidase antiperoxidase stain; diaminobenzidine. ×500. Intense labeling of outer aspect of tubular basement membranes and staining in vessel wall. Staining for λ light chains was negative.*

venous, are frequently thickened and may contain eosinophilic material in their walls corresponding to light chain deposits.

Immunofluorescence Microscopy/Immunohistochemistry. In LCDD, as its name indicates, deposition of monotypical light chains along the glomerular basement membranes, in the mesangium, along the tubular basement membranes, in the interstitium proper, and in the vasculature, represent the pathognomonic finding in these disorders (Figure 10.23) [2–8]. The amount of monotypical light chain deposits in the various renal compartments is variable; therefore, the manifestations may be somewhat different. Glomerular staining may be along peripheral capillary walls and/or in mesangium. Depending on the case, the distribution of the staining varies, but in most cases, both peripheral walls and mesangial areas reveal staining [6]. Staining for the nonpertinent light chain is invariably negative.

The preferred methodology to demonstrate the deposition of light chains is immunofluorescence, as nonspecific staining is generally not present, in comparison to immunohistochemistry where background staining may be a problem. However, there are cases where immunohistochemistry can be used to convincingly demonstrate the deposition of monoclonal light chains in the various renal compartments (Figure 10.24). There is no staining for immunoglobulins, complement components, fibrinogen or albumin in LCDD. Demonstration of monoclonal light chains using immunofluorescence and/or immunohistochemistry is not always possible, as the commercially available antibodies may not be able to detect the light chain deposits in tissues which are composed of physicochemical abnormal light chains or fragmented light chains that lack the epitopes detected by the antibodies or have covered epitopes.

In HCDD, stains for both κ and λ light chains are negative. Staining for one of the immunoglobulins is the main finding with peripheral capillary wall and mesangial fluorescence. Gamma (IgG) and mu (IgM) represent the most commonly involved heavy chains [6–8,44]. Staining for the remaining immunoreactants in the typical renal battery is negative with the exception of staining for C1. Glomerular C1q staining varies from granular to pseudogranular and can be a subtle, or a striking finding. Demonstration of lack of the CH1 (most common), CH2 or hinge region epitopes of the heavy chains in the renal glomeruli, using specific antibodies to these regions, can further confirm the diagnosis of HCDD [6,42,44].

Electron Microscopy. Granular, punctate to powdery electron-dense material can be seen in all renal compartments in both LCDD and HCDD. In glomeruli, it is typically noted in subendothelial and mesangial locations (Figure 10.25) but can also be seen in Bowman's capsule [2–8,44–46,48]. The lamina rara interna of the glomerular basement membrane is obliterated early, and as the disease process advances, deposits may extend into the lamina densa. When the light chain deposits locate on top of the lamina densa of the glomerular basement membrane, obliterating it along segments, an appearance that can be easily confused with dense deposit disease occurs [51]. The amounts of peripheral capillary wall versus mesangial deposits are variable, but peripheral deposits are more common and easier to identify than those restricted to the mesangium.

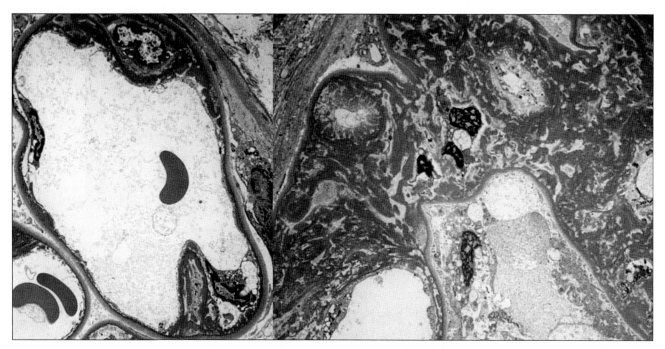

FIGURE 10.25: LCDD. Transmission electron microscopy. Uranyl acetate and lead citrate. Left: ×7,500; right: ×7,500. Fluffy, slightly electron-dense material in subendothelial zone (left panel) along peripheral capillary wall, and in the mesangium (right panel), totally obliterating the normal mesangial matrix. In some cases, light chain deposits are difficult to identify and a high degree of suspicion, as well as correlation with immunofluorescence findings is needed to make a definitive diagnosis.

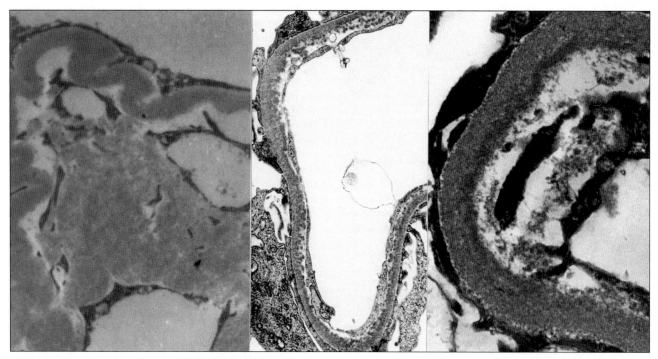

FIGURE 10.26: LCDD. Transmission electron microscopy. Uranyl acetate and lead citrate. Left: ×7,500; middle: ×5,600; and right: ×7,500. Different ultrastructural appearances of the light chain deposits in glomeruli. Note the variation in electron density of the light chain deposits, and subtle powdery deposits in middle panel.

Deposits in both compartments are seen in the great majority of the cases [2–8,43–45,47]. The appearance of the light chain deposits can be quite heterogeneous, as their electron density and overall texture may be variable (granular, finely granular electron-dense material or merely increased electron density, punctuate – distinct point-like granular electron-dense material,

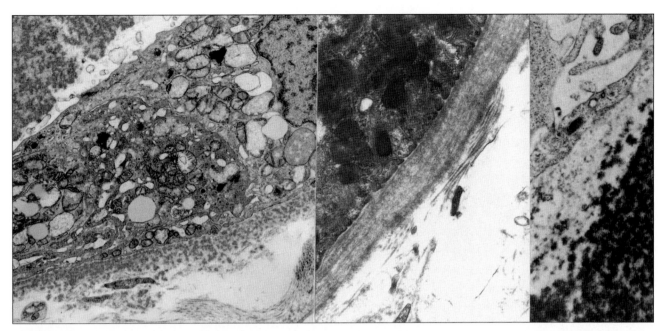

FIGURE 10.27: *LCDD. Transmission electron microscopy. Uranyl acetate and lead citrate. Left: ×5,600; middle: ×7,500; and right: ×8,500. Light chain deposits along the tubular basement membranes (left and middle panels), and in the interstitium proper (right panel.)*

or powdery – fluffy variably dense electron-dense material) depending on the light chain that is involved, and the amount of light chain deposition in the various renal compartments (Figure 10.26). Depending on the electron density of the light or heavy chain deposits, they may or may not stand out when they merge with the mesangial matrix.

In the tubular interstitial compartment, the light and heavy chain deposits are found on the outer aspect of the tubular basement membranes (Figure 10.27) and in the interstitium proper (Figure 10.27). Also noted is similar material in vessel walls, both arteries and veins of various calibers, as well as in surrounding peritubular capillaries [2–8]. There is significant variability from case to case regarding the amount of light chain deposited in the various compartments, and the specific distribution within the renal parenchyma. In some cases, pristine light chain deposits are very difficult to detect ultrastructurallly. In a few cases, light chain deposits cannot be identified ultrastructurally, in spite of a striking linear fluorescence for monoclonal light chains. There is an unusual variant of LCDD, which mimics an immune complex-mediated glomerulopathy because the light chain deposits assemble in a peculiar manner resembling immune complexes [52].

Differential Diagnosis. When the advanced disease, nodular glomerulosclerosis, is the pattern under consideration, diabetic nephropathy must be ruled out. The differences at the light microscopic level can be subtle. The mesangial nodules in diabetic nephropathy are spread through the peripheral part of the glomeruli and are seldom seen near the hilum or in the central part of the glomeruli [6]. In the advanced lesion associated with LCDD, all glomeruli contain mesangial nodules, not varying in size between and within the glomeruli, which contrasts with the appearance of the nodular glomerulosclerosis in diabetic nephropathy. Hyaline caps and capsular drops, which represent insu-

dative and exudative lesions composed of plasma proteins, are seen in diabetic nephropathy, and not in LCDD. Furthermore, prominent hyalinosis of both afferent and efferent arterioles represent a typical finding in diabetic nephropathy, and is absent in LCDD. In diabetic nephropathy, thickening of the lamina densa of the glomerular basement membranes represents the typical finding; this finding is absent in LCDD. In most cases, the demonstration of monotypical light or heavy chains in the glomeruli provides unequivocal evidence to make a diagnosis of LCDD or HCDD. There are cases of nodular glomerulosclerosis that have been described unassociated with diabetes, LCDD, or HCDD [53]. The pathogenesis of these disorders remains speculative, but the combined effect of smoking and hypertension appear to play a main role [53].

If the patterns present in the biopsy specimens are those primarily associated with proliferative glomerulopathies, the differential diagnosis can be quite broad and includes all conditions characterized by mesangioproliferative and membranoproliferative patterns [5,12]. In the great majority of these cases, immunofluorescence/immunohistochemistry and/or electron microscopy provide unequivocal diagnostic evidence. There are cases, however, in which the differential diagnosis may not be able to be easily resolved. The use of immunoelectron microscopy to address these cases has been proposed, and it has indeed proven to be a helpful ancillary diagnostic technique to address challenging cases [12,13]. Subendothelial immune complexes can sometimes be difficult to differentiate from light chain deposits especially when they are continuous rather than well-delimited (Figure 10.28); the final interpretation in these instances rests on the evaluation of the data obtained from all three diagnostic modalities. For example, a demonstration of light or heavy chain restriction or staining for both light chains in subendothelial glomerular areas where the electron-dense deposits are identified represent an important differentiating feature.

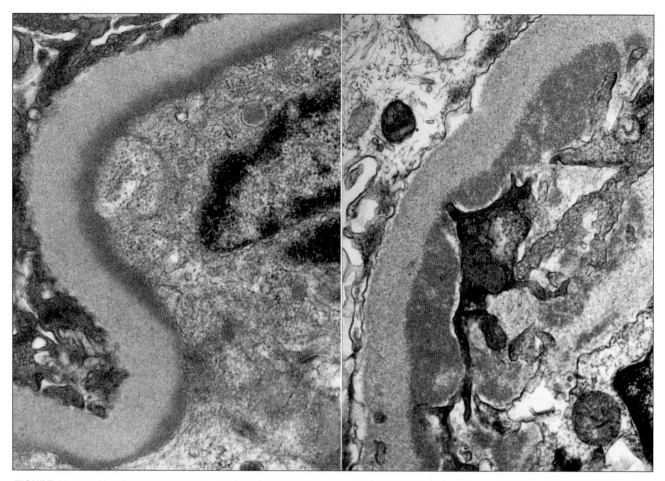

FIGURE 10.28: *Membranoproliferative glomerulonephritis with subendothelial immune complexes mimicking light chain deposits. Transmission electron microscopy. Uranyl acetate and lead citrate. Left: ×12 500; and right: ×15 500. Subendothelial immune complexes may mimic light chain deposits in some instances. Some immune complexes are not as organized in discrete electron-dense structures as they generally are, and can be a source of confusion with light chain deposits.*

Light (AL) and Heavy (AH) Chain-Related Amyloidosis

Clinical Presentation. Amyloidosis is a rare disorder of elderly individuals. Amyloidosis associated with light chains (AL-type) is the most common type in the western world. Heavy chain-associated amyloidosis (AH) is a rare disorder. Only a few cases have been documented in the literature [14,54] and awareness of AH-amyloidosis is still limited. All types of amyloidosis share the same light and ultrastructural features, and cannot be differentiated on the basis of morphologic findings. Detection of the precursor protein in association with the amyloid tissue deposits is essential to properly characterize the type of amyloidosis (see "Amyloid Typing").

Clinically, the patients typically present with nonspecific findings, most commonly fatigue and weight loss. Proteinuria with or without nephrotic syndrome is the most common clinical finding, at time in association with renal insufficiency. There are numerous other manifestations of this disease, including peripheral neuropathy, congestive heart failure, cardiac arrhythmias, carpal tunnel syndrome, orthostatic hypotension, and hepatomegaly among others [7,8,14,54–56].

Gross Pathology. The kidneys in patients with amyloidosis of all types are generally enlarged. Interestingly, the weight of the kidneys did not correlate with renal function or the site of amyloid deposition, and was generally inversely proportional to the amount of renal amyloid in the study by Dickman et al. [56]. The average weight of the kidneys in patients with AL-amyloidosis was 200 g in a recent autopsy study [25].

Light Microscopy. The characteristic finding is the presence of amorphous, eosinophilic material in the glomeruli, interstitium proper and vascular walls (Figure 10.29). This material is first noted in the mesangium and then extends into peripheral capillary walls [2–8]. The mesangium shows loss of silver positivity as the mesangial matrix is replaced by amyloid fibrils (Figure 10.30). The material is weakly PAS-positive, blue with the trichrome stain, and negative with the silver stain. Spicules are sometimes noted with the silver stain along the peripheral capillary walls and in the mesangial areas. In the early cases, subtle mesangial amyloid deposition can be easily missed. The amyloid deposition results in nodular (Figure 10.29) and diffuse (Figure 10.31) patterns of glomerular deposition [56]. Amyloid deposits can be seen in any of the renal compartments (Figure 10.32). There is a rare subset of these patients that, at presentation, only reveal vascular amyloid deposits [12], and may represent a diagnostic challenge. The amyloid deposits are Congo red positive

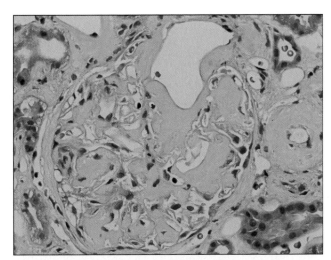

FIGURE 10.29: *AL-amyloidosis. Hematoxylin and eosin. × 500. Amorphous eosinophilic material present in mesangial areas and focally extending into peripheral capillary walls represents the typical appearance of amyloidosis. Also, note similar material in an adjacent arteriolar wall.*

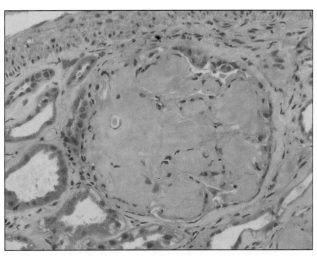

FIGURE 10.31: *AL-amyloidosis, diffuse pattern. Hematoxylin and eosin. × 500. Amyloid deposition has also extended into peripheral capillary walls and the entire glomerular architecture has been obliterated. Note the glomerular enlargement, a finding that may be helpful in the differential diagnosis with a sclerosed (often shrunken) glomeruli.*

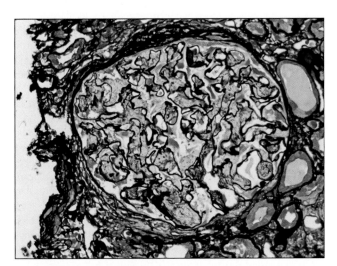

FIGURE 10.30: *AL-amyloidosis. Silver methenamine. × 500. The mesangial areas have been replaced by amyloid fibrils, and as a result, the mesangium has lost its argyrophilia.*

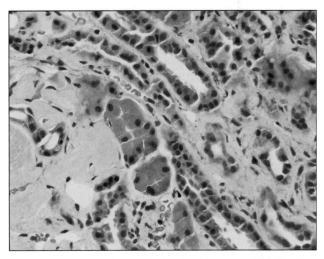

FIGURE 10.32: *AL-amyloidosis, interstitial. Hematoxylin and eosin. × 350. Focal deposition of eosinophilic, amorphous material in the interstitium most consistent with amyloid.*

(Figure 10.33) and fluoresce with Thioflavin T or S (Figure 10.34) [4–8].

Immunofluorescence Microscopy/Immunohistochemistry. Interpretation of the renal pattern of immunofluorescence stains routinely used in diagnostic renal biopsies allows depiction of some types of amyloid such as light and heavy chain and fibrinogen-associated. Immunohistochemistry is used to identify other precursor proteins and therefore characterize the type of amyloid present, as is the case in the diagnosis of AA-amyloidosis. Monotypical light chain staining in association with the eosinophilic amorphous material is diagnostic of AL-amyloidosis (Figure 10.35A,B). The majority of these cases are associated with λ light chains (λVI predominantly). Staining for the other light chain is negative in the great majority of the

cases. Likewise, staining for immunoglobulins, complement components, fibrinogen, and albumin are all negative. The absence of staining of amyloid deposits for both light chains does not necessarily rule out AL-amyloidosis [57]. In cases of heavy chain amyloidosis, the amyloid deposits stain for one of the heavy chains (γ or μ usually) [14,54]. No staining for light chains or any other immunoreactants is present in AH-amyloidosis.

Electron Microscopy. Amyloid is characterized by randomly disposed nonbranching fibrils, which measure 8–10 nm in diameter. There are no morphologic differences between the fibrils in light or heavy chain-associated amyloidosis [2–8]. Initially, the amyloid fibril aggregates are noted in focal mesangial areas (Figure 10.36). In the advanced stages of the

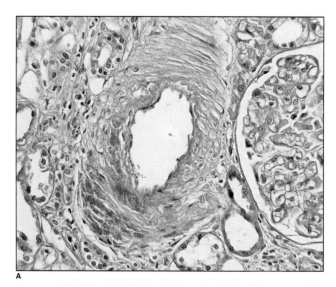
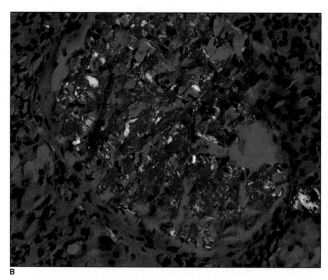

FIGURE 10.33: *AL-amyloidosis. A: Strong Congo red positivity is seen in the wall of an interlobular artery. Note the subtle mesangial staining in the glomerulus corresponding to early glomerular involvement by amyloidosis (×200). B: Polarized microscopy displays extensive Congo red staining of the glomerulus.*

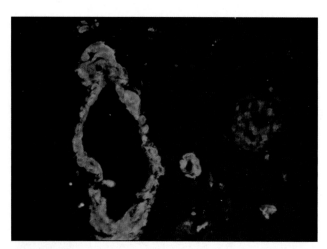

FIGURE 10.34: *AL-amyloidosis. Thioflavin T fluorescence. ×350. Prominent staining of vessel walls and focal glomerular staining, predominantly mesangial is shown.*

disease process, amyloid fibrils virtually replace the entire mesangium and extend into peripheral capillary walls sometimes replacing the glomerular basement membranes (Figures 10.37 and 10.38). It has been proposed that when this finding is present, amyloidosis is associated with a faster progression and a worse prognosis [56]. The mesangial fibrils are sometimes arranged in spicules (Figure 10.38). Atypical amyloid deposition in electron-dense aggregates resembling immune complexes has also been reported in one case in the literature [58]. Ultrastructural immunogold labeling can be used to detect the precursor protein associated with the amyloid fibrils (Figure 10.39).

Differential Diagnosis. Early amyloidosis should be differentiated from minimal change glomerulopathy [12]. A careful exami-

nation of the light microscopic sections to detect focal, early, and subtle amyloid deposition is a must (Figure 10.40). Likewise, the electron microscopy grids must be carefully scrutinized to identify focal mesangial and vascular areas with amyloid fibrils. In advanced cases, the challenge is at times to differentiate amyloidosis from glomerulosclerosis. Congo red and Thioflavin T stains as well as electron microscopy are conclusive in establishing the correct diagnosis. Differentiation from other glomerulopathies associated with mesangial nodularity (nodular glomerulosclerosis) such as LCDD, HCDD, and diabetes may also be needed in selected cases, especially in the nodular form of amyloidosis. Generally, the mesangial amyloid deposits result in mesangial nodularity. The weak positivity for PAS and the absence of silver staining in the nodules is helpful to differentiate these lesions. Congo red and Thioflavin T or S stains generally provide unequivocal support for the diagnosis of amyloidosis. Furthermore, ultrastructurally amyloidosis will show fibrils whereas the deposits in light or heavy chain deposition disease are granular, punctuate to powdery [2–8]. Amyloid-P component is only present in association with amyloidosis but not LCDD, or HCDD.

Amyloidosis must also be differentiated from fibrillary glomerulopathy at the ultrastructural level. The latter is Congo red and Thioflavin T negative, and shows similarly randomly disposed fibrils which are thicker than amyloid measuring 25 to 30 nm in diameter. Fibrillary glomerulonephritis also has a characteristic immunofluorescence pattern with pseudolinear "smudged" staining for IgG and C3 which is quite unique (see "Fibrillary Glomerulonephritis" section).

Amyloid Typing. Once a definitive diagnosis of amyloidosis is made, proper typing is required for proper patients' management. Proper identification of the type of amyloid is performed by detecting the precursor protein associated with the amyloid. In essence, there are three broad types of amyloidosis that need to be differentiated: AL (the most common in the western world), AA, and hereditary. The latter are rare and generally

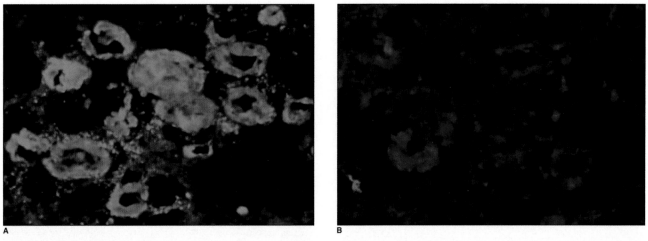

FIGURE 10.35: AL-amyloidosis. A: Strong lambda light chain staining is seen in multiple arterial cross sections. B: Corresponding arterial cross sections are negative with kappa light chain (Direct immunofluorescence, × 400).

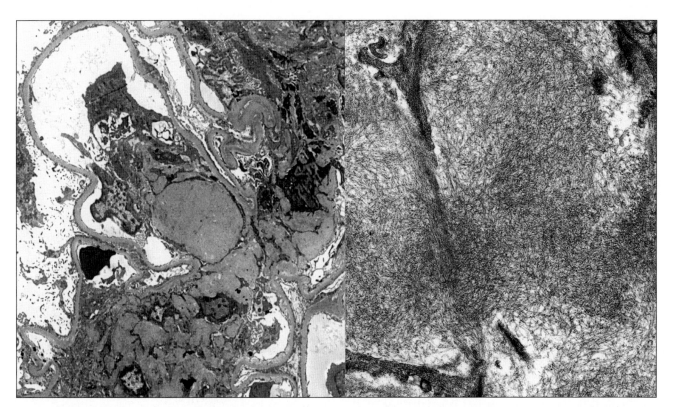

FIGURE 10.36: AL-amyloidosis. Transmission electron microscopy. Uranyl acetate and lead citrate. Left: × 3,500; right: × 10,500. Note the small nodule in mesangium (left panel) which when examined on high power reveals its fibrillary composition (right panel). The fibrils have typical diameter and disposition of amyloid fibrils.

autosomal dominant diseases related to mutation of a number of amyloid precursor proteins.

The routine immunofluorescence battery of stains will help identify AL-amyloidosis cases, the majority of which will be λ light chain-associated. Negative stains for κ and λ light chains do not exclude a diagnosis of AL-amyloidosis. There are cases in which the monotypical protein deposited in tissues is so abnormal or truncated that the idiotypic epitopes detected by commercially available antibodies may not be present [57]. The routine battery

of immunofluorescence stains will also depict the rare fibrinogen A α-chain (AFib)-associated and heavy chain-related amyloidosis.

There are also commercially available antibodies to identify other amyloid precursor proteins such as AA protein, transthyretin (TTR), lysozyme, calcitonin (Figure 10.41), and beta 2 microglo-bulin-associated amyloids. The detection of these proteins is only possible by light microscopy using immunohistochemical techni-ques, as there are no fluorescent-tagged commercially available antibodies to detect these. Sometimes, only glomerular amyloid

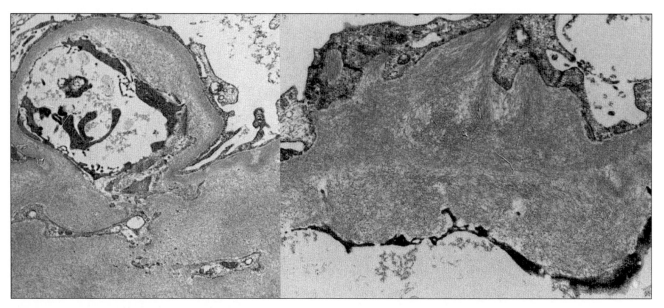

FIGURE 10.37: AL-amyloidosis. Transmission electron microscopy. Uranyl acetate and lead citrate. Left: ×7,500; right: ×13,500. Left panel: mesangial and peripheral capillary wall deposition of amyloid fibrils. Right panel: note that the fibrils are located transmembranously in B. Amyloid spikes are also present.

deposition is present (Figure 10.42). At the ultrastructural level, immunogold labeling may also be used to type the amyloid present; this technique is very sensitive and exquisitely elegant.

General recommendations and pitfalls pertaining to amyloid typing can be found in the referenced editorial [59]. It should also be remembered that combinations of different types of amyloid can occur, and that a high index of suspicion is needed to depict these and address situations that arise as a consequence of the complexity associated with amyloid typing in some instances [59].

Etiology and Pathogenesis of Monoclonal Light Chain Related Renal Diseases

To understand the pathogenesis of light chain-related renal pathology, it is helpful to review first the renal handling of normal light chains.

Catabolism of Light Chains in Normal Individuals

Circulating free light chains are found in the serum in very small quantities and delivered to the kidneys in normal individuals. It is because of their low molecular weight (approximately 20–25 kDa) that they are filtered through the capillary walls and delivered to the proximal tubules. Once they reach the proximal tubules, the light chains are endocytosed using the megalin/cubilin receptor present in the microvillus borders and catabolized by an endosomal/lysosomal pathway [60,61]. These normal light chains are not at all attracted to the mesangium and do not interact with mesangial cells.

What Happens with Structurally Abnormal Light Chains?

The situation is quite different with some pathologic light chains. The specific physicochemical abnormalities present in these abnormal light chains essentially determine the type of renal damage that will occur. As previously mentioned, tubulopathic light chains are more frequent than glomerulopathic ones. While understanding the patterns of renal damage centered in proximal and distal tubules in light chain-associated renal diseases is not difficult because of the way light chains are handled by the kidneys, it is perhaps more difficult to conceptualize how glomerular damage occurs.

Monotypical light chains can produce proximal tubular damage as a consequence of direct toxicity. Physicochemically abnormal light chains are reabsorbed in the proximal tubules. Marked expansion of the lysosomal compartment typically occurs, and abnormal (sometimes markedly) lysosomes are detected in the cytoplasm of the proximal tubular cells. These lysosomes are enlarged and assume atypical forms. Ultrastructural labeling demonstrates that they are packed with monotypical light chains that cannot be properly catabolized. As a result, lysosomal breakdown eventually occurs with spillage of their contents into the cytoplasm with the resultant vacuolization and damage [5,13]. Eventually, fragmentation, desquamation, and even frank necrosis of tubular cells occur.

The inflammatory tubular interstitial lesion seen in association with monotypical light chains occurs likely as a result of binding of the monotypical light chains to the tubular basement membranes, altering intrinsic tissue antigens, and promoting the release of cytokines, resulting in chemoattraction of inflammatory cells [40]. Light chains may reach the tubular basement membranes by transcytosis after they are taken in by the proximal tubular cells.

The distal tubular lesion (light chain cast nephropathy) is characterized by delivery of large concentrations of monotypical light chains to the distal nephron where, interacting with Tamm-Horsfall protein, they engage in the formation of casts, resulting in nephron obstruction. The binding site in both κ and λ light chains resides within complementarity-determining region-3 (CDR-3) [62,63].

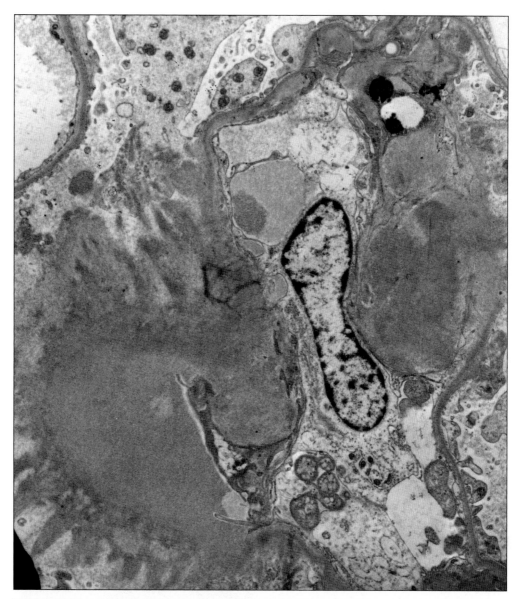

FIGURE 10.38: *AA-amyloidosis. Transmission electron microscopy. Uranyl acetate and lead citrate. ×5,600. Note spicular arrangement of the amyloid fibrils in the mesangium.*

A group of structurally abnormal light chains actively interact with mesangial cells where they find a receptor on the mesangial cell membranes that engages them. The presence of purported receptors on mesangial cells facilitate and likely control this interaction, and lead to a series of alterations that culminate in either formation of mesangial nodules with increased extracellular matrix material, or replacement of the mesangium by amyloid fibrils. Interplay of two growth factors plays a fundamental role in the development of the lesions in these two diseases. In LCDD, initial activation of PDGF-β with mesangial cell proliferation is followed by activation of TGF-β, which is associated with deposition of mesangial matrix rich in tenascin [64]. The resultant glomerular appearance will depend on whether the action of PDGF-β (which resulting in various proliferative patterns such as mesangial proliferative and membranoproliferative types), or TGF-β predominates (resulting in

the nodular glomerulosclerosis) (Figure 10.43) [65,66]. Activation of TGF-β also results in inhibition of mesangial cell proliferation. In contrast, in AL-amyloidosis, initial PDGF-β activation is followed by a series of different events governed by the formation of amyloid and deposition in the mesangium resulting in activation of metalloproteinases and destruction of the native mesangium, which is eventually replaced by amyloid fibrils [67]. The results in the extracellular matrix are diametrically different in the LCDD than in the amyloidoses. While in the first instance, activation of TGF-β leads to the formation of an excess of extracellular matrix in the mesangium, in the case of amyloidoses, amyloid deposition exerts an inhibitory effect on TGF-β, and results in the activation of metalloproteinases which eventually destroy the native matrix. Since TGF-β is inhibited, no repair of the mesangium is possible (Figure 10.1). In both conditions, apoptosis of mesangial cells results in cell deletion, which

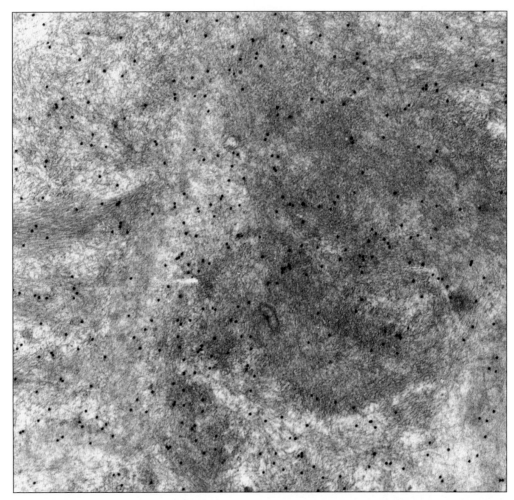

FIGURE 10.39:   *AL-amyloidosis. Transmission electron microscopy. Immunogold labeling for λ light chains. Gold particles: 10 nm. Uranyl acetate and lead citrate. ×12,500. Gold particles localize on top of amyloid fibrils indicating their association with λ light chains.*

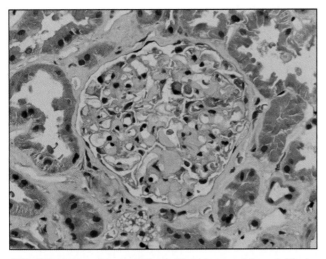

FIGURE 10.40:   *AA-amyloidosis. Early mesangial amyloidosis. Hematoxylin and eosin. ×500. Note early deposition of eosinophilic, amorphous material in some mesangial areas.*

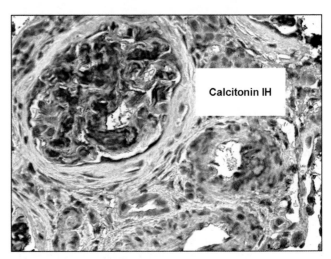

FIGURE 10.41:   *Calcitonin-associated amyloidosis in patient with metastatic medullary carcinoma of thyroid. Immunohistochemical stain for calcitonin (×350). Distinct staining of mesangial areas in glomerulus and focal staining of arteriolar wall.*

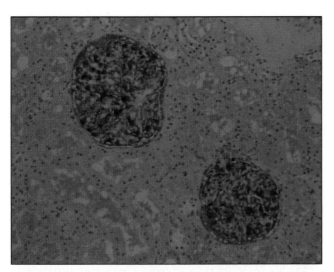

FIGURE 10.42: AA-amyloidosis. Immunohistochemical stain for AA-protein (×175). Selective glomerular (mesangial) staining for AA-protein in association with amyloid deposits.

explains why in the advanced stages of both conditions (deposition diseases and amyloidosis), the mesangium hardly contains any cells. Ronco et al. have accurately stated that LCDD represents a model of glomerulosclerosis at the molecular level [45].

The main extracellular matrix protein that deposits in the mesangial nodules in light and heavy chain deposition diseases is tenascin (Figure 10.44) [64] produced by TGF-β [63]. Tenascin

is a rather interesting protein with a peculiar configuration that allows it to interact by means of tentacle-like extensions with a variety of surrounding extracellular matrix components. It is mainly catabolized by metalloproteinase 7, but also by MMPs-1 and 3. In this condition, there is a problem with the release of MMP7 from mesangial cells, so that once the tenascin is deposited, it cannot be efficiently destroyed [68].

Structural Abnormalities in Light and Heavy Chains Responsible for Pathogenicity

Much work has been done in the last two decades elucidating how the structural characteristics of immunoglobulin light chains influence the renal pathology that is seen in patients with plasma cell dyscrasias and renal involvement. Only fundamental concepts will be reviewed here, as work on the subject continues, and currently, the information is somewhat preliminary in some areas. Host factors may also be of significance in the pathogenesis of these diseases [69], but these have not been studied in detail.

Only a few monoclonal immunoglobulin light chains involved in proximal tubulopathies have been studied at the molecular level with their structures documented. The most elegant work has been done in Fanconi syndrome-associated proximal tubular injury [70]. The great majority of cases of Fanconi syndrome is associated with VκI subgroup and emanates from two germ lines: LCO 2 and LCO 12. In this condition, the partially digested light chains form the cytoplasmic inclusions characteristic of this disorder. The inclusions contain a truncated NH-terminal fragment, which corresponds to the variable domain of the light chain that is necessary for crystallization to

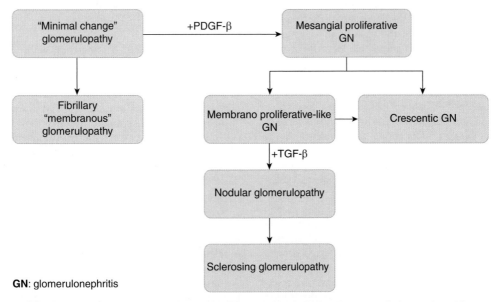

GN: glomerulonephritis

FIGURE 10.43: *Proposed sequence of molecular events in the development of glomerulopathies associated with light chain deposition. Early manifestations of light chain deposition disease are characterized by essentially unremarkable glomeruli by light microscopy. Upon the activation of PDGF-β, mesangial cell proliferation occurs and a mesangial proliferative pattern becomes manifest. Further PDGF-β activation results in more pronounced proliferative glomerular lesions, including membranoproliferative and crescentic lesions. Once TGF-β activation is on board, proliferative activities are controlled and matrix deposition prevails giving rise to the nodular glomerulosclerosis pattern, characteristic of LCDD. Further glomerular damage and matrix deposition produces a sclerosing glomerulopathy.*

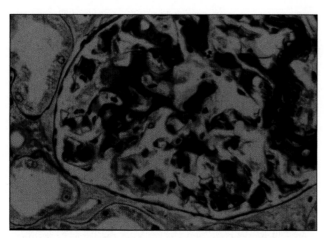

FIGURE 10.44: *LCDD. Immunohistochemistry for tenascin. Avidin-biotin complex; diaminobenzidine as marker, methyl green counterstain. × 750. Note intense staining for tenascin in expanded mesangial areas.*

occur. The main defect occurs in position 30 of the variable portion of the light chain molecule where there is an unusual hydrophobic residue, likely accounting for the resistance of the light chain to cathepsin proteolysis fostering crystalization. Primary structure analysis of these peculiar light chains have also demonstrated substitutions in residues 28 and 31 of the complementarity determining region (CDR1), which additionally has been proposed to alter the proper catabolism of the light chains in the proximal tubules. Clearly, the light chains involved in this unique type of tubulopathy most often belong to the VkI family, but it appears that variations in the sequence of the proteins involved may tune the severity of the disease, and change its morphological manifestations. An animal model of this condition has been created and manipulated which has provided unequivocal evidence for pathogenesis of this disorder [70].

The CDR3 of particular light chains is responsible for binding to the Tamm-Horsfall protein initiating cast formation. Variations in the CDR3 sequences of the light chains determine the propensity for binding. The amino acid sequence of the CDR3 region, along with the other possible contributing factors, modulates the binding of Tamm-Horsfall protein to the light chains, and subsequent development of cast nephropathy. Differences in the CDR3 region accounts for the variability in affinity of various light chains to Tamm-Horsfall protein, and their propensity to develop light chain cast nephropathy [62,63]. Thus, the amino acid sequence of the light chain molecules and CDR3 region, and some host-related factors among others, control the binding of Tamm-Horsfall protein to light chains, and the subsequent development of clinical manifestation and renal failure as a result of cast nephropathy. Other factors such as poor hydration, hypercalcemia, contrast media material administration, and the use of certain diuretics could act as potentiating factors for cast formation in the proper setting [38].

Amino acid substitutions in the variably region of abnormal light chains associated with LCDD and AL-amyloidosis result in alterations in their primary, and at times, tertiary conformation [71]. These substitutions introduce hydrophobic residues in the exposed portions of the variable region of the light chains. Posttranslational modifications can also be responsible for the glomerulopathic properties of some light chains [72].

Amino acid substitutions introducing hydrophobic residues in the variable region of the light chains usually in the CDR 1 and CDR 3, and less often in the CDR 2 and FR regions, regardless of light chain subtype, but more often in κ light chains, are associated with LCDD [73,74]. The light chains involved in LCDDs exhibit a restricted usage of three κ-germline genes with an overexpression of VκIV subgroup, abnormal size, and a striking ability to polymerize, glycosylation, high isoelectric point, and clustering of hydrophobic residues mainly in the CDRs [74]. The exposed hydrophobic residues may be responsible for destabilization of the light chains leading to its aggregation, and for hydrophobic interactions between V domains or the V domains with extracellular matrix proteins explaining their precipitation in the various renal compartments.

Studies of the structure of heavy chains from two patients with HCDD have shown striking abnormalities in the variable segment, especially in the framework regions [75].

Glycosylated light chains are four times more frequently associated with AL-amyloidosis than those light chains that are not glycosylated [72]. Lambda 6 light chains exhibit a unique tropism for renal amyloidosis [76]. Proteins encoded by the λ germline gene (IGLV6SI) accounts for a large part of this predominance due to the virtually 100 percent association of these proteins with fibril formation. It remains unknown whether this fact reflects specific structural features of these light chains that make them more prone to fibrillogenesis.

Other Types of Amyloidosis

AA-amyloidosis

AA-amyloidosis occurs in association with chronic inflammatory conditions, including tuberculosis, rheumatoid arthritis, ankylosing spondylitis, chronic inflammatory bowel disease, infections, periodic fevers, and malignancies. The fibrillary protein in these conditions is derived from serum amyloid A protein (SAA). Although the majority of the cases of AA-amyloidosis have no hereditary component, a small number of hereditary conditions associated with recurrent inflammation with deposition of AA-amyloid in tissues have been recognized. The best example of familial AA amyloidosis is Familial Mediterranean fever.

AA amyloidosis is diagnosed in patients of various age groups. The age range (11–87 years) in the published series is quite broad. Familial Mediterranean fever must be considered in the differential diagnosis of younger patients affected by AA-amyloidosis. When associated with chronic diseases, the conditions have generally been present for many years and have been categorized as severe. In the western world, rheumatoid arthritis followed by ankylosing spondylitis is the most common conditions associated with AA-amyloidosis [77].

Proteinuria and nephrotic syndrome represent the most common presentations for all types of AA-amyloidosis, including when associated with Familial Mediterranean Fever [77]. In the latter, proteinuria may be massive and renal vein thrombosis can complicate the disease process. Some of the most severe cases of proteinuria and nephrotic syndrome described in the literature have been in patients with amyloidosis. Although it is rare to find patients with AA-amyloidosis without significant proteinuria, there are cases in the literature that have advanced renal failure without significant proteinuria throughout the course of the disease.

The five-year survival in patients with AA-amyloidosis has been reported to be 40 percent [77]. If the underlying disorder can be controlled, the survival rate can be improved considerably. There are new therapies for AA-amyloidosis that appear promising (see section on therapy).

Hereditary Amyloidosis

This group of amyloidosis continues to expand, but it remains a small percentage of all cases with amyloidosis. The low incidence of these conditions, however, may be a reflection of underdiagnosis. They occur from mutations of amyloid precursor proteins and represent a rather diverse group of diseases. Diagnosis may be challenging as their clinical presentation, and pathological findings may be similar to those of the better known types of amyloidosis. Family history is not always present. In some cases, these particular conditions are concentrated in certain geographic areas where they should be suspected. Differential diagnosis in cases from these regions should always consider the hereditary type of amyloidosis as a possibility. The most common type of hereditary amyloidosis in the United States is transthyretin-associated (ATTR), while in England, A-Fib is the most common.

Amyloid derived from TTR is associated with more than one hundred mutations of the precursor protein. The most frequent mutation in the TTR molecule is in position 30 where there is a valine-methionine substitution (Met30). While this disease is most commonly seen in Portugal, Sweden, and Japan, 4 percent of African-Americans carry an abnormal TTR gene. The disease is usually not clinically apparent until middle or later life, and family history is sometimes not present. Varying degrees of amyloid deposition have been reported in the kidney with involvement of all compartments. However, the amyloid deposits may be restricted to the interstitium in the medulla [78].

Amyloid derived from a mutant of fibrinogen Aα (AFib) shows striking renal tropism causing renal disease unassociated with cardiac involvement or neuropathy. The amyloid in the kidney is characteristically deposited in glomeruli, sparing the other renal compartments, and this appearance should be considered suspicious for this type of amyloid [79], but not pathognomonic.

Miscellaneous Types of Amyloidosis

Other types of familial systemic amyloidoses include those derived from apolipoprotein I (AApoI), apolipoprotein II (AApoII), lysozyme (ALys), gelsolin (AGel), and cystatin (ACys). They can all be associated with the amyloid deposition in the renal parenchyma.

Dialysis-related amyloidosis derived from β2-microglobulin occurs in patients with end-stage renal disease and long-term hemodialysis. This type of amyloid may be detected in end-stage kidneys with little if any clinical significance. Deposition of amyloid typically occurs in bones, joints, and synovium [80].

This section will be divided into two, one for monoclonal immunoglobulin deposition diseases and the other for amyloidosis.

Monoclonal Immunoglobulin Deposition Diseases

The treatment for LCDD is far more advanced than that of the heavy chain-associated counterpart, mainly because the latter disease has been around for much less time. Combined nephrological and hematological management is important. Treatment strategies must take into consideration renal manifestations and the plasma cell clone involved. One of the most fundamental aspects in predicting prognosis is the stage at which the disease process is diagnosed. In many cases, renal damage is quite pronounced at the time the diagnosis is established precluding much improvement with treatment. A significant number of these patients fail to show definitive evidence of myeloma at the time of diagnosis, but up to 33 percent develop overt myeloma during the course of the disease, negatively affecting prognosis [81]. Extrarenal involvement in this condition is variable but common, and it may be of significance in altering response to therapy and prognosis, and in preventing some therapeutic approaches.

Treatment should essentially begin with controlling the amount of light or heavy chain, produced by the neoplastic plasma cells. High-dose chemotherapy with melphalan and prednisone is generally used [82]. There is significant controversy as to whether chemotherapy should be used in cases that fail to meet diagnostic criteria for myeloma in the bone marrow aspirate/biopsy specimens. Current approaches suggest that earlier and more aggressive treatment is indicated. Chemotherapy is far more useful when the serum creatinine is less than 2 mg/dl. The severity of the plasma-cell dyscrasia and the degree of renal failure represent key factors in response to therapy and prognosis. The majority of these patients, however, progress to end-stage renal disease [6,8,81–83]. Patients with overt myeloma do worse than the others. Bone marrow transplantation should be considered in appropriate candidates before irreversible damage to organs, such as the heart, occurs. Aggressive chemotherapy and bone marrow transplant are indicated in the younger patients (less than 65 years old), but this is not yet standard therapy. A few cases with resolution of nodular glomerulosclerosis after therapy have been reported in the literature [84,85]. Renal transplantation represents a viable therapeutic modality especially in patients with the disease process restricted to the kidneys [86,87]. Although recurrence may occur, it is not always associated with rapid loss of the allograft [87]. Complete control of the plasma cell dyscrasia is generally not possible, so the risk for disease recurrence is real. In general, transplantation can be used to improve quality of life in selected patients, but does not appear to be a long-term solution for most.

Amyloidsis

Prognosis varies according to the type of amyloidosis, but is generally poor. AL-amyloidosis has the worst prognosis. Only rare patients with long-term survival have been documented in

AL-amyloidosis [88]; only 7 percent of the patients survive five years after the diagnosis, and less than 1 percent is alive at ten years postdiagnosis [89]. The median survival for these patients is 14–21.5 months, depending on the series [89,90].

In cases with an early detection of amyloidoses, the chances for survival is better. Cardiac involvement remains a predictor of poor survival. Even in AA-amyloidosis, which is characterized by rare cardiac involvement, prognosis is adversely affected when it occurs. Kidney involvement is a key finding in most types of amyloidoses. As the disease progresses, an increase in proteinuria and renal insufficiency occurs with dialysis being the outcome in virtually all cases [91]. Dialysis typically starts at 13.8 months after diagnosis. The approach to therapy in amyloidosis depends on the amyloid type. In the cases of light or heavy chain-associated amyloidosis, control of the plasma cell dyscrasia is crucial [8,92]. High-dose melphalan followed by autologous blood stem-cell transplantation has resulted in an overall increase in survival rate in AL-amyloidosis with accompanying beneficial effect on renal function [93]. One of the main drawbacks of this treatment protocol is early mortality associated with stem-cell transplantation (up to 40 percent), making it a risky treatment modality [94]. In AA-amyloidosis, elimination or control of the underlying disease is crucial for an improvement to occur. New therapeutic measures for AA-amyloidosis are being used with promising results. Agents designed to block the formation of amyloid fibrils by inhibition of glycosaminoglycan binding have shown to be effective in this condition [95]. Colchicine is used in Familial Mediterranean Fever and although it may cause remissions, it does not seem to affect progression of the renal damage. In many patients with hereditary amyloidosis, liver transplantation has been performed to eliminate the source of the precursor protein with reasonably good results. In several patients with hereditary amyloidosis, liver transplantation has been combined with heart and/or kidney transplantation to replace organs that have been irreversibly damaged as a result of the disease process. In some patients with hereditary amyloidosis only affecting kidneys, renal transplantation has been performed. The best results have occurred in patients with AFib and TTR-amyloidosis that have had hepatorenal transplants [96].

Renal transplantation in systemic AL-amyloidosis has had relatively good outcomes with five-year organ survival rates in the 60–65 percent range [97,98], in spite of an increased incidence of early posttransplantation complications, mostly related to infections and sepsis. It has been estimated that recurrence of AL-amyloidosis in the kidney occurs in approximately 20 percent of the transplant patients [97,98]. Severe systemic complications are responsible for a significant percentage of posttransplant morbidity and mortality. It is because of these facts that renal transplantation should be performed preferentially in patients in whom control of their plasma cell dyscrasia has been achieved. The patient's heart should not be involved, and the patient should be in a relatively good shape to be able to withstand the often stormy posttransplantation period.

The majority of renal transplants have been performed in patients with AA-amyloidosis. Outcomes in renal transplantation for AA-amyloidosis are even better with approximately 92 and 89 percent patients and graft survival rates, respectively (National Amyloid Centre Database, United Kingdom). Car-

diac involvement remains a contraindication for renal transplantation. De novo amyloidosis has been reported in the transplanted kidneys in patients with AL and other types of amyloidosis [99,100].

WALDENSTROM MACROGLOBULINEMIA (WM)

Clinical Presentation

WM is a rare, usually slowly progressive disease more common in Caucasians than in blacks, and approximately twice more common in men than in women. The incidence for this condition is much lower than for multiple myeloma, and rise sharply with age. It is an extremely uncommon disease for people below forty-five years of age. It usually affects individuals in their seventies [101]. The disease was originally described by Jan Waldenstrom who initially reported two patients with generalized lymphadenopathy, anemia and a markedly elevated erythrocyte sedimentation rate [102]. Their bone marrow evaluations showed increased numbers of lymphoplasmacytic cells. A significant number of these patients have a monoclonal IgM gammopathy without symptoms, signs or evidence of bone marrow abnormalities. Eventually, they may develop overt manifestations of WM. It may take years for a patient with a monoclonal IgM gammopathy to develop overt clinical manifestations.

The clinical manifestations of this disease relate to direct tumor infiltration in various organs, and to the amount and characteristics of the monoclonal IgM. One particular phenomenon associated with this disorder is a reflection of the ability of the IgM molecules to form complexes among themselves, and occlude the lumens of vessels in various organs, including skin and glomeruli. These patients may have neurologic (10 percent), pulmonary, cutaneous-urticaria, ocular, and gastrointestinal manifestations. Clinical signs and manifestations include fatigue, weakness, recurrent bleeding, lymphadenopathy, splenomegaly, anemia, elevated sedimentation rate, high serum viscosity, and decreased fibrinogen. A hyperviscosity syndrome occurs in a significant percentage of these patients. They may also exhibit lytic bone lesions, although infrequently (less than 5 percent) and amyloidosis develops in approximately 2 percent of patients with this disorder with deposition of fibrils in the heart, kidneys, liver and lungs. Renal involvement occurs infrequently [103,104].

Gross Pathology

One report of giant kidneys associated with infiltration of the renal parenchyma by neoplastic plasma cells is documented in the literature [105]. Renal and perirenal infiltrates of plasma cells [106] and masses containing a monotonous population of plasma cells have also been described. Other studies have shown no apparent gross pathology attributable to WM in the kidneys of these patients.

Light Microscopy

Although there is variability in the morphological manifestations of renal involvement by WM, the most commonly described alteration is glomerular subendothelial deposits or intracapillary protein thrombi which are PAS positive (Figure 10.45 & 10.46) [106–108]. In some cases, thrombi within

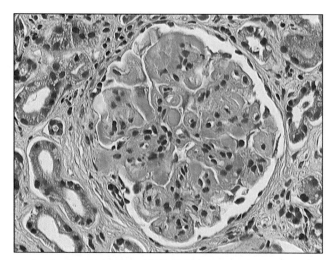

FIGURE 10.45: *Waldenstrom macroglobulinemia. The glomerulus reveals large subendothelial deposits and intracapillary protein thrombi without significant hypercellularity (H&E, ×400, Courtesy of Dr. T. Nadasdy).*

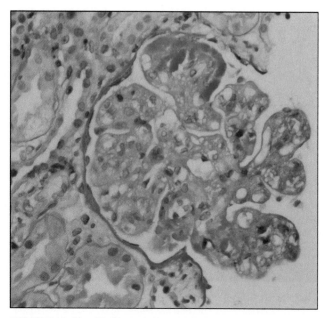

FIGURE 10.46: *Waldenstrom macroglobulinemia. Periodic acid Schiff. ×500. PAS stain highlights segmental glomerular alterations (seen at the top) which include large subendothelial deposits and a capillary thrombus.*

capillary spaces are noted, and in rare instances, it is associated with segmental glomerular necrosis. The glomerular alterations may be focal and segmental (Figure 10.46). Cryoglobulins may be present in the capillary thrombi. Morphologic overlap may occur between cryoglobulinemic nephropathy and WM. Patients with cryoglobulinemia I and II may have underlying WM. Amyloidosis has been described associated with WM in rare cases [108,109]. In three of the sixteen cases, patients with WM, reported by Morel-Maroger et al. had renal amyloidosis [108]. Interstitial plasma cell infiltrates with strong PAS positivity are not uncommon [108]. Although cast nephropathy is extremely unusual in patients with WM, it has also been described [110]. Additional uncommon renal manifestation of WM include diffuse infiltration of the renal parenchyma by plasma cells-producing kidney enlargement (which can be detected with imaging techniques) [105], and the presence of focal aggregates of neoplastic lymphoplasmacytic cells forming discrete renal masses.

Immunofluorescence Microscopy

The glomerular deposits generally stain for IgM and quite frequently IgG as well. The staining pattern may be granular or amorphous, depending on the amounts of IgM and IgG present. Some of the peripheral capillary wall deposits are accompanied by C3 or C4 staining. Capillary thrombi, when present, may also show striking fluorescence for the above immunoreactants, most commonly IgM (Figure 10.47). A rather peculiar distribution of intense staining at the periphery of the thrombi with central latency is occasionally noted. Even normal-appearing glomeruli may exhibit some granular peripheral capillary wall, or mesangial staining for IgM. Arterioles and small arteries are occasionally associated with granular IgM staining. The large amounts of circulating IgM in these patients may be responsible for some of the staining detected in the various renal compartments [106–108]. In some cases, there is also light chain restriction.

Electron Microscopy

The deposits are variably electron-dense, and located in various renal compartments such as subendothelium, within glomerular capillary spaces, or in the extraglomerular vasculature (Figure 10.48) [106–108]. The capillary thrombi have no identifiable substructure, unless they contain cryoglobulins. In some cases, there are inflammatory cells within capillary spaces. If associated cryoglobulinemia is present, the glomerular and vascular deposits may contain cryoglobulins exhibiting their typical appearance.

Differential Diagnosis

There are significant similarities between the nephropathy that is typically seen in WM, and those seen in cryoglobulinemic nephropathy. The proliferative and exudative glomerular changes and the presence of thrombi are shared by both conditions. Cryoglobulins may be present in the nephropathy seen in association with WM. Clinical information becomes essential to make the correct diagnosis. The finding of IgM with or without light chain restriction in association with the deposits and capillary thrombi is also of great value in confirming the diagnosis of WM [108].

Etiology and Pathogenesis

Patients with monoclonal IgM in their serum do not always develop full-blown WM. This only occurs in 17 to 26 percent of these patients [103,104,109]. The ability of IgM molecules to form intravascular complexes resulting in vascular occlusion represents a crucial event in the pathogenesis of this disease. A high viscosity syndrome resulting from the high molecular

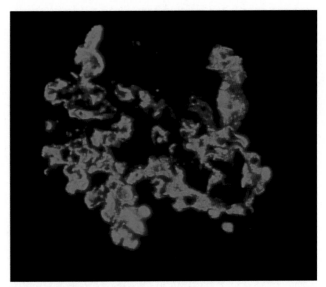

FIGURE 10.47: *Waldenstrom macroglobulinemia. Immunofluorescence microscopy shows intense subendothelial and intracapillary staining for IgM (Direct immunofluorescence, ×400, Courtesy of Dr. T. Nadasdy).*

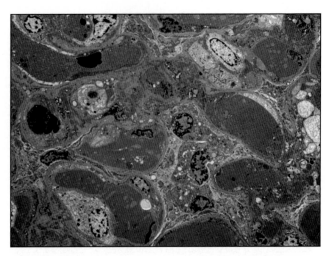

FIGURE 10.48: *Waldenstrom macroglobulinemia. Electron photomicrograph reveals part of glomerular tuft with numerous large subendothelial and intra-luminal electron dense deposits (Courtesy of Dr. T. Nadasdy).*

weight of the IgM molecules results in increased plasma osmotic pressure and plasma volume.

Clinical Course, Prognosis, Treatment, and Clinical Correlation

Then the patients with WM do not present symptoms related to the hypergammaglobulinemia, it is appropriate to monitor them without instituting treatment. Studies have proven that there is no benefit in starting treatment at diagnosis when compared with waiting until clinical manifestations develop. Renal abnormalities do not occur often in patients with WM. Mild or moderate renal functional impairment occurs in 15 to 20 percent of these patients. Glomerular abnormalities are more common than tubulointerstitial manifestations [105–109], contrasting with plasma cell dyscrasias. Occasional patients develop nephrotic or nephritic syndrome. Acute renal failure is rare, and usually a result of extensive vascular occlusion by IgM complexes, dehydration, massive renal infiltration by neoplastic cells or distal nephron obstruction, but the latter is extremely uncommon [110].

Older patients (greater than 60 years of age), male sex, anemia, and neutropenia at presentation are associated with poorer prognosis. Treatment is not needed until complications, associated with this condition, appear.

In essence, treatment is aimed at reducing the tumor load and clearing the circulating IgM. Renal manifestations rarely require dialysis. Plasma exchange has a role in those patients with an extensive vascular occlusion, renal failure, failure to respond, or becoming refractory to standard therapy. Repeated plasmapheresis may be used to delay catatonic therapy. Occlusive vascular lesions in various organs should be treated accordingly. Oral alkylating agents are often used. Chlorambucil at low doses or intermittently at higher doses is also employed [111,112]. Combination therapy

including the use of rituximab, alkylating agents, and purine nucleoside analogues such as fludarabine yields results at least as good, if not better than the use of single agents [111]. Stem-cell bone marrow transplantation is a feasible therapeutic alternative in Waldestrom macroglobulinemia, but used rarely [112].

The median survival for all patients is about five years from the time that clinical manifestations become obvious. If amyloidosis is found complicating the clinical picture in this disease, survival decreases to about half the period, and if cardiac involvement is present associated with amyloidosis, the survival period is even shorter [109]. Gastrointestinal hemorrhage is the most common cause of death. A small percentage of these patients die as a consequence of renal failure.

DISEASES WITH ORGANIZED DEPOSITS

Introduction

Renal disorders with organized deposits can be divided into two fundamental categories: Congo red positive diseases, which encompass all types of amyloidoses, and Congo red negative disorders, which include all other diseases with organized deposits. Another way to conceptualize these conditions is whether the deposits are related to immunoglubulins or not. With the exception of the large category occupied by non-AL-amyloidosis, most of the conditions with organized deposits are immunoglobulin-derived [113,114].

These conditions manifest generally in glomeruli by the expanded mesangial areas. An algorithm for diagnosis of these conditions is shown in Figure 10.49. The organized deposits in the diseases that will be discussed in this chapter are extracellular, and primarily located in the mesangium in most of the diseases discussed.

The separation of amyloidosis from these conditions can be accurately performed in the great majority of the cases using the Congo red and/or Thioflavin T or S stains, which are only

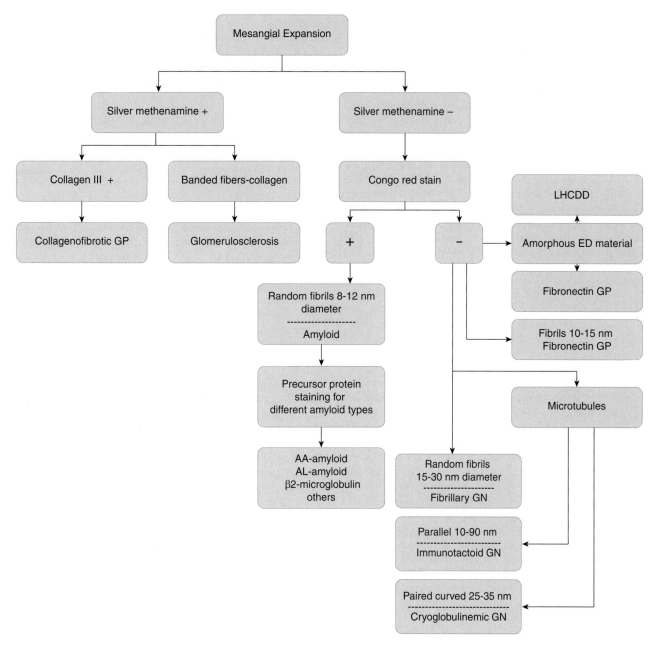

GP = glomerulopathy; **ED** = electron dense; **LHCDD** = light & heavy chain deposition disease; **GN** = glomerulonephritis

FIGURE 10.49: Algorithmic approach to the interpretation of glomerular diseases with organized deposits.

positive in amyloidosis. However, small amounts of amyloid may not be detected by these stains, as their sensitivity is limited. Rarely, spurious positivity for Congo red and Thioflavin T has also been reported representing an important source of confusion in diagnosis; this is often a result of technical mishaps.

Ultrastructural evaluation can be of crucial value in appropriately diagnosing these diseases, and sometimes the only way to make a definitive and final diagnosis. These organized deposits take a variety of forms, which can be divided into several general categories: fibrils of various types, some with character-istic periodicity, hollow cylinders or microtubules, and spheres. The specific features of the organized deposits and how they organize themselves represent crucial finding to characterize the various disorders, and, therefore, the correct characterization of the electron microscopic manifestations is the key for an accurate diagnosis (Figure 10.49). Organized deposits must be distinguished from artifacts, features of the extracellular matrix which are normally present, or which occur as a consequence of disease processes, and debris resulting from cellular damage [114]. Organized deposits derived from immunoglobulins include cryoglobulinemia, fibrillary and immunotactoid glomerulopathies, and dysproteinemias. These typically show fluorescence for various immunoglobulin-associated immunoreactants and, therefore, immunofluorescence evaluation is important in their characterization and diagnosis. A second group of these diseases are not derived from immunoglobulins, including those seen in fibronectin, nail-patella syndrome, and collagenofibrotic glomerulopathies.

Diseases with organized deposits represent specific entities with important clinico-pathologic correlates, but some are of unclear pathogenesis. In the literature, some authors still dispute whether fibrillary and immunotactoid glomerulopathies should be considered different entities, or part of the spectrum of one disease process [115]. It is because there are definitive clinicopathologic reasons to separate these two entities, and most consider them as two distinct entities that they will be treated separately in this chapter [115–118].

Fibrillary Glomerulonephritis (FG)

Clinical Presentation. FG is characterized by the deposition of Congo red negative fibrils in the renal parenchyma, most commonly in glomeruli. These fibrils are randomly disposed and nonbranching; however, their diameter is wider than that of amyloid fibrils. This entity was first documented in the literature in 1977 under the rubric of Congo-red-negative amyloid-like fibrillary deposits [119], but FG was recognized as a specific disease process by Duffy et al [120]. It is an uncommon disease which typically accounts for approximately 1 percent of all renal biopsies accessioned in busy renal pathology practices. It was Alpers et al. in 1987 who coined the term fibrillary glomerulonephritis when he described seven cases with glomerular deposition of fibrils ranging in size from 10 to 20 nm [121] associated with monoclonal κ deposition. A number of other designations for FG have been given in the literature including "non amyloid fibrillary glomerulonephritis" and "Congo-red-negative amyloidosis-like glomerulopathy". These terms although quite descriptive are not acceptable at present. This disease does not have a specific clinical profile. There is a mild female preponderance and the disease appears to be far more common in Caucasians than in any other race. The mean age at presentation is the fifth decade of life. Virtually, all the patients present with proteinuria, most often in the nephrotic range, and more than half of the patients exhibit microscopic hematuria (70 percent); approximately, half of the patients show renal insufficiency, and more than half of the patients exhibit hypertension (65 percent) at the time of presentation. Patients with FG may have a number of underlying systemic conditions, including systemic lupus erythematosus, cutaneous T cell lymphoma, chronic lymphocytic leukemia, diabetic mellitus, malignant hypertension, scleroderma, human immunodeficiency-associated infection, gastric adenocarcinoma, and Rifampin therapy for tuberculosis, but many of the cases are single case reports without an association with the described systemic disorders. Chain restriction, usually κ has been noted, and a small number of patients with FG have been found to have an underlying plasma cell dyscrasia. Renal insufficiency is generally present at the time of presentation in the majority of these patients, and the mean serum creatinine is 3 mg/dl [116,117,122].

Light Microscopy. The light microscopic features of this condition are quite heterogeneous. Mesangial matrix expansion is the most reproducible finding and probably the first abnormality noticeable in patients with FG. In the initial stages of the disease process, this finding may be very subtle, or rather nonspecific with mild segmental mesangial expansion and/or segmental glomerular collapse (Figure 10.50). The mesangial matrix is generally PAS positive which contrasts with amyloid that is typically associated with weak PAS staining. In most cases, there is also segmental or diffuse capillary wall thickening. Cellular proliferation is often present in mesangial areas mimicking mesangial proliferative glomerulonephritis (Figure 10.51) and, in some instances, the degree of proliferation is much more marked, and accentuated lobularity is the result. In the latter cases, a membranoproliferative pattern becomes prominent. Crescent formation occurs in as many as 27 percent of the cases[113,114,116,117,122]. Segmental glomerular collapse and associated sclerosis, a pattern indistinguishable from focal segmental glomerulosclerosis, may also be identified. The expanded mesangium usually appears glassy to amorphous, and is generally PAS-positive (Figure 10.52), purple blue on trichrome stain, and nonargyrophilic due to replacement of the normal mesangial matrix (Figure 10.53). Congo red and Thioflavin T or S stains are negative. Changes in the tubular interstitial and vascular compartments consisting of fibrosis, tubular atrophy and drop-out, and vascular sclerosis follows the progression of the glomerular process as the disease advances and glomerulosclerosis occurs.

Immunofluorescene Microscopy. The pattern of immunoreactivity is generally quite characteristic in this condition. Mesangial staining is seen in virtually all the cases, and this staining, along with the staining invariably present along the peripheral capillary walls, creates the diagnostic pattern for this condition. When fluorescence is only detected in the mesangium (a small number of cases), the staining-pattern can be comma-like. Likewise, if only peripheral capillary-wall staining is noted, it may be confused with antiglomerular basement membrane disease. There is ribbon-like, linear or pseudolinear, at times interrupted staining for IgG, C3, κ and λ light chains with variable intensities (Figure 10.54) [113,114,122]. C4 is also detected in the majority of these cases. The appearance of the fluorescence staining can be somewhat subdued, and has been described as "smudged" in some cases. The most common subtype of IgG detected in association with the fibrils is IgG4, which is the dominant IgG in the majority of the cases. Kappa, but not λ staining, is noted in a subset of patients with FG. Staining for other immunoglobulins and C1q is usually negative, but has been reported positive in occasional cases. Amyloid-P component colocalizes with the fibrils and can be identified by either using immunofluorescence or immunohistochemistry techniques [113,114,124]. In the cases with κ restriction, the pattern is similar to a membranous nephropathy with regularly disposed epimembranous deposits [121].

Electron Microscopy. Ultrastructural evaluation provides the conclusive evidence for substantiating a diagnosis of FG. The finding of randomly aligned fibrils with a diameter in the range of 15–30 nm represents the characteristic finding. In most reported studies, the mean fibril diameter is around 15–20 nm.

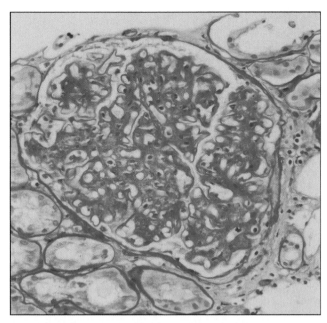

FIGURE 10.50: *Fibrillary glomerulonephritis. Periodic acid Schiff. ×500. Mild alterations are noted with subtle segmental mesangial expansion and thickening of some peripheral capillary walls.*

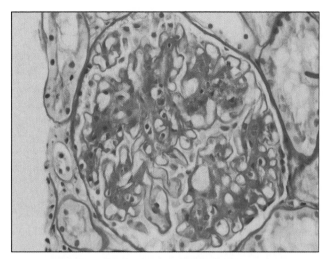

FIGURE 10.52: *Fibrillary glomerulonephritis. Periodic acid Schiff. ×500. Well-defined mesangial expansion and segmental thickening of peripheral capillary walls are identified in this case.*

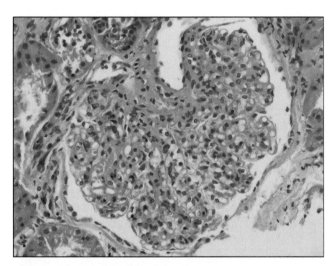

FIGURE 10.51: *Fibrillary glomerulonephritis. Hematoxylin and eosin. ×500. Mesangial proliferative pattern with subtle segmental mesangial expansion.*

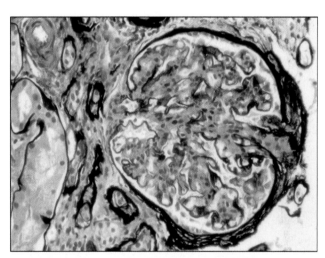

FIGURE 10.53: *Fibrillary glomerulonephritis. Silver methenamine. ×500. Note absence of mesangial staining indicating that the normal mesangial matrix is no longer present.*

These fibrils are similar to those seen in amyloids in that they do not branch and are haphazardly arranged. They are always found in the mesangium (Figure 10.55), but in the great majority of the cases they are also found along the peripheral capillary walls (Figure 10.56), accounting for the immunofluorescence pattern described above. Subepithelial, subendothelial, and transmembranous fibrils can be seen along the capillary walls with variable distribution documented [113,114,122,123]. In a subgroup of patients with FG, the fibrillary material is noted in intimate association with deposits which have the appearance of immune complexes; this appearance is most commonly seen in

cases with "membranous" distribution of the deposits (Figure 10.57) [121,125,126]. In some cases, partially empty areas along the peripheral capillary walls, mimicking stage IV membranous nephropathy, alternate with others that contain fibrils (Figure 10.58). In a few cases, fibrils with features as noted above can be demonstrated around peritubular capillaries and surrounding tubular basement membranes.

Differential Diagnosis. From a clinical standpoint, this condition is essentially never suspected, as the clinical manifestations are entirely nonspecific. It is because the findings in FG include different degrees of a combination of hypercellularity, matrix expansion, and thickening of peripheral capillary walls, as well as crescent formation that the light microscopic manifestations can be quite variable and heterogeneous [116–123]. If the light microscopic and immunofluorescence data is taken

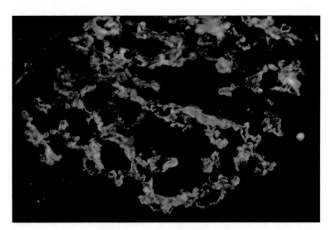

FIGURE 10.54: Fibrillary glomerulonephritis. Direct immunofluorescence stain for IgG; fluorescein isothiocyanate. ×500. Pseudolinear or ribbon-like fluorescence staining of capillary walls and contiguous mesangial staining are the characteristic finding in this condition.

into account, the differential diagnosis commonly includes membranous nephropathy because of the peripheral fluorescence staining for IgG, C3, κ, and λ light chains and the thickening of peripheral capillary walls that is often present; the ribbon-like character of the staining should alert the observer

to a possible diagnosis of FG [113,114,122]. Mesangial proliferative and membranoproliferative glomerulonephritis can also be in the differential diagnosis of those cases associated with significant cellular proliferation. It is because crescents can be seen in some cases that crescentic glomerulonephritis may also be in the differential diagnosis. If the fluorescence pattern of staining is restricted to the peripheral capillary wall, confusion may arise in this crescentic pattern with antiglomerular basement membrane disease. If mesangial expansion is the predominant finding at the light microscopic level, the possibility of amyloidosis is often entertained; the negative Congo red and Thioflavin T stains are very useful in this situation, but the ultrastructural findings provide the definitive answer. At the ultrastructural level, the main differential diagnosis is amyloid, and although the disposition and overall appearance of the fibrils is similar, the distinction lies in the diameter of the fibrils [113,114,122].

Etiology and Pathogenesis. Much discussion has taken place regarding the etiology and pathogenesis of this condition. While there may be more than one specific pathogenetic mechanism involved in this condition, it appears that, in the majority of the cases, FG is the result of an immune complex mediated process in which the complexes are polymerized into fibrils [117]. It is theorized by some that the relative homogeneity in the immune deposits is responsible for the fibrillary appearance in those cases. Amyloid-P component has been identified in

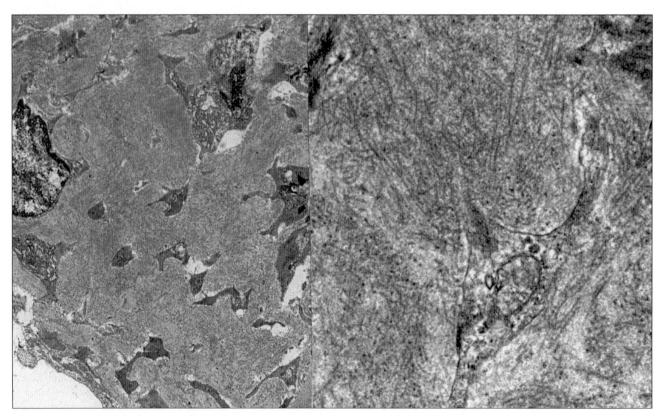

FIGURE 10.55: Fibrillary glomerulonephritis. Transmission electron microscopy. Uranyl acetate and lead citrate. Left: ×8,500; right: ×16,500. The entire mesangium is replaced by randomly disposed, nonbranching fibrils which measure 15–25 nm in diameter. These fibrils extend into peripheral capillary walls.

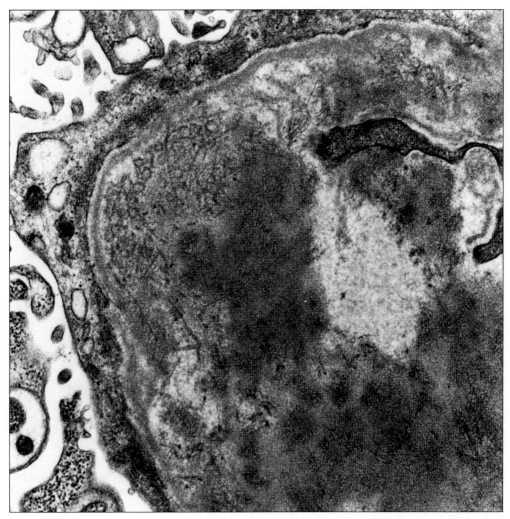

FIGURE 10.56: *Fibrillary glomerulonephritis. Transmission electron microscopy. Uranyl acetate and lead citrate. ×13 500. Peripheral capillary walls with fibrils predominantly located subendothelially.*

association with the fibrillary deposits, suggesting a possible role in the genesis of the fibrils [124].

The reasons for chronic immune stimulation in patients with FG can be variable. Some of these patients have an underlying collagen vascular disease, most commonly systemic lupus erythematosus, others harbor a hepatitis C infection, and some have a variety of chronic inflammatory conditions that may be associated with robust stimulation of the immune system. A few cases with FG associated with an underlying lymphoplasmacytic disorder may result from polymerization of monotypical light chains [2,5]. Since there is no experimental model to study FG, the theories regarding pathogenesis of this condition cannot be entirely substantiated at this time.

Clinical Clourse, Prognosis, Treatment and Clinical Correlation. Unfortunately, most of these patients present late in the course of their disease with significant renal functional impairment. There is a high risk of progression to end-stage renal disease in patients with FG. Approximately, half of the patients with FG develop end-stage renal disease within two to four years after diagnosis [117,118,122]. In a study of fifty-six

patients with FG, 45 percent developed end-stage renal disease [117] within that timeframe. According to one reported series, the pattern of involvement (as detected by light microscopy) correlated with the clinical features and severity of renal insufficiency, the amounts of proteinuria, the presence or absence of a full-blown nephrotic syndrome at presentation, as well as the clinical outcomes [117].

Although a variety of therapeutic interventions have been tested in these patients, results have been poor. Patients have been treated with a variety of immunosuppressants including steroids, cyclophosphamide, and cyclosporine [117,122,123]. In some instances, the therapy has been tailored to the pattern of glomerular involvement that has been noted. Although some responses were noted with therapy initially, resulting in a decrease in proteinuria and serum creatinine, the response only lasted for a limited amount of time and a progression of the disease eventually occurred [117]. Patients with associated monoclonal gammopathies have been treated for their hematologic condition with Melphalan and prednisone and/or immuran usually without significant improvement in renal parameters.

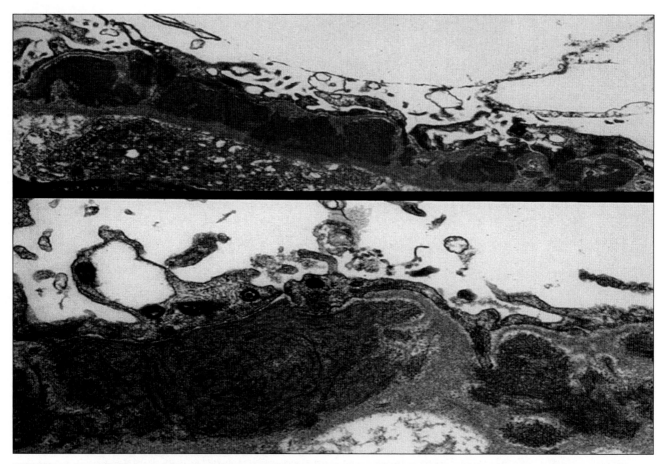

FIGURE 10.57: *Fibrillary glomerulonephritis, membranous pattern. Transmission electron microscopy. Uranyl acetate and lead citrate. Top: ×3,500; bottom: ×9,500. On the top panel, intramembranous electron densities are noted in a pattern reminiscent of membranous glomerulopathy. On the bottom panel, the electron densities are noted to be associated with randomly oriented fibrils similar to those seen in Figure 10.56.*

Renal transplantation in these patients has resulted in recurrence in approximately 50 percent of the cases but allograft loss has not always occurred following the diagnosis of recurrence in the transplanted kidney [127]. De-novo FG has been described in the transplanted kidney of a patient, with systemic lupus erythematosus, who developed biopsy-proven end-stage renal disease as a consequence of lupus nephritis [128].

Diabetic Fibrillosis

Clinical Presentation. This entity was first described by Sohar et al. in 1970 who described deposits of PAS positive, colloidal iron and Congo-red-negative material in the blood vessels of virtually all the organs examined in the autopsies from three patients with diabetes mellitus [129]. The blood vessels involved included capillaries, venules, arterioles, and large size arteries. This material was fibrillary measuring approximately 10 nm in diameter. The authors at the time interpreted the findings as indicative of a systemic disease of connective tissue resembling amyloidosis [129]. Since then, the appellation has also been used to designate the accumulation of fibrils in the

mesangium of patients with diabetic nodular glomerulosclerosis [130].

Light Microscopy. The typical findings of diabetic nephropathy (nodular glomerulosclerosis) are present in these patients. The mesangial nodules stain generally intensely with silver, and the peripheral capillary walls are thickened. The mesangium stains PAS-positive, and is blue with the trichrome stain [130]. Tubular interstitial fibrosis, tubular atrophy, and dropout are typically present. Vascular sclerosis and hyaline arteriolosclerosis are the characteristic findings in these patients. Congo red stain is negative.

Immunofluorescence Microscopy. The immunofluorescence profile of these cases is identical to that seen in other patients with nodular diabetic glomerulosclerosis . Linear staining for both IgG and albumin is clearly seen along the peripheral capillary walls, and the other immunoreactants are typically negative in glomeruli, with the exception of nonspecific trapping of IgM and C3, as it often occurs in diabetic nephropathy with nodular glomerulosclerosis. Linear fluorescence of tubular basement membranes for albumin and at times IgG is also a striking finding.

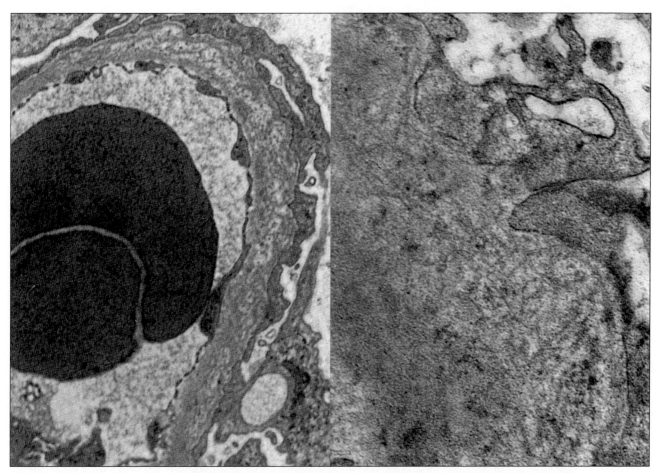

FIGURE 10.58: *Fibrillary glomerulonephritis. Transmission electron microscopy. Uranyl acetate and lead citrate. Left: ×5,600; and right: ×9,500. Left: Fibrils are present along peripheral capillary wall predominantly in an intramembranous location. Right: a subepithelial aggregate of similar fibrils is shown.*

Electron Microscopy. The characteristic finding is the presence of randomly distributed fibrils which vary in diameter from 10 to 25 nm in the mesangial nodules with a marked increase in extracellular matrix (Figure 10.59). These fibrils are restricted to the mesangium and are not found along peripheral capillary walls [130].

Differential Diagnosis. The differential diagnosis includes amyloidosis and fibrillary glomerulonephritis. The absence of staining for Congo red and Thioflavin stains rules out amyloidosis. The differential diagnosis with fibrillary glomerulonephritis is based on the usual bundle-like arrangement of the fibrils and mesangial restriction in diabetic fibrillosis, and the absence of the typical fluorescence profile present in FG, as well as the smaller diameter of the non branching fibrils [113,114, 129–131].

Clinical Course, Prognosis, Treatment, and Clinical Correlations. No detailed studies addressing the significance of this lesion are documented in the literature. The presence of diabetic fibrillosis does not seem to alter the prognosis of what represents the otherwise classical diabetic nodular glomerulosclerosis. There are no therapeutic implications associated with the diagnosis of diabetic fibrillosis,and nor are there any established specific clinical correlations. It is generally diagnosed in advanced cases of diabetic nephropathy.

Immunotactoid Glomerulopathy

Clinical Presentation. There has been considerable debate regarding the relationship, if any, between FG and immunotactoid glomerulopathy. The latter is characterized by the deposition in glomeruli, mainly in the mesangial areas, of microtubules measuring generally more than 30 nm in diameter with a hollow center and arranged in a parallel fashion, and less frequently in tacked arrays. Therefore, morphologically speaking, immunotactoid glomerulopathy is a distinct entity clearly separable from FG. The supporters of a single entity have argued that the differences in morphology are related to fibril diameter and the resolution of the electron microscope rather than a result of different pathogenetic mechanisms or patients profile [115]. Recent publications have made a convincing case for separating these two entities [113, 116–118].

Immunotactoid glomerulopathy is a significantly less common disease than FG (in the neighborhood of 100 times less common). Patients with immunotactoid glomerulopathy are

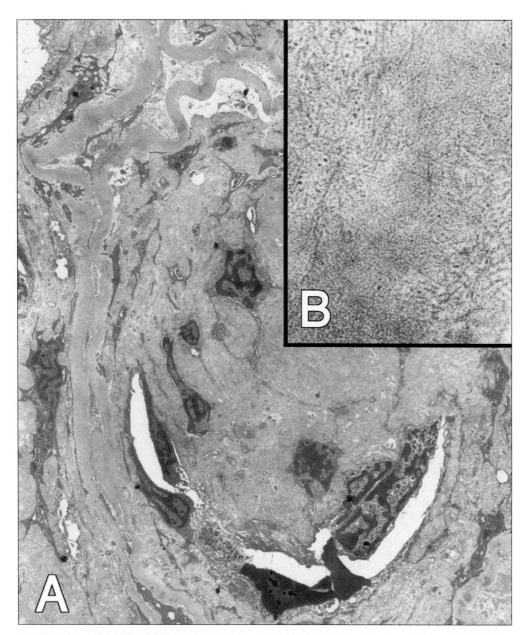

FIGURE 10.59: *Diabetic fibrillosis. Transmission electron microscopy. Uranyl acetate and lead citrate. A: ×8,500; and B: ×15,500. Patient with diabetic nephropathy, nodular glomerulosclerosis with deposition of fibrils which measure about 20 nm in diameter in mesangial nodules.*

generally ten years older than those with FG (in their late fifties or early sixties) [115,123]. Their clinical manifestations, however, are rather similar. These patients typically have, at presentation, proteinuria in the nephrotic range with nephrotic syndrome present in approximately half of the patients. Two characteristics separate these patients from those with FG: a higher incidence of serum or urine monoclonal proteins with underlying lymphoproliferative disorders and hypocomplementemia, both statistically significant in the several series reported in the literature where these parameters have been carefully analyzed [115–117, 127]. These patients also have an increased propensity for detection of serum cryoglo-

bulins when searched for, creating some questions as to whether there may be some association between cryoglobulinemia and immunotactoid glomerulopathy. Therefore, a diagnosis of immunotactoid glomerulopathy should generate a clinical search for an underlying dysproteinemia, or occult cryoglobulinemia.

Light Microscopy. The light microscopic patterns in this condition are also quite diverse. Making the diagnosis of immunotactoid glomerulopathy on light microscopy is not possible. Proliferative glomerular changes can be the predominant morphologic finding, and a diagnosis of mebranoproliferative or diffuse proliferative glomerulonephritis may be rendered on the basis of the light microscopic features. In contrast, other cases may exhibit "membranous-like" or "focal segmental sclerosis-like" features (Figure 10.60) [113–115,122,123,127]. Glomerular inflammatory cells are typically absent and necrotizing glomerular changes, capillary thrombi and crescents are not characteristic findings in this disorder. The expanded mesangial areas, when present, are nonargyrophilic and variably PAS-positive.

Immunofluorescence Microscopy. The typical glomerular staining pattern is coarsely granular and often restricted to the mesangium, although peripheral capillary wall staining is also present in a significant number of these cases. The most commonly positive immunoglobulins are IgG (invariably present), IgM (about half of the cases), and IgA (about one third of the cases). C3 staining is a classical finding (Figure 10.61) and glomerular staining for C4 and C1q is only detected sporadically [113,114,123]. Light chain restriction with κ predominance may be seen, but it is not unusual for cases to show staining for both light chains with almost equal intensity. The cases with light chain monoclonality are commonly associated with an underlying lymphoplasmacytic disorder. Monoclonal IgG is present in approximately 60 percent of the patients with immunotactoid glomerulopathy.

Electron Microscopy. The material deposited in the glomeruli is composed of hollow cylinders (microtubule) with a mean diameter of 40 nm, but with a variation in diameter that can be from 10 to 90 nm with the microtubules generally in the range of 20–60 nm (Figure 10.62). It is the finding of microtubules, rather than fibrils that segregates this group of cases into a homogeneous group as there may be some overlap in the diameter of the structures identified in deposits. The appearance of the structures that are identified should take precedence over the diameter of the structures. The microtubular structures may arrange in tightly bundled groups or exhibit a looser arrangement. All cases show mesangial deposits and in a significant number of the cases either subendothelial or subepithelial microtubular aggregates are noted [113,114,123]. It is not as common for the microtubules to display the transmembrane

deposition that is so commonly seen with fibrils in FG. No microtubular aggregates have been described in any other renal compartment or any other organs.

Etiology and Pathogenesis. The strong association with an underlying neoplastic lymphoplasmacytic disorder suggests that the disease may occur as a result of a peculiar polymerization of monotypical light chains. There is no experimental model to study this disease.

Differential Diagnosis. From the light microscopic point of view, the glomerular changes in this condition can mimic a variety of diseases as the mesangium is usually expanded, and thickening of peripheral capillary walls, segmental glomerulosclerosis, and even some mesangial proliferation may be present. Diseases that manifest with these rather nonspecific findings have to be considered in the differential diagnosis. These include mesangial proliferative glomerulonephritis of various etiologies, including IgA nephropathy and mesangial lupus nephritis. Sometimes, the mesangial expansion resembles amyloidosis at the light microscopic level [113,114]. Those cases with focal and segmental glomerulosclerosis need to be segregated from those of primary or secondary glomerulosclerosis. Immunofluorescence is very helpful in separating some of the above mentioned disorders from immunotactoid glomerulopathy, but ultrastructural evaluation represents the diagnostic modality that allows proper recognition of this entity. Degenerative cellular changes resulting in cellular debris, deposited in the mesangium, should not be misdiagnosed as immunotactoid glomerulopathy (Figure 10.63).

Clinical Course, Prognosis, Treatment, and Clinical Correlation. In contrast to FG, these patients have better prognosis with progression to renal disease occurring not as fast, and as often [116–118]. However, in a study of six patients with immunotactoid glomerulopathy followed for a mean of ten months (two to twenty months), the mean renal survival was only 17.2 months [118].

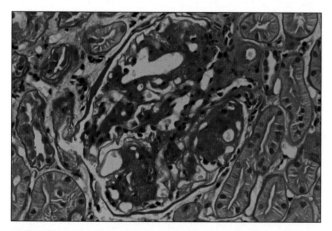

FIGURE 10.60: *Immunotactoid glomerulopathy. Periodic acid Schiff. ×500. Expanded mesangial areas and a segmental area of glomerular collapse characterize one of the morphologic patterns that can be seen in this condition.*

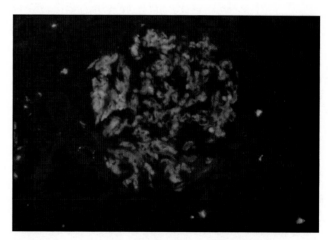

FIGURE 10.61: *Immunotactoid glomerulopathy. Direct immunofluorescence stain for C3; fluorescein isothiocyanate. ×500. Coarsely granular mesangial and peripheral capillary wall C3 staining is the classical fluorescence staining pattern in this disease.*

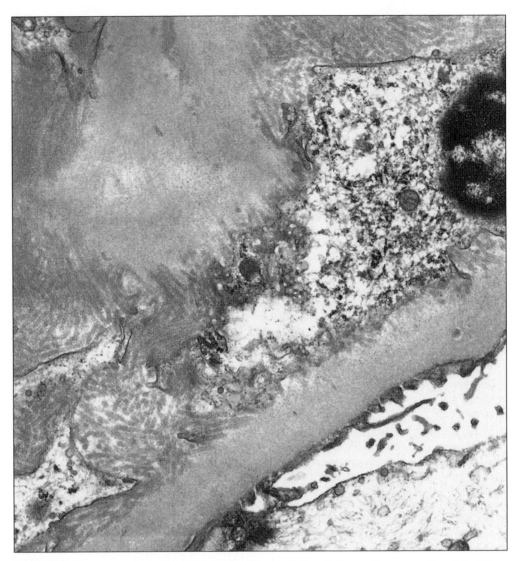

FIGURE 10.62: *Immunotactoid glomerulopathy. Transmission electron microscopy. Uranyl acetate and lead citrate. × 19,500. Hollow cylindrical structures with an average diameter of 40–50 nm located subendothelially and in the mesangium represents the typical ultrastructural finding in this condition.*

Patients with immunotactoid glomerulopathy are treated for their hematologic condition (underlying plasma cell dyscrasia) when it can be substantiated. Although response to therapy is generally poor, one patient with chronic lymphocytic leukemia had significant decreases in proteinuria and serum creatinine when treated with a course of fludarabine [118]. Unfortunately, there are not many studies addressing the treatment in this condition, and the fact that some authors combine this disorder with FG in their studies, further confuses the issues and makes evaluation of the effect of various treatment protocols very difficult.

Cryoglobulinemic Glomerulonephritis

Clinical Presentation. Cryoglobulinemia is more prevalent in females. Renal involvement in cryoglobulinemia may be associated with low-grade proteinuria, nephrotic or nephritic syn-

drome, and/or hypertension. Overall, approximately 20 percent of patients with cryoglobulinemia develop renal manifestations. Other systemic clinical features of this condition include purpura, Raynaud's phenomenon, neuropathy, hepatosplenomegaly, arthralgias, and vasculitis. A marked decrease in serum C4 associated with normal C3 levels should raise the possibility of cryoglobulinemia in the proper clinical setting [132–134].

Cryoglobulins are peculiar immunoglobulins that remain soluble at 37°C, but precipitate at 4°C. There are three well-recognized types of cryoglobulins, the immunomorphologic manifestations of which can be somewhat different when associated with renal disease. A classification of cryoglobulins was accepted in 1974 and is still in use. Type I cryoglobulins are monoclonal and usually of the IgM class. These are normally associated with B-cell neoplasms. Types II are those in which the cryoglobulins are complexes of monoclonal IgM and polyclonal IgG. Currently, these are most commonly associated with hepatitis C infection. Type III are cryoglobulins in which

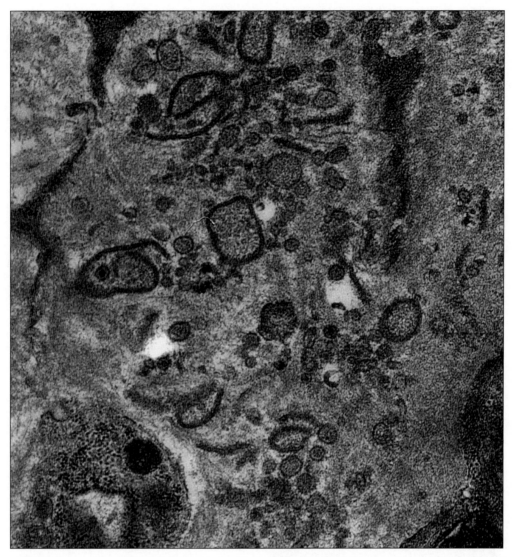

FIGURE 10.63: *Mesangial cellular debris. Transmission electron microscopy. Uranyl acetate and lead citrate. ×22,500. Mesangial cellular debris such as illustrated in this electron micrograph should not be misdiagnosed as immunotactoid glomerulopathy.*

polyclonal IgM is reactive with the Fc fragment of polyclonal IgG. Most Type III cryoglobulins are also associated with hepatitis C, attesting to the fact that most cases with cryoglobulinemia today are related to the underlying hepatitis C infection [135]. Mixed cryoglobulins represent mixtures of the above with combinations of Types II and III being the most common; these are generally found in association with infections, connective tissue diseases, and neoplasms. A percentage of cryoglobulins are not associated with a recognized underlying disorder and are referred to as "essential." This percentage has been gradually decreasing throughout the years, as new associations and disease processes are discovered. For example, since the recognition of hepatitis C, cases of "essential" cryoglobulinemia have been reduced considerably, and only a small percentage of cryoglobulins remain in that category [135].

Monoclonal IgM has an affinity for the mesangium where it is deposited, and then leads to IgG binding in situ. In other instances, complexes of IgG and IgM with or without hepatitis C virus forms in the circulation, and are eventually delivered to the glomerulus. Renal disease is most commonly seen in association with Type II cryoglobulinemia, which results from the above-described pathogenetic pathway.

Light Microscopy. The renal manifestations in this disorder are primarily in the glomerular and vascular compartments, and they are quite variable. The spectrum of morphologic manifestations is quite heterogeneous and the findings depend to some degree on the type of circulating cryoglobulins. In some cases, only mild mesangial hypercellularity is present. In other cases, the cellular proliferation is far more pronounced with increased glomerular lobularity, exudative inflammatory changes, and segmental duplication of peripheral capillary walls by mesangial cell cytoplasm interposition and are best seen in the silver stained section. These are findings that recapitulate the

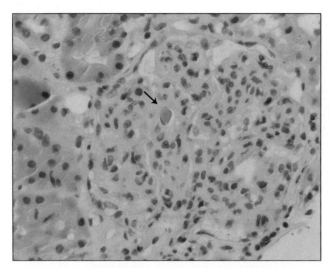

FIGURE 10.64: *Cryoglobulinemic glomerulonephritis. Hematoxylin and eosin. ×500. Mesangial proliferative changes accompanied by a single thrombus (arrow) in a glomerular capillary. Subtle findings like this can be easily missed.*

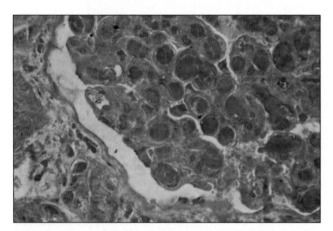

FIGURE 10.65: *Cryoglobulinemic glomerulonephritis. Trichrome. ×500. Numerous thrombi in capillary spaces in this case of cryoglobulinemic glomerulonephritis, Type II.*

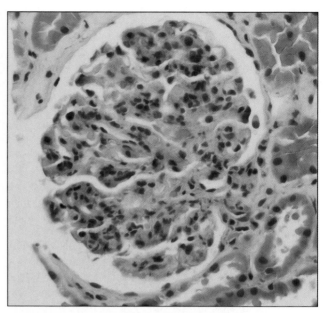

FIGURE 10.66: *Cryoglobulinemic glomerulonephritis. Hematoxylin and eosin. ×500. In addition to the capillary thrombi, evidence of intraglomerular cellular proliferation and exudative changes, as seen in this figure, provide additional morphological evidence to support the diagnosis.*

morphologic appearance associated with membranoproliferative glomerulonephritis, Type I (Figures 10.64 to 10.66). An exudative element may also be present. Monocytes are sometimes present in the partially obliterated capillary spaces. Hyalin thrombi in glomerular capillaries, which may be a very focal and subtle finding (Figure 10.64) or easily identifiable (Figures 10.65), represent an important finding that should immediately place the diagnosis of cryoglobulinemic glomerulonephritis in the differential diagnosis. Segmental glomerular necrosis may also be seen. Subendothelial deposits in glomeruli may be highlighted on the PAS stain. Cryoglobulin thrombi can also be seen in arterioles and even in the larger vessels. Vasculitis with endothelial fibrinoid necrosis may be seen in intra- or extrarenal vessels, but this a relatively uncommon finding in biopsy specimens [135–140].

Immunofluorescence Microscopy. The fluorescence patterns associated with cryoglobulinemic glomerulopathy are also quite variable. In those instances in which capillary thrombi are present, they may stain monoclonally for one type of immunoglobulin and/or one of the two light chains (Figure 10.67). The same is true of the subendothelial deposits. Kappa light chain restriction is far more common than λ restriction in cryoglobulinemic glomerulonephritis. Staining can also be spotty in subendothelium and mesangium (Figure 10.67), and usually for the same immunoglobulin as found in the circulation [135–138].

Electron Microscopy. Cryoglobulins can be detected in any of the glomerular compartments, but most commonly are seen in subendothelial locations and in capillary thrombi (Figure 10.68). The classical appearance is characterized by subendothelial, mesangial, or intracapillary deposits consisting of paired, curved microtubular to annular structures with spokes that measure 25–40 nm in diameter (Figures 10.68 and 10.69). Which of the two appearances predominates depends on whether the structures have been sectioned longitudinally or cross-sectionally. This appearance is most commonly seen in mixed cryoglobulins. In the monoclonal cryoglobulins, either straight fibrils forming bundles, which may appear cross-hatched on cross section or tubular structures in a fingerprint array, represent the characteristic ultrastructural appearance. The ultrastructural features associated with cryoglobulins can be varied (Figures 10.68 and 10.69) [138,139]. Fingerprints have also been described in cryoglobulinemic deposits [141]. In my experience, the most characteristic ultrastructural findings in the cryoglobulins that allow an unequivocal diagnosis are found in the capillary thrombi, so these should be examined carefully.

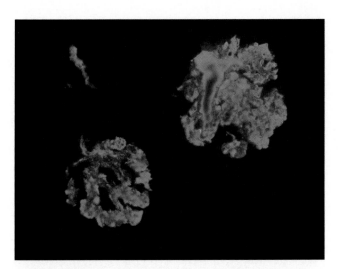

FIGURE 10.67: *Cryoglobulinemic glomerulonephritis. Direct immunofluorescence stain for κ light chains; fluorescein isothiocyanate. ×350. Intense staining in glomeruli and capillary thrombi represents one of the immunofluorescence patterns that can be seen in this disease. There was no staining for λ light chain, confirming the presence of monoclonal cryoglobulins.*

Cryoglobulin deposits may coexist with classical immune complexes in a number of entities such as lupus nephritis. The diagnosis of cryoglobulinemia may be unsuspected and the ultrastructural identification of the classical ultrastructural features associated with cryoglobulins allows a definitive diagnosis. In other cases, a clinical suspicion of cryoglobulinemia prompts the renal biopsy, and the challenge is to either link the renal disease with the systemic process, or to rule out an association.

In addition, varying degrees of mesangial and endocapillary proliferation can be seen in most cases, while mesangial interposition along peripheral capillary walls is present in some of the cases [139,140]. The latter is only absent in instances when the proliferative activity is minor, and such is not common in the spectrum of these diseases. Monocytes can participate in the genesis of the peripheral capillary wall-splitting or tramtrack appearance. An exudative inflammatory component is seen in some cases, and it can be quite pronounced. Effacement of foot processes correlates with the degree of proteinuria.

Etiology and Pathogenesis. Precipitation of cryoglobulins resulting in vascular occlusion is associated with hypoperfusion and necrosis of segmental glomerular areas and, in rare cases, even renal parenchymal infarcts, if the thrombotic process involves large vessels.

Clinical Course, Prognosis, Treatment, and Clinical Correlations. Clinically, patients with cryoglobulinemia are characterized by exacerbations and remissions, and clinical and histologic findings do not directly correlate with the detection of circulating cryoglobulins, or the amount detected in the serum [132,142].

Cryoglobulins can be identified in patients with a variety of renal diseases, most commonly in membranoproliferative glo-

merulonephritis Type I, and lupus nephritis. Alternatively, approximately 21–29 percent of the patients with cryoglobulinemia exhibit renal disease, which is more common in Type II cryoglobulinemia. The overall renal prognosis in this condition is excellent with only approximately 10 percent of the cases ending in end-stage renal disease that require dialysis [132,135,143]. Hypertension may be difficult to control, making cerebrovascular and cardiovascular complications common and the most challenging clinical problems in these patients [143]. Treatment is primarily symptomatic.

Difficult cases that cannot be adequately controlled with symptomatic treatment may require the use of immunosuppressive therapy, steroids, and/or plasmapheresis [132,143]. Response of the renal manifestations to therapy is rather unpredictable, except in cases with acute renal failure secondary to cryoglobulinemic nephropathy which is a rare occurrence where aggressive intervention produces excellent results [143]. Renal transplantation in these patients is uncommon and recurrent cryoglobulinemic glomerulonephritis may occur in the transplanted kidney.

Fibronectin Glomerulopathy

Clinical Presentation. This is a very rare disease. The pattern of inheritance in most of the affected families has been determined to be autosomal dominant [144]. This entity was first reported by Burgin in 1980 when he documented three siblings and one first-degree cousin [145] affected by the same condition. A few other families have since been reported. Clinically, these patients present with proteinuria, often nephrotic range, microhematuria, and hypertension. The patients' age at presentation can be quite variable. Renal function is characteristically compromised at presentation in less than 50 percent of the patients. Slowly, progressive deterioration of renal function typically occurs. No systemic manifestations have been documented in these patients.

Light Microscopy. The glomeruli are enlarged and accentuation of the lobular architecture is often noted [113,144–146]. No significant glomerular hypercellularity or duplication of peripheral capillary walls by mesangial cell cytoplasm interposition has been described in these cases. However, expansion of mesangial areas and segmental thickening of peripheral capillary walls are the most common findings. The expanded mesangium may be strikingly PAS positive (Figure 10.70), red with the trichrome stain (Figure 10.71), and fails to stain with the silver methenamine stain [144–146]. There are no specific tubular interstitial or vascular changes noted. Interstitial fibrosis and vascular sclerosis occurs as the glomerular process advances.

Immunofluorescence Microscopy/Immunohistochemistry. Focal, segmental sparse deposits containing immunoglobulins and complement components have been described with a rare patient showing more significant staining for immunoglobulins (IgG and M), C3 and fibrinogen. The typical finding is striking immunoreactivity for fibronectin in mesangial areas [144–146]. No staining for other extracellular matrix proteins typically present in the mesangium, including collagen IV is detected in these cases.

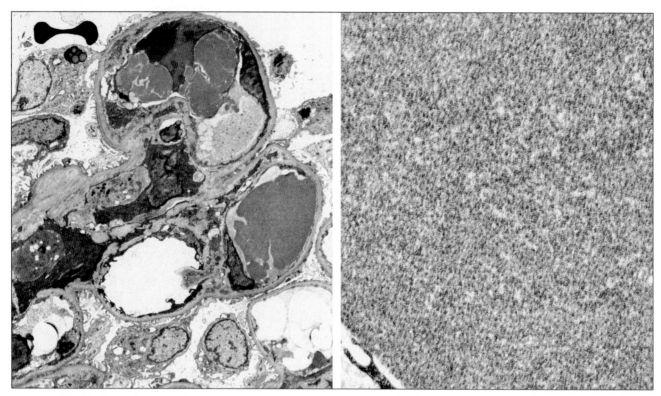

FIGURE 10.68: *Cryoglobulinemic glomerulonephritis. Transmission electron microscopy. Uranyl acetate and lead citrate. A: ×2,500; B: ×35,000. Capillary thrombi are illustrated in A and in B, the appearance of the thrombus confirms the presence of cryoglobulins.*

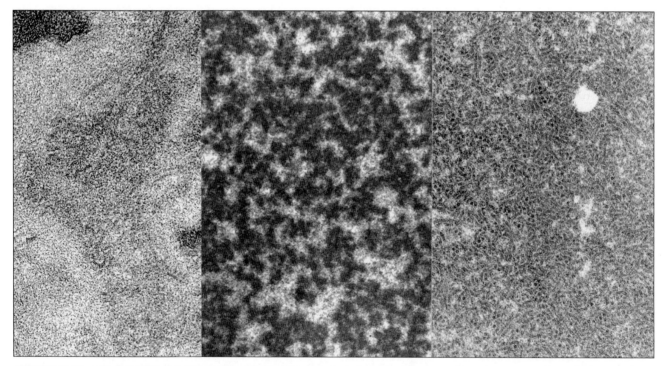

FIGURE 10.69: *Cryoglobulinemic glomerulonephritis. Transmission electron microscopy. Uranyl acetate and lead citrate.*
Left: ×25,500; middle: ×37,500; and right: ×30,500. Capillary thrombi in cryoglobulinemic glomerulonephritis illustrating variability in ultrastructural appearance of cryoglobulins.

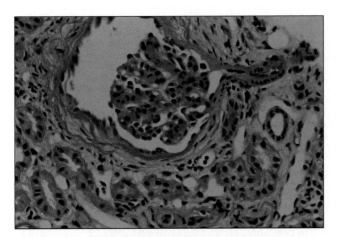

FIGURE 10.70: *Fibronectin glomerulopathy, early changes. Periodic acid Schiff. ×350. Mild expansion of mesangial areas represents the first alteration generally seen in this disease.*

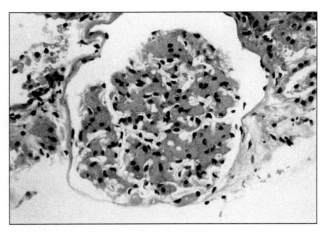

FIGURE 10.71: *Fibronectin glomerulopathy. Trichrome. ×500. Note intense the red staining in expanded mesangial areas (Courtesy of Dr. D. Sedmak).*

Electron Microscopy. Varying degrees of effacement of the foot processes of the visceral epithelial cells is noted. No immune complexes are identified. The crucial finding is the presence of abundant deposition of markedly electron-dense, generally granular (Figure 10.72) but sometimes fibrillary material in subendothelial and mesangizzal areas. Admixtures of granular and fibrillary material has been described in some cases. Massive deposits may be seen in thze mesangium (Figure 10.72) [113,144,146]. In the families in which fibrillary material has been found, the fibrils are reported to measure 10–14 to 16 nm in diameter [144]. No increase in mesangial matrix per se is present. The peripheral capillary walls are usually not involved, but in one family, subepithelial and intramembranous deposits were described. Extraglomerular deposits are rare but have been documented along the Bowman's capsule and tubular basement membranes.

Etiology and Pathogenesis. The fibronectin that is deposited in the glomeruli does not appear to be produced locally, but rather results from circulating fibronectin that deposits in the mesangium. It is believed that this disorder occurs because of a defect in a factor involved in the catabolism of fibronectin. This factor remains elusive at the present time. It can be concluded with the information available at the present time that abnormalities in the metabolism of fibronectin may play a fundamental pathogenetic role in this disease of probable autosomal dominant inheritance [144]. However, genetic analysis has failed to show a definitive pathogenetic role for fibronectin, desmin, and villin [147].

Clinical Course, Prognosis, Treatment, and Clinical Correlations. No specific treatment is available for this condition at the present time. Hypertension associated with progressive renal function deterioration over a period of about ten to fifteen years has been reported to occur in the majority of the cases reported in the literature [148]. Although excellent results have been noted after renal transplantation, in one case, fibronectin deposits appeared in the allograft twenty-seven months after transplantation, and the renal allograft was eventually lost [148].

Collagenofibrotic Glomerulopathy (Collagen III Glomerulopathy)

Clinical Presentation. Less than fifty patients with this condition have been documented in the literature. Dombros and Katz published the first case of this entity in 1982 [149], and since then approximately thirty cases have been published in the English literature. A number of synonyms have been used for this entity including primary glomerular fibrosis and the two already mentioned names. The patients with this disorder have been between 6 and 72 years of age and no sex predilection has become apparent. The first symptoms may appear in early childhood, or in late adulthood. The clinical presentation includes proteinuria with associated edema, hematuria, hypertension, and renal insufficiency. Hypertension is documented at the time of presentation in approximately one-third of these patients, and the proteinuria may or may not be in the nephrotic range. The nail and bone alterations typical of the nail-patella syndrome are not present in these patients. No evidence of systemic involvement has been described [150–152].

Light Microscopy. The glomeruli in these cases typically appear enlarged and sometimes resemble the appearance of membranoproliferative glomerulonephritis on light microscopy. Eosinophilic material is present in mesangial areas resulting in their expansion and is responsible for imparting the glomeruli their accentuated lobular appearance (Figure 10.73). As a result, the surrounding capillary spaces are variably compressed, and partially obliterated. The mesangial material is weakly PAS positive, and most commonly also silver positive; however, a loss of the normal mesangial argyrophilia has been described in some cases [152–155]. The altered mesangium is usually red with the trichrome stain. In adults, mesangial nodularity may be present, sometimes with a focal, segmental pattern and in some cases, with a diffuse, generalized distribution. There is no evidence of overt significant glomerular hypercellularity, necrosis or crescent formation. However, a mild

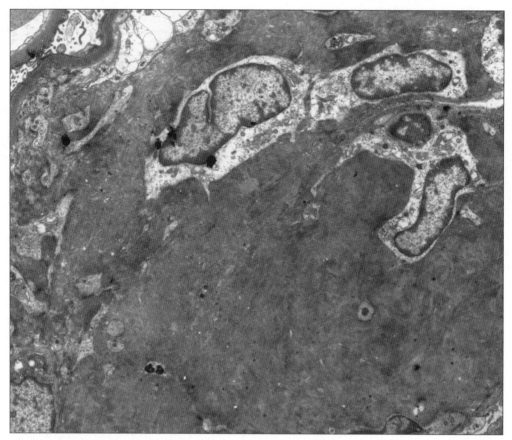

FIGURE 10.72:   Fibronectin glomerulopathy. Transmission electron microscopy. Uranyl acetate and lead citrate. ×22,500. Expanded mesangial area containing massive accumulations of electron-dense material corresponding to fibronectin (Courtesy of Dr. D. Sedmak).

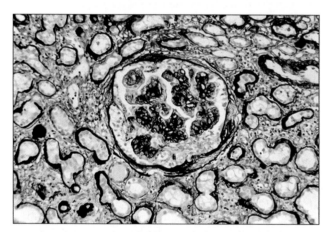

FIGURE 10.73:   Collagenofibrotic glomerulopathy. Silver methenamine. ×350. Accentuated glomerular lobularity associated with an increase in mesangial silver staining is the most common finding in this disorder (Courtesy of Dr. C. Jennette).

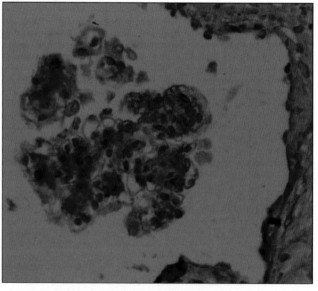

FIGURE 10.74:   Collagenofibrotic glomerulopathy. Immunohistochemical stain for collagen III. Peroxidase antiperoxidase stain; diaminobenzidine. ×500. Strong immunoreactivity for collagen III in mesangial areas confirms the diagnosis in this condition.

increase in mesangial cells may be detected, especially in cases diagnosed early in their clinical course. Sometimes subendothelial expansion and even double-contoured glomerular basement membranes may be detected with the silver methenamine stain.

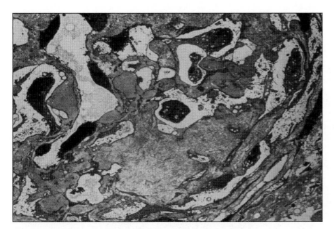

FIGURE 10.75: *Collagenofibrotic glomerulopathy. Transmission electron microscopy. Uranyl acetate and lead citrate. ×5,500. Note variable degrees of mesangial expansion with readily identifiable collagen fibrils.*

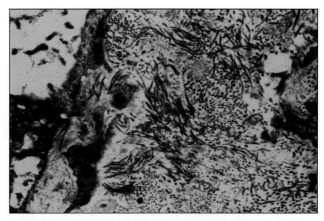

FIGURE 10.76: *Collagenofibrotic glomerulopathy. Transmission electron microscopy. Uranyl acetate and lead citrate. ×9,500. The collagen III fibrils are typically abnormal in their morphological appearance in this disorder.*

Immunofluorescence Microscopy/Immunohistochemistry. The crucial confirming test for a diagnosis of collagenofibrotic glomerulopathy is to demonstrate the presence of collagen III in the expanded mesangial areas (Figure 10.74). This can be done by using either immunofluorescence or immunohistochemistry techniques. The staining detected is usually abundant and readily identifiable as an abnormal finding. Normally, there should be no collagen III in the glomerular mesangium. The antibody to collage III is commercially available, and works well in tissue sections. For the most part, the usual immunofluorescence workup that is used for renal biopsies is negative. Nonspecific IgG, IgM, and C1q staining has been described in some cases [149]. It appears from the descriptions in the publications that this glomerular staining is focal and segmental, mostly a result of trapping, and clearly of no pathogenetic significance. The normal collagen IV that is present in mesangial areas is either displaced to the periphery of the accentuated mesangial zones or markedly decreased, as it appears to be replaced by collagen III. The collagen III deposition is usually rather diffuse and generalized, not focal as seen in some cases with glomerulosclerosis in a variety of diseases [156,157] (Figure 10.74). Some mesangial collagen I may also be detected, but in much less concentration in these cases.

Electron Microscopy. The characteristic finding in this condition is deposition of collagen fibers with unusual ultrastructural features in the mesangium, resulting in its expansion (Figure 10.75) [152–154]. The peripheral capillary walls are spared. The expanded mesangial areas with the collagenous material may be focal and segmental (Figure 10.75). These fibers can be highlighted if the ultrathin sections are treated with phosphotungstic acid. The collagen fibrils appear abnormal, sometimes uniquely curved, frayed, bent, curled or spiral-shaped in longitudinal sections, and in some cases, the collagen fibrils have been described as worm-like in transverse section (Figure 10.76). They then arrange in peculiar bundles different from ordinary collagen III fibers that can be seen in the interstitium, which are typically straight and circular in longitudinal

and transverse sections, respectively (Figure 10.77). The overall appearance of the collagen fibers may also be altered; their diameter may be wider than typical fibrillary collagen and the individual fibers may display a fusiform appearance (Figure 10.77, inset). Also, the periodicity of the collagen fibrils has been variably measured at 430, 480, and 560 nm, also attesting to the abnormal appearance of the collagen fibers. There are cases with collagen identified with normal periodicity (640 nm), but these are typically admixed with collagen fibrils with abnormal periodicity [149–153]. Although subendothelial deposition of abnormal fibers may be seen in a few cases, no deposition of these unusual fibers in intimate association with the glomerular basement membranes or in any other renal compartments has been described. No electron-dense deposits of the immune complex type are present in any of the renal compartments.

Differential Diagnosis. The main differential diagnosis is membranoproliferative glomerulonephritis, Type I, especially in children. The main differentiating point is that cellular proliferation is not a feature of collagenofibrotic glomerulopathy. Ultrastructurally, as the differential diagnoses is under consideration, the finding of the abnormal fibrils, as already described, and the absence of immune complexes would provide more than sufficient evidence to rule out membranoproliferative glomerulonephritis. Likewise, the absence of a positive immunofluorescence indicating an immune complex-mediated process would provide additional supporting evidence. Other conditions where there is marked expansion of mesangium such as diabetic nephropathy, light or heavy chain deposition disease, or the idiopathic type of nodular glomerulosclerosis also need to be considered in the differential diagnosis. In diabetic nephropathy, characteristic glomerular basement membrane thickening and subepithelial lamellation should be present. The absence of monoclonal deposits of light or heavy chains by immunofluorescence and punctuate to powdery light/heavy chain deposits by electron microscopy should suffice to make a distinction. The abnormal collagen fibers are not disposed

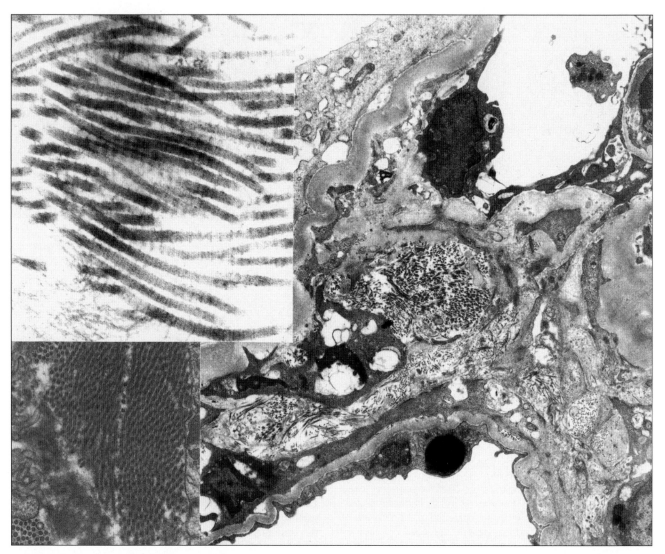

FIGURE 10.77: *Mesangial fibrillary collagen deposition in segmental glomerulosclerosis. Transmission electron microscopy. Uranyl acetate and lead citrate. Right: ×7,500; top left: ×45,000; and bottom left: ×32,500. Longitudinally (top left) and cross sectioned (bottom left) collagen fibers usually display an orderly arrangement and maintain the expected collagen periodicity (640 nm). These fibers should be distinguished from those illustrated in Figure 10.76, characteristic of collagenofibrotic glomerulopathy.*

along the glomerular basement membranes as is the case in the nail-patella syndrome, which helps in differentiating these two conditions at the ultrastructural level. Furthermore, the abnormal-appearing collagen fibers described in collagenofibrotic glomerulopathy are not present in the nail-patella syndrome where the collagen is unremarkable ultrastructurally.

Ultrastructurally, collagen should not be confused with other structures with periodicity. For example, fibrin may occasionally exhibit a striking periodicity and be a source of confusion (Figure 10.78). Likewise, deposition of fibrillary collagen in the mesangium can be seen in a number of advanced glomerulopathies, most notably focal segmental glomerulosclerosis and diabetic nephropathy-nodular glomerulosclerosis, as part of the general process of glomerulosclerosis [155–157]. Collagen deposition is characterized by a parallel arrangement of collagen fibers with characteristic periodicity (640 nm). The

parallel deposition of fibers in this situation is quite helpful in properly characterizing the pathological process (Figure 10.77).

Etiology and Pathogenesis. There is no indication that a specific etiology for this condition exists. However, since the majority of the cases have been described in Japan, genetic, racial, and/or geographical factors may be associated with this disease. Inheritance follows an autosomal recessive pattern with variable gene penetrance, as illustrated by the fact that the majority of cases in Japan have been reported in adults and the cases from Europe, reported in children. There has been one documented case associated with factor H deficiency [154].

It has been speculated that synthesis and/or degradation of skeletal collagen may be deranged in these cases with increased

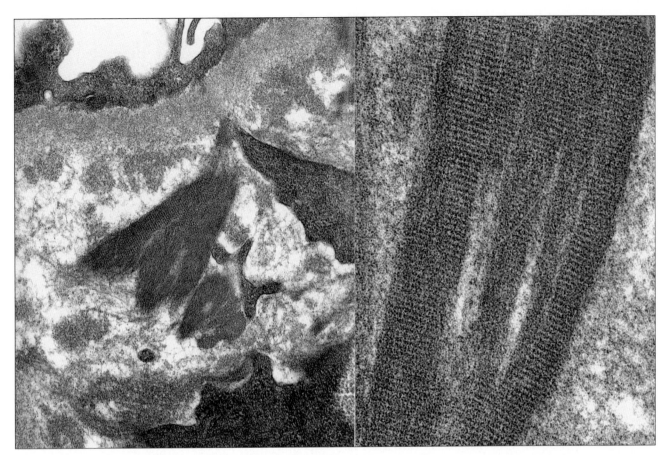

FIGURE 10.78: *Fibrin in capillary thrombus. Transmission electron microscopy. Uranyl acetate and lead citrate. Left: ×22,500; right:× 60,000. Typical ultrastructural appearance of fibrin with its characteristic periodicity. This should not be confused with fibrillary collagen.*

quantities of collagen III precursors, or fragments of mature collagen III released into the circulation and entrapped in the glomeruli. Several patients have been documented in the literature to have a marked increase in serum levels of procollagen III [150,158]; however, no source for an extrarenal source for these peptides has been found. Elevated procollagen III peptide has been regarded as an indicator of stimulated collagen synthesis in a variety of diseases, including some renal disorders. Whether this finding is of importance in terms of the etiology of this disorder is controversial. Measurements of serum precollagen levels may be helpful in supporting a diagnosis of collagenofibrotic glomerulopathy in difficult cases. Striker et al. proposed that perhaps interstitial type of collagen III could migrate into glomeruli, but no breaks in Bowman's capsule have been demonstrated in these cases [157].

Mesangial cells are capable of producing collagen III, so this disorder may occur as a result of overproduction of collagen III locally in the mesangium. It appears that most of the available evidence supports the hypothesis that the overproduction of collagen III is by the mesangial cells which may be genetically programmed to do so, but there are no definitive studies that can confirm that this is the case.

Clinical Course, Prognosis, Treatment, and Clinical Correlations. There is no treatment for this condition. It is because of the apparent autosomal recessive genetic inheritance pattern that has been identified in children that genetic counseling may be recommended once this diagnosis is made. The disease exhibits a sporadic pattern in adults.

The natural history of this condition is not clear at the present time, partly due to the small number of confirmed patients with this disease. Also, the age at presentation, the severity and the rate of progression of the disease are quite variable. In at least a group of patients with this condition, the disease is progressive. In some cases, progression to end-stage renal disease may be quite fast. A case has been reported by Ikeda et al. in which progression to renal failure occurred three years after the diagnosis [150]. Other cases have been reported with increasing proteinuria and development of renal failure occurring rather rapidly after diagnosis [152–155].

Nail-Patella Syndrome

Clinical Presentation. The nail-patella syndrome, also referred to as osteo-onychodysplasia, is a very rare hereditary disorder characterized by a variety of bone lesions and renal

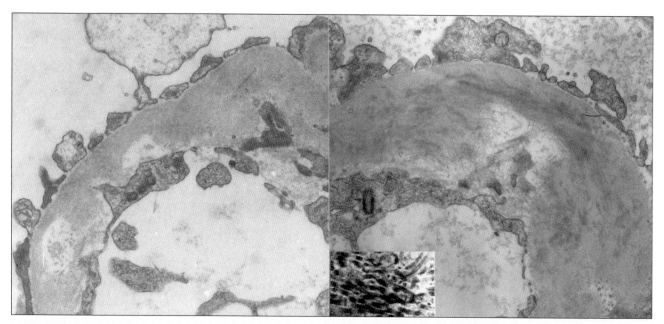

FIGURE 10.79: *Nail-patella syndrome. Transmission electron microscopy. Uranyl acetate and lead citrate. Left: × 5,500; right: × 15,500. Left panel: Note relatively empty spaces in the lamina densa of the glomerular basement membrane and a suggestion of some structures in the empty spaces. Right panel: High power magnification (and in some cases phosphotungstic acid treatment to the sections) is needed to reveal the typical appearance of collagen fibers and make a definitive diagnosis.*

disease [158–162]. This syndrome was first recognized by Little in 1897 [159]. It was many years later that the renal lesion in these patients was characterized. Hoyer and coworkers published seminal papers in the early 1970s [158].

Gross Pathology. The gross evaluation of these kidneys is of limited importance in regards of the main disease process, as nonspecific scarring occurs as the disease advances. However, these patients may also have urinary tract abnormalities detected by radiographic evaluation, including cortical scarring, dilatation of the pelvocalyceal system, and features of vesicoureteral reflux. Unilateral renal hypoplasia associated with bifid ureter, a variety of calyceal abnormalities, and contralateral double kidneys have also been reported in these patients [162].

Light Microscopy. In many cases, the glomeruli appear normal or may show segmental basement membrane thickening that can be observed with the PAS and silver stains. Generally, no specific alterations of the glomerular basement membranes can be noted. Varying degrees of focal and segmental and global glomerulosclerosis may be found in the more advanced stages of the disease process [160–162]. The tubular interstitial and vascular changes relate to the degree of glomerular damage, and are entirely nonspecific.

Immunofluorescence Microscopy. The panel of immunofluorescence stains is entirely negative in cases with nonsclerosed glomeruli. Trapping of various immunoglobulins, primarily IgM, C1q and C3 is identified in those cases in which

segmental and global glomerulosclerosis have occurred, as expected.

Electron Microscopy. The pathognomonic finding is the presence of mottled and lucent rarefactions of the lamina densa of the glomerular basement membranes creating a "moth-eaten" appearance [160]. When the ultrathin sections are stained using lead citrate and uranyl acetate, the lamina densa are sometimes found to contain banded-collagen fibrils with their expected periodicity (Figure 10.79). The collagen fibrils do not appear morphologically abnormal. In some cases, staining of the sections with phosphotungstic acid is needed to bring out the collagen fibers. Therefore, in cases where the "moth-eaten" appearance is the only abnormality noted, staining with phosphotungstic acid should be performed. The fibers are most commonly located in focal areas of the glomerular basement membranes but have been described as widespread along the peripheral capillary walls in some cases. The glomerular basement membranes usually appear variably thickened. The mesangium is sometimes expanded as well, and may contain some of the same collagen fibers, sometimes with lucencies appreciated when the thin sections are routinely stained. There are no alterations similar to those already described in any other membrane other than the glomerular basement membranes. Effacement of the foot processes of the visceral epithelial cells may be seen in cases with significant proteinuria.

Interestingly, the changes along the glomerular basement membranes may be detectable even in patients without overt clinical manifestations, and in some cases in patients without the bone manifestations usually associated with this disorder [161].

Differential Diagnosis. There are no specific light microscopic features that allow the diagnosis of this condition. Likewise, immunofluorescence data is noncontributory. The ultrastructural findings are very definitive, as discussed above. The subset of patients with "moth-eaten" appearance of the lamina densa of the glomerular basement membranes may generate a differential diagnosis that includes stage IV membranous nephropathy; in that situation, empty spaces where the immune complexes were located may be found along the glomerular basement membranes. In most cases of advanced membranous nephropathy, a careful electron microscopic search reveals at least a few capillary walls with identifiable immune complexes providing a solid base for a diagnosis of a late stage of membranous nephropathy.

Etiology and Pathogensis. Overall, the pathogenesis of this disorder is unclear. The pattern of inheritance is autosomal dominant and the gene locus for this syndrome is linked to chromosome 9 and found in the distal end of the long arm of this chromosome [163]. This is linked also to the ABO blood group locus. The main disorder may be based on a currently poorly defined abnormality in collagen metabolism. It has also been suggested that the *COLA5* gene may be involved in the genesis of this disorder. The nail-patella locus has been located to 9q34. The *COLA5* gene has been linked to the 9q34.2–9q34.3 regions, thus suggesting a relationship [164].

Clincial Course, Prognosis, Treatment, and Clinical Correlation. The majority of the patients with the nail-patella syndrome have no apparent clinical renal manifestations. Those with clinical findings present with abnormal urinary sediment, difficulty in concentrating or acidifying the urine, nephrotic or nonnephrotic range proteinuria with edema, microhematuria, renal stones, or hypertension. The manifestations of this syndrome include nail alterations in approximately 80–90 percent of all the patients and most commonly in the fingernails. These include discoloration, koilonychias, ridges, and triangular lunulae. The nails may also be dystrophic or entirely absent. The changes are generally symmetric. The patella may be absent or hypoplastic. A number of other skeletal manifestations may be identified including prominent anterior horns of the iliac crests which are considered by some as pathognomonic of this syndrome, even more than the patellar findings. There are also elbow changes, which include aplasia, hypoplasia, and posterior processes at the distal end of the humerus. Finally, hypoplastic radial heads, abnormalities of the radioulnar joint and iliac horns have also been reported [162].

Approximately 30 percent of the patients progress to renal failure. There is no treatment for the progressive renal disease, and dialysis is the final outcome in these patients. The mean age at end-stage renal failure was thirty-three years in one series. Some of these patients have been transplanted and, as expected, the basement membrane changes have not been recurred in the allografts. However, it has been reported that some of the skeletal manifestations may improve and even revert to normal in some transplanted patients. Genetic counseling is indicated for the affected families [163].

RENAL PATHOLOGY ASSOCIATED WITH SICKLE CELL DISEASE

Clinical Presentation

Sickle cell disease encompasses all individuals carrying at least one sickle gene. Therefore, the renal pathology that can be seen in patients both with the heterozygote (AS) and homozygous (SS) conditions. In the United States, approximately 8–10 percent of all African-Americans have AS, and 0.15 percent of black American children have SS (1 in approximately 600) [165]. The incidence of SS is lower in African-American adults because of death occurring early in life as a consequence of the disease. It should also be noted that combinations of the sickle gene with other abnormal hemoglobin genes may result in significant pathologic alterations, some with renal manifestations. The most marked and best understood manifestations (including those affecting the kidneys) occur in the patients with the fullest manifestations of sickle cell disease (SS), also known as those with sickle cell anemia, followed by those with combinations with other genes such as that of hemoglobin C which further produce difficulties in oxygen saturation of the blood. Both tubular interstitial and glomerular alterations can occur in these patients and are responsible for renal damage. In some cases, the clinical manifestations are primarily or exclusively functional. In this chapter, the focus is on those renal manifestations that have well-defined morphologic correlates.

The renal functional alterations that may be seen in these patients with sickle cell disease include hyposthenuria (inability to concentrate the urine), which is the most common, and often the earliest abnormality noted. Hyposthenuria can lead to polyuria and the risk of dehydration with associated acute tubular necrosis increases considerably in these patients. Impaired renal acidification and potassium excretion and supranormal proximal tubular function may also be present in these patients, mostly in young individuals. Other renal manifestations include papillary necrosis, hematuria, proteinuria, renal insufficiency, and renal failure. Asymptomatic hematuria is one of the most frequently noted features of the disease and has been reported in as many as 3 to 4 percent of patients with AS, and less common in SS. Although hematuria disappears spontaneously in the majority of these patients, it recurs in approximately 50 percent of the patients, and may be severe enough to require transfusions. The reasons for hematuria are several including papillary necrosis and malignancy with medullary carcinoma representing a type of renal carcinoma that occurs most frequently in this population. Mild to moderate proteinuria may be found in occasional AS patients, but is reported in approximately 31 percent of individuals with SS. In about one-half of these patients, the proteinuria is in the nephrotic range. Asymptomatic bacteriuria and pyelonephritis are also increased in sickle cell disease. Hypertension is unusual with only 2–6 percent of these patients with documented elevated blood pressure [166–171].

Nephrotic syndrome is reported not infrequently in patients with SS disease. A number of pathological entities may be associated with this, including minimal change glomerulopathy, focal segmental glomerulosclerosis (classic variant), membranous nephropathy, lupus nephritis, postinfectious glomerulonephritis, and an immune complex-mediated membranoproliferative glomerulonephritis Type I or membranoproliferative-like glomerulonephritis, mimicking chronic thrombotic microangiopathy. While the first five types of glomerulopathies appear to represent coexistent disease processes, the last entity has been linked directly to the primary disease process with a proposed etiology discussed below [172–174]. There are also single reports of FG [reported as "immunotactoid GN"] [175] and collapsing glomerulonephritis [176] associated with sickle cell disease.

While renal failure has been noted in 5–18 percent of the total population of patients with sickle cell disease, end-stage renal disease as a cause of death occurs in approximately 9–12 percent of patients with sickle cell anemia (SS). In adults, end-stage renal disease accounts for 20 percent of all deaths in these patients [177–179].

Gross Pathology

In patients with sickle cell trait, no significant gross pathological alterations are reported. If any findings are present, they are usually subtle and rather insignificant. Petechial hemorrhages in the cortical and medullary portions of the kidneys have been reported in patients with sickle cell trait and hematuria. A percentage of these patients reported by Mostofi et al. had papillary necrosis (14 percent), 73 percent revealed hemorrhage in the renal pelvis and clots in 14 percent of the cases [180]. In sickle cell anemia, small cortical infarcts may be found in subcapsular locations. Cortical scars may be seen in some instances, more prominent in older patients. In the most severely involved kidneys, the scars are large and depressions of the cortex are easily identifiable grossly. Distorted and variably altered renal papillae, often blunted, are seen in those cases with previous episodes of papillary necrosis. Active papillary necrosis associated with hemorrhage may also be identified [181–184].

In cases with end-stage renal disease, the kidneys are small and atrophic with surface scars and granularity and the cortex becomes thin and sometimes almost nonexistent. In the absence of prominent changes in the pelvis, as described above, the gross findings are indistinguishable from kidneys from patients with end-stage renal disease as a consequence of a variety of primary renal disorders [179].

Light Microscopy

As expected, the findings in patients with sickle cell trait are much less significant than those in patients with sickle cell disease. In the latter case, the renal alterations may be found along the entire length of the nephron from the glomerulus to the papillary tip.

Sickle Cell Trait

A series of nephrectomies from patients with sickle cell trait with intractable hematuria has been reported in the literature. The findings noted in this condition are generally limited to the medulla where the environment, characterized by acidosis, hypertonicity, and hypoxia predisposes to red cell sickling and hemoglobin S polymerization, sickle cell-endothelial cell interactions and vaso-occlusion-induced hypoxia. The findings listed below are, therefore, easy to conceptualize. There are severely congested peritubular capillaries with sickled erythrocytes and extravasated red blood cells in the interstitium. In 23

percent of the cases, there were tubular red blood cell casts. In the majority of the cases (77 percent), there was hemosiderin deposition in tubular cells. In 91 percent of the cases, there were scars in the medulla [180]. Renal papillae showed focal lesions including vascular engorgement, small hemorrhages, papillary necrosis and denudation and regeneration of the transitional epithelium lining the pelvis. Papillary necrosis resulting primarily from occlusion of the microvasculature of the vasa rectae, medullary ischemia and infarction can also be seen in these patients [182–185]. If bilateral sloughing of renal papillae occurs, renal failure may result from obstruction to urine outflow at the level of the ureters.

Sickle Cell Anemia

There are a variety of morphological changes that can be noted in the kidneys from these patients. The findings are subtle in those with no evidence of clinical renal disease or minimal manifestations. Congestion of glomerular capillaries with sickled red blood cells (Figure 10.80), glomerulomegaly, slight glomerular hypercellularity, hemosiderin pigmentation in visceral and epithelial cells, focal and global glomerulosclerosis are common findings of doubtful or no clinical significance in the great majority of these patients. Patchy interstitial fibrosis and tubular atrophy are also common. Other relatively minor changes included acute tubular necrosis in various stages of evolution (often with no significant clinical manifestations), and medullary pyramids with abnormalities varying from edema to myxoid change to fibrosis. Hemosiderin pigment at deposition in the cytoplasm of tubular cells is commonly noted.

The situation is quite different in those patients that present significant clinical manifestations. In these patients, the most typical finding is that of a glomerulopathy that mimics membranoproliferative glomerulonephritis but may also exhibit a component of segmental glomerulosclerosis [173,176] (Figure 10.81). Glomerular hypercellularity with accentuation of their lobularity, splitting, or duplication of the peripheral capillary walls clearly seen on the silver stained section (Figure 10.82), and varying degrees of capillary obliteration represent the most striking changes.

There is significant variability in the degree of alterations with a number of cases only showing relatively subdued proliferative manifestations (these can be referred to as membranoproliferative-like glomerulopathy). Some authors have indicated that the sclerosing changes are far more prominent that the membranoproliferative type of alterations, and that the term membranoproliferative glomerulonephritis probably should not be applied to these cases [176,185,186]. Cases of sickle cell disease with focal glomerulosclerosis without proliferative component may also be found [187]. Microangiopathic glomerulopathy can also occur in these patients and be a source of diagnostic difficulty [188]. Iron deposits are invariably present in tubular cells (Figure 10.83A and B) and evidence of tubular damage may accompany this finding.

Some patients with long-standing sickle cell disease develop amyloidosis [189]. Renal medullary carcinoma represents a highly malignant renal neoplasm arising in patients with sickle cell disease (Figure 10.84) [190–193]. Any patient with sickle cell and hematuria should be screened for the possibility of harboring this very malignant renal tumor [193].

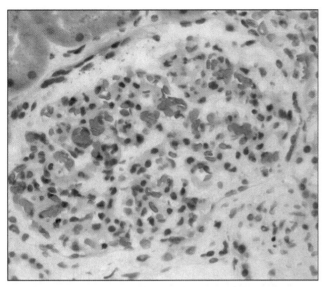

FIGURE 10.80: *Sickle cell disease-associated nephropathy. Hematoxylin and eosin ×750. Glomerular capillaries filled with sickled erythrocytes.*

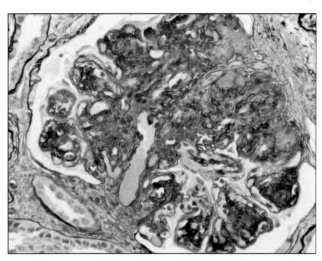

FIGURE 10.81: *Sickle cell disease-associated nephropathy. Silver methenamine. ×750. Accentuated glomerular lobularity reminiscent of membranoproliferative glomerulonephritis and a segmentally collapsed glomerular area in the same glomerulus. These findings in the proper clinical context are most consistent with this entity.*

Immunofluorescene Microscopy

In the great majority of the patients with sickle cell disease and renal manifestations, no immune complexes are noted and the immunofluorescence battery of stains is entirely negative in glomeruli, tubular, interstitial, and vascular compartments. In cases with focal and segmental sclerosing glomerular changes, trapping of C3 and IgM can be noted in the segmentally and globally sclerosed glomeruli and sometimes, in focal, segmental mesangial areas with a granular pattern of staining [194,195]. There have been reports in the literature showing that patients with the membranoproliferative pattern may exhibit focal and segmental deposits containing predominantly IgG and C3, but also containing kappa and lambda light chains; the subdued fluorescence positivity reflects the scattered immune complexes noted ultrastructurally.

Electron Microscopy

In cases with membranoproliferative pattern, there are variable degrees of mesangial cell proliferation and matrix expansion, resulting in accentuation of the glomerular lobularity, splitting or reduplication of peripheral capillary wall basement membranes by mesangial cell cytoplasm interposition (Figure 10.85). Segmental wrinkling and collapse of glomerular basement membranes may be identified. In the type of membranoproliferative disease that is indistinguishable from MPGN, Type I, scattered subendothelial and mesangial electron-dense deposits are identified (Figure 10.85, right panel) [195]. In the MPGN-like pattern, no immune complexes are present but subendothelial expansion is commonly identified (Figure 10.84, left panel) [173,175,176].

Occasional intracellular membrane-bound vesicles containing granular electron-dense material can be identified in mesan-

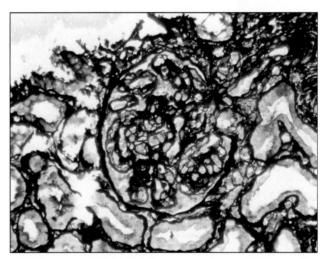

FIGURE 10.82: *Sickle cell disease-associated nephropathy. Silver methenamine. ×500. Extensive reduplication of glomerular peripheral capillary walls is illustrated.*

gial cells; this has been considered to represent iron-containing material.

Differential Diagnosis

It is because of the varied morphologic manifestations in these cases that discussion of the differential diagnosis requires focusing on the various patterns. For example, a patient with focal, segmental glomerulosclerosis requires distinction from other glomerulopathies with identical morphology [187].

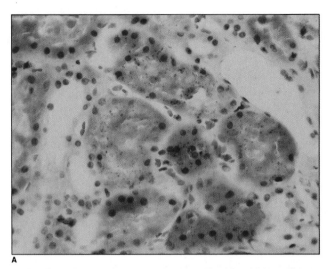
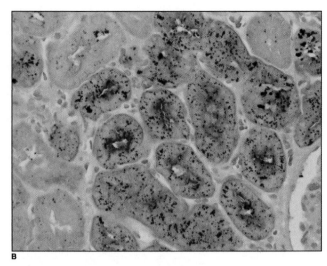

A   **B**

FIGURE 10.83:   Sickle cell disease-associated nephropathy. A: Hematoxylin and eosin; B: Pearls' ieon stain. A×500, B×500. Iron deposition noted in A as yellowish pigmentation in the cytoplasm of tubular cells and in B iron stains blue.

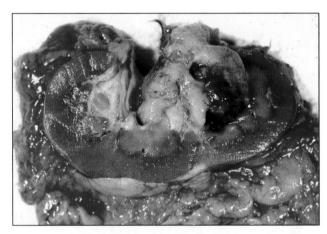

FIGURE 10.84:   Medullary carcinoma in a patient with sickle cell disease. Gross photo. Partially necrotic and hemorrhagic tumor mass in the medulla, the classical appearance of medullary carcinoma.

In patients exhibiting the membranoproliferative pattern, the differential diagnosis includes other diseases that share this morphologic expression. There are a number of systemic disorders, as well as primary membranoproliferative glomerulonephritis, Type I that show morphologic findings virtually indistinguishable from the sickle cell disease-associated MPGN, Type I [178,194,195]. As previously noted, frequently the immune complexes are few, and sometimes even difficult to identify in spite of other morphologic features consistent with MPGN, Type I.

Etiology and Pathogenesis

The enhanced glomerular and tubular function that has been noted in young patients with sickle cell anemia result from increased renal blood flow, and glomerular filtration rate. Renal plasma flow increases proportionally more than the glomerular filtration rate, resulting in a decreased filtration fraction. The increased blood flow has been proposed to be related to the anemia; however, a couple of studies have shown that it remains increased even after transfusions, so this issue remains unsettled. Hyperperfusion from shunting of blood from medulla to cortex accounts for the glomerular enlargement, and the congestion that is found invariably in sickle cell anemia patients. Alterations in renal hemodynamics may also be responsible for proteinuria and focal glomerulosclerosis in some of these patients [169].

Increased renal blood flows together with medullary hypoperfusion provide an explanation for the presence of dilated glomerular capillaries in the renal pelvis. Shunting of blood to the vessels in the renal pelvis resulting in dilatation, congestion, and eventual rupture of these vascular structures provides a pathophysiologic reason for the hematuria that is often present in these patients.

Patients with sickle cell disease and structural abnormalities are generally adults. The more severe morphologic manifestations are present in young adults, so years of hyperperfusion may be needed for structural damage to be noticeable and lead to renal functional manifestations. It is also of importance that nephrotic syndrome and irreversible glomerular damage occurs far more frequent in patients with sickle cell anemia than trait, providing support to the theory that hyperperfusion may be key in the genesis of the progressive glomerular damage. Patients with sickle cell trait have no glomerular hyperperfusion, but exhibit predominantly medullary hypoperfusion, providing a sound pathogenetic explanation for the lesions that they most often present including failure to properly concentrate urine, renal tubular acidosis, and papillary necrosis. Chronic sickling underlies several mechanisms responsible for renal injury in patients with sickle cell disease: structural papillectomy, urine-concentrating defects, hyperfiltration, glomerular enlargement, damage, and sclerosis [185]. The hypertonicity and low pH of the renal medulla promote sickle cell formation

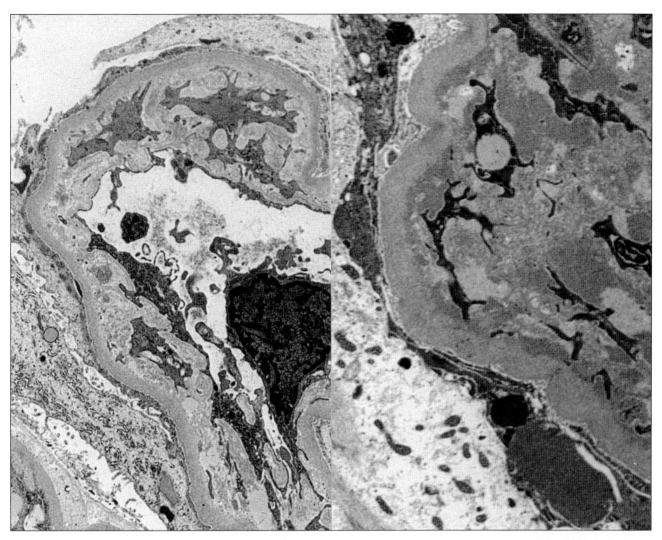

FIGURE 10.85: *Sickle cell disease-associated nephropathy. Transmission electron microscopy. Uranyl acetate and lead citrate. Left: ×5,600; right:×10,500. Duplication of glomerular basement membranes by mesangial cell cytoplasm interposition is clearly seen in both left and right panels. In the left panel, there are no associated immune complexes, while in the right panel subendothelial immune complexes are easily identifiable.*

resulting in an increase in blood viscosity, venous engorgement, interstitial edema, and resultant ischemia and infarction [185].

Pardo and associates in 1975 postulated that the immune complex-mediated glomerulopathy (membranoproliferative glomerulonephritis, Type I) that is seen in some patients with sickle cell anemia is linked to the presence of immune complexes containing renal tubular epithelial antigen released by the tubular cells as a result of ischemia or other hemodynamic reasons directly related to sickling of red blood cells and vascular stagnation [195]. Although the above pathogenetic hypothesis has been questioned, a better accepted explanation has not been provided as of yet. Some authors do not believe that an immune complex mediated glomerulopathy is part of the spectrum of conditions seen in association with sickle cell disease.

Clinical Course, Prognosis, Treatment, and Clinical Correlation

There is ample literature on the treatment of the various manifestations of sickle cell trait and disease. The emphasis of the treatment is on the particular manifestation/s of the disease process that is/are present.

It is because the pathogenesis of sickle cell nephropathy remains controversial the treatment protocols are not based on solid understanding of what the management of these patients requires. No consistent benefit of immunosuppressive drugs has been demonstrated in the treatment of sickle cell nephropathy [196]. Reduction of proteinuria using short-term angiotensin converting enzyme inhibitors is generally considered beneficial.

Maintenance hemodialysis and renal transplantation are used in the management of patients with sickle cell nephropathy that progress into end-stage renal disease [197]. Renal survival after transplantation in these patients is similar to that of the nonsickle recipients, but this modality of treatment has only been used selectively. In a report of thirty-four transplants on thirty sickle cell patients issued in 1980, one- year patient and graft survival were 87 percent and 67 percent, respectively [198]. In 1987, a subsequent report of forty-five transplants into forty recipients reported 88 percent one-year overall patient survival, and 82 percent one-year graft survival rate in living related donors, and 62 percent in cadaveric transplant recipients [199]. More recent series by Warady et al. in 1998 and Ojo et al. in 1999, the one-year survival was similar to that of transplanted nonsickle cell patients but the three-year cadaveric graft survival was diminished among patients with sickle cell nephropathy [200,201]. Survival in patients with sickle cell nephropathy was also significantly lower than for others both at one year and three years [200,201]. The high mortality rate in transplanted patients with sickle cell nephropathy was most likely a result of complications associated with the underlying disease, rather than as a consequence of the transplantation. An increase in the frequency of crisis has been reported after renal transplantation [202]. Crises tend to be more frequent the first year after renal transplantation. In addition, recurrent sickle cell nephropathy has been reported in transplanted kidneys [203,204]. In summary, the information available indicates that results from renal transplantation in patients with sickle cell disease are similar to those in patients from other etiologies, leading to end-stage renal disease, for age and race-matched cohorts. Higher death rates in transplanted patients with sickle cell disease are most likely the result of the primary disease process with transplantation not playing a significant role in explaining the difference. Renal transplantation has become an acceptable viable alternative to chronic dialysis in patients with this disease who develop renal failure.

Bone marrow transplantation with the potential for cure of the disorder has emerged as a treatment modality for sickle cell [205]. Whether sickle cell nephropathy can be reversed or progression of the renal damage can be stopped after bone marrow transplantation is unknown at the present time. Additional studies are required to determine whether the renal alterations may reverse after the disease process is controlled.

REFERENCES

1. Kyle RA. Multiple Myeloma: How did it begin? *Mayo Clin Proc* 1994; 69:680–3.
2. Sanders PW, Herrera GA, Kirk KA, Old CW, Galla JH.The spectrum of glomerular and tubulointerstitial renal lesions associated with monotypical immunoglobulin light chain deposition. *Lab Invest* 1991; 64:527–37.
3. Buxbaum JN, Chuba JV, Hellman C, Solomon A, Gallo GR. Monoclonal immunoglobulin deposition disease: light chain and light and heavy chain deposition diseases and their relation to light chain amyloidosis. *Ann Int Med* 1990; 112:455–64.
4. Sanders PW, Herrera GA. Monoclonal immunoglobulin light chain-related renal diseases. *Sem Nephrol* 1993; 13:324–41.
5. Herrera GA. Renal manifestations on plasma cell dyscrasias: an appraisal of the patients' bedside to the research laboratory. *Annals Diagn Pathol* 2000; 4:174–200.
6. Lin J, Markowitz GS, Valeri AM, Kambham N, Sherman WH, Appel GB, D'Agati VD. Renal monoclonal immunoglobulin deposition disease: the disease spectrum. *J Am Soc Nephrol* 2001; 12:1482–92.
7. Markowitz GS. Dysproteinemia and the kidney. *Adv Anat Pathol* 2004; 11:49–63.
8. Korbet SM, Schwartz MM. Multiple myeloma. *J Am Soc Nephrol* 2006; 17:2533–45.
9. Kyle RA, Therneau TM, Rajkumar SV, Larson DR, Plevak MF, Offord JR, Dispenzieri A, Katzmann JA, Melton LJ. Prevalence of monoclonal gammopathy of undetermined significance. *N Engl J Med* 2006; 354:1362–9.
10. Kyle RA. Monoclonal gammopathy of undetermined significance: natural history in 241 cases. *Am J Med* 1978; 64: 814–26.
11. Kyle RA, Therneau TM, Rajkumar SV. A long-term study of prognosis in monoclonal gammopathy of undetermined significance. *N Engl J Med* 2002; 346:564–9.
12. Herrera GA, Sanders PW, Reddy BV, Hasbargen JA, Hammond WS, Brook JD. Ultrastructural immunolabeling: a unique diagnostic tool in monoclonal light chain related renal diseases. *Ultrastruct Pathol* 1994; 18:401–16.
13. Herrera GA. The contributions of electron microscopy to the understanding and diagnosis of plasma cell dyscrasia-related renal lesions. *Med Elect Mic* 2001; 34:1–18.
14. Eulitz M, Weiss DT, Solomon A. Immunoglobulin heavy-chain-associated amyloidosis. *Proc Natl Acad Sci USA* 1990; 87:6542–6.
15. Randall RE, Williamson WC, Mullinax F, Tung MY, Still WJS: Manifestations of systemic light chain deposition. *Am J Med* 60:293–299, 1976.
16. Copeland JN, Kouides PA, Grieff M, Nadasdy T. Metachronous development of nonamyloidotic lambda light chain deposition disease and IgG heavy chain amyloidosis in the same patient. *Am J. Surg Pathol* 2003; 27: 1477–82.
17. Nasr SH, Colvin R, Markowitz GS. IgG1 lambda light and heavy chain renal amyloidosis. *Kidney Int* 2006; 70:7.
18. Cohen AH: The kidney in plasma cell dyscrasias: Bence-Jones cast nephropathy and light chain deposit disease. *Am J Kidney Dis* 1998; 32:529–32.
19. Stokes MG, Aronoff B, Siegel D, D'Agati VD. Dysproteinemia-related nephropathy associated with crystal-storing histiocytosis. *Kidney Int* 2006; 70:597–602.
20. Kyle RA, Beard CM, O'Fallen WM, Kurland LT. Incidence of multiple myeloma in Olmsted County, Minnesota: 1978 through 1990, with review of trend since 1945. *J Clin Oncol* 1994; 12: 1577–83.
21. Rayner HC, Haynes AP, Thompson JR.Perspectives in multiple myeloma: survival, prognostic factors and disease complications in a single center between 1975 and 1988. *QJ Med* 1991; 79:517–25.

22. Blade J, Kyle RA. Nonsecretory myeloma, immunoglobulin D myeloma and plasma cell leukemia. *Hematol Oncol Clin North Am* 1999; 13:1259–72.

23. Kapadia SB. Multiple myeloma: a clinicopathic study of 62 consecutively autopsied cases. *Medicine (Baltimore)* 1980; 59:380–92.

24. Ivanyi B.Frequency of light chain deposition nephropathy relative to renal amyloidosis and Bence Jones cast nephropathy in a necropsy study of patients with myeloma. *Arch Pathol Lab Med* 1990; 114:986–7.

25. Herrera GA, Joseph L, Gu X, Hough A, Barlogie B. Renal pathologic spectrum in an autopsy series of patients with plasma cell dyscrasias. *Arch Pathol Lab Med* 2004; 128: 875–9.

26. Cai G, Sidhu GS, Wieczorek R, Gu X, Herrera GA, Cubukcu-Dimopulo O, Kahn T. Plasma cell dyscrasia with kappa light chain crystals in proximal tubular cells: a histological, immunofluorescence and ultrastructural study. *Ultrastruct Pathol* 2006; 30:315–19.

27. Decort C, Bridoux F, Touchard G, Cogne M. A monoclonal Vκl light chain responsible for incomplete proximal tubulopathy. *Am J Kidney Dis* 2003; 41:497–504.

28. Ronco PM, Aucouturier P. The molecular basis of plasma cell dyscrasia-related renal diseases. *Nephrol Dial Transplant* 1999; 14(S): 4–8.

29. Carstens HB, Woo D. Crystalline glomerular inclusions in multiple myeloma. *Am J. Kidney Dis* 1989; 14:56–60.

30. Maldonado JE, Velosa JA, Kyle RA, Wagoner RD, Holley KE, Salassa R. Fanconi synbrome in adults: a manifestation of a latent form of myeloma. *Am J Med* 1975; 58:354–64.

31. Haas M, Spargo BH, Wit EJC, Meehan SM. Etiologies and outcome of acute renal insufficiency in older adults: a renal biopsy study of 259 cases. *Am J Kid Dis* 2000; 35:433–47.

32. Alpers CE, Magil AB, Gown AM. Macrophage origin of the multinucleated cells of myeloma cast nephropathy. *Am J Clin Pathol* 1989; 92:662–5.

33. Start DA, Silva FG, David LD, D'Agati V, Pirani CL. Myeloma cast nephropathy: immunohistochemical and lectin stidies. *Mod Pathol* 1988; 1:336–47.

34. Uribe-Uribe NO, Herrera GA. Ultrastructure of tubular casts. *Ultrastruct Pathol* 2006; 30:159–66.

35. Soffer O, Nassar VH, Campbell WG, Burke E. Light chain cast nephropathy and acute renal failure associated with Rifampin therapy. *Am J Med* 1987; 82:1052–6.

36. Said, SM, Nasr, SH, Samsa, R, Markowitz, GS, D'Agati, VD. Nephrotoxicity of antivretroviral therapy in an HIV-infected patient. *Kidney Int* 2007; 71: 1071–5.

37. Misiani R, Tiraboschi G, Mingardi G, Mecca G. Management of myeloma kidney: an antilight chain approach. *Am J Kidney Dis* 1987; 10:28–33.

38. Gertz MA. Managing myeloma kidney. *Ann Intern Med* 2005; 143:835–7.

39. Madore F.Does plasmapheresis have a role in the management of myeloma cast nephropathy? *Nat Clin Pract (Nephrology)* 2006; 2:406–7.

40. Gu X, Herrera GA. Light chain-mediated acute tubular interstitial nephritis: a poorly recognized pattern of renal disease in patients with plasma cell dyscrasia. *Arch Pathol Lab Med* 2006; 130:165–9.

41. Venkataseshan VS, Faraggiana T, Hughson MD, Buchwald D, Olesnicky L, Goldstein MH. Morphologic variants of light chain deposition disease in the kidney. *Am J Nephrol* 1988; 8:272–9.

42. Aucouturier P, Khamlichi AA, Touchard G. Brief report: heavy chain deposition disease. *N Engl J Med* 1993; 329:1389–93.

43. Bhargava P, Rushin JM, Rusnock EJ, Hefter LG, Franks TJ, Sabnis SG, Travis WD. Pulmonary light chain deposition disease: report of five cases and review of the literature. *Am J Surg Pathol* 2007; 31:267–76.

44. Kambham N, Markowitz GS, Appel GB, Kleiner MJ, Aucouturier P, D'Agati VD. Heavy Chain Deposition Disease: the Disease Spectrum. *Am J Kidney Dis* 1999; 33:954–62.

45. Ronco PM, Alyanakian M-A, Mougenot B, Aucouturier P: Light chain deposition disease: a model of glomerulosclerosis defined at the molecular level. *J Am Soc Nephrol* 2001; 12:1558–65.

46. Buxbaum JN. Abnormal immunoglobulin synthesis in monoclonal immunoglobulin light chain and light and heavy chain deposition disease. *Amyloid* 2001; 8:84–93.

47. Herrera G, GU X. Lesions associated with plasma cell dyscrasias in renal biopsies: a 10 year retrospective study. *(Abstract) Lab Invest* 86:262A.

48. Yasuda T, Fujita K, Imai H, Morita K, Nakamoto Y, Miura AB. Gamma-heavy chain deposition disease showing nodular glomerulosclerosis. *Clin Nephrol* 1995; 44:394–9.

49. Cheng IKP, Ho SKN, Chan DTM, Chan KW. Crescentic nodular glomerulosclerosis secondary to truncated immunoglobulin heavy chain deposition. *Am J Kidney Dis* 1996; 28:283–8.

50. Silva FG, Meyrier A, Morel-Maroger L, Pirani C. Proliferative glomerulonephropathy in multiple myeloma. *J Pathol* 1980; 130:229–36.

51. Knobler H, Kopolovic J, Kleinman Y, Rubinger D, Silver J, Friedlaender MM, Popovtzer MM. Multiple myeloma presenting as dense deposit disease. Light chain nephropathy. *Nephron* 1983; 34:58–63.

52. Chang A, Peutz-Kootstra CJ, Richardson CA, Alpers CE. Expanding the pathologic spectrum of light chain deposition disease: a rare variant with clinical follow-up of 7 years. *Modern Pathology* 2005; 18:998–1004.

53. Markowitz GS, Lin J, Valeri AM, Avila C, Nasr SH, D'Agati V. Idiopathic nodular glomerulosclerosis is a distinct clinicopathologic entity linked to hypertension and smoking. *Hum Pathol* 2002; 33:837–45.

54. Mai, HL, Sheikh-Hamad D, Herrera GA, Gu X, Truong L. Immunoglobulin heavy chain can be amyloidogenic: morphologic characterization, including immunoelectron microscopy. *Am J Surg Pathol* 2003; 27:541–5.

55. Dember LM. Amyloidosis-associated kidney disease. *J Am Soc Nephrol* 2006; 17:3458–71.

56. Dikman SH, Churg J, Kahn T. Morphologic and clinical correlates in renal amyloidosis. *Human Pathol* 1981; 12: 160–6.

57. Novak L, Cook WJ, Herrera GA, Sanders PW. AL-amyloidosis is underdiagnosed in renal biopsies. *Nephrol Dial Transplant* 2004; 19:3050–3.

58. Veeramachaneni R, Gu X, Herrera GA. Atypical amyloidosis: diagnostic challenges and the role of immunoelectron microscopy in diagnosis. *Ultrastruct Pathol* 2004; 28: 75–82.

59. Picken M, Herrera GA. The burden of "sticky" amyloid typing challenges. *Arch Pathol Lab Med* 2007; 131:850–1.

60. Batuman V, Verroust PJ, Navar GL. Myeloma light chains are ligands for cubilin (gp 280). *Am J Phys Renal Physiol* 1998; 275:F246–F254.

61. Herrera GA. Low molecular weight proteins and the kidney. Physiological and pathological considerations. *Ultrastruct Pathol* 1994;18:89–98.

62. Huang Z-Q, Sanders PW. Localization of a single binding site for immunoglobulin light chains on human Tamm-Horsfall glycoprotein. *J Clin Invest* 1997; 99:732–8.

63. Ying WZ, Sanders PW. Mapping the binding domain of immunoglobulin light chains for Tamm-Horsfall protein. *Am J Pathol* 2001; 158:1859–66.

64. Zhu L, Herrera GA, Murphy-Ullrich JE, Huang ZQ, Sanders PW. Pathogenesis of glomerulosclerosis in light chain deposition disease: role for transforming growth factor-β. *Am J Pathol* 1995; 147:375–85.

65. Turbat-Herrera EA, Isaac J, Sanders PW, Truong LD, Herrera GA. Integrated expression of glomerular extracellular proteins and β1 integrins on monoclonal light chain-related renal diseases. *Mod Pathol* 1997; 10:485–95.

66. Herrera GA, Schultz J, Soong S, Sanders PW. Growth factors in monoclonal light chain-related renal diseases. *Hum Pathol* 1994; 25:883–9.

67. Keeling J, Herrera GA. Matrix metalloproteinases and mesangial remodeling in light chain-related glomerular damage. *Kidney Int* 2005; 68:1590–603.

68. Keeling J, Herrera GA. An in vivo model of light chain deposition disease. *Kidney Int* 2008 Oct 15 [Epub ahead of print]

69. Solomon A, Weiss DT. Protein and host factors implicated in the pathogenesis of light chain amyloidosis (AL-amyloidosis). *Int J Exp Clin Invest* 1995; 2:269–79.

70. Sirac C, Bridoux F, Carrion C, Devuyst O, Fernandez B, Goujon JM, El Hamel C, Aldigier JC, Touchard G, and Cogné M. Role of the monoclonal Kchain V domain and reversibility of renal damage in a transgenic model of acquired Fanconi syndrome. *Blood* 2006; 108:536–43.

71. Bellotti V, Mangione P, Merlini G. Review: immunoglobulin light chain amyloidosis – the archetype of structural and pathogenic variability. *J Struct Biol* 2000; 130:280–9.

72. Omtvedt LA, Bailey D, Renouf DV. Glycosylation of immunoglobulin light chains associated with amyloidosis. *Amyloid* 2000; 7:227–44.

73. Khamlichi AA, Aucouturier P, Silvain C, Bauwens M, Touchard G, Preud'homme JL, Nau F, Cogne M. Primary structure of a monoclonal kappa chain in (FRA) myeloma with light chain deposition disease. *Clin Exp Immunol* 1992; 87:122–6,.

74. Decourt C, Touchard G, Preud'homme JL, Vidal R, Beaufils H, Diemert MC, Cogne M. Complete primary sequences of two (lambda) immunoglobulin light chains in myelomas with nonamyloid (Randall-Type) light chain deposition disease. *Am J Pathol* 1998; 153:313–18.

75. Khamlichi AA, Aucoturer P, Preud'Homme JL, Cogne M. Structure of abnormal heavy chains in human heavy chain deposition disease. *Eur J Biochem* 1995; 229:54–60.

76. Comenzo RL, Zhang Y, Martinez C, Osman K, Herrera GA. The tropism of organ involvement in primary systemic amyloidosis: contributions of Ig VL germline gene use and clonal plasma cell burden. *Blood* 2001; 98:714–20.

77. Rocken C, Shakespeare A. Pathology, diagnosis and pathogenesis of AA amyloidosis. *Virchows Arch* 2002; 440: 111–22.

78. Lobato I. Portuguese-type amyloidosis (transthyretin amyloidosis ATTR V30M). *J Nephrol* 2003; 16:438–42.

79. Benson MD. Ostertag revisited: the inherited systemic amyloidosis without neuropathy. *Amyloid* 2005;12:75–87.

80. Gejyo F, Narita I. Current clinical and pathogenetic understanding of β2-M amyloidosis in longterm dialysis patients. *Nephrology* 2003; 8:S45–49.

81. Heilman RL, Velosa JA, Holley KE, Offord KP, Kyle RA. Long-term follow-up and resonse to chemotherapy in patients with light chain deposition disease. *Am J Kidney Dis* 1992; 20:34–41.

82. Royer B, Arnulf B, Martinez F, Roy L, Flageril B, Etienne I, Ronco P, Brouet FC, Fermand JP. High dose chemotherapy in light and heavy chain deposition disease. *Kidney Int* 2004; 65:642–8.

83. Montseny JJ, Kleinkuecht D, Meyrier A, Vanhille P, Simon P, Pruna A, Eladari D. Long-term outcome according to renal histological lesions in 118 patients with monoclonal gammopathies. *Nephrol Dial Transplant* 1998; 13:1438–45.

84. Komatsuda A, Wakui H, Ohtani H, Kodama T, Miki K, Imai H, Miura AB. Disappearance of nodular mesangial lesions in a patient with light chain nephropathy after long-term chemotherapy. *Am J Kidney Dis* 2000; 35:1–5.

85. Hotta O, Taguma Y. Resolution of nodular glomerular lesions in a patient with light-chain nephropathy. *Nephron* 2002; 91:504–5.

86. Leung N, Lager DJ, Gertz MA, Wilson K, Kanakiriya S, Fervenza FC. Long-term outcome of renal transplantation in light chain deposition disease. *Am J Kidney Dis* 2004; 43:147–53.

87. Short AK, O'Donoghill DJ, Ried HN, Short CD, Roberts IS. Recurrence of light chain nephropathy in a renal allograft. A case report and review of the literature. *Am J Nephrol* 2001; 21:237–40.

88. Goldsmith DJA, Sandooran D, Short MD, Mallick NP, Johnson RWG. Twenty-one years survival with systemic AL-amyloidosis. *Am J Kidney Dis* 1996; 28:278–82.

89. Kyle RA, Gertz MA. Primary systemic amyloidosis. *Sem Haematol* 1995; 32:45–59.

90. Gertz MA, Kyle RA, Greipp PR. Response rates and survival in primary systemic amyloidosis. *Blood* 1991; 77: 257–62.

91. Gertz MA, Kyle RA, O'Fallon M. Dialysis support of patients with primary systemic amyloidosis. *Arch Intern Med* 1992; 152:2245–50.

92. Dember, LM, Sanchorwala, V, Comenzo RL, Seldin, DC, Wright DG, LaValley M, Berk JL, Falk RH, Sinner M. Effect of dose-intensive intravenous melphalan and autogous blood stem cell transplantation in AL-amyloidosis-

associated renal disease. *Ann Intern Med* 2001; 134: 746–53.

93. Skinner M, Sauchoranala V, Seldin DC. High-dose intravenous melphalan and autologous stem cell transplantation in patients with AL-amyloidosis: an eight year study. *Ann Intern Med* 2004; 40:85–93.

94. Schonlaud SO, Lockhorst H, Buzyn A, Leblond V, Hegenbart U, Bandini G, Campbell A, Carreras E, Ferrant A, Grommisch L, Jacobs P, Kroger N, La Nasa G, Russell N, Zachee P, Goldschmidt H, Iacobelli S, Niederwieser D, Gahrton G. Allogenic and syngeneic hematopoetic cell transplantation in patients with amyloid light-chain amyloidosis: a report from the European Group for Blood and Marrow Transplantation. *Blood* 2006; 107:2578–84.

95. Hauck, W, Dember LM, Hawkins PN, Hazenberg, BPC, Skinner M, Bouwmeester MC, Briand R, Chicoine É, Gurbindo C, Hughes L, Garceau D, on behalf of the Fibrillex Amyloidosis Secondary Trial (FAST) group. A prospective analysis of demography, etiology, and clinical findings of AA amyloidosis patients enrolled in the International Clinical Phase II/III Fibrillex study. In: Grateau C, Kyle RA Skinner M, eds. *Amyloid and Amyloidosis.* Boca Raton, FL: CRC Press; 2005: pp 179–81.

96. Lobato I, Ventura A, Beirao I. End-stage renal disease in familial amyloidosis. ATTR Val 30 Met: A definite indication to combined liver-kidney transplantation. *Transplant Proc* 2003; 35:1116–20.

97. Hartmann A, Holdaas H, Fauchald P, Nordal KP, Berg KJ, Talseth L, Leivestad T, Brekke IB, Flatmark A. Fifteen years experience with renal transplantation in systemic amyloidosis. *Transplant Int* 1992; 5:15–18.

98. Pasternack A, Ahonen J, Kuhlback B. Renal transplantation in 45 patients with amyloidosis. *Transplantation* 1986; 42:598–601.

99. Harrison KL, Alpers CE, Davis CL. De novo amyloidosis in a renal allograft: a case report and review of the literature. *Am J Kidney Dis* 1993; 22:468–76.

100. Le QC, Wood TC, Alpers CE. De novo AL amyloid in a Renal Allograft. *Am J Nephrol* 1998; 18:67–70.

101. Herrinton LJ, Weiss NS. Incidence of Waldenstrom's macroglobulinemia. *Blood* 1993; 82:3148–50.

102. Waldenstrom J. Incipient myelomatosis or "essential" hyperglobulinemia with fibrinogenopenia –a new syndrome? *Acta Med Scandinav* 1944; 117:216–47.

103. Kyle RA, Garton JP. The spectrum of IgM monoclonal gammopathy in 430 cases. *Mayo Clin Proc* 1987; 62:719–31.

104. Dimopoulos MA, Galani E, Matsouka C. Waldenström's macroglobulinemia. *Hem/Onc Clin N Amer* 1999; 13:1351–66.

105. Grossman ME, Bria MJ, Goldwein MI, Hill G, Goldberg M. Giant kidneys in Waldenstrom's macroglobulinemia. *Arch Intern Med* 1977; 137:1613–15.

106. Dutcher TF, Fahey JL. The histopathology of the macroglobulinemia of Waldenstrom. *J Natl Cancer Inst* 1959; 22:887–901.

107. Argani I, Kipkie GF. Macroglobulinemic nephropathy. *Am J Med* 1964; 36:151–7.

108. Morel-Maroger L, Bash A, Danon F, Verroust P, Richet G. Pathology of the kidney in Waldenstrom's macroglobulinemia. Study of sixteen cases. *N Engl J Med* 1970; 283:123–9.

109. Gertz MA, Kyle RA, Noel P. Primary systemic amyloidosis: a rare complication of immunoglobulin monoclonal gammopathies and Waldenstrom's macroglobulinemia. *J Clin Oncol* 1993; 11:914–20.

110. Isaac J, Herrera GA. Cast nephropathy in a case of Waldenstrom's macroglobulinemia. *Nephron* 2002; 91:512–15.

111. Gertz MA. Waldenstrom macroglobulinemia: a review of therapy. *Am J Hematol* 2005; 79:147–57.

112. Anagnostopoulos A, Giralt S. Stem cell transplantation (SCT) for Waldenstrom's macroglobulinemia (WM). *Bone Marrow Transplant* 2002; 29:943–7.

113. Iskandar SS, Herrera GA. Glomerulopathies with organized deposits. *Sem Diag Pathol* 2002; 19:116–32.

114. Howell D, Gu X, Herrera GA. Organized deposits and lookalikes. *Ultrastruct Pathol* 2003; 27:295–312.

115. Schwartz MM, Korbet SM, Lewis EJ. Immunotactoid glomerulopathy. *J Am Soc Nephrol* 2002; 13:1390–7.

116. Alpers C. Fibrillary glomerulonephritis and immunotactoid glomerulopathy: two entities, not one. *Am J Kidney Dis* 1993; 22:448–51.

117. Fogo A, Qureshi N, Horn RG. Morphologic and clinical features of fibrillary glomerulonephritis versus immunotactoid glomerulopathy. *Am J Kidney Dis* 1993; 22:367–77.

118. Rosenstock JL, Markowitz GS, Valeri AM, Sacchi G, Appel GB, D'Agati VD. Fibrillary and immunotactoid glomerulonephritis: distinct entities with different clinical and pathologic features. *Kidney Int* 2003; 63:1450–61.

119. Rosenmann E, Eliakim M. Nephrotic syndrome associated with amyloid-like glomerular deposits. *Nephron* 1977; 18:301–8.

120. Duffy JL, Khurana E, Susin M, Gomez-Leon G, Churg J. Fibrillary renal deposits and nephritis. *Am J Pathol* 1983; 113: 279–90.

121. Alpers CE, Rennke HG, Hopper J, Biava CG. Fibrillary glomerulonephritis: an entity with unusual immunofluorescence features. *Kidney Int* 1987; 31:781–9.

122. Iskandar SS, Falk RJ, Jennette C. Clinical and pathologic features of fibrillary glomerulonephritis. *Kidney Int* 1992;42:1401–7.

123. Korbet SM, Schwartz MM, Lewis EJ. The fibrillary glomerulopathies. *Am J Kidney Dis* 1994; 23:751–65.

124. Yang GCH, Nieto R, Stachura I, Gallo GR. Ultrastructural immunohistochemical localization of polyclonal IgG, C3, and amyloid P component on the congo-red-negative amyloid-like fibrils of fibrillary glomerulopathy. *Am J Pathol* 1992; 141:409–19.

125. Olesnicky L, Doty SB, Bertani T, Pirani CL. Tubular microfibrils in the glomeruli of membranous nephropathy. *Arch Pathol Lab Med* 1984; 108:902–5.

126. Rosenmann E, Brisson ML, Bercovitch DD, Rosenberg A. Atypical membranous glomerulonephritis with fibrillary subepithelial deposits in a patient with malignant lymphoma. *Nephron* 1988; 48:226–30.

127. Samanigo M, Nadasdy GM, Laszik Z. Outcome of renal transplantation in fibrillary glomerulonephritis. *Clin Nephrol* 2001; 55:159–66.

128. Isaac J, Herrera GA, Shihab FS. De-novo fibrillary glomerulopathy in the renal allograft of a patient with systemic lupus erythematosus. *Nephron* 2001; 87:365–8.

129. Sohar E, Ravid M, Ben-Shaul Y, Reshef T, Gafni J. Diabetic Fibrillosis. *Am J Med* 1970; 49:64–9.

130. Gonul II, Gough J, Jim K, Benediktsson H. Glomerular mesangial fibrillary deposits in a patient with diabetes mellitus. *Int Urol Nephrol* 2006; 38:767–72.

131. Kronz JD, Neu AM, Nadasdy T. When noncongophilic glomerular fibrils do not represent fibrillary glomerulonephritis: nonspecific mesangial fibrils in sclerosing glomeruli. *Clin Nephr* 1998; 50:218–23.

132. Dispenzieri A, Gorevic PD. Cryoglobulinemia. *Hematol/Oncol Clinics North Am* 1999; 13:1315–49.

133. Porush JG, Grishman E, Alter AA, Mandelbaum H, Churg J. Paraproteinemia and cryoglobulinemia associated with atypical glomerulonephritis and the nephrotic syndrome. *Am J Medicine* 1969; 47:957–64.

134. Karras A, Noel, LH, Droz, D, Delansorne D, Saint-Andre JP, Aucouturier P, Alyanakian MA, Grunfeld JP, Lesavre P. Renal involvement in monoclonal (Type I) cryoglobulinemia: two cases associated with IgG3κ cryoglobulin. *Am J Kidney Dis* 2002; 40:1091–6.

135. D'Amico G. Renal involvement in human hepatitis C infection: cryoglobulinemic glomerulonephritis. *Kidney Int* 1998; 54:650.

136. Golde D, Epstein W. Mixed cryoglobulins and glomerulonephritis. *Ann Int Med* 1968; 69:1221–7.

137. Pais B, Panadés MJ, Ramos J, Montoliu J. Glomerular involvement in Type I monoclonal cryoglobulinema. *Nephrol Dial Transplant* 1995; 10:130–2.

138. Verroust P, Mery JP, Morel-Maroger L, Clauvel JP, Richet G. Glomerular lesions in monoclonal gammopathies and mixed essential cryoglobulinemias IgG-IgM. *Adv Nephrol* 1971; 1:161–94.

139. Tornroth T, Skrifvars B. Ultrastructural changes in acute nonstreptococcal glomerulonephritis associated with mixed cryoglobulinemia. *Exp Mol Pathol* 1973; 19:160–7.

140. Feiner H, Gallo G. Ultrastructure in glomerulonephritis associated with cryoglobulinemia. *Am J Path* 1977; 88:145–55.

141. Ogihara T, Saruta T, Saito I, Abe S, Ozawa Y, Kato E, Sakaguchi H. Finger print deposits of the kidney in pure monoclonal IgG kappa cryoglobulinemia. *Clin Nephr* 1979; 12:186–90.

142. Cordonnier D, Martin H, Groslambert P, Micouin C. Mixed IgG-IgM cryoglobulinemia with glomerulonephritis. *Am J Medicine* 1975; 59:867–72.

143. Tarantino A, Campise M, Banfi G, Confalonieri R, Bucci A, Montoli A, Colasanti G, Damilano I, D'Amico G, Minetti L, Ponticelli C. Long-term predictors of survival in essential mixed cryoglobulinemic glomerulonephritis. *Kidney Int* 1995; 47:618–23.

144. Strøm, EH, Banfi G, Krapf R, Abt A, Mazzucco G, Monga G, Gloor F, Neuweiler J, Riess R, Stosiek P, Hebert LA, Sedmak DD, Gudat F, Mihatsch M. Glomerulopathy associated with predominant fibronectin: a newly recognized hereditary disease. *Kidney Int* 1995; 48:163–70.

145. Burgin M, Hoffmann E, Reutter FW. Familial glomerulopathy with giant fibrillary deposits. *Virchows Arch A Pathol Anat Histol* 1980; 388:313–26.

146. Assman KJM, Loene RAP. Familial glomerulonephritis characterized by massive deposits of fibronectin. *AM J Kidney Dis* 1995; 25:781–91.

147. Hilderbrandt F, Strahm B, Prochoroff A. Glomerulopathy associated with predominant fibronectin deposits: exclusion of the genes for fibronectin, villin and desmin as causative genes. *Am J med Genet* 1996; 63:323–7.

148. Gemperle O, Neuweiler J, Reutter FW. Familial glomerulopathy with giant fibrillary (fibronectin positive) deposits: 15-year follow-up on a large kindred. *Am J Kidney Dis* 1996; 28:668–75.

149. Dombros N, Katz A. Nail patella-like renal lesion in the absence of skeletal abnormalities: report of a kindred. *Am J Kidney Dis* 1982; 1:237–40.

150. Ikeda K, Yokoyama H, Tomosugi N, Kida H, Ooshima A, Kobayashi K. Primary glomerular fibrosis: a new nephropathy caused by diffuse intraglomerular increase in atypical Type III collagen fibers. *Clin Nephrol* 1990; 33:155–59.

151. Salcedo JR. An autosomal recessive disorder with glomerular basement membrane abnormalities similar to those seen in the nail patella syndrome: report of a kindred. *Am J Med Genet* 19:579–84.

152. Imbasciati E, Gherardi G, Morozumi K, Gudat F, Epper R, Basler V, Mihatsch MJ. Collagen Type III glomerulopathy: a new idiopathic glomerular disease. *Am J Nephrol* 1991; 11:422–9.

153. Gubler MC, Dommergues JP, Foulard M, Bensman A, Leroy JP, Broyer M, Habib R. Collagen Type III glomerulopathy: a new type of hereditary nephropathy. *Pediatr Nephrol* 1993; 7:354–60.

154. Vogt BA, Wyatt RJ, Burke BA, Simonton S, Kashtan CE. Inherited factor H deficiency and collagen Type III glomerulopathy. *Pediatr Nephrol* 1995; 9:11–15.

155. Tamura H, Matsuda A, Kidoguchi N, Matsumura O, Mitarai T, Isoda K. A family with two sisters with collagenofibrotic glomerulonephropathy. *Am J Kidney Dis* 1996; 27:558–95.

156. Yoshioka K, Takemura T, Tohda M, Akano N, Miyamoto H, Ooshima A, Maki S. Glomerular localization of Type III collagen in human kidney disease. *Kidney Int* 1989; 35:1203–11.

157. Striker MML, Killen PD, Chi E, Striker GE. The composition of glomerulosclerosis I. Studies in focal sclerosis, crescentic glomerulonephritis and membranoproliferative glomerulonephritis. *Lab Invest* 1984; 51:181–92.

158. Hoyer JR, Michael AP, Vermer RL. Renal disease in nail-patella syndrome: clinical and morphologic studies. *Kidney Int* 1972; 2:231–8.

159. Little EM. Congenital absence in delayed development of the patella. *Lancet* 1897; 2:781–4.

160. Ben-Bassat M, Cohen L, Rosenfield J. The glomerular basement membrane in the nail-patella syndrome. *Arch Pathol* 1971; 92:350–5.

161. Bennett WM, Musgrave JE, Campbell RA, Elliot D, Cox R, Brooks RE, Lovrien EW, Beals RK, Porter GA. The nephropathy of the nail-patella syndrome: clinicopathologic analysis of 11 kindreds. *Am J Med* 1973; 54:304–19.

162. Hawkins CF, Smith OE. Renal dysplasia in a family with multiple hereditary abnormalities, including iliac horns. *Lancet* 1950; 1:803–8.

163. Looij BJ, TeSlaa RL, Hogewind BL, Van de Kamp JJP. Genetic counseling in hereditary osteo-onychodysplasia (HOOD, nail-patella syndrome) with nephropathy. *J Med Genet* 1988; 25:682–6.

164. Schleutermann DA, Bias WB, Murdoch JL, McKusick VA. Linkage of the loci for the nail-patella syndrome and adenylate kinase. *Am J Hum Genet* 1969; 21:606–30.

165. Steinberg MH, Brugnara C. Pathophysiological-based approaches to treatment of sickle cell disease. *Ann Rev Med* 2003; 54:89–112.

166. Ataga KI, Orringer EP. Renal abnormalities in sickle cell disease: *Am J Hematol* 2000; 63:205–11.

167. Flanagan G, Packham DK, Kincaid-Smith P. Sickle cell disease and the kidney. *Am J Kidney Dis* 1993; 21:325–7.

168. Pham P-TT, Pham P-CT, Wilkinson AH, Lew SQ. Renal abnormalities in sickle cell disease. *Kidney Int* 2000; 57:1–8.

169. Scheinman JI. Sickle cell disease and the kidney. *Semin Nephrol* 2003; 23:66–76.

170. Wigfall DR, Ware RE, Burchinal MR, Kinney TR, Foreman JW. Prevalence and clinical correlates of glomerulopathy in children with sickle cell disease. *J Pediatr* 2000; 136:749–53.

171. Wong WY, Elliott-Mills D, Powars D. Renal failure in sickle cell anemia. *Hematol Oncol Clin North Am* 1996; 10:1321–31.

172. Bhathena DB, Soundheimer JH. The glomerulopathy of homozygous sickle hemoglobin (SS) disease: morphology and pathogenesis. *J Am Soc Nephrol* 1991; 1:1241–52.

173. Iskandar SS, Morgann RG, Browning MC, Lorentz WB. Membranoproliferative glomerulonephritis associated with sickle cell disease in two siblings. *Clin Nephrol* 1991; 35: 47–51.

174. Balal M, Paydas S, Seyrek N and Karayaylali I. Different glomerular pathologies in sickle cell anemia. *Clin Nephrol* 2004; 62:400–1.

175. Aviles DH, Craver R, Warrier RP. Immunotactoid glomerulopathy in sickle cell anemia. *Pediatric Nephrol* 2001; 16: 82–4.

176. Nasr SH, Markowitz GS, Sentman RL, D'Agati VD. Sickle-cell disease, nephrotic syndrome, and renal failure. *Kidney Int* 2006; 69:1276–80.

177. Platt OS, Brambilla DJ, Rosse WF, Milner PF, Castro O, Steinberg MH, Klug PP. Mortality In Sickle Cell Disease. *Life Expectancy and Risk Factors for Early Death* 1994; 330:1639–44.

178. Falk RJ, Jennette JC. Sickle cell nephropathy. *Adv Nephrol Necker Hosp* 1994; 23:133–47.

179. Naicker S. Secondary glomerulonephritides. *Ethn Dis.* 2003; 13:S125–30.

180. Mostofi, FK, Vorder Bruegge, CF, Diggs, LW. Lesions in kidneys removed for unilateral hematuria insickle-cell disease. *Arch Pathol* 1957; 63:336–51.

181. Jung DC, Kim SH, Jung SI, Hwang SI, Kim SH: Renal papillary necrosis: review and comparison of findings at multi-director row CT and intravenous urography. *Radiographics* 2006; 26:1827–36.

182. Griffin MD, Bergstralhn EJ, Larson TS. Renal papillary necrosis – a sixteen-year clinical experience. *J Am Soc Nephrol* 1995; 6:248–56.

183. Ahmed SG, Ibrahim UA. Haemoglobin-0S in sickle cell trait with papillary necrosis. *Br J Haematol* 2006; 135:415–16.

184. Alebiousu CO. Renal papillary necrosis as first presentation of a Nigerian sickle cell patient *West Afr J Med* 2002; 21:168–9.

185. Saborio P, Scheinman JI Sickle cell nephropathy. *J Am Soc Nephrol* 1999; 10:187–92.

186. Guasch A, Navarrete J, Nass K, Zayas CF. Glomerular involvement in adults with sickle cell hemoglobinopathies: prevalence and clinical correlates of progressive renal failure. *J Am Soc Nephrol* 2006; 17:2228–35.

187. Verani RR, Conley SB. Sickle cell glomerulopathy with focal segmental glomerulosclerosis. *Child Nephrol Urol* 1991; 11:206–8.

188. Vogler C, Wood E, Lane P, Ellis E, Cole B, Thorpe C. Microangiopathic glomerulopathy in children with sickle cell anemia. *Pediatr Pathol Lab Med* 1996; 16:275–84.

189. Simsek B, Bayazit AK, Ergin M, Soran M, Dursun H, Kilinc Y. Renal amyloidosis in a child with sickle cell anemia. *Pediatr Nephrol* 2006;n21:877–9.

190. Pickhardt PJ. Renal medullary carcinoma: an aggressive neoplasm in patients with sickle-cell disease. *Nat Clin Pract Urol* 2006; 3:279–83.

191. Sathyamoorthy K, Teo A, Atallah M. Renal medullary carcinoma in a patient with sickle-cell disease. *Nat Clin Pract Urol* 2006; 3:279–83.

192. Patel K, Livni N, MacDonald D. Renal medullary carcinoma, a rare cause of haematuria in sickle-cell disease. *(Images in Hematology). Br J Haematol* 2006; 132:1.

193. Johal NS, Desai D, Cuckow PM. Renal medullary carcinoma: beware of diagnosing a urinary tract infection in a young sickle cell patient. *Hosp Med* 2005; 66:114–15.

194. Seyrek N, Paydas S, Karayaylali I, Tuncer I Sagliker Y. Nephrotic syndrome in two cases with sickle cell nephropathy. *Nephron* 1996; 74:218.

195. Pardo V, Strauss J, Kramer H, Ozawa T, McIntosh RM. Nephropathy associated with sickle cell anemia: an autologous immune complex nephritis. II. Clinicopathologic study of seven patients. *Am J Med* 1975; 59:650–9.

196. Martin H, Steinberg MD. Management of sickle cell disease. *N Engl J Med* 1999; 340:1021–30.

197. Ribot S. Kidney transplant in sickle cell nephropathy. *Int J Artif Organs* 1999; 22:61–3.

198. Chatterjee SN. National study on natural history of allografts in sickle cell disease or trait. *Nephron* 1980; 25:199–201.

199. Chatterjee SN. National study in natural history of renal allograft in sickle disease or trait: a second report. *Transplant Proc* 1987; 19(Suppl): 33–5.

200. Warady BA, Sullivan EK. Renal transplantation in children with sickle cell disease: a report of the North American Pediatric Transplant Cooperative Study (NAPRTCS). *Pediatr Transplant* 1998; 2:130–3.

201. Ojo AO, Govaerts TC, Schmouder RL, Leichtman AB, Leavy SF, Wolfe RA, Held PJ, Port FK, Agodoa LY. Renal transplantation in end-stage sickle cell nephropathy. *Transplantation* 1999; 67:291–5.

202. Spector D, Zachary JB, Steriott S, Milan J. Painful crises following renal transplantation in sickle cell anemia. *Am J Med* 1978; 64:835–9.

203. Montgomery R, Zibari G, Hill GS, Ratner LE. Renal transplantation in patients with sickle cell nephropathy. *Transplantation* 1994; 58:618–20.

204. Miner DJ, Jorkasky DK, Perloff LJ, Grossman RA, Tomaszewski JE. Recurrent sickle cell nephropathy in a transplanted kidney. *Am J Kidney Dis* 1987; 10:306–13.

205. Iannone R, Ohene-Frempong K, Fuchs EJ, Casella JF, Chen AR 2005. Bone marrow transplantation for sickle cell anemia: progress and prospects. *Pediatric Blood Cancer* 2005; 44: 436–40.

CHAPTER 11

Tubulointerstitial diseases

Shane M. Meehan, MD, and Tibor Nadasdy, MD

INTRODUCTION

Tubular and interstitial diseases are considered together since injury to one of these compartments almost invariably leads to injury of the other. Lesions affecting these compartments arise in a wide variety of renal and systemic diseases. Tubular injury and tubulointerstitial inflammatory processes can be primary lesions of the tubulointerstitial compartment, or may arise secondary to glomerular or vascular disease of the kidney. This chapter focuses on tubulointerstitial injury in the absence of glomerular or vascular disease. Injury to the tubules and interstitium can be caused directly by cellular injury or indirectly by ischemia and immune-mediated inflammation. In many instances, etiologic diagnosis on the basis of biopsy pathology is difficult because a limited morphologic spectrum of lesions may be induced by many different injurious agents.

TUBULAR DISEASE

Acute Tubular Necrosis

Acute tubular necrosis (ATN) may be defined simply as acute deterioration of renal function associated with tubular epithelial cell injury. Common causes of tubular injury include ischemia and nephrotoxins. Acute tubular injury is a synonym used to convey the idea that necrosis is cellular rather than geographic, focal, and limited to a small percentage of epithelial cells. Most cells have sublethal injury. There is also consistent microvascular injury, including vasoconstriction with endothelial activation, in the setting of acute tubular necrosis, leading some to adopt the nonspecific, all-encompassing term "acute kidney injury" to define pathophysiologic events in this disorder [1].

Epidemiology and Clinical Presentation

The incidence of ATN is approximately 1 percent of hospital admissions and up to 50 percent of patients undergoing high-risk surgical procedures such as cardiac bypass, or aortic aneurysm repair [1]. ATN is the commonest cause of established acute renal failure, accounting for more than 80 percent of cases. There is acute deterioration of renal function, in the setting of blood loss, extracellular fluid loss, sepsis, cardiac failure, or exposure to renal toxins of endogenous or exogenous origin. Deterioration is observed to occur over hours to days. Typically, there is oliguria at presentation. Acute renal failure is confirmed by elevated serum creatinine, blood urea nitrogen,

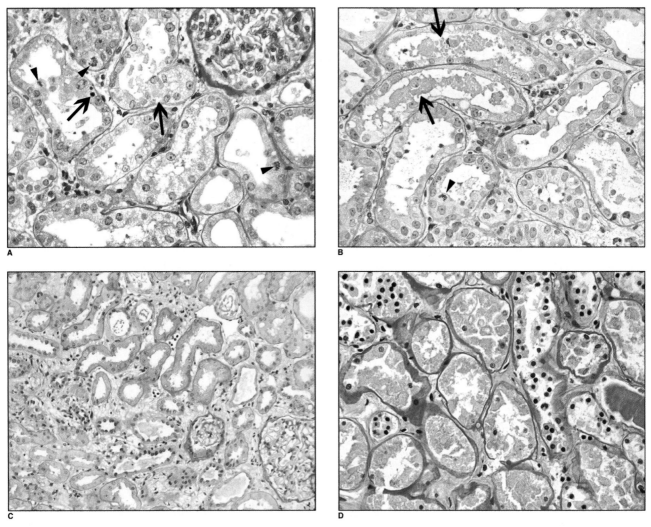

FIGURE 11.1: *Ischemic ATN. A. Tubular profiles with flattened epithelium, diminished brush border, apoptotic bodies (arrow, left), single cell necrosis (arrow, right), and regeneration with mitoses (arrowheads) (PAS, 400×). B. Attenuated epithelium with necrotic luminal debris (arrows) and mitosis (arrowhead) (PAS, 400×). C. ATN with focal interstitial edema and mild mononuclear infiltrate (PAS, 200×). D. Autolysis with loss of cellular adhesion and loss of nuclear basophilia (PAS, 400×).*

and serum potassium levels. Urine microscopy reveals sloughed epithelial cells and muddy brown casts.

Approach to Interpretation

Grossly, the kidneys are enlarged with an increase in weight of up to 30 percent of normal. The cut surface reveals a pale turgid cortex and a red congested medulla. By light microscopy, single epithelial cell necrosis, apoptosis, and segmental coagulative necrosis of tubules may be apparent (Figure 11.1A) [2]. Tubular basement membranes may have segmental denudation. Injured epithelial cells lose adhesion for the tubular basement membrane, and accumulate in the lumens as necrotic cellular casts (Figure 11.1B). Degenerated cells in casts may have abundant lipofuscin giving a brown appearance, most readily apparent in distal nephron segments. Dystrophic calcium phosphate or apatite deposits may be apparent in tubules. The interstitium may have mild edema with sparse mononuclear cell and neutrophilic

infiltrates (Figure 11.1C). Tubulitis is absent or minimal. Vasa recta may have clusters of intraluminal mononuclear cells, consisting of hematopoietic precursors (erythroblast and myeloblast), megakaryocytes, and endothelial progenitors (CD34+). Even in early biopsies, evidence of epithelial regeneration, with flattened, simplified epithelium and prominent proximal tubular lumens is apparent at low power, in contrast with the solid, narrow lumens observed in immersion-fixed normal kidney tissue (Figures 11.2A,B). The epithelial cytoplasm loses the usual eosinophilic, granular, voluminous appearance to become more basophilic with a loss of granularity and apical cytoplasm. Periodic acid-Schiff (PAS) staining reveals a characteristic diminished or absent brush border (Figures 11.1 and 11.2). Further evidence of tubular regeneration includes epithelial mitoses and a crowding of nuclei in proximal segments [2]. Bowman's capsule show transformation of the normally flat parietal epithelium to cuboidal cells, a feature termed tubularization. Immunofluorescence (IF) microscopy is nonspecific. Electron

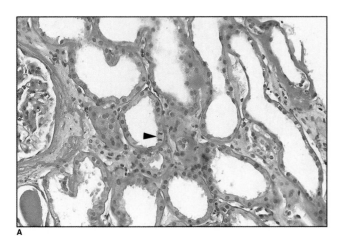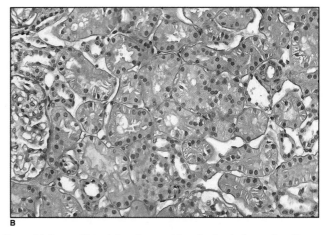

FIGURE 11.2: *Ischemic ATN. A. Flattened proximal tubular epithelium with loss of brush borders and focal mitosis (arrowhead) (PAS, 200×). B. Normal kidney with high cuboidal epithelium and PAS-positive brush borders (PAS, 200×).*

microscopy (EM) reveals a diminished number and length of epithelial surface microvilli, and reduced complexity of basolateral membrane folds with cytoplasmic swelling, and disarray of the organelles. There may also be single cell necrosis with a loss of cell-to-cell and cell-to-basement membrane adhesion (Figure 11.3). EM is not necessary for diagnosis of ATN.

Differential Diagnosis

Tubular autolysis may be difficult to distinguish from ATN in autopsy specimens. Kidney weight is normal in autolysis in contrast to heavy kidneys in ATN. Loss of cell-to-cell and cell-to-basement membrane adhesion, are seen in all segments of the nephron in autolysis (Figure 11.1D). Nuclei are preserved, or have uniformly reduced basophilia in proximal segments in autolysis. Granular casts in distal nephron segments may help to identify true ATN. Immunohistochemistry may reveal the kidney injury molecule 1 (KIM-1) expression in tissue with ATN, and an absence of expression of this molecule in autolysis [3].

ATN is a morphologic diagnosis with a variety of etiologies. Specific features of ATN are occasionally helpful in resolving

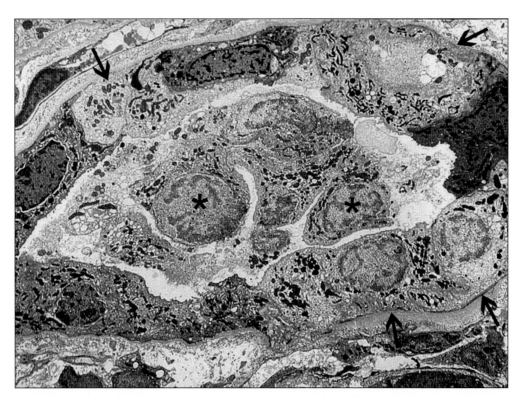

FIGURE 11.3: *Ischemic ATN. EM reveals focal epithelial necrosis of tubular lining cells (arrows) and necrotic cell clusters in the lumen (asterisks). (Uranyl acetate, lead citrate, 4290×).*

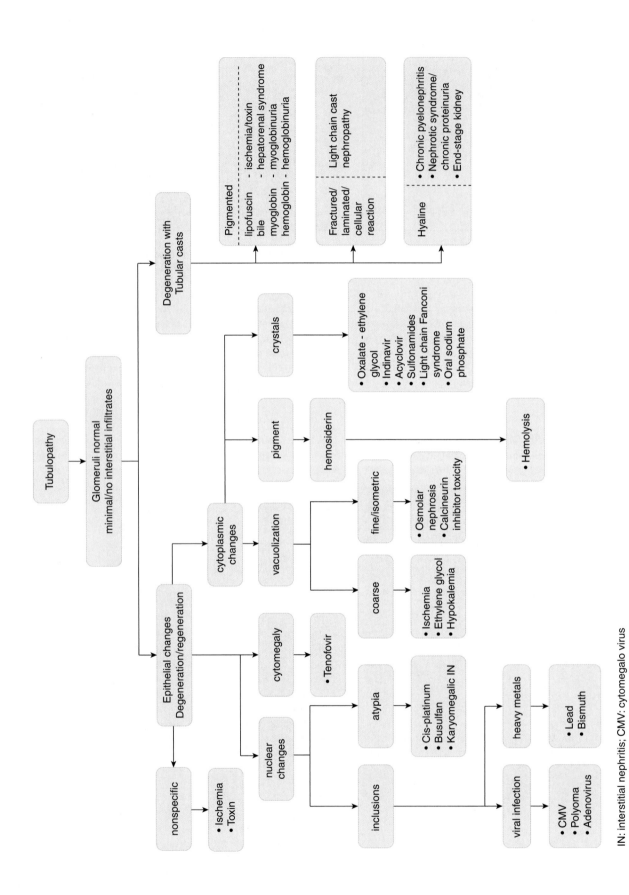

IN: interstitial nephritis; CMV: cytomegalo virus

Algorithm 1: Approach to Differential Diagnosis of Tubular Disease.

410

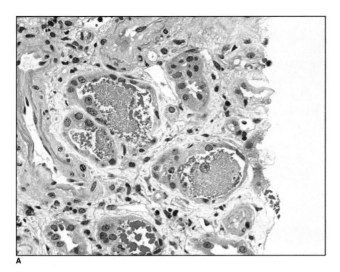
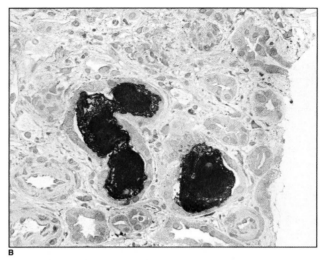

FIGURE 11.4: *ATN with myoglobin casts. A. Tubules with granular eosinophilic casts, epithelial injury, interstitial edema, and slight mononuclear infiltrate (H&E, 400×). B. Myoglobin is identified by immunohistochemistry. (Immunoperoxidase with daiminobenzidine chromogen, 400×).*

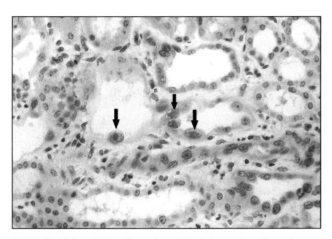

FIGURE 11.5: *ATN with eosinophilic intranuclear inclusions (arrows) typical of lead toxicity (H&E, 400×).*

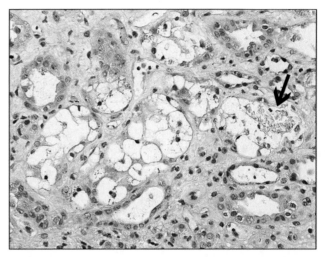

FIGURE 11.6: *Ethylene glycol toxicity with large cytoplasmic vesicles and focal calcium oxalate crystals (arrow) (H&E, 400×).*

the differential diagnosis. Algorithm 1 presents a diagnostic approach to tubular disorders. Globular eosinophilic tubular luminal casts may indicate myoglobinuria, and myoglobin may be confirmed by immunohistochemistry (Figures 11.4A,B). Heavy metal toxicity (lead and bismuth) has characteristic eosinophilic, PAS, and acid-fast-positive tubular epithelial intranuclear inclusions (Figure 11.5). Coarse epithelial vacuolization and birefringent calcium oxalate crystal deposition in distal and/or proximal tubules raise the possibility of ethylene glycol toxicity (Figure 11.6). Certain toxic agents, for example, mercuric chloride, exert their toxic effects on specific tubular segments, with other segments remaining relatively unaffected; however, this may be difficult to identify in biopsy specimens. Tubular vacuolization may be coarse or isometric, and the distinction may have diagnostic implications. Coarse vacuolization is nonspecific, and can be a feature of ischemic or toxic

injury. Isometric vacuolization (Figure 11.7) may be seen in osmotic nephrosis attributable to hyperosmolar solutions such as dextran, mannitol, hydroxyethyl starch, and possibly radiocontrast agents. Osmotic agents are used as plasma expanders or as stabilizers in intravenous immunoglobulin (IVIG) solutions. Epithelial cells of the proximal tubules are typically swollen rather than flattened in this setting and changes are usually diffuse. Calcineurin inhibitors including cyclosporine and tacrolimus, are commonly used as immunosuppressive agents in a variety of immunologic disorders, and in transplantation. Calcineurin inhibitor-associated acute tubular injury has isometric vacuolization of principally the straight portions of the proximal tubules, and tends to be more focally distributed than osmotic lesions. Megamitochondria and calcium phosphate deposits may also be evident in calcineurin inhibitor toxicity,

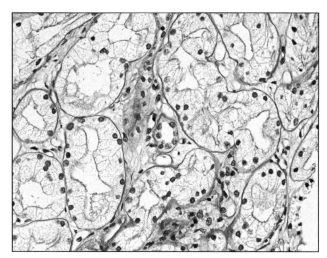

FIGURE 11.7: Osmotic nephrosis. Proximal segments have voluminous foamy cytoplasm with isometric vacuolization and preservation of the brush border (PAS, 400×).

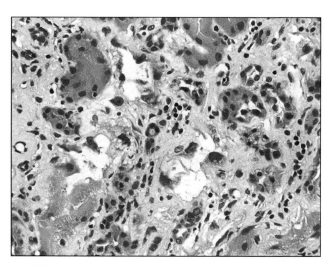

FIGURE 11.8: Acute tubular injury with nuclear atypia in a patient with a history of cis-platinum exposure. Note interstitial fibrosis with mild mononuclear cell infiltrates (H&E, 400×).

but are not specific. Antiviral agents tenofovir, adefovir, and cidofovir have been associated with the development of acute tubular injury with mitochondrial abnormalities [4]. Although reports are limited, the tubular injury associated with these agents mainly involves the proximal segments and consists of cellular necrosis, epithelial flattening or simplification, and marked nuclear enlargement with pleomorphism and cytomegaly. EM reveals increased numbers, enlargement, dilation, and clustering of mitochondria with loss of cristae [4,5]. The proximal tubular epithelial cytosegrosomes with myeloid bodies (also called gentamicin bodies) may be identified ultrastructurally in toxic ATN attributable to gentamicin or other aminoglycosides.

Pathogenesis

Ischemic ATN is thought to arise from hypoxic renal injury and is propagated by vascular alterations via afferent arteriolar vasoconstriction and tubuloglomerular feedback, each of which reduces the glomerular filtration rate. Renal dysfunction is compounded by back-leak of glomerular filtrate, including nitrogenous waste, through the injured tubule wall, and by intrarenal tubular obstruction by cellular casts [6]. The kidney is particularly susceptible to toxic injury for a variety of reasons that include (i) high blood flow increasing the likelihood of exposure to circulating injurious agents, (ii) glomerular filtration facilitating direct exposure of tubular epithelium to these injurious agents, (iii) a large surface area of proximal tubules for exposure to toxins, (iv) concentration of agents in tubular lumens as a result of water reabsorption in proximal tubules, and (v) utilization of epithelial surface specific transport mechanisms that allow increased intraepithelial concentration of injurious agents.

Clinical Course and Prognosis

The recovery of function depends on the severity of initial renal failure and the underlying disease. The recovery of renal func-

tion may take weeks to months after initiation of hemodialysis. In ischemic acute renal failure, 5 to 16 percent of patients have irreversible renal failure. Mortality exceeds 50 percent in the hospitalized patients, who require dialysis. Large cohort analysis indicates that acute renal failure is an independent predictor of mortality [7].

Tubulointerstitial Diseases Associated with Exposure to Metals

These are a group of disorders characterized by direct renal toxicity of mainly heavy metals. Other metals like iron and copper are also included. Exposure is environmental and often occupational, and can be acute or chronic. Toxic agents in this category of renal tubulointerstitial disease include lead, mercury, chromium, bismuth, arsenic, antimony, and cis-platinum.

Epidemiology and Clinical Presentation

In general, exposure to these agents is environmental, and may be occupational since these agents are used in a variety of manufacturing processes. Inhalation or oral ingestion of vapors and dusts are the usual routes of entry of these toxins. Acute exposure may be associated with acute renal failure. Chronic toxic exposure usually results in chronic renal failure, and/or Fanconi syndrome since many have toxic effects on proximal tubules. Up to 50 percent of patients with chronic lead toxicity have hyperuricemia or gout. Nephrolithiasis may be associated with cadmium toxicity.

Approach to Interpretation

ATN may be seen as a result of exposure to toxic quantities of lead, mercury, arsenic, bismuth, antimony, copper, iron, and cis-platinum. Distinctive differential diagnostic features associated with ATN include tubular nuclear inclusions in proximal tubules, and loops of Henle (eosinophilic, irregular size and shape, acid fast, and PAS-positive) in lead toxicity (Figure 11.5). Bismuth toxicity has similar, but regular and rounded inclusions. Copper and iron deposits are detectable using Rubeanic acid and Prussian blue stains respectively. Bizarre reactive nuclear features in the straight portions of proximal tubules are seen in experimental, and rarely in clinical cis-platinum toxicity (Figure 11.8). Peripheral blood levels of specific toxic agents may be elevated.

The chronic exposure to these toxic compounds is associated with bilateral grossly shrunken kidneys with a granular subcapsular surface. Cadmium toxicity may be associated with calcium phosphate stones. Histologically, there is a nonspecific chronic interstitial nephritis. Lead, cadmium, mercury, arsenic, and gold exposures may all be associated with chronic interstitial nephritis. Nuclear inclusions are rare and difficult to detect, and there may be gouty tophi in the renal medulla in chronic lead nephropathy.

IF is generally noncontributory, but may reveal membranous glomerulopathy in mercury and gold toxicity. EM reveals that tubular nuclear-lead inclusions have circumscribed, rounded clusters of electron-dense, irregular-branching fibrils with central, granular electron density, in contrast to the well-defined round inclusions in bismuth toxicity. Gold spicules can be identified in the cytoplasm of tubular epithelium and in the interstitium.

Differential Diagnosis

With the exceptions of lead and bismuth, the morphologic features of ATN due to these agents are not distinctive. Tubular nuclear atypia has been observed in busulphan exposure, and in karyomegalic-chronic interstitial nephritis [8]. Segmental tubular injury and necrosis in the pars recta may be identifiable in mercuric chloride toxicity. Viral infections should be considered in tissues with tubular nuclear inclusions, or with nuclear atypia. Chronic tubulointerstitial nephritis (TIN) has a lengthy differential diagnosis because of a lack of specific features on histology. Spectroscopy may be necessary to identify toxic elements in tissue. Identification of elevated tissue-levels of a heavy metal does not necessarily implicate toxicity from environmental exposure, since there may be retention of elemental metals due to a failure of excretion in advanced renal failure.

Etiology and Pathogenesis

Most heavy metals cause toxicity by a direct injury to cell membranes and mitochondria in proximal tubular segments. Cadmium interferes with calcium metabolism resulting in hypercalciuria and nephrolithiasis.

Clinical Course and Prognosis

The outcome of ATN depends on the severity and duration of toxic exposure. Ethylene diamine tetraacetic acid (EDTA) is used as a lead chelator in acute lead toxicity, and may be effective in reversal of acute renal failure. Chronic toxic nephropathy with the development of chronic interstitial nephritis may stabilize after withdrawal of the offending agent. The risk of progressive renal failure may be related to the extent of renal scarring at the time of diagnosis.

TUBULOINTERSTITIAL NEPHRITIS (TIN)

Introduction

TIN is a histologic response by the kidney to injury from a variety of agents, and may be acute, chronic, or both. Acute lesions are characterized by interstitial edema, exudation of inflammatory cells to the interstitium with tubular invasion, and acute tubular injury. Tubular intraepithelial inflammatory cells define tubulitis, and these lesions are usually evident in the absence of tubular basement membrane rupture. Tubular inflammation colocalized with basement membrane rupture may be seen in TIN, but is not a specific lesion. The acute lesions are usually associated with acute renal dysfunction, and in the absence of scarring are potentially clinically reversible.

Chronic TIN is characterized by interstitial fibrosis and tubular atrophy with variable inflammatory infiltrates. In early interstitial fibrosis, there is tubular separation by myxoid matrix with plump interstitial spindle cells. There is progressive collagen deposition, with a change from matrix basophilia to eosinophilia in later stages, with progressive, irreversible tubular atrophy. Tubular atrophy has four main appearances: (i) Classic – characterized by diminished tubular diameter, wrinkling, and lamination of the basement membrane, with simplification and loss of epithelial cells. Progressive cellular loss results in progressive shrinkage of tubular cross-sectional area, with eventual loss of the tubular epithelial population in the affected tubular segments. (ii) "Thyroidization" – a form of microcystic change where the affected tubules are rounded, and have attenuated tubular epithelium with luminal hyaline casts. This is characteristic of chronic pyelonephritis, but not specific. (iii) "Endocrine" – small, solid, or hollow tubules, with clear epithelium, and very thin basement membranes. The term "endocrine" comes from the uniform, rounded appearance of the epithelial nuclei, resembling, for example, the parathyroid or anterior pituitary cells. (iv) "Super" tubules – enlarged with dilated lumens, irregular profiles, and enlarged epithelial cells, often with apical "snouts." These are found in association with extensive interstitial fibrosis, and often glomerulomegaly, and are indicative of nephron hypertrophy. Types (i) and (iv) express immunochemical markers of proximal tubular segments, in contrast with distal segment markers expressed by type (ii) lesions. Endocrine tubules (type (iii) express immunochemical markers of distal segments mainly; however, proximal markers are also identifiable in this type of atrophy [9]. These chronic lesions are usually associated with chronic renal failure, and irreversible clinical dysfunction.

Infectious Tubulointerstitial Nephritis

Acute Pyelonephritis

A pathologic disorder characterized by acute suppurative inflammation of the renal parenchyma, and the pelvicalyceal system attributable to direct infection by microorganisms. There are two possible routes of infection of the kidney parenchyma: (a) ascending from the lower urinary tract and (b) hematogenous spread.

Epidemiology and Clinical Presentation. In infancy and early childhood, infection is predominantly by the ascending route, and males are the most commonly affected. Infection arises in association with urinary tract abnormalities that predispose to reflux or urinary obstruction. In adults, ascending infection is much more common in females of childbearing age. In older age groups, ascending infection is often associated with obstructive lesions of the lower urinary tract associated with nodular prostatic hyperplasia, carcinoma of the cervix and urothelium, and nephrolithiasis. Classical presentation is with fever, chills, flank pain, urinary frequency, and dysuria. Urinalysis reveals white cells and white cell casts (pyuria). Urinary culture reveals more than 100,000 colony-forming units per mL. Blood cultures may be positive for microorganisms.

Approach to Interpretation. Grossly, kidneys are enlarged with dilation of the pelvicalyceal system and pyramidal blunting, if there is obstruction. The cut surface in the ascending renal infection may have linear abscesses in the medulla and cortex, most notably at the poles. There may be papillary necrosis. Abscess formation in the pelvis, pyonephrosis, may be evident. Hematogenous infection is characterized by multiple small cortical abscesses.

Microscopically, there is segmental involvement of the cortex by interstitial edema with predominantly neutrophilic infiltrates (Figure 11.9). Neutrophils can be seen in direct contact circumferentially with tubular basement membranes (tagging), within the epithelium (tubulitis), and in tubular luminal casts (Figures 11.9A,B). There may be an accompanying infiltrate of mononuclear cells, including macrophages, lymphoid cells, and plasma cells, depending on the duration of the infection. Abscesses (Figure 11.9C) may involve glomeruli in hematogenous infection. IF and EM are noncontributory.

Differential Diagnosis. The presence of peritubular neutrophil tagging with neutrophilic tubulitis, luminal pus, and microabscesses are characteristic of infectious TIN. Tubular casts with clusters of apoptotic cells may be observed in ATN, and may be mistaken for neutrophils; however, these are distinguishable by careful inspection. Scattered interstitial neutrophils and neutrophilic tubulitis may be associated with calcium oxalate deposits in tubular epithelium in ATN in the absence of infection. Focal neutrophilic inflammation may be a nonspecific feature of tubular rupture. Drug-induced acute tubulointerstitial nephritis (ATIN) and light chain cast nephropathy may occasionally have tubular or interstitial neutrophils, without demonstrable infection. Special stains including Gram, PAS, or Gomori methenamine silver stains may be used for detection of microorganisms, with low sensitivity, however. Urine and blood cultures are necessary to

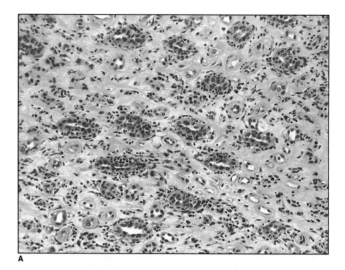

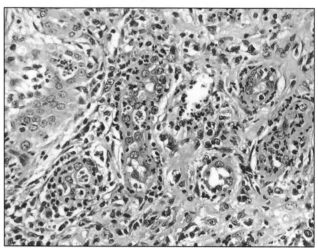

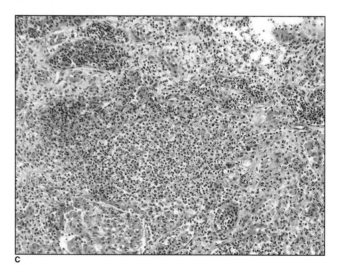

FIGURE 11.9: *Acute pyelonephritis. A. Neutrophil tagging and tubulitis in medullary collecting ducts (H&E, 200×). B. Neutrophilic tagging, tubulitis, and luminal casts (H&E, 400×). C. Cortical abscess with neutrophil casts in surrounding tubules (H&E, 100×).*

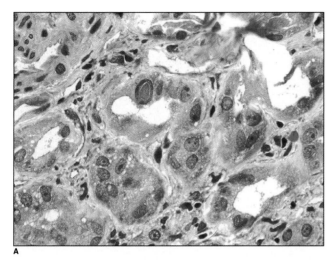 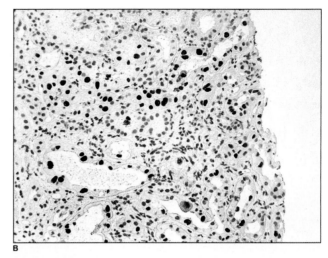

A **B**

FIGURE 11.10: *PV nephropathy in a patient who received an autologous hematopoietic stem cell transplantation 1-year prior to the biopsy with: A. Classical nuclear inclusions (H&E, 400×) and B. PV large-T antigen expression in epithelial cell nuclei (immunoperoxidase, 200×).*

determine the bacterial or fungal species involved. Polyoma virus (PV) nephropathy (Figure 11.10A) can have considerable neutrophilic infiltration with subtle viral cytopathic changes. Immunohistochemical detection of SV40-T antigen in biopsy tissue (Figure 11.10B), and detection of BK, JC, or SV40 viral DNA in peripheral blood confirms the diagnosis. Differentiation of ascending from hematogenous acute pyelonephritis can be difficult or impossible on biopsy, and requires clinical correlation.

Etiology and Pathogenesis. The commonest organisms in ascending infection are Gram-negative coliform species including *Escherichia coli*, Proteus, Klebsiella, and Enterobacter. Urinary tract abnormalities with obstruction and reflux predispose to renal parenchymal infection. Staphylococcal species and *E. coli* are the commonest organisms associated with hematogenous infection. Organisms associated with direct infection of the renal parenchyma are many, and those more commonly encountered are summarized in Table 11.1.

Clinical Course and Prognosis. Treatment of acute infection requires antibiotic therapy, and if necessary, surgical intervention to correct obstruction or vesicoureteral reflux. Complications of acute pyelonephritis include recurrent infection, local spread of infection with perinephric abscess, pyonephrosis, and papillary necrosis. Recurrent infection may lead to chronic pyelonephritis. Persistent or recurrent infection may rarely lead to malakoplakia or xanthogranulomatous pyelonephritis.

Other Causes of Infectious Tubulointerstitial Nephritis (Table 11.1)

A wide variety of direct infections are associated with acute or chronic TIN. Bacterial infections due to mycobacteria and

Table 11.1 Infectious Tubulointerstitial Nephritis

Direct Infection of the Kidney
Bacteria
Acute pyelonephritis
    Ascending – *E. coli*, Proteus, Klebsiella, Enterobacter
    Hematogenous – *E. coli*, Staphylococcus
Chronic pyelonephritis
    Obstructive
    Nonobstructive/reflux associated
    Xanthogranulomatous
    Malakoplakia
Specific infections – M. tuberculosis, M. leprae, T. pallidum, others
Fungi – Candida, Cryptococcus, Histoplasma, Blastomyces, others
Rickettsia – R. rickettsia, Typhus
Viruses – Polyoma, Cytomegalovirus, Adenovirus, Hantavirus

Reactive TIN associated with extrarenal/systemic infection
Bacteria – beta-hemolytic streptococci, C. diphtheriae,
    L. pneumophilia, others
Viruses – Influenza, Epstein-Barr, HIV-1, Rubeola, others
Parasites – Leishmania donovani, Toxoplasma gondii

Brucella, and fungal infections including coccidioidomyces and cryptococcus tend to have granulomas with necrosis. Abscesses are seen in many additional infections including Salmonella, Staphylococcus and many other bacteria, nocardiosis [10], candidiasis [11], aspergillosis, actinomycosis, and other organisms [10]. Suppurative granulomas may be seen in nocardiosis, cryptococcosis, and blastomycosis. Lymphoplasmacytic and eosinophilic infiltrates may be seen in Toxoplasmosis, Leptospirosis, Legionella infection, and other spirochetal infections. Viral infections including Hantavirus and Flaviviruses

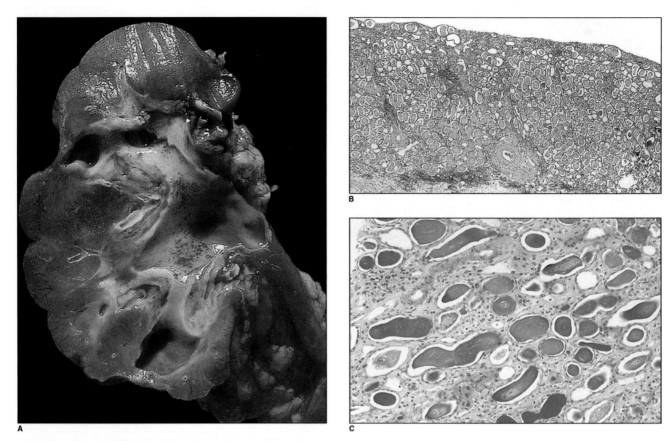

FIGURE 11.11: *A. Chronic obstructive pyelonephritis, with dilated ureter, pelvis and calyces, blunted medullary pyramids, and segmental marked cortical thinning with retraction of the capsular surface. B, C. Chronic pyelonephritis with diffuse tubular microcystic change with luminal casts, reminiscent of thyroid tissue (B, H&E, 40×; C, PAS, 200×).*

have mononuclear infiltrates with interstitial hemorrhage, and some organisms may be identified using specific antibodies [12]. Cytomegalovirus (CMV) and PV infections have mainly mononuclear cells with viral inclusions in endothelium (CMV), and tubules (PV, CMV). Many of these agents are associated with tubulointerstitial disease in the native kidneys of immuno-suppressed patients, and may also be observed in the transplanted kidney.

Chronic Pyelonephritis

This is chronic tubulointerstitial inflammation and scarring with involvement of the pelvis and calyces, attributable to recurrent or persistent infection, urinary reflux, or obstruction. There are two main types: designated chronic obstructive pyelonephritis, and chronic nonobstructive pyelonephritis or reflux nephropathy. Obstructive chronic pyelonephritis is chronic pyelonephritis associated with urinary obstruction. Nonobstructive chronic pyelonephritis is mainly associated with vesicoureteral reflux.

Epidemiology and Clinical Presentation. Obstructive pyelonephritis accounts for the majority of cases of chronic pyelo-

nephritis. Reflux nephropathy is associated with congenital patency of the vesicoureteral junction that permits vesicoureteral reflux on micturition, and is comparatively uncommon. The incidence of obstructive chronic pyelonephritis was 1.4 percent and that of reflux nephropathy was 0.23 percent in one autopsy series [13]. Reflux nephropathy is evident in up to 20–40 percent of children investigated for persistent urinary infection. The majority of patients with nonobstructive chronic pyelonephritis have vesicoureteral reflux with urinary infection. Clinically, the majority of these patients have a history of urinary tract infections. Clinical findings are nonspecific and include proteinuria, chronic renal insufficiency, and hypertension. There may be bacteriuria and pyuria. Radiologic evaluation by intravenous pyelogram reveals coarse parenchymal scarring with blunted medullary pyramids, and calyceal dilation. These findings may be localized to the upper and lower poles in reflux nephropathy. Micturating cystourethrogram reveals vesicoureteral reflux.

Approach to Interpretation. A gross examination is essential for accurate diagnosis. The kidney size is variable and may be enlarged or shrunken, depending on the duration of disease, and the extent of scarring. The capsular surface has coarse segmental scars that are typically asymmetrical in cases with bilateral involvement. The parenchyma between the scars may be smooth, or may have fine granularity. The cut surface reveals cortical scars overlying blunted or effaced pyramids (Figure 11.11A). These areas have dilated and distorted calyces. Calyceal dilation may be more extensive in obstructive disease. The calyces, pelvis and ureter may be dilated (Figure 11.11A) with mural thickening and granularity of the urothelial surface.

Microscopically, there is segmental scarring most often at the renal poles. Scar may alternate with noninflamed tissue, giving a segmental appearance. The cortex has prominent tubular atrophy with microcysts lined by attenuated epithelium, and hyaline luminal casts. The appearance is often designated thyroidization because of its superficial resemblance to thyroid tissue (Figures 11.11B,C). The interstitium has mononuclear infiltrates with fibrosis. The infiltrates are composed of lymphoid cells, often forming follicles, with plasma cells and macrophages. Some neutrophils with tubular luminal neutrophil casts may be evident. There may be focal tubular rupture with extrusion of Tamm-Horsfall protein (also called uromodulin) into the interstitium, a nonspecific finding. Tubular protein extrusion may be associated with localized, nonspecific neutrophilic, eosinophilic, and mononuclear inflammation (Figure 11.12). Glomeruli are closely approximated to each other due to interstitial fibrosis, and atrophy of the tubules. There may be periglomerular fibrosis often associated with ischemic glomerular collapse. In severe parenchymal scarring with significant nephron loss, there may be compensatory hypertrophy of the remnant nephrons, and glomerulomegaly with secondary focal segmental glomerular sclerosis. In advanced disease, there may be extensive glomerular sclerosis rendering the differentiation of tubulointerstitial from glomerular disease impossible. Arteriosclerosis and arteriolosclerosis may be prominent and secondary to hypertension. IF and EM have no significant role to play in the diagnosis of chronic pyelonephritis. EM is helpful, however, in making the distinction of primary from secondary focal segmental glomerular sclerosis.

Differential Diagnosis. The diagnosis of chronic pyelonephritis cannot be made reliably on renal biopsy. Chronic tubulointerstitial inflammation with scarring, as observed in chronic pyelonephritis, is a nonspecific pattern that can be seen in a variety of circumstances including chronic ischemia, chronic drug-induced, or toxic nephropathy.

Etiology and Pathogenesis. Obstruction of urinary outflow can be structural or functional. Structural causes include congenital strictures, posterior urethral valves, calculi, prostatic hyperplasia and neoplasms of urothelial, prostatic, cervical, and periureteral origin. Functional causes include bladder and ureteral dysmotility associated with neurogenic disorders.

Repeated or persistent bacterial infection of the renal parenchyma associated with intrarenal reflux or urinary obstruction results in chronic inflammation, and scar formation. Compound papillae, located at the renal poles, are thought to pre-

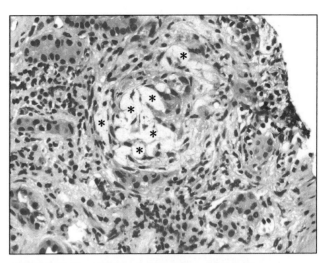

FIGURE 11.12: *Tubular rupture with extrusion of Tamm-Horsfall protein (asterisks), peritubular mononuclear cells, eosinophils, and rare neutrophils in a young male with malignant hypertension and proteinuria (H&E, 400×).*

dispose to intrarenal reflux more than simple papillae resulting in polar scars. Renal parenchymal scar formation typically occurs predominantly in infancy and early childhood before the age of 6 years [14]. The acquisition of new parenchymal scars attributable to infection is rare in adulthood, and associated with severe reflux. Reflux may cease spontaneously after years.

When there is advanced parenchymal scarring with nephron loss, the remnant nephrons undergo hypertrophy. There is increased glomerular hydrostatic pressure with hyperfiltration. Over the years, there is podocyte senescence with loss of protein selectivity of the glomerular filtration barrier, proteinuria, and eventual development of focal segmental scars.

Clinical Course and Prognosis. Antibiotic therapy and surgical correction of structural abnormalities may be necessary for the treatment of active infection. Most children with vesicoureteral reflux outgrow the condition. Progression to end-stage disease depends on bilateral involvement, and on the extent of renal scarring at the time of initial presentation. Thirty to 50 percent of patients progress to end-stage disease over many years. Chronic pyelonephritis accounts for end-stage renal failure in up to 25 percent of children and young adults, and in approximately 10 percent of adults. Complications include papillary necrosis, and xanthogranulomatous pyelonephritis when there is nephrolithiasis, secondary focal segmental glomerular sclerosis, and hypertension.

Chronic Pyelonephritis Variants

(Xanthogranulomatous Pyelonephritis)

This variant of pyelonephritis is characterized by xanthogranulomas and is frequently associated with nephrolithiasis, and urinary tract obstruction.

Epidemiology and Clinical Features. A study from Britain estimated the incidence of this disorder at 1.4 per 100,000 per annum [15]. Adult females are the most commonly affected, but the disease is well recognized in males and may present at all ages, most commonly between 50 and 70 years. Clinically, patients have flank pain, weight loss, fever, nausea, and vomiting. Urinalysis reveals pyuria, proteinuria, and rarely hematuria. Urine culture reveals *E. coli*, Klebsiella sp., *Proteus* sp., *Pseudomonas aeruginosa*, and *Enterococcus faecalis* in a descending order of frequency [16]. Radiologic studies reveal unilateral renal enlargement with pelvicalyceal dilation, and staghorn calculi. Struvite stones (magnesium ammonium phosphate] are evident in 80 percent of cases.

Approach to Interpretation. A gross examination reveals unilateral renal enlargement. Bilateral involvement is exceptional. In diffuse renal involvement, there is a replacement of the parenchyma by tan-yellow nodules (Figure 11.13A), which may have focal central yellow softening. The capsule is thickened, and the process may extend into the perirenal adipose tissue. In focal disease, there is localized involvement of the parenchyma. The pelvicalyceal system is dilated with effacement of the medullary pyramids (Figure 11.13A). Staghorn calculi and viscous yellow fluid may be identified in the pelvis.

Microscopic examination reveals nodules composed of large aggregates of foamy macrophages, replacing the renal parenchyma (Figure 11.13B). A second nonfoamy, macrophage population has PAS-positive cytoplasmic granules, and there may be multinucleated foreign body-type giant cells. Neutrophils, lymphocytes, and plasma cells are also prominent. Intra- and extracellular hemosiderin may be abundant. Focal abscesses and necrosis with cholesterol clefts may be evident. The parenchyma between nodules has chronic pyelonephritis, and may have marked coarse fibrosis. Renal vein thrombi are seen in 20 percent of cases. Gram stains reveal Gram-negative bacilli in exudates and in neutrophils, but only rarely in macrophages. Bacilli may also be demonstrated using the Dieterle stain and by EM [17]. IF staining is nonspecific.

Differential Diagnosis. Focal xanthogranulomatous pyelonephritis may grossly resemble renal cell carcinoma Microscopically, the distinction of macrophages from epithelial tumor cells is straightforward, and can be confirmed using CD68 and cytokeratin immunohistochemical stains. Malakoplakia of the kidney can be distinguished by the presence of von Hansemann cells, and Michaelis-Gutmann bodies. Foam cells are absent in malakoplakia and megalocytic interstitial nephritis. Discrete clusters of foamy macrophages may be seen in Mycobacterium avium-intracellulare. Mycobacteria are identifiable using Ziehl-Neelsen stains. Table 11.2 provides a list of disorders to consider in the differential diagnosis of interstitial foam cells.

Pathogenesis. The pathogenesis is unclear. Urinary obstruction, with infection by Gram-negative organisms, and extensive tissue-necrosis results in massive accumulation of foam cells, hemosiderin, and cholesterol crystals.

Clinical Course and Prognosis. Extrarenal spread of xanthogranulomatous pyelonephritis may result in perirenal abscess, or sinus formation with the small intestine, colon, or skin. Progressive renal destruction results in eventual cessation of function. Antibiotics are ineffective. Nephrectomy is often curative.

(Malakoplakia)

This is a chronic granulomatous disorder that mainly affects the urinary bladder, and rarely, the kidney parenchyma.

Etiology and Clinical Presentation. This disorder is uncommon and involves predominantly the lower urinary tract. Kidney parenchymal involvement is rare. Women are affected more frequently than men and with a peak incidence in the fifth decade. Flank pain, fever, rigors, and a history of recurrent urinary tract infection are typical findings. Urinalysis reveals pyuria, proteinuria, and hematuria. Bacterial microorganisms are isolated from the urine.

Approach to the Diagnosis. Grossly, the renal parenchyma has multiple tan-brown discrete nodules from 0.1 to 2 cm distributed primarily in the renal cortex. Nodules are frequently multifocal and bilateral [18], and uncommonly, localized. Nodules are firm, well-circumscribed, and may have central yellow softening. The pelvis and calyces may be dilated and have brown plaques on the mucosal surface. Microscopically, the nodules are composed of sheets of large macrophages with abundant granular PAS-positive material in the cytoplasm. These cells are known as von Hansemann cells (Figure 11.14). Many of these cells have well-circumscribed, 5–10 μm, cytoplasmic inclusions that stain for calcium (von Kossa-positive), iron (Prussian blue-positive), and by PAS (Figure 11.14). These inclusions are designated Michaelis-Gutmann bodies, and may also be evident in extracellular locations. Occasionally, these inclusions have a laminated appearance. There may be infiltrates of neutrophils, lymphoid cells, and plasma cells. IF is nonspecific. EM is used to identify laminated Michaelis-Gutmann bodies, and bacilli may be identified in the macrophage cytoplasm.

Differential Diagnosis. Other infectious granulomatous disorders need to be excluded. Rarely, the lesions may resemble primary or metastatic carcinoma, or melanoma. Michaelis-Gutmann bodies are pathognomonic of malakoplakia. Megalocytic interstitial nephritis has similar sheets of macrophages without PAS-positive cytoplasmic granules or Michaelis-Gutmann bodies, leading many to consider these different phases of the same disease-process (reviewed in Ref. [19]).

Pathogenesis. The disorder is a granulomatous response to Gram-negative bacteria, specifically *E. coli, Proteus vulgaris,*

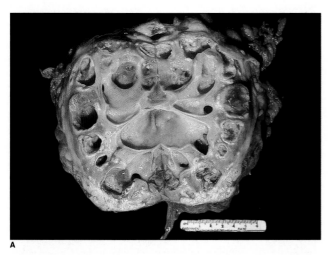 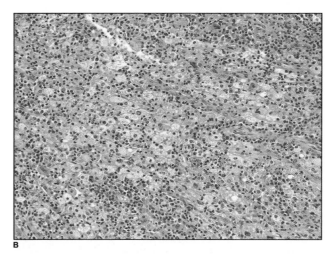

FIGURE 11.13: *A. Xanthogranulomatous pyelonephritis showing dilated pelvis and calyces with effacement of medullary pyramids, parenchymal tan-yellow nodules (lower pole), and a marked thickening of the renal capsule. B. Xanthogranulomatous pyelonephritis with foamy macrophages admixed inflammatory infiltrates including neutrophils and plasma cells (H&E, 200×).*

Aerobacter aerogenes, and *Klebsiella pneumoniae*. The pathogenesis is unclear. Defective lysosomal killing of microorganisms in macrophages has been proposed, but is not proven. Increased frequency in patients receiving immunosuppression has been observed.

Clinical Course and Prognosis. An extensive renal involvement may result in end-stage kidney disease. Early diagnosis and treatment using fluoroquinolone antibiotics may allow resolution [20].

Noninfectious Tubulointerstitial Nephritis

Acute Tubulointerstitial Nephritis (ATIN)

ATIN is focal or diffuse acute inflammation with fluid and cellular exudates in the tubulointerstitial compartment associated with tubular epithelial injury. ATIN is thought to be an immune-mediated reaction to a variety of agents, and is also known as acute allergic tubulointerstitial nephritis. Inflammation arises as a reaction to antigens or haptens derived from extrinsic agents, including antigenic products of drugs and infectious agents.

Table 11.2 Disorders Associated with Tubulointerstitial Foam Cells

Xanthgranulomatous pyelonephritis
M. avium-intracellulare infection
Nephrotic syndrome and chronic heavy (nonselective) proteinuria
Cholesterol granulomas
Alport nephropathy
Whipple disease
Metabolic disorders – Fabry, Lysosomal storage diseases

Epidemiology and Clinical Features. A Finnish study of young men disclosed an incidence of 0.7 per 100,000 biopsied for hematuria or proteinuria [21]. Renal biopsy series have observed ATIN in 2–3 percent of biopsies [22]. In unselected patient-cohorts with TIN on biopsy of the kidney, pharmacologic agents account for 63–71 percent of cases [23,24]. The classical clinical presentation of fever, a maculopapular rash, eosinophilia, and acute renal failure is observed together, or as individual findings in only a minority of instances [24]. Some patients have eosinophiluria. More typically, there is an acute renal dysfunction with an elevation of the serum creatinine temporally related to the intake of the offending agent, or to an extrarenal infection. Urinalysis reveals sterile pyuria and hematuria. There may be low-grade proteinuria, with Fanconi syndrome, and loss of urinary concentrating ability. Radiologic studies reveal diffuse bilateral kidney enlargement.

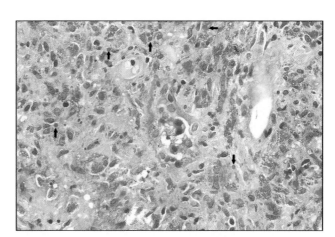

FIGURE 11.14: *Malakoplakia with cytoplasmic granules in macrophages (von Hansemann cells) and numerous Michaelis-Gutmann bodies stained by PAS (arrows) (PAS, 400×).*

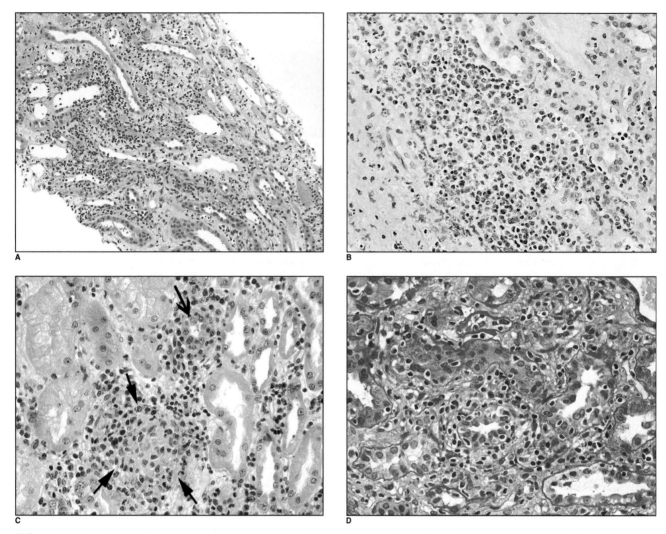

FIGURE 11.15: *A. TIN with eosinophils, lymphoid cells, and macrophages in the outer medulla (H&E, 200×). B. Eosinophil microabscess (H&E, 400×). C. Small noncaseating granuloma (solid arrows) with tubulitis (upper arrow). Note acute tubular injury (right), compared with normal tubules (upper left) (H&E, 400×). D. Tubulitis with intraepithelial lymphoid cells (PAS, 400×).*

Approach to Interpretation. Grossly, the kidneys are uniformly enlarged, pale and heavy, with distinct corticomedullary junctions. Microscopically, there is focal, multifocal, or diffuse interstitial expansion with edema including inflammatory mononuclear cells, and variable numbers of eosinophil granulocytes (Figure 11.15A). Eosinophils may be absent, sparse, or abundant, and may form focal aggregates or rarely eosinophilic microabscesses (Figure 11.15B). The mononuclear cell population is composed of lymphocytes in various stages of activation. Macrophages may form small noncaseating granulomas (Figure 11.15C). The granulomas may be tubulocentric, with or without foci of tubular basement membrane rupture. Lymphoid, plasmacytic, granulomatous, and eosinophilic infiltrates may be seen in the same renal biopsy specimens, or there may be a predominance of one cell type. Plasma cells may be abundant. The tubules have acute tubular epithelial injury (Figure 11.15C), with

or without colocalized inflammation. Tubulitis with intraepithelial mononuclear inflammation is typically mild and focal (Figure 11.15D). Severe lesions may have tubular basement membrane rupture. Immunophenotyping reveals an abundance of T cells and macrophages, with lesser amounts of B cells (Figures 11.16A,B). Infiltrating cells in tubulitis are mainly of T cell phenotype (Figure 11.16C) [25,26]. Defining the etiology of these infiltrates is difficult, and requires clinicopathologic correlation. Glomeruli and blood vessels are typically unremarkable, with the exception of ATIN due to nonsteroidal antiinflammatory agents, which may have diffuse podocytopathy resembling minimal change disease, or features of membranous glomerulopathy. IF and EM are helpful in excluding immune complex causes of ATIN, like SLE, Sjogren syndrome (SS) and hypocomplementemic TIN, that may have inflammatory infiltrates indistinguishable from other causes. IF may reveal subtle glomerular

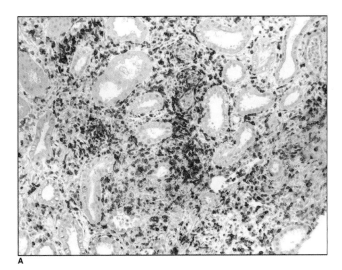

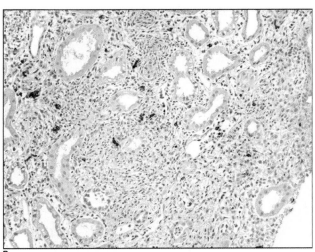

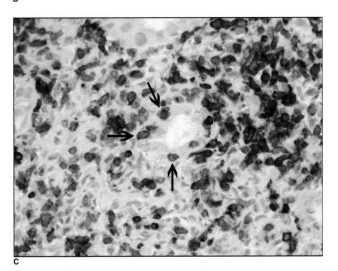

FIGURE 11.16: *ATIN immunophenotyping. A. Abundant CD3+ T cells (immunoperoxidase, 200×). B. Few CD20+ B cells (immunoperoxidase, 200×). C. CD3+ T cells in a focus of tubulitis (arrows) (immunoperoxidase, 600×).*

disease, such as membranous nephropathy, associated with ATIN.

Differential Diagnosis. Morphologic features of mononuclear and eosinophilic infiltrates are nonspecific patterns of tissue injury. Algorithm 2 presents an approach to the differential diagnosis of acute tubulointerstitial inflammation based on the predominant type of the inflammatory cell. The resolution of the differential diagnosis requires detailed clinical information. The distinction from an acute ischemic or toxic tubular necrosis is based on the extent and severity of inflammation. If there is more than a slight interstitial inflammation, and more than an occasional focus of tubulitis, then ATIN is likely. If there is a predominance of tubulointerstitial neutrophils, ascending or hematogenous bacterial infection should be considered. Eosinophils may indicate an allergic reaction to drugs especially diuretics and antibiotics [27,28]. Other idiopathic disorders such as TIN and uveitis (TINU, also called Dobrin syndrome) may have lymphocytes, plasma cells, macrophages, eosinophils, and granulomas in the inflammatory infiltrate [29]. Interstitial hemorrhage with ATIN may indicate Hantavirus infection, which can be identified using specific antibodies. Other organisms such as viruses, Leptospira, and Rickettsiae can be identified using special stains, specific antibodies, or EM. Tubular viral inclusions are evident in PV nephropathy in immunocompromised individuals (Figure 11.10). The differential diagnosis of granulomatous interstitial nephritis is given in Table 11.6, and will be discussed in a later section of this chapter.

Etiology and Pathogenesis. ATIN is a histologic pattern of injury that arises in response to a wide variety of injurious agents the commonest of which are drugs and infection. The causes of ATIN include drugs (71 percent), infection (15 percent), TIN with uveitis (5 percent), sarcoidosis (1 percent), and of unknown cause (8 percent), from a recent review [24]. Antibiotics are responsible for about one-third of drug-induced disease, and many other agents have been implicated in this disorder (Table 11.3). Infections at sites outside the kidney, attributable to streptococci, pneumococci, and Yersinia species, are a cause of reactive ATIN, and these infections are more commonly observed in children [30,31]. Currently, ATIN is more likely to be attributable to the agents used for treatment of the infection than to the infection itself. The principal pathogenetic mechanisms involved in ATIN include cell-mediated and less commonly antibody-mediated immune injury. Biopsies only rarely have evidence of immunoglobulin deposits; however, interstitial infiltrates have abundant T cells, admixed with macrophages, which may form granulomas. Tubular epithelium has increased expression of class I and II major histocompatibility antigens, a feature which may contribute to localization of inflammation [32]. The inflammation may arise in response to antigens derived directly from the offending agent, or from a metabolite, or a hapten, that localize to the tubular epithelium, basement membrane, or interstitium. The reaction is idiosyncratic, not dose dependent, and may take months to develop after an initial exposure to the inciting agent. A recurrence of ATIN occurs on reexposure to the agent, or to related compounds. Other mechanisms may include inflammation in response to tubular

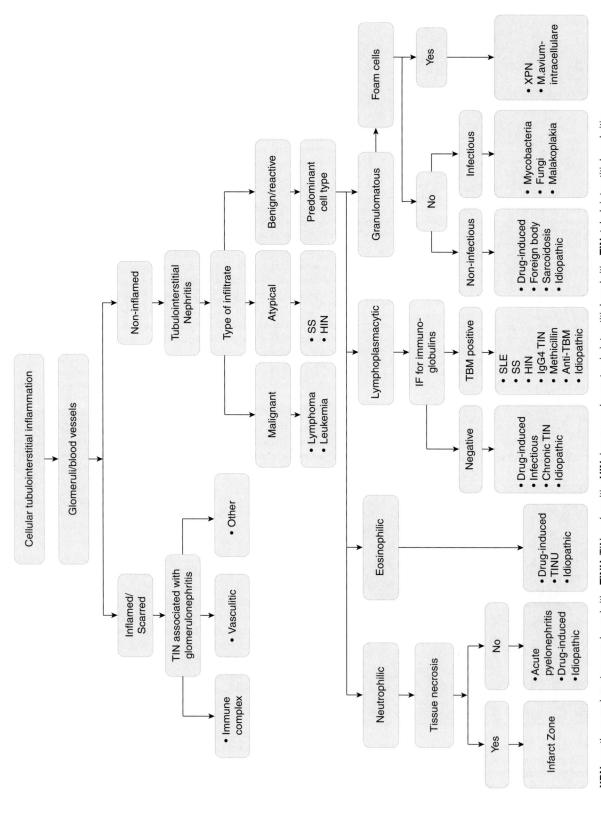

XPN: xanthogranulomatous pyelonephritis; **TINU**: TIN and uveitis; **HIN**: hypocomplementemic interstitial nephritis; **TIN**: tubulointerstitial nephritis; **TBM**: tubular basement membrane; **SS**: Sjogren Syndrome

Algorithm 2: Approach to Differential Diagnosis of Tubulointerstitial Nephritis.

Table 11.3: Common causes of ATIN

Drugs
NSAIDs including COX-2 inhibitors
Antibiotics including penicillin and cephalosporins, rifampicin, ciprofloxacin
Sulfonamides including trimethoprim-sulfamethoxazole
Thiazide diuretics – furosemide, bumetanide
Cimetidine
Allopurinol
Proton pump inhibitors – omeprazole, lansoprazole
Antiretrovirals – indinavir
5-aminosalicylates – mesalamine

Infectious agents (direct and reactive)
Streptococcal sp
Corynebacterium diphtheriae
Yersinia
Legionella
Leptospira
Cytomegalovirus
Polyoma virus

ATIN with immune mechanisms (see Table 11.7)
Humoral - anti-TBM disease, Immune complex mediated
Cell mediated-TIN with uveitis

Sarcoidosis

Idiopathic

injury, and an alteration of local prostaglandin synthesis in the case of nonsteroidal antiinflammatory agents [33].

Treatment and Prognosis. The removal of the inciting agent may allow a reversal of acute inflammation and a recovery of the renal function. Drug-induced lesions usually respond in days to weeks after removal of the offending agent; however, recovery of the renal function may take months, and may require steroid therapy. One study [34] examined the risk factors for the outcome in ATIN attributable to drugs, infection, and idiopathic

Table 11.4 Tubulointerstitial disease with crystal deposits

Pharmacologic Agents
Oral sodium phosphate purgatives
Antiviral agents – acyclovir, indinavir, foscarnet
Antibiotics – sulfonamides (sulfadiazine, sulfamethoxazole), ciprofloxacin
Diuretics – triamterene
Antimetabolites – methotrexate
Miscellaneous – pyridoxylate, vitamin C, primidone, methoxyflurane (oxalate)

Metabolic
Hypercalcemic nephropathy
Oxalate nephropathy – enteric hyperoxaluria
Urate nephropathy
Cystinosis
Hemosiderosis
Light chain Fanconi syndrome and cast nephropathy

disease. Histologic predictors of irreversible renal failure included diffuse interstitial inflammation, granulomas, and diffuse tubular atrophy [34]. Clinical predictors of irreversible renal failure included duration of exposure of more than one month, and depended on the nature of the inciting agent, with the highest frequency of irreversibility in nonsteroidal antiinflammatory agent-associated disease, and with lesser frequency in ATIN due to antibiotics.

Tubulointerstitial Nephropathy with Crystal Deposits

Only disorders associated with pharmacologic agents are discussed in this section. Metabolic disorders such as oxalate nephropathy, and cystinosis are discussed in the chapter on metabolic diseases. Disorders associated with tubulointerstitial nephropathy, and crystal deposits are summarized in Table 11.4.

(Acute Calcium Phosphate Nephropathy Associated with Oral Sodium Phosphate)

This is a recently described disorder defined by (i) acute and chronic tubulointerstitial injury with abundant calcium phosphate deposition; (ii) recent exposure to oral sodium phosphate as bowel-cleansing preparation for colonoscopy; (iii) acute renal failure; (iv) absence of hypercalcemia; (v) no other significant renal disease [35]. Biopsy findings indicate nephrocalcinosis, characterized by calcium phosphate, or hydroxyl-apatite concretions in tubular epithelium, lumens, basement membranes, and interstitium. The resultant nephropathy has tubular injury, tubular atrophy, and interstitial fibrosis.

Epidemiology and Clinical Presentation. The proportion of patients undergoing colonoscopy who develop this disorder is unknown. The largest series includes twenty-one patients identified in a single center from a series of 7,349 biopsies (0.3 percent) [35]. Most of the affected patients were Caucasian females with a mean age of 64 years. Most had a history of hypertension, treated with angiotensin converting enzyme inhibitors, or angiotensin receptor blockers. Clinically, these patients present with acute renal failure within days, weeks, or months after colonoscopy, and give a history of exposure to oral sodium phosphate solution, or a tablet form of this compound. There may be mild proteinuria (mean 24-hour protein 256 mg), and urinalysis reveals a bland sediment. These patients are, by definition, normocalcemic. There may be demonstrable hyperphosphatemia in the early acute stages of the disease.

Approach to Interpretation. The early changes include ATN with diffuse calcium phosphate deposits. Tubular injury affects all tubular segments. Von Kossa-positive calcium phosphate deposits are evident in the tubules, with lesser amounts in the interstitium (Figures 11.17A,B). The calcium phosphate concretions are observed in distal tubules and collecting ducts, and in the medullary tubular segments. Later stages of the disease have persistent acute tubular injury and, in addition, progressive tubular atrophy with interstitial fibrosis. Extensive calcium phosphate deposits persist. Mononuclear infiltrates are absent in the early stages, and tend to be mild to moderate, and localized to the scarred parenchyma in the later stages. Tubulitis is not prominent. Vessels and glomeruli have features of arterionephrosclerosis. IF is nonspecific. EM reveals laminated concretions in

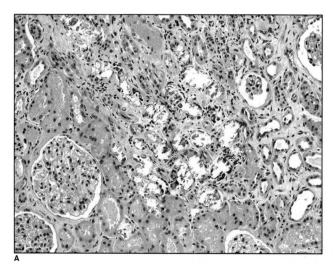
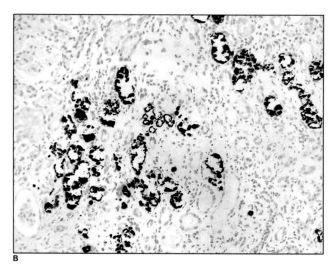

A   B

FIGURE 11.17:   A.Oral sodium phosphate nephropathy with extensive tubular calcium phosphate deposits, tubular injury, and focal interstitial fibrosis (H&E, 200×). B. Von Kossa stain demonstrating calcium phosphate deposits (200×). (Courtesy of Dr. Glen Markowitz, MD, Columbia University, New York,).

intratubular, intraepithelial and interstitial locations, and severe epithelial cell injury.

Differential Diagnosis. The differential diagnosis of nephrocalcinosis includes hypercalciuria, hyperparathyroidism, hypercalcemia of malignancy, sarcoidosis, vitamin D toxicity, and distal renal tubular acidosis. Medullary nephrocalcinosis has been described in long-term furosemide abuse [36], and in analgesic nephropathy [37].

Clinical Course and Prognosis. Acute renal failure is immediate, but detection may be delayed. Some patients have latency periods of weeks to months before the detection of renal failure, depending on when interval tests of renal function are performed. Patients presenting early with acute renal failure may benefit from hemodialysis to reduce hyperphosphatemia. Nineteen percent of the patients developed end-stage renal failure, and the remaining 81 percent of patients developed persistent elevation of the serum creatinine [35]. None had a return of serum creatinine to baseline levels.

(Other Pharmacologic Agents Associated with Crystal Deposition)

Sulfadiazine

This is a sulfonamide used as first-line treatment of central nervous system (CNS) toxoplasmosis in patients with HIV infection. It is one of the first agents known to cause crystal nephropathy.

Epidemiology and Clinical Presentation. Acute renal failure occurs in 1–29 percent of patients receiving this agent [5,38]. Isolated crystalluria has been described in up to 45 percent of patients with HIV. Most patients are asymptomatic, but some complain of back, flank, or abdominal discomfort. There is typically an oliguric acute renal failure. The urinary sediment typically reveals variably sized and shaped (needle-like, dumb-bell, rounded, and rhomboid), birefringent crystals, distributed singly, in rosette-like clusters, or in larger clusters resembling sheaves of wheat, and often admixed with erythrocytes.

Approach to Interpretation. Gross findings are not described. Microscopically, there is crystal deposition in the distal nephron, typically in the collecting ducts. Crystals may be admixed with tubular protein, or cellular debris. The tubules may have features of ATN, with obstructive ectasia. There may also be acute interstitial nephritis often with eosinophils and occasionally with granulomas. Lithiasis may be observed in the calyces.

Differential Diagnosis. Other crystal nephropathies including gout and antiviral agent-associated nephropathies have to be excluded with the help of clinical correlation. Definitive identification of crystals may require spectroscopic analysis.

Pathogenesis. Most sulfadiazine (66 percent) is excreted in the urine as the parent compound, and as acetylsulfadiazine metabolite. Sulfadiazine is weakly acidic and relatively insoluble in acidic urine, with a tendency to precipitate when the urinary pH falls below 5.5. Precipitation is observed in the collecting ducts. High doses of the agent, over 4 g per day, increase the likelihood of precipitation.

Clinical Course and Prognosis. The removal of the offending agent, hydration, urinary alkalinization using sodium bicarbonate, all help to ensure solubilization of crystals and recovery of renal function.

Antiviral agents

Acyclovir and indinavir are agents used in the treatment of various viral infections, and each has been linked to the development of renal dysfunction. Crystal deposition in the renal tubules causes intrarenal tubular obstruction, and acute renal

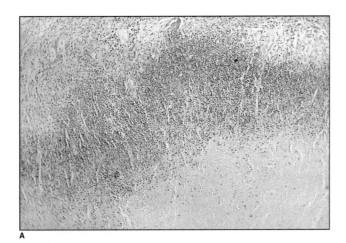

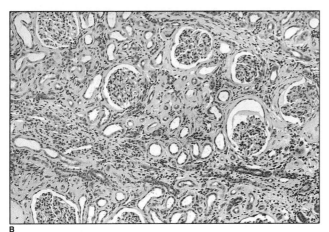

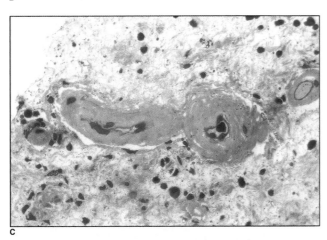

FIGURE 11.18: *A.Papillary necrosis with viable parenchyma and neutrophil rich infiltrates at the junction of viable and necrotic tissue (H&E, 100×). B. Chronic interstitial nephritis associated with papillary necrosis (H&E, 200×). C. Capillary sclerosis in renal pelvis (toluidine blue, 400×). (Courtesy of Dr. Cyril Abrahams, MD, University of Chicago, Chicago, IL).*

failure. Most of these agents have limited solubility in urine at physiologic pH. Underlying renal disease, dehydration, and the use of high doses of the specific agents appear to be the important risk factors.

Epidemiology and Clinical Features. The incidence of acyclovir-associated renal failure is 12–48 percent after rapid intravenous bolus administration [5,38]. The use of slower administration has decreased the frequency of this complication. Acute and subacute renal failure are the predominant modes of clinical presentation. The urinalysis reveals polarizable crystals.

Approach to Interpretation. The gross features are not described. Histologically, there may be ATN or interstitial nephritis with mononuclear cells and noncaseating granulomas. Specific features associated with these agents are based on anecdotal evidence. Acyclovir is associated with deposition of birefringent crystalline material in collecting ducts. Indinavir has been associated with accumulation of needle-like, fan-shaped, and plate-like clusters of nonpolarizable crystals, residing in the cytoplasm of macrophages, in cortical and medullary collecting duct lumens [39]. There may be lithiasis with indinavir sulfate stones with or without calcium phosphate. The renal parenchyma may have severe interstitial fibrosis and tubular atrophy.

Clinical Course and Prognosis. Acyclovir toxicity is associated with complete recovery of the renal function in 38–50 percent of cases on withdrawal of the agent with appropriate hydration. Indinavir toxicity may be associated with chronic renal impairment.

Chronic Tubulointerstitial Nephritis

This is chronic tubulointerstitial inflammation with fibrosis often attributable to specific agents that includes analgesic nephropathy and lithium nephropathy. Heavy metal-associated chronic TIN is considered under toxic ATN. Other rare disorders, such as Balkan nephropathy (possibly associated with ochratoxin A), and Chinese herbs (aristolochic acid) nephropathy, are not discussed in detail.

(Analgesic Nephropathy)

This is an increasingly uncommon disorder characterized pathologically by bilateral renal papillary necrosis, chronic interstitial nephritis with cortical atrophy, capillary sclerosis of the renal medulla and urothelium, and clinically by a history of the use of phenacetin containing analgesic agents.

Epidemiology and Clinical Features. This disorder has been estimated to account for 20–25 percent of cases of end-stage renal failure in the European and Australian studies in 1980 [37]. Autopsy studies had a frequency of analgesic nephropathy of 4 percent in 1980. A ban on the sales of phenacetin in many countries has greatly reduced the frequency of this disorder to 0.2 percent in autopsies in 2000 in one study [40]. U.S. Renal Data Systems data for 2003 indicate that analgesic nephropathy accounted for 0.2 percent of cases of end-stage renal failure in the United States. The clinical features include nocturia and polyuria because of a loss of the concentrating ability, with chronic renal failure. Classical analgesic nephropathy is infrequently seen nowadays probably because of the withdrawal of phenacetin from the market; however, other analgesic agents

Table 11.5 Causes of Renal Medullary Papillary Necrosis

Diabetic nephropathy
Acute obstructive pyelonephritis
Fungal infection – candidiasis, aspergillosis, mucormycosis
Nonsteroidal antiinflammatory agent nephropathy
Analgesic (phenacetin) nephropathy
Sickle cell nephropathy
Renal vein thrombosis
Vasculitis – Wegener's granulomatosis, microscopic polyangiitis

(e.g., NSAID) most likely aggravate the underlying renal injury, and cause progressive renal insufficiency.

Approach to Interpretation. The gross examination, in the early phases of disease, reveals only yellow-white papillary streaks. In the advanced stages, the kidneys have bilateral shrinkage with retracted surface scars, and cortical atrophy over necrotic papillae. All papillae tend to have focal or diffuse softening and brown discoloration. In advanced necrosis, there may be complete detachment of the papillae imparting a concave appearance to the remaining medullary surface. The mucosal surface of the pelvis and calyces may have brown discoloration.

Light microscopy reveals medullary coagulation necrosis (Figure 11.18A) that may involve the entire pyramid, or more frequently focal necrosis involving the papillary tip, or central portion of the papilla. The necrotic areas may have dystrophic calcification, and less frequently ossification. The overlying cortex has tubulointerstitial mononuclear inflammation with lymphoid cells and plasma cells, interstitial fibrosis, and tubular atrophy (Figure 11.18B). These cortical changes probably arise secondary to papillary necrosis. Medullary, pelvicaliceal, and ureteral capillary sclerosis is also an important diagnostic finding (Figure 11.18C). This lesion is characterized by marked thickening of the capillary basement membranes by PAS-positive material, and is the earliest recognizable lesion in this disorder. IF reveals nonspecific findings only. EM reveals multilayering of the basal lamina of capillary walls in the medulla and pelvis.

Differential Diagnosis. The other causes of papillary necrosis have to be excluded, including diabetic nephropathy, acute pyelonephritis, sickle cell nephropathy, and nonsteroidal antiinflammatory agent-associated disease (Table 11.5). Less common causes of papillary necrosis include renal vein thrombosis, which may have hemorrhagic necrosis: Wegener's granulomatosis, with necrotizing glomerulonephritis and medullary vasculitis; and fungal infections attributable to candidiasis [41], aspergillosis, and mucormycosis. Fungal organisms are identifiable using the Gomori methenamine silver stain. Capillary sclerosis may be a feature of analgesic nephropathy and diabetic nephropathy; however, other features of diabetic nephropathy such as mesangial sclerosis, glomerular capillary basement membrane thickening, and hyaline arteriolosclerosis should be evident, in the correct clinical context, to attribute changes to diabetic nephropathy. An acute tubulointerstitial inflammation with neutrophil-casts raises the possibility of acute pyelonephritis. Sickled erythrocytes in vasa recta, tubular hemosiderosis,

and glomerular capillary double contours suggest sickle-cell nephropathy.

Etiology and Pathogenesis. Epidemiologic observations support a link between the use of mixed analgesic compounds containing phenacetin, paracetamol, codeine, and caffeine, or combinations of these ingredients in the pathogenesis of analgesic nephropathy. The removal of phenacetin from the market has been associated with a decrease in the incidence of analgesic nephropathy despite the availability of other mixed compounds. There is an argument in favor of a central role for phenacetin or its metabolites in this disease. Toxic injury of capillary walls in the medulla and lamina propria of urothelial lined structures by phenacetin or its metabolites is thought to be an important early step in the pathogenesis of papillary necrosis. Necrosis of the medulla is initially focal and may become diffuse with eventual detachment of the papilla. Chronic TIN develops secondary to papillary necrosis.

Clinical Course and Prognosis. A cessation of analgesic abuse may allow long-term renal survival with an impaired function. There is an increased frequency of urothelial carcinoma and of renal cell carcinoma in this patient population. The detachment of papillae may result in obstruction with hydronephrosis.

(Lithium Nephropathy)

Lithium chloride is an agent used for the treatment of bipolar disorder. An acute lithium intoxication is associated with acute renal failure. The prolonged use of this agent is associated with the impairment of urinary concentrating ability, nephrogenic diabetes insipidus, and TIN with chronic renal failure.

Epidemiology and Clinical Presentation. Approximately 20 percent of patients on long-term lithium therapy have polyuria. Other manifestations include reversible concentrating defects, distal renal tubular acidosis, nephrotic syndrome, and chronic renal failure [42]. The true incidence of lithium nephropathy is unknown.

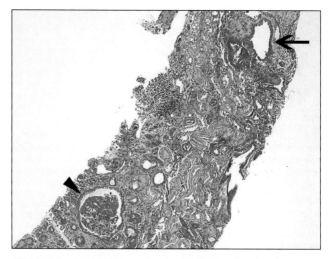

FIGURE 11.19: *Lithium nephropathy with collecting duct cysts (one highlighted by arrow), interstitial scarring, mononuclear infiltrates, and FSGS (arrowhead) (PAS, 100×).*

Approach to Interpretation. The kidneys are grossly shrunken with cortical microcysts visible on the cut surface. Microscopically, the glycogen accumulation in distal tubules and collecting ducts may be observed days after the initiation of lithium therapy [43]. Later, there is focal interstitial fibrosis with tubular atrophy, and scant mononuclear inflammatory infiltrates. Characteristically, there is ectasia of the distal tubule and cortical collecting duct segments (Figure 11.19). Up to 50 percent of biopsies have focal segmental glomerulosclerosis (Figure 11.19) [44]. Minimal-change disease has also been reported in the setting of lithium therapy. Biopsies obtained in the setting of acute renal failure may reveal ATN [45]. IF studies are nonspecific. EM confirms distal tubular and collecting-duct epithelial glycogen deposits. Podocytopathy of minimal-change disease and focal segmental glomerulosclerosis may also be identified by EM.

Differential Diagnosis. Distal tubular and collecting ductal ectasia with interstitial fibrosis are nonspecific features of renal scarring. PAS-positive glycogen deposits in ectatic tubules are said to be specific for lithium-induced disease.

Etiology and Pathogenesis. Lithium induces downregulation of the aquaporin-2 water channel on principal cells of the cortical collecting ducts. This downregulation is a possible explanation for polyuria and diabetes insipidus. The mechanisms of the development of glycogen accumulation and ductal ectasia are unknown.

Clinical Course and Prognosis. Chronic TIN is an irreversible lesion that does not regress after the cessation of lithium therapy. In one recent series, 29.2 percent of the patients progressed to end-stage failure despite cessation of therapy, after a mean duration of 13.6 years [44].

(Chronic Tubulointerstitial Nephritis from Other Causes)

ATIN from drug-induced and other causes is not always reversible, especially in the case of nonsteroidal antiinflammatory agents. Reversibility is often related to the duration of the exposure to the injurious agent. Epstein–Barr virus infection of proximal tubules has recently been suggested in idiopathic chronic interstitial nephritis [46], although this association is not proven. Balkan endemic nephropathy is an uncommon disorder with geographic distribution largely confined to the Balkan states. Histologically, the disorder is characterized by interstitial fibrosis with tubular atrophy affecting the outer cortex predominantly. The inciting agent is unclear and a role for ochratoxin A or other mycotoxins has been suggested. These patients have an increased risk of urothelial carcinoma. Chinese herbs nephropathy (more appropriately called aristolochic acid nephropathy [47]) is a cause of rapidly progressive renal failure, and Fanconi syndrome. Pathologically, the kidneys are asymmetrically shrunken, and there is marked interstitial fibrosis, and tubular atrophy most prominent in the outer cortex (Figure 11.20). Aristolochic acid is thought to be the inciting agent, and these patients are at increased risk of urothelial carcinoma. Drugs and toxic agents such as cisplatin, cyclosporin, nitrosoureas, and heavy metals may be associated with chronic interstitial nephritis.

Systemic karyomegaly with chronic TIN has been described in small case series [8,48]. Clinically, there is chronic renal failure, mild proteinuria, microscopic hematuria, and in many instances, abnormal hepatic transaminases, arising in patients in the third or fourth decades of life (range 9–51 years old). Histologically, there is mononuclear infiltration by lymphocytes, plasma cells and macrophages, with interstitial fibrosis and tubular atrophy. Characteristically, the proximal tubular epithelium has enlarged, pleomorphic, hyperchromatic nuclei (Figure 11.21). Distal tubular epithelium, atrophic tubular segments, glomeruli, vascular endothelium, smooth muscle, and interstitial cells may have similar atypical nuclei. Mesenchymal cells of other organs such as the liver, lungs, and rectum may have similar nuclear changes. Evidence of viral infection has not been observed. High DNA ploidy values are evident in affected cells [48]. The renal dysfunction is irreversible.

Hereditary disorders such as autosomal recessive, familial hypokalemic nephropathy [49,50] or nephropathy associated with

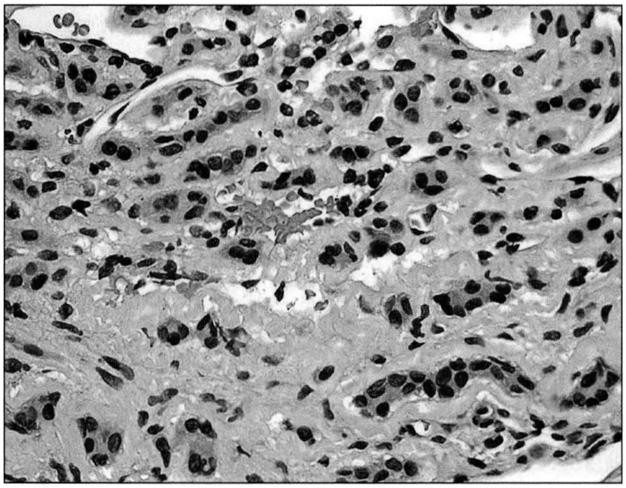

FIGURE 11.20: *Chinese herbs nephropathy with diffuse interstitial fibrosis and severe tubular atrophy with no inflammatory infiltrate (H&E, 400×).*

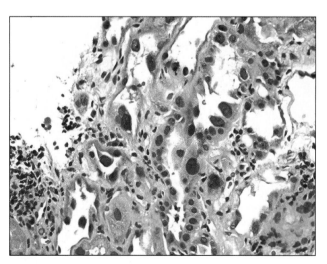

FIGURE 11.21: *Karyomegalic interstitial nephritis with enlarged hyperchromatic tubular epithelial nuclei (H&E, 400×).*

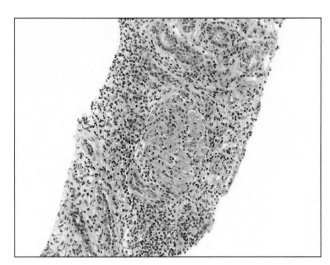

FIGURE 11.22: *Interstitial nephritis with a nonnecrotizing granuloma attributable to sarcoidosis (H&E, 100×).*

mitochondrial DNA abnormalities [51,52] have nonspecific chronic TIN by light and IF microscopy. Ultrastructurally, hypokalemic nephropathy may have mitochondrial enlargement with electron-dense inclusions. In nephropathy associated with mitochondrial DNA abnormalities, the mitochondria are large and dysmorphic, with stacked parallel crista in some instances [53]. These findings are suggestive of these disorders, but are not diagnostic. Metabolic disorders such as cystinosis, hyperuricemia, and hyperoxaluria are also causes of chronic interstitial nephritis; however, these disorders are discussed in a separate chapter.

Granulomatous Tubulointerstitial Nephritis

This is defined by the presence of clustered epithelioid macrophages in the interstitium in the absence of glomerulonephritis. Many different etiologic agents give rise to this pattern of injury [54]. Lesions range from subtle interstitial microscopic granulomas to large confluent masses of macrophages in malakoplakia, and of foam cells in xanthogranulomatous pyelonephritis.

Epidemiology and Clinical Presentation

Large biopsy series cite a frequency of granulomatous inflammation in 5.9–6.7 percent of all renal biopsies [54,55]. Clinically, there is an acute or subacute renal failure.

Approach to Interpretation

Grossly, there may be diffuse enlargement with an increase in kidney weight and visible nodules on the cut surface. Microscopically, there is a range of appearances from a few focal, circumscribed, clusters of epithelioid macrophages, less than the size of a glomerulus (Figure 11.22), to large confluent masses of these cells obliterating the renal parenchyma. There is typically an accompanying infiltrate of lymphocytes and plasma cells with or without eosinophils. Multinucleated giant cells are nonspecific, and are frequently observed. Granulomas may have central necrosis. Tubules have epithelial injury, tubu-

litis, and rupture of the basement membrane. Granulomas may be tubulocentric, and associated with tubular rupture. In isolation, this may be an entirely nonspecific phenomenon, but such changes can be observed in conjunction with viral or bacterial infection, and in drug-induced interstitial nephritis. The glomeruli and blood vessels are unremarkable. Special stains for microorganisms and urinary culture are essential for identification of infectious agents. IF is nonspecific. EM may help in the identification of infectious microorganisms.

Differential Diagnosis

Table 11.6 provides a list of broad categories of diseases associated with granulomatous interstitial nephritis in the absence of glomerulonephritis or vasculitis. Granulomas in sarcoidosis tend to be well formed, discrete, and nonnecrotizing (Figure 11.22), with numerous giant cells, in contrast to drug-induced granulomas, which tend to be poorly formed (Figure 11.15C) in many instances [56], but with a few exceptions [57]. Infectious agents may be occasionally identified on special stains and, more importantly, by culture of the urine or blood. Macrophages in confluent sheets with eosinophilic cytoplasm suggest malakoplakia. Von Kossa stain for calcium phosphate, and PAS stains are helpful in identifying Michaelis–Gutmann bodies, and cytoplasmic granules stain for PAS in malakoplakia. Other special stains may be needed to detect microorganisms. Severe crescentic glomerulonephritis and necrotizing vasculitis should be carefully excluded. If no underlying etiology is identified, lesions are classified as idiopathic granulomatous TIN [58].

Etiology and Pathogenesis

A hypersensitivity reaction is suggested by a latency of days to months after an initial exposure to the inciting agent, coexistence of fever, arthralgia and rash, and interstitial granulomas. Immunophenotyping of the infiltrating cell populations reveals CD4- positive T cells, and CD68-positive macrophages consistent with a delayed type hypersensitivity reaction.

Clinical Course and Prognosis

Since this category of disease is a heterogenous group of disorders, a typical course of disease cannot be prescribed. Prognosis depends on the removal of the offending agent, and the degree of tubulointerstitial scarring evident in the biopsy. In an unselected series [55] of twenty-four patients with tubulointerstitial granulomatous inflammation, only five of nine patients with drug-induced lesions demonstrated return of the serum creatinine to baseline, in twenty to sixty days after the cessation of the offending agent. The remaining drug-induced lesions and lesions associated with sarcoidosis, tuberculosis, and idiopathic disease had persistent chronic renal dysfunction. In another study, granulomatous inflammation was a predictor of irreversible renal dysfunction [34].

Granulomatous Tubulointerstitial Nephritis
Associated with Mycobacterium tuberculosis

TIN develops as a result of a direct renal infection by *M. tuberculosis*. There are two principal types of renal tuberculosis:

Table 11.6 Causes of Granulomatous Interstitial Nephritis

Infection
Mycobacteria
Brucella
Histoplasma
Candida
Polyoma virus
Adenovirus

Drug hypersensitivity
Antibiotics – ampicillin, methicillin, vancomycin, sulfonamides,
  rifampicin, ciprofloxacin
Diuretics – thiazides, triamterene
Antiinflammatory agents – indomethacin, ketoprofen, fenoprofen
Other agents – acyclovir, allopurinol, captopril

Foreign body reactions
Tubular rupture
Gout
Calcium oxalate – enteric hyperoxaluria
Intravenous drug abuse

Sarcoidosis

Immune mediated disease – TIN with uveitis syndrome (Dobrin),
  anti-TBM disease

Primary unclassified (idiopathic)

(i) cavitary – arising as a late manifestation of prior infection of the lung or gastrointestinal tract and (ii) miliary tuberculosis.

Epidemiology and Clinical Presentation

Renal involvement by tuberculosis is now rare in developed countries; however, it remains a problem in developing countries. Approximately 5 percent of the patients with tuberculosis have clinical involvement of the kidneys [59]. The interval between the primary infection and manifestations of renal disease is typically 15–25 years. In reactivation infection, the interval is shorter, typically 4–8 years [59]. Most patients have dysuria, flank pain, nocturia, hematuria, and pyuria. A minority has fever, night sweats, weight loss, anorexia, and evidence of pulmonary disease. About 25 percent of patients are asymptomatic. Repeated culture of early morning urine specimens may be necessary for identification of organisms because bacilluria tends to be intermittent. Urinary PCR using mycobacterial probes may be a more sensitive method of detection. Intravenous pyelography identifies cavitary, destructive lesions in later stages of disease.

Approach to Interpretation

A gross examination may reveal multiple firm nodules with central softening measuring 0.5–2.0 cm, and distributed in the cortex and medulla. A progressive enlargement may result in cavitary masses replacing the parenchyma (Figure 11.23). At autopsy, 75 percent of patients have bilateral involvement. The calyces, pelvis, and ureter may have mural thickening with multiple, circumscribed, surface nodules. Miliary tuberculosis

Table 11.7: TIN with Immune Complex Deposits

Without glomerulopathy
Idiopathic hypocomplementemic interstitial nephritis
IgG4 TIN with autoimmune pancreatitis
Polyoma virus nephropathy (transplant kidney)
Sjogren syndrome
Rarely – SLE

With glomerulopathy
SLE
Sjogren syndrome
Cryoglobulinemia – mixed
Hepatitis B (membranous nephropathy)
Syphilis
Nonsteroidal antiinflammatory agents (glomerulopathy may be
  absent)
Childhood membranous nephropathy with tubulointerstitial
  deposits
Idiopathic

---

has bilateral diffuse yellow-tan 0.1–0.2 cm nodules, or tubercules, distributed predominantly in the cortex. Granulomas with caseous necrosis are characteristic. These are typically admixed with noncaseous lesions. Granulomas may be glomerulocentric or tubulocentric [60]. Mononuclear inflammatory infiltrates composed of lymphocytes, plasma cells, and macrophages, with interstitial fibrosis, and tubular atrophy are also evident. Ziehl-Neelsen or auramine rhodamine stains may detect the organisms in necrotic zones of granulomas in kidney tissue. Granulomas may heal giving rise to circumscribed, fibrous nodules often with focal calcification [60].

Differential Diagnosis

Disorders included in the differential diagnosis are listed in Table 11.6. Demonstration of mycobacteria by special stains, culture or PCR, establishes the diagnosis. Other mycobacteria can also cause renal infection, including *Mycobacterium bovis*, *Mycobacterium kansasii*, *Mycobacterium avium-intracellulare*, and *Mycobacterium leprae*.

Etiology and Pathogenesis

Mycobacteria incite immune reactions that are prototypical delayed-type hypersensitivity reactions. Organisms reach the kidney by hematogenous spread from the primary source of infection. The establishment of infection leads to granuloma formation, and these are often localized to glomeruli. Organisms may remain dormant in these foci for years. If there is severe local inflammation, there may be rupture of glomerular capillaries with spread to Bowman's space, and thereafter to the tubules where a nidus of infection may be established in loops of Henle with localized granuloma formation.

Clinical Course and Prognosis

Complications include secondary bacterial infection (12–50 percent) [61], nephrolithiasis (7–18 percent) [62], and hypertension.

Standard treatment is triple therapy with isoniazid, rifampicin, and ethambutol. Increasingly, resistant mycobacteria are encountered. Without treatment, renal tuberculosis has a high mortality (50–85 percent).

Tubulointerstitial Nephritis Associated with Immune Disorders

This is a heterogenous group of uncommon disorders associated with either immune deposits in the tubular basement membranes and in the interstitium [some SS, SLE, idiopathic hypocomplementemic interstitial nephritis (HIN), and anti-TBM disease], or with cell-mediated mechanisms (most SS and TINU). Mixed cryoglobulinemia may also have tubulointerstitial immune deposits; however, glomerulonephritis is invariably also present.

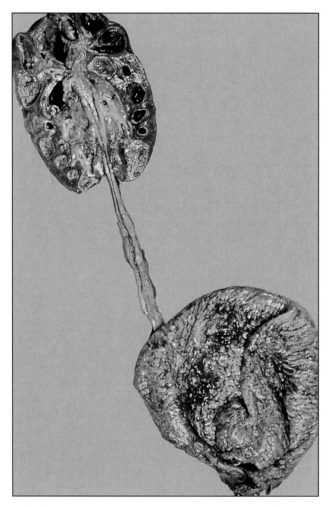

FIGURE 11.23: *Urinary tract infection by Mycobacterium tuberculosis with involvement of the renal parenchyma by cavitary nodules and with marked nodularity of the bladder mucosa. (Courtesy of Dr Jenö Ormos, MD, Szent-Gyorgi Albert Medical University, Szeged, Hungary).*

Epidemiology and Clinical Presentation

Approximately, one-third of patients with SS have renal disease. Renal involvement in SS includes the following: renal tubular acidosis with nephrocalcinosis, nephrogenic diabetes insipidus, Fanconi syndrome, interstitial nephritis, and glomerulonephritis. Idiopathic HIN is a disorder characterized by TIN with extensive tubulointerstitial immune deposits, and hypocomplementemia, of which there are eleven reported cases [63,64]. Antitubular basement membrane disease (ATBMD) is a rare disorder characterized by (1) primary TIN; (2) linear tubular basement membrane staining for IgG and C3, with absence of immune deposits by EM; (3) circulating antitubular basement membrane antibodies, or detectable antitubular basement membrane antibodies in eluates of renal tissues. Antibody reactivity can be detected by indirect IF using the patient's serum. Secondary forms of ATBMD are also recognized. Clinically, there may be chronic renal insufficiency, with mild proteinuria, impaired concentrating ability, Fanconi syndrome, and renal tubular acidosis. Serum complement components C3 and C4 are reduced in HIN. TINU (Dobrin syndrome [29]) is a disorder almost exclusively identified in young women characterized by TIN with eosinophils and granulomas, bone marrow granulomas, and uveitis. Autoimmune/sclerosing pancreatitis with TIN has been observed predominately in males, in the seventh decade, associated with mild chronic renal failure, increased serum IgG4 levels, tissue infiltration by IgG4 containing plasma cells [65–67], and possibly circulating autoantibodies to carbonic anhydrase II [68].

Approach to Interpretation

In the early phases of disease, the kidneys may be enlarged, and with progressive scarring, the kidneys become small and firm. Microscopically, there is interstitial mononuclear inflammation that contains lymphoid cells, plasma cells, and macrophages, with or without eosinophils (Figures 11.24 and 11.25A). Tubulitis may be prominent (Figure 11.25B). SS and HIN may have

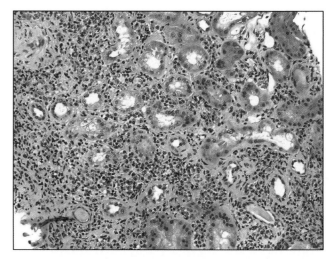

FIGURE 11.24: *SS interstitial nephritis with extensive plasma cell and lymphoid infiltrates, and mild interstitial fibrosis (H&E, 200×).*

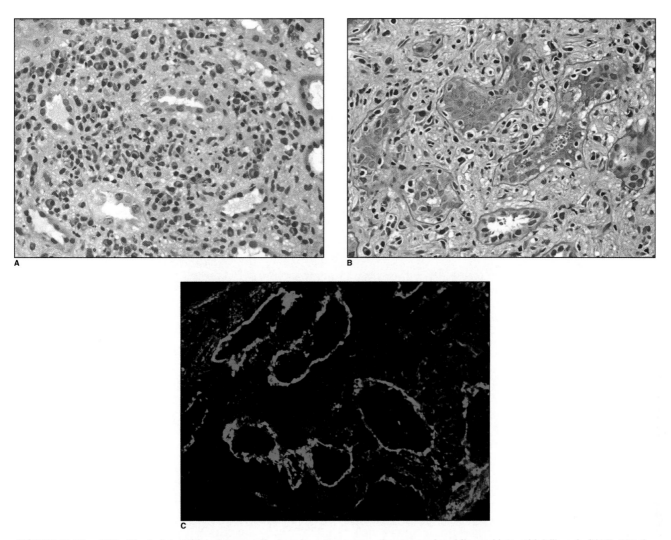

FIGURE 11.25: *HIN with: A. Interstitial plasma cells, lymphocytes, macrophages, eosinophils, and interstitial fibrosis (H&E, 400×).*
B. HIN with tubulitis and interstitial fibrosis (PAS, 400×). C. Direct IF revealed IgG along tubular basement membranes (400×).

atypical lymphoid cells with enlarged centrocytoid blastic nuclei, described as atypical lymphoid infiltrates or pseudolymphoma. Immunophenotyping reveals a preponderance of plasma cells and B cells, with abundant T cells, in SS and in HIN. Tubular atrophy is prominent, and may be associated with thickened hyalinized basement membranes in HIN [64]. In contrast, in ATBMD, mononuclear infiltrates have an abundance of macrophages and multinucleated giant cells, with lesser populations of lymphoid cells, eosinophils, and neutrophils. TINU is indistinguishable histologically from other forms of ATIN. Interstitial fibrosis and tubular atrophy is variable in these disorders. Glomeruli and blood vessels are unremarkable. IF reveals granular, and rarely linear, deposits of IgG and C3 along the tubular basement membranes in SS and HIN (Figure 11.25C). EM reveals granular immune deposits along the tubular basement membranes (Figure 11.25D). Deposits in the tubular basement membranes may have organized substructure in SS and HIN. ATBMD has band-like

linear deposits containing IgG, and usually C3, along the TBM [69,70,71]. IF studies are nonspecific in TINU.

Differential Diagnosis

Interstitial nephritis with atypical lymphoid infiltrates needs to be reliably distinguished from lymphoma. The finding of granular or linear, tubular, basement-membrane-immune deposits by IF in the absence of glomerulopathy, narrows the differential diagnosis of inflammatory disorders to SLE, idiopathic HIN, TIN with IgG4 deposits and autoimmune pancreatitis, and anti-TBM disease. SLE typically has immune deposits in glomeruli and peritubular capillaries in addition to tubular basement membranes and interstitium. Isolated tubulointerstitial inflammation with immune deposits in SLE, is very rare. TIN with autoimmune pancreatitis has IgG4 deposits along the tubular basement membrane, and cytoplasmic IgG4 in infiltrating plasma cells [65,66]. Band-like replacement of tubular basement membranes by electron-dense material, containing C3 alone, is observed in

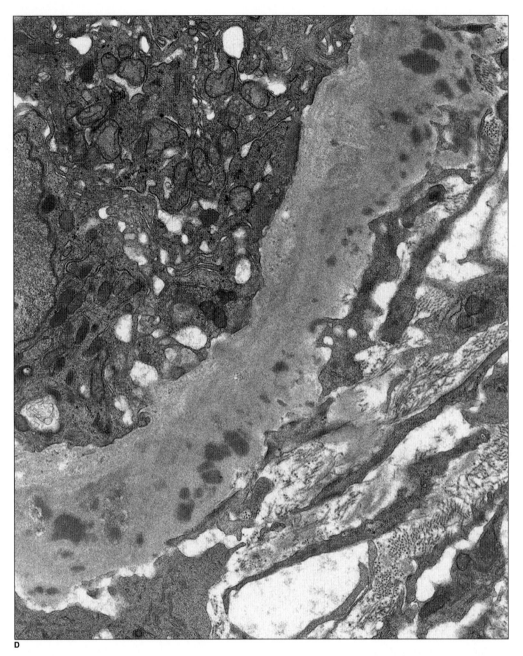

FIGURE 11.25: *D. Electron-dense deposits along thickened basement membranes (uranyl acetate, lead citrate, 17186×).*

dense-deposit disease. Fluffy dense deposits in a band-like pattern along the tubular (and glomerular) basement membranes, containing monotypic light chains, are observed in light chain deposition disease. Secondary ATBMD may be observed in anti-GBM disease with linear staining for IgG along the glomerular basement membranes. Anti-TBM antibodies have also been observed in membranous nephropathy in children [70–72], methicillin-associated TIN, lupus nephritis, poststreptococcal glomerulonephritis, and in renal allografts. Linear staining of the glomerular and tubular basement membranes for IgG may be observed in many proteinuric states and in diabetic nephropathy; however, a similar pattern of staining is observed for albu-

min in these circumstances. Granular C3 deposition may be observed along tubular basement membranes as a nonspecific finding, typically in atrophic tubular segments. Atrophic tubules may have electron-dense material embedded within the basement membrane by EM. Careful inspection reveals variable microspherical and lamellar membranous structures, which should not be mistaken for immune complex deposits.

Etiology and Pathogenesis

The etiology of these immune disorders is unknown. Three autoantigens of 48–70 kD, have been identified from collagenase digests of human TBMs, and are believed to be important in the pathogenesis of ATBMD. These antigens are distributed along the proximal tubules and Bowman's capsule. Immune complex accumulation in the tubules or interstitium may trigger local inflammation with tubular injury and cellular infiltration. Persistence of immune complex deposits is associated with persistent inflammation and scar development. Removal of the inciting antigen(s) is critical to resolution of TIN.

Clinical Course and Prognosis

Patients with renal involvement by immune-mediated TIN may benefit from treatment with prednisone. Many patients have persistent chronic renal failure and progress to end-stage renal disease.

REFERENCES

1. Lamiere N, Van Biesen W, Vanholder R. Acute renal failure. *Lancet* 2005; 365: 417–30.
2. Solez K, Morel-Maroger L, Sraer JD. The morphology of "acute tubular necrosis" in man: analysis of 57 renal biopsies and a comparison with the glycerol model. *Medicine (Baltimore)* 1979; 58: 362–76.
3. Zhang PL, Lin F, Han WK, Blasik TM, Bonventre JV. Kidney injury molecule-1 is a specific biomarker, which enables diagnosis of premortem acute tubular necrosis in the presence of autolytic artefacts in cadaver kidneys. *Mod Pathol* 2007; 20; 10A.
4. Izzedine H, Launay-Vacher V, Deray G. Antiviral drug-induced nephrotoxicity. *Am J Kidney Dis* 2005; 45: 804–17.
5. Markowitz GS, Perazella MA. Drug-induced renal failure: a focus on tubulointerstitial disease. *Clin Chim Acta* 2005; 351: 31–47.
6. Solez K. Pathogenesis of acute renal failure. *Int Rev Exp Pathol* 1983; 24: 277–328.
7. Levy EM, Viscoli CM, Horwitz RI. The effect of acute renal failure on mortality. *JAMA* 1996; 275: 1489–94.
8. Mihatsch MJ, Gudat F, Zollinger HU, Heierli C, Reutter FW. Systemic karyomegaly associated with chronic interstitial nephritis. A new disease entity? *Clin Nephrol* 1979; 12: 54–62.
9. Nadasdy T, Laszik Z, Blick KE, Johnson DL, Silva FG. Tubular atrophy in the end-stage kidney. *Hum Pathol* 1994; 25: 22–8.
10. Raghavan R, Date A, Bhaktaviziam A. Fungal and nocardial infections of the kidney. *Histopathology* 1987; 11: 9–20.
11. Ramsay AG, Olesnicky L, Pirani CL. Acute tubulointerstitial nephritis from Candida albicans with oliguric renal failure. *Clin Nephrol* 1985; 24: 310–14.
12. Kim S, Kang ET, Kim YG, Han JS, Lee JS, Kim YI, Hall WC, Dalrymple JM, Peters CJ. Localization of Hantaan viral envelope glycoproteins by monoclonal antibodies in renal tissues from patients with Korean hemorrhagic fever H. *Am J Clin Pathol* 1993; 100: 398–403.
13. Farmer ER, Heptinstall RH. Chronic nonobstructive pyelonephritis – a reappraisal. In: Kincaid-Smith P, Fairley KF, eds. *Renal infection and renal scarring*. Melbourne: Mercedes Publishing; 1971, pp. 233–6.
14. Hodson CJ, Wilson S. Natural history of chronic pyelonephritis scarring. *Br Med J* 1965; 2: 191–4.
15. Parsons MA, Harris SC, Longstaff AJ, Grainger RG. Xanthogranulomatous pyelonephritis: a pathological, clinical and aetiological analysis of 87 cases. *Diagn Histopathol* 1983; 6: 203–19.
16. Grainger RG, Longstaff AJ, Parsons MA. Xanthogranulomatous pyelonephritis: a reappraisal. *Lancet* 1982; 1:1398–401.
17. Khalyl-Mawad J, Greco A, Schinella RA. Ultrastructural demonstration of intracellular bacteria in xanthogranulomatous pyelonephritis. *Hum Pathol* 1982; 13: 41–7.
18. Cadnapaphornchai P, Rosenberg BF, Taher S, Prosnitz EH, McDonald FD. Bilateral renal parenchymal malakoplakia. *New Engl J Med* 1978; 299: 1110–13.
19. Dobyan DC, Truong LD, Eknoyan G. Renal malakoplakia reappraised. *Am J Kid Dis* 1993; 22: 243–52.
20. Tam VKK, Kung WH, Li R, Chan KW. Renal parenchymal malakoplakia: a rare cause of ARF with a review of the literature. *Am J Kidney Dis* 2003; 41: E21.
21. Pettersson E, Bonsdorff M, Tornroth T, Lindholm H. Nephritis among young Finnish men. *Clin Nephrol* 1984; 22: 217–22.
22. Alpers CE. The evolving contribution of renal pathology to understanding interstitial nephritis. *Renal Failure* 1998; 20: 763–71.
23. Laberke HG, Bohle A. Acute interstititial nephritis: correlations between clinical and morphological findings. *Clin Nephrol* 1980; 14; 263–73.
24. Baker RJ, Pusey CD. The changing profile of acute tubulointerstitial nephritis. *Nephrol Dial Transplant* 2004; 19: 8–11.
25. D'Agati VD, Theise ND, Pirani CL, Knowles DM, Appel GB. Interstitial nephritis related to nonsteroidal antiinflammatory agents and beta-lactam antibiotics: a comparative study of the interstitial infiltrates using monoclonal antibodies. *Mod Pathol* 1989; 2(4): 390–6.
26. Boucher A, Droz D, Adafer E, Noël LH. Characterization of mononuclear cell subsets in renal cellular interstitial infiltrates. *Kidney Int* 1986; 29: 1043–49.
27. Baldwin DS, Levine BB, McCluskey RT, Gallo GR. Renal failure and interstitial nephritis due to penicillin and methicillin. *New Engl J Med* 1968; 279: 1245–52.
28. Galpin JE, Shinaberger JH, Stanley TM, Blumenkrantz MJ, Bayer AS, Friedman GS, Montgomerie JZ, Guze LB, Coburn JW, Glassock RJ. Acute interstitial nephritis due to methicillin. *Am J Med* 1978; 65: 756–65.
29. Dobrin RS, Vernier RL, Fish AL. Acute eosinophilic interstitial nephritis with bone marrow-lymph node granulomas and anterior uveitis. *Am J Med* 1975; 59: 325–33.
30. Kobayashi Y, Honda M, Yoshikawa N, Ito H. Acute tubulointerstitial nephritis in 21 Japanese children. *Clin Nephrol* 2000; 54: 191–7.
31. Ellis D, Fried WA, Yunis EJ, Blau EB. Acute interstitial nephritis in children: a report of 13 cases and a review of the literature. *Pediatrics* 1981; 67: 861–70.
32. Cheng H_F, Nolasco F, Cameron JS, Hildreth G, Neild G, Hartley B. HLA DR display by renal tubular epithelium and phenotype of infiltrate in interstitial nephritis. *Nephrol Dial Transplant* 1989; 4: 205–15.

33. Rossert J. Drug-induced acute interstitial nephritis. *Kidney Int* 2001; 60: 804–17.

34. Schwarz A, Krause PH, Kunzendorf U, Keller F, Distler A. The outcome of acute interstitial nephritis: risk factors for the transition from acute to chronic interstitial nephritis. *Clin Nephrol* 2000; 54: 179–90.

35. Markowitz GS, Stokes MB, Radhakrishnan J, D'Agati VD. Acute phosphate nephropathy following oral sodium phosphate bowel purgative: an unrecognized cause of chronic renal failure. *J Am Soc Nephrol* 2005; 16: 3389–96.

36. Kim Y-G, Kim B, Kim M-K, Chung S-J, Han H-J, Ryu J-A, Lee Y-H, Lee K-B, Lee JY, Huh W, Oh H-Y. Medullary nephrocalcinosis associated with long-term furosemide abuse in adults. *Nephrol Dial Transplant* 2001; 16: 2303–9.

37. Brunner FP, Selwood NH. End-stage renal failure due to analgesic nephropathy, its changing pattern and cardiovascular mortality. *Nephrol Dial Transplant* 1994; 9: 1371–6.

38. Perazella MA. Crystal induced acute renal failure. *Am J Med* 1999; 106: 459–65.

39. Tashima KT, Horowitz JD, Rosen S. Indinavir nephropathy. *New Engl J Med* 1997; 336: 138–40.

40. Mihatsch MJ, Khanlari B, Brunner FP. Obituary to analgesic nephropathy – an autopsy study. *Nephrol Dial Transplant* 2006; 21: 3139–45.

41. Brunner FP, Selwood NH. End-stage renal failure due to analgesic nephropathy, its changing pattern and cardiovascular mortality. *Nephrol Dial Transplant* 1994; 9: 1371–6.

42. Walker RG, Bennett WM, Davies BM, Kincaid-Smith P. Structural and functional effects of long-term lithium therapy. *Kidney Int* 1982; 21(S11); S13–S19.

43. Walker RG, Dowling JP, Alcorn D, Ryan GB, Kincaid-Smith P. Renal pathology associated with lithium therapy. *Pathology* 1983; 15: 403–11.

44. Markowitz GS, Radhakrishnan J, Kambham N, Valeri AM, Hines WH, D'Agati. Litihium nephrotoxicity: a progressive combined glomerular and tubulointerstitial nephropathy. *J Am Soc Nephrol* 2000; 11: 1439–48.

45. Olsen S. Renal histopathology in various forms of acute anuria in man. *Kidney Int* 1976; 10: S2–S8.

46. Becker JL, Miller F, Nuovo GJ, Josepovitz C, Schubach WH, Nord EP. Epstein-Barr virus infection of proximal renal tubule cells: possible role in chronic interstitial nephritis. *J Clin Invest* 1999; 104: 1673–81.

47. Nortier JL, Vanherweghem JL. For patients taking herbal therapy – lessons from aristolochic acid nephropathy. *Nephrol Dial Transplant* 2007; 22: 1512–17.

48. Bhandari S, Kalowski S, Collet P, Cooke BE, Kerr P, Newland R, Dowling J, Horvath J. Karyomegalic nephropathy: an uncommon cause of progressive renal failure. *Nephrol Dial Transplant* 2002; 17: 1914–20.

49. Cremer W, Bock KD. Symptoms and course of chronic hypokalemic nephropathy in man. *Clin Nephrol* 1977; 7: 112–19.

50. Potter WZ, Trygstad CW, Helmer OM, Nance WE, Judson WE. Familial hypokalemia associated with renal interstitial fibrosis. *Am J Med* 1974; 57: 971–7.

51. Zsurka G, Ormos J, Ivyani B, Turi S, Endreffy E, Magyari M, Sonkodi S, Venetianer P. Mitochondrial mutation as a probable causative factor in familial progressive tubulointerstitial nephritis. *Human Genet* 1997; 99: 484–7.

52. Rotig A, Goutieres F, Niaudet P, Rustin P, Chretien D, Guest G, Mikol J, Gubler MC, Munnich A. Deletion of mitochondrial DNA in patients with chronic tubulointerstitial nephritis. *J Pediatr* 1995; 126: 597–601.

53. Tzen C-Y, Tsai J-D, Wu T-Y, Chen B-F, Chen M-L, Lin S-P, Chen S-C. Tubulointerstitial nephritis associated with a novel mitochondrial point mutation. *Kidney Int* 2001; 59: 846–54.

54. Viero RM, Cavallo T. Granulomatous interstitial nephritis. *Hum Pathol* 1995; 26: 1347–53.

55. Mignon F, Mery JPH, Mougenout B, Ronco P, Roland J, Morel-Maroger L. Granulomatous interstitial nephritis. *Adv Nephrol* 1984; 13: 219–45.

56. Magil AB. Drug-induced acute interstitial nephritis with granulomas. *Hum Pathol* 1983; 13:36–41.

57. Schwarz A, Krause PH, Keller F, Offermann G, Mihatsch MJ. Granulomatous interstitial nephritis after antiinflammatory drugs. *Am J Nephrol* 1988; 8: 410–16.

58. Robson MG, Banerjee D, Hopster D, Cairns HS. Seven cases of granulomatous interstitial nephritis in the absence of extrarenal sarcoid. *Nephrol Dial Transplant* 2003; 18: 280–4.

59. Alvarez S, McCabe WR. Extrapulmonary tuberculosis revisited: a review of experience at Boston City and other hospitals. *Medicine (Baltimore)* 1984; 63: 25–55.

60. Medlar EM. Cases of renal infection in pulmonary tuberculosis. *Am J Pathol* 1926; 2: 401–13.

61. Cinman AC. Genitourinary tuberculosis. *Urology* 1982; 20: 353–8.

62. Christiansen WI. Genitourinary tuberculosis: review of 102 cases. *Medicine (Baltimore)* 1974; 53: 377–90.

63. Kambham N, Markowitz GS, Tanji N, Mansukhani MM, Orazi A, D'Agati V. Idiopathic hypocomplementemic interstitial nephritis with extensive tubulointerstitial deposits. *Am J Kidney Dis* 2001; 37; 388–99.

64. Vaseemuddin M, Schwartz MM, Dunea G, Kraus MA. Idiopathic hypocomplementemic immune-complex-mediated tubulointerstitial nephritis. *Nat Clin Pract Nephrol* 2007; 3; 50–8.

65. Takeda S, Haratake J, Kasai T, Takaeda C, Takazakura E. IgG4-associated idiopathic tubulointerstitial nephritis complicating autoimmune pancreatitis. *Nephrol Dial Transplant* 2004; 19; 474–6.

66. Cornell LD, Chicano SL, Deshpande V, Collins AB, Selig MK, Lauwers GY, Colvin RB. Pseudotumors due to IgG4 immune complex tubulointerstitial nephritis associated with autoimmune pancreatocentric disease. *Am J Surg Pathol* 2007; 31: 1586–97.

67. Watson SJW, Jenkins DAS, Bellamy COS. Nephropathy in IgG4-related systemic disease. *Am J Surg Pathol* 2006; 30: 1472–7.

68. Nishi H, Tojo A, Onoxato ML, Jimbo R, Nangaku M, Uozaki H, Hirano K, Isayama H, Omata M, Kaname S. Anticarbonic anhydrase II antibody in autoimmune pancreatitis and tubulointerstitial nephritis. *Nephrol Dial Transplant* 2007; 22: 1273–4.

69. Orfila C, Rokotoavirony J, Durand D, Suc JM. A correlative study of immunofluorescence, electron and light microscopy in immunologically mediated renal tubular disease in man. *Nephron* 1979; 23: 14–22.

70. Ivyani B, Haszon I, Endreffy E, Szenohradszky P, Petri IB, Kalmar T, Butkowski RJ, Charonis AS, Turi S. Childhood membranous nephropathy, circulating antibodies to the 58-kD TIN antigen, and antitubular basement membrane nephritis: an 11-year follow-up. *Am J Kidney Dis* 1998; 32: 1068–74.

71. Markowitz GS, Seigle RL, D'Agati VD. Three-year-old boy with partial Fanconi syndrome. *Am J Kidney Dis* 1999; 34: 184–8.

72. Levy M, Guesry P, Loirat C, Dommergues JP, Nivet H, Habib R. Immunologically mediated tubulointerstitial nephritis in children. *Contrib Nephrol* 1979; 16: 132–40.

CHAPTER 12

Hypertension and Vascular Diseases of the Kidney

Michael D. Hughson, MD

Hypertension and diseases of the large renal arteries are covered in this chapter. The topics are related to each other from two perspectives. First, hypertension is a major risk factor for atherosclerosis, and atherosclerosis is the most common cause of large artery disease of the kidney. Second, renal artery stenosis competes with renal parenchymal disease as the most common cause of secondary hypertension, and renovascular hyperten-

sion secondary to atherosclerosis of the main renal arteries is becoming increasingly prevalent in aging populations throughout the world [1].

Renal biopsy is not usually indicated for the diseases described in this chapter. Nevertheless, some patients with primary hypertension have significant proteinuria that can clinically mimic a primary glomerular disease, particularly nonnephrotic focal segmental glomerulosclerosis (FSGS) or IgA nephropathy. In such cases, the pathology of hypertension must be appreciated in order to avoid misclassifying the disease. In addition, evidence of renal damage due to hypertension is frequently seen in biopsies of primary and systemic diseases affecting the kidney, and an understanding of the changes attributable to hypertension will allow the person interpreting the biopsy to more fully appreciate the role of hypertension in the progression of all forms of kidney disease. The vascular changes that may be seen in a renal biopsy or autopsy and the differential diagnosis of clinical conditions causing those changes are shown as an algorithm in Figure 12.1.

ANATOMY OF THE RENAL ARTERIES

The kidney is supplied by medium-, to small-size muscular arteries (Figure 12.2 A–D). These begin with the renal artery that arises from the aorta and branches into anterior and posterior divisions. At the next level, the interlobar arteries enter the kidney between the renal pyramids (synonym, renal lobes). At the corticomedullary junction, arcuate arteries branch from the interlobar arteries parallel to the capsular surface of the kidney. From the arcuate arteries, interlobular arteries penetrate the cortex in a radial manner and give rise to afferent arterioles that perfuse the 900,000 ± 300,000 glomeruli that are normally found in each kidney [2].

The muscular arteries of the kidney have an internal and an external elastic lamina that is demonstrated with elastic tissue stains. An external elastic lamina is poorly formed in the interlobular arteries and is not seen in afferent arterioles. The afferent arteriole has an internal elastic lamina up to the level of the juxtaglomerular apparatus. At this point, endothelium sits on a periodic acid-Schiff (PAS) positive but elastic tissue-negative basal lamina. The efferent arteriole, a thin-walled vessel that frequently lacks a muscular coat, exits the glomerulus, and gives rise to the peritubular capillary bed.

The juxtaglomerular apparatus consists of modified granular and agranular smooth muscle cells in the wall of the afferent arteriole just before it enters the glomerulus. Opposite the glomerulus, the juxtaglomerular smooth muscle cells and a group of extraglomerular mesangial cells, termed lacis cells or the polar cushion, lie in contact with the macula densa, the initial segment of the distal convoluted tubule (Figure 12.3). Juxtaglomerular granular cells contain specific and nonspecific granules. Nonspecific granules represent lipofuscin pigment. Specific granules contain renin and can be demonstrated with PAS, Luxol fast blue, Bowie stains, and by immunocytochemistry with renin specific antibodies.

HYPERTENSION

Introduction

The definition of hypertension is somewhat arbitrary, since there is no clear division between normal and elevated blood pressure [3]. Blood pressure is a continuous variable having a unimodal distribution that differs by age, ethnicity, and gender [2,3]. In the United States, at about 30 years of age, blood pressure begins to increase, as the population gets older. This increase in blood pressure has a steeper slope for African Americans than Caucasians. By the middle of the sixth decade of life, 53 percent of women and 44 percent of men have developed hypertension, and rates of hypertension are 37 percent higher for African American men and 49 percent higher for African American women compared to Caucasians of the respective gender [4].

In 1978, the World Health Organization (WHO) recommended defining hypertension as a blood pressure of 160/95 mmHg or above and a normal blood pressure as below 140/90 mmHg [5]. There is a clear reduction in cardiovascular disease risk when blood pressure in reduced below 140/90 mmHg and blood pressure at or above this level has become the standard definition of hypertension [2]. Nevertheless, cardiovascular disease risk increases when systolic blood pressure rises above 115 mmHg, and in the United States, the latest guidelines adopted by the Joint National Committee on Hypertension (JNC-7) recommends that normal blood pressure be defined as 120/80 mmHg or below, and hypertension as 140/90 mmHg or above [6].

Blood pressure between normal and hypertension is considered prehypertension. Hypertension is further divided into stage 1 and stage 2 (Table 12.1). These guidelines do not separately distinguish severe (stage 3) hypertension at a blood pressure of greater than 180/110 mmHg and very severe (stage 4) hypertension at greater than 210/120 mmHg that were represented in previous JNC recommendations [7]. It also does not mention malignant hypertension.

Clinical Presentation

Hypertension is a notoriously silent disease until it is complicated by stroke, cardiac disease, or chronic renal failure. Hypertension is termed benign when blood pressure is elevated but is stable or increases slowly over time. Hypertension is regarded as accelerated when a very high blood pressure is associated with the grade 3 hypertensive retinal changes of hemorrhages and exudates; and malignant when a very high blood pressure (diastolic blood pressure usually greater than 120 mmHg) is combined with a hypertensive encephalopathy and grade 3 plus the grade 4 hypertensive retinal changes of papilledema [8]. The syndromes of accelerated and malignant hypertension are complicated by acute renal vascular damage, proteinuria, and renal failure.

Etiology and Pathogenesis

Hypertension is essential or primary if it cannot be attributed to an underlying condition. When an underlying cause can be identified, the hypertension is termed secondary. Secondary hypertension is estimated to be responsible for 5 to 20 percent of hypertension [8–12]. Table 12.2 lists the more common causes of hypertension and their relative frequency. There is little data on the actual prevalence of the different causes of secondary hypertension, and the broad range of estimates is

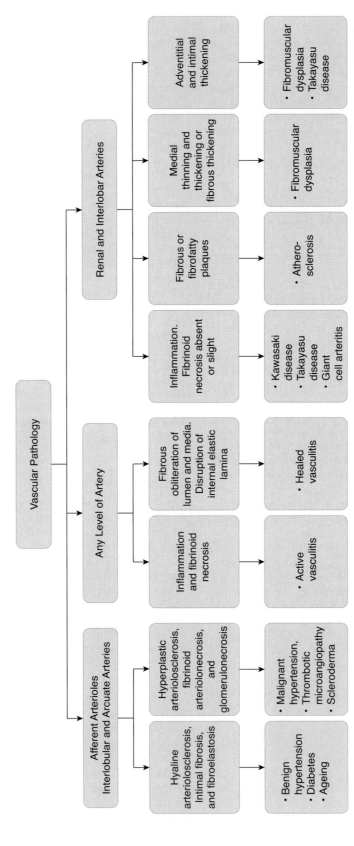

FIGURE 12.1: *Algorithm of the vascular changes that can be seen in renal biopsies or autopsies and the differential diagnosis of the clinical conditions causing those changes.*

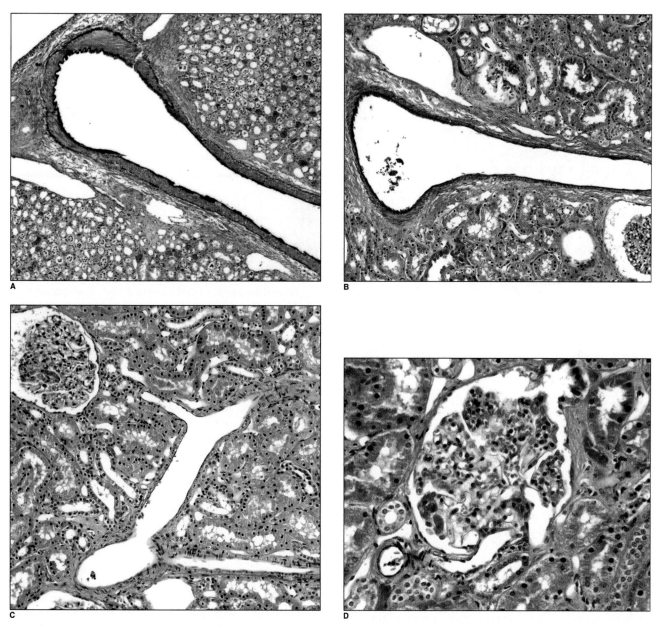

FIGURE 12.2: *Renal arteries in the normal kidney of an 18-year-old female. A: Interlobar artery branching into an arcuate artery. The arteries at this level have well developed external elastic lamina. (Verhoef, Van Gieson, ×40) B: Interlobular artery branching from an arcuate artery. The interlobular artery has a poorly developed external elastic artery. (Verhoef, Van Gieson, ×100) C: Afferent arterioles dividing from an interlobular artery. (Verhoef, Van ×Gieson, ×100) D: Afferent arteriole entering a glomerulus. A thin elastic lamina is seen in the afferent arteriole proximal to but not at the level of the macular densa. (Verhoef, Van Gieson, ×200).*

due to the different criteria applied for diagnoses, particularly for primary aldosteronism, and renovascular hypertension [9,11].

Blood pressure is regulated by the balance between cardiac output and peripheral vascular resistance, and hypertension is the result of the increase in one or both of these physiological factors. The kidney plays a central role in the long-term regulation of blood pressure by means of the renin-angiotensin-aldosterone system and pressure natriuresis [13]. The role of the renin-angiotensin-aldosterone system will be described more fully in the section of this chapter on renovascular hypertension.

Pressure natriuresis is the physiological mechanism whereby sodium is excreted at a rate that is determined by the perfusion pressure of the kidney [13]. Increased salt intake expands extracellular fluid volume and elevates systemic arterial pressure. The higher renal perfusion pressures result in natriuresis that lowers body sodium content and returns blood pressure toward normal.

Some individuals are unusually prone to develop high blood pressure when consuming high salt diets and are identified as having "salt-sensitive hypertension." It is a form of "low-renin" hypertension that is conceptually regarded as a resetting of the threshold for sodium excretion curves in which higher blood

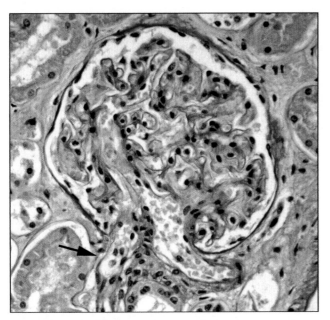

FIGURE 12.3: Modified smooth muscle cells of the polar cushion sit in contact with the macula densa of the distal tubule between the afferent and the efferent (arrow) arteriole. (PAS, hematoxylin, ×200).

Table 12.2 Estimated Prevalence of Causes of Hypertension [8–12]

A. Primary, essential 80–95%
B. Secondary 5–20%
   1. Renal parenchymal 2–5%
   2. Renovascular 2–5%
   3. Primary aldosteronism 0.5–13%
   4. Obstructive sleep apnea 1–3%
   5. Phaeochromocytoma < 1%
   6. Single-gene defects < 1%

pressures are needed to excrete a particular level of sodium intake [13]. Affected individuals retain sodium unless blood pressure increases.

Hypertension tends to be familial, but blood pressure is also influenced by acquired factors such as obesity, alcohol intake, diet, smoking, stress, and has both a genetic and environmental basis. Hypertension resulting from single gene mutations is extremely uncommon, and the familial basis for essential hypertension is considered to be polygenetic with polymorphisms being identified in genes related to the renin-angiotensin-aldosterone system that regulate renal sodium transport [14,15]. The importance of the kidney and sodium retention in the pathogenesis of essential hypertension is emphasized by the fact that the known single-gene mutations that cause hypertension do so by increasing renal sodium reabsorption [16].

Renal parenchymal disease is generally considered the most common cause of secondary hypertension with blood pressure becoming elevated in 75 to 90 percent of chronic kidney disease (CKD) patients as they progress to end-stage renal disease (ESRD) [9]. This is usually a renoprival form of hypertension

Table 12.1 Classification of Blood Pressure for Adults ⩾ 18 years of age (JNC-7)

Classification	Blood Pressure (mmHg)
Normal	<120/80
Prehypertension	120/80 to 139/89
Stage 1 hypertension	140/90 to 159/99
Stage 2 hypertension	⩾160/100

Does not separately classify: severe hypertension 180/110 to 209/119 or malignant hypertension ⩾ 210/120 mmHg (when combined with grade 3 and 4 retinal changes and hypertensive encephalopathy).

with patients having an expanded extracellular volume caused by the loss of the normal excretory function of the kidney. In view of the fact that atherosclerosis is found in such a large proportion of their aging populations, renal vascular disease may now be the most common cause of secondary hypertension in Western countries. The U.S. Renal Data System currently lists large vessel disease and hypertension as a single etiologic cause of ESRD [1].

The frequency of secondary hypertension increases with the severity of the elevation of the blood pressure. With mild hypertension, the index of suspicion for secondary hypertension is low and testing for an underlying cause is not recommended [9]. With accelerated or malignant hypertension, 10 to 45 percent of patients may have an underlying condition that is most commonly renal parenchymal disease or renovascular hypertension [9,17].

Hypertension due to single-gene mutations should be considered in young individuals with a strong family history of hypertension [16]. These single gene defects cause low-renin hypertension as a result of abnormalities that increases mineralocorticoid activity at the level of the distal tubule. The best characterized, but still very rare, examples of these genetic disorders are (1) glucocorticoid remedial aldosteronism (GRA) or familial hyperaldosteronism type 1 and (2) Liddle syndrome [16]. GRA is an autosomal dominant condition that is the result of a mutation that fuses the aldosterone synthetase and 11-hydroxylase genes and places aldosterone synthesis under the control of adrenocorticotropic hormone (ACTH). Glucocorticoid levels are low and ACTH is elevated resulting in excessive aldosterone synthesis and secretion. Treatment with glucocorticoids reduces ACTH levels, decreases aldosterone synthesis, and lowers blood pressure. Liddle syndrome is the result of mutations in the gene for the sodium channel in the distal tubule. The mutation causes excessive numbers of channels to accumulate in the cell membranes resulting in increased sodium reabsorption.

Approach to Interpretation

Benign Hypertension

Arteriolosclerosis, the sclerotic thickening of arterioles and small arteries, is attributed to benign hypertension but also increases with age, and is found in patients who have never been known to have elevated blood pressure [18]. Although prevailing scientific opinion regards renal arteriolosclerosis as being a hypertrophic response to elevated pressures, another view suggests that it represents premature aging of the arteries and may be the cause of hypertension [18–23]. Benign hypertension is associated with two types of pathology of small arteries or arterioles:

1. Hyaline arteriolosclerosis,
2. Intimal fibrosis (synonym, intimal fibroplasia).

Gross pathology. Kidneys showing these vascular changes can be normal in size and appearance, or the cortex can be uniformly to somewhat irregularly thinned from the normal thickness of 0.6 to 0.7 cm and have a finely to coarsely granular subcapsular surface [18–20]. A few to several simple cysts may be present. The cortical atrophy results from a reduction in blood flow through the sclerotic small arteries and arterioles and is termed benign arteriolonephrosclerosis or simply nephrosclerosis (synonym, arteriolar nephrosclerosis) (Figure 12.4). In benign essential hypertension, the kidney volume is not usually reduced by more than 30 percent, although some kidneys may weigh one-half of normal [18,20].

Patients with advanced arteriosclerosis, in addition, have irregularly pitted and contracted kidneys with deep V-shaped cortical scars. These deeper scars are caused by arteriosclerosis of larger arteries, generally proximal to the arcuates [24]. Usually a combination of large and small artery disease is present and "arterio-arteriolonephrosclerosis" may be the preferred term (Figure 12.5).

Light microscopy. The granular subcapsular appearance of benign arteriolonephrosclerosis is the result of small scars in

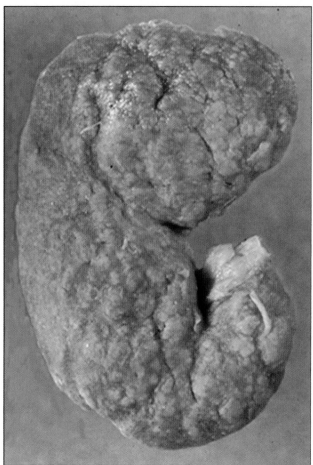

FIGURE 12.5: *Benign nephrosclerosis with a marked reduction in kidney size. The cortical surface of the kidney is coarsely granular and also contains deep, V-shaped scars. The latter are attributed to arteriosclerosis involving the large renal arteries (arterio-arteriolonephrosclerosis).*

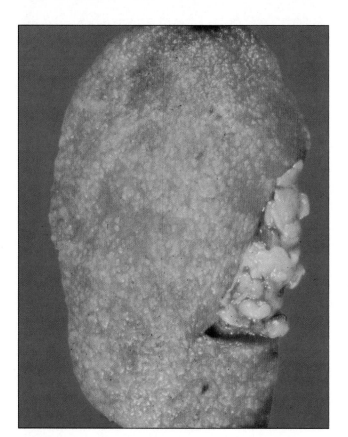

FIGURE 12.4: *Benign nephrosclerosis. The subcapsular surface of this kidney is finely granular.*

the outer cortex that are somewhat wedge-shaped and have their base on the subcapsular surface of the kidney. They contain obsolete glomeruli and atrophic tubules, and alternate with normal to hypertrophied cortex, producing the granularity of the cortical surface (Figure 12.6). The hyaline arteriolosclerosis of essential hypertension affects afferent arterioles. In more severely involved kidneys, the hyaline change can be seen in interlobular arteries. The walls of the hyalinized arterioles are thickened by homogeneous (or glassy), eosinophilic staining material that frequently contains lipid droplets. The hyaline stains slightly PAS positive, blue with Masson's trichrome stain, and is unstained with the PAS-methenamine-silver method. Mild degrees of arteriolosclerosis show partial thickening of the vessel wall with hyaline material that first accumulates under the endothelium (Figure 12.7). With severe changes, the better part of the arteriolar wall is hyalinized and the lumen is narrowed (Figure 12.8). Hyaline arteriolosclerosis occurs in diabetic patients with and without hypertension [25]. In diabetic nephropathy (DNP), hyalinization is found in efferent as well as afferent arterioles. This can be appreciated when both vessels are cut in the same plane of section at the hilum of a glomerulus.

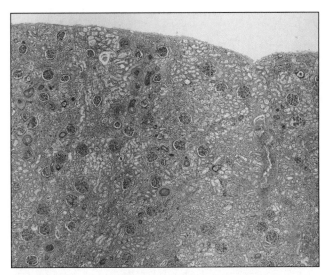

FIGURE 12.6: *Benign nephrosclerosis with a mild reduction in kidney size. The granular appearance of the subcapsular surface of the kidney is due to cortical scarring that contains obsolete glomeruli and atrophic tubules and alternates with normal to hypertrophied cortex. (PAS, hematoxylin, ×20).*

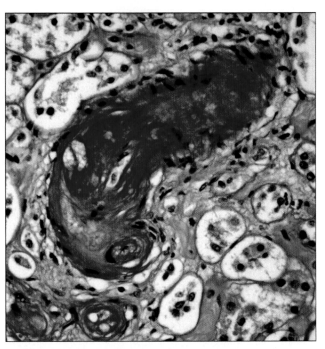

FIGURE 12.8: *Benign nephrosclerosis. Hyaline arteriolosclerosis in a patient with severe hypertension. The entire arteriolar wall is hyalinized and the vessel lumen is narrowed. (PAS, hematoxylin, ×200).*

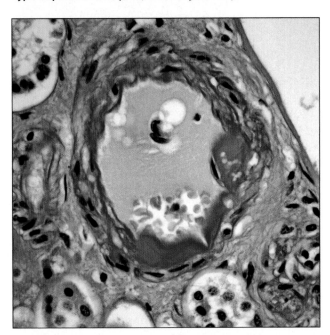

FIGURE 12.7: *Benign nephrosclerosis. Hyaline arteriolosclerosis in which there is partial thickening of the arteriolar wall by hyaline material containing lipid droplets accumulating under the endothelium. (PAS, hematoxylin, ×200).*

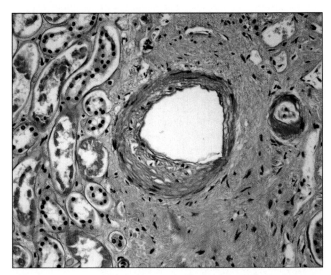

FIGURE 12.9: *Mild intimal fibrosis in an interlobular artery that eccentrically thickens the intima. (PAS, hematoxylin, ×200).*

Efferent arteriolar hyalinization is rarely, if ever, seen in essential hypertension [20].

Intimal fibrosis involves arcuate and interlobular arteries, and consists of collagenous connective tissue that thickens the intima and narrows the lumens of the affected vessels. In early stages, the process is somewhat eccentric (Figure 12.9), but as it becomes more severe the intima are concentrically thickened (Figure 12.10). Between collagen fibers, the intima contains relatively sparse numbers of spindle cells (myointimal cells) that ultrastructurally have plasma membrane vesicles and cytoplas-

mic condensations of thin filaments. These ultrastructural features are typical of smooth muscle; by immunocytochemistry, myointimal cells can be stained with antibodies specific for smooth muscle actin. The internal elastic lamina is reduplicated in arteries showing intimal fibrosis. The increase in intimal elastic tissue can be relatively inconspicuous, or there can be pronounced concentric fibroelastic thickening (Figure 12.11). With mild degrees of intimal fibrosis, the media of small arteries may be thickened. When there is advanced intimal fibrosis, the media focally has reduced numbers of smooth muscle cells that are replaced by fibrous tissue (Figure 12.12). The

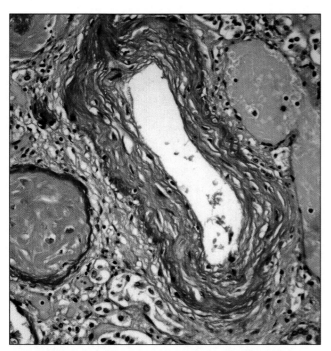

FIGURE 12.10: *Benign nephrosclerosis. Marked intimal fibrosis in an interlobular artery of a patient with severe hypertension that concentrically thickens the intima. (PAS, hematoxylin, × 200).*

reduction in smooth muscles cells is considered to be the result of these cells migrating from the media into the intima where they proliferate and subsequently become fixed myointimal cells that synthesize collagen and elastic tissue [26]. The severity of intimal fibrosis has been related more clearly to elevated blood pressure than has hyaline arteriolosclerosis [22]. Arteriolar hyalinization may correlate better with glucose intolerance, hyperlipidemia, and coronary heart disease than with hypertension [27].

A type of glomerulosclerosis, termed glomerular obsolescence, develops in association with arteriolosclerosis (Figure 12.13 A–D). Glomerular obsolescence is thought to be caused by a reduction in glomerular blood flow and is also referred to as ischemic glomerular obsolescence [28]. In early stages, the affected glomeruli reveal wrinkling and thickening of the glomerular basement membranes. Subsequently the glomerular tuft contracts toward the vascular pole, and as it contracts, the glomerular tuft becomes simplified into fewer and smaller capillary loops. Collagenous connective tissue gradually builds up on the inner side of the basement membrane of Bowman's capsule. In some glomeruli, this process, termed intracapsular fibrosis, begins at the vascular pole adjacent to the glomerular stalk. Intracapsular fibrosis eventually fills Bowman's space over a collapsed remnant of the glomerular tuft. The PAS stain colors the contracted glomerular capillary basement membranes a bright magenta. The PAS reaction additionally outlines the basement membrane of Bowman's capsule where it encircles the intracapsular fibrosis. The basement membrane of Bowman's capsule can be identified, although with increasing degrees of fragmentation, until very late stages of obsolescence. In very late stages, obsolete glomeruli become infiltrated with lymphocytes (Figure 12.14), basement membranes are resorbed, and the sclerotic glomeruli eventually disappear from the kidney.

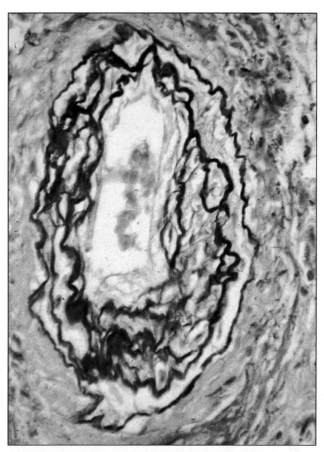

FIGURE 12.11: *Benign nephrosclerosis. Marked intimal fibrosis with reduplication of the internal elastic lamina in an interlobular artery. (Verhoef, Van Gieson, × 200).*

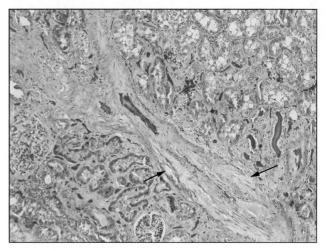

FIGURE 12.12: *Benign nephrosclerosis. Marked intimal fibrosis of an interlobular artery showing focal loss of medial smooth muscle (arrows). (Masson's trichrome, × 200).*

Another pattern of glomerulosclerosis termed glomerular solidification also occurs with hypertension [20,24]. Glomerular solidification is less frequently seen than glomerular obsolescence and consists of an expansion of the glomerular tuft by increased mesangial matrix in which the expanded tuft tends to

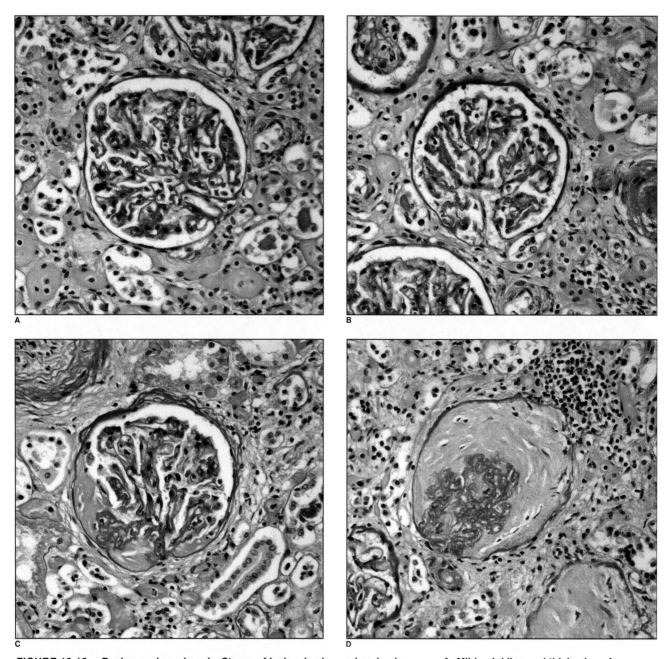

FIGURE 12.13: *Benign nephrosclerosis. Stages of ischemic glomerular obsolescence. A: Mild wrinkling and thickening of glomerular capillary basement membranes. B: Thickening and wrinkling of glomerular capillary basement membranes, contraction of the glomerular tuft toward the vascular pole, and simplification of the glomerular tuft into fewer and smaller capillary loops. C: Shrinking of the glomerular tuft and intracapsular fibrosis beginning at the vascular pole adjacent to the glomerular stalk. D: The obsolete glomerular tuft is a contracted knot of basement membranes. Bowman's space is filled with acellular fibrous tissue surrounded by an intact Bowman's capsular basement membrane. (PAS, hematoxylin, ×200).*

fill Bowman's space (Figure 12.15 A–D). Hyalinosis lesions are commonly found in the solidified tuft, and Bowman'capsule is often fragmented. Solidified glomeruli are accompanied by some segmentally sclerotic glomeruli that appear to be an early stage of solidification. Solidified glomeruli are more frequently found in the kidneys of African Americans than Caucasians [29]. Their development has been attributed to a loss of afferent arteriolar autoregulatory tone and glomerular hyperperfusion

in which there is a rapid loss of renal function termed decompensated benign nephrosclerosis [24].

Immunofluorescent microscopy. IgM, C3, and frequently properdin are routinely identified in hyalinized arterioles and may represent plasma proteins that become entrapped in the vessel wall (Figure 12.16) [30]. IgM and C3 are also frequently found in glomeruli in a mesangial distribution and in the

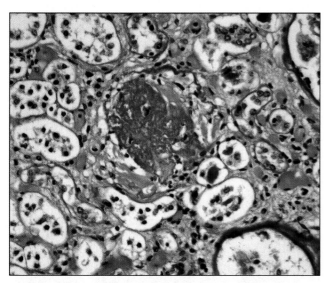

FIGURE 12.14: *Benign nephrosclerosis. Late stage of glomerular obsolescence in which there is infiltration of the sclerostic glomerulus by lymphocytes and partial resorption of basement membranes. (PAS, hematoxylin, ×200).*

collapsing segments of capillary loops during the development of glomerular obsolescence (Figure 12.17) [24]. Small amounts of weakly staining glomerular mesangial and arteriolar IgG and IgA may also be seen and should not be misinterpreted as evidence for an IgA nephropathy [20].

Electron microscopy. Hyalinized arterioles reveal thickened basement membranes beneath the endothelium and surrounding smooth muscle together with homogeneous, electron-dense material (Figure 12.18) [20,24]. The latter appears to correspond to the glassy, eosinophilic material seen by light microscopy and is probably derived from plasma proteins [24]. Glomeruli undergoing ischemic obsolescence reveal thickening and wrinkling of the glomerular capillary basement membranes (Figure 12.19) [31]. Immune-type electron-dense deposits should be absent.

Differential Diagnosis. In benign arteriolonephrosclerosis, the immunofluorescent finding of glomerular IgM and C3 in a mesangial pattern and even small amounts if IgA and IgG is usually nonspecific and does not indicate an immune complex disease. The presence of moderate to marked amounts of mesangial IgG and IgA with dominant or codominant IgA would indicate an underlying IgA nephropathy as a primary renal disease, especially if dense deposits are found by electron microscopy.

Albuminuria that is usually less than 1.0 g/day is seen in many patients with high blood pressure [32]. Nephrotic syndrome has been reported in patients with benign essential hypertension, but high levels of proteinuria should prompt a search for an alternate diagnosis such as primary FSGS. Similarly, if more than a few sclerotic glomeruli are of the solidified rather than the obsolete type, and if segmental glomerulosclerosis is frequently encountered, idiopathic FSGS rather than essential hypertension should be considered [20].

Accelerated and Malignant Hypertension

Gross pathology. The kidneys may be normal in size, or if there is prior benign hypertension and significant arteriolosclerosis, they can be smaller than normal and show varying degrees of nephrosclerosis. The cortices and mucosal surfaces of the renal pelvis display widespread petechial hemorrhages in cases without advanced chronic parenchymal disease. Petechial hemorrhages are absent or are not prominent in end-stage kidneys removed from dialysis patients because of malignant hypertension [33].

Light microscopy. Accelerated and malignant hypertension are characterized by two renal vascular lesions [34–36]:

1. Hyperplastic arteriolosclerosis, or "onion-skinning" (synonyms, hyperplastic arteriolitis, endarteritis fibrosa, mucoid intimal edema).
2. Fibrinoid necrosis.

A hyperplastic arteriolosclerosis is most prominent in the afferent arterioles and interlobular arteries; whereas, fibrinoid necrosis is found in the afferent arterioles (fibrinoid arteriolar necrosis) and glomeruli (fibrinoid glomerular necrosis) and infrequently in interlobular arteries. These vascular lesions are also seen without hypertension in the group of disorders termed the thrombotic microangiopathies (Chapter 9). When they are the result of hypertension, fibrinoid arteriolar and glomerular necrosis probably do not occur unless diastolic blood pressure reaches 120 mmHg [36].

Hyperplastic arteriolosclerosis consists of concentric thickening of the intima by mucoid ground substance, myointimal cells, and loosely arranged connective tissue fibers (Figure 12.20). This produces an onionskin appearance that markedly constricts the vessel. Red blood cells and red blood cell fragments are usually present in the thickened intima, and fibrin thrombi frequently occlude the narrowed lumen. The internal elastic lamina may be focally attenuated but not reduplicated unless the prior changes of benign hypertension are present. In fibrinoid arteriolar necrosis, the wall of the arteriole is effaced by an insudate of fibrillar to granular appearing eosinophilic material that has the staining properties of fibrin (Figure 12.21) [24,36]. Fibrinous insudates may sometimes be present in the interlobular arteries within the thickened mucoid intima (Figure 12.22).

Fibrinoid glomerular necrosis often involves the vascular pole of the glomerulus in continuity with fibrinoid arteriolar necrosis. Fibrinoid necrosis of the glomerular tuft is often segmental (Figure 12.23), but a large part of the glomerulus can be necrotic. Crescents can be found in association with glomerular necrosis (Figure 12.24 A,B). Glomeruli may also display afferent arteriolar or glomerular capillary thrombosis, mesangiolysis, or a marked congestion with red blood cells (Figure 12.25). Additional light microscopic changes that may be seen are focal acute renal tubular necrosis and small cortical infarcts.

Immunofluorescent microscopy. In approximately one-half of the cases, immunofluorescent microscopy discloses fibrinogen, complement, and immunoglobulins (usually IgM but occasionally IgG and IgA) in glomerular capillary walls and in small arteries and arterioles (Figure 12.26) [34,37]. The plasma

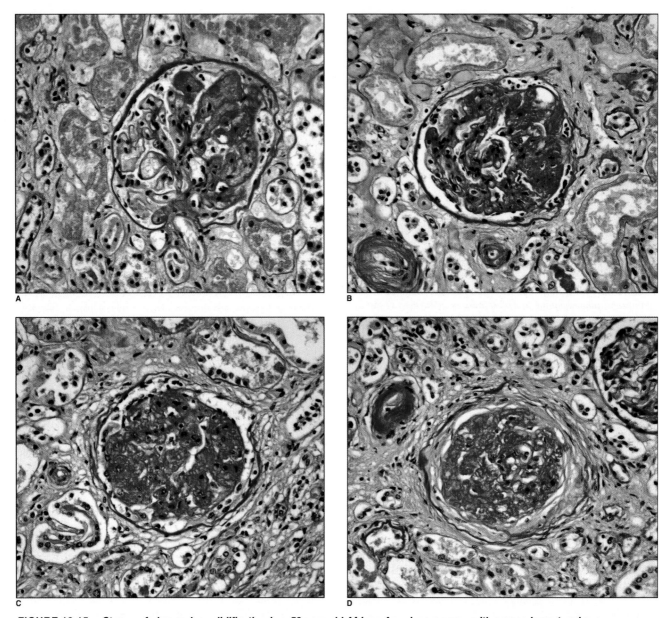

FIGURE 12.15: *Stages of glomerular solidification in a 53-year-old African American woman with severe hypertension.*
A: Increased mesangial matrix effaces glomerular capillary loops in a segment of a glomerular tuft producing segmental glomerulosclerosis with a capsular adhesion. B: Expansion of mesangial matrix in more the one-half of a glomerular tuft. C: The glomerular tuft is globally solidified and expands to fill Bowman's space. D: The solidified glomerulus is surrounded by fibrous tissue containing fragmented remnants of the basement membrane of Bowman's capsule. (PAS, hematoxylin, × 200).

proteins are thought to have leaked into these vascular structures as the result of increased permeability.

Electron microscopy. By electron microscopy, glomerular capillary basement membranes often show varying degrees of wrinkling and folding. Glomeruli may reveal endothelial swelling and a widened subendothelial space containing electron-lucent, "fluffy" acellular material (Figure 12.27). In examples of fibrinoid glomerular necrosis, capillary lumens contain swollen endothelium, thrombi, red blood cells, and red blood cell fragments (Figure 12.28) [34,37].

Differential diagnosis. Hyperplastic arteriolosclerosis, fibrinoid arteriolar and glomerular necrosis, and the ultrastructural and immunofluorescent findings just described for malignant hypertension are also seen in hemolytic uremic syndrome (HUS), thrombotic thrombocytopenic purpura (TTP), postpartum acute renal failure, and scleroderma. HUS, TTP, and postpartum acute renal failure comprise the thrombotic microangiopathies [38]. Fibrinoid arteriolar necrosis is probably a misnomer, and in these settings, including malignant hypertension, there is little evidence that any arteriolar cells are necrotic. The effacement of arteriolar structure appears to be the result of the local accumulation of

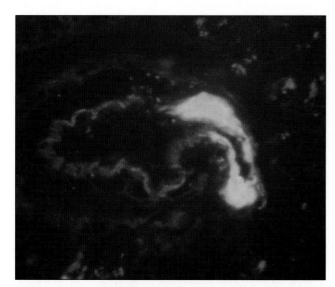

FIGURE 12.16: *Benign nephrosclerosis. Direct immunofluorescence demonstrates IgM in a hyalinized arteriole branching from an interlobular artery. C3 was present in addition to IgM. (×100).*

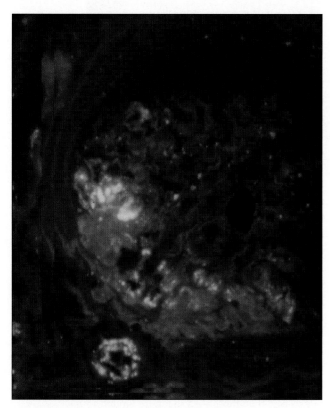

FIGURE 12.17: *Benign nephrosclerosis, direct immunofluorescence. Glomerulus showing mesangial C3 and C3 in an underlying arteriole (×400).*

fibrin-related proteins caused by coagulation occurring in the vascular lumen and within the vessel wall itself [34,38].

The close morphologic resemblance of malignant hypertension to scleroderma has been attributed to the fact that patients with scleroderma are commonly severely hypertensive at or near the time tissues are obtained. Nevertheless, patients with scleroderma who have never been hypertensive develop the characteristic pathologic changes [38,39]. It has been suggested that the vascular lesions of malignant hypertension as well as the thrombotic microangiopathies and scleroderma are caused by microvascular injury. Thrombosis and increased permeability are thought to follow the loss of the inhibitory control on clotting that is associated with normal vascular integrity [38–40].

The fibrinoid glomerular necrosis of malignant hypertension also resembles the focal necrotizing glomerulonephritis seen in systemic vasculitis (Chapter 6), and in neither case will immune complex deposits be found [41]. The association of segmental glomerular necrosis with fibrinoid arteriolar necrosis and a hyperplastic arteriolosclerosis and the involvement of relatively few glomeruli are features of malignant hypertension rather than systemic vasculitis.

Clinical course, prognosis, and clinical correlation. Untreated malignant hypertension will cause the death of all or nearly all patients. In a 1959 British study of untreated severe hypertension, 55 percent of patients with papilledema became uremic, 30 percent had fatal strokes, and 15 percent died of cardiovascular disease within one to three years [42].

While malignant hypertension frequently leads to uremia, ESRD is an uncommon complication of benign hypertension. The Multiple Risk Factor Intervention Trail (MRFIT) followed 332,544 men for a mean follow-up of sixteen years and found a graded relationship between blood pressure and risk of ESRD [43]. The proportion of patients and the adjusted relative risk (RR) of ESRD with 95 percent confidence intervals (CI) for different levels of hypertension were as follows:

A. Prehypertension, 22 percent of patients, RR 1.9 (CI, 1.4–2.7).

B. Stage 1 hypertension, 26 percent of patients, RR 3.1 (CI, 2.3– 4.3).

C. Stage 2 hypertension, 7 percent of patients, RR 6.0 (CI, 4.3–8.4).

D. Stage 3 hypertension, 1.6 percent of patients, RR 11.2 (CI, 7.7–16.2).

E. Stage 4 hypertension, 0.4 percent of patients, RR 22.1 (CI, 14.2–34.3).

Although overall rates of renal failure are fairly low, the large number of individuals in the United States that have high blood pressure accounts for essential hypertension being exceeded only by diabetes as a cause of ESRD. Of patients who enter ESRD programs, 27 percent have a diagnosis of hypertensive nephrosclerosis [1].

The U.S. Joint National Committee has recommended that all patients with hypertension should have their blood pressure lowered [6,7]. If diet and lifestyle modifications are not successful, or if the blood pressure is more than mildly elevated, hypertension should be controlled pharmacologically.

The morbidity and mortality of hypertension is related to end-organ damage produced by arteriosclerosis in arteries supplying the brain, heart, and kidney. The treatment of severe hypertension reduces morbidity and mortality by two-thirds or more [44 – 46]. The treatment of mild and moderate hypertension reduces deaths due to cardiovascular disease and stroke

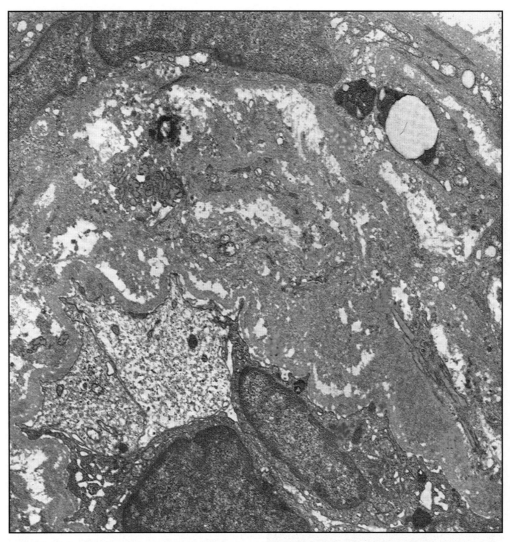

FIGURE 12.18: *Electron photomicrograph of a hyalinized arteriole. Basement membranes beneath the endothelium and surrounding smooth muscle are thickened. There is also extracellular homogeneous electron dense material, cell debris, and intracellular lipid in the arteriolar wall. (×5,800).*

by 20 to 30 percent and prevents blood pressure from rising to progressively higher levels [47,48].

Although the treatment of malignant hypertension can preserve renal function, many patients with benign hypertension progress to ESRD despite adequate blood pressure control [49–52]. A decline in renal function has been observed in 15 percent of patients with treated essential hypertension who were followed from one to more than ten years. The deterioration in renal function was found to occur twice as frequently in African Americans as whites and to be associated with increased proteinuria. It did not seem to be related to a lack of adequate blood pressure control or to an increased prevalence of severe hypertension [49–51].

SCLERODERMA

Introduction and Clinical Presentation

Scleroderma usually has its onset between 45 to 64 years of age and affects women at a ratio of as much as 8:1 over men [53].

Scleroderma is classified into limited, intermediate, and diffuse cutaneous forms of the disease [53]. Limited scleroderma consists of Raynaud's phenomenon, sclerosis of the skin of the fingers, and in some cases sclerosis of the armpits, face, and neck. Intermediate scleroderma affects the skin of the limbs, neck, and face, but not the trunk. Diffuse scleroderma produces fibrosis of the skin of the extremities, face, and trunk. Patients with diffuse cutaneous scleroderma are more prone to develop visceral involvement consisting of esophageal sclerosis, pulmonary fibrosis, pulmonary hypertension, and myocardial and kidney disease than those with the more limited forms.

An acute renal crisis consisting of acute oliguric renal failure commonly with an abrupt elevation of blood pressure, often at levels of malignant hypertension, occurs in approximately 10 percent of all scleroderma patients [54]. The acute renal crisis is seen in 1 percent of patients with limited and in 20 to 25 percent of patients with diffuse scleroderma with the onset occurring less than four years after the initial symptoms of scleroderma in 75 percent of cases [54].

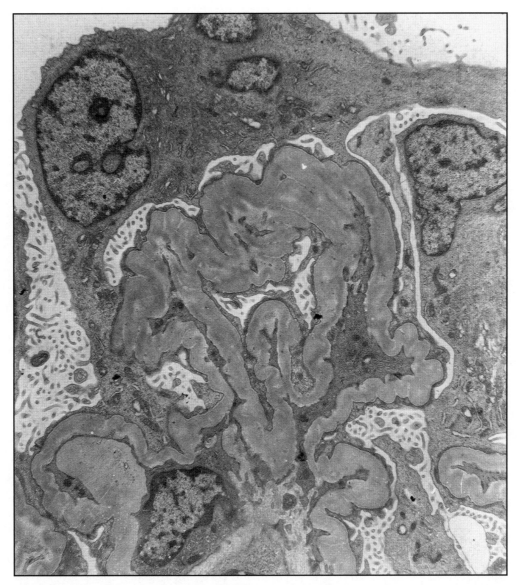

FIGURE 12.19: *Benign nephrosclerosis. Glomerulus undergoing ischemic glomerular obsolescence. This electron photomicrograph reveals thickenining and wrinkling of the glomerular capillary basement membranes. (×3,800).*

Etiology and Pathogenesis

The cause of scleroderma is unknown, but it appears to be primarily a disorder of cellular immunity [55,56]. Activated CD4 T-cells accumulate in the skin and other affected organs and release cytokines or promote the secretion of proteins including TGFβ that stimulate the growth of fibroblast and the accumulation of extracellular matrix and collagen. Microchimerism is a proposed source of the activated lymphocytes. These are thought to be fetal lymphocytes retained after pregnancy in the mother's tissues that become sensitized by maternal antigens [56]. Endothelial damage by proteins such as granzyme B released by activated lymphocytes or by antibodies may be an early manifestation of the disease. In such damage, the fibrosis that is so characteristic of the disease may be secondary to ischemia that follows microvascular injury [55]. Exposures to organic solvents and taxane chemo-

therapy have been implicated as environmental risks for scleroderma.

Immunologic tests are helpful in the diagnosis of scleroderma, and the frequent positive results suggest that an abnormality in humoral immunity is important in the pathogenesis of the disease [53]. High-titer antinuclear ribonucleoprotein (anti-nRNP) antibodies are found in patients with mixed connective tissue disease that often has features of scleroderma. Anticentromere antibodies are found in 90 percent of patients with limited, and in 10 percent of patients with generalized scleroderma. Anti-Scl-70 (anti-DNA-topoisomerase I) and antinucleolar antibodies are found, respectively, in 20 and 40 percent of scleroderma patients and are highly specific for the disease. An IgG antinucleolar staining pattern can sometimes be seen in the direct immunofluorescence microscopy of kidney sections from patients with high antinucleolar antibody titers.

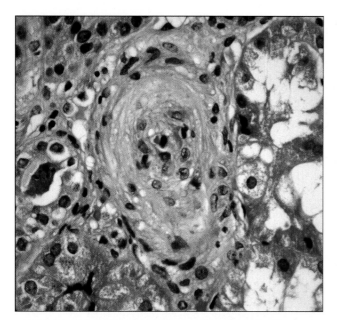

FIGURE 12.20:   Malignant hypertension. Hyperplastic arteriolosclerosis with concentric intimal thickening of an interlobular artery by mucoid ground substance and loosely arranged connective tissue fibers. (PAS, hematoxylin, ×200).

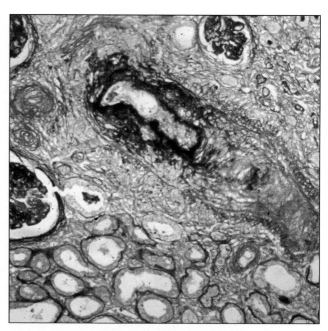

FIGURE 12.22:   Malignant hypertension. Fibrinoid necrosis in an interlobular artery involved by a hyperplastic arteriolosclerosis. A fibrinous insudate dissects along the mucoid intima. (PAS, luxol fast blue, ×150).

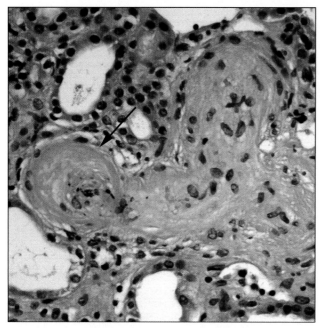

FIGURE 12.21:   Malignant hypertension. Fibrinoid arteriolonecrosis of an afferent arteriole (arrow) branching from an interlobular artery involved by a hyperplastic arteriolosclerosis. (PAS, hematoxylin, ×200).

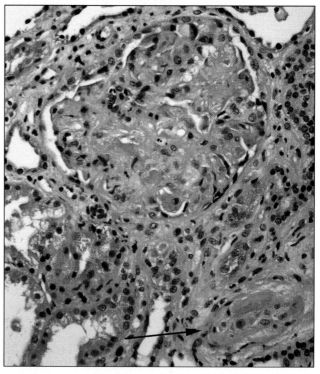

FIGURE 12.23:   Malignant hypertension. Fibrinoid glomerulonecrosis. Fibrinoid arteriolonecrosis is seen in the underlying arteriole (arrow). (PAS, hematoxylin, ×200).

Approach to Interpretation

Gross pathology. The kidneys can be normal or slightly reduced in size and the cortex smooth or granular. Petechial hemorrhages and small infarcts are present when patients have died in an acute renal crisis.

Light microscopy. The characteristic feature of the renal crisis of generalized scleroderma is mucoid intimal thickening of interlobular arteries and afferent arterioles (Figure 12.29). The vascular lumens are markedly narrowed and frequently

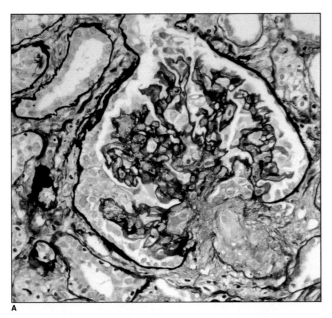

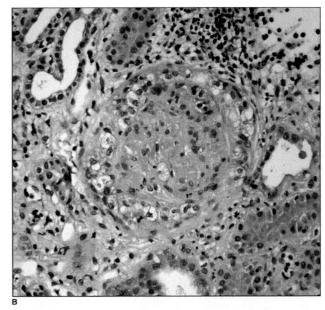

A

B

FIGURE 12.24: *Malignant hypertension. A: Segmental crescent in a glomerulus showing fibrinoid necrosis in the afferent arteriole. B: Global glomerulonecrosis with a circumferental crescent. (PAS, hematoxylin, ×200).*

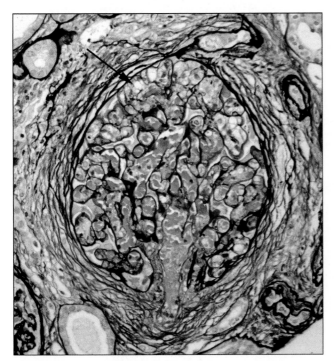

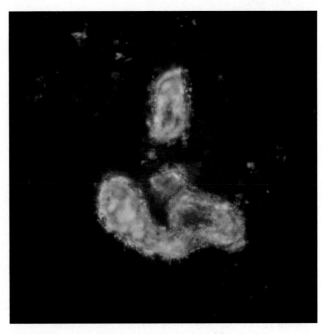

FIGURE 12.26: *Malignant hypertension. Direct immunofluorescence reveals IgM in an interlobular artery and arterioles. (×100).*

FIGURE 12.25: *Malignant hypertension. Marked congestion of glomerular capillaries with mesangiolysis (arrow). There is fibrinoid necrosis of the afferent arteriole. (Periodic acid methenamine silver, ×200).*

thrombosed. Fibrin, red blood cells, and red blood cell fragments may be found in the mucinous intima [54,57]. Afferent arterioles frequently show fibrinoid necrosis that often extends into glomeruli, resulting in fibrinoid glomerular necrosis. Glomeruli reveal hyperplasia of the juxtaglomerular apparatus and

reflect the high plasma renin activity found in an acute renal crisis [54,57]; this histologic picture resembles malignant hypertension. In many cases of scleroderma, periarterial fibrosis will be pronounced [54,57]. Periarterial fibrosis will not be conspicuous in primary malignant hypertension and, when well developed, can help distinguish between the pathology of the two diseases (i.e., scleroderma and primary malignant

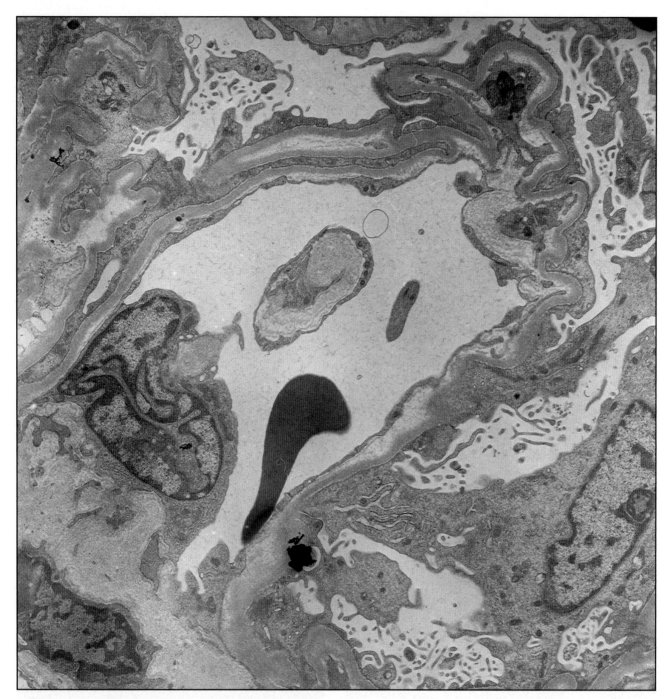

FIGURE 12.27: *Malignant hypertension. Electron photomicrograph demonstrating widening of the subendothelial space and subendothelial electron-lucent material. (×3,800).*

hypertension). In addition to vascular disease, the kidneys in scleroderma will show chronic interstitial inflammation and may contain small infarcts that will be accompanied by acute inflammation.

The kidneys of patients with chronic limited or diffuse scleroderma display fibrous arterial intimal thickening, interstitial fibrosis, and tubular atrophy [57]; these are findings expected with chronic benign hypertension or aging and their signifi-

cance needs to be correlated with the patient's age and blood pressure.

Immunofluorescence and electron microscopy. In the acute disease, glomerular capillary walls, arterioles, and interlobular arteries demonstrate the presence of fibrinogen, immunoglobulins, and complement [54,57]. The immune proteins consist mainly of IgM and C3 and are probably passively entrapped

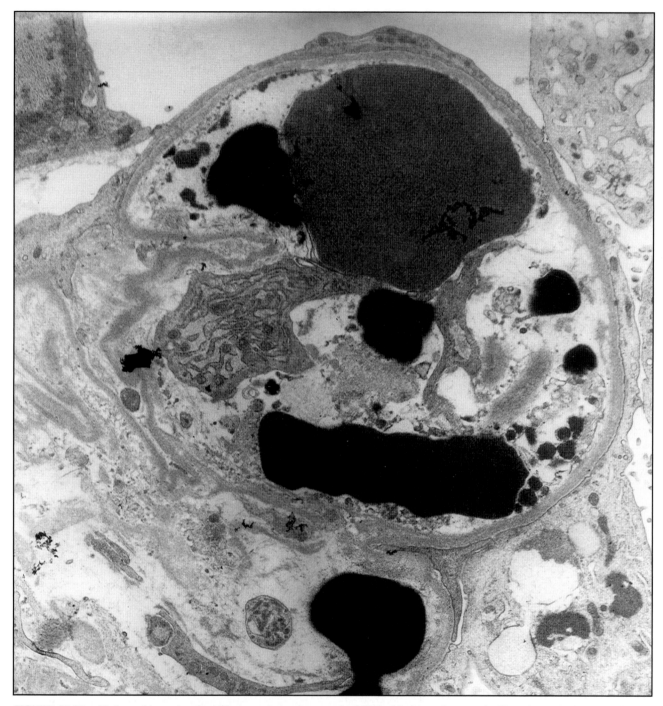

FIGURE 12.28: *Malignant hypertension. Electron photomicrograph of fibrinoid glomerulonecrosis. There is marked endothelial swelling in a capillary loop containing thrombotic material, red blood cells, and red blood cell fragments. (×3,800).*

in the capillary walls because of an increase in local vascular permeability. Electron microscopy discloses widening of the subendothelial space, as well as subendothelial electron-lucent material beneath glomerular capillary basement membranes (Figure 12.30). The immunofluorescence and electron microscopic abnormalities correspond to those seen in the other thrombotic microangiopathies and support an abnormality in

coagulation as being important in the pathogenesis of the vascular changes [54,57].

Clinical course, prognosis, and treatment. The clinical course of scleroderma is determined by renal, heart, and lung involvement. Without visceral disease, ten-year survival is approximately 85 percent [53]. Patients who develop an acute

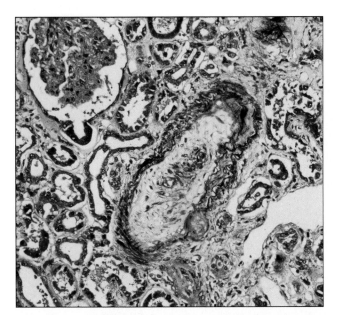

FIGURE 12.29: *Scleroderma, acute renal crisis. An interlobular artery shows a hyperplastic arteriolosclerosis with marked mucoid intimal edema. The cortical interstitium is edematous. (Phosphotungstic acid, hematoxylin, ×100).*

renal crisis have a one-year survival rate of 15 percent if they are untreated [53]. Treatment of the acute renal disease with angiotensin converting enzyme inhibitors has improved one-year survival to 76 percent, and ten-year survival rates are 35 percent [53,54]. Patients with a normotensive renal crisis do worse that those who are hypertensive. Presumably, this is because the normotensive crisis is more difficult to recognize and treatment is delayed [54].

DISEASES OF THE MAIN RENAL ARTERY

Introduction

Diseases of the main renal artery are causes of secondary hypertension and renal failure that may be potentially correctable. Most renovascular hypertension is the result of unilateral or bilateral renal artery stenosis due to atherosclerosis, but it is also seen with fibromuscular dysplasia and large vessel vasculitis. Neurofibromatosis is a rare cause of renovascular disease. Renal artery stenosis is responsible for approximately 0.2 percent of cases of mild hypertension. At higher levels of blood pressure, the percentage of patients with renovascular hypertension increases, accounting for an estimated 5 to 15 percent of cases of moderate and more than 30 percent of cases of malignant hypertension [58,59].

Atherosclerosis

Epidemiology and Clinical Presentation

Atherosclerosis of the renal arteries is often bilateral, and enlarging plaques that progressively obstruct renal blood flow

can be responsible for an unexpected rapid loss of renal function [60–62]. Patients with renal artery atherosclerosis invariably have some degree of renal microvascular pathology as a result of hypertension or diabetes. Determining whether any underlying chronic renal failure is caused by large vessel or small vessel disease is often problematic [62]. In one highly selected elderly Caucasian population, 12 to 15 percent of dialysis patients were considered to have developed ESRD as a result of bilateral atherosclerotic occlusion of the renal arteries [61]. A broader survey using the US Renal Data System database from 1991 to 1997 found that large vessel disease was the indicated cause of renal failure in 2.1 percent of ESRD patients, but it was also noted that as a cause of ESRD large vessel disease was increasing faster than other etiologies, including diabetes [63].

Embolization of cholesterol crystals from an atherosclerotic aorta or renal artery can cause an abrupt rise in blood pressure, and widespread showers of emboli can precipitate acute renal failure. This clinical situation may occur spontaneously but usually follows the repair of an abdominal aortic aneurysm or other invasive vascular procedures that disturb atheromatous plaques.

Approach to Interpretation

Gross pathology. After the fifth decade, the ostia of the renal arteries are frequently narrowed by atherosclerosis of the aorta (Figure 12.31). Less frequently, atherosclerotic plaques develop in the renal artery [64]. In autopsy studies, severe atherosclerosis of the renal arteries was found in 57 percent of patients who had a history of hypertension [65]. Severe stenosis was also found in patients who had normal blood pressures but at a lesser prevalence of 17 percent. Atherosclerotic plaques have been found distal to the main renal artery in 6.6 percent of patients being screened by arteriography for renal artery stenosis [66]. Yellowish plaques can be identified up to the level of the arcuate arteries in diabetics and in patients with hypercholesterolemia. The atherosclerotic plaque is composed of a fibrous cap overlying an inner core of foam cells and extracellular fatty debris containing cholesterol clefts (Figure 12.32). When plaques are ulcerated or physically disrupted, it is this fatty material that produces cholesterol emboli after being released into the circulation.

Microscopic pathology. Atherosclerotic vascular disease can cause acute or chronic renal failure as a result of bilateral stenosis of the renal arteries, renal artery thrombosis, or cholesterol emboli. Renal biopsies that are performed on patients who have atheromatous emboli frequently show cholesterol clefts within arcuate and interlobular arteries (Figure 12.33) and more rarely within glomerular capillaries [67]. Patchy acute tubular necrosis and, less commonly, renal infarcts may be seen in patients with acute renal failure. In early vascular lesions, fresh thrombi are formed around the atheromatous debris, and there is an accompanying polymorphonuclear inflammatory reaction. More often, cholesterol clefts are surrounded by multinucleated giant cells, mononuclear inflammatory cells, and fibrous tissue. The adjacent cortex usually demonstrates interstitial fibrosis, tubular atrophy, and ischemic glomerular changes that can be the result of embolization, atherosclerotic narrowing of the renal artery, or intrarenal arteriolosclerosis. Deep subcapsular scars representing old infarcts may be present.

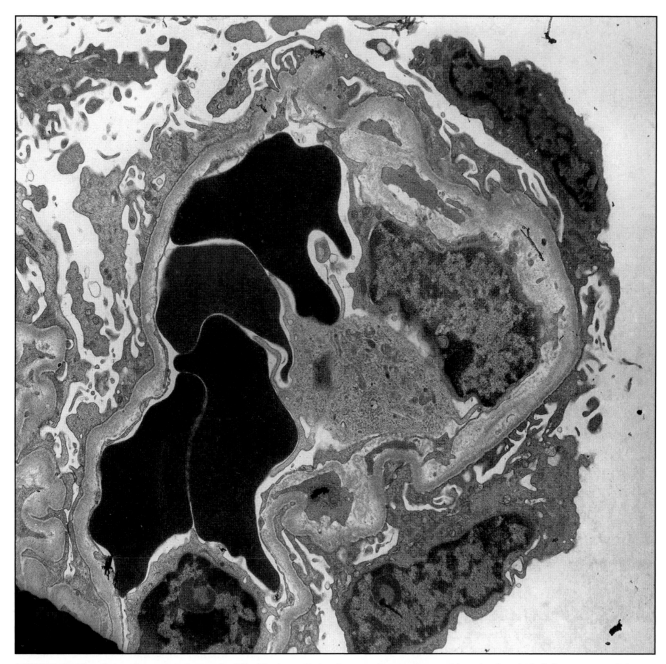

FIGURE 12.30: *Scleroderma, acute renal crisis. Electron photomicrograph revealing a widened subendothelial space containing granular to fibrillar electron-lucent material. (×3,800).*

Cholesterol crystals are removed by lipid solvents during the routine processing of histologic sections, leaving behind empty biconcave clefts. Although it is not usually needed for their identification, cholesterol crystals can be demonstrated by their birefringence of polarized light in cryostat sections obtained for immunofluorescence microscopy.

Renal Artery Dysplasia

The cause of renal artery dysplasia is not known. It is not clear whether it is a congenital or acquired abnormality [68,69]. Medial fibroplasia occurs with the Ehlers-Danlos syndrome,

and there are reports of fibromuscular dysplasia with Alport's and Marfan's syndromes that may indicate a defect in connective tissue synthesis at least in those clinical settings. Some cases may be difficult to distinguish from large vessel vasculitis, and it has been suggested that periarterial fibroplasia is a form of idiopathic retroperitoneal fibrosis [68,69].

Approach to Interpretation

Gross and microscopic pathology. Renal artery dysplasia is divided into several categories, all of which display an abnormal distribution of smooth muscle or collagenous connective tissue

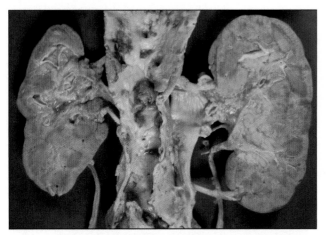

FIGURE 12.31: *Atherosclerotic renal artery stenosis. The kidney on the left (right kidney) is reduced to less than two-thirds the size of the opposite kidney because of atherosclerotic narrowing of the main and accessory renal arteries.*

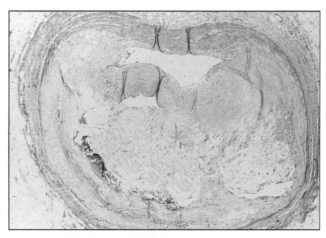

FIGURE 12.32: *Atherosclerosis of a renal artery. There is an inner core of necrotic, extracellular fatty material containing cholesterol clefts (H&E, × 20).*

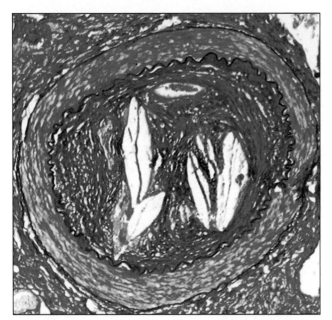

FIGURE 12.33: *Atheromatous embolus. Angular, biconcave cholesterol clefts occlude an interlobular artery. The cholesterol clefts are surrounded by intimal fibrous tissue. (Aldehyde fuchsin, Van Gieson, × 100).*

within the wall of the main renal artery and its major branches [68,69]. Five categories of renal artery dysplasia are presented in Table 12.3.

In order to study the pathology of renal artery dysplasia, it is necessary to take tissue blocks that sample the arteries both longitudinally and in cross-section. Trichrome and elastic tissue stains are also needed to evaluate abnormalities in the distribution of smooth muscle, collagen, and elastic tissue. Two of the most common forms of fibromuscular dysplasia are illustrated in (Figure 12.34 A,B). The most common is medial fibroplasia that shows segments of medial attenuation alternating with segments of medial thickening creating a series of sacculations described in renal arteriograms as a "string of beads." The next most common

is medial fibroplasia that consists of the replacement of the outer media by fibrous and sometimes vascularized fibrous tissue.

Dissecting renal artery aneurysms are found in 5 to 10 percent of cases of renal artery stenosis [68]. Dissections commonly extend from dissecting aortic aneurysms but can be limited to the renal artery. Limited dissections of the renal artery can be seen in association with renal artery dysplasia. This seems to be most common with intimal and perimedial fibroplasia [68].

Neurofibromatosis

The renal arteries of approximately 50 percent of neurofibromatosis patients are obstructed by nodules of myointimal cells (Figure 12.35). The condition affects arteries of all sizes and can cause renovascular hypertension [70]. Neurofibromatosis type 1 (NF1) represents the majority of cases of the disease and is characterized by café au lait spots, multiple neurofibromas, occasional sarcomas, and renovascular hypertension, among other findings. It is caused by a mutation in the NF1 gene that maps to chromosome 17q11.2, and can be diagnosed by molecular genetic methods [71]. Patients with neurofibromatosis frequently have pheochromocytomas, which should be considered in the differential diagnosis of their hypertension [72].

Renovascular Hypertension

Clinical and Laboratory Diagnosis

The methods for diagnosing renovascular hypertension have their origins in the studies of the Goldblatt kidney [9,59]. Blood flow is diminished to a kidney that has a narrowed renal artery. The lowered perfusion pressure at the level of the afferent arteriole causes hyperplasia of the juxtaglomerular apparatus and the increased secretion of renin (Figure 12.36).

Renin is an enzyme that acts on the renin substrate angiotensinogen to produce angiotensin I. Angiotensin-converting enzyme (ACE) cleaves two peptides from angiotensin I to produce angiotensin II. Angiotensin II is a potent vasoconstrictor

TABLE 12.3 Categories of Fibromuscular Dysplasia [68,69]

Category (% Affected Patients)	Sex Predilection	Age at Diagnosis	Extrarenal Disease	Pathologic Changes
Medial fibroplasia (60-80%)	Female/male ratio 8:1	20–50 yrs	Carotid, coronary, mesenteric, hepatic, iliac arteries	Marked medial thinning that alternates with medial segments thickened by irregularly distributed smooth muscle bundles. Produces multiple aneurysmal sacculations of the renal artery and its main branches.
Perimedial fibroplasia (10-25%)	Female	< 30 yrs	None	Smooth muscle of outer media of midportion of renal artery replaced by collagenous and sometimes neovascularized connective tissue. Frequently bilateral. Often complicated by thrombosis.
Medial hyperplasia (1–5%)	None	Adolescence to late middle age	None	Short segments of renal artery narrowed by markedly thickened media composed of increased smooth muscle cells. No fibrosis.
Intimal fibroplasia (1–5%)	Female in childbearing age	Childhood and adult forms	Cerebral, mesenteric arteries; arteries to limbs.	Lumina narrowed by concentrically or eccentrically thickened intima containing ground substance, collagen fibers, and myointimal cells.
Periarterial fibroplasia (<1%)	None	15–30 yrs	None	Chronic inflammation and fibrous tissue surrounds adventitia and extends into periarterial fat.

and, in addition, promotes aldosterone synthesis and secretion by the zona glomerulosa of the adrenal cortex. High renin levels contribute to hypertension by means of both vasoconstriction and the expansion of extracellular volume by aldosterone-mediated salt retention. Screening tests for renovascular hypertension that are useful for primary care patients are the plasma renin assay; and the measurement of plasma renin activity and blood pressure after the administration of an ACE inhibitor (the captopril test) [9,59].

Patients with positive screening tests and patients who have clinical findings or a clinical history suspicious of renovascular hypertension can be subjected to more costly and more invasive procedures. Moderate and severe hypertension or a recent increase in blood pressure is more likely to be associated with renal vascular stenosis than stable mild hypertension. A hypertensive patient older than 50 years with generalized atherosclerosis has a high likelihood of having atherosclerotic narrowing of a renal artery; hypertension in children and young adults is frequently associated with renal artery dysplasia.

Renal scintigraphy is frequently used to screen patients with a high suspicion of renovascular hypertension [17]. The procedure radiographically visualizes the renal cortex and provides a measure of glomerular filtration rate. Bilateral renal artery stenosis is present in 29 percent of patients with renovascular hypertension [59]. Reduction in perfusion is not equal in the two kidneys, and excretory differences can be brought out by scintigraphy following a dose of captopril (captopril scintigraphy), which is estimated to have a 90 percent sensitivity and a

95 percent specificity for the diagnosis of renovascular hypertension.

Intrarenal arteriograms are the gold standard for identifying a stenotic renal artery [17]. A narrowed renal artery having a reduced pressure gradient across the stenotic segment of greater than 10 to 15 mmHg suggest the presence of renovascular hypertension. A lower pressure gradient indicates that a stenosis is not physiological significance. More recently, magnetic resonance angiography and computed axial tomography have become the preferred methods for evaluating renal artery stenosis [17].

Renal vein renin assays can be used to determine whether stenosis is functionally significant [17]. An ischemic kidney produces high renin levels, and renin levels are suppressed in the contralateral nonischemic kidney. A renin ratio of greater than 1.5 between the sample from the renal vein of an ischemic kidney and the renal vein of the contralateral kidney has a reported sensitivity of 80 percent and specificity of 62 percent for the diagnosis of renovascular hypertension. Because of the low predictive value, renal vein renin assays are not a routinely recommended procedure [17].

Treatment and Prognosis

Patients with renovascular hypertension can be successfully treated pharmacologically [9,17]. The intensity of the therapy and its duration over the lifetime of the patient will weigh in the decision to undertake a revascularizing procedure, either surgery or percutaneous transluminal angioplasty.

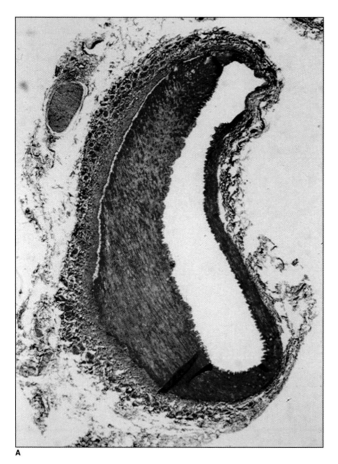
A

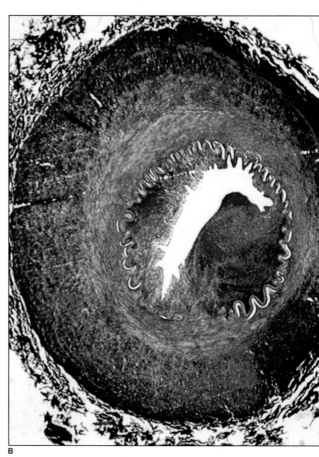
B

FIGURE 12.34: *Renal artery dysplasia. A:Medial fibroplasia showing thinning of the media along the half of the artery wall on the right side of the photomicrograph. B: Perimedial fibroplasia in which there is replacement of the outer media by collagenized connective tissue. (Masson trichrome, × 20).*

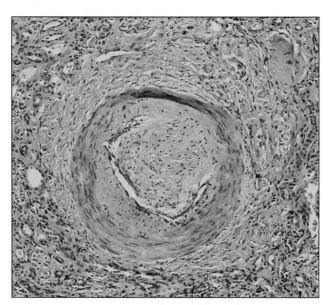

FIGURE 12.35: *Neurofibromatosis Type 1. A nodule of myointimal cells obstructs an interlobular artery. (H&E, × 200).*

Revascularization is reported to cure hypertension in 27 percent and to lower blood pressure in 75 percent of patients with fibromuscular dysplasia [73]. With atherosclerotic reno-vascular hypertension, hypertension is rarely cured, but blood pressure is reported as being improved in 29 percent to as many as 75 percent of patients [74]. Although blood pressure may not be corrected, revascularization of atherosclerotic arteries may still be beneficial. The procedures can be used to restore or improve renal function in patients who develop renal failure because of renal artery obstruction [60]. Atherosclerotic reno-vascular disease has a poor prognosis that reflects the advanced age of the patients and the presence of comorbid coronary and cerebral artery disease. Perioperative and late postprocedural deaths are most frequently caused by myocardial infarction, and the ten-year survival rate is approximately 25 percent [75].

LARGE VESSEL VASCULITIS

Introduction

The Chapel Hill Consensus Conference has defined ten clinical and pathologic types of vasculitis that can involve the kidney [76,77]:

1. Wegener's granulomatosis
2. Microscopic polyangiitis
3. Churg–Strauss syndrome
4. Essential cryoglobulinemic vasculitis

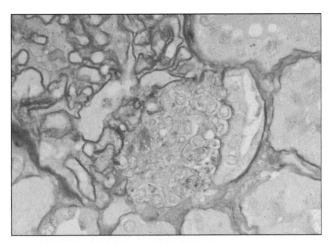

FIGURE 12.36: *Renovascular hypertension. A glomerulus from an ischemic kidney reveals hyperplasia of the juxtaglomerular apparatus. (Alcian blue PAS, × 400).*

5. Henoch–Schonlein purpura
6. Cutaneous leukocytoclastic vasculitis
7. Classic polyarteritis nodosa
8. Giant cell (temporal) arteritis
9. Takayasu's arteritis
10. Kawasaki disease

The first six of these forms of vasculitis affect small arteries, arterioles, capillaries, and venules. The first three are strongly associated with antineutrophil cytoplasmic antibodies (ANCA) that current evidence indicates are pathogenetically related to the vascular injury [77]. A glomerulonephritis usually occurs with Wegeners granulomatosis, microscopic polyangitiis, essential cryoglobulinemic vasculitis, and Henoch–Schonlein purpura and is sometimes seen with a cutaneous leukocytoclastic glomerulonephritis and Churg–Strauss syndrome. All of the small vessel vasculitides may be associated with a pulmonary-renal syndrome. It is the presence of glomerulonephritis, pulmonary involvement, and ANCA in microscopic polyangiitis (older synonym: microscopic polyarteritis) that has allowed the distinction of microscopic polyangiitis from classical polyarteritis in which these findings are characteristically absent.

The small vessel vasculitides are described in Chapter 6. This section covers vasculitis that affects large and medium-size arteries. It includes polyarteritis nodosa and Kawasaki disease that affect medium-sized arteries and giant cell (temporal) arteritis and Takayasu's arteritis that involve large and medium sized arteries.

Epidemiology and Clinical Presentation

Polyarteritis nodosa is most common between the ages of 40 and 60 years and occurs at a 2:1 ratio of males over females [78,79]. A chronic hepatitis B infection is found in approximately 10 percent of patients. The clinical course begins with fever, myalgia, and weight loss. The kidneys, heart, liver, GI tract, and peripheral nerves are commonly affected; symptoms or findings can include subcutaneous nodules, gastrointestinal pain, peripheral neuropathies, congestive heart failure, and

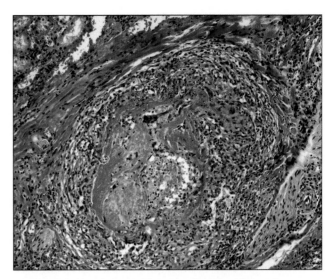

FIGURE 12.37: *Polyarteritis nodosa. Active phase of a vasculitis. There is an infiltrate composed predominantly of lymphocytes, monocytes, and plasma cells throughout the wall of an interlobar artery. (H&E, × 400).*

myocardial infarction. Testicular or leg pain are frequently experienced as a result of vasculitis in these parts of the body. Hypertension, sometimes at malignant levels, is seen in approximately 40 percent of patients with polyarteritis nodosa.

Kawasaki disease (synonym, mucocutaneous lymph node syndrome) is a disease of unknown but possible infectious etiology of infants or young children [80,81]. It is characterized by high temperatures and an erythematous mucocutaneous rash that lasts about ten days. Twenty to fifty percent of patients develop a vasculitis and aneurysms of the coronary arteries.

Giant cell arteritis is a disease of the elderly, and the majority of patients are more than 75 years old [79,82]. The condition most commonly involves the large and medium-sized extracranial arteries of the head and neck, but it can affect any site of the body. The usual symptoms are throbbing headache, skin tenderness localized to the temporal region of the head, and visual disturbances. Temporary or permanent blindness can occur with involvement of the ophthalmic arteries. Visual loss is the most critical problem; temporal artery biopsies are frequently performed to evaluate headache and visual abnormalities. In approximately 50 percent of patients, giant cell arteritis overlaps with polymyalgia rheumatica (a syndrome of hip, thigh, neck, and shoulder pain) that can precede, follow, or coexist with the vasculitis.

Takayasu's arteritis is a panarteritis with a predilection for young women that produces constricting adventitial and intimal fibrosis of the aorta and its main branches [79,83]. Symptoms are the result of ischemia that causes limb claudication, intestinal angina, and central nervous system symptoms.

Approach to Interpretationy

Polyarteritis Nodosa

In the acute phase, polyarteritis nodosa displays fibrinoid necrosis of the involved arteries and an early cellular infiltrate of neutrophils with variable numbers of eosinophils that later

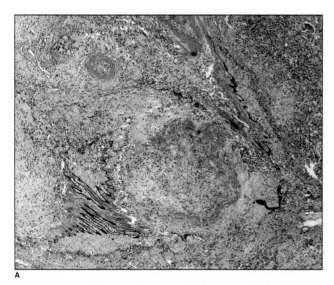

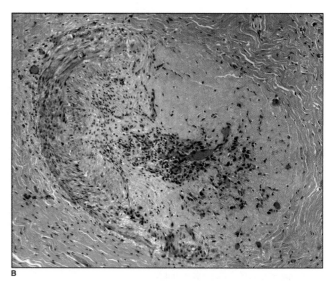

A

B

FIGURE 12.38: *Polyarteritis nodosa. A: Healing vasculitis. The amount of inflammation is reduced. Some fibrinous exudate remains and the wall of the artery is disrupted by fibrous tissue (Verhoef, Van Gieson; x400). B: Healed vasculitis. There is little remaining inflammation. The lumen of the artery is replaced by hemosiderin containing fibrous tissue. (H&E, × 400).*

becomes predominantly composed of lymphocytes, plasma cells, and monocytes (Figure 12.37). The vascular lesions progress through acute, healing, and healed phases [79]. Inflammation begins to disappear from the healing and healed vasculitis (Figure 12.38 A,B), eventually leaving lumina and media replaced by hemosiderin-containing fibrous tissue. In the kidney, the vasculitis produces renal infarcts and renal artery aneurysms. Elastic tissue stains are essential for identifying the disrupted elastic lamina in the destroyed segments of artery, and such findings or the presence of aneurysms may provide the only evidence of vasculitis in treated patients.

Kawasaki Disease

The vasculitis of Kawasaki disease affects coronary, axillary, subclavian, and renal arteries [80,81]. The renal arteries are involved in 50 to 75 percent of cases [79]. Microscopically, the arteries display transmural edema and inflammation but with less fibrinoid necrosis than is seen with the vasculitis of polyarteritis nodosa [79]. The infantile form of polyarteritis nodosa can enter the differential diagnosis although most of these cases appear to have been examples of Kawasaki disease [79]. Cases of Kawasaki disease examined after the acute stage of the illness usually reveal a healed vasculitis with thrombosis or aneurysms.

Giant Cell (Temporal) Arteritis

Arteries involved by giant cell arteritis show an infiltrate of lymphocytes, histiocytes, and giant cells that is associated with disruption of the internal elastic lamina and intimal thickening (Figure 12.39). The inflammation can involve all layers of the vessel, or it may be concentrated in the inner media where giant cells are clustered along a fragmented internal elastic lamina. Giant cell arteritis is typically segmental in its distribution along an artery, and step sectioning of multiple blocks of tissue may be necessary to show inflammation or giant cells.

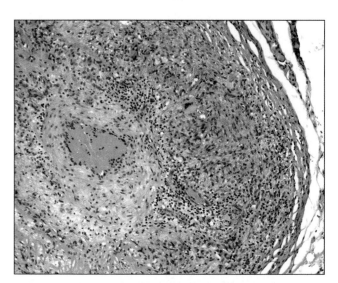

FIGURE 12.39: *Giant cell arteritis. Vasculitis composed of mononuclear inflammatory cells without fibrinoid necrosis in a temporal artery. The inflammation tends to concentrate adjacent to the internal elastic lamina where giant cells are found. (H&E, × 100).*

Giant cell arteritis is a chronic vasculitis that does not produce a notable amount of fibrinoid necrosis [79,84]. The presence of granulomatous inflammation with pronounced fibrinoid necrosis should raise the differential diagnosis of Wegener's granulomatosis. In some cases of polyarteritis nodosa, the inflammation has a granulomatous appearance, and both polyarteritis and Wegener's vasculitis can involve the temporal arteries. Sometimes, a granulomatous arteritis is identified that cannot be classified clinically or histopathologically as temporal arteritis, Wegener's granulomatosis, or polyarteritis nodosa [82]. Some of these cases have been associated with phenytoin hypersensitivity. In other cases, the pathogenesis is unknown.

Takayasu's Arteritis

Takayasu's arteritis rarely involves the intrarenal arteries. It is mainly a disease of the aorta and its main branches [79,83]. Narrowing of the renal artery is common, and renovascular hypertension is seen in the majority of patients. Takayasu's arteritis affects all layers of the arterial wall. In early stages, inflammation composed of lymphocytes, plasma cells, histiocytes, and multinucleated giant cells is concentrated in the outer media and adventitia. Later, when inflammation subsides, the media is disrupted and marked intimal and adventitial fibrosis thickens artery walls and narrows their lumens. Thrombosis often complicates stenosis of the aortic branches.

Clinical Course, Prognosis, and Treatment

Classic polyarteritis nodosa is treated with corticosteroids and cyclophosphamide. Results have been excellent with three-year survival rates of 90 percent. Therapeutic failures usually occur within the first year with deaths being the result of opportunistic infections or uncontrolled vasculitis attributed to undertreatment [85]. Kawasaki disease is an acute illness that is treated at its onset with high-dose intravenous gammaglobulin and aspirin, the latter initially at high dose to inhibit inflammation and then at low dose as an antiplatelet agent [80]. Most early deaths and long-term morbidity are the result of cardiac involvement [86]. Glucocorticoids are contraindicated because their use has been associated with the development of aneurysms.

Glucocorticoids are the mainstay for the treatment of giant cell arteritis and Takayasu's arteritis. Giant cell arteritis is a self-limited illness that usually lasts two years or less [87]. Takayasu's arteritis has an indolent but typically progressive course with a five-year survival of 83 percent in one major series [88].

RENAL VEIN THROMBOSIS

Introduction

Renal vein thrombosis occurs most often in one of three clinical settings: (1) with the nephrotic syndrome, (2) in dehydrated infants, and (3) with trauma to, or compression of, the kidneys. Compression may be due to such conditions as abdominal aortic aneurysms or neoplastic enlargement of lymph nodes. Renal vein thrombosis has been found with several types of renal diseases including the antiphospholipid syndrome, but it is especially common with membranous glomerulonephropathy [89,90]. Acute renal vein thrombosis presents as gross hematuria, flank pain, and a rapid deterioration in renal function, but vein obstruction is more often chronic and patients are asymptomatic.

Clinical Presentation

Experimental and clinical data have shown that the nephrotic syndrome is the cause, not the result, of renal vein thrombosis. Nephrotic syndrome is associated with hypercoaguability that may be secondary to the urinary loss of the plasma anticoagulants antithrombin III, protein C, or protein S [90,91]. Elevated fibrinogen levels, enhanced platelet aggregation, and increased inhibition of fibrinolysis due to urinary plasminogen loss have been demonstrated and may contribute to the clotting tendency. Thrombosis of extrarenal veins is prone to develop, and deep vein thrombosis with pulmonary thromboemboli is a common cause of death in nephrotic syndrome patients who have renal vein thrombosis [91,92].

Gross and Microscopic Pathology

Thrombi in different stages of organization are found in the main renal vein, its lobar branches, and in the smaller intrarenal veins [92]. In some cases, it is thought that thrombi form first in the small veins and spread to the main renal vein. In other cases, only the lobar or main renal veins are thrombosed (Figure 12.40A,B). Histologically, interstitial edema, and glomerular capillary congestion with margination of neutrophils have been associated with renal vein thrombosis (Figure 12.41). These changes are nonspecific and are not generally helpful findings, and venous thrombi, themselves, are only rarely seen in renal biopsies. Clinical diagnosis is best established by renal vein doppler ultrasonography [93].

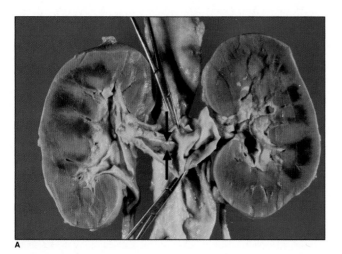

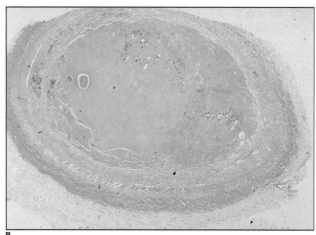

A   B

FIGURE 12.40: *Renal vein thrombosis in a 21 year old patient with minimal change nephrotic syndrome associated with Hodgkins Disease. A: A thrombus is shown in the main renal vein (arrow). B: The thrombus occludes the renal vein and is organized to the vein wall. (H&E, ×20).*

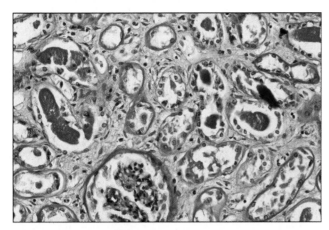

FIGURE 12.41: *The renal cortex of the patient with the renal vein thrombosis shown in the previous illustration. There is marked interstitial edema and degenerative tubular changes.*

Prognosis and Treatment

Patients can be successfully treated by anticoagulation. Prophylactic anticoagulation with low-molecular-weight heparin has been advocated for patients with membranous nephropathy that have levels of proteinuria at or exceeding 20 grams per day [93,94]. Prognosis is related to the risk of pulmonary emboli and the success of preventing their development.

REFERENCES

1. United States Renal Data Service 2003 Annual Data Report *Am J Kidney Dis* 2003;42(suppl.5):S1–S230.
2. Hughson MD, Douglas-Denton R, Bertram JF, Hoy WE. Hypertension, glomerular number, and birth weight in African American and white subjects in the southeastern United States. *Kidney Int* 2006;69:671–8.
3. Textor SC, Bakris GL. Hypertension. *NephSAP* 2006; 5(No.5):288–96.
4. Fields LE, Burt VL, Cutler JA, Hughes J, Roccella EJ, Sorlie P. The burden of adult hypertension in the United States 1999 to 2000. A rising tide. *Hypertension* 2004;44:398–404.
5. World Health Organization. Arterial hypertension: report of a WHO expert committee. *WHO* Technical Report Series No. 1978;628:1.
6. Chobanian AV, Bakris GL, Black HR, Cushman WC, Green LA, Izzo JL, Jones DW, Materson BJ, Oparil S, Wright JT, Rocella EJ. Seventh report of the National Joint Committee on Prevention, Detection, Evaluation, and Treatment of High Blood Pressure. *Hypertension* 2003;42:1206–52.
7. Joint National Committee on Detection, Evaluation, and Treatment of High Blood Pressure. The Fifth Report of the Joint National Committee on Detection, Evaluation, and Treatment of High Blood Pressure (JNCV). *Arch Intern Med* 1993;153:154–83.
8. Oparil S, "Arterial hypertension" in CJ Bennett, , F Plum(eds.), *Cecil Textbook of Medicine* (Philadelphia, PA: W.B. Sanders Co, 1996), pp. 256–71.
9. Segura J, Ruilope LM, "Renal parenchymal hypertension, posttransplant hypertension, Renovascular hypertension" in EJ Battegay, GY Lip, GL Bakris (eds.), *Hypertension. Principles and Practice* (Boca Raton, FL: Taylor & Francis, 2005), pp.713–32.
10. Gami AS, Somers VK, "Obstructive sleep apnea" in S Oparil, MA Weber (eds.), *Hypertension. Companion to Brenner & Rector's The Kidney* (Elsevier, 2005) pp. 765–773.
11. Young WF. "Adrenal cortex hypertension" in S Oparil, MA Weber (eds.), *Hypertension. Companion to Brenner & Rector's The Kidney* (Elsevier Inc., 2005), pp.792–806.
12. Wofford MR, Jones DW, "Pheochromocytoma: detection and management" in S Oparil, , MA Weber (eds.), *Hypertension. Companion to Brenner & Rector's The Kidney* (Elsevier Inc., 2005), pp. 807–12.
13. Bie P, Wamberg S, Kjolby M. Volume natriuresis vs. pressure natriuresis. *Acta Physiol Scand* 2004;181:495–503.
14. Bianchi G, Tripodi G. Genetics of hypertension: the adducing paradigm. *Ann NY Acad Sci* 2003;986:660–8.
15. Zakrzewski-Jakubiak M, de Denus S, Dube MP, Belanger F, White M. Ten renin-angiotensin system-related gene polymorphisms in maximally treated Caucasian patients with heart failure. *Brit J Clin Pharmacol* 2008;65:925–32.
16. Garovic VD, Hilliard AA, Turner ST. Monogenic forms of low-renin hypertension. Review. *Nat Clin Pract Nephrol* 2006;2:624–30.
17. Spitalewitz S, Reiser IW, "Renovascular hypertension: diagnosis and management" in S Oparil, Weber MA (eds.): *Hypertension. Companion to Brenner & Rector's The Kidney* (Elsevier Inc., 2005) pp. 774–791.
18. Bell, ET. *Renal Diseases*. 2nd Ed (Lea & Febigera, 1950)
19. Blythe WB, Maddux FW. Hypertension as causative diagnosis of patients entering end-stage renal disease programs in the United States from 1980 to 1986. *Am J Kidney Dis* 1991;18:33.
20. Heptinstall RH, "Hypertension I: essential hypertension"in RH Heptinstall (ed,), *Pathology of the Kidney*, 4th edition. (Boston, MA: Little, Brown,1993) p. 951.
21. Kasiske BL. Relationship between vascular disease and age associated changes in the human kidney. *Kidney Int* 1987;31:1153.
22. Tracy RE, Bhandaru SY, Oalmann MC et al. Blood pressure and nephrosclerosis in black and white men and women aged 25 to 54. *Mod Pathol* 1991;4:602.
23. Tracy RE. Blood pressure related separately to parenchymal fibrosis and vasculopathy of the kidney. *Am J Kidney Dis* 1992;20:124–31.
24. Olson JL, "Renal disease caused by hypertension" in JC Jennette, JL Olson, MM Schwartz, FG Silva (eds.), *Heptinstall's Pathology of the Kidney*, 6th edition. (Philadelphia, PA: Lippincott, Williams & Wilkins, 2006), p. 937.
25. Thomsen OF, Anderson AR, Christensen JS et al. Renal changes in long-term type I (insulin-dependent) diabetic patients with and without clinical nephropathy: a light microscopy, morphometric study of autopsy material. *Diabetologia* 1984;26:361.
26. Ross R. The pathogenesis of atherosclerosis-an update. *N Engl J Med* 1986;314:488–500.
27. Tracy RE, Malcom GT, Oalmann MC et al. Nephrosclerosis, glycohemoglobin, cholesterol and smoking in subjects dying of coronary heart disease. *Mod Pathol* 1994;7:301.
28. Hughson MD, Johnson K, Young RL, et al. Glomerular size and glomerulosclerosis. Relationships to disease categories,

glomerular solidification, and ischemic obsolescence. *Am J Kidney Dis* 2002;39:649–88.

29. Marcotoni C, Ma L-T, Federspeil C, Fogo A. Hypertensive nephrosclerosis in African Americans versus Caucasians. *Kidney Int* 2002;62:172.

30. Valenzuela R, Gogate PA, Deodhar SD et al. Hyalin arteriolar nephrosclerosis. Immunofluorescent findings in the vascular lesions. *Lab Invest* 1980;43:530.

31. Nagle RB, Kohnen PW, Bulger RE et al. Ultrastructure of human renal obsolescent glomeruli. *Lab Invest* 1969;21:519.

32. Narvarte J, Prive M, Saba SR et al. Proteinuria in hypertension. *Am J Kidney Dis* 1987;10:408.

33. McManus JFA, Hughson MD, Fitts CT et al. Studies in end-stage kidneys. I. Nodule formation in intrarenal arteries and arterioles. *Lab Invest* 1977;37:339.

34. Jones DB. Arterial and glomerular lesions associated with severe hypertension. *Lab Invest* 197;31:303.

35. Pitcock JA, Johnson JG, Share L et al. Malignant hypertension due to musculomucoid intimal hyper plasia of intrarenal arteries. *Circ Res, suppl.* 1975;1, 36:S133.

36. Heptinstall RH. Malignant hypertension: a study of fifty-one cases. *J Pathol Bacteriol* 1953;65:423.

37. Bohle A, Helmchen U, Grund RE et al. Malignant nephrosclerosis in patients with hemolytic uremic syndrome (primary malignant nephrosclerosis). *Curr Top Pathol* 1977;65:81.

38. Kincaid-Smith P: The Kidney. *A Clinico-pathological Study.* Blackwell Scientific, Oxford, 1975.

39. Cannon PJ, Hassar M, Case DB et al. The relationship of hypertension and renal failure in scleroderma (progressive systemic sclerosis) to structural and functional abnormalities of the renal cortical circulation. *Medicine (Baltimore)* 1974;53:1.

40. Esmon CT: Cell mediated events that control blood coagulation and vascular injury. *Annu Rev Cell Biol* 1993;9:1.

41. Jennette JC, Falk RJ. Current concepts in renal pathology. The pathology of vasculitis involving the kidney. *Am J Kidney Dis* 1994;24:130.

42. Leishman AWD. Observations on prognosis in hypertension. *BMJ* 1953;1:1131–5.

43. Klag MJ, Whelton PK, Randall BL, Neaton JD, Brancati FL, Ford CE, Shulman NB, Stamler J. Blood pressure and end-stage renal disease in men. *N Eng J Med* 1996;334:13–18.

44. Leishman AWD. Hypertension-treated and untreated-a study of 400 cases. *BMJ* 1961;1:1361–8.

45. Hamilton M, Thomson EN, Wisniewski TKM. The role of blood pressure control in preventing complications of hypertension. *Lancet* 1964;1:235–8.

46. Veterans Administration Cooperative Study Group on Antihypertensive Agents. Effects of treatment on morbidity in hypertension. Results in patients with diastolic blood pressures averaging 115 through 129 mmHg. *JAMA* 1967;202:1028.

47. Hypertension Detection and Follow-up Program Cooperative Group. Five year findings of the hypertension and detection follow-up program. I. Reduction in mortality of persons with high blood pressure, including mild hypertension. *JAMA* 1979;242:2562.

48. Hypertension Detection and Follow-up Cooperative Group. The effect of treatment on mortality in "mild" hypertension. Results of the Hypertension Detection and Follow-up Program. *N Engl J Med* 1982;307:976.

49. Blyth WB, Maddux FW. Hypertension as a causative diagnosis of patients entering end-stage renal disease programs in the United States from 1980 to 1986. *Am J Kidney Dis* 1981;18:33.

50. McClellan W, Tuttle E, and Issa A. Racial differences in the incidence of hypertensive end-stage renal disease (ESRD) are not entirely explained by differences in the prevalence of hypertension. *Amer J Kidney Dis* 1988;12:285.

51. Segura J, Campoc C, Gil P et al. Development of chronic kidney disease and cardiovascular prognosis in essential hypertensive patients. *J Am Soc Nephrol* 2004;15:1616–22.

52. Rostand SG, Brown G, Kirk KA et al. Renal insufficiency in treated essential hypertension. *N Engl J Med* 1989;320:684.

53. Ferri C, Valentini G, Cozzi F et al. Systemic sclerosis: demographic, clinical, and serologic features and survival in 1,012 Italian patients. *Medicine (Baltimore)* 2002;81:139–53.

54. Steen VD, "Organ involvement: Renal" in PJ Clements, and DE Furst (eds.), *Systemic Sclerosis* (Baltimore, MD: Williams & Wilkins, 1996), pp. 425–39.

55. Jiminez SA, Derk CT: Following the molecular pathways toward an understanding of the pathogenesis of systemic sclerosis. *Ann Intern Med* 2004;140:37–50.

56. Bianchi DW. Fetal maternal cell trafficking: a new cause of disease? *Am J Med Genet* 2000;91:22–8.

57. D'Agati VD, Cannon PJ, Scleroderma (systemic sclerosis). in E Grishman, J Churg, MA Needle, VS Venkataseshan (eds.); *The Kidney in Collagen Vascular Diseases.* (New York, NY:Raven, 1993), p. 21.

58. Davis BA, Crook JE, Vestal RA et al. Prevalence of renovascular hypertension in patients with grade III or grade IV hypertensive retinopathy. *N Engl J Med* 1979;301:1273.

59. Mann SJ, Pickering TG: Detection of renovascular hypertension. State of the art: 1992, review. *Ann Intern Med* 1992;117:845.

60. Rimmer JM, Gennari FJ. Atherosclerotic renovascular disease and progressive renal failure. *Ann Intern Med* 1993;118:712.

61. Mailloux LV, Napolitano B, Bellucci AG et al. Renal vascular disease causing end-stage renal disease, incidence, clinical correlates, and outcomes: a 20 year experience. *Am J Kidney Dis* 1994;24:622.

62. Textor SC. Ischemic nephropathy: where do we go from here? *J Am Soc Nephrol* 2004;15:1974–82.

63. Fatica RA, Port FK, Young EW. Incidence trends and mortality in end-stage renal disease attributed to renovascular disease in the United States. *Am J Kidney Dis* 2001;37:1184–90.

64. Vidt DG. Geriatric hypertension of renovascular origin: diagnosis and clinical management. *Geriatrics* 1987;42:59.

65. Holley KE, Hunt JC, Brown AL et al. Renal artery stenosis. A clinical-pathologic study in normotensive and hypertensive patients. *Am J Med* 1964;37:14–22.

66. Bookstein JJ, Abrams HL, Buenger RE et al. Radiographic aspects of renovascular hypertension. Part 3. Appraisal of arteriography. *JAMA* 1972;221:368.

67. Lajoie G, Laszik Z, Nadasdy T, Silva FG. The renal-cardiac connection: renal parenchymal alterations in patients with heart disease. *Semin Nephrol* 1994;14: 441.

68. Luscher TF, Keller HM, Imhof HG et al. Fibromuscular hyperplasia: extension of the disease and therapeutic outcome. Results of the University Hospital Zurich Cooperative Study on Fibromuscular Hyperplasia. *Nephron, suppl.* 1986;1, 44:S109.

69. Slovut DP, Olin JW. Fibromuscular dysplasia. Current concepts. *N Eng J Med* 2004;350:1862–71.

70. Salyer WR, Salyer DC. The vascular lesions of neurofibromatosis. *Angiology* 1974;25:510.

71. Kayes LM, Burke W, Riccardi VM, et al. Deletions spanning the neurofibromatosis I gene: identification and phenotype of five patients. *Am J Hum Genet* 1994;54:424.

72. Kalif V, Shapiro B, Lloyd R et al. The spectrum of phaeochromocytoma in hypertensive patients with neurofibromatosis. *Arch Intern Med* 1982;142:2092.

73. Carmo M, Bower TC, Mozes G, et al. Surgical management of renal fibromuscular dysplasia: challenges in the endovascular era. *Ann Vasc Surg* 2005;19:208–217.

74. Garovic VD, Textor SC. Renovascular hypertension and ischemic nephropathy. *Circulation* 2005;112:1362–74.

75. Lawrie GM, Morris GC, Glaeser DH et al. Reno-vascular reconstruction: factors affecting long-term prognosis in 919 patients up to 31 years. *Am J Cadiol* 1989;63:1085.

76. Jennette JC, Falk RJ, Andrassy K et al. Nomenclature of systemic vasculitis. Proposal of an international consensus conference. *Arthritis Rheum* 1994;37:187.

77. Jennette JC, Thomas DB, "Pauci-immune and anti-neutrophil cytoplasmic antibody-mediated crescentic glomerulonephritis and vasculitis" in JC Jennette, JL Olson, MM Schwartz, FG Silva (eds.), *Heptinstall's Pathology of the Kidney*, 6th edition. (Philadelphia, PA: Lippincott, Williams & Wilkins, 2006), p. 643.

78. Lightfoot RW, Michel BA, Bloch DA et al.The American College of Rheumatology 1990 criteria for the classification of polyarteritis nodosa. *Arthritis Rheum* 1990;33:1108.

79. Jennette JC, Singh HK, "Renal involvement in polyarteritis nodosa, Kawasaki disease, Takayasu arteritis, and giant cell arteritis" in JC Jennette, JL Olson, MM Schwartz, FG Silva (eds.), *Heptinstall's Pathology of the Kidney*, 6th edition. (Philadelphia,PA:Lippincott, Williams & Wilkins, 2006) p.675.

80. Melish ME, Hicks RV. Kawasaki's syndrome: clinical features, pathophysiology, etiology and therapy. *J Rheumatol suppl.* 1990;24:2–10.

81. Wortman DW, Nelson AM: Kawasaki's syndrome. *Rheum Dis Clin North Am* 1990;16:363.

82. Hunder GG, Bloch DA, Michel BA et al. The American College of Rheumatology 1990 criteria for the classification of giant cell arteritis. *Arthritis Rheum* 1990;33:1122.

83. Arend WP, Michel BA, Bloch DA et al. The Ameri can College of Rheumatology 1990 criteria for the classification of Takayasu's arteritis. *Arthritis Rheum* 1990;33:1129.

84. Lie JT. Subcommittee on the Classification of Vasculitis: illustrated histopathological classification criteria for selected vasculitis syndromes. *Arthritis Rheum* 1990;33:1074.

85. Bourgarit A, Toumelin Pl, Pagnoux C, et al. for the French Vasculitis Study Group: Deaths occurring during the first year after treatment onset for polyarteritis nodosa, microscopic polyangiitis, and Churg-Straus syndrome: a retrospective analysis of causes and factors predictive of mortality based on 595 patients. *Medicine (Baltimore)* 2005;84:323–330.

86. Nakamura Y, Yanagawa H, Kawasaki T. Mortalityamong children with Kawasaki's disease in Japan. *N Engl J Med* 1992;326:1246.

87. Huston KA, Hunder GG, Lie JT et al. Temporal arteritis: a 25 year epidemiologic, clinical, and pathologic study. *Ann Intern Med* 1978;88:162.

88. Subramanyan R, Joy J, Bolokrishnan KG. Natural history of aortoarteritis (Takayasu's disease). *Circulation* 1989;*80:429.*

89. Uthman I, Khamashta M. Antiphospolipidsyndrome and the kidney. *Semin Arthritis Rheum* 2006;35:360.

90. Llach F. Hypercoaguability, renal vein thrombosis, and other thrombotic complications of nephrotic syndrome. *Kidney Int* 1985;28:429.

91. Harris RC, Ismail N: Extrarenal complications of the nephrotic syndrome. *Am J Kidney Dis* 1994;23:477.

92. Wagoner RD, Stanson AW, Holley KE et al: Renal vein thrombosis in idiopathic membranous glomerulopathy and nephrotic syndrome: incidence and significance. *Kidney Int* 1983;23:368.

93. Rostoker G, Durand-Zaleski I, Petit-Phar M, et al.: Prevention of the thrombotic complications of the nephrotic syndrome by the low-molecular-weight heparin enoxaparin. *Nephron* 1995;69:20.

94. Wu CH, Ko SF, Lee CH, et al. Successful outpatient treatment of renal vein thrombosis by low-molecular weight heparins in 3 patients with nephrotic syndrome. *Clin Nephrol* 2006;65:433.

CHAPTER 13

Cystic and Developmental Diseases

Arthur G. Weinberg, MD

INTRODUCTION

Cystic and developmental diseases of the kidney comprise a large group of diverse etiology (Table 13.1). Most are not encountered in renal biopsies, but may come to attention as nephrectomy specimens or at postmortem examination. Recent advances in molecular biology have provided important new insights into understanding the pathogenesis and nosology of these disorders [1–4]. Many of the genes that cause renal cystic

Table 13.1 Classification of Renal Cystic Disease

Dysplasia
Polycystic kidney disease (PKD)
    Autosomal dominant polycystic kidney disease (ADPKD)
    Autosomal recessive polycystic kidney disease (ARPKD)
Nephronophthisis/Medullary cystic disease complex
    Nephronophthisis (NPHP) – autosomal recessive
    Medullary cystic kidney disease (MCKD) – autosomal dominant
Glomerulocystic kidney disease (GCKD)
Medullary Sponge kidney (MSK)
Acquired renal cystic disease (see Chapter 15)

and developmental disease encode proteins that localize to the primary cilia/centrosome/basal body complex and are referred to as cystoproteins [5,6]. The terms polycystic kidney and polycystic kidney disease are usually reserved for autosomal dominant (ADPKD) and autosomal recessive polycystic kidney disease (ARPKD) and should not be applied to the various forms of renal dysplasia.

Gross examination of a kidney or a renal segment with cysts should include careful attention to the distribution of the cysts. Cortical cysts often distort the normally smooth renal surface, but small cysts can be obscured by the external renal capsule. Dilatation of the ureter and/or pelvicaliceal system suggestive of obstruction or reflux should be noted, and the drainage system opened along its entire length with a scissors. Initial examination of the cut surface of the kidney is best accomplished by a single vertical cut that extends from the lateral surface toward the hilum and bivalves the specimen. After bivalving the kidney, the external renal capsule should be stripped from one or both halves of the specimen to better assess the external renal surface and suggest areas for microscopic sampling. Stripping the capsule will not compromise microscopic evaluation of the outer renal cortex, but secondary scarring can cause the outer renal capsule to adhere tightly to the kidney and frustrate this effort. The size and distribution of cysts within the kidney are important in the differential diagnosis and should be documented. Some forms of cystic renal disease predispose to renal neoplasia and care should be taken to sample any suspicious solid areas.

The algorithmic approach to interpretation of cystic and developmental diseases of the kidney is illustrated in (Figure 13.1). When formulating a differential diagnosis for renal cystic disease, it is important to consider the age of the patient. Renal dysplasia and its variants are, by far, the most likely diagnosis in an infant or young child, particularly if there is an abnormality of urinary drainage or the disease is unilateral. Bilateral, large, cystic kidneys in an infant may also represent dysplasia, even in the absence of obstruction, but ADPKD, ARPKD, and glomerulocystic kidney disease (GCKD) can also present in this manner. Radial oriented elongate cysts are diagnostic of ARPKD; only microscopic evaluation can help to distinguish the other disorders.

The kidneys of older children and adults with ADPKD are large with cysts that involve both cortex and medulla. In most other forms of cystic disease in adults, the kidneys are of normal size or small. Cysts at the corticomedullary junction occur in nephronophthisis (NPHP) and medullary cystic kidney disease (MCKD), while cysts limited to the renal papillae are the hall-

mark of medullary sponge kidney. Adults with ARPKD can also have medullary cysts.

AUTOSOMAL DOMINANT POLYCYSTIC KIDNEY DISEASE

Epidemiology and Clinical Presentation

ADPKD in Adults

Autosomal dominant polycystic kidney disease (ADPKD) has a prevalence of approximately 1:1000. It is the third most common cause of end-stage renal disease (ESRD) in adults [3]; less than 5 percent of patients are identified in infancy and childhood. ADPKD is caused by mutation of the *PKD1* (85 percent) or *PKD2* (15 percent) genes, which encode polycystin 1 and polycystin 2 on chromosomes 16p and 4q, respectively. Approximately 10 percent of patients represent new mutations. A third genetic locus has been sought without success to explain rare families that lack identifiable *PKD1* or *PKD2* mutations. The principal clinical symptoms are hematuria, abdominal and flank pain, and hypertension. Urinary tract infection and urolithiasis are additional clinical problems. Progressive enlargement of the cysts gradually impairs function of the noncystic parenchyma and leads to renal insufficiency. Factors that correlate with more rapid disease progression include PKD1, male sex, disease onset before age 30 years, large renal size at diagnosis, hypertension before age 35 yars, early onset of gross hematuria, more than three pregnancies, and moderate proteinuria [7].

Renal disease evolves more slowly in PKD2 than PKD1. PKD1 patients become symptomatic at approximately 40 years of age and PKD2 patients a decade later. The median age of death or ESRD in PKD1 is 53 years; 10–15 years earlier than PKD2 [8]. Cysts enlarge at a relatively constant rate in individual patients and the rate of enlargement correlates with the total renal volume at presentation, independent of age [9]. PKD1 is clinically more severe than PKD2 because more cysts are present and develop earlier than in PKD2; not because the cysts in PKD1 grow at a faster rate [10]. The rate of cyst expansion is usually the same in both kidneys, but asymmetric disease evolution occurs in some children. Disease severity is highly variable within the same family. Renal function is inversely related to renal size and progression to renal failure is more rapid in patients with a renal volume >1500 ml, as measured by magnetic resonance imaging (MRI) [9].

ADPKD in Infancy and Childhood

While ADPKD is usually a disease of adults, it can be identified in utero and become symptomatic in infancy and childhood [11,12]. Oligohydramnios may accompany severely affected fetuses [13]. Sixty percent of children who carry *PKD1* mutations have sonographically detectable cysts by 5 years of age. By 18 years of age, cysts are detectable in 75 to 80 percent of PKD1 patients. ADPKD usually affects both kidneys symmetrically, but up to 17 percent of children present with apparently unilateral disease. Most children younger than 12 years have mild disease (less than ten cysts). Those with more than ten cysts at the time of initial evaluation have more rapid renal enlargement over time than children with mild disease, a pattern of

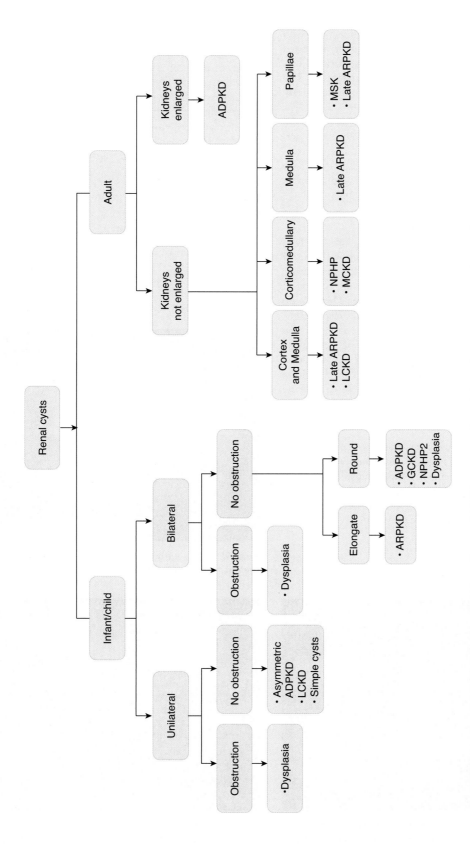

ADPKD : autosomal dominant polycystic kidney disease; **ARPKD** : autosomal recessive polycystic kidney disease; **GCKD** : glomerulocystic kidney disease; **NPHP** : nephronophthisis; **MCKD** : medullary cystic kidney disease; **MSK** : medullary sponge kidney; **LCKD** : localized cystic kidney disease

FIGURE 13.1: Algorithmic approach to the interpretation of cystic diseases of the kidney.

progression similar to adults. Hypertension, pain, and proteinuria occur in children with more numerous cysts. However, renal function is usually well preserved in childhood with the exception of rare children born with enlarged kidneys and who have early-onset hypertension. Previous reports that suggested a high rate of early mortality for patients with prenatally diagnosed disease may have reflected a bias of ascertainment. The long-term prognosis for children with ADPKD and adverse risk factors for disease progression remains unclear.

A rare form of severe ADPKD in childhood is associated with a chromosomal deletion that involves both *PKD1* and *TSC2*, the gene that causes tuberous sclerosis and which is contiguous with *PKD1* on chromosome 16. These patients have extrarenal manifestations of tuberous sclerosis in addition to renal cystic disease [14].

Extrarenal Manifestations of ADPKD

Hepatic cysts develop in the majority of patients with ADPKD, the prevalence increasing from 20 to 70 percent from the third to the seventh decade (Figures 13.2 and 13.3). They are larger and more numerous in females, but are usually not of clinical consequence except in a small minority of patients who develop severe hepatic dysfunction. The cysts are usually macroscopically evident, but microscopic bile duct hamartomas (von Meyenburg complexes) also occur. The majority of portal tracts are normal, in contrast to the diffuse ductal plate malformation (congenital hepatic fibrosis) that characterizes ARPKD. However, ductal plate malformation does occur in some patients with ADPKD [15]. Autosomal dominant polycystic disease of the liver is a genetically unrelated disorder in which renal cysts are absent.

Asymptomatic pancreatic cysts are detectable in up to 10 percent of ADPKD patients and cysts are sometimes present in the seminal vesicles. The most common noncystic manifestations of ADPKD are mitral-valve prolapse (25 percent) and intracranial aneurysms (8 to 10 percent). Aneurysms can also develop at other sites and colonic diverticula are more prevalent.

Gross Pathology

The cysts in early ADPKD are small and widely scattered with no abnormality of the intervening parenchyma. The typical kidney of advanced ADPKD is markedly enlarged yet maintains a reniform shape (Figure 13.4). A prominently bosselated external surface results from numerous thin-walled cysts that present beneath the renal capsule and vary from several mm. to several cm. in diameter. Most are translucent and straw-colored, but many are deep red or purple due to intracystic hemorrhage. The kidneys can exceed 40 cm in length, and weigh up to 8 kg. The cut surface recapitulates the external appearance with innumerable cysts of various size and color that obliterate the cortico-medullary architecture and leave little intervening parenchyma (Figure 13.5) The cysts impinge upon and distort, but do not obstruct the pelvicaliceal system. There is no morphologic distinction between PKD1 and PKD2 disease.

Light Microscopy

Small cysts are lined by cuboidal epithelium that becomes flattened as the cysts enlarge. Global glomerulosclerosis, tubular

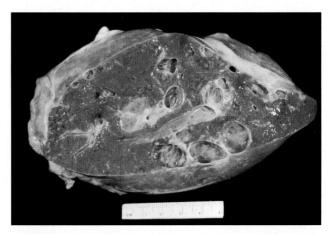

FIGURE 13.3: *Large spherical cysts are scattered through the cut surface of the liver.*

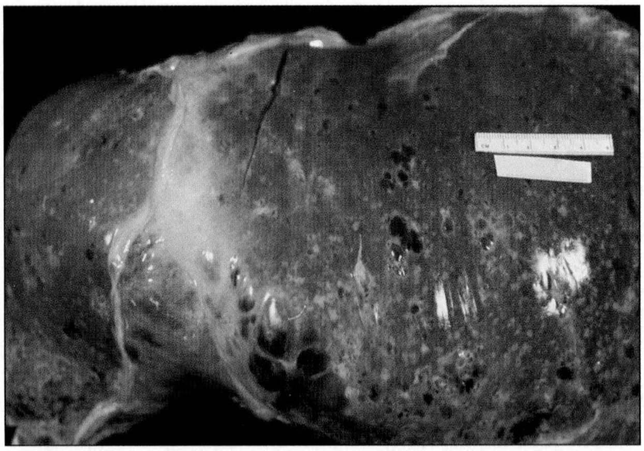

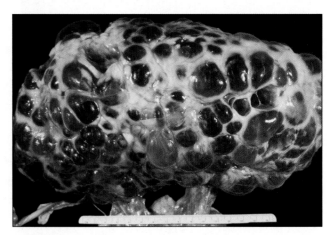

FIGURE 13.4: *ADPKD in a 50 year old female. Numerous cysts of various sizes produce marked nephromegaly and a bosselated external renal surface.*

FIGURE 13.2: *Liver of a 54-year-old female with ADPKD. Thin-walled cysts filled with clear fluid are visible beneath the hepatic capsule.*

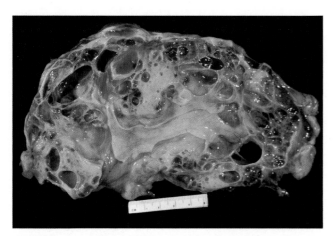

FIGURE 13.5: *The renal parenchyma in ADPKD is replaced by round cysts filled with translucent fluid that varies from clear to maroon. The pelvicaliceal system is distorted, but widely patent.*

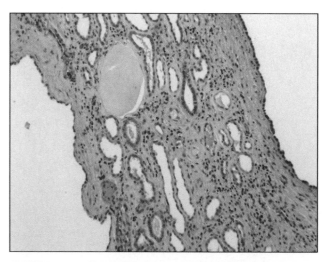

FIGURE 13.6: *Septa between the cysts of ADPKD are fibrotic with tubular atrophy and mild chronic inflammation (× 200).*

atrophy, thickened tubular basement membranes, interstitial fibrosis, and chronic inflammation are present in the intervening parenchyma and correlate with the severity of clinical renal disease (Figure 13.6) Cystic dilatation of Bowman's space is often present in non sclerotic glomeruli and glomerulocystic change can be the predominant finding in infants with ADPKD (Figures 13.7 and 13.8) [13]. Affected infants also have small renal medullae with a cellular interstitium that may condense into peritubular fibromuscular collars and resemble medullary dysplasia. Arterial and arteriolar sclerosis is a prominent feature of advanced disease and reflects the frequent occurrence of significant hypertension in ADPKD patients.

Epithelial hyperplasia and micropolyps with fibrovascular cores are frequent within the cysts, even in patients with early disease and no history of dialysis [16] (Figure 13.9). Microscopic adenomas occur in approximately 20 percent of patients with advanced disease [17]. These epithelial lesions reflect underlying dysregulation of cell proliferation that is intrinsic to the molecular pathobiology of ADPKD. Adenocarcinoma is a relatively uncommon complication and its prevalence is similar to the general population. However, adenocarcinoma in ADPKD occurs at a younger age and is more often bilateral, multicentric, and sarcomatoid [18].

Differential Diagnosis

No other cystic renal disease produces the massive bilateral renal enlargement found in adults with ADPKD. The diagnosis may be more problematic in a young child with precocious onset of ADPKD or when the disease presents asymmetrically in the absence of a positive family history. Distinguishing late presentation of ARPKD from early presentation of ADPKD can also be problematic in the absence of a family history, however, renal enlargement is typically more pronounced in ADPKD and ductal plate malformation of the liver is usually absent. Neonatal ADPKD can be distinguished from ARPKD by the absence of radially arrayed elongate cysts in the kidneys and the presence of normal portal tracts in the liver. In the absence of obstruction, extrarenal disease or a family history of ADPKD, distinction of neonatal ADPKD from diffuse bilat-

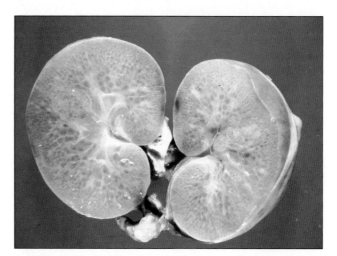

FIGURE 13.7: *Kidney from the fetus of a mother with ADPKD. Small round cysts are present throughout the kidney. The kidney somewhat resembles ARPKD, but the cysts are spherical rather than elongate. (Courtesy of Dr. Laura Finn., Children's Hospital and Regional Medical Center, Seattle, Washington).*

eral renal dysplasia or from glomerulocystic kidney disease (GCKD) may not be possible. In this situation, the risk for cystic disease in a subsequent pregnancy is as high as 50 percent, regardless of the precise diagnosis. Infantile nephronophthisis (NPHP2) should also be included in the differential diagnosis.

A lesion that can be confused with unilateral presentation of ADPKD in the absence of a positive family history is unilateral cystic renal disease, also referred to as localized or segmental cystic kidney disease (LCKD) [19]. Cysts are limited to one kidney except for an occasional small cyst in the contralateral side. The cysts can be segmental or diffusely involve the kidney with little intervening residual normal parenchyma (Figure 13.10). The gross and microscopic appearance of the cysts is similar to ADPKD. In addition to the negative family history, which alone does not exclude ADPKD, LCKD is

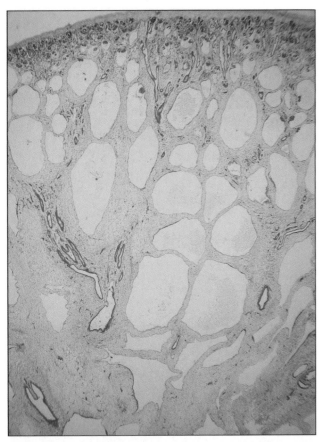

FIGURE 13.8: *Numerous spherical cysts are present throughout the cortex and medulla. Many of the cortical cysts contain glomerular tufts. The medullae are slender and poorly developed (×20). (Courtesy of Dr. Laura Finn., Children's Hospital and Regional Medical Center, Seattle, Washington).*

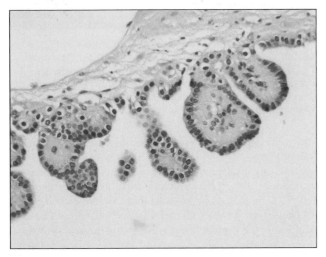

FIGURE 13.9: *Focus of intracystic papillary hyperplasia of the tubular epithelium in an adult with ADPKD (×200).*

nonprogressive and is not associated with cysts in other organs. Both adults and children are affected, but only in an adult can one be confident that the lesion is not the initial presentation of ADPKD. Included in the clinical differential diagnosis are

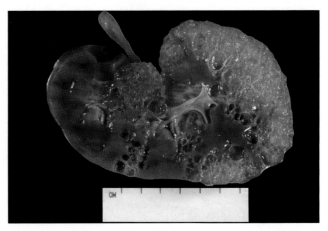

FIGURE 13.10: *Localized cystic kidney disease in an 11 year old female with a negative family history of renal disease. Clusters of thin-walled spherical cysts are separated by large areas of uninvolved kidney.*

benign multilocular cystic nephroma, segmental dysplasia, and a cluster of simple cysts. The cysts in a cystic nephroma are not separated by normal parenchyma and the lesion is sharply demarcated from the adjacent kidney. Dysplasia has its own set of distinctive histologic features. However, a cluster of simple cysts is indistinguishable from LCKD.

Etiology and Pathogenesis

ADPKD is caused by mutation of either *PKD1* on chromosome 16p, which encodes polycystin-1, or *PKD2* on chromosome 4p, which encodes polycystin-2. Both are membrane glycoproteins. They colocalize to primary monocilia that are present on almost all cells of the body, including the apex of each renal tubular epithelial cell [20]. Polycystin-1 has a mechanosensory function in the ciliary membrane and is closely linked to polycystin-2, a Ca^{2+}-permeable nonselective cation channel. Mechanical sheer applied to the cilium induces increased calcium ion flux through the polycystin-2 channel. The polycystins also colocalize in the cell membrane at the cell-matrix focal adhesion complex and at cell-cell junctions and polycystin-2 is present in the endoplasmic reticulum [3,21]. The polycystins play an important role in maintaining cell differentiation and polarization, determining transmembrane fluid flow, and controlling cell proliferation and apoptosis, all of which are abnormal in ADPKD. Altered calcium flux is likely central to this process, but the exact mechanisms involved in the complex subcellular interactions associated with the polycystins are still incompletely understood.

Cysts in ADPKD form as outpouchings anywhere along the nephron, with a propensity for the collecting ducts and the loops of Henle. As the cysts enlarge, they detach from the nephron and continue to expand due to cell proliferation and a net influx of fluid into the lumen independent of flow within the nephron [3,21]. Although the physical effect of enlarging cysts probably plays an important role in the progressive decline of renal function in ADPKD, other factors might also contribute to nephron injury in the noncystic parenchyma.

The number and size of the cysts increase steadily with age, but cysts develop from only a small minority of nephrons, despite the fact that all renal epithelial cells harbor the same germ line mutation; haploinsufficiency alone does not explain the initiation of cystogenesis in human ADPKD. Epithelial cells derived from cysts show clonal loss of heterozygosity for the polycystin gene indicating that a second genetic hit to the complementary polycystin allele is required to reduce or disrupt polycystin function sufficiently to enable cystogenesis [22]; the *PKD* genes appear to act in a recessive manner at the cellular level. While the two hit hypothesis is attractive, the mechanism underlying cystogenesis is complex and loss of heterozygosity for the polycystin gene may not be the only explanation for the initiation of cyst formation.

Modifier genes and/or epigenetic factors in addition to disrupted polycystin signal transduction likely explain the wide intrafamilial variability of disease severity in patients with the same germ line mutation, including a more variable course in siblings than in monozygous twins [23]. Various hormones and growth factors such as epidermal growth factor (EGF), transforming growth factor alpha (TGF-alpha), and cyclic AMP may affect the rate of epithelial cell proliferation and intracystic fluid accumulation and are possible targets for therapeutic intervention [24,25].

AUTOSOMAL RECESSIVE POLYCYSTIC KIDNEY DISEASE (ARPKD)

Epidemiology and Clinical Presentation

ARPKD has a prevalence of 1:20,000 live births and is caused by mutation of *PKHD1* (polycystic kidney and hepatic fibrosis 1) on chromosome 6p [24]. In contrast to ADPKD, renal cysts are almost always present in utero and oligohydramnios caused by reduced fetal urine is a frequent complication. This results in pulmonary hypoplasia with consequent neonatal respiratory insufficiency. Most deaths occur in the first month of life and are due to respiratory rather than renal failure. However, the clinical spectrum of ARPKD is broad with presentation ranging from infancy to adulthood, depending on the extent of cyst formation. In a large cohort of patients diagnosed after 1990, overall patient survival was 86 percent at 1 month of age [26]. Five- and twenty-year survival rates after the first month of life may be as high as 90 percent [26–28], a much better prognosis than once thought. Hypertension is frequent and renal insufficiency evolves in many patients. The risk for developing hypertension and renal insufficiency correlates inversely with the age at diagnosis. Nephrocalcinosis, while not usually thought of as a component of ARPKD, is often present in imaging studies and can sometimes produce the radiologic appearance of medullary sponge kidney (MSK) [28].

All patients with ARPKD have dysgenesis of the intrahepatic bile ducts termed ductal plate malformation or congenital hepatic fibrosis. Normal imaging studies of the liver do not completely exclude its presence [28]. The lesion develops in utero and infants may have hepatomegaly, but liver dysfunction does not usually manifest clinically until later in childhood or in adults, when portal hypertension and/or cholangitis develop in approximately half of ARPKD patients [28]. Portal hypertension often dominates the clinical course in older patients and may be the clinical presentation of patients with minimal or no evidence of renal disease. One-third of patients with hepatic disease as the principal manifestation of ARPKD present after

20 years of age. Grossly evident spherical hepatic cysts are uncommon, but cystic dilatation of the intrahepatic bile ducts (Caroli's disease) does occur and is relatively common in older patients [28].

Approach to Interpretation

Gross Pathology

The gross appearance of the kidneys varies with patient age. Infants who succumb in the neonatal period have bilateral, symmetric, marked nephromegaly (Figure 13.11). The kidneys maintain a reniform shape with smooth external surfaces, but numerous small translucent cysts are visible through the renal capsule (Figure 13.12). The pelvicaliceal system is widely patent with little distortion. The cut surface reveals innumerable, elongate, fusiform cysts several mm in diameter that extend in radial array from the medulla to the outer cortex (Figure 13.13). These represent dilated collecting ducts and produce a distinctive sponge-like appearance with loss of corticomedullary definition. Some medullary cysts can assume a more spherical shape.

Kidneys of patients who survive the neonatal period or present at an older age are smaller and contain fewer, but larger, more spherical cysts that can be cortical and/or medullary [29–31]. Interstitial fibrosis and parenchymal atrophy develop over time in those patients who progress to renal insufficiency. The kidneys can resemble ADPKD, but they do not undergo progressive massive cystic transformation typical of ADPKD, and may even decrease in size [28,32].

Light Microscopy

Elongate, dilated profiles of medullary and cortical collecting ducts are the microscopic hallmark of ARPKD in early infancy (Figures 13.14 and 13.15). Intact nephrons are present between the dilated ducts, which are lined by cuboidal epithelial cells (Figure 13.16). Glomerular cysts are absent and fibrosis is inconspicuous except for increased cellularity of the medullary stroma that can sometimes be prominent and resemble medullary dysplasia (Figure 13.17). Survival beyond the neonatal period correlates with the presence of fewer cysts or mildly ectatic cortical and/or medullary collecting ducts (Figure 13.18), sometimes

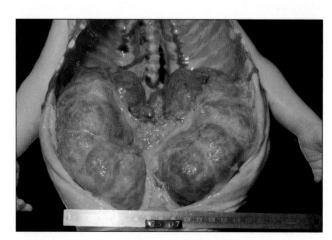

FIGURE 13.11: *Markedly enlarged kidneys fill the retroperitoneum of a neonate with ARPKD.*

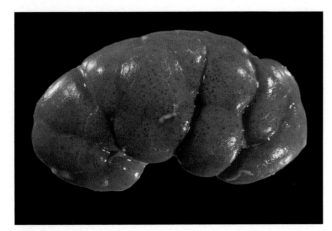

FIGURE 13.12: *Numerous small cysts are visible through the renal capsule in ARPKD.*

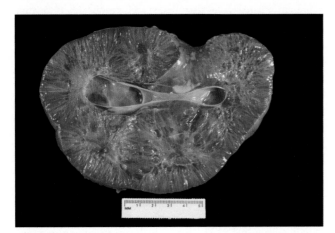

FIGURE 13.13: *Innumerable elongate cysts arrayed perpendicular to the renal capsule are characteristic of the infantile form of ARPKD.*

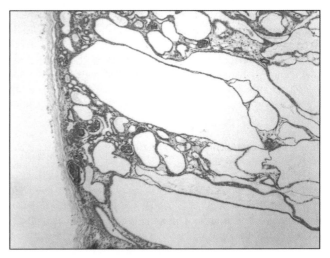

FIGURE 13.14: *ARPKD. Intact parenchyma without significant fibrosis separates markedly dilated collecting ducts (×40).*

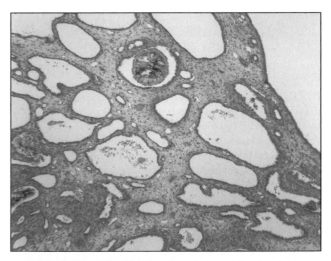

FIGURE 13.15: *ARPKD. Dilated medullary collecting ducts are separated by increased stroma. A urate crystal is present in one of the ducts (×40).*

referred to as medullary ductal ectasia. Kidneys removed for renal failure in older patients have extensive interstitial fibrosis and associated parenchymal atrophy.

Portal tracts in the liver are expanded by fibrous tissue (Figure 13.19) and contain arcuate or more complex profiles of small bile ducts with patent lumens that are often situated at the periphery of the tracts (Figures 13.20 and 13.21). All portal tracts are affected, in contrast to the focal lesions of ADPKD. Secondary changes caused by recurrent cholangitis can alter the microscopic appearance in older patients. Ductal plate malformation is not unique to ARPKD. It occurs in other hereditary syndromes including Meckel-Gruber syndrome, nephronophthisis (NPHP), Jeune's asphyxiating thoracodystrophy, Ivemark syndrome (renal-hepatic-pancreatic dysplasia) and rarely in ADPKD [33].

Differential Diagnosis

The differential diagnosis of diffuse cystic renal disease in infancy includes ARPKD, ADPKD, NPHP2, GCKD, and diffuse multicystic renal dysplasia. The distinction of typical examples of ARPKD in infancy from ADPKD in older adults should not be difficult. However, neonatal or childhood presentation of ADPKD can pose a diagnostic challenge if evaluation is limited to imaging studies. The presence of diffuse ductal plate malformation of the liver and the absence of renal cysts in the parents strongly favor the diagnosis of ARPKD. Infantile NPHP, though rare, must also be included in the differential diagnosis of diffuse cystic disease in an infant or young child with bilateral nephromegaly; the liver is normal and interstitial disease is more prominent than in ADPKD. Renal dysplasia has distinctive histologic features and clinical associations that should not be confused with ARPKD. Other forms of syndromic renal cystic disease should be distinguishable on the basis of associated extrarenal abnormalities.

Etiology and Pathogenesis

ARPKD is caused by mutation of *PKHD1*, which is located on chromosome 6p and encodes the protein fibrocystin/polyductin

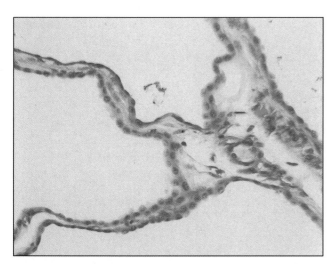

FIGURE 13.16: *ARPKD. The collecting duct cysts in the outer cortex are lined by cuboidal cells and interstitial fibrosis is absent (×200).*

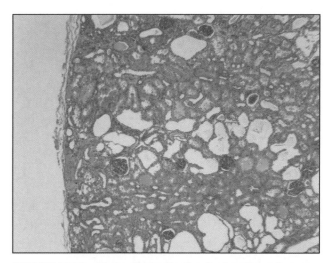

FIGURE 13.18: *The cortical collecting duct cysts in a 3 year old child with ARPKD are fewer and there is more intact cortical tissue between cysts. Small foci of early parenchymal fibrosis are also present (×40).*

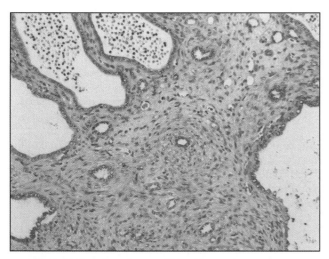

FIGURE 13.17: *Stroma can sometimes encircle medullary collecting ducts in a manner resembling medullary dysplasia, but the typical changes in the overlying cortex should allow recognition of ARPKD (×100).*

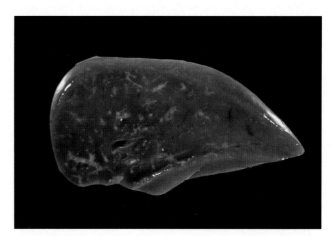

FIGURE 13.19: *The liver of a neonate with ARPKD shows increased prominence of portal tracts without gross cysts.*

[34]. The gene is large and most patients are compound heterozygotes with private mutations. Fibrocystin/polyductin is a multifunctional integral membrane protein that is involved in regulation of cell adhesion and proliferation, signal transduction and cell–matrix interactions. During embryogenesis, it is expressed in the ureteric bud, from which the collecting ducts develop, and is also expressed in biliary epithelium. Like other cystoproteins, it colocalizes in centrosomes, basal bodies, and primary cilia. It is also present at other sites in the cell and may be involved in Ca^{2+} signaling. It is likely that many of the same cellular mechanisms involved in ADPKD are relevant to ARPKD. Epidermal growth factor receptor (EGFR) and c-AMP mediated pathways appear to play an important role and are potential targets for therapeutic intervention [34].

There is some evidence of genotype/phenotype correlation in ARPDK. Patients with truncating mutations in both *PKHD1*

alleles have severe perinatal disease, while patients surviving the neonatal period have a missense rather than a truncating mutation in at least one of the alleles [27]. Siblings usually have a similar clinical course, but disease expression in approximately 20 percent of families varies significantly between siblings.

NEPHRONOPHTHISIS AND RELATED DISORDERS

Epidemiology and Clinical Presentation

NPHP comprises a group of genetically distinct, but clinically overlapping, autosomal recessive disorders in which there is progressive tubulointerstitial disease with the formation of small cysts at the corticomedullary junction late in the course [5, 35–37]. NPHP is the most frequent genetic cause of end stage renal disease in childhood and adolescence, although the prevalence is only 1:50,000 live births. The juvenile form is most common and presents in childhood with anemia and

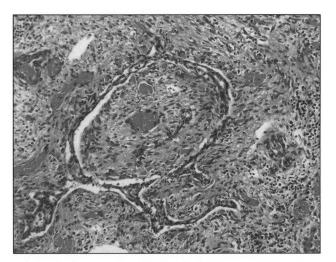

FIGURE 13.20: *Ductal plate malformation in ARPKD. Small bile ducts form an arcuate pattern at the periphery of a portal tract (×100).*

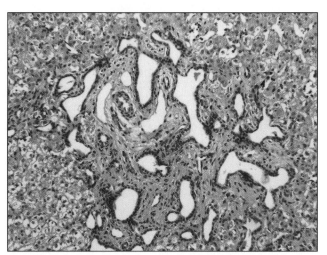

FIGURE 13.21: *Ductal plate malformation of the liver in ARPKD can also appear as a more irregular network of small ducts that extends throughout an expanded portal tract (×100).*

renal tubular dysfunction manifested by polyuria and polydipsia. This is accompanied by growth retardation and progresses to renal failure at a median age of 13 years. Proteinuria and hypertension are usually absent and there is renal salt wasting. The adolescent form is similar in all respects except that the median age of renal failure is 19 years. Infantile NPHP (NPHP2) differs significantly from both juvenile and adolescent disease in having bilateral nephromegaly caused by numerous cortical cysts with progression to renal failure by 1–3 years of age [35].

Extrarenal manifestations are present in 10 to15 percent of patients with NPHP [5,36,37]. The eponym Senior-Loken syndrome applies to patients with tapetoretinal degeneration (retinitis pigmentosa) and Cogan syndrome to those with oculomotor apraxia. There are other autosomal recessive syndromes in which NPHP-like renal disease is variably expressed. These include Joubert, Bardet-Biedl, Arima, COACH, and Alstrom syndromes [38]. Features that occur in these various syndromes include maldevelopment of the cerebellar vermis, anosmia, mental retardation, hepatic fibrosis, infertility, obesity, diabetes mellitus, congenital amaurosis, and cone-shaped epiphyses with some degree of phenotypic overlap between syndromes. Situs inversus is present in some infants with NPHP2 [39].

Approach to Interpretation

Gross Pathology

All but the infantile form of NPHP are morphologically similar and also share morphologic features of medullary cystic kidney disease (MCKD). The kidneys are normal or reduced in size. The cortical surface is granular and the cut surface is firm and pale. Small round cysts are usually present at the corticomedullary junction and can sometimes involve the medulla, but they are sometimes absent [40] (Figure 13.22). Caliectasis with calyceal blunting and diverticula are often present in Bardet-Biedl syndrome.

Light Microscopy

While cysts are a feature of NPHP, the histologic findings are dominated by tubular atrophy with thickened, split, disrupted tubular basement membranes (Figure 13.23), prominent interstitial fibrosis, and chronic inflammation that is best characterized as chronic sclerosing tubulointerstitial nephropathy. Glomerular disease is minimal early in the course, but glomerulosclerosis evolves in advanced disease. Tubular basement membranes show lamellation and lucencies similar to Alport syndrome, but the glomerular basement membranes do not. Some examples of renal dysplasia described in patients with NPHP variants, such as Arima and Joubert syndromes, represent imprecise use of that term and morphologically fall within the spectrum of NPHP [38].

Infantile nephrophthisis (NPHP2) differs morphologically from other forms of NPHP in having large kidneys with numerous small cysts lined by cuboidal epithelium scattered in the cortex, in addition to cysts in the corticomedullary region. Cysts become less numerous as the disease progresses. There is interstitial fibrosis and tubular atrophy with chronic inflammation, but tubular basement membranes are not thickened and glomerular cysts can be prominent [39]. Liver disease is absent.

The hepatic disease in NPHP and related syndromes is sometimes referred to as congenital hepatic fibrosis. However, it consists of portal fibrosis with or without increased small ducts and/or cholangioles and differs from the network of dilated small ducts within the portal tracts that constitute the ductal plate malformation characteristic of ARPKD [41].

Differential Diagnosis

The pathologic appearance of NPHP is identical to MCDK, which is why the term nephronophthisis–medullary cystic disease complex is sometimes used to encompass both disorders. Their clinical distinction is based on the pattern of inheritance, age of onset, and presence or absence of hyperuricemia or extrarenal syndromic features. Other forms of chronic tubulointerstitial nephropathy may have similar morphologic features, but corticomedullary cysts are

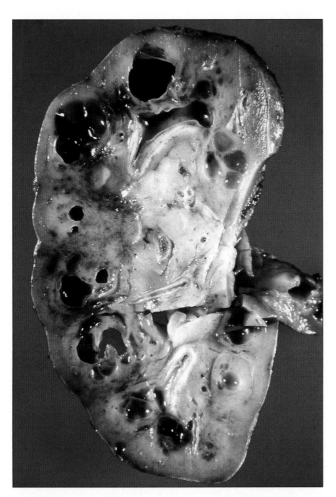

FIGURE 13.22: *Kidney from a 13 year old girl with ESRD due to medullary cystic kidney disease. Cysts are located at the corticomedullary junction. (Courtesy of Dr. Laura Finn., Children's Hospital and Regional Medical Center, Seattle, Washington).*

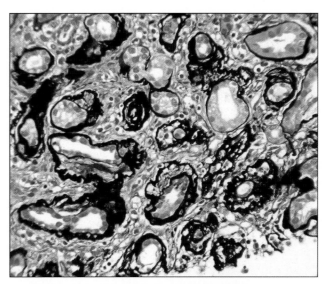

FIGURE 13.23: *The tubular basement membranes in 9 year old girl with nephronophthisis associated with COACH syndrome show prominent splitting/duplication. This abnormality is a characteristic but non-specific finding (Jones stain × 400). (Courtesy of Dr. Laura Finn., Children's Hospital and Regional Medical Center, Seattle, Washington).*

absent. The diagnosis of NPHP can be missed if cysts are absent and there is no clinical suspicion of the disease. Infantile NPHP has its own distinctive morphology with a differential diagnosis that includes other forms of diffuse cystic renal disease in infancy.

Etiology and Pathogenesis

All of the genes so far associated with NPHP and its related syndromes are autosomal recessive and encode proteins that localize to primary cilia, basal bodies, or centrosomes of renal epithelial cells or associate with other cystoproteins [5]. This likely explains their convergent renal phenotype. These proteins are also present at other intracellular sites and have complex interactions beyond ciliary function including cell-cell and cell-matrix adhesion and signaling. Their widespread distribution in extrarenal tissues explains their pleiotropic, sometimes overlapping, clinical manifestations when mutated.

Six different NPNP genes are known, but mutations in these six genes are not detected in a large proportion of affected patients, suggesting that additional loci will be found [42]. *NPHP1* and *NPHP3-6* encode their respective nephrocystin

proteins. Most cases of juvenile disease are caused by *NPHP1* and some by *NPHP4* mutations. *NPHP3* mutations are infrequent and are associated with adolescent disease. *NPHP5* mutations result in juvenile disease with a high incidence of tapetoretinal degeneration (Senior-Loken syndrome). However, there is phenotypic overlap between these groups and the genotype does not necessarily correlate with the extrarenal phenotype, even in the same sibship [36]. *NPHP2*, the gene mutated in infantile NPHP, encodes inversin [39]. Inversin colocalizes with nephrocystin-1 and beta-tubulin in the cilia–centrosome complex and is important in both ciliary function and left–right patterning in the embryo, which explains the occurrence of situs inversus in some patients.

NPHP1 (JBTS4) and *NPHP6* mutations are found in some patients with Joubert syndrome (hypoplasia of cerebellar vermis, retinopathy, polydactyly, hepatic fibrosis), but Joubert syndrome is both phenotypically and genetically heterogenous with a low incidence of clinical renal disease [43]. Bardet-Biedl syndrome (mental retardation, obesity, retinopathy, coloboma, polydactyly) is also genetically heterogenous with at least twelve loci, many of which are known to encode proteins associated with the basal body and/or ciliary axoneme [44]. NPHP-like renal disease occurs in more than 70 percent of patients with Bardet-Biedl syndrome [45], although renal insufficiency is usually delayed until adulthood.

MEDULLARY CYSTIC DISEASE

Epidemiology and Clinical Presentation

MCKD comprises two genetically distinct autosomal dominant disorders, MCKD1 and MCKD2, whose clinical and morphologic features overlap with NPHP and with each other, including tubulointerstitial nephropathy and cysts at the corticomedullary junction. In contrast to NPHP, the age of onset in MCKD is usually in adulthood; the median age of ESRD is 62 years in MCKD1 and 32 years in MCKD2, but the onset can be in childhood [46]. Impaired urinary concentrating ability and hyperuricemia with hypouricosuria are characteristic features of MCKD. They are more severe in MCKD2, but can also occur in MCKD1. The disorder termed familial juvenile hyperuricemic nephropathy (FJHN) is now recognized as an allelic variant of MCKD2 with no unique distinguishing clinical features except for the apparent absence of cysts in FJHN, but patients with cysts and without cysts can occur in the same family [47]. Although patients with MCKD can have anemia, renal tubular dysfunction and/or salt wasting, others have only slowly progressive renal failure. In contrast to NPHP, corticomedullary cysts are often absent on imaging studies in MCKD and there are no extrarenal phenotypic associations.

Approach to Interpretation

Gross Pathology

The kidneys in MCKD are of normal size in early disease, but become smaller as parenchymal atrophy progresses. The gross appearance is not distinctive except for cysts at the corticomedullary junction, a feature that appears late in the disease and is absent in many patients (Figure 13.22).

Light Microscopy

MCKD1 and MCKD2 are histologically similar and indistinguishable from NPHP. Thickened and split tubular basement membranes, tubular dilatation and/or atrophy, prominent interstitial fibrosis and nonspecific chronic inflammation are the principal histologic findings [40,47]. Advanced disease is associated with glomerulosclerosis. Tubular cysts, when present, display no distinctive features aside from their corticomedullary location. Glomerular cysts are present rarely [48]. Immunohistochemical studies demonstrate intracytoplasmic accumulation of uromodulin in epithelial cells lining cysts derived from the thick ascending loop of Henle [49]. The ultrastructural correlate is distension of the endoplasmic reticulum by fibrillary material that is presumed to be uromodulin [48].

Differential Diagnosis

The diagnosis of MCKD and its distinction from the various forms of NPHP and unrelated causes of chronic sclerosing tubulointerstitial nephropathy is based almost entirely on clinical and genetic associations. The morphology is largely nonspecific and the diagnosis can be missed in the absence of strong clinical suspicion of the disease. The absence of cysts does not exclude the diagnosis of MCKD, and cysts are unlikely to be present in a biopsy of the renal cortex. Conversely, examination of the excised kidney may reveal cysts not appreciated by imaging studies.

Etiology and Pathogenesis

MCKD1 links to 1q21, but no specific disease-associated gene has yet been identified [50]. Most cases of MCKD2 result from mutation of *UMOD* at 16p12, which encodes uromodulin, also known as Tamm-Horsfall protein [46,51]. Uromodulin is expressed normally only in the ascending limb of the loop of Henle and distal convoluted tubules. Reduced urinary excretion of uromodulin is typical of MCKD2, but also occurs in some patients with MCKD1 and in families with no demonstrable linkage to either 1p21 or16p12 [52], making it likely that there are additional unrecognized genetic loci that impact uromodulin function. Ultrastructural and immunohistochemical evidence of uromodulin accumulation within the endoplasmic reticulum of renal tubular cells in MCKD2 suggests that altered intracellular trafficking of uromodulin, possibly due to abnormal protein folding, is central to the pathophysiology of the disease [53].

GCKD with hyperuricemia and severe impairment of urine concentrating ability is another disorder in which *UMOD* mutation has been demonstrated [48]. The terms uromodulin-associated kidney disease and uromodulin storage disease have been proposed to encompass the spectrum of renal disease caused by uromodulin mutations (MCKD2, FJHN, and GCKD with hyperuricemia) [51,54].

MEDULLARY SPONGE KIDNEY

Epidemiology and Clinical Presentation

Medullary sponge kidney (MSK) is usually a nonprogressive, sporadic disease of adults, but also occurs in children and can rarely be familial [55,56]. It is present in up to 1 percent of patients without renal stones who undergo intravenous pyelography and up to 20 percent of adults with stones [57]. Females are more frequently affected than males. A patient with radiographic features of MSK is described in a family with well-documented ARPKD and rare reports of the association of MSK with Caroli disease or congenital hepatic fibrosis might be additional examples of ARPKD, as hepatic disease is not expected in MSK [28]. MSK occurs with increased frequency in patients with hemihypertrophy and Beckwith-Wiedemann syndrome, both of which can be subtle and easily overlooked.

MSK is usually bilateral, but can be unilateral or segmental. Hematuria, urinary tract infection and urolithiasis are the principal clinical presentations. Renal function is not usually disturbed, although mild renal tubular acidosis, hypercalcuria, and/or mildly impaired concentrating ability are often present and there may be reduced excretion of citrate and magnesium [56]. The diagnosis is based on a characteristic radiographic appearance utilizing intravenous pyelography. The lesion is variously described as medullary tubular ectasia, or a paint brush or bouquet-like pattern limited to the renal pyramids with or without nephrolithiasis. The overlying cortex is normal unless there is secondary chronic pyelonephritis

Pathology

The kidney is of normal size unless chronic pyelonephritis has caused cortical scarring. The ectatic tubules are located in the renal papillae and are usually <0.5 cm in diameter, but can be larger. Diffuse dilatation of the intrapapillary aspect of the collecting ducts is the histologic correlate for the gross and radiographic findings. The dilated ducts often contain calcific deposits and inflammatory changes may be superimposed.

Differential Diagnosis

The only other renal disorders with medullary tubular ectasia are ARPKD and infantile ADPKD. There is no likelihood that the neonatal or infantile presentation of ARPKD or ADPKD would be confused with MSK. ARPKD presenting in an older child or adult could be more problematic, but the liver is always abnormal in ARPKD and should be normal in MSK.

Etiology and Pathogenesis

MSK is thought to be congenital, but the pathogenesis of most cases is unknown. Hypercalcuria with reduced citrate and magnesium excretion and impaired urinary acidification may contribute to nephrolithiasis. Hyperparathyroidism is not more prevalent in MSK than in patients with renal stones who do not have MSK [58]. Abnormal development of the renal medullae, sometimes referred to as medullary dysplasia, is a characteristic histologic feature of Beckwith-Wiedemann syndrome and is likely the substrate for the evolution of MSK in this syndrome.

GLOMERULOCYSTIC KIDNEY DISEASE AND GLOMERULAR CYSTS

Glomerular cysts represent a two- to threefold enlargement of Bowman's space and are usually <2–3 mm in diameter. The descriptive term glomerulocystic kidney (GCK) is used when at least 5 percent of the cysts in a kidney contain glomerular tufts [13]. Glomerular cysts occur in a wide variety of clinical contexts that can be roughly grouped into four categories (Table 13.2): 1) GCKD, in which cystic renal disease is the principle clinical manifestation of the disorder, 2) GCK as a major or minor aspect of a heritable syndrome, 3) Glomerular cysts as a component of renal dysplasia, 4) Acquired glomerular cysts in medical renal disease.

Glomerulocystic Kidney Disease

Most examples of GCKD are infants from families with ADPKD and represent a morphologic variant of the latter (Figure 13.7 and 13.8). The kidneys are enlarged with multiple cysts that can involve tubules as well as glomeruli. The renal medullae are small and narrow and contain dilated collecting ducts with periductal fibrosis that may condense into fibromuscular collars [13]. Radiographic demonstration of medullary collecting duct ectasia can lead to confusion with ARPKD. Some infants have asymmetric or segmental disease and 10 percent have a mild form of hepatic ductal plate malformation. A negative family history does not exclude ADPKD, as approximately 10 percent of ADPKD patients represent new mutations. Oligohydramnios with neonatal death occurs in some affected infants. Older children and adults with typical ADPKD can also have glomerular cysts, but they are overshadowed by cystic renal tubules. Glomerular cysts are rare in ARPKD and the

---

Table 13.2 Glomerular Cysts [13, 65, 93]

Glomerulocystic kidney disease (GCKD)
- Autosomal dominant polycystic kidney disease (ADPKD)
- Sporadic and autosomal dominant GCKD of undetermined etiology
- Autosomal dominant glomerulocystic disease with hyperuricemia
- Familial hypoplastic glomerulocystic disease with HNF-1β mutation with or without diabetes (MODY5)
- Infantile Nephronophthisis (NPHP2)

Syndrome-associated glomerulocystic kidneys
- Oro-facial-digital syndrome, type 1
- Tuberous sclerosis
- Brachymesomelia-renal syndrome
- Glutaric aciduria, type 2
- Short rib-polydactyly syndrome
- Chromosomal trisomy (9, 13, 18, 21)
- Asphyxiating thoracodystrophy (Jeune syndrome)
- Zellweger syndrome
- Hemihypertrophy
- Various others

Renal dysplasia
- Obstruction
- Meckel-Gruber and related syndromes
- Renal-hepatic-pancreatic dysplasia (Ivemark syndrome)
- Other forms of diffuse non-obstructive renal dysplasia

Acquired glomerular cysts
- Systemic lupus erythematosus
- Hemolytic-uremic syndrome
- Thrombotic microangiopathy

---

associated elongate collecting duct cysts characteristic of ARPKD should dispel any confusion [13].

Syndrome-Associated Glomerulocystic Kidney

Numerous hereditary syndromes can display glomerular cysts. Dysplasia can also occur in many of these syndromes, as can large and small nondescript cortical cysts unrelated to glomeruli. Cystic renal disease is usually a minor component, but is sometimes a dominant abnormality; as in oro-facial-digital syndrome type 1 (OFD1) [59]. OFD1 comprises facial dysmorphism, oral defects and distal limb anomalies. It is an X-linked dominant disorder that is lethal to males in utero. Sporadic new mutations account for up to 75 percent of cases. Cystic renal disease is present in at least 15 percent of affected females and may progress to renal failure. The kidneys are usually normal or reduced in size with numerous cysts that are smaller than those of ADPKD. Many cysts involve glomeruli, but tubules are also affected. The OFD1 protein localizes to the cell centrosome/basal body, as do many other cystoproteins.

Other Nonsyndromic Glomerulocystic Kidney Disease

After ADPKD, renal dysplasia, and the numerous syndromes associated with glomerular cysts are excluded, some GCKD patients remain. The kidneys of these patients are usually of normal size or small and the clinical course is varied. One recently-identified cause for autosomal dominant or sporadic GCKD is mutation of *HNF-1β*, also known as *TCF2* [60]. Type

5 maturity onset diabetes of the young (MODY5) is present in many, but not all patients [61,62]. Affected patients manifest a broad spectrum of renal maldevelopment that includes hypoplastic GCKD, dysplasia, aplasia, oligomeganephronic hypoplasia, atypical juvenile hyperuricemic nephropathy with tubular cysts, horseshoe kidney, and diffuse cystic disease without dysplasia [61,63,64]. One-third to one-half has de novo mutations and there is no clear genotype–phenotype correlation, even within families [60,62].

Another mutation that causes nonsyndromic familial GCKD affects *UMOD* (uromodulin), the same gene that underlies autosomal dominant MCKD2. The clinical features in patients with this allelic *UMOD* mutation overlap those of hyperuricemic MCKD2. However, there are numerous small cysts that involve 40 percent of the glomeruli with only mild interstitial fibrosis in contrast to the corticomedullary cysts and severe tubulointerstitial disease that typifies MCKD2 [48]. The cause for other examples of nonsyndromic autosomal dominant GCKD remains unknown.

Acquired Glomerular Cysts

Glomerular cysts occur in some patients with various systemic disorders, including systemic lupus erythematosus, hemolytic uremic syndrome, and thrombotic microangiopathy. They are not usually of clinical significance and the mechanism of their development is not well understood.

TUBEROUS SCLEROSIS

The tuberous sclerosis complex (TSC) is an autosomal dominant disorder with a broad spectrum of lesions that affect many organ systems. Mutations of tumor suppressor genes *TSC1* on chromosome 9q and *TSC2* on chromosome 16p underlie the disorder. Renal manifestations include cysts, angiomyolipomas, metanephric hamartomas, and vascular dysplasia. Cysts occur in approximately one third of patients. They may be few or innumerable and can involve one or both kidneys (Figure 13.24). All segments of the nephron are affected, including the glomeruli [65]. Cysts are more prevalent, larger, and more numerous in TSC2 [66,67]. The cysts of TSC are distinguished from other

renal cysts by a distinctive lining of hypertrophic, deeply eosinophilic epithelial cells that sometimes produce hyperplastic tufts, and may display nuclear atypia (Figure 13.25) [68].

A severe form of cystic renal disease occurs in some infants and young children with TSC and rarely in adults [69]. It can present unilaterally and may precede the diagnosis of TSC. This variant results from a large chromosomal deletion that involves both *TSC2* and *PKD1*, which lie contiguous on chromosome16p, and is termed TSC2/PKD1 contiguous gene syndrome [14]. The gross and microscopic features are similar to ADPKD, except for the distinctive eosinophilic cells that line the cysts. Cysts larger than 2 cm and clinically significant polycystic kidney disease are unique to patients with TSC2 and severe, progressive cystic renal disease is largely confined to those with TSC2/PKD1 contiguous deletion syndrome [66]. Tuberin, the gene product of *TSC2*, is important for normal intracellular trafficking of polycystin-1, the cystoprotein that is disrupted in ADPKD. This may help to explain cystogenesis in TSC, even in the absence of *PKD1* involvement [70].

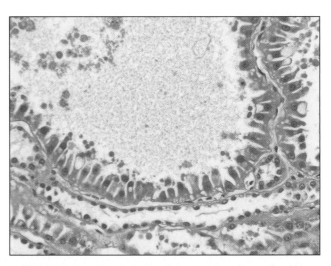

FIGURE 13.25: *The cysts in tuberous sclerosis are lined by distinctive enlarged eosinophilic epithelial cells (×200).*

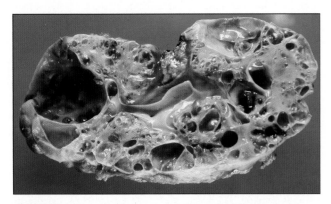

FIGURE 13.24: *Numerous cysts distort the kidney of a 13 year old child with tuberous sclerosis and renal angiomyolipomas. (Courtesy of Dr. Laura Finn., Children's Hospital and Regional Medical Center, Seattle, Washington).*

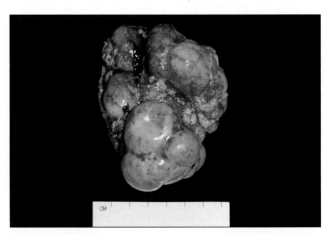

FIGURE 13.26: *The external contour of a multicystic dysplastic kidney lacks a reniform shape due to distortion by numerous large and small cysts.*

VON HIPPEL LINDAU SYNDROME

Von Hippel-Lindau syndrome is an uncommon autosomal dominant disorder characterized by unusual cystic and solid tumors at various sites including the brain, spinal cord, retina, pancreas, epididymis, broad ligament and inner ear. It is caused by germline mutation of the tumor suppressor gene *VHL*, which resides on chromosome 3p and encodes pVHL. Subsequent somatic mutations in the second allele result in loss of heterozygosity for *VHL*, and the development of cysts and tumors. Renal lesions occur in up to two-thirds of patients and can be the presenting manifestation. They span a spectrum that includes simple cysts, atypical cysts (lining 2–3 cells thick), and cystic or solid carcinomas [71]. Cystic and solid lesions often coexist in the same kidney. The cysts are usually small (<1.5 cm) and few (mean 7.8 per kidney) so that the kidneys are not typically enlarged unless adenocarcinoma has supervened. Larger cysts can be present and are sometimes multilocular. Enlarged polycystic kidneys resembling ADPKD occur rarely [72]. The epithelial cells comprising all of these renal lesions are highly distinctive clear cells that coexpress cytokeratins 8 and19

and vimentin [73]. In addition to having a clear cell lining, the cysts are surrounded by a rim of highly vascularized tissue that is not found in other forms of renal cystic disease. This likely reflects overproduction of vascular endothelial growth factor mediated by inactivation of the *VHL* gene. Both cysts and tumors have a similar cellular phenotype suggesting that the cysts are neoplastic from inception. The presence of renal cysts in a patient with clear cell carcinoma of the kidney should prompt consideration of Von Hippel-Lindau syndrome.

CONGENITAL ANOMALIES OF THE KIDNEY AND URINARY TRACT (CAKUT)

CAKUT is an acronym proposed for the spectrum of congenital anomalies of the kidney and urinary tract that include duplicated collecting system, ureteropelvic junction obstruction, vesicoureteral reflux, ectopic ureter, and the many forms of renal dysplasia, aplasia, hypoplasia, and agenesis [74]. Various combinations of these lesions often occur together in an individual or within a family and may share common developmental

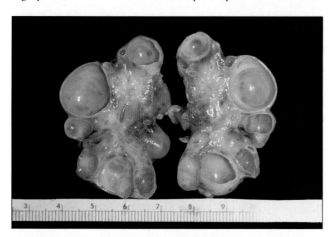

FIGURE 13.27: *The cysts of a multicystic dysplastic kidney vary widely in size, are separated by fibrous tissue and have thick walls. There is no recognizable corticomedullary delineation or residual intact parenchyma.*

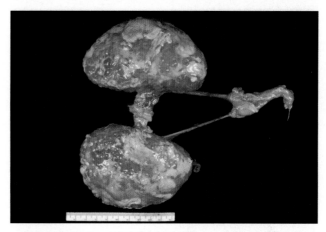

FIGURE 13.29: *Diffuse cystic dysplasia in a neonate with Ivemark syndrome (renal, hepatic and pancreatic cysts). The enlarged kidneys are similar in size and maintain a reniform contour.*

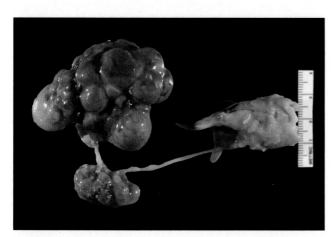

FIGURE 13.28: *A multicystic dysplastic kidney with atretic ureter on one side and contralateral hypoplastic dysplastic kidney.*

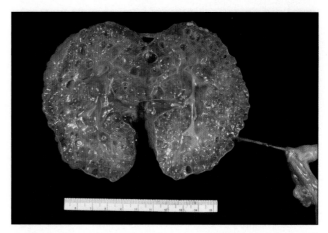

FIGURE 13.30: *The cut surface of one of the kidneys depicted in Fig.13.29 displays more uniform, smaller cysts than in a typical multicystic dysplastic kidney.*

mechanisms. CAKUT is the most common cause of ESRD in patients less than 21 years of age.

Dysplasia

Introduction

Renal dysplasia is the most common form of cystic renal disease in childhood and infrequently comes to attention in adults. Dysplasia in this context is used in a developmental rather than a neoplastic sense. It should be the first diagnosis considered when examining a cystic kidney in a child and the term multi-cystic renal dysplasia is applicable in most cases. Obstruction to urine flow at the level of the ureter, urinary bladder or urethra is a frequent association. Diffuse bilateral dysplasia without obstruction is unusual and is likely to be part of a systemic malformation syndrome, however, there are rare examples of apparently isolated diffuse bilateral dysplasia and these can be familial [75]

Gross Pathology

The gross appearance of renal dysplasia is highly variable and depends on its extent and clinical context. In many cases, the kidney is so distorted as to completely lose its reniform shape (Figures 13.26 to 13.28). In other cases, some semblance of corticomedullary architecture is preserved. Cysts range from microscopic to several centimeters in diameter. They may be few or numerous and bilateral, unilateral or segmental. The ureter and pelvicaliceal system are often markedly distorted or atretic, but can be dilated if obstruction is at or distal to the ureteropelvic junction or if intrauterine ureterovesical reflux is a contributing factor. Urologists sometimes use the term multi-cystic kidney when cysts of various sizes produce a multilobate mass that lacks a reniform shape with no distinct pelvicaliceal system and an atretic proximal ureter. The cysts of nonobstructive diffuse bilateral dysplasia are usually more uniform in size and distribution than those of multicystic dysplasia (Figures 13.29 and 13.30).

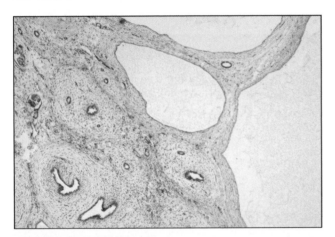

FIGURE 13.31: *Dysplastic cortex contains large fibrous-walled cysts and non-cystic dysplastic tubules. A rare immature-appearing glomerulus is also present in the fibrotic stroma (×40).*

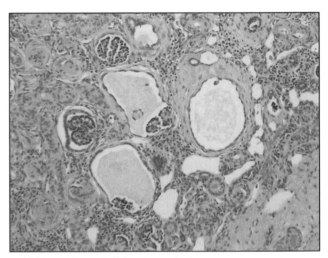

FIGURE 13.33: *Glomerular cysts in a dysplastic kidney (×100).*

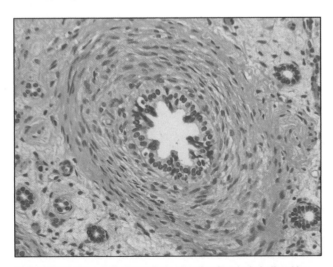

FIGURE 13.32: *A characteristic dysplastic tubule is lined by crowded columnar tubular epithelium and cuffed my loose, cellular mesenchymal tissue (×200).*

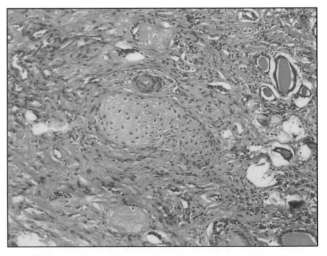

FIGURE 13.34: *Cartilage can occur in a dysplastic kidney, but is often absent (×200).*

Light Microscopy

Primitive ducts and tubules lined by crowded cuboidal or columnar epithelial cells and surrounded by cuffs of cellular mesenchyme are the histologic hallmark of renal dysplasia (Figures 13.31 and 13.32). Larger cysts are lined by flattened or cuboidal epithelium and often have fibrous rather than cellular walls. Clusters of small dysplastic ducts are commonly found and resemble maldeveloped medullae. The dysplastic ducts and larger cysts are disorganized and separated by fibrous stroma that may contain scattered glomeruli, which can appear immature or cystic (Figure 13.33). The ratio of stroma to cysts is highly variable. Islands of hyaline cartilage (Figure 13.34) and less commonly, smooth muscle (Figure 13.35) or other mesenchymal tissues are additional histologic features, but are often absent and are not required for diagnosis.

Hypoplastic Dysplasia, Aplasia, and Agenesis

Hypoplastic dysplasia refers to a dysplastic kidney that is smaller than normal and should be distinguished pathologically from renal hypoplasia in which the histologic architecture of the renal parenchyma is intact and cysts are absent (see "Hypoplasia"). Renal aplasia represents a small fibrous nubbin with scattered dysplastic tubules with or without an associated remnant of ureter (Figure 13.36). A few small cysts may be present. Renal agenesis applies when there is complete absence of any renal remnant and partial or complete absence of the ureter.

Renal agenesis, aplasia, and hypoplasia are often sonographic diagnoses without pathologic confirmation, which makes it difficult to draw accurate clinicopathologic correlations. Serial sonographic studies show that multicystic kidneys regress substantially before or after birth in a majority of patients and may sonographically disappear [76]. Most examples of apparent renal agenesis likely represent renal aplasia [77].

Medullary Dysplasia

Medullary dysplasia, also called obstructive dysplasia, is a form of renal dysplasia in which the medullary collecting ducts are separated by cellular stroma that condenses concentrically around them in a manner typical of dysplasia (Figure 13.37). The number of medullary ducts/tubules in the dysplastic medullae is reduced. Cysts are often present in the subcapsular region of the overlying cortex, which can be hypoplastic and/or have dysplastic features (Figure 13.38), but corticomedullary delineation is usually maintained. Because medullary and multicystic dysplasia can both result from obstruction, the two patterns are often intermingled in the same kidney. Medullary dysplasia is most commonly found when obstruction of the upper or lower urinary tract is incomplete and multicystic dysplasia when obstruction is complete, but the degree of dysplasia does not always parallel the severity of obstruction. Medullary dysplasia is the pattern usually seen in the upper pole of a kidney drained by a duplex collecting system in which the upper pole ureter terminates in an ectopic distal location, often accompanied by an ureterocele.

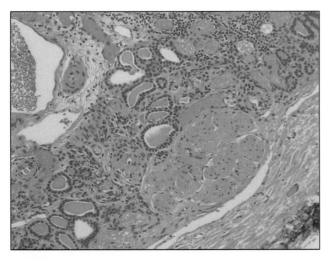

FIGURE 13.35: *Smooth muscle beneath the capsule of a dysplastic kidney. The tubules are atrophic, but are not dysplastic in this field (×200).*

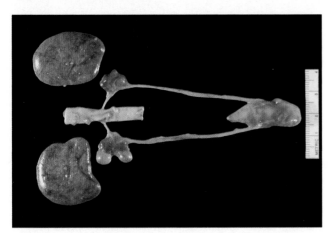

FIGURE 13.36: *Bilateral renal aplasia. The adrenal glands dwarf the small nubbins of dysplastic renal tissue in which there are several small cysts.*

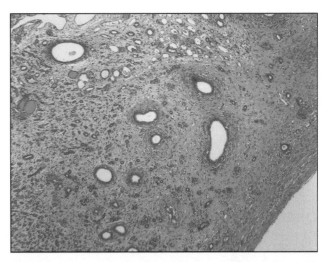

FIGURE 13.37: *Medullary dysplasia in a child with lower tract obstruction. A dilated calyx lies at the lower right. There is a paucity of medullary ducts and the residual ducts have prominent mesenchymal cuffs (×40).*

Hypoplasia

The term renal hypoplasia should be reserved for abnormally small kidneys that weigh less than 50 percent of expected weight and are histologically normal or show only nephron hypertrophy with or without secondary glomerulosclerosis. One or both kidneys can be affected. When only one kidney is hypoplastic, the contralateral side may display some other aspect of the CAKUT spectrum. Hypoplasia reflects deficient branching of the ureteral bud and/or insufficient induction of nephrons in the overlying metanephric blastema. Renal lobes and papillae are reduced in number (normal; ≥ 10), with unipapillary kidney at the extreme end of the spectrum (Figure 13.39). When nephron hypertrophy is absent, as is the case in infants and young children with hypoplastic kidneys, the unmodified terms hypoplasia or simple hypoplasia are appropriate. Hypoplasia should not be used for kidneys that are structurally normal but small because of acquired renal disease such as diffuse chronic pyelonephritis; atrophy is a more appropriate term in that context.

The extent to which renal mass is reduced determines clinical outcome. If renal hypoplasia is bilateral and the parenchymal mass is sufficiently small, there is compensatory nephron hypertrophy with markedly enlarged glomeruli of increased complexity associated with dilated tubules lined by hypertrophic epithelial cells termed oligomeganephronic renal hypoplasia or oligomeganephronia (Figure 13.40). Polyuria and polydipsia are the principal early clinical manifestation [78]. Renal function often remains stable for a long period before secondary focal segmental glomerulosclerosis produces renal insufficiency, likely consequent to glomerular hyperfiltration [79]. Oligomeganephronia can be sporadic or familial and mutations of various genes that affect ureteric bud development are an important cause of the disorder.

Syndromic associations of renal hypoplasia include branchio-oto-renal syndrome, acro-renal syndrome, and renal-coloboma syndrome [78]. Extrarenal manifestations of these syndromes can sometimes be minimal or absent. A more subtle reduction in nephron number affecting both kidneys and not appreciated grossly as renal hypoplasia may be a significant contributor to the development of essential hypertension in adults and may have its origins in prematurity [80].

A lesion sometimes referred to as segmental hypoplasia or Ask-Upmark kidney is a small kidney with one or more sharply demarcated areas of parenchymal atrophy that overlie elongate blunt calyces (Figure 13.41). Hypertension is the principal clinical finding. The affected segments are fibrotic and contain atrophic tubules, occasional small sclerotic glomeruli, and prominent vessels. Inflammation is minimal or absent. Residual tubules may have dysplastic features and there is sometimes complete absence of residual parenchyma (Figure 13.42). Ask-Upmark kidney is now considered to be a form of reflux nephropathy with postnatal parenchymal atrophy [81] . However, some cases likely develop in utero and impaired parenchymal growth in addition to secondary parenchymal atrophy contributes to the lesion.

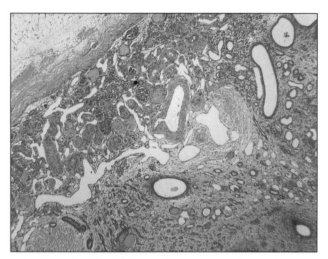

FIGURE 13.38:   The cortex immediately overlying the papilla shown in Fig. 13.37 contains prominent vessels and a paucity of nephrons, but no dysplastic tubules or significant fibrosis (×40).

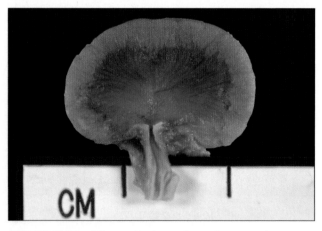

FIGURE 13.39:   The most extreme form of pure renal hypoplasia is represented by a unipapillary kidney.

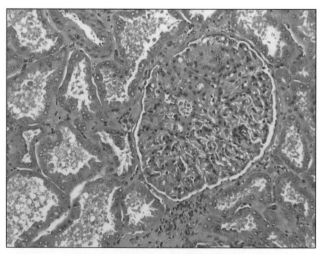

FIGURE 13.40:   Oligomeganephronic renal hypoplasia in a 12 year old child. The glomerulus is large and complex and adjacent tubules are dilated. The glomerulus shows focal segmental glomerulosclerosis. (×400).

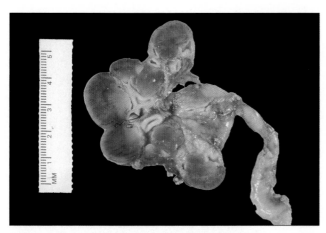

FIGURE 13.41: *Ask-Upmark kidney, a form of reflux nephropathy, has sharply demarcated areas of parenchymal atrophy//hypoplasia overlying elongated calyces.*

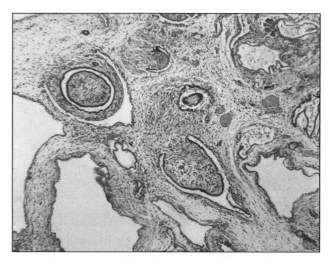

FIGURE 13.43: *Dysplastic tubules in Meckel syndrome often contain distinctive intratubular polyp-like structures (×40).*

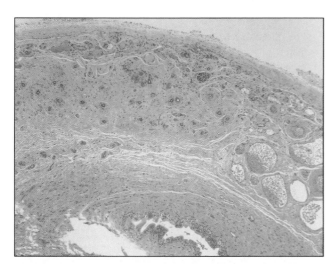

FIGURE 13.42: *Renal parenchyma overlying a calyx shows marked parenchymal atrophy on the left with fibrous collars around the atrophic tubules. The parenchyma on the right lacks any recognizable residual nephrons and may represent an area of hypoplasia (×40).*

Etiology and Pathogenesis of CAKUT

Recent advances in molecular embryology have provided better understanding of the close interrelationship between the various lesions of CAKUT [1,2,4,82–84]. Each ureter develops from a ureteric bud that originates from the proximal aspect of the mesonephric (Wolffian) duct in the lateral wall of the urogenital sinus. The ureteric bud is capped by metanephric blastema within which nephrogenesis is induced in association with successive branching at the apex of the bud. The process involves complex signaling under the control of numerous genes, many of which have multiple roles in the process. This may explain why the morphologic expression of a single mutation can vary widely, even within a single family.

The human *PAX2* gene, located on chromosome 10q24-25, is highly expressed in embryonic kidney, as well as in the eye, cochlea, pancreas, and central nervous system (CNS). It is important both in the development of the ureteric bud and in differentiation of metanephric blastema. *PAX2* mutations in man cause renal-coloboma syndrome (renal malformations and optic nerve dysplasia) [78,85]. Urinary tract lesions that occur in this syndrome include unilateral and bilateral renal hypoplasia, unilateral renal agenesis, ureteropelvic junction obstruction, vesicoureteral reflux, and multicystic dysplasia. There can be considerable morphologic variation in a kindred and the optic nerve abnormality can be subtle and easily overlooked [86].

There are numerous other syndromes associated with CAKUT, including many with specific genetic mutations. The latter include branchio-oto-renal syndrome (hearing defects, preauricular pits, branchial clefts defects, renal abnormalities) due to mutations in *EYA1* or *SIX1*; renal cysts, and diabetes mellitus (MODY5) due to mutations in *HNF-1β*, and Towne-Brocks syndrome (imperforate anus, triphalangeal thumb, rocker bottom feet, hearing defects, and hypospadias) related to *SALL1* mutations. The spectrum of renal abnormalities is similar to that caused by *PAX2*. Mutations were detected in 17 percent of 100 unrelated children with nonobstructive renal hypoplasia/dysplasia and reduced renal function who were screened for mutations in these genes [4]. *PAX2* and *HNF-1β* mutations were the most frequent and phenotypic abnormalities were limited to the urinary tract in almost half of the affected children. *HNF-1β* mutations were found in 31 percent of 80 children with renal cysts, renal hyperechogenicity, renal hypoplasia or a single kidney [61]. There was no correlation between the specific mutation and the renal phenotype. Uroplakin IIIa mutation is another recently recognized cause for renal adysplasia [87].

Meckel-Gruber syndrome is a severe autosomal recessive multisystem malformation disorder in which bilateral renal dysplasia is a cardinal feature. Omphalocele, polydactyly, cleft lip, and CNS malformations including occipital encephalocele are additional features. The kidneys are large and contain innumerable cysts that display histologic features of dysplasia and there is ductal plate malformation of the liver. A distinctive feature of the renal lesion is polypoid structures within the renal cysts

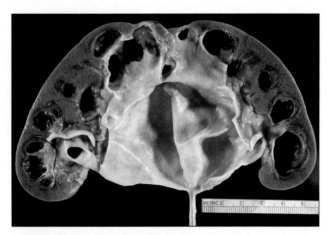

FIGURE 13.44: *Ureteropelvic junction obstruction is part of the CAKUT spectrum of renal maldevelopment.*

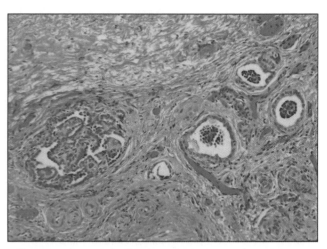

FIGURE 13.45: *Small sclerosing perilobar nephrogenic rest in a dysplastic kidney. Immature-appearing glomeruli are also present (×100).*

(Figure 13.43). Three genes have been linked to the syndrome and at least one of these is a cilioprotein [88].

Because renal dysplasia is often associated with obstruction to urinary flow, it is possible that increased hydrostatic pressure in the developing kidney plays a role in its development. Experimental models, particularly in sheep, confirm that ureteral ligation in the fetus can produce at least some of the histologic features of dysplasia [89]. Dysregulation of *PAX2* and *TGF-β,1* induced by increased hydrostatic pressure is one possible explanation for dysplasia in the context of obstruction [1].

Clinical Correlation

The spectrum of clinical disease associated with CAKUT is broad. Survival of infants in the immediate postnatal period with any combination of bilateral renal dysplasia, aplasia, or agenesis is more dependent upon impaired pulmonary function than renal insufficiency. Amniotic fluid is formed principally from fetal urine in the last half of pregnancy and low fetal urine output results in oligohydramnios with consequent pulmonary hypoplasia. Spontaneous bilateral pneumothorax in a neonate should raise concern for pulmonary hypoplasia caused by severe bilateral renal disease.

Beyond the newborn period, the clinical course of patients with CAKUT varies widely and depends largely on the amount of intact renal parenchyma and the character of the urinary tract anomalies. Those patients with unilateral or localized segmental disease, including those with unilateral renal aplasia/agenesis, may never come to medical attention. Those with abnormalities of the lower urinary tract that predispose to reflux and pyelonephritis and those with significantly reduced intact nephrons, may develop progressive renal insufficiency over the course of many years that culminates in ESRD.

Isolated multicystic renal dysplasia and its variants are usually sporadic. However, sonographic examination of parents and siblings of infants with unilateral renal agenesis and dysplasia of the contralateral kidney or bilateral renal agenesis demonstrates a tenfold increase of occult renal disease, most commonly unilateral renal agenesis [90]. The familial association of bilateral renal agenesis, unilateral renal agenesis, and renal dysplasia is often referred to as hereditary renal adysplasia.

The spectrum of renal adysplasia in some families includes ureteropelvic junction (UPJ) obstruction (Figure 13.44) and ureterovesical reflux. The empiric risk for recurrence of renal adysplasia in a subsequent pregnancy is approximately 3.5 percent, but increases to 15–20 percent if renal anomalies are detected in a parent or sibling [91].

Nephrogenic rests occur with increased frequency in dysplastic kidneys (Figure 13.45). The estimated frequency is approximately 5 percent, a fivefold increase over the general population. Although there are rare examples of Wilms' tumor and renal carcinoma developing in dysplastic kidneys, this small risk is not considered to be clinically significant [92].

REFERENCES

1. Woolf AS, Price KL, Scambler PJ et al. Evolving concepts of renal dysplasia. *J Am Soc Nephrol* 2004;15:998–1007.

2. Glassberg KI. Normal and abnormal development of the kidney: a clinician's interpretation of current knowledge. *J Urol* 2002;167(6): 2339–50; discussion 2350–1.

3. Torres VE, Harris PC. Mechanisms of disease: autosomal dominant and recessive polycystic kidney diseases. *Nat Clin Pract Nephrol* 2006;2:40–55.

4. Weber S, Moriniere V, Knuppel T, Charbit M et al. Prevalence of mutations in renal developmental genes in children with renal hypodysplasia: results of the ESCAPE study. *J Am Soc Nephrol* 2006;17(10):2864–70.

5. Hildebrandt F, Otto E. Cilia and centrosomes: a unifying pathogenic concept for cystic kidney disease? *Nat Rev Genet* 2005;6(12):928–40.

6. Guay-Woodford LM. Renal cystic diseases: diverse phenotypes converge on the cilium/centrosome complex. *Pediatr Nephrol* 2006;21:1369–76.

7. Johnson AM, Gabow PA. Identification of patients with autosomal dominant polycystic kidney disease at highest risk for end-stage renal disease. *J Am Soc Nephrol* 1997;8(10): 1560–7.

8. Hateboer N, v Dijk MA, Bogdanova N, Coto E et al. Comparison of phenotypes of polycystic kidney disease types 1

and 2. European PKD1-PKD2 Study Group. *Lancet* 1999; 353(9147):103–7.

9. Grantham JJ, Torres VE, Chapman AB, Guay-Woodford LM et al. Volume progression in polycystic kidney disease. *N Engl J Med* 2006;354(20):2122–30.

10. Grantham JJ, Cook LT, Torres VE, Bost JE et al. Determinants of renal volume in autosomal-dominant polycystic kidney disease. *Kidney Int* 2008;73(1):108–16.

11. Fick-Brosnahan GM, Tran ZV, Johnson AM, Strain JD et al. Progression of autosomal-dominant polycystic kidney disease in children. *Kidney Int* 2001;59(5):1654–62.

12. Shamshirsaz A, Bekheirnia R, Kamgar M, Johnson AM et al. Autosomal-dominant polycystic kidney disease in infancy and childhood: progression and outcome. *Kidney Int* 2005;68(5): 2218–24.

13. Bernstein J. Glomerulocystic kidney disease–nosological considerations. *Pediatr Nephrol* 1993; 7(4):464–70.

14. Brook-Carter PT, Peral B, Ward CJ, Thompson P et al. Deletion of the TSC2 and PKD1 genes associated with severe infantile polycystic kidney disease–a contiguous gene syndrome. *Nat Genet* 1994;8(4):328–32.

15. Cobben JM, Breuning MH, Schoots C, ten Kate LP et al. Congenital hepatic fibrosis in autosomal-dominant polycystic kidney disease. *Kidney Int* 1990;38(5):880–5.

16. Bernstein, J, Evan AP, Gardner KD, Jr. Epithelial hyperplasia in human polycystic kidney diseases. Its role in pathogenesis and risk of neoplasia. *Am J Pathol* 1987;129(1):92–101.

17. Gregoire JR, Torres VE, Holley KE, Farrow GM. Renal epithelial hyperplastic and neoplastic proliferation in autosomal dominant polycystic kidney disease. *Am J Kidney Dis* 1987; 9(1): 27–38.

18. Keith DS, Torres VE, King BF, Zincki H et al. Renal cell carcinoma in autosomal dominant polycystic kidney disease. *J Am Soc Nephrol* 1994; 4(9):1661–9.

19. Bisceglia M, Creti G. AMR series unilateral (localized) renal cystic disease. *Adv Anat Pathol* 2005;12(4): 227–32.

20. Nauli SM, Zhou J. Polycystins and mechanosensation in renal and nodal cilia. *Bioessays* 2004;26(8):844–56.

21. Wilson PD. Polycystic kidney disease. *N Engl J Med* 2004;350(2):151–64.

22. Nauli SM, Rossetti S, Kolb RJ, Alenghat FJ et al. Loss of polycystin-1 in human cyst-lining epithelia leads to ciliary dysfunction. *J Am Soc Nephrol* 2006;17(4):1015–25.

23. Fain PR, McFann KK, Taylor MR, Tison M et al. Modifier genes play a significant role in the phenotypic expression of PKD1. *Kidney Int* 2005;67(4):1256–67.

24. Avner ED, Sweeney WE Jr. Renal cystic disease: new insights for the clinician. *Pediatr Clin North Am* 2006;53(5):889–909.

25. Chang MY, Ong AC. Autosomal dominant polycystic kidney disease: recent advances in pathogenesis and treatment. *Nephron Physiol* 2008;108(1):1–7.

26. Guay-Woodford LM and Desmond RA. Autosomal recessive polycystic kidney disease: the clinical experience in North America. *Pediatrics* 2003;111(5 Pt 1):1072–80.

27. Bergmann C, Senderek J, Windelen E, Kupper F et al. Clinical consequences of PKHD1 mutations in 164 patients with autosomal-recessive polycystic kidney disease (ARPKD). *Kidney Int* 2005;67(3):829–48.

28. Adeva M, El-Youssef M, Rossetti S, Kamath PS et al. Clinical and molecular characterization defines a broadened spectrum of autosomal recessive polycystic kidney disease (ARPKD). *Medicine (Baltimore)* 2006;85(1):1–21.

29. Blyth H, Ockenden BG. Polycystic disease of kidney and liver presenting in childhood. *J Med Genet* 1971;8(3):257–84.

30. Dehner LP, *Pediatric Surgical Pathology*,2nd ed. (Baltimore, MD: Williams and Wilkins, 1987), pp.598–602.

31. Lieberman E, Salinas-Madrigal L, Gwinn JL, Brennan LP et al. Infantile polycystic disease of the kidneys and liver: clinical, pathological and radiological correlations and comparison with congenital hepatic fibrosis. *Medicine (Baltimore)* 1971;50(4):277–318.

32. Blickman JG, Bramson RT, Herrin JT. Autosomal recessive polycystic kidney disease: long-term sonographic findings in patients surviving the neonatal period. *AJR Am J Roentgenol* 1995; 164(5):1247–50.

33. Johnson CA, Gissen P, Sergi C. Molecular pathology and genetics of congenital hepatorenal fibrocystic syndromes. *J Med Genet* 2003;40(5):311–9.

34. Sweeney WEJr., Avner ED. Molecular and cellular pathophysiology of autosomal recessive polycystic kidney disease (ARPKD). *Cell Tissue Res* 2006;326(3):671–85.

35. Hildebrandt F, Omram H. New insights: nephronophthisis-medullary cystic kidney disease. *Pediatr Nephrol* 2001;16(2): 168–76.

36. Saunier S, Salomon R, and C. Antignac C, Nephronophthisis. *Curr Opin Genet Dev*, 2005. ;15(3): p. 324–31.

37. Hildebrandt F, Zhou W. Nephronophthisis-associated ciliopathies. *J Am Soc Nephrol* 2007;18(6): 1855–71.

38. Kumada S, Hayashi M, Arima K, Nakayama H et al., Renal disease in Arima syndrome is nephronophthisis as in other Joubert-related Cerebello-oculo-renal syndromes. *Am J Med Genet A* 2004;131(1):71–6.

39. Otto EA, Schermer B, Obara T, O'Toole JF et al. Mutations in INVS encoding inversin cause nephronophthisis type 2, linking renal cystic disease to the function of primary cilia and left-right axis determination. *Nat Genet* 2003;34(4): 413–20.

40. Waldherr R,Lennert T, Weber HP, Fodisch HJ et al. The nephronophthisis complex. A clinicopathologic study in children. *Virchows Arch A Pathol Anat Histol* 1982;394(3):235–54.

41. Witzleben CL, Sharp AR. "Nephronophthisis-congenital hepatic fibrosis": an additional hepatorenal disorder. *Hum Pathol* 1982;13(8):728–33.

42. O'Toole JF, Otto EA, Hoefele J, Helou J et al. Mutational analysis in 119 families with nephronophthisis. *Pediatr Nephrol* 2007;22(3):366–70.

43. Parisi MA, Doherty D, Eckert ML, Shaw DW et al., AHI1 mutations cause both retinal dystrophy and renal cystic disease in Joubert syndrome. *J Med Genet* 2006;43(4):334–9.

44. Stoetzel C, Muller J, Laurier V, Davis EE et al. Identification of a novel BBS gene (BBS12) highlights the major role of a vertebrate-specific branch of chaperonin-related proteins in Bardet-Biedl syndrome. *Am J Hum Genet* 2007;80(1):1–11.

45. Parfrey PS, Davidson WS, Green JS. Clinical and genetic epidemiology of inherited renal disease in Newfoundland. *Kidney Int* 2002;61(6):1925–34.

46. Wolf MT, Beck BB, Zaucke F, Kunze A et al. The Uromodulin C744G mutation causes MCKD2 and FJHN in children and adults and may be due to a possible founder effect. *Kidney Int* 2007;71(6):574–81.

47. Dahan K, Fuchshuber A, Adamis S, Smaers M et al. Familial juvenile hyperuricemic nephropathy and autosomal dominant medullary cystic kidney disease type 2: two facets of the same disease? *J Am Soc Nephrol* 2001;12(11):2348–57.

48. Rampoldi L, Caridi G, Santon D, Boaretto F et al. Allelism of MCKD, FJHN and GCKD caused by impairment of uromodulin export dynamics. *Hum Mol Genet* 2003;12(24): 3369–84.

49. Dahan K, Devuyst O, Smaers M, Vertommen D et al., A cluster of mutations in the UMOD gene causes familial juvenile hyperuricemic nephropathy with abnormal expression of uromodulin. *J Am Soc Nephrol* 2003;14(11):2883–93.

50. Wolf, M.T, Mucha BE, Hennies HC, Attanasio M et al. Medullary cystic kidney disease type 1: mutational analysis in 37 genes based on haplotype sharing. *Hum Genet* 2006;119(6):649–58.

51. Hart TC, Gorry MC, Hart PS, Woodard AS et al. Mutations of the UMOD gene are responsible for medullary cystic kidney disease 2 and familial juvenile hyperuricaemic nephropathy. *J Med Genet* 2002;39(12):882–92.

52. Hodanova K, Majewski J, Kublova M, Vyletal P et al. Mapping of a new candidate locus for uromodulin-associated kidney disease (UAKD) to chromosome 1q41. *Kidney Int* 2005;68(4): 1472–82.

53. Bernascone I, Vavassori S, Di Pentima A, Santambrogio S et al. Defective intracellular trafficking of uromodulin mutant isoforms. *Traffic* 2006;7(11):1567–79.

54. Scolari F, Caridi G, Rampoldi L, Tardanico R et al. Uromodulin storage diseases: clinical aspects and mechanisms. *Am J Kidney Dis* 2004;44(6):987–99.

55. Patriquin HB, O'Regan S. Medullary sponge kidney in childhood. *AJR Am J Roentgenol* 1985; 145(2):315–9.

56. Indridason OS, Thomas L, Berkoben M. Medullary sponge kidney associated with congenital hemihypertrophy. *J Am Soc Nephrol* 1996;7(8):1123–30.

57. Ginalski JM, Portmann L, Jaeger P. Does medullary sponge kidney cause nephrolithiasis? *AJR Am J Roentgenol* 1990;155(2):299–302.

58. Yagisawa T, Kobayashi C, Hayashi T, Yoshida A et al. Contributory metabolic factors in the development of nephrolithiasis in patients with medullary sponge kidney. *Am J Kidney Dis* 2001;37(6):1140–3.

59. Feather SA, Winyard PJ, Dodd S, Woolf AS. Oral-facial-digital syndrome type 1 is another dominant polycystic kidney disease: clinical, radiological and histopathological features of a new kindred. *Nephrol Dial Transplant* 1997;12(7):1354–61.

60. Edghill EL, Bingham C, Ellard S, Hattersley AT. Mutations in hepatocyte nuclear factor-1beta and their related phenotypes. *J Med Genet* 2006;43(1):84–90.

61. Ulinski T, Lescure S, Beaufils S, Guigonis V et al. Renal phenotypes related to hepatocyte nuclear factor-1beta (TCF2) mutations in a pediatric cohort. *J Am Soc Nephrol* 2006;17(2):497–503.

62. Decramer S, Parant O, Beaufils S, Clauin S et al. Anomalies of the TCF2 gene are the main cause of fetal bilateral hyperechogenic kidneys. *J Am Soc Nephrol* 2007;18(3):923–33.

63. Bingham C, Ellard S, Cole TR, Jones KE et al. Solitary functioning kidney and diverse genital tract malformations associated with hepatocyte nuclear factor-1beta mutations. *Kidney Int* 2002; 61(4):1243–51.

64. Bellanne-Chantelot C, Chauveau D, Gautier JF, Dubois-Laforgue D et al. Clinical spectrum associated with hepatocyte nuclear factor-1beta mutations. *Ann Intern Med* 2004;140(7):510–17.

65. Bisceglia M, CA Galliani, C Senger, C Stallone et al. Renal cystic diseases: a review. *Adv Anat Pathol* 2006;13(1):26–56.

66. Dabora SL, Jozwiak S, Franz DN, Roberts PS et al. Mutational analysis in a cohort of 224 tuberous sclerosis patients indicates increased severity of TSC2, compared with TSC1, disease in multiple organs. *Am J Hum Genet* 2001;68(1): 64–80.

67. Rakowski SK, Winterkorn EB, Paul E, Steele DJ et al. Renal manifestations of tuberous sclerosis complex: Incidence, prognosis, and predictive factors. *Kidney Int* 2006;70(10): 1777–82.

68. Bernstein J., Renal cystic disease in the tuberous sclerosis complex. *Pediatr Nephrol* 1993;7(4): 490–5.

69. Martignoni G, Bonetti F, Pea M, Tardanico R et al. Renal disease in adults with TSC2/PKD1 contiguous gene syndrome. *Am J Surg Pathol* 2002;26(2):198–205.

70. Kleymenova E., Ibraghimov-Beskrovnaya O, Kugoh H, Everitt J et al. Tuberin-dependent membrane localization of polycystin-1: a functional link between polycystic kidney disease and the TSC2 tumor suppressor gene. *Mol Cell* 2001;7(4):823–32.

71. Truong LD, Choi YJ, Shen SS, Ayala G et al. Renal cystic neoplasms and renal neoplasms associated with cystic renal diseases: pathogenetic and molecular links. *Adv Anat Pathol* 2003; 10(3):135–59.

72. Chatha RK, Johnson AM, Rothberg PG, Townsend RR et al. Von Hippel-Lindau disease masquerading as autosomal dominant polycystic kidney disease. *Am J Kidney Dis* 2001; 37(4):852–8.

73. Paraf, F, Chauveau D, Chretien Y, Richard S et al., Renal lesions in von Hippel-Lindau disease: immunohistochemical expression of nephron differentiation molecules, adhesion molecules and apoptosis proteins. *Histopathology* 2000;36(5): 457–65.

74. Nishimura H, E. Yerkes K. Hohenfellner, Y. Miyazaki, et al., Role of the angiotensin type 2 receptor gene in congenital anomalies of the kidney and urinary tract, CAKUT, of mice and men. *Mol Cell* 1999;3(1):1–10.

75. Sase M, Tsukahara M, Oga A, Kaneko N et al. Diffuse cystic renal dysplasia: nonsyndromal familial case. *Am J Med Genet* 1996;63(2):332–4.

76. Rottenberg GT, Gordon I, De Bruyn R. The natural history of the multicystic dysplastic kidney in children. *Br J Radiol* 1997;70(832):347–50.

77. Hiraoka M, Tsukahara H, Ohshima Y, Kasuga K et al. Renal aplasia is the predominant cause of congenital solitary kidneys. *Kidney Int* 2002;61(5):1840–4.

78. Salomon R, Tellier AL, Attie-Bitach T, Amiel J et al. PAX2 mutations in oligomeganephronia. *Kidney Int* 2001;59(2): 457–62.

79. Suzuki H, Tokuriki T, Kamita H, Oota C et al. Age-related pathophysiological changes in rat oligomeganephronic hypoplastic kidney. *Pediatr Nephrol* 2006;21(5):637–42.

80. Keller G, Zimmer G, Mall G, Ritz E et al. Nephron number in patients with primary hypertension. *N Engl J Med* 2003;348(2):101–8.

81. Shindo S, Bernstein J, Arant BS Jr. Evolution of renal segmental atrophy (Ask-Upmark kidney) in children with vesicoureteric reflux: radiographic and morphologic studies. *J Pediatr* 1983; 102(6):847–54.

82. Pope JCt, Brock JW 3rd, Adams MC, Stephens FD et al. How they begin and how they end: classic and new theories for the development and deterioration of congenital anomalies of the kidney and urinary tract, CAKUT. *J Am Soc Nephrol* 1999;10(9):2018–28.

83. Woolf AS, PJ Winyard. Molecular mechanisms of human embryogenesis: developmental pathogenesis of renal tract malformations. *Pediatr Dev Pathol* 2002;5(2):108–29.

84. Thomas JC, DeMarco RT, Pope JCt. Molecular biology of ureteral bud and trigonal development. *Curr Urol Rep* 2005;6(2):146–51.

85. Dziarmaga A, Quinlan J, Goodyer P. Renal hypoplasia: lessons from Pax2. *Pediatr Nephrol* 2006; 21(1):26–31.

86. Fletcher J, Hu M, Berman Y,Collins F et al. Multicystic dysplastic kidney and variable phenotype in a family with a novel deletion mutation of PAX2. *J Am Soc Nephrol* 2005;16(9): 2754–61.

87. Jenkins D, Bitner-Glindzicz M, Malcolm S, Hu CC, et al. De novo Uroplakin IIIa heterozygous mutations cause human renal adysplasia leading to severe kidney failure. *J Am Soc Nephrol* 2005;16(7):2141–9.

88. Smith UM, Consugar M, Tee LJ, McKee BM et al. The transmembrane protein meckelin (MKS3) is mutated in Meckel-Gruber syndrome and the wpk rat. *Nat Genet* 2006;38(2):191–6.

89. Kitagawa H, Pringle KC, Zuccolo J, Stone P et al. The pathogenesis of dysplastic kidney in a urinary tract obstruction in the female fetal lamb. *J Pediatr Surg* 1999;34(11):1678–83.

90. Roodhooft AM, JC Birnholz, LB Holmes. Familial nature of congenital absence and severe dysgenesis of both kidneys. *N Engl J Med* 1984;310(21):1341–5.

91. McPherson E, Carey J, Kramer A, Hall JG et al. Dominantly inherited renal adysplasia. *Am J Med Genet* 1987;26(4):863–72.

92. Narchi H. Risk of Wilms' tumour with multicystic kidney disease: a systematic review. *Arch Dis Child* 2005;90(2):147–9.

93. Woolf AS, Feather SA, Bingham C. Recent insights into kidney diseases associated with glomerular cysts. *Pediatr Nephrol* 2002:17(4):229–35.

CHAPTER 14

The Aging Kidney

Xin J. Zhou MD, Dinesh Rakheja MD, and Fred G. Silva MD

INTRODUCTION AND EPIDEMIOLOGY

Improvements in prevention and medical treatment of diseases have led to increased life expectancies all over the world, resulting in an absolute increase in the number of elderly people. In addition, the lower population growth rates in the developed world have led to a relative increase in the elderly, leading to an inversion of the population pyramid. The growth in the number and proportion of older adults is unparalleled in the history of the United States. Longer life spans and aging baby boomers will double the population of Americans aged 65 years and older during the next twenty-five years. By 2030, there will be 71 million older adults accounting for approximately 20 percent of the U.S. population [1]. Similarly, in the European Union, the population aged 60 years and over comprises 21 percent of the population, and is projected to increase to 27 percent by 2022, and 33 percent by 2050 [2]. Aging is accompanied by a higher rate of morbidity, with a consequent impact on the economic and human resources. Compared to younger individuals, it costs three to five times more to provide health care for an American older than 65 years. As a result, by 2030, the nation's health care spending is projected to increase by 25 percent [1].

The increased incidence of renal diseases in the elderly is a result of the increased life expectancy, and the predisposition of the aging kidney to injury. According to the U.S. Renal Data System (USRDS), between 1995 and 2005, the adjusted point-prevalence rates per million population of reported end-stage renal disease increased from 70.5 to 82.1 (16 percent increase) in the age group 0–19 years, from 730.6 to 858.2 (17 percent increase) in the age group 20–44 years, from 2333.3 to 3150.4 (35 percent increase) in the age group 45–64 years, from 3627.5 to 5500.6 (51 percent increase) in the age group 65–74 years, and from 2762.4 to 4795.8 (73 percent increase) in the age-group $\geq$75 years [3]. This increase in the numbers of older patients on dialysis and on renal transplant lists has obvious social and economic implications, and underscores the need for stronger research initiatives directed to the causes of renal diseases in the elderly [4].

It is important to realize that, although structural and functional changes of the kidney occur ubiquitously with aging, there is no specific disease confined only to the geriatric population. In general, the types of renal diseases seen in the elderly are similar to those encountered in the general population, although certain disorders may have an increased prevalence (i.e., renal disease secondary to type 2 diabetes mellitus, hypertension, and amyloidosis, among others). Therefore, the approach to the interpretation of renal biopsies in the elderly is similar to that of the general population as detailed throughout this book. Thus, the first step is to study each individual component (i.e., glomeruli, tubules, interstitium, and vessels) of the kidney, and to sort out which renal compartment is primarily involved by the disease process. Given the high prevalence of type 2 diabetes mellitus and hypertension in the elderly, these two disorders should be ruled out before ascribing any

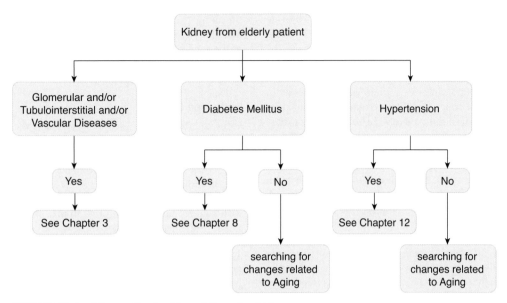

FIGURE 14.1: *Diagnostic algorithm of the aging kidney.*

morphologic changes to aging, although aging is often intricately intertwined with hypertension and/or diabetes. Figure 14.1 provides a simplified algorithmic approach for the interpretation of renal biopsy from the elderly patients.

CLINICAL PRESENTATION

Functional Changes of the Aging Kidney

Glomerular Function

Inulin clearance, an excellent measure of the glomerular filtration rate (GFR), is about 20 mL/min at birth, and gradually rises to 120 mL/min by the age of 30 years. It is a generally accepted dogma that the GFR declines with increasing age after the age of about 30 years, when it starts dropping at an average rate of 1 mL per year [5], which calculates to an inulin clearance of 60 mL/min at the age of 90 years. However, in the Baltimore longitudinal study of aging among 254 "normal" subjects, although the mean decline in creatinine clearance was 0.75 mL/min/year, 36 percent of the subjects showed no aging-related decrease in creatinine clearance, and a few of these subjects actually showed an increase in their creatinine clearance [6]. Creatinine clearance, of course, is influenced by the nutritional status, protein intake, and muscle mass, and is therefore, an inferior method to estimate GFR in the elderly. Healthy, elderly subjects with daily ingestion of more than 1 g of protein/kg body weight had a creatinine clearance of 90–100 mL/min/1.73 m² body surface area, while those with diets, poorer in protein, had lower creatinine clearances [7]. In addition, the creatinine production gradually declines with age in proportion with the decreasing muscle mass and body weight. Therefore, the urinary creatinine output also shows a corresponding decline. This is the reason why the plasma creatinine does not increase with increasing age, despite the aging-related reduction in the creatinine clearance [8]. It follows that a modestly elevated plasma creatinine may be of greater significance in the elderly than in a younger patient.

Several formulas have been developed to calculate GFR, using serum creatinine, and taking variable parameters such as age, gender, body weight, and height into consideration. To this end, the Modification of Diet in Renal Disease Study Group (MDRD) formula [9] for calculating GFR is superior to the Cockroft-Gault formula [10], which underestimates creatinine clearance in older subjects. However, the MDRD formula has not been validated in population older than 70 years [9]. More recently, serum cystatin C measurement, especially when compared to the reference values adjusted for age, has become a promising index of renal function in the elderly [11].

Cockroft-Gault formula [10]:

$$C_{Cr}(mL/\min) = \frac{(140 - Age \times Weight)}{72 \times S_{Cr}} \times (0.85 \ if \ female)$$

MDRD formula [9]:

$$GFR(mL/\min \ per \ 1.73m^2) = 186 \times (S_{Cr})^{-1.154}$$
$$\times (Age)^{-0.203} \times (0.742 \ if \ female)$$
$$\times (1.210 \ if \ African\text{-}American)$$

Tubular Function

Several tubular functions are altered in the aging kidney (Table 14.1) [12–15]. The kidneys in the elderly show an attenuated decline

Table 14.1 Altered Tubular Functions in the Aging Kidney

Inability to conserve and/or excrete sodium chloride
Inability to maintain other electrolyte balances
Inability to concentrate and/or dilute urine
Impaired distal tubular acidification
Blunted tubular transport capacities and delayed response
Decreased 1,25 Vitamin D production and impaired response to various hormones

in sodium excretion in response to dietary sodium chloride deprivation. In healthy subjects (free of cardiovascular, renal, or adrenal disease) on diets restricted to 230 mg of sodium, the reduction in urine sodium occurred significantly earlier in subjects under 30 years compared to subjects aged 30 to 59 years; and the delay in reduction in urine sodium was even greater in subjects over 60 years of age [16]. On the other hand, on a diet containing 4,000 mg of sodium, there were no significant differences in mean 24-hour urinary sodium excretion and fractional excretion of sodium between the healthy young (26 ± 3 years), the healthy elderly (68 ± 7 years), the elderly with treated and untreated hypertension (70 ± 6 years), and the elderly with compensated mild to moderate heart failure (69 ± 6 years). Compared to the healthy young subjects, the mean lithium clearance, an indicator of proximal tubular function, was significantly lower in all the three groups of elderly subjects. Accordingly, the fractional proximal sodium reabsorption was significantly higher in the elderly subjects, but this was offset by the lower distal fractional reabsorption of sodium in the elderly [17].

The elderly are predisposed to developing drug-induced hyperkalemia with a variety of drugs such as potassium supplements, potassium-sparing diuretics, nonsteroidal antiinflammatory drugs, angiotensin-converting enzyme inhibitors, beta-blockers, heparin, digoxin, and trimethoprim. Potassium is freely filtered across the glomerular capillaries into the proximal convoluted tubules, where it is actively reabsorbed. Urine potassium is derived from active transtubular transport from the blood across the "principal cells" in the distal nephron and collecting duct. This potassium secretion is linked to the reabsorption of sodium across the aldosterone-modulated Na-K ATPase transporters in the principal cells. Thus, impaired potassium secretion may occur because of tubular atrophy or tubulointerstitial scarring as a result of prior pyelonephritis or ongoing glomerulosclerosis, hyporeninemic hypoaldosteronism associated with diabetes mellitus or renal insufficiency, normoreninemic hypoaldosteronism of unknown cause, and decreased water and sodium delivery to the distal nephron due to dehydration and reduced intravascular volume. All these conditions are common in the elderly, predisposing them to develop hyperkalemia in response to drugs that challenge the already compromised potassium secreting ability of their kidneys [18].

The ability of the kidney to both maximally concentrate and dilute the urine diminishes with age. Compared to healthy subjects aged 20–39 years and 40–59 years, the healthy subjects aged 60 to 79 years had an approximately 20 percent reduction in maximum urine osmolality, a 100 percent increase in minimal urine flow rate, and a 50 percent decrease in the ability to conserve solute [19]. The otherwise healthy elderly subjects had a higher rate of nocturia, and a higher nocturnal excretion of water, sodium, and potassium than their younger counterparts [20]. Compared to the young, the elderly had lower plasma vasopressin than the young, and a reduced maximum free water clearance, but similar overall ability to excrete the water-load [21]. Based on these results, the authors suggested that the elderly subjects were in a state similar to partial cranial diabetes insipidus, which may predispose them to dehydration and hypernatremia; on the other hand, the reduction in maximum free water clearance may predispose them to hyponatremia if excess fluid is administered [21]. The reduced concentrating and diluting abilities of the aged kidneys may be related to the aging-related decline in GFR. While a relative increase in medullary blood flow may also impair the concentrating ability of the aged kidney, a functional impairment of the diluting segment of the thick ascending loop of Henle may also account for the diminished diluting ability.

Endocrine Function

While there are many causes of anemia in the elderly, normocytic normochromic anemia may be related to the reduced erythropoietin (EPO) production by the kidney [22]. The InCHIANTI study showed an association between advancing age, declining renal function, reduced EPO production, and anemia. After adjusting for confounding variables, the subjects with a creatinine clearance of ≤ 30 mL/min had a higher prevalence of anemia compared to those with a creatinine clearance ≥ 90 mL/min. Subjects with a creatinine clearance of ≤ 30 mL/min had significantly lower age- and hemoglobin-adjusted endogenous EPO levels. After excluding men and women with a creatinine clearance of ≤ 30 mL/min and adjusting for confounders, the authors found a trend toward an increase in the prevalence of anemia with a decreasing renal function [23]. Serum EPO levels rise with age in healthy subjects, perhaps a compensation for aging-related subclinical blood loss, increased red blood cell turnover, or increased EPO resistance of red cell precursors [24]. On the other hand, the serum EPO levels are unexpectedly lower in elderly with anemia compared to the young subjects with anemia, suggesting a blunted response to low hemoglobin [25].

A low creatinine clearance of less than 65 mL/min is reported to be an independent risk factor for falls and associated fractures in the elderly with osteoporosis [26]. In a recent study, elderly women with osteoporosis and low creatinine clearance (< 60 mL/min) had lower calcium absorption, lower serum 1,25-dihydroxyvitamin D, and normal serum 25-hydroxyvitamin D, suggesting a decreased conversion of 25-hydroxyvitamin D to 1,25-dihydroxyvitamin D by the aging kidney. Furthermore, calcitriol therapy reduced the number of falls by 50 percent, which was postulated by the authors to be related to an increase in serum 1,25-dihydroxyvitamin D, in addition to an upregulation of vitamin D receptors in muscle, and an improvement in muscle strength [27].

Predisposition of the Aging Kidney to Diseases

The aging kidney may be affected by a myriad of diseases, some of which are more prevalent in the elderly. However, there is no specific disease confined exclusively to the elderly population. These disorders (Table 14.2) [12–15] are discussed elsewhere in this book.

APPROACH TO INTERPRETATION

Gross Pathology

The average kidney weight increases from birth to about age 40–50 years, and then progressively declines with a dramatic decrease of 20–30 percent occurring between 70 and 90 years of age. This loss of kidney mass affects the renal cortex more than the medulla, leading to thinning of the renal cortical parenchyma [12]. On gross examination, the kidneys from elderly subjects are symmetrically contracted with a finely granular texture of the subcapsular surface. In addition to the loss of renal mass, almost 50 percent of the subjects over the age of

Table 14.2 Diseases that Commonly affect the Aging Kidney

Systemic diseases

Hypertension
Diabetes mellitus
Dyslipidemia
Atherosclerosis
Atheroemboli
Myeloma cast nephropathy
Amyloidosis
Light chain deposition disease
Vasculitides

Glomerular diseases

Membranous glomerulopathy
Mesangial proliferative GN (including IgA nephropathy)
Pauci-immune crescentic GN
Anti-GBM disease
Minimal change disease
Focal segmental glomerulosclerosis

Acute renal failure

Hypovolemic and cardiovascular shock
Septic shock
Nephrotoxic injury
Nonsteroidal anti-inflammatory agents
Antibiotics (penicillins, cephalosporins, sulfonamides, rifampin, ciprofloxacin)
Diuretics (furosemide, potassium-sparing diuretics)
Contrast media
Cancer chemotherapy
Allopurinol
Cimetidine
Captopril

Interstitial nephritis

Urinary tract infection

Renal stones

Obstructive uropathy

Benign Causes
Nodular hyperplasia of prostate
Neurogenic bladder
Renal stones
Obstructive pyelonephritis/papillary necrosis
Urethral stricture
Malignant Causes
Prostate cancer
Bladder cancer
Pelvic tumors
Colonic tumors
Retroperitoneal tumors

Renal tumors

Primary
Metastatic

Simple renal cysts

From: Zhou XJ, Rakheja D, Yu XQ, Saxena R, Vaziri ND, Silva FG. *Kidney Int* 2008; 74(6):710–20 (with permission).

40 years have one or more acquired renal cysts [28,29]. The cysts are usually round to oval and unilocular, contain clear yellowish fluid, and are believed to arise either from dilated tubules or glomeruli, or from tubular diverticula that are found in an increasing incidence with aging.

Light Microscopy

Aging Glomerulus

Many morphologic changes have been noted in the human glomerulus with aging (Table 14.3) [12,14,15,29]. The numbers of glomeruli (and therefore, nephrons) in each kidney vary from 333,000 to 1,100,000 with a mean of 620,000 ± 250,000 (25th percentile at 500,000 and 75th percentile at 740,000) [30]. An even greater variation in normal glomerular numbers was found by Hughson et al. who found that the total number of glomeruli was normally distributed and ranged from 227,327 to 1,825,380 in autopsy kidneys from thirty-seven African-Americans and nineteen Caucasians [31]. The average female has 15 percent fewer glomeruli than the average male [32]. The mean glomerular number is significantly lower in Australian aborigines, but is not significantly different between Caucasians and African-Americans [32]. Consistent with the decrease in the kidney-weight and thinning of the cortical ribbon with increasing age, the glomeruli also decrease in number with aging [30,32]. At birth, the number of nephrons is directly and linearly

Table 14.3 Morphological Changes of the Aging Kidney

Glomerulus

• Progressive decline in the number of intact/normal glomeruli
• Increased number of globally sclerotic glomeruli, especially the glomeruli in the outer cortical regions initially
• Abnormal glomeruli with shunts between the afferent and efferent arterioles, especially those in the juxtamedullary region
• Progressive decrease, and then later increase, in the size of intact glomeruli
• Focal or diffuse thickening of the glomerular basement membranes[a]
• Increased mesangial volume and matrix (i.e., mesangial sclerosis)[a]

Tubulointerstitium

• Decreased tubular volume, length and number
• Increased number of tubular diverticula, especially the distal convoluted tubules
• Tubular atrophy, often with simplification of the tubular epithelium and thickening of the tubular basement membranes
• Increased interstitial volume with interstitial fibrosis, and sometimes even inflammatory cells
• Decreased peritubular capillary density

Vasculature

• "Fibroelastic hyperplasia" of the arcuate arteries
• Tortuous/spiraling interlobar arteries with thickening of the medial muscle cell basement membrane
• Intimal fibroplasia of the interlobular arteries
• "Hyaline" change/plasmatic insudation of the afferent arterioles
• Vascular "simplification" with direct channels forming between the afferent and efferent arterioles

[a] Not all agreed.

proportional to the birth weight, with regression coefficient analysis predicting an increase of 257,426 glomeruli per kilogram increase of birth weight [31]. There is an up to eightfolds variation in the adult glomerular volume, which shows a strong inverse correlation with the number of glomeruli [33].

Interestingly, while there were no significant relationships between the glomerular number, mean arterial blood pressure (MAP), and birth weights in African-Americans from the southeastern United States, the glomerular number directly correlated with birth weight and inversely with MAP in the White adults [32]. These intriguing data suggest that the low nephron number, and possibly low birth weight may play a role in the development of hypertension in the Whites, but not in the African-Americans. African-Americans also show significantly larger glomerular volume compared to the Whites, and this difference is most marked in the juxtamedullary zone and is independent of age, body surface area (BSA), and glomerular number. There are no significant zonal differences in the glomerular volumes in the young (ages 20–30 years), or those with BSA ≤ 2.11 m^2. On the other hand, the superficial glomeruli in the older age-group (ages 51–69 years), in those with BSA > 2.11 m^2, and in Caucasians were significantly larger than the juxtamedullary glomeruli [34].

Four types of glomeruli have been described in aging kidneys: normal, hypertrophic, focal segmental sclerotic (FSGS-type), and ischemic. The hypertrophic and FSGS-type glomeruli are significantly larger whereas the ischemic glomeruli are significantly smaller than the normal glomeruli [35]. Small glomeruli may also be secondary to tubulointerstitial damage, and a loss of connection of the glomeruli to the proximal tubules. These "atubular glomeruli" are smaller in volume, contain fewer capillaries, and do not contribute to glomerular filtration [36]. Besides primary tubulointerstitial diseases, atubular glomeruli may occur in diabetes mellitus, and may represent a mechanism for the gradual nephron loss associated with aging [37,38]. Many studies have shown that the development of focal

segmental glomerulosclerosis and the percentage of glomeruli showing global glomerulosclerosis increases with age. Standard morphometric techniques and multiple linear regression analysis have shown a direct correlation between the number/percentage of globally sclerotic glomeruli and increasing age as well as intrarenal vascular disease, especially outer cortical vascular disease; and an inverse correlation between global glomerulosclerosis and intrarenal arterial lumen area [39]. In this study, the glomerular size was best directly correlated with heart weight and coronary artery atherosclerosis, rather than with global glomerulosclerosis. The latter correlated directly with aortic atherosclerosis [39].

One has to keep in mind that the different appearances of globally sclerosed glomeruli may be related to different etiopathogenesis. In the solidified globally sclerosed glomeruli, the sclerotic tuft fills the entirety of the Bowman's space with hyaline lesions often recognizable, representing the sclerosis of the FSGS-type glomeruli (Figure 14.2) [35]. If a globally sclerosed glomerulus appears larger than usual, then an infiltrative process such as amyloidosis or diabetes mellitus should be considered (Figure 14.3). The glomerulosclerosis secondary to ischemic vascular disease (obsolescent sclerotic glomeruli) displays initial shrinkage of the glomerular tuft, with wrinkling and thickening of the glomerular basement membrane (GBM), and collagen deposition internal to Bowman's capsule, near the vascular hilum; subsequently, the progressive collagen deposition fills the entire Bowman's space (Figure 14.4) [12,29]. Another route to glomerulosclerosis is via glomerular inflammation, such as that happens after an extensive crescent formation. This type of glomerulosclerosis may be identified with breaks in the basal lamina of Bowman's capsule [12,29] (Figure 14.5). It can occur in numerous diseases such as IgA nephropathy, antineutrophil cytoplasmic antibody (ANCA)-associated disease, and lupus, and as such, these conditions should be carefully excluded before ascribing global glomerulosclerosis to aging. In addition, the percentage of globally sclerosed glomeruli that can be considered "normal" depends on the patient's age. Thus,

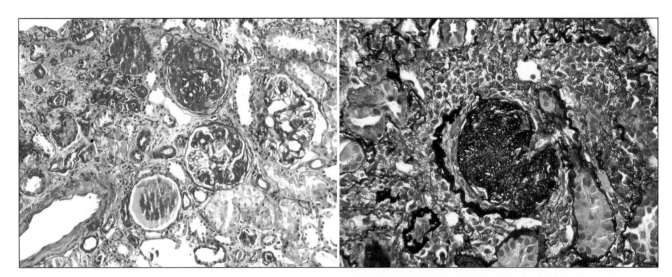

FIGURE 14.2: Focal segmental and global glomerulosclerosis in aging kidney. (left) There are two globally sclerotic glomeruli and one glomerulus showing segmental sclerosis. There is also tubular atrophy, interstitial fibrosis, and chronic inflammation. The interlobular artery has significant intimal fibrosis (PAS; × 200). (right). Solidified global glomerulosclerosis. The entire glomerular tuft is solidified (Jones methenamine silver; × 400).

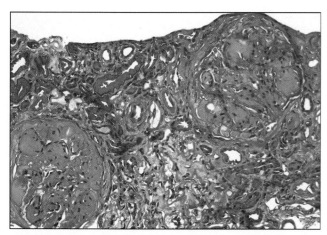

FIGURE 14.3: *Advanced nodular diabetic glomerulosclerosis. The two globally sclerotic glomeruli remain relatively large with a nodular appearance (Trichrome; × 200).*

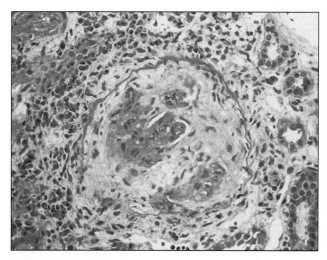

FIGURE 14.5: *Globally sclerotic glomerulus with fibrous/ fibrocellular crescent. The glomerular tuft is fragmented due to an intervening crescent with disruption of the Bowman's capsule (PAS; × 400).*

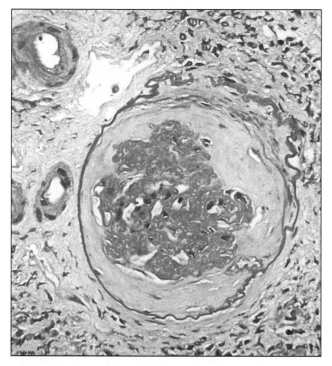

FIGURE 14.4: *Ischemic glomerular obsolescence. The glomerular tuft is shrunken and globally wrinkled and thickened with loss of most cells. The Bowman's space is filled with collagenous material that stains less intensely than the capillary tuft. The Bowman's capsule is intact (PAS; × 400).*

up to 10 percent of the glomeruli may be globally sclerotic in a subject younger than 40 years; beyond 40 years, the estimation of "normal" sclerosed glomeruli is difficult as the effects of diseases such as diabetes, hypertension, and vascular disease confound such estimation [40]. It has been suggested that the renal pathologist should seriously consider "pathologic" glomerulosclerosis when the number of globally sclerosed glomeruli exceeds the number calculated by the formula: (patient's age/2) – 10 [41].

It is important to note that the search for globally sclerosed glomeruli in kidney biopsies may be problematic, and that globally sclerosed glomeruli may be underestimated on single section examinations using the routine hematoxylin and eosin (H&E) stain. Special histochemical stains, such as periodic acid Schiff (PAS), silver methenamine, and Masson trichrome, are helpful in recognizing shrunken globally sclerosed glomeruli that may merge imperceptibly with the adjacent, usually scarred, and sometimes inflamed interstitium. Globally sclerotic glomeruli can also be resorbed over time, leading to underestimates of the proportion of sclerotic glomeruli.

The pathogenesis of aging-associated focal segmental and global glomerulosclerosis is not completely understood and likely multifactorial. Dysautoregulation of the afferent and efferent arterioles of the glomerulus may lead to increased glomerular plasma flow, increased glomerular intracapillary pressures, and subsequent "hyperperfusion" glomerular injury with mesangial matrix accumulation [42,43]. The vascular adaptations to functional or structural nephron loss may help preserve GFR by producing hyperperfusion and hyperfiltration in the surviving functional nephrons. This local glomerular hypertension and hypertrophy may lead to cytokine-mediated mesangial matrix increase, and eventually glomerulosclerosis. Such hyperperfusion glomerular injury is seen with oligomeganephronia, diabetic nephropathy, morbid obesity, and reflux nephropathy. It has been suggested that the vascular/ischemic changes seen in the aging kidneys first cause cortical glomerulosclerosis, and consequently, juxtamedullary glomerular hypertrophy, followed by juxtamedullary glomerulosclerosis. However, another study noted that the superficial cortical glomeruli were 20 percent larger than the juxtamedullary glomeruli in twelve adult males aged 51 to 69 years, suggesting that the loss of glomeruli in the superficial cortex might shift perfusion to adjacent functional glomeruli within the peripheral vascular supply of the superficial cortex, and promote their enlargement [34].

Besides segmental or global glomerulosclerosis, the aging glomeruli may show mesangial sclerosis and thickening of GBM, which are nonspecific changes that may also be seen in

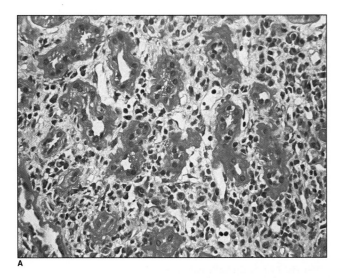

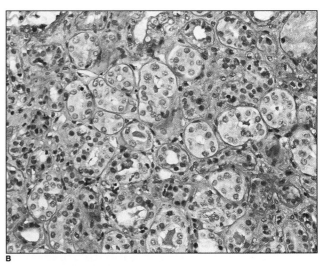

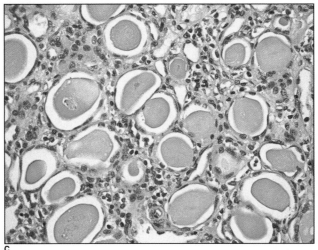

FIGURE 14.6:   Tubular atrophy. A. Classic type: there is severe tubular atrophy with thickening and lamellation of the tubular basement membranes (PAS; × 400). B.Endocrine type: often seen in vascular ischemia, these monotonous small tubules show cuboidal cells with pale-staining cytoplasma (containing abundant mitochondria) and virtually no lumens, reminiscent of endocrine glands (PAS; × 200, courtesy of Dr Tibor Nadasdy). C. Thyroidization type: the atrophic tubules have thin epithelium and contain homogeneous casts, resembling thyroid tissue. This change is characteristic, but not pathognomonic of chronic pyelonephritis (H&E; × 400).

many conditions including hypertension and diabetes mellitus. On the other hand, some studies do not show consistent mesangial sclerosis, or GBM thickening with aging [44].

Aging Tubules and Interstitium

Many parameters of renal function such as serum creatinine, creatinine clearance, and urine osmolality correlate with changes in the tubulointerstitium rather than with changes in the glomeruli or vessels [45,46]. Several such tubulointerstitial changes have been noted in the aging kidney (Table 14.3) [12,29].

Morphologically, three types of tubular atrophy have been described. These are: the "classic form" with wrinkling and thickening of the tubular basement membranes and simplification of the tubular epithelium (Figure 14.6A); the "endocrine form" with simplified tubular epithelium, thin basement membranes, and numerous mitochondria (Figure 14.6B); and the "thyroidization form" with hyaline cast-filled dilated tubules (Figure 14.6C) [47]. Although there is an overlap, the "endocrine

form" is classically seen with vascular ischemia, and the "thyroidization form" with chronic pyelonephritis, although this is not pathognomonic of this disorder. The distal renal tubules develop diverticula that increase in number with increasing age. As mentioned earlier, the diverticula in distal and collecting tubules may be precursors of simple cysts seen in the aging kidney. These diverticula may promote bacterial growth and contribute to the frequent renal infections in the elderly.

The tubular atrophy in the aging kidney is accompanied by an increased degree of interstitial fibrosis, and an influx of infiltrating macrophages and myofibroblasts. The fibrosis is caused, at least in part, by the deposition of collagen types I and III, mediated by the local expression of transforming growth factor-β.

Aging Renal Vasculature

A number of changes in the renal vasculature have been documented in the aging human kidney (Table 14.3) [12,29], none of which is specific for aging.

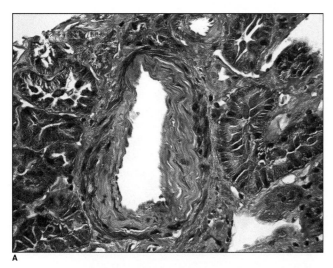

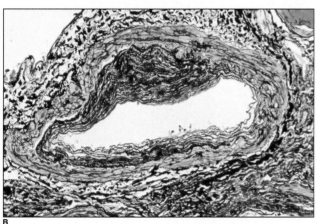

FIGURE 14.7: *Arteriosclerosis (intimal fibrosis). A. An interlobular artery with fibrous thickening and migration of medial muscle cells into the intima with an atrophic muscle layer (Trichrome; × 400). B. An interlobular artery showing reduplication of the internal elastic lamina (Jones methenamine silver; × 400).*

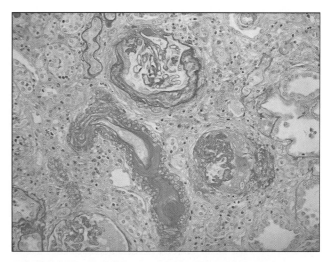

FIGURE 14.8: *Arteriolar hyalinosis. An arteriole discloses extensive subendothelial hyaline deposit with narrowing of the lumen and atrophy of the muscularis. There are two glomeruli showing severe ischemic changes and one glomerulus with global sclerosis. There is also tubular atrophy, interstitial fibrosis and chronic inflammation (PAS; × 200).*

Arterial intimal fibrosis (or fibroplasia), sometimes termed "arteriosclerosis", denotes thickening of the arterial wall and narrowing of the vascular lumen produced by fibrotic intimal thickening and replication of the internal elastic lamina (Figure 14.7A). This lesion may be seen with hypertension, diabetes mellitus, and aging, and its frequency increases with increasing age [12,29,48]. The intima is expanded by myofibroblasts and fibroblasts and an accumulation of collagenous matrix coupled with concentric collagenous laminae that are best seen with elastic stains (Figure 14.7B). Intimal fibrosis/fibroplasia may be associated with the thinning of the media, and is found uniformly in the older kidneys with or without underlying cardiovascular disease. Intimal fibroplasia is seen primarily in arteries that are 80–300 μm in diameter such as the interlobular arteries. The regional heterogeneity of intimal hyperplasia may account for the heterogeneity of ischemic nephrons. While the etiology of aging-associated intimal fibroplasia is not entirely clear, it starts early in life, and is accelerated by hypertension. Intimal hyperplasia in the interlobular arteries may allow the transmission of the pulse wave abnormally into the smaller distal branches leading to

arteriolar hyaline changes, which may themselves accelerate the proximal intimal fibrosis. Global glomerulosclerosis appears to be associated with arterial intimal fibrosis than with arteriolar hyaline change [49–52].

Another common feature of the aging kidney is hyaline arteriolosclerosis that refers to plasmatic insudation, or pushing of plasma proteins into the afferent arteriolar walls (vessel 10–30 μm in diameter), a change that is better correlated with arterial intimal fibrosis than with systemic hypertension in most, but not in all studies. The hyaline material is eosinophilic, strongly PAS-positive, Jones methenamine silver-negative, and fuchsinophilic with trichrome stain (Figure 14.8). It may also be seen with diabetes mellitus; in fact, it is most striking and severe in patients with uncontrolled diabetes mellitus with or without hypertension [12,29]. Hyaline arteriolosclerosis increases rapidly from ages 15 to 34 years, but stabilizes from ages 35 to 102 years, indicating that it is neither a cause nor a consequence of hypertension because it emerges early in life when hypertension is rare, and fails to progress later in life when hypertension becomes increasingly common [53]. It is tempting to speculate that the lack of correlation between hyaline arteriolosclerosis and renal injury/hypertension may be partially related to the fact that with perfusion fixation, the hyaline masses encroaching on the vascular lumen flatten out into the thinned media with consequent restoration of the lumen. Indeed, detailed morphometric analysis has shown that the lumens of hyaline arterioles are substantially larger than those of arterioles without hyalinosis. Interestingly, the glomeruli served by the hyaline arterioles are hypertrophic (not ischemic), with lesions of segmental glomerulosclerosis eventually ensuing [35].

The aging kidney is also associated with a high percentage of afferent and efferent arterioles that communicate directly with each other because of loss of glomeruli, particularly the juxtamedullary glomeruli ("aglomerular arterioles") [29,48] (Figure 14.9). As mentioned previously, the dysautoregulation of arteriolar blood flow may be a causative factor for aging-related glomerulosclerosis. A morphometric study of the aging

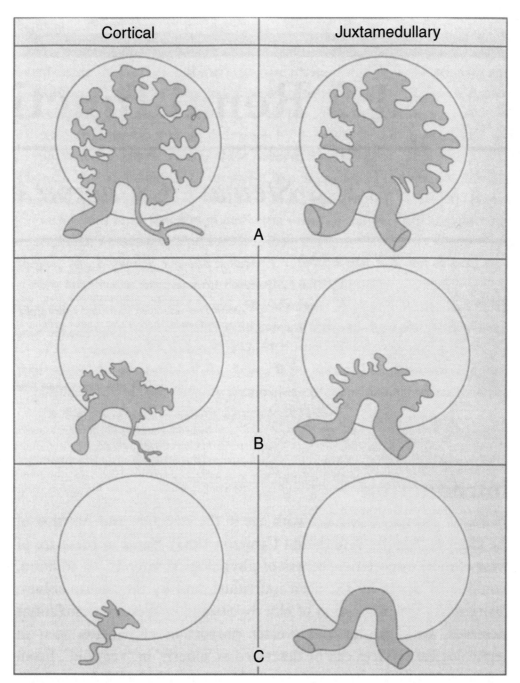

FIGURE 14.9: *Microangiography demonstrates important differences in the vascular consequences of glomerular degeneration in juxtamedullary (right) and the more peripheral nephrons (left). Changes are shown progressing from top to bottom (A–C). In healthy peripheral nephrons, the afferent arteriole forms glomerular capillaries, which then join to become efferent arterioles; in juxtamedullary nephrons, the glomerular capillaries more closely resemble side branches of a continuous afferent-efferent arteriolar unit. When peripheral glomeruli degenerate, afferent arterioles end blindly; degeneration of juxtamedullary glomeruli results in direct communication between afferent and efferent arterioles (McLachlan, M. Anatomic structural and vascular changes in aging kidney. In: Cameron, JS, Macias Nunez JF, eds. Renal Function and Disease in the Elderly. Butterworth-Heinemann, 1987; pp. 3–26. Courtesy of Elsevier and Dr. Macias Nunez JF.)*

kidneys showed dilatation of the afferent arterioles and glomerular capillary lumens (especially hilar), and enlarged glomeruli that suggested a dysregulation between the afferent and efferent arterioles [42].

The gross appearance of granularity and pitting of renal surface (nephrosclerosis) is secondary to the underlying vascular disease, which leads to small regions of the outer renal cortex undergoing global glomerulosclerosis, tubular atrophy, and interstitial fibrosis. These features are best correlated with intimal fibrosis of the interlobular arteries associated with hypertension, diabetes mellitus, and/or aging [12,29].

The aging-related vascular changes of intimal fibrosis and hyaline arteriolosclerosis are accentuated by hypertension, and probably diabetes mellitus as well. On the other hand, it has been suggested that aging-related interlobular arterial sclerosis may precede rather than follow systemic hypertension. Mean blood pressure rises by 1.6 mmHg for each 1 μm increase in intimal thickness in a 100 μm diameter artery because of microischemia in scattered nephrons. This source of hypertension may account for the rise of blood pressure with age. The rate of decrease of renal plasma flow is accelerated by hypertension. Mean arterial blood pressure is directly proportional to the rate of decline of creatinine clearance. Increase in hypertension is a strong independent risk factor in end-stage renal disease, especially in African-Americans. Thus, hypertension and morphological vascular changes are not easily separable at this time [12,14,15,29,49–53].

Although the term "arterionephrosclerosis of aging" has been widely used by pathologists and clinicians to describe pathologic changes (both vascular and parenchymal) observed in the senescent kidney, it is not a well-defined entity because no specific morphologic finding is pathognomonic of the aging kidney, and as such, arterionephrosclerosis of aging is a diagnosis of exclusion. It is generally believed that arterionephrosclerosis of aging is qualitatively similar, but quantitatively less severe than hypertensive arterionephrosclerosis.

ETIOLOGY AND PATHOGENESIS

As described in the previous section, the chief histological features of renal aging are glomerulosclerosis, tubular atrophy, interstitial fibrosis, and arterial intimal fibrosis. While kidneys of the elderly are affected by diseases like hypertension, diabetes mellitus, and sporadic insults such as infections, which may themselves accelerate the "natural" process of aging, it appears that renal aging does occur in the absence of systemic or local diseases. The molecular basis of the phenomenon of renal aging is poorly understood but under active investigation, especially in animal models. In general, the theories of senescence include genomic instability and telomere loss, oxidative damage, endothelial dysfunction, glomerular hypertension and hyperfiltration, genetic programming, and cell death [14,15,54]. Here, we review some of the promising results from the investigations directed specifically at renal aging.

Telomeres

DNA-protein complexes located at the ends of chromosomes, called telomeres, protect the chromosomes from fusing with each other. The enzyme telomerase synthesizes the telomeric DNA, which are repeats of the sequence TTAGGG. However, most somatic cells do not synthesize telomerase, and therefore, telomeres shorten with each cell division. Ultimately, the cells are left with chromosomes that have critically shortened telomeres. The cellular machinery senses the short telomeres as DNA strand-breaks, which leads to the activation of p53 and p16, and the induction of cell-cycle arrest and replicative senescence [55]. It has been shown that telomeres shorten with increasing age in the

kidney, especially in the renal cortex, where 0.24 percent to 0.25 percent telomere shortening occurs every year [56].

Oxidative Stress

Cumulative oxidative stress is believed to play a major role in the process of cellular aging. The increase in oxidative stress and lipid peroxidation in the aging kidney correlates with an increase in the advanced glycosylation end-products and their receptors (AGE and RAGE) that can cross-link adjacent proteins. This, along with reactive oxygen species that can activate ubiquitin-proteasome, may degrade hypoxia inducible factor-1-alpha (HIF-1alpha), and limit the capacity of the aging cells to form hypoxia inducible factor-1 (HIF-1)-DNA hypoxia-responsive recognition element (HRE) complexes (HIF-1-HRE complexes) [4,57]. In the kidney, the consequent decrease in the ability of the cells to respond to hypoxia could explain the attenuated anemia-induced secretion of EPO as well as the decreased hypoxia-induced production of vascular endothelial growth factor leading, respectively, to reduced erythropoiesis and angiogenesis. In addition, oxidative stress causes telomere shortening [58] and lowers nitric oxide (NO) bioavailability, further accelerating the process of renal aging.

Nitric Oxide Deficiency and Intrarenal Activation of Rennin Angiotensin System

NO deficiency also has a role in the renal changes of aging [59]. NO deficiency could be caused by several mechanisms: (a) accumulation of endogenous NO synthase (NOS) inhibitors such as asymmetric dimethyl arginine; (b) reduced abundance or activity of NOS enzymes; and (c) oxidative stress that lowers NO bioavailability. It has been shown that both endothelial and neuronal NOS are reduced in the aging kidney, and the latter is associated with renal injury. The renin-angiotensin system, via its effects on the angiotensin receptor AT1, may induce the synthesis of reactive oxygen species and transforming growth factor-β1 (TGF-β1) that produce fibrosis. Indeed, angiotensin-converting enzyme inhibitors (ACE inhibitors) and angiotensin receptor blockers ameliorated the aging-related renal damage in rats leading to a decline in glomerular sclerosis and mesangial expansion, tubular atrophy, interstitial fibrosis, and mononuclear infiltration [60]. The effect of ACE inhibitors may be mediated by their positive modulation of aging-related dysfunction and ultrastructural changes in the mitochondria, the cell organelles involved in energy metabolism and production of reactive oxygen species [61].

Klotho, the Anti-Aging Gene

A defect in the expression of the gene klotho leads to the development of aging-like syndrome in mice, while overexpression of the Klotho protein leads to suppression of age-related organ degeneration and elongation of the lifespan in mice. The hormonal action of Klotho is mediated by binding to a cell-surface receptor, and repressing the intracellular signals of insulin and insulin-like growth factor 1 (IGF-1) [62]. It appears that the antiaging effect of the Klotho-induced inhibition of insulin/IGF-1 signaling is associated with increased resistance to oxidative stress. It has been shown that Klotho induces the expression of manganese superoxide dismutase, an antioxidant enzyme that confers protection against oxidative stress by facilitating the removal of reactive oxygen species [63]. On the other hand, hydrogen peroxide-induced oxidative stress led to a reduced expression of klotho in the murine inner medullary collecting duct (mIMCD3) cell line [64]. In addition, angiotensin II can downregulate the renal expression of klotho, an effect that was mitigated by iron chelation and free radical scavenging in a rat model [65]. Klotho may also be involved in vitamin D, calcium, and phosphate metabolism via its proposed enzymatic β-glucuronidase action on steroid β-glucuronides, and the calcium channel transient receptor potential vallinoid-5 (TRPV5). In addition, Klotho may also be an essential cofactor for the stimulation of fibroblast growth factor (FGF) receptor by FGF23 [66]. Pertinently, Klotho is highly expressed in the human kidney, where it colocalizes with TRPV5 in the distal tubular cells [67]. Klotho gene polymorphisms have been associated with variations in bone mineral density in women [68], and decreased longevity [69]. Recently, a homozygous missense mutation in the Klotho gene was reported in a 13-year-old girl with severe tumoral calcinosis with dural and carotid artery calcifications [70].

Other Genes and Mechanisms

Using global gene expression by cDNA microarray analyses, Melk et al. identified more than 500 genes that were differentially expressed among human kidney samples from young (8 weeks to 8 years), adult (31 to 46 years), and old (71 to 88 years) subjects. Genes that showed declining expression in the old kidneys included those associated with cellular and metabolic processes like respiratory electron transport chain; glucose and lipid metabolism; and protein, amino acid, and nucleotide turnover. Other aging-related changes included: altered expression of cytoskeletal genes; increased expression of genes associated with extracellular matrix synthesis and turnover; reduced expression of genes associated with collagen catabolism; reduced expression of genes encoding transporters involved in tubular transport of electrolytes, ions, glucose, amino acids, and organic acids; reduced expression of glutathione-related enzymes; and an increased expression of genes encoding immune response and inflammatory mediators [71].

In the preceding paragraphs, we have provided a brief overview of the current concepts of the molecular basis of renal aging, which is an ongoing fascinating story that is far from complete. However, it should be noted that most of the data addressing the molecular mechanisms of renal aging comes from animal studies. Caution should be exercised in extrapolating these findings to humans, given the interspecies differences.

ELDERLY AS DONORS OR RECIPIENTS OF RENAL TRANSPLANTATION

As stated in the introduction, the number of elderly requiring dialysis has increased substantially in the United States and Europe. Amongst more than 300,000 U.S. patients currently on dialysis, the prevalence rates are the highest amongst the patients in their seventh and eighth decades [5]. The adjusted point prevalence rate per million population of reported end-stage renal disease in patients older than 65 years is more than 10,000 per million population, about two and half times higher than in younger patients [3]. Consequently, the number of patients with end-stage kidney disease who could potentially

benefit from renal transplantation is the greatest in the older age-groups. Given the perennial shortage of donor-kidneys, and the long waiting list for a kidney transplant, kidney transplantation in the elderly with end-stage renal failure, not surprisingly, raises questions related to ethics and optimal cost-benefit ratio. Should a donor-kidney be transplanted to an elderly patient with comorbidities and an average life expectancy of 10–15 years in preference to a younger patient with a higher average life expectancy? However, studies have clearly shown that the elderly patients with end-stage renal failure do benefit from kidney transplantation. Thus, for patients over the age of 60 years, the annual death rate per 100 patient–years was 23.2 for those on dialysis, and only 7.4 for those who received a renal transplant, with the renal transplantation adding 3–5 years to the life expectancy in the latter group [5,72]. In fact, the relative risk of renal graft failure, adjusted for comorbidities, is statistically similar for renal transplant recipients older than 65 years and their younger counterparts [73]. Similarly, for end-stage renal failure patients over the age of 75 years, the five-year survival was 59.9 percent in recipients of a live donor-kidney, 40.3 percent in recipients of a deceased donor-kidney, 29.7 percent in dialysis patients waiting for transplant, and 12.5 percent in dialysis patients not selected for a kidney transplantation. In this study, the elderly with hypertension and diabetes mellitus as a cause of end-stage renal failure also benefited from the transplant [74]. The most common cause of graft loss in the elderly transplant recipient is the comorbidities-related death of the patient. A careful screening of the elderly patients for comorbidities such as cancer, cardiovascular disease, peripheral vascular disease, diabetes mellitus, and chronic obstructive pulmonary disease may help minimize early posttransplant morbidity and mortality [5]. Therefore, it is not surprising that there is currently no age limit for access to renal transplantation in the United States [75]. While initially considered a risky procedure in the elderly with end-stage renal disease, patients older than 65 years now comprise 13 percent of all recipients of cadaveric donor-kidneys [5].

It is interesting that the average age of the cadaveric kidney donors has also been rising, in parallel with the decreasing mortality rate of the younger populace. While the ideal donor is a young individual with excellent hemodynamic and renal function, given the long waiting period for receiving a deceased donor-kidney, "expanded criteria donor" kidneys are now offered; these kidneys are from donors over the age of 60 years or donors over the age of 50 years with two comorbidities from amongst hypertension, death from cerebrovascular accident, or terminal serum creatinine levels greater than 1.5 mg/dL [76]. At present, in the United States, there are two renal transplant lists: one list for standard criteria donors, and the other for expanded criteria donors. Most centers across the nation recommend the following potential recipients to be listed on the expanded criteria list: older patients, patients with diabetes mellitus as the primary cause for renal failure, and patients with difficult vascular access. The expanded criteria donor-kidneys now comprise 17 percent of the deceased donor transplants in the United States [77]. Similarly, in Europe, there is a comparable Eurotransplant Senior Program that allows for local allocation of kidneys from donors over 65 years of age to recipients over the age for 65 years, so-called old-for-old kidney allocation. However, it appears that kidney transplantation from older donors do have an increased risk of allograft failure. As discussed earlier, older kidneys have aging-related decline in renal function. In addition, older renal allografts are more prone to ischemia and drug toxicity, have a reduced capacity for repair, and may demonstrate a higher degree of immunogenecity. Thus, the 5-year graft survival was 50 percent for the deceased kidney allografts from donors over the age of 60 years and 70 percent for the deceased kidney allografts from donors between 19 and 45 years [78]. Similarly, kidney allografts from living donors older than 55 years also have a greater risk of failure compared to younger kidneys [79]. On the other hand, most allograft failures in older recipients are the result of unrelated death with a functioning allograft, and therefore "old-for-old" kidney allocation makes a lot of sense. Another strategy for obtaining maximal benefit from expanded criteria donor-kidneys is the use of dual renal transplants that allows for the use of two marginal kidneys into one recipient in the hope of providing adequate number of functioning nephrons. Thus, dual kidney transplants from donors older than 54 years of age, when compared to single kidney transplants from the same age-group, were shown to have a significantly decreased incidence of delayed graft function, and lower serum creatinine levels up to two years after transplant [80]. Further, for the older recipients who underwent dual kidney transplants from expanded criteria donors, the eight-year actuarial patient and graft survivals were equivalent to those who underwent standard single kidney transplantation [81]. Preimplantation histologic evaluation of the expanded criteria donor-kidney further optimizes their use. In a histologic scoring schema, with 0 representing no lesions and 12 representing marked changes in the renal parenchyma (vessels/glomeruli/tubules/connective tissue), kidneys with score of 3 or less should have enough viable nephrons for single kidney transplants, those with scores 4–6 should have enough viable nephrons for dual kidney transplants, and kidneys with higher scores are not suitable for transplantation [82–84].

REFERENCES

1. CDC. The State of aging and health in America 2007 Report. 2007 [cited November 1, 2007]; Available from: http://www.cdc.gov/aging/saha.htm.

2. Csiszar A, Toth J, Peti-Peterdi J, and Ungvari Z. The aging kidney: role of endothelial oxidative stress and inflammation. *Acta Physiol Hung* 2007; 94(1–2): 107–15.

3. USRDS. USRDS 2007 Annual data report: atlas of chronic kidney disease and end-stage renal disease in the United States. 2007[cited November 1, 2007]; Available from: http://www.usrds.org/reference.htm.

4. Buemi M, Nostro L, Aloisi C, Cosentini V, Criseo M, and Frisina N. Kidney aging: from phenotype to genetics. *Rejuvenation Res* 2005; 8(2): 101–9.

5. Morrissey PE and Yango AF. Renal transplantation: older recipients and donors. *Clin Geriatr Med* 2006; 22(3): 687–707.

6. Lindeman RD, Tobin J, and Shock NW. Longitudinal studies on the rate of decline in renal function with age. *J Am Geriatr Soc* 1985; 33(4): 278–85.

7. Kimmel PL, Lew SQ, and Bosch JP. Nutrition, ageing and GFR: is age-associated decline inevitable? *Nephrol Dial Transplant* 1996; 11 Suppl. 9: 85–8.

8. Musch W, Verfaillie L, and Decaux G. Age-related increase in plasma urea level and decrease in fractional urea excretion: clinical application in the syndrome of inappropriate secretion of antidiuretic hormone. *Clin J Am Soc Nephrol* 2006; 1(5): 909–14.

9. Levey AS, Coresh J, Balk E, Kausz AT, Levin A, Steffes MW, Hogg RJ, Perrone RD, Lau J, and Eknoyan G. National Kidney Foundation practice guidelines for chronic kidney disease: evaluation, classification, and stratification. *Ann Intern Med* 2003; 139(2): 137–47.

10. Cockcroft DW and Gault MH. Prediction of creatinine clearance from serum-creatinine. *Nephron Exp Nephrol* 1976; 16(1): 31–41.

11. Ognibene A, Mannucci E, Caldini A, Terreni A, Brogi M, Bardini G, Sposato I, Mosconi V, Salvadori B, Rotella CM, and Messeri G. Cystatin C reference values and aging. *Clin Biochem* 2006; 39(6): 658–61.

12. Silva FG. The aging kidney: a review – part I. *Int Urol Nephrol* 2005; 37(1): 185–205.

13. Silva FG. The aging kidney: a review–part II. *Int Urol Nephrol* 2005; 37(2): 419–32.

14. Zhou XJ, Rakheja D, Yu XQ, Saxena R, Vaziri ND, and Silva FG. The aging kidney. *Kidney Int* 2008; 74(6):710–20.

15. Zhou XJ, Saxena R, Liu ZH, Vaziri ND, and Silva FG. Renal senescence in 2008: progress and challenges. *Int Urol Nephrol* 2008; 40(3): 823–39.

16. Epstein M and Hollenberg NK. Age as a determinant of renal sodium conservation in normal man. *J Lab Clin Med* 1976; 87(3): 411–7.

17. Fliser D, Franek E, Joest M, Block S, Mutschler E, and Ritz E. Renal function in the elderly: impact of hypertension and cardiac function. *Kidney Int* 1997; 51(4): 1196–204.

18. Perazella MA and Mahnensmith RL. Hyperkalemia in the elderly: drugs exacerbate impaired potassium homeostasis. *J Gen Intern Med* 1997; 12(10): 646–56.

19. Sands JM.Urine-concentrating ability in the aging kidney. *Sci Aging Knowledge Environ* 2003; 2003(24): PE15.

20. Kirkland JL, Lye M, Levy DW, and Banerjee AK. Patterns of urine flow and electrolyte excretion in healthy elderly people. *Br Med J (Clin Res Ed)* 1983; 287(6406): 1665–7.

21. Faull CM, Holmes C, and Baylis PH. Water balance in elderly people: is there a deficiency of vasopressin? *Age Ageing* 1993; 22(2): 114–20.

22. Eisenstaedt R, Penninx BW, and Woodman RC. Anemia in the elderly: current understanding and emerging concepts. *Blood Rev* 2006; 20(4): 213–26.

23. Ble A, Fink JC, Woodman RC, Klausner MA, Windham BG, Guralnik JM, and Ferrucci L. Renal function, erythropoietin, and anemia of older persons: the InCHIANTI study. *Arch Intern Med* 2005; 165(19): 2222–7.

24. Ershler WB, Sheng S, McKelvey J, Artz AS, Denduluri N, Tecson J, Taub DD, Brant LJ, Ferrucci L, and Longo DL. Serum erythropoietin and aging: a longitudinal analysis. *J Am Geriatr Soc* 2005; 53(8): 1360–5.

25. Ferrucci L, Guralnik JM, Bandinelli S, Semba RD, Lauretani F, Corsi A, Ruggiero C, Ershler WB, and Longo DL. Unexplained anaemia in older persons is characterised by low erythropoietin and low levels of proinflammatory markers. *Br J Haematol* 2007; 136(6): 849–55.

26. Dukas L, Schacht E, and Stahelin HB. In elderly men and women treated for osteoporosis a low creatinine clearance of < 65 ml/min is a risk factor for falls and fractures. *Osteoporos Int* 2005; 16(12): 1683–90.

27. Gallagher JC, Rapuri P, and Smith L. Falls are associated with decreased renal function and insufficient calcitriol production by the kidney. *J Steroid Biochem Mol Biol* 2007; 103(3–5): 610–3.

28. Tada S, Yamagishi J, Kobayashi H, Hata Y, and Kobari T. The incidence of simple renal cyst by computed tomography. *Clin Radiol* 1983; 34(4): 437–9.

29. Zhou XJ, Laszik ZG, and Silva FG. Anatomical changes in the aging kidney. In: Macias-Nunez JF, Cameron JS, and Oreopoulos DG, eds. *The Aging Kidney in Health and Disease.* Springer; 2007, pp. 39–54.

30. Nyengaard JR and Bendtsen TF. Glomerular number and size in relation to age, kidney weight, and body surface in normal man. *Anat Rec* 1992; 232(2): 194–201.

31. Hughson M, Farris AB, 3rd, Douglas-Denton R, Hoy WE, and Bertram JF. Glomerular number and size in autopsy kidneys: the relationship to birth weight. *Kidney Int* 2003; 63(6): 2113–22.

32. Hughson MD, Douglas-Denton R, Bertram JF, and Hoy WE. Hypertension, glomerular number, and birth weight in African-Americans and white subjects in the southeastern United States. *Kidney Int* 2006; 69(4): 671–8.

33. Keller G, Zimmer G, Mall G, Ritz E, and Amann K. Nephron number in patients with primary hypertension. *N Engl J Med* 2003; 348(2): 101–8.

34. Samuel T, Hoy WE, Douglas-Denton R, Hughson MD, and Bertram JF. Determinants of glomerular volume in different cortical zones of the human kidney. *J Am Soc Nephrol* 2005; 16(10): 3102–9.

35. Hill GS, Heudes D, Jacquot C, Gauthier E, and Bariety J. Morphometric evidence for impairment of renal autoregulation in advanced essential hypertension. *Kidney Int* 2006; 69(5): 823–31.

36. Marcussen N. Tubulointerstitial damage leads to atubular glomeruli: significance and possible role in progression. *Nephrol Dial Transplant* 2000; 15 Suppl. 6: 74–5.

37. Najafian B, Crosson JT, Kim Y, and Mauer M. Glomerulotubular junction abnormalities are associated with proteinuria in type 1 diabetes. *J Am Soc Nephrol* 2006; 17(4 Suppl. 2): S53-60.

38. Gibson IW, Downie TT, More IA, and Lindop GB. Atubular glomeruli and glomerular cysts – a possible pathway for nephron loss in the human kidney? *J Pathol* 1996; 179(4): 421–6.

39. Kasiske BL. Relationship between vascular disease and age-associated changes in the human kidney. *Kidney Int* 1987; 31(5): 1153–9.

40. Kaplan C, Pasternack B, Shah H, and Gallo G. Age-related incidence of sclerotic glomeruli in human kidneys. *Am J Pathol* 1975; 80(2): 227–34.

41. Smith SM, Hoy WE, and Cobb L. Low incidence of glomerulosclerosis in normal kidneys. *Arch Pathol Lab Med* 1989; 113(11): 1253–5.

42. Hill GS, Heudes D, and Bariety J. Morphometric study of arterioles and glomeruli in the aging kidney suggests focal loss of autoregulation. *Kidney Int* 2003; 63(3): 1027–36.

43. Brenner BM. Hemodynamically mediated glomerular injury and the progressive nature of kidney disease. *Kidney Int* 1983; 23(4): 647–55.

44. Steffes MW, Barbosa J, Basgen JM, Sutherland DE, Najarian JS, and Mauer SM. Quantitative glomerular morphology of the normal human kidney. *Lab Invest* 1983; 49(1): 82–6.

45. Nath KA. Tubulointerstitial changes as a major determinant in the progression of renal damage. *Am J Kidney Dis* 1992; 20(1): 1–17.

46. Eknoyan G, McDonald MA, Appel D, and Truong LD. Chronic tubulo-interstitial nephritis: correlation between structural and functional findings. *Kidney Int* 1990; 38(4): 736–43.

47. Nadasdy T, Laszik Z, Blick KE, Johnson DL, and Silva FG. Tubular atrophy in the end-stage kidney: a lectin and immunohistochemical study. *Hum Pathol* 1994; 25(1): 22–8.

48. Takazakura E, Sawabu N, Handa A, Takada A, Shinoda A, and Takeuchi J. Intrarenal vascular changes with age and disease. *Kidney Int* 1972; 2(4): 224–30.

49. Tracy RE and Ishii T. What is 'nephrosclerosis'? Lessons from the US, Japan, and Mexico. *Nephrol Dial Transplant* 2000; 15(9): 1357–66.

50. Tracy RE, Malcom GT, Oalmann MC, Qureshi U, Ishii T, and Velez-Duran M. Renal microvascular features of hypertension in Japan, Guatemala, and the United States. *Arch Pathol Lab Med* 1992; 116(1): 50–5.

51. Tracy RE, Newman WP, 3rd, Wattigney WA, Srinivasan SR, Strong JP, and Berenson GS. Histologic features of atherosclerosis and hypertension from autopsies of young individuals in a defined geographic population: the Bogalusa Heart Study. *Atherosclerosis* 1995; 116(2): 163–79.

52. Tracy RE, Parra D, Eisaguirre W, and Torres Balanza RA. Influence of arteriolar hyalinization on arterial intimal fibroplasia in the renal cortex of subjects in the United States, Peru, and Bolivia, applicable also to other populations. *Am J Hypertens* 2002; 15(12): 1064–73.

53. Tracy RE. Age trends of renal arteriolar hyalinization explored with the aid of serial sections. *Nephron Clin Pract* 2007; 105(4): c171–7.

54. Johnson FB, Sinclair DA, and Guarente L. Molecular biology of aging. *Cell* 1999; 96(2): 291–302.

55. Jiang H, Ju Z, and Rudolph KL. Telomere shortening and ageing. *Z Gerontol Geriatr* 2007; 40(5): 314–24.

56. Melk A, Ramassar V, Helms LM, Moore R, Rayner D, Solez K, and Halloran PF. Telomere shortening in kidneys with age. *J Am Soc Nephrol* 2000; 11(3): 444–53.

57. Frenkel-Denkberg G, Gershon D, and Levy AP. The function of hypoxia-inducible factor 1 (HIF-1) is impaired in senescent mice. *FEBS Lett* 1999; 462(3): 341–4.

58. Houben JM, Moonen HJ, van Schooten FJ, and Hageman GJ. Telomere length assessment: biomarker of chronic oxidative stress? *Free Radic Biol Med* 2007.

59. Baylis C. Changes in renal hemodynamics and structure in the aging kidney; sexual dimorphism and the nitric oxide system. *Exp Gerontol* 2005; 40(4): 271–8.

60. Basso N, Paglia N, Stella I, de Cavanagh EM, Ferder L, del Rosario Lores Arnaiz M, and Inserra F. Protective effect of the inhibition of the renin-angiotensin system on aging. *Regul Pept* 2005; 128(3): 247–52.

61. de Cavanagh EM, Piotrkowski B, Basso N, Stella I, Inserra F, Ferder L, and Fraga CG. Enalapril and losartan attenuate mitochondrial dysfunction in aged rats. *Faseb J* 2003; 17(9): 1096–8.

62. Kurosu H, Yamamoto M, Clark JD, Pastor JV, Nandi A, Gurnani P, McGuinness OP, Chikuda H, Yamaguchi M, Kawaguchi H, Shimomura I, Takayama Y, Herz J, Kahn CR, Rosenblatt KP, and Kuro-o M. Suppression of aging in mice by the hormone Klotho. *Science* 2005; 309(5742): 1829–33.

63. Kuro-o M. Klotho as a regulator of oxidative stress and senescence. *Biol Chem* 2008; 389(3): 233–41.

64. Mitobe M, Yoshida T, Sugiura H, Shirota S, Tsuchiya K, and Nihei H. Oxidative stress decreases klotho expression in a mouse kidney cell line. *Nephron Exp Nephrol* 2005; 101(2): e67–74.

65. Saito K, Ishizaka N, Mitani H, Ohno M, and Nagai R. Iron chelation and a free radical scavenger suppress angiotensin II-induced downregulation of klotho, an anti-aging gene, in rat. *FEBS Lett* 2003; 551(1–3): 58–62.

66. Razzaque MS and Lanske B. The emerging role of the fibroblast growth factor-23-klotho axis in renal regulation of phosphate homeostasis. *J Endocrinol* 2007; 194(1): 1–10.

67. Torres PU, Prie D, Molina-Bletry V, Beck L, Silve C, and Friedlander G. Klotho: an antiaging protein involved in mineral and vitamin D metabolism. *Kidney Int* 2007; 71(8): 730–7.

68. Yamada Y, Ando F, Niino N, and Shimokata H. Association of polymorphisms of the androgen receptor and klotho genes with bone mineral density in Japanese women. *J Mol Med* 2005; 83(1): 50–7.

69. Arking DE, Krebsova A, Macek M, Sr., Macek M, Jr., Arking A, Mian IS, Fried L, Hamosh A, Dey S, McIntosh I, and Dietz HC. Association of human aging with a functional variant of klotho. *Proc Natl Acad Sci U S A* 2002; 99(2): 856–61.

70. Ichikawa S, Imel EA, Kreiter ML, Yu X, Mackenzie DS, Sorenson AH, Goetz R, Mohammadi M, White KE, and Econs MJ. A homozygous missense mutation in human KLOTHO causes severe tumoral calcinosis. *J Clin Invest* 2007; 117(9): 2684–91.

71. Melk A, Mansfield ES, Hsieh SC, Hernandez-Boussard T, Grimm P, Rayner DC, Halloran PF, and Sarwal MM. Transcriptional analysis of the molecular basis of human kidney aging using cDNA microarray profiling. *Kidney Int* 2005; 68(6): 2667–79.

72. Wolfe RA, Ashby VB, Milford EL, Ojo AO, Ettenger RE, Agodoa LY, Held PJ, and Port FK. Comparison of mortality in all patients on dialysis, patients on dialysis awaiting transplantation, and recipients of a first cadaveric transplant. *N Engl J Med* 1999; 341(23): 1725–30.

73. Oniscu GC, Brown H, and Forsythe JL. How old is old for transplantation? *Am J Transplant* 2004; 4(12): 2067–74.

74. Macrae J, Friedman AL, Friedman EA, and Eggers P. Live and deceased donor-kidney transplantation in patients aged 75 years and older in the United States. *Int Urol Nephrol* 2005; 37(3): 641–8.

75. Rao PS, Merion RM, Ashby VB, Port FK, Wolfe RA, and Kayler LK. Renal transplantation in elderly patients older than 70 years of age: results from the Scientific Registry of Transplant Recipients. *Transplantation* 2007; 83(8): 1069–74.

76. Metzger RA, Delmonico FL, Feng S, Port FK, Wynn JJ, and Merion RM. Expanded criteria donors for kidney transplantation. *Am J Transplant* 2003; 3 Suppl 4: 114–25.

77. Schold JD, Kaplan B, Baliga RS, and Meier-Kriesche HU. The broad spectrum of quality in deceased donor-kidneys. *Am J Transplant* 2005; 5(4 Pt 1): 757–65.

78. Nyberg SL, Baskin-Bey ES, Kremers W, Prieto M, Henry ML, and Stegall MD. Improving the prediction of donor-kidney quality: deceased donor score and resistive indices. *Transplantation* 2005; 80(7): 925–9.

79. Bunnapradist S, Daswani A, and Takemoto SK. Graft survival following living-donor renal transplantation: a comparison of tacrolimus and cyclosporine microemulsion with mycophenolate mofetil and steroids. *Transplantation* 2003; 76(1): 10–5.

80. Lu AD, Carter JT, Weinstein RJ, Stratta RJ, Taylor RJ, Bowers VD, Ratner LE, Chavin KD, Johnson LB, Kuo PC, Cole EH, Dafoe DC, and Alfrey EJ. Outcome in recipients of dual kidney transplants: an analysis of the dual registry patients. *Transplantation* 2000; 69(2): 281–5.

81. Tan JC, Alfrey EJ, Dafoe DC, Millan MT, and Scandling JD. Dual-kidney transplantation with organs from expanded criteria donors: a long-term follow-up. *Transplantation* 2004; 78(5): 692–6.

82. Remuzzi G, Cravedi P, Perna A, Dimitrov BD, Turturro M, Locatelli G, Rigotti P, Baldan N, Beatini M, Valente U, Scalamogna M, and Ruggenenti P. Long-term outcome of renal transplantation from older donors. *N Engl J Med* 2006; 354(4): 343–52.

83. Ruggenenti P, Perico N, and Remuzzi G. Ways to boost kidney transplant viability: a real need for the best use of older donors. *Am J Transplant* 2006; 6(11): 2543–7.

84. Saxena R, Yu X, Giraldo M, Arenas J, Vazquez M, Lu CY, Vaziri ND, Silva FG and Zhou XJ. Renal transplantation in the elderly. *Int Urol Nephrol* 2009; 41: 195–210.

CHAPTER 15

End-Stage Renal Disease

Steven A Bigler, MD, and Michael D. Hughson, MD

INTRODUCTION

Chronic kidney disease (CKD) is defined by the National Kidney Foundation (Kidney Disease Outcomes Quality Initiative, K/DOQI) as structural or functional abnormalities in the kidneys lasting for three months or longer [1]. CKD can be divided into five stages based on the level of renal function as identified by glomerular filtration rate (GFR). Although GFR is a continuous variable, arbitrary cut-offs have been employed to classify patients into groups (stages) and provide an indication of the severity of impairment in kidney function (Table 15.1). Kidney damage can be recognized as either pathologic changes in the kidney or abnormalities in the blood or urine composition due to kidney dysfunction, or abnormal imaging studies of the kidneys. Proteinuria is an important marker of kidney damage, which may or may not be associated with decreased GFR.

Kidney failure (or renal failure) is defined as either GFR of <15 ml/min/1.73 m^2 body surface area, or the need to initiate renal replacement therapy (dialysis or transplantation) to treat symptoms of decreased renal function [2–4]. Most patients with GFR less than 15 ml/min will have signs and symptoms of uremia. End-stage renal disease (ESRD) is a term that applies specifically to patient eligibility under the Medicare ESRD program in the United States. ESRD is closely related to kidney failure, but differs in two important ways: (1) not all patients with GFR < 15 ml/min will be treated with dialysis or transplantation, as for example some patients with acute renal failure due to acute tubular necrosis (hence renal failure, but not end-stage renal disease as the term is used by the Medicare program) and (2) transplant patients with a functioning transplanted kidney who have GFR > 15 ml/min and have not resumed dialysis have

ESRD but should not be considered in renal failure. ESRD implies chronic renal failure (three months or longer with GFR ≤ 15 ml/min/1.73 m^2) requiring dialysis or transplantation.

EPIDEMIOLOGY AND UNDERLYING ASSOCIATIONS

The most common cause of CKD in the United States and other developed countries is diabetes mellitus (Table 15.2), accounting for 45 percent of patients entering dialysis in the United States [5]. Diabetes is particularly prevalent as a cause of end stage kidney disease among Native Americans (accounting for 72 percent) and Hispanics (59 percent) [6,7].

It is commonly stated that diabetes mellitus and hypertension cause approximately two-thirds of all cases of ESRD; however, hypertension is frequently associated with CKD, without necessarily being the primary cause of the renal disease [8,9]. Hypertension contributes to the renal injury in patients with progressive renal disease, and worsening renal insufficiency leads to blood pressure elevations [10], setting the stage for a vicious cycle of declining renal function, and elevating blood pressure.

Frasinetti, et al [6] found that the etiology of CKD is more commonly attributed to hypertension in African-Americans, and that on further review the proportion of CKD attributable to hypertension appeared to be overstated in African-Americans. In their study, there were 19 percent of cases of ESRD in African-Americans, which had originally been attributed to hypertension, and this was reduced to 10 percent after review. The proportion of cases attributable to hypertension was also reduced after review of Caucasian patients, but to a lesser degree. Even after

Table 15.1 Stages of Chronic Kidney Disease

Stage	Description	GFR (ml/min/1.73 m^2)
1	Kidney damage with normal or ↑ GFR	≥90
2	Kidney damage with mild ↓ GFR	60–89
3	Moderate ↓ GFR	30–59
4	Severe ↓ GFR	15–29
5	Kidney failure	<15 or dialysis

Source: From K/DOQI, with permission [1].

their review, the proportion of cases attributable to hypertension was considerably higher in the African-American patients than in Caucasian patients among whom only 3.5 percent were attributed to primary hypertension.

Other common causes of ESRD include glomerulonephritis, interstitial nephritis/pyelonephritis, and cystic/hereditary/congenital diseases of the kidneys. Among the glomerular diseases, focal segmental glomerulosclerosis is the most common cause of ESRD, and accounts for 3.6 percent of patients with end stage kidney disease. Other important glomerular causes of end stage kidney disease include IgA nephritis (1.1 percent), membranous glomerulopathy (0.7 percent), membranoproliferative glomerulonephritis (0.7 percent), rapidly progressive glomerulonephritis (0.5 percent), and Goodpasture syndrome (0.2 percent). Fewer than one percent of patients begin dialysis in the United States as a complication of neoplasms [3].

In the developing world, CKD is most commonly caused by chronic glomerulonephritis and interstitial nephritis, in contrast with the relatively low prevalence of these causes in the developed world, reflecting a high incidence of bacterial, viral, and parasitic infections involving the kidneys. Histologic types of glomerulonephritis vary geographically with IgA predominating in Asia and the Pacific region (accounting for 35 to 45 percent of cases of glomerulonephritis) but appearing uncommonly in Africa (only 3-4 percent of cases), and focal segmental glomerulosclerosis being prevalent in South America, India, Saudi Arabia, and the native populations of Africa. Diabetes accounts for 9.1 to 29.9 percent of CKD in various developing countries [11,12].

END-STAGE RENAL DISEASE IN CHILDREN

ESRD in children differs from adult end stage kidney disease in the spectrum and frequency of etiologies (Table 15.3). The causes of end stage kidney disease in children depend on the populations studied, and distinct geographic differences are due, in part, to racial, environmental, genetic, and cultural (consanguinity) differences [13,14].

ESRD is much less frequent in children with an annual incidence of 13 per million age-related population (MARP) in patients less than 20 years of age in the 1988 cohort of the U.S. Renal Data System (USRDS) and 15 per MARP in the 2003 cohort compared with 119 per MARP in the 20–44-year age group and 518 per MARP in the 45–64-year age range in the 2003 cohort [15].

In developed countries, including the United States, chronic renal insufficiency is frequently due to congenital causes especially obstructive uropathy (22 percent), aplasia/hypoplasia/dysplasia (18 percent), and reflux nephropathy (8 percent) which together

Table 15.2 Incidence of Various Primary Diagnoses among Patients with End-Stage Kidney Disease

Primary Diagnosis	Percent Incidence
Diabetes	36.7
Type I (juvenile)	
Type II (adult onset or unspecified)	
Hypertension/large vessel disease	24.4
Hypertension (no primary renal disease)	
Renal artery stenosis or occlusion	
Cholesterol emboli, renal emboli	
Glomerulonephritis	16.1
Focal glomerulosclerosis, focal GN	3.6
Membranous GN	0.7
Membranoproliferative GN, types I & II	0.7
IgA nephropathy (Berger disease)	1.1
Rapidly progressive GN	0.5
Goodpasture syndrome	0.2
GN not otherwise specified	8.6
Others	0.7
Cystic diseases	6.7
Polycystic kidneys, adult (dominant)	4.4
Alport's/other hereditary/familial	0.6
Congenital obstructive uropathy	0.7
Renal hypoplasia, dysplasia	0.6
Others	0.4
Interstitial nephritis/pyelonephritis	4.6
Chronic interstitial nephritis	1.7
Nephrolithiasis/obstruction/gouty	1.3
Chronic pyelonephritis/reflux nephritis	0.8
Analgesic abuse	0.2
Others	0.6
Secondary GN/Vasculitis	3.3
SLE nephritis	2.0
Wegener granulomatosis	0.3
Vasculitis and its derivatives	0.3
Hemolytic uremic syndrome	0.2
Others	0.5
Neoplasms/tumors	0.9
Renal or urological neoplasm	
Multiple myeloma	
Light chain nephropathy	
Amyloidosis	
Miscellaneous conditions	3.2
Tubular necrosis (no recovery)	1.0
AIDS nephropathy	0.6
Complications postbone marrow or other transplant	0.3
Postpartum failure, others	1.3
Etiology uncertain	4.1
Missing	2.8

The data reported here have been supplied by the U.S. Renal Data System (USRDS). The interpretation and reporting of these data are the responsibility of the author(s) and in no way should be seen as an official policy or interpretation of the U.S. government. [3]

account for approximately half of cases of ESRD in children [based on data from the North American Paediatric Renal Trials and Collaborative Studies (NAPRTCS)] [15]. In less developed countries, the presentation of chronic renal insufficiency is at later stages and infectious or acquired diseases predominate.

Table 15.3 Incidence of Treated ESRD in Pediatric Patients (Age <20 years) with Median Age in the United States, Puerto Rico, and Territories 1993–97

Primary Disease Group	Total # of Patients	Median Age	% of Total
Glomerulonephritis (GN)	*1,620*	*16*	*29.8*
Focal glomerulosclerosis, focal GN	555	15	10.2
Membranous nephropathy	29	16	0.5
Membranoproliferative GN	138	16	2.5
IgA nephropathy, Berger's disease	86	17	1.6
Rapidly progressive GN	113	14	2.1
Goodpasture syndrome	37	16	0.7
Unspecified GN	562	16	10.3
Other proliferative GN	81	16	1.5
Cystic/congenital/hereditary iseases	*1,410*	*10*	*26.0*
Polycystic, adult (dominant)	110	10	2.0
Polycystic, infantile (recessive)	52	4	1.0
Medullary cystic, nephronophthisis	60	13	1.1
Alport's, other hereditary/familial disease	148	16	2.7
Cystinosis	38	12	0.7
Primary oxalosis	19	3	0.3
Congenital nephrotic syndrome	64	2	1.2
Congenital obstructive uropathy	362	11	6.7
Renal hypoplasia/dysplasia	481	8	8.9
Prune belly syndrome	61	7	1.1
Other cystic/hereditary/congenital disease	15	18	0.3
Interstitial nephritis/pyelonephritis	*494*	*14*	*9.1*
Chronic pyelonephritis/reflux nephropathy	147	14	2.7
Nephropathy caused by other agents	48	15	0.9
Nephrolithiasis, Obstruction, Gout	176	12	3.2
Chronic interstitial nephritis	106	15	2.0
Secondary GN/Vasculitis	*485*	*15*	*8.9*
Lupus erythematosus	252	17	4.6
Wegener's granulomatosis	40	16	0.7
Henoch-Schonlein syndrome	45	14	0.8
Hemolytic uremic syndrome	106	8	2.0
Hypertensive/Large vessel disease	*262*	*17*	*4.8*
Hypertension, (no primary renal disease)	244	18	4.5
Renal artery stenosis or occlusion	18	10	0.3
Diabetes	*89*	*16*	*1.6*
Neoplasms/Tumors	*38*	*7*	*0.7*
Renal or urologic neoplasms	37	6	0.7
Miscellaneous conditions	*204*	*12*	*3.8*
Sickle cell disease/anemia or trait	17	19	0.3
AIDS nephropathy	23	16	0.4
Tubular necrosis (no recovery)	55	7	1.0
Etiology uncertain	*387*	*15*	*7.1*
Missing	*442*	*13*	*8.1*

The data reported here have been supplied by the United States Renal Data System (USRDS). The interpretation and reporting of these data are the responsibility of the author(s) and in no way should be seen as an official policy or interpretation of the U.S. government. [93]

Of the glomerular lesions, focal segmental glomerulosclerosis (FSGS) accounts for 10.2 percent of childhood CKD, while all other glomerulonephritides combined account for 19.6 percent of CKD. FSGS is particularly prevalent among African American adolescents with CKD, with a three-fold difference between African-American children and Caucasian children.

Other important causes of chronic renal insufficiency in patients younger than 20 years of age in the NAPRTCS data included polycystic disease (4 percent), prune belly (2.8 percent), renal infarct (2.4 percent), hemolytic uremic syndrome (2 percent), and lupus nephritis (1.5 percent). Diabetic nephr-

opathy accounted for only 11 out of 6,405 cases (0.17 percent) of chronic renal insufficiency in the NAPRTCS data [15].

MORPHOLOGIC EVALUATION OF END-STAGE KIDNEYS

General features

Gross and histologic studies of end-stage kidneys allows us to recognize basic patterns of injury which correlate with general

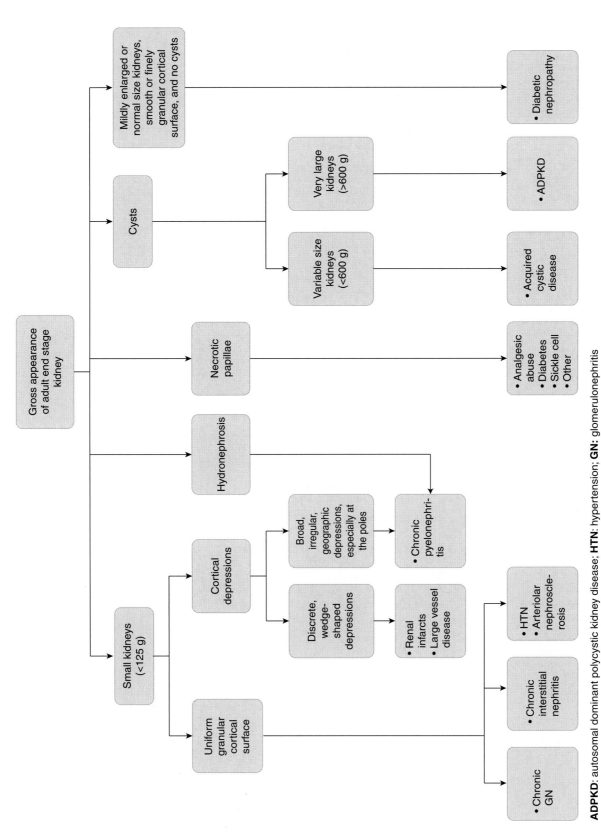

ADPKD: autosomal dominant polycystic kidney disease; **HTN**: hypertension; **GN**: glomerulonephritis

FIGURE 15.1: *Algorithm for determination of etiology in end-stage kidney disease, based on gross examination.*

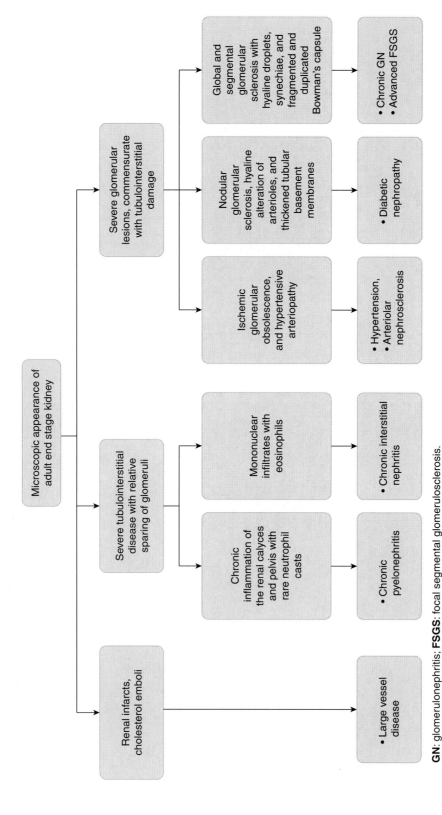

GN: glomerulonephritis; FSGS: focal segmental glomerulosclerosis.

FIGURE 15.2: *Algorithm for determination of etiology of end-stage kidney disease based on histologic evaluation.*

causes of renal impairment [16–18]. Routine gross examination and histology can be used to identify end stage kidney disease secondary to primary hypertension, diabetes mellitus, glomerulonephritis, chronic pyelonephritis, polycystic kidney disease, large vessel disease including thromboembolism, and renal papillary necrosis (see Figures 15.1 and 15.2).

The ability to recognize a particular type of primary disease process in the end stage setting depends on the adequacy of sampling and the chronicity of the end-stage status. In current surgical technique, native kidneys are usually not removed at the time of renal transplantation, and so one does not generally have the entire kidney to evaluate at this stage. After many years of dialysis and/or transplantation, the kidneys often develop secondary changes, including acquired cystic change and features of hypertensive renal damage. These secondary changes may obscure the underlying disease process and the associated morphologic patterns when the kidneys are examined after years of renal replacement therapy. Gross inspection of the kidneys is often very helpful in determining the underlying disease process. Imaging studies of the kidneys can substitute for gross examination when biopsy samples of end-stage kidneys are to be evaluated. A biopsy sample may not be representative, especially with regard to the renal pelvis and the vasculature. Recognizing these limitations, it is generally possible to identify the underlying category of renal injury in most end-stage kidneys which can be adequately studied.

The importance of correlating morphologic data with clinical history cannot be overstated in the evaluation of end-stage kidneys.

Certain features of end-stage kidney disease are common to many etiologies, especially in the later fibrogenic and destructive phases of the process. Acquired cystic renal disease is one such nonspecific pattern, which will be discussed below. The degree of tubular atrophy generally correlates with increasing interstitial collagen deposition, and the combination of tubular atrophy and interstitial fibrosis often correlates with the baseline level of renal function in a given kidney. Accumulation of interstitial collagen can be demonstrated with trichrome stains (Figure 15.3). Atrophic tubules can assume one of at least three morphologic patterns. Tubules can become shrunken with thickened, wrinkled, and reduplicated basement membranes (Figure 15.4). They may become dilated and accumulate protein rich material in the lumens, rendering a pattern that has been coined "thyroidization" because of its resemblance to colloid in thyroid follicles (Figure 15.5). Some atrophic tubules have been termed "endocrine tubules" not because of any demonstrated endocrine function but because they somewhat resemble endocrine units in other organs, presenting as clusters of very small tubules with absent or tiny lumens and thin delicate basement membranes, lined by cuboidal epithelial cells with bland round nuclei (Figure 15.6). Calcium deposits in tubules are common in end-stage kidneys (Figure 15.7). Extensive deposition of calcium oxalate crystals may be seen in some cases of end stage kidney disease (Figure 15.8), including rare cases of primary hyperoxaluria [19], cases of chronic pyelonephritis, and patients with hyperparathyroidism.

Obsolescent glomeruli vary in their appearance. Two important patterns, which should be noted, are ischemic glomerular

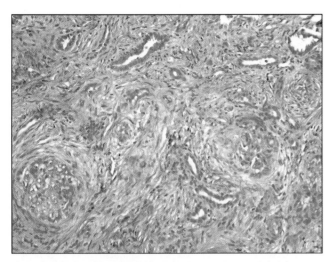

FIGURE 15.3: *End-stage kidney disease with abundant interstitial collagen demonstrated with this trichrome stain.*

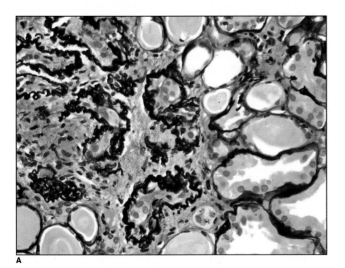

A

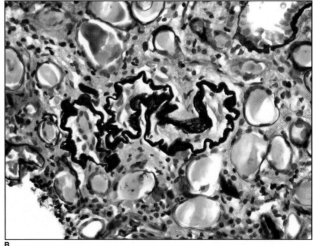

B

FIGURE 15.4: *(A&B) End-stage kidney disease with typical atrophy of the renal tubules, characterized by wrinkling, duplication, and thickening of the tubular basement membranes. (PAMS stain).*

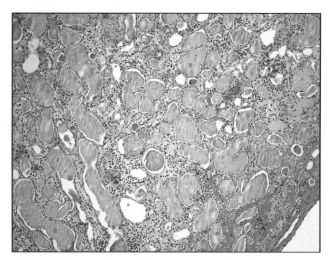

FIGURE 15.5: "Thyroidization" pattern of tubular atrophy in end-stage renal disease. Atrophic tubules are distended and contains protein rich material in the lumens.

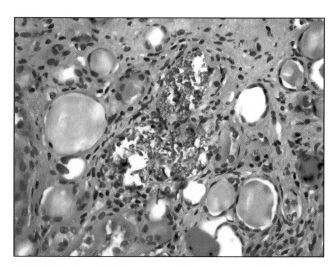

FIGURE 15.7: Calcifications in renal tubules in end-stage kidney disease.

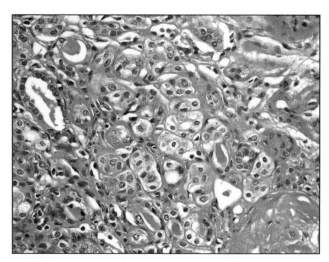

FIGURE 15.6: Tubular atrophy with a pattern of "endocrine tubules" characterized by small tubular structures with absent or very narrow lumens and delicate basement membranes.

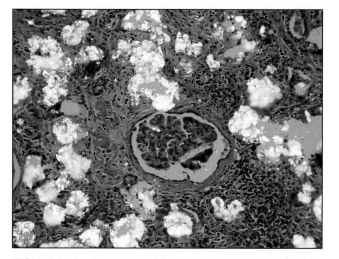

FIGURE 15.8: Abundant calcium oxalate crystal deposition in this patient with end-stage kidney disease, demonstrated with polarized light.

obsolescence and global glomerular sclerosis. Ischemic glomerular obsolescence is typical of hypertensive arteriolar nephrosclerosis, but can also be seen in other causes of end stage kidney disease as hypertension complicates the underlying cause of renal injury. It is characterized by a pattern where the capillary tufts are wrinkled and collapsed into a tight ball near the vascular pole, and the Bowman's space is filled with a bland, layered deposition of mature collagen (Figure 15.9) [20,21]. In contrast, global sclerosis is the pattern most commonly seen in glomeruli damaged by primary glomerulonephritis. It is characterized by consolidation of the capillary tufts that fill the space to Bowman's capsule (Figure 15.10). There is often fragmentation and duplication of the basement membrane of Bowman's capsule, and the capillary loops form attachments or synechiae with Bowman's capsule.

End-stage kidneys often demonstrate a proliferation of small cells at the periphery of obsolete glomeruli in the region of the parietal epithelium (Figure 15.11) [22]. This phenomenon has

been termed "embryonal hyperplasia of Bowman's capsular epithelium." These cells initially form pseudotubular or linear structures, oriented parallel to the Bowman's capsule, but they may produce large solid aggregates, which may require step sections in order to identify the association with a glomerulus. These structures have been particularly noted in the end-stage kidneys of children, but they are also commonly encountered in adults. Similar structures have been described in association with renal tubules in children, sometimes with a branching pattern in the interstitium. Some have suggested that the cells proliferating in embryonal hyperplasia of Bowman's capsule are the same as those seen in metanephric adenoma, with which they share histologic similarities (Figure 15.12).

Hypertension/Ischemia

End-stage kidneys secondary to primary hypertension and arteriolar nephrosclerosis are typically small and shrunken

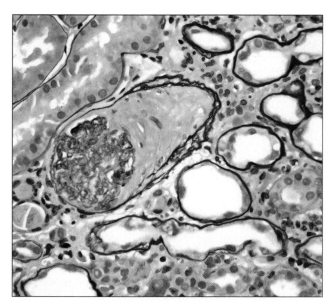

FIGURE 15.9: *Ischemic glomerular obsolescence. The glomerular capillary tufts are wrinkled and collapsed down to the vascular pole and Bowman's space is filled with collagen. (PAMS stain)*

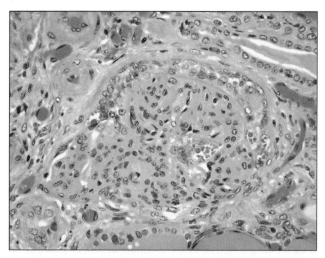

FIGURE 15.11: *End-stage kidney disease with global sclerosis of this glomerulus, which demonstrates "embryonal hyperplasia" of the epithelial cells adjacent to Bowman's capsule.*

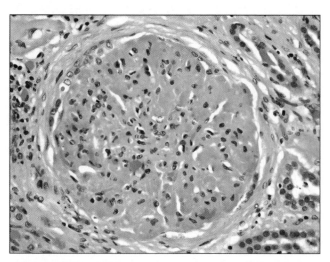

FIGURE 15.10: *Global glomerulosclerosis and solidification in a patient with end-stage glomerulonephritis. The glomerular capillary tufts are not shrunken and collapsed, but fill the space out to Bowman's capsule.*

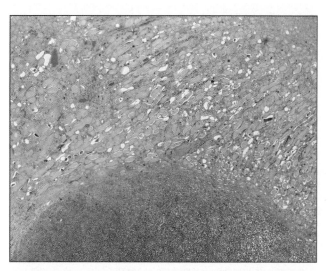

FIGURE 15.12: *End-stage renal disease with a metanephric adenoma-like nodule and marked tubular atrophy. These nodules are thought to be related to the pattern of embryonal hyperplasia commonly seen in globally sclerosed glomeruli.*

(Figure 15.13). They may weigh as little as 30–40 g in some cases (normal is 150–175 g). The external surface of the kidney has a highly characteristic, granular appearance. Generally, the process is bilateral and uniform; however, in patients with unilateral or asymmetric renal artery stenosis the features of hypertensive/ischemic renal damage will be much more severe on the side with stenosis. The cut-surface of the kidney demonstrates thinning of the cortex, which may be only 1–2 mm thick (Figure 15.14).

Histologically, end-stage kidneys due to hypertension (Figures 15.15 and, 15.16) can be shown to have prominently thickened arteries and arterioles with muscular hyperplasia of the arterial tunica media and concentric or eccentric intimal fibrosis with myointimal cellular proliferation [23–26]. There is prominent tubular atrophy and interstitial fibrosis, but these findings are relatively nonspecific and are seen in patients with end stage kidney disease from a variety of causes. The interstitium in such kidneys generally includes a nonspecific infiltrate of lymphocytes. The glomeruli are small with a typical pattern of ischemic glomerular obsolescence. Typically, the glomerular changes are most pronounced in the outer cortex, sometimes with a zone of sparing immediately under the capsule due to vascular supply via the adrenal arteries in this location. In patients with hyper-reninemic hypertension, one can often identify prominence and hyperplasia of the rennin producing cells in the afferent arterioles at the glomerular hila.

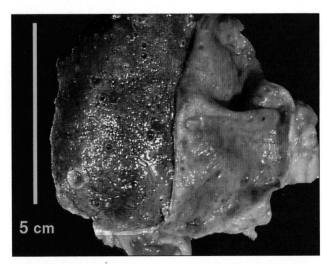

FIGURE 15.13: *End-stage kidney disease in a patient with hypertension and severe chronic arteriolar nephrosclerosis. Note the granular surface of this small kidney.*

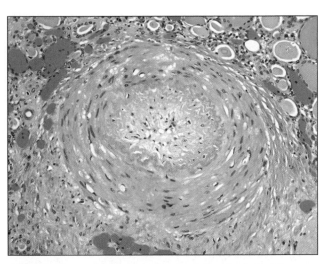

FIGURE 15.15: *Typical pattern of arteriopathy in end-stage kidney disease with marked luminal narrowing, intimal fibrosis, and medial smooth muscle hyperplasia.*

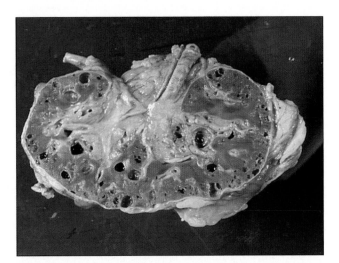

FIGURE 15.14: *Acquired cystic renal disease in a patient with end-stage kidney disease and many years of dialysis. There are numerous small cysts throughout the renal parenchyma.*

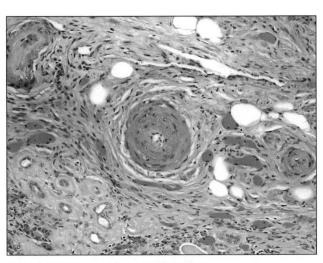

FIGURE 15.16: *A small muscular artery with typical arteriopathy of end-stage kidney disease with marked luminal narrowing, medial smooth muscle hyperplasia, and periarterial fibrosis.*

Diabetes Mellitus

End-stage kidneys secondary to diabetic nephropathy are larger than end-stage kidneys due to other causes. The external surface of the diabetic kidney is often granular due to associated vascular disease, but the prominence of the granularity is generally less than that seen in primary hypertensive nephrosclerosis. There are typically no depressions or indentations of the kidney surface, unless there has been superimposed embolic disease or pyelonephritis. The cut section of the kidney shows that the renal cortex is relatively thick compared to kidneys with other causes of end-stage injury. Patients with diabetes mellitus are prone to development of renal papillary necrosis (Figure 15.17).

The histology of end-stage diabetic nephropathy has a number of characteristic findings (Figure 15.18). The glomeruli are relatively large and demonstrate nodular expansion of the mesangial matrix (Kimmelstiel-Wilson nodules, Figure 15.19)

[21]. Hyalinosis lesions are commonly identified in end-stage diabetic glomeruli. The basement membranes of the glomerular capillaries, the renal tubules, and the afferent and efferent arterioles are typically thickened, prominently wrinkled, and reduplicated with deposition of hyaline material (Figure 15.20). Electron microscopy will also demonstrate thickening and wrinkling of glomerular capillary, tubular, and vascular basement membranes typical of diabetic nephropathy.

Glomerulonephritis

The kidneys from patients with end-stage glomerulonephritis vary with the acuity of the disease process, the particular type of glomerulonephritis, and the duration of renal replacement therapy. Grossly, the kidneys of advanced glomerulonephritis may

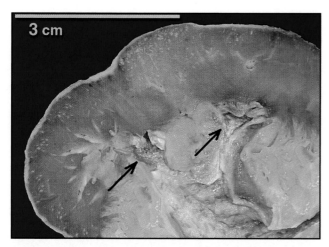

FIGURE 15.17: *End-stage diabetic kidney with papillary necrosis. Note the loss of the papillary tips with friable granular necrotic remnants.*

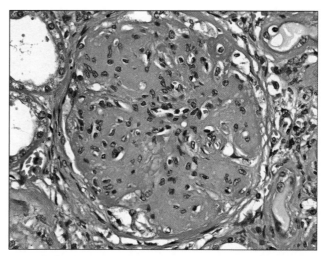

FIGURE 15.19: *Typical nodular glomerulosclerosis in a patient with end-stage diabetic nephropathy.*

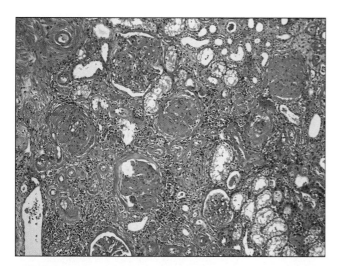

FIGURE 15.18: *End-stage diabetic nephropathy with typical nodular glomerular sclerosis.*

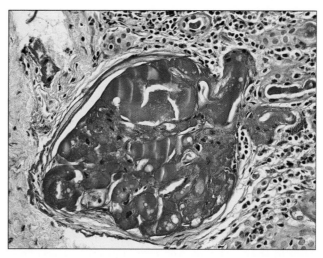

FIGURE 15.20: *End-stage diabetic nephropathy with hyalinosis lesions of the capillary tufts and the afferent and efferent arterioles.*

be very small, and demonstrate a granular surface, which is often somewhat coarser than the uniform fine granularity of small vessel arteriolar nephrosclerosis seen in primary hypertension. The cut surface may demonstrate an indistinct corticomedullary junction, but in our experience, this finding is not very reliable or helpful.

By light microscopy, cases of advanced glomerulonephritis often show predominance of glomerular lesions (Figure 15.21) which are more extensive than the associated tubular atrophy and interstitial fibrosis which always accompanies end-stage kidneys [16,17,21]. Patients with rapidly progressive glomerulonephritis may have cellular crescents in the best-preserved glomeruli, but after renal replacement therapy, these crescents disappear or become fibrotic. Fibrous crescents must be distinguished from the bland acellular collagen deposition seen in ischemic glomerular obsolescence by identifying residual cells in the collagenous matrix filling Bowman's space. Periodic acid Schiff (PAS) and silver stains often demonstrate fragmentation

and duplication of the glomerular basement membranes including the basement membrane of Bowman's capsule. The glomeruli often show segmental, nonuniform injury or scarring (Figure 15.22). Glomerular capillary tufts often demonstrate formation of segmental synechia with attachment to Bowman's capsule. There may be hyaline deposits present, particularly in cases of end-stage FSGS (Figure 15.23). These glomerular hyaline deposits must be distinguished from hyaline accumulations in diabetic glomerular lesions. Hyalinosis lesions in patients with glomerulonephritis tend to be focal and segmental, less widespread than in diabetes, and are often associated with hyaline protein accumulations identified in visceral epithelial cells. Also, hyaline changes in diabetes characteristically involve the afferent and efferent arterioles prominently and are associated with diffuse mesangial expansion. Immunofluorescence studies may demonstrate residual immune complexes in cases of immune complex associated glomerulonephritis (such as IgA

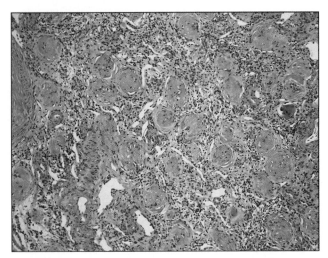

FIGURE 15.21:   Numerous globally sclerosed, obsolescent glomeruli in a patient with end-stage glomerulonephritis.

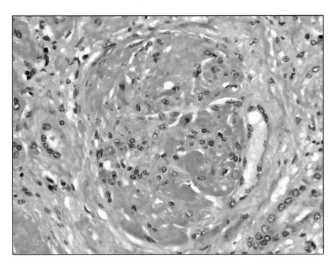

FIGURE 15.23:   Global glomerulosclerosis in a patient with end-stage glomerulonephritis. There is early pseudotubule formation of the parietal epithelial cells and focal hyaline accumulation in the sclerosed capillary tufts.

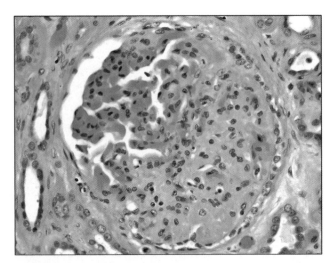

FIGURE 15.22:   Segmental glomerulosclerosis in a patient with end-stage focal segmental glomerulosclerosis. There is early "embryonal" hyperplasia of epithelial cells in adjacent to the Bowman's capsule.

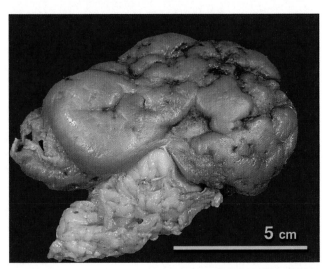

FIGURE 15.24:   Chronic pyelonephritis with irregular scarring, which in this case is most pronounced in the upper pole.

nephritis), even years after the acute process. On the other hand, scarred glomeruli often show nonspecific "trapping" of immune products, especially IgM and C3, and it is important when examining end-stage kidneys by immunofluorescence to focus on the best preserved glomeruli and the least scarred capillary loops. Immune complexes may also be identified by electron microscopy, but the discrete dense deposits may be difficult to distinguish in a background of advanced glomerular sclerosis with irregular density of the mesangial matrix material.

Pyelonephritis and Chronic Interstitial Nephritis

Grossly, the kidneys of patients with end-stage pyelonephritis often demonstrate irregular areas of scarring represented by geographic regions of depression (Figure 15.24). In chronic, nonobstructive pyelonephritis the poles of the involved kidney are prone to injury because the renal lobes at the poles are fused and form compound papillae which are subject to reflux [18]. The cut surface reveals variable degrees of hydronephrosis, especially deep to the depressed cortical scars (Figure 15.25). Calculi may be present in the renal pelvis.

Histologically, there is prominent chronic inflammation of the stroma adjacent to the renal pelvis and reactive/reparative cytologic changes in the urothelial cells lining the pelvis, very frequently with formation of lymphoid follicles beneath the uroepithelium (Figure 15.26). The glomeruli are relatively spared and there is a prominent interstitial inflammatory infiltrate which may be out of proportion to the degree of tubular atrophy and interstitial fibrosis present (Figure 15.27). In pyelonephritis, neutrophils are commonly noted in the lumens of collecting ducts and renal tubules, and microabscesses may be present in the interstitium (Figure 15.28). The "thyroidization"

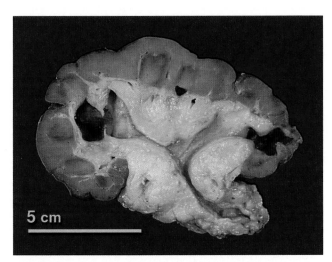

FIGURE 15.25: *Chronic obstructive pyelonephritis. The pelvicalyceal system is dilated and there is loss of cortical parenchyma, especially in the upper and lower pole.*

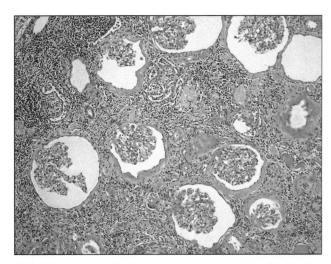

FIGURE 15.27: *End-stage chronic pyelonephritis with relative preservation of the glomeruli and prominent tubular atrophy, inflammation of the interstitium and tubules, and interstitial fibrosis.*

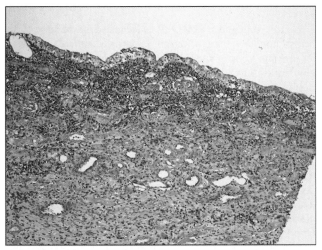

FIGURE 15.26: *Chronic pyelonephritis with chronic inflammation in the subepithelial region of the renal pelvis.*

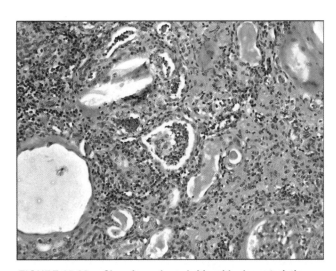

FIGURE 15.28: *Chronic pyelonephritis with characteristic inflammatory debris in tubules, interstitial inflammation and fibrosis. Intratubular inflammatory debris can also be seen in other causes of end-stage kidney disease.*

pattern of tubular atrophy is very common in end-stage kidneys secondary to pyelonephritis, but can also be seen in patients with other etiologies. The glomerular changes in patients with chronic pyelonephritis may be relatively minor or nonspecific with global and segmental sclerosis [27].

End-stage kidney disease secondary to chronic interstitial nephritis is similar to chronic pyelonephritis in that there is relative sparing of the glomeruli (Figure 15.29). Neutrophil casts are less likely in chronic interstitial nephritis and the interstitial infiltrates often include eosinophils.

Renal Papillary Necrosis

Grossly, renal papillary necrosis is generally apparent on cut section, with the soft, gray to white or yellow necrotic papillae contrasting with the normal appearance of renal papillae. Sloughed papillae may be seen in the renal pelvis or at the

ureteropelvic junction. Sometimes the necrotic papillae have sloughed entirely, and one can only identify the ragged, gray, and hemorrhagic medullary remnant.

Histologically, there is characteristic coagulation necrosis of the involved renal papillae (Figure 15.30). Correlation with the clinical history and other morphologic features may demonstrate associated conditions, including pyelonephritis, diabetes mellitus, sickle cell disease, and analgesic abuse [28].

Thromboembolic Disease

Thromboemboli from vegetations of endocarditis, cardiac mural thrombi, or aortic atherosclerotic plaques cause wedge

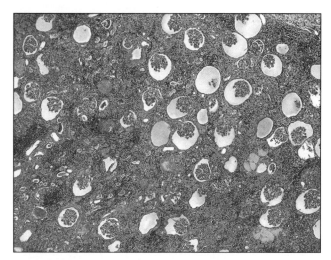

FIGURE 15.29: *End-stage chronic interstitial nephritis. The glomeruli are relatively well-preserved with prominent loss of tubules, interstitial fibrosis, and chronic inflammation.*

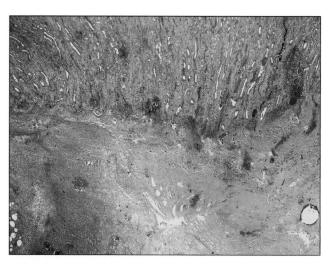

FIGURE 15.30: *Papillary necrosis in a patient with diabetes mellitus and chronic pyelonephritis. A zone of inflammation and hyperemia demarcates the viable tissue from the necrotic papillary tip.*

shaped infarctions of the renal cortex. Long-standing infarcts will demonstrate glomerular obsolescence and loss of tubules with scarring and retraction of the interstitium, which, will be identified as a V-shaped scar on cross section during gross examination. Sometimes cholesterol emboli will be identified in arcuate or interlobular renal arteries near the apex of the infarct.

PATHOGENESIS OF END-STAGE RENAL DISEASE

The initial injury in patients who develop end stage kidney disease may include hypertensive/ischemic injury, diabetes mellitus, glomerulonephritis, pyelonephritis, chronic interstitial nephritis, autosomal dominant polycystic kidney disease, renal involvement in systemic autoimmune diseases such as lupus erythematosus, or a variety of other insults. Some patients may have a combination of factors contributing to the initiation or progression of renal disease. Indeed, at some point in the disease process of virtually every patient who develops end stage kidney disease hypertension develops and can contribute to the progression of renal failure irrespective of the initiating injury.

Most experts agree that when GFR has been reduced by 50 to 70 percent renal function subsequently declines along a final common pathway, which is independent of the initiating renal injury [29–31]. Preventing or treating the factors that contribute to this final common pathway may extend renal function in patients with underlying impairments and delay or prevent the need for renal replacement therapy [32,33]. Morphologically the final common pathway is characterized by increasing glomerular sclerosis, tubular atrophy, and interstitial fibrosis.

Glomerular alteration in the setting of declining numbers of functioning nephrons, is initially characterized by enlargement or hypertrophy of perfused glomeruli associated with increased hydrostatic pressure in glomerular capillary loops. Elevated capillary pressure results in increased filtration in individual glomeruli while the overall GFR is decreased due to large numbers of nonfunctioning nephrons. Eventually, elevated glomerular pressure leads to visceral epithelial cell injury and segmental glomerulosclerosis. Reactive mesangial cell changes and deposition of extracellular mesangial matrix material are mediated by the elaboration of growth factors, including transforming growth factor-beta (TGF-β) and lead to segmental and ultimately global sclerosis [34,35]. The rate of progression of glomerular sclerosis and ischemic glomerular obsolescence in CKD is critically dependent on systemic blood pressure, and control of hypertension has been shown to be crucial in slowing the rate of progression to ESRD. Although systemic blood pressure control is vital, it is important to remember that individual glomerular capillary pressure may increase independently of systemic blood pressure [36]. Treatment with inhibitors of the renin-angiotensin system reduces glomerular capillary pressure and systemic blood pressure, and interferes with TGF-β, helping to preserve functioning nephrons [34,37].

Tubular atrophy and interstitial fibrosis is often a better histologic predictor of baseline renal function than glomerular obsolescence. Eddy [33] has divided the progression of interstitial fibrosis in the development of end-stage kidney disease into four arbitrary but sequential stages, recognizing that the process of destructive interstitial fibrosis is complex, integrating multiple molecular and cellular targets and events. These four stages are: (1) cellular activation and injury, (2) fibrogenic signaling, (3) fibrogenesis, and (4) the destructive phase.

Glomerular protein leak is fundamental in the initial stage of cellular activation and injury, and protein in the proximal renal tubules appears to be a mediator of epithelial cell injury, possibly through the actions of reactive oxygen species or through the actions of complement and complement activation. Complement C3a and C5a are potent chemoattractants. Also, monocyte chemoattractant protein-1 (MCP-1) is produced by tubular epithelial cells in response to proteinuria. These factors and others lead to the accumulation of monocytes and T-lymphocytes into the interstitium. Renal epithelial cells in the setting of proteinuria produce endothelin-1 a potent vasoconstrictor and together with the effects of angiotensin II can result in ischemic tubular epithelial cell injury. Interstitial fibroblasts transform into myofibroblasts with cytoplasmic production of alpha smooth muscle actin filaments. Transformation of interstitial fibroblasts into myofibroblasts depends on the presence of TGF-β [30,33,35]. Some authors have suggested that renal tubular epithelial cells can transform into myofibrobasts as a response to injury and the action of growth factors (especially TGF-β) via a mechanism termed "epithelial-to-mesenchymal transformation." This process of transformation is potentially critical in the development of renal interstitial fibrosis, and is the subject of active research and debate [30,38,39].

Molecular mediators characterize the stage of fibrogenic signaling leading to increased deposition of collagen and other extracellular matrix products adjacent to renal tubules and in the interstitium [33]. TGF-β is considered the key factor responsible for renal fibrosis [40,41]. TGF-β can be produced by resident cells in the kidney or infiltrating inflammatory cells, and its production is increased by a large number of stimuli, including angiotensin II, insulin, endothelin-1, atrial natriuretic factor, platelet activating factor, insulin-like growth factor-1, and ischemia. TGF-β acting through its transmembrane receptors phosphorylates various cytoplasmic proteins including members of the SMAD family of proteins. Eventually, these phosphorylated proteins activate transcription of genes encoding for matrix proteins including collagen. Connective tissue growth factor (CTGF) is a very important downstream mediator of the effects of TGF-β. The profibrotic effects of these mediators are balanced against antifibrotic factors including interferon γ, and hepatocyte growth factor/scatter factor. Insulin-like growth factor can have both pro-fibrotic and antifibrotic effects [30,31,35].

The phase of fibrogenesis is characterized by an increase in the production of normal interstitial matrix proteins, proteoglycans and glycoproteins, polysaccharides, normal tubular basement membrane components, and novel matrix proteins [33]. There is inadequate and generally decreased production of factors which degrade matrix proteins including plasminogen activators and metalloproteinases (MMPs). Tissue inhibitor of metallopreinase-1 (TIMP-1) is markedly increased in renal fibrosis, and TIMP-2 and TIMP-3 may also play important roles in inhibiting the degradation and remodeling of the interstitial matrix. TGF-β is a potent inducer of plasminogen activator inhibitor-1 (PAI-1) which is an important inhibitor of protein catabolism produced by tubular epithelial cells, interstitial fibroblasts, and myofibroblasts. Animals genetically deficient in PAI-1 develop significantly less interstitial fibrosis in experimental models of CKD [42].

The destructive phase of interstitial fibrosis is characterized by tubular atrophy, and eventually reabsorption of nephron segments, sometimes leaving behind relatively normal appearing, but nonfunctioning "atubular" glomeruli. Ischemia is probably a major factor in ongoing tubular injury. Apoptosis of tubular epithelial cells appears to be important, and apoptosis of endothelial cells in peritubular capillaries has also been demonstrated in CKD. The end-result of the destructive phase of interstitial fibrosis is the loss of renal volume and loss of function.

CLINICAL COURSE AND SYSTEMIC COMPLICATIONS OF END-STAGE RENAL DISEASE

Systemic complications of ESRD are diverse and depend on the effectiveness of renal replacement therapy.

Hypertension is very common in patients with ESRD, and is characterized by sensitivity to salt and fluid intake between dialysis sessions and is often associated with high plasma renin levels. Patients may respond to the acute decline in intravascular fluid volume associated with dialysis treatments with an exaggerated production of renin and develop episodic hypertension as a reflex to dialysis, requiring careful monitoring and control of blood pressure during and after dialysis.

Secondary hyperparathyroidism is common in ESRD [43], and is due in large part to decreased phosphate excretion in the urine. Retention of phosphate leads to deposition of calcium phosphate salts, lowering ionized calcium levels and stimulating the parathyroid glands. Also, the diseased kidney is ineffective in converting 25(OH)-vitamin D_3 into the potent 1,25 $(OH)_2$-vitamin D_3 which is largely responsible for the intestinal absorption of calcium, resulting in further depression of plasma calcium levels. Generally, all four parathyroid glands are enlarged and show nodular hyperplasia of chief cells (Figure 15.31).

The effects of chronic hyperparathyroidism include the development of osteitis fibrosa or renal osteodystrophy (Figure 15.32), characterized by high bone turnover [44,45]. The cortex of long bones becomes relatively porous and weak. Histologically, there are numerous osteoclasts with active resorption lacunae, and irregularly thickened bony trabeculae formed of nonmineralized woven bone or osteoid. In addition to high turnover bone disease patients with ESRD also develop low turn-over or adynamic bone disease [46].

Beta-2-microglobulin is an 11,800 Da protein of the class I HLA antigens which accumulates in patients with ESRD [47]. It is frequently deposited as amyloid in the femur and other bones, resulting in cysts and an unusually high prevalence of femoral neck fractures in hemodialysis patients [48,49]. Beta-2-microglobulin amyloid also deposits in the soft tissue of the wrist resulting in carpal tunnel syndrome, in nerve sheaths, and in the heart in the endocardium, around small cardiac blood vessels, and in the myocardium [50]. Amyloid tumors may accumulate in the tongue, buttocks, breast, or other soft tissue locations [51–55].

ESRD is associated with diverse, important cardiovascular complications including cardiomyopathy, atherosclerotic coronary artery disease, cardiac valvular calcifications, and calcemic uremic arteriopathy (formerly referred to as "calciphylaxis") [56]. Cardiomyopathy may be either dilated or hypertrophic [57,58]. Hypertrophic cardiomyopathy (Figure 15.33) is found in 27 percent of patients beginning dialysis and confers a marked increase in mortality. Calcemic uremic arteriopathy is characterized by calcification of small arteries in the dermis and subcutaneous soft tissue, resulting in painful red skin nodules, especially on the thighs, buttocks and abdomen. Calcemic uremic arteriopathy is associated with approximately 30 percent mortality rates in patients with nonulcerated lesions, but this rises to more than 80 percent mortality in patients with ulcerated lesions [59,60]. Patients with uremia may develop fibrinous pericarditis resulting in chest pain and possibly even tamponade [61,62]. In the long term, constrictive pericarditis and heart

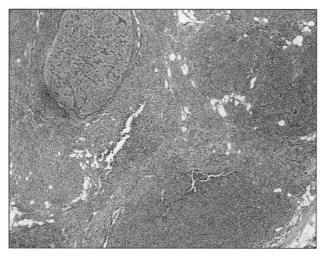

FIGURE 15.31: Secondary parathyroid hyperplasia in a patient with end-stage kidney disease. Note the nodular growth and depletion of fat cells.

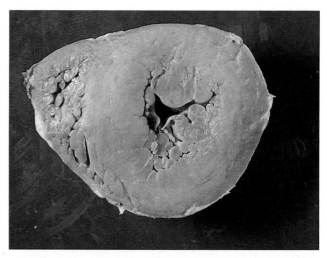

FIGURE 15.33: Hypertrophic cardiomyopathy in a patient with end-stage renal disease and acquired cystic disease. Note the markedly thickened wall of the left ventricle in this cross section of the heart.

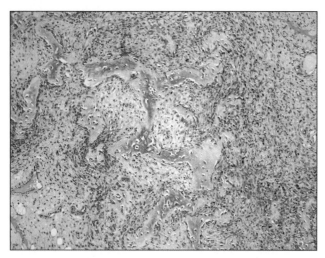

FIGURE 15.32: Hyperdynamic bone disease (osteitis fibrosa cystica or brown tumor) in a patient with end-stage kidney disease and secondary parathyroid hyperplasia. There is abundant osteoblastic activity associated with irregular osteoid production.

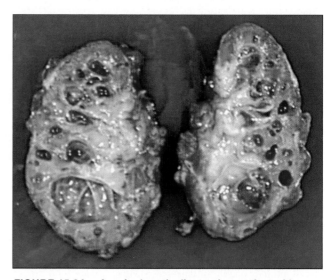

FIGURE 15.34: Acquired cystic disease in a patient with end-stage kidney disease. The renal parenchyma contains numerous, variably sized cysts in this patient with many years of dialysis.

failure may result from organized fibrinous pericarditis [63]. Cardiac conditions are the most commonly identified cause of death in patients with ESRD in the United States.

Chronic renal insufficiency and ESRD are associated with hypoplastic anemia, due in large part to erythropoietin deficiency [64]. Platelet dysfunction is also caused by renal dysfunction and predisposes to bleeding in the gastrointestinal tract and elsewhere, exacerbating anemia in some patients.

ESRD is associated with central nervous system abnormalities [65] including cerebrovascular disease, uremic encephalopathy, and dialysis disequilibrium syndrome. Careful control of aluminum exposure in dialysis patients has essentially eliminated the phenomenon of dialysis dementia. Five percent of

deaths in patients with ESRD are attributed to cerebrovascular disease.

Acquired Renal Cystic Disease

Acquired renal cystic disease is a condition seen in patients with long-standing dialysis (Figure 15.34). The condition was described in 1977 by Dunnill, and occurs in patients with hemodialysis or peritoneal dialysis [66]. The incidence is quite variable depending on the definition used and the patient population studied. Radiologic criteria for acquired renal cystic disease have been proposed as three or more cysts per kidney by some investigators, and as five or more cyst per kidney by others, and pathologic criteria have been proposed as greater

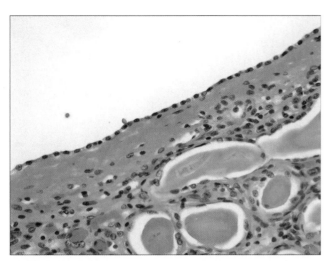

FIGURE 15.35: *Renal cyst formation in early acquired cystic disease in a dialysis patient. The cyst is lined by bland cuboidal or flattened epithelium.*

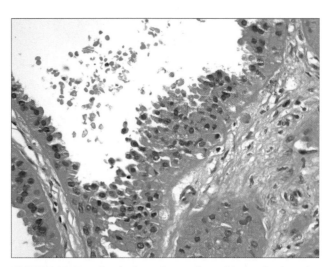

FIGURE 15.36: *Atypical cyst in a patient with acquired cystic disease. The epithelium is piled up, with nuclear enlargement and atypical cytologic features.*

than 40 percent replacement of the renal parenchyma with cysts [67]. This variation in defining criteria may account for some of the differences in reported incidence of acquired renal cystic disease. Within the first three years of dialysis, approximately 10–20 percent of patients will develop acquired renal cystic disease, by five years approximately 50 percent will have developed the condition, and after ten years 90 percent or more will have acquired renal cystic disease [68–71]. The condition can also be seen in patients with renal transplants, but the risk in these patients seems to be driven by the length of time that they were on dialysis prior to transplantation. Indeed, following successful transplantation there is likely to be no progression of acquired renal cystic disease and in some patients there appears to be regression [72–74]. If the transplanted kidney fails, there will be progression of the cystic change. It is clear that the changes of acquired cystic renal disease can precede dialysis in patients surviving long-term with uremia, and it is suspected that acquired cystic renal disease is caused by long-standing uremia, which in the case of dialysis patients may be episodic. The rate of development of acquired renal cystic disease may be lower in diabetic patients than other patients with ESRD and males have higher rates of acquired renal cystic disease than females in the first ten years following transplant. After fifteen years of dialysis, the rates of acquired renal cystic disease are approximately equal between men and women.

The appearance of acquired renal cystic disease should be clearly distinguished from a single or rare parenchymal cyst in a patient with advanced kidney disease. In some cases of acquired cystic disease the kidneys can develop numerous simple cysts, and the kidneys may enlarge to a degree somewhat resembling autosomal dominant polycystic kidney disease; however, the two conditions are generally readily distinguished by history and the fact that kidneys in acquired renal cystic disease rarely exceed 800 g, while kidneys from patients with renal failure secondary to autosomal dominant polycystic kidney disease typically weigh from 2,000 to 4,000 g.

Histologically, the kidneys from patients with acquired renal cystic disease demonstrate numerous cysts, generally lined by

flattened, nondescript epithelium or bland cuboidal epithelial cells (Figure 15.35). The lining cells have been shown to include distal tubular epithelial cells and cells from the proximal tubules by lectin histochemistry techniques, and the cysts are derived from all levels of the nephron. Some cysts are lined by tall epithelial cells, which tend to pile up and form intraluminal pseudopapillae (Figure 15.36), and such cysts have been designated "atypical" cysts because of nuclear enlargement, hyperchromasia, and loss of polarity. The kidneys of acquired cystic renal disease demonstrate typical features of advanced renal disease with glomerular obsolescence, tubular atrophy, interstitial fibrosis and thickened vessel walls in the remaining parenchyma between the cysts. It is common for oxalate crystals to accumulate in the interstitium or in the cysts.

Renal Cell Carcinoma in End-Stage Renal Disease

Patients with ESRD have an increased incidence of malignant neoplasms including renal cell carcinoma [75–79]. Renal cortical neoplasms have been identified in 17 percent of end-stage kidneys and are multiple in 9 percent. Kidneys with acquired renal cystic disease are particularly prone to the development of renal cell carcinoma [80–82]. There is a 100-fold increase in the incidence of renal cell carcinoma in the native kidneys of renal transplant recipients over the general population [83,84].

Most studies have indicated that the renal cell carcinomas seen in patients with end stage kidney disease are similar to those seen in patients with functioning kidneys (Figures 15.37 and, 15.38). However, Tickoo, et al. reported on a series of 261 tumors from 66 end-stage kidneys (52 patients) and noted that the majority of tumors could not be classified easily by conventional criteria [85]. They proposed two new categories of renal cell carcinoma, which they felt were specifically associated with end-stage kidneys. They classified the dominant nodule in the end-stage kidneys that they studied as having usual classic morphology in 27 of the 66 kidneys (41 percent), including 12 clear cell, 10 papillary, and 5 chromophobe carcinomas. The other tumors were classified as one of two types: "acquired cystic

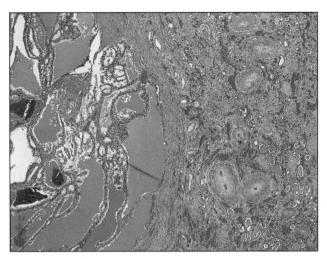

FIGURE 15.37: *Cystic renal cell carcinoma in a patient with end-stage kidney disease.*

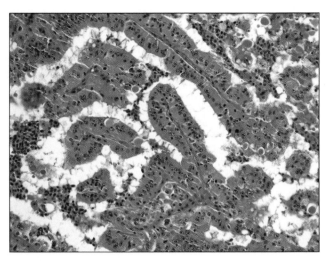

FIGURE 15.39: *Papillary renal cell carcinoma in a patient with end-stage kidney disease.*

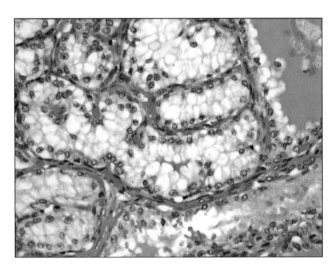

FIGURE 15.38: *Conventional (clear cell) pattern of renal cell carcinoma in a patient with end-stage kidney disease.*

disease associated RCC" or "clear-cell papillary RCC of the end-stage kidney." Acquired cystic disease associated RCC is characterized by a microcystic growth pattern of cells with abundant eosinophilic cytoplasm and nuclear grade 3 out of 4 [86], often with focal areas of papillary growth, and focal cells with clear cytoplasm. These tumors frequently contained abundant oxalate crystals, were seen only in kidneys with acquired renal cystic disease, and accounted for the dominant tumor in 24 cases (36 percent overall). Fifteen of the tumors (23 percent) were designated as "clear cell papillary renal cell carcinoma" and were characterized by cystic neoplasms with prominent diffuse papillary architecture and purely clear-cell cytology. In their study, only two patients had lymph node metastases, and two had sarcomatoid features. All of these occurred in patients with the acquired cystic disease associated renal cell carcinoma pattern, and one of the patients with sarcomatoid morphology died within 34 months of the nephrectomy. They concluded that the acquired cystic disease associated RCC was more aggressive than clear cell papillary RCC.

Most investigators have reported a mixture of tumor types resembling the neoplasms seen sporadically in functioning kidneys, with a relative overrepresentation of papillary renal cell carcinoma in the end stage setting. Papillary renal cell carcinomas of the end-stage kidneys generally demonstrate abundant eosinophilic cytoplasm (Figure 15.39) and would qualify as type II papillary carcinoma in the classification of Delahunt and Eble [87].

The molecular events associated with tumors in the end stage kidney are somewhat unclear. Approximately half of patients with end-stage kidneys and conventional clear cell carcinoma have deletions of 3p, and Yoshida et al found VHL gene mutations in three of seven conventional clear cell carcinomas from end-stage kidneys [88]. Mutations in the VHL gene, deletions of 3p, and loss of heterozygosity of 3p are much more commonly demonstrated in sporadic conventional clear cell carcinoma in functioning kidneys. Hughson, et al detected trisomy of chromosome 7 or 17 or both by microsattelite analysis in 5 of 14 (36 percent) papillary tumors in end-stage kidneys, fewer than one would expect based on the experience of sporadic tumors in functioning kidneys [89]. Mutations of the c-met oncogene are common in patients with familial papillary renal cell carcinoma and are seen in 13 percent of patients with sporadic papillary renal cell carcinoma [90], but Yoshida et al did not find any mutations of the tyrosine kinase region of the MET oncogene in seven papillary renal cell carcinomas from end-stage kidneys [88]. This may be a reflection of the fact that c-met oncogene mutations are associated with papillary renal cell carcinomas with type I histology which is less common in the end-stage setting. Overall, the findings suggest that additional or different factors are involved in the development of renal cell carcinoma in end-stage kidneys, compared to sporadic renal cell carcinoma in functioning kidneys.

The behavior of renal cell carcinoma in the setting of ESRD is thought to be less aggressive than in sporadic renal cell carcinoma in functioning kidneys [79,91,92]. Metastases have been observed in up to 17 percent of ESRD patients with renal cell carcinoma. Two percent to ten percent of patients with renal cell carcinoma in the setting of end stage kidney disease have died as a result of renal cell carcinoma. Improved survival may be due to close clinical follow-up of patients with ESRD, resulting in earlier stage tumors and thus improved survival, or there may be biologic factors specific to tumors in the end stage kidney, which are inherently more indolent.

REFERENCES

1. *National Kidney Foundation.* Kidney Disease Outcome Quality Initiative (K/DOQI). Part 4. Definition and classification of stages of chronic kidney disease. *Am. J. Kidney Dis* 2002; 39 (Suppl 1):S46–S75

2. Coresh, J, Astor, B.C., Greene, T., Eknoyan G, Levy AS. Prevalence of chronic kidney disease and decreased kidney function in the adult US population: Third National Health and Nutrition Examination Survey. *Am. J. Kidney Dis* 2003; 41:1–12.

3. United States Renal Data System. USRDS 2004 Annual Data Report: Atlas of End-Stage Renal Disease in the United States, National Institutes of Health. *NIDDK* 2004; Bethesda MD, Table B.7 p. 53–54.

4. Nickolas TL, Frisch GD, Opotowsky AR, Arons R, Radhakrishnan J. Awareness of kidney disease in the US population: Findings from the national health and nutrition examination survey (NHANES) 1999 to 2000. *Am J Kidney Dis* 2004; 44:185–197.

5. Centers for Disease Control and Prevention (CDC). Prevalence of chronic kidney disease and associated risk factors– United States, 1999–2004. *MMWR Morb Mortal Wkly Rep* 2007; 56(8):161–5.

6. Frasinetti FP, Ellis PA, Roderick PJ, Cairns HS, Hicks JA, Cameron JS. Causes of end-stage renal failure in black patients starting renal replacement therapy. *Am J Kidney Dis* 2000; 36:301–309.

7. Marcantoni C, Ma LJ, Federspiel C, Fogo AB. Hypertensive nephrosclerosis in African-Americans versus Caucasians. *Kidney Int* 2002; 62:172–180.

8. Luke RG. Hypertensive nephrosclerosis: pathogenesis and prevalence: essentially hypertension is an important cause of end-stage renal disease. *Nephrol Dial Transplant* 1999; 14:2271–2278.

9. Kincaid-Smith P. Hypothesis: obesity and the insulin resistance syndrome play a major role in end-stage renal failure attributed to hypertension and labeled 'hypertensive nephrosclerosis'. *J Hypertens* 2004; 22:1051–1055.

10. Hill GS, Heudes D Jacquot C, Gauthier E, Bariety J Morphometric evidence for impairment of real autoregulation in advanced essential hypertension. *Kidney Int* 2006; 69:823–831.

11. Kher V. End-stage renal disease in developing countries. *Kidney Int* 2002; 62:350–362, 2002.

12. Barsoum RS. Chronic kidney disease in the developing world. *New England J Med* 2006; 354:997–999.

13. Ardissino G, Daccò V, Testa S, Bonaudo R, Claris-Appiani A, Taioli E, Marra G, Edefonti A, Sereni F. Epidemiology of chronic renal failure in children: data from the ItalKid project. *Pediatrics* 2003; 111:e382–e387. URL: http://www.pediatrics.org/cgi/content/full/111/4/e382

14. Groothoff JW. Long-term outcomes of children with end-stage renal disease. *Pediatr Nephrol* 2005; *online publication accessed 3/4/2007 online at URL:* http://www.springerlink.com/content/h550x482t416942u/fulltext.html

15. Warady BA, Chadha V. chronic kidney disease in children: the global perspective. Pediatr Nephrol, 2007; e-publication ahead of print, accessed 3/18/2007 online at URL: http://www.springerlink.com/content/b420808077043774/fulltext.pdf

16. Heptinstall RH. Pathology of end-stage kidney disease. *Am J Med* 1968;44:656–663.

17. Schwartz MM, Cotran RS. Primary renal disease in transplant recipients. *Hum Pathol* 1976;7:455–9.

18. Hughson MD, Fox M, Garvin AJ. Pathology of the end-stage kidney after dialysis. Progress. *Reproductive Urinary Tract Pathol* 1990;2:157.

19. Raju DL, Cantarovich M, Brisson ML, Tchervenkov J, Lipman ML. Primary hyperoxaluria: clinical course, diagnosis, and treatment after kidney failure. Am J Kidney Dis. 2008; 51:e1–e5, 2008.

20. Heptinstall RH, Hypertension I. essential hypertension. In R.H. Heptinstall (Ed.), *Pathology of the Kidney*1993; (4th ed.). Boston: Little Brown & Co., p. 951.

21. Hughson MD, Johnson K, Young RJ, Hoy WE, Bertram JF. Glomerular size and glomerular sclerosis: relationship to disease categories, glomerular solidification, and ischemic obsolescence. *Am J Kidney Dis.* 2002;39:679–688.

22. Hughson MD, McManus JFA, Hennigar GR. Studies on end-stage kidneys. II. Embryonal hyperplasia of Bowman's capsular epithelium. *Am J Pathol* 1978; 91:71–84.

23. McManus JFA, Hughson MD, Fitts CT, Williams AV. Studies on end-stage kidneys. I. Nodule formation in intrarenal arteries and arterioles. *Lab. Invest* 1977; 37:339.

24. Kasiske, BL. Relationship between vascular disease and age associated changes in the human kidney. *Kidney Int* 1987; 31:1153–1159.

25. Tracy, RE). Blood pressure related separately to parenchymal fibrosis and vasculopathy of the kidney. Am J Kidney Dis 1992; 20:124–131.

26. Heptinstall RH. End-stage renal disease. In R.H. Heptinstall (Ed.), *Pathology of the Kidney* 1993; (4th ed.). Boston: Little Brown & Co., p. 713.

27. Cotran, R.S. Glomerulosclerosis in reflux nephropathy. *Kidney Int*1982; 21:528.

28. Buckalew VM Jr., Shey HM. Renal disease from habitual antipyretic analgesic consumption: an assessment of the epidemiological evidence. *Medicine* 1986; 11:291.

29. Fogo AB. Progression and potential regression of glomerulosclerosis. *Kidney Int* 2001; 59:804–819.

30. Zeisberg M, Kalluri R. The role of epithelial-to-mesenchymal transition in renal fibrosis. *J Mol Med* 2004;82:175–181.

31. Iwano M, Neilson EG. Mechanisms of tubulointerstitial fibrosis. *Curr Opin Nephrol Hypertens* 2004; 13:279–284.

32. Remuzzi G, Benigni A, Remuzzi A. Mechanisms of progression and regression of renal lesions of chronic nephropathies and diabetes. *J Clin Invest* 2006; 116:288–296.

33. Eddy AA. Molecular basis of renal fibrosis. *Pediatr Nephrol* 2000 15:290–301.

34. Aldigier JC, Kanjanbuch T, Ma LJ, Brown NJ, Fogo AB. Regression of existing glomerulosclerosis by inhibition of aldosterone. *J Am Soc Nephrol* 2005;16:3306–3314.

35. Schena FP, Strippoli GFM, Wankelmuth P. Renal growth factors: past present and future. *Am J Nephrol* 1999; 19:308–312.

36. Fogo AB. Mechanisms in nephrosclerosis and hypertension-beyond hemodynamics. *J Nephrol supp* 2001;14:S63–S69.

37. Epstein, M. Aldosterone and the hypertensive kidney: its emerging role as a mediator of progressive renal dysfunction: a paradigm shift. *J Hypertens* 2001;19:829–842.

38. Yang J, Liu Y. Dissection of key events in tubular epithelial to myofibroblast transition and its implications in renal interstitial fibrosis. *Am j Pathol* 2001;159:1465–1475.

39. Copeland JW, Beaumont BW, Merrilees MJ, Pilmore HL. Epithelial –to-mesenchymal transition of human proximal tubular epithelial cells; effects of rapamycin, mycophenolate, cyclosporine, azathioprine, and methylprednisolone. *Transplantation* 2007; 83:809–814.

40. Zeisberg M, Strutz F, Müller GA. Renal fibrosis: an update. *Curr Opin Nephrol Hypertens* 2001;10:315–320.

41. Zoja C, Abbate M, Remuzzi G. Progression of chronic kidney disease: insights form animal models. *Curr Opin Nephrol Hypertens* 2006; 15:250–257.

42. Fogo AB. Renal fibrosis: not just PAI-1 in the sky. *J Clin Invest* 2003;112:326–328.

43. Alphonso S, Santamaria I, Guinsburg ME, Gomez AO, Miranda JL, Jofre R, Menarguez J, Cannata-Andia J, Cigudosa JC. Chromosomal aberrations, the consequence of refractory hyperparathyroidism: its relationship with biochemical parameters. *Kidney Int* 2003;(Suppl 85):S32–S38.

44. Hruska KA, Teitelbaum SL. Renal osteodystrophy. *N Engl J Med* 1995; 333:166–174.

45. Lund RJ, Davies MR, Matthew S, Hruska KA. New discoveries in the pathogenesis of renal osteodystrophy. *J Bone Miner Metab* 2006; 24:169–171.

46. Davies MR, Lund RJ, Matthew S, Hruska KA. Low-turnover osteodystrophy and vascular calcification are amenable to skeletal anabolism in an animal model of chronic kidney disease and the metabolic syndrome. *J Am Soc Nephrol* 2005; 16:917–928.

47. McCarthy JT, Williams AW, Johnson WJ. Serum beta-2-microglobulin concentration in dialysis patients: Importance of intrinsic renal function. *J Lab Clin Med* 1994; 123:495

48. Onishi S, Andress DL, Maloney NA, Coburn JW, Sherrard DJ. Beta-2-microglobulin deposition in bone in chronic renal failure. *Kidney Int* 1991; 39:990–995.

49. Manske CL. Dialysis-related amyloidosis. *J Lab Clin Med* 1994; 123:458.

50. Takayama F, Miyazaki S, Morita T, Hirasawa Y, Jiwa T. Dialysis related amyloidosis of the heart in long-term dialysis patients. *Kidney Int* 2001;78:8172–8176.

51. Yusa H, Yoshida H, Kikuchi H, Onizawa K. Dialysis-related amyloidosis of the tongue. *J Oral Maxillofacial Surg* 2001; 59:947–950.

52. Bandini S, Bergesio F, Conti P, Mancini G, Cerretini C, Cirami C, Rosati A, Caselli GM, Arbustini E Merlini G, Ficarra G, Salvadori M. Nodular macroglossia with combined light chain and β-2 microglobulin deposition in a long-term dialysis patient. *J Nephrol* 2001; 14:128–131.

53. Mount SL, Eltabbakh GH, Hardin NJ. β-2-microglobulin amyloidosis presenting as bilateral ovarian masses: a case report and review of the literature. *Am J Surg Pathol* 2002; 26 :130–133.

54. Shimizu S, Yasui C, Yasukawa K, Nakamura H, Shimizu H, Tsuchia K. Subcutaneous nodules on the buttocks as a manifestation of dialysis related amyloidosis: a clinicopathologic entity? *Brit J Dermatopathol* 2003; 149:400–404.

55. Fleury AM, Buetens OW, Campassi C, Argani P.. Pathologic quiz case: A 77 year-old woman with bilateral breast masses. Amyloidosis involving the breast. *Arch Pathol Lab Med 2004*; 128:e67–69, 2004.

56. Briese S, Wiesner S, Will JC, Lembcke A, Opgen-Rheim B, Nissel R, Wernecke KD, Andreae J, Haffner D, Querfeld U. Arterial and cardiac disease in young adults with childhood-onset end-stage renal disease — impact of calcium and vitamin D therapy. *Nephrol Dial Transplant* 2006; 21:1906–1914.

57. Parfrey PS, Hartnett JD, Barre PE. The natural history of myocardial disease in dialysis patients. *J Am Soc Nephrol* 1991; 2:2–12.

58. Foley RN, Parfrey PS, Hartnett JD, Kent GM, Martin CJ, Murray DC, Bare PE. Clinical and echocardiographic disease in patients starting end-stage renal disease therapy. *Kidney Int* 1995; 47:186–192.

59. Duh Q-Y, Lim RC, Clark OH. Calciphylaxis in secondary hyperparathyroidism. Diagnosis and parathyroidectomy. *Arch Surg* 1991; 126:1213.

60. Moe SM). Calcemic uremic arteriopathy: a new look at an old disorder. *NephSAP* 2004;3:77–83.

61. Rutsky EA, Rostand SG. Pericarditis in end-stage renal disease: Clinical characteristics and management. *Semin Dialysis* 1989; 2:25.

62. Rostand SG, Rutsky EA. Pericarditis in end-stage renal disease. *Cardiol Clin* 1990; 8:701.

63. Weiss SW, Taw RL, Hutchins GM. Constrictive uremic pericarditis following hemodialysis for acute renal failure. *Johns Hopkins Med J* 1973; 132:301.

64. Eschbach JW, Adamson JW. Anemia of endstage renal disease (ESRD). *Kidney Int* 1985; 28:1–5.

65. Fraser CL, Arieff AL. Nervous system manifestations of renal failure. In R.W. Schrier, (Ed.), *Diseases of the Kidney* 2001;(7th ed.). Philadelphia: Lippincott Williams & Wilkins, p. 2769.

66. Dunnill MS, Millard PR, Oliver D. Acquired cystic disease of the kidneys: A hazard of long-term intermittent maintenance haemodialysis. *J Clin Pathol* 1977; 30:868.

67. Feiner HD, Katz LA, Gallo GR. Acquired cystic disease of the kidney in chronic dialysis patients. *Urology* 1981; 17:260–264.

68. Matson MA, Cohen EP. Acquired cystic kidney disease: occurrence, prevalence, and renal cancers. *Medicine* 1990; 69:217–226.

69. Gagnon RF, Kintzen Gm, Kaye M. Acquired cystic kidney disease: rapid progression from small to enlarged kidneys simulating adult polycystic kidney disease. *Clin Nephrol* 2000; 53:307–311.

70. Choyke PL. (2000). Acquired cystic kidney disease. *Eur Radiol*; 2000; 10:1716–1721.

71. Ishikawa I, Saito Y, Asaka M, Tomosugi N, Yuri T, Watanabe M, Honda R. Twenty-year follow-up of acquired renal cystic disease. *Clin Nephrol* 2003; 59:153–9.

72. Ishikawa I, Yuri T, Kitada H, Shinoda A. Regression of acquired cystic disease of the kidney after successful renal transplantation. *Am J Nephrol* 1983; 3:310–314.

73. Ishikawa I, Saito A, Chikazawa Y, Asaka M, Tomosugi N, Yuri T, Suzuki K, Ueda Y, Ozaki M. Cystic renal cell carcinoma, suspected because of lack of regression of renal cysts after renal transplantation in a dialysis patient with acquired renal cystic disease. *Clin Exp Nephrol* 2003; 7:81–4.

74. Jenkins DA, Temple RM, Winney RJ, Allan PL, Notgi A, Wild SR. Effect of treatment mode on the natural history of acquired cystic renal disease of the kidney in patients on renal replacement therapy. *Nephrol dial transplant* 1992; 7:613–617.

75. Kliem V, Koditz M, Behrend M, Ehlerding G, Pichlmayr R, Koch KM, Brunkhorst R. Risk of renal cell carcinoma after kidney transplantation. *Clin Trnasplant* 1997; 11:255–258.

76. Ondrus D, Pribylincová V, Breza J, Bujdák P, Miklosi M, Resnícek J, Zvarva V. The incidence of tumors in renal transplant recipients with long-term immunosuppressive therapy *Int Urol Nephrol* 1999; 31:417–422.

77. Denton MD Magee CC, Ovuworie C, Mauiyyedi S, Pascual M, Colvin RC, Cosimi AB, Tolkoff-Rubin N. Prevalence of renal cell carcinoma in patients with ESRD pre-transplantation: a pathologic analysis. *Kidney Int* 2002; 61:2201–2209.

78. Petrolla AA, MacLennan. Renal cell carcinoma associated with end stage renal disease. *J Urol* 2006;176:345.

79. Kojima Y, Takahara S, Miyake O, Nonomura N, Morimoto A, Mori H. Renal cell carcinoma in dialysis patients: a single center experience. *Int J Urol* 2006; 13:1045–1048.

80. Hughson MD, Hennigar GR, McManus JF.Atypical cysts, acquired renal cystic disease, and renal cell tumors in end-stage dialysis kidneys. *Lab Invest* 1980; 42:475–480.

81. Hughson MD, Buchwald D, Fox M. Renal neoplasia and acquired cystic disease in patients receiving long-term dialysis. *Arch. Pathol. Lab. Med.* 1986; 110:592–601.

82. Heinz-Peer G, Schoder M, Rand T, Mayer G, Mostbeck GH. Prevalence of acquired cystic kidney disease and tumors in native kidneys of renal transplant recipients: a prospective US study. *Radiology* 1995; 195:667–71.

83. Moudouni SM, Lakmichi A, Tligui M, Rafii A, Tchala K, Haab F, Gattegno B, Thibault P, Doublet JD. Renal cell carcinoma of native kidney in renal transplant recipients. *BJU Int* 2006; 98:298–302

84. Neuzillet Y, Lay f, Luccioni A, Daniel M, Berland Y, Coulange C, Lechevallier E. De novo renal cell carcinoma of native kidney in renal transplant recipients. *Cancer* 2005; 103:251–257.

85. Tickoo SK, deParalta-Venturina MN, Harik LR, Worcester HD, Salam ME, Young AN, Moch H, Amin M. Spectrum of epithelial neoplasms in end-stage renal disease: an experience from 66 tumor bearing kidneys with emphasis on histologic patterns distinct from those in sporadic adult renal neoplasia. *Am J Surg Pathol* 2006; 30:141–153.

86. Fuhrman SA, Laski LC, Limas C. Prognostic significance of morphologic parameters in renal cell carcinoma. *Am J Surg Pathol* 1982; 6:655–663.

87. Delahunt B, Eble JN. Papillary renal cell carcinoma: a clinicopathologic and immunohistochemical study of 105 tumors. *Mod Pathol* 1997; 10:537–544.

88. Yoshida M, Yao M, Ishikawa I, Kishida T, Nagashima Y, Kondo K, Nakaigawa N, Hosaka M. Somatic von Hippel-Lindau disease gene mutation in clear-cell renal carcinomas associated with end-stage renal disease/acquired cystic disease of the kidney. *Genes Chromosomes Cancer* 2002; 35:359–64.

89. Hughson MD, Bigler S, Dickman K, Kovacs G. (Renal cell carcinoma of end-stage renal disease: an analysis of chromosome 3, 7, and 17 abnormalities by microsatellite amplification. *Mod Pathol* 1999; 12:301–309.

90. Lubensky IA, Schmidt L, Zhuang Z, Weirich G, Pack S, Zambrano N, wlathier MM, Choyke P, Linehan WM, Zbar B. Hereditary, and sporadic papillary renal cell carcinomas with *c-met* mutations share a distinct morphologic phenotype. *Am J Pathol* 1999; 155:517–526.

91. Farivar-Mohseni H, Perlmutter AE, Wilson S, Shingleton WB, Bigler SA, Fowler JEJr. Renal cell carcinoma and end stage renal disease. *J Urol* 2006; 175:2018–2020.

92. Peces R, Martínez-Ara J, Miguel JL, Arrieta J, Costero O, Górriz JL, Picazo ML, Fresno M. Renal cell carcinoma coexistent with other renal disease: clinico-pathological features in re-dialysis patients and those receiving dialysis or renal transplantation. *Nephrol Dial transplant* 2004; 19:2789–2796.

93. United States Renal Data System. *USRDS 1999 Annual Data Report: Chapter VIII Pediatric End-Stage Renal Disease*, National Institutes of Health, NIDDK 1999; Bethesda MD, p. 117.

CHAPTER 16

Pathology of Renal Transplantation

Tibor Nadasdy, MD, Anjali Satoskar, MD, and Gyongyi Nadasdy, MD

INTRODUCTION

Renal transplantation is the treatment of choice for end stage renal disease. According to the U.S. Renal Data system (USRDS), graft survival half-life was between 10.5 and 11.1 years for deceased donor transplant kidneys and living donor transplant kidneys, respectively [1]. The annual cost of transplant maintenance is a fraction of the cost of continuous dialysis; therefore, it is obvious that renal transplantation not only provides a much better quality of life for patients, but it is also considerably less expensive than dialysis treatment. The surgical pathologist's main role in managing renal transplant patients is diagnosing rejection or other conditions, affecting the transplant kidney, in renal allograft biopsies. The most important question is to decide whether the graft is rejecting or not. Many years ago, the acute rejection rate was between 40 and 50 percent in the first year, now this is between 5 and 20 percent in most transplant centers. Acute rejection rate in compliant patients is even less common after the first year. This is the consequence of more and more effective antirejection treatment regimens. On the other hand, these immunosuppressive medications may also give rise to a variety of novel pathologies, which should be recognized by the pathologist. Therefore, in recent years we clearly see a shift in the pattern of pathologic changes seen in renal allograft biopsy specimens; we see less and less cases of classic acute rejection episodes and more cases of other changes, including drug toxicities, infections, and recurrent and de novo diseases.

In spite of efforts to find reliable and easy laboratory tests for diagnosing acute rejection and other conditions causing graft dysfunction, the gold standard of the diagnosis is still the renal allograft biopsy. Therefore, it is not surprising that in renal pathology laboratories, renal transplant biopsies comprise a large proportion of renal biopsies, averaging between 30 and 50 percent in most centers. Therefore, every pathologist who interprets renal biopsies should be prepared to diagnose rejection and other conditions leading to graft failure. This chapter is intended to be a short practical guide for pathologists and residents who are interested in renal allograft pathology and need to read renal allograft biopsies. Because of space limitations, we cannot discuss pathogenesis in detail in this chapter. The interested reader is referred to in-depth reviews and papers on pathogenesis [2].

We provide two simplified algorithmic approaches on the light microscopic evaluation of renal allograft biopsies from patients with early and late graft dysfunction (Figures 16.1 and 16.2). However, we would like to emphasize that these algorithms provide only a rough guidance for the novice in renal allograft pathology. The morphologic patterns of injury frequently overlap and correct interpretation can only be achieved after considering the entire "gestalt" of findings, including immunofluorescence/immunoperoxidase (C4d and in many cases the antibodies used in native renal biopsy evaluation) and, if necessary, electron microscopy. Careful correlation of the morphology with the clinical history, treatment, and laboratory findings is crucial in the evaluation of every renal allograft biopsy, taken for an indication. At the end of the chapter, in the Appendix, we provide a more detailed but still simplified differential diagnostic approach on the interpretation of basic morphologic patterns seen in renal allograft biopsies.

Handling and Processing of Renal Transplant Biopsies

Having a quick turnaround time is imperative for renal allograft biopsies performed for graft dysfunction. The shorter the delay, the more effectively the rejection or other conditions can be treated and this can influence graft outcome. Therefore, renal allograft biopsies (except for protocol biopsies) should undergo rapid processing. This can be done by performing rapid processing using automated dehydration, allowing paraffin embedded sections to be prepared within 4–5 hours of biopsy [3]. Recently, the introduction of microwave processing technology further cut down the turnaround time [4]. At our institution, we can provide a diagnosis within 2 or 3 hours of taking the renal biopsy. Frozen sections could provide the fastest diagnosis; however, we do not recommend this practice because the quality of the frozen sections depends on numerous factors, including the experience of the histotechnologist preparing the frozen sections.

We submit the bulk of the specimen in formalin for routine processing and paraffin embedding. We routinely perform the same stains we apply to every renal biopsy (H&E, Periodic acid Schiff [PAS]), Trichrome, and methenamine silver). However, the methenamine silver stain is usually not important unless the patient has glomerular disease. The PAS stain is relevant for the correct examination of the renal tubules for tubulitis and for the identification of arteriolar hyalin. The trichrome stain is helpful to determine the degree of interstitial fibrosis and the presence of fibrin thrombi or fibrinoid necrosis in the vasculature.

The introduction of C4d staining in tissue sections has provided a powerful tool for diagnosis of antibody mediated rejection. We routinely perform C4d immunofluorescence on every allograft biopsy specimen (see section on "Humoral Rejection"); therefore, a small piece of the tissue, preferably renal cortex, is submitted for immunofluorescence. If the biopsy is small, a 2–3 mm piece of viable cortex is sufficient to perform adequate C4d staining. C4d staining is not only present in the cortical peritubular capillaries, but also in the vasa recta in the renal medulla; however, in our experience, the staining in the medullary vasa recta and the cortical peritubular capillaries may occasionally be discordant. Antibodies to C4d that work on formalin fixed paraffin-embedded sections are also available and the results are comparable to those with immunofluorescence [5]. Therefore, some centers prefer not to submit tissue for immunofluorescence, but to perform C4d immunoperoxidase stain on paraffin sections. This is acceptable; however, we prefer performing immunofluorescence because of the much faster turnaround time. This could be relevant, particularly at transplant centers performing renal transplantation in presensitized patients following a desensitization protocol.

We routinely submit a small piece of renal cortex for electron microscopy from every biopsy specimen taken after the first twelve months following transplantation (such practices vary between centers). In these cases, we also perform a full panel immunofluorescence with antibodies that we routinely apply to native kidney biopsies (antibodies to IgG, IgA, IgM,

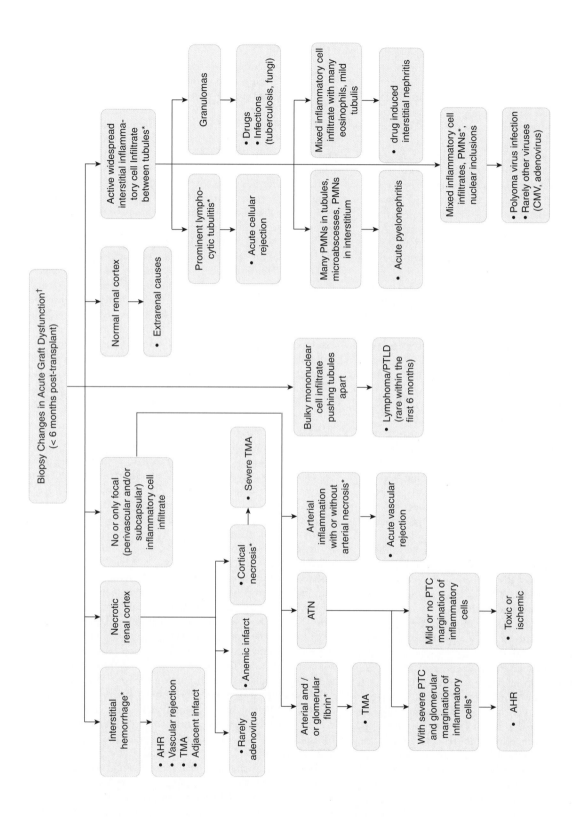

AHR: acute humoral rejection; **ATN:** acute tubular necrosis; **CMV:** cytomegalo virus; **PMNs:** poly morphonuclear leukocytes; PTC: peritubular capillary; PTLD: post-transplant lymphoproliferative disorder.

*May occur in AHR (C4d + PTC)

† These morphologic patterns frequently overlap. For more details on individual morphologic patterns and associated conditions, see Appendix

FIGURE 16.1: Biopsy changes in early graft dysfunction (<6 months posttransplant).

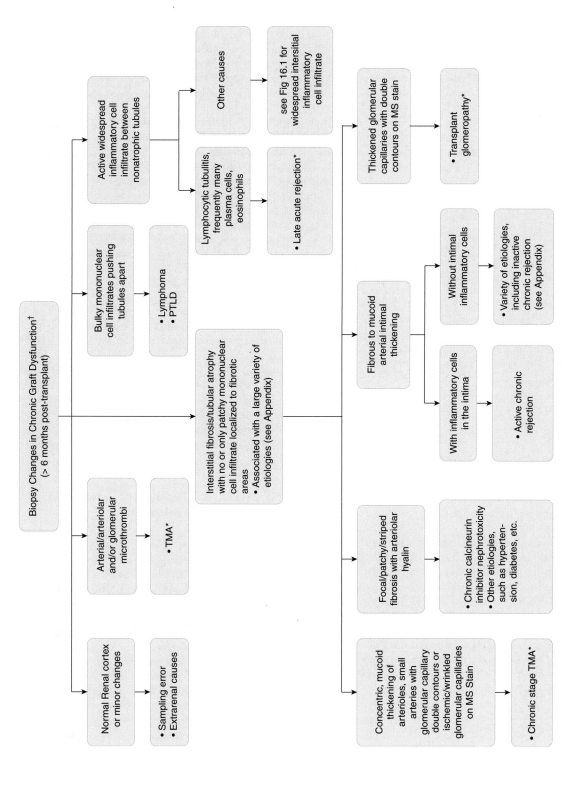

†: Causes of acute graft dysfunction can also cause chronic graft dysfunction. These morphologic patterns frequently overlap. For more details on individual morphologic patterns and associated conditions, see Appendix.

*Diffuse PTC C4d staining is not uncommon (rarely, C4d PTC staining may occur with any of the above patterns of injury).

MS: methenamine silver; **PTC:** peritubular capillary; **PTLD:** post-transplant lymphoproliferative disorder; **TMA:** thrombotic microangiopathy;

FIGURE 16.2: Biopsy changes in Late graft dysfunction (>6 months posttransplant).

kappa and lambda light chains, C3, C1q, fibrinogen, and albumin). If the immunofluorescence is negative, if the light microscopy of the glomeruli is unremarkable, and if the clinical history does not indicate glomerular disease, we only prepare semithin sections from the resin embedded tissue for electron microscopy and do not perform ultrastructural examination. If the immunofluorescence is positive in the glomeruli, if the light microscopic morphology of the glomeruli is abnormal, or if the patient has symptoms of glomerular disease, we perform electron microscopy.

Electron microscopy and routine immunofluorescence with the antibodies used in the workup of native renal biopsies are not contributory in many renal transplant biopsies. Therefore, we will only discuss immunofluorescence and electron microscopy findings where they are relevant to the diagnosis.

Representativeness of the Allograft Biopsy

It is difficult to determine reliable criteria for the representativeness of the specimen. The Banff classification proposes that the tissue has to contain at least seven glomeruli and at least one arterial cross section (preferably an arcuate artery) [6]. Obviously, if diagnostic lesions are present, even a small biopsy may be sufficient to make a definitive diagnosis. However, particularly if the lesions are zonal and focal, even a larger biopsy specimen may not be adequate for diagnosis. In our and others' opinion, the adequate allograft biopsy specimen should consist of at least two cores, containing renal cortex [7]. Still, the adequacy should be determined by the examining pathologist, depending on the presence or absence of diagnostic lesions in the specimen.

BIOPSY CHANGES ASSOCIATED WITH REJECTION

There are two major ways to classify the rejection process in renal allografts. One of them is the conventional classification, which is based on the pattern of injury [8]. The other is based primarily on a scoring system, which was introduced by a group of pathologists and nephrologists in Banff, Canada; hence the name Banff classification [6,9–12]. The most recent updates of the Banff classification also take the underlying pathogenesis into consideration [10–12]. We use both classifications in our renal allograft biopsy reporting. The Banff classification (Banff scoring system) is best considered a working classification because it is being continuously updated at consecutive Banff conferences. The first (1991) Banff classification was published in 1993 [6], which was modified in 1997 [7], 2003 [10], 2005 [11], and most recently in 2007 [12].

Conventional Classification of Rejection

Hyperacute Rejection

Hyperacute rejection is the consequence of circulating preformed antidonor antibodies in the recipient. Today this form of rejection is extremely rare because pretransplant cross matching methodologies detect the antibodies [2,8]. Hyper-

acute rejection is the most aggressive form of antibody mediated rejection. Typically, the characteristic gross changes already appear on the operating table immediately after the circulation of the transplant kidney has been reconstituted. The kidney turns dusky and cyanotic. (Figure 16.3). Light microscopy reveals accumulation of leukocytes in the glomerular and peritubular capillaries as well as in arterioles. (Figure 16.4). This is commonly associated with congestion and fibrin thrombi. If the transplant kidney is not removed, the graft will undergo complete necrosis. If one performs immunofluorescence in hyperacute rejection, complement (C3, C4d) and occasionally even immunoglobulins are often detectable in the glomerular and peritubular capillaries (PTC). There is no effective treatment for hyperacute rejection.

Disseminated intravascular coagulation (DIC) in the donor kidney can cause differential diagnostic problem if an immediate post-transplant biopsy is taken. DIC is not uncommon in deceased donor kidneys, particularly if the donor expired because of head trauma. The absence of relevant accumulation of leukocytes in the peritubular and glomerular capillaries and the absence of severe congestion are histologic signs, indicating that the glomerular microthrombi are not secondary to hyperacute rejection. Immunofluorescence for C4d is negative. Also, the surgeon usually does not see the characteristic dusky, cyanotic discoloration of the graft. These donor microthrombi usually dissolve very quickly following transplantation and do not influence graft outcome [12].

Glomerular capillary (sometimes even arteriolar) thrombosis secondary to severe preservation injury may occasionally cause a differential diagnostic dilemma. In such cases, there is evidence of severe tubular injury and the C4d staining in the PTC is negative. Of note is that margination of inflammatory cells and congestion of PTC is common in severe preservation injury.

Acute Cellular (Acute Cell-Mediated, Acute Interstitial, or Acute Tubulointerstitial) Rejection

The terminology of this type of rejection is somewhat confusing in the literature. In the past, many investigators refrained using the term "acute cellular rejection" because it implicated pathogenesis and in some cases not only cellular but also antibody mediated antidonor responses were evident. Other investigators simply called it acute interstitial rejection because the hallmark lesion is infiltration of the renal interstitium by inflammatory cells. Because the majority of the infiltrating inflammatory cells are T cells, the 2005 and 2007 revisions of the Banff classification calls it acute T cell mediated rejection (types 1A and 1B) [11,12]. Since the inflammation also involves the tubules, acute tubulointerstitial rejection is the best descriptive terminology.

Acute tubulointerstitial (cellular) rejection usually develops after the first week of transplantation. This is the most frequent type of acute rejection, but as mentioned previously, because of the effective immunosuppressive medications, we see it less and less frequently. Acute cellular rejection in compliant patients is rare after the first month, but it can happen anytime, particularly if immunosuppressive drug levels become low (diarrhea, vomiting, changes in medication and, in particular, noncompliance).

Gross Pathology

Grossly, the kidney is swollen with a pale edematous appearing cortex. (Figure 16. 5).

Light Microscopy

The hallmark of acute tubulointerstitial rejection is the infiltration of the interstitium and tubules by mononuclear cells, primarily lymphocytes, but also macrophages. (Figure 16.6). Most infiltrating cells are T cells (Figure 16.7), primarily CD8+ effactor cells, but CD4+ cells and macrophages are also common [13]. Plasma cells, eosinophils, and polymorphonuclear leukocytes may also occur, but usually not in large numbers, unless the rejection develops late following transplantation [14, 15]. In occasional biopsies, B cell aggregates/nodules are present. [Figure 16.8]. The relevance of these is debated, but some investigators believe that these B cell aggregates indicate a more aggressive form of rejection [16]. A variable degree of interstitial edema is usually associated with the inflammatory cell infiltrate. Another hallmark of acute cellular rejection is tubulitis. (Figure 16.6C).

Tubulitis means the infiltration of the renal tubular epithelium by inflammatory cells. The inflammatory cells in the renal epithelium usually reflect the composition of the interstitial inflammatory cell infiltrate (mostly T cells and macrophages). The Banff scoring system is used to determine the severity of the interstitial inflammatory cell infiltrate and tubulitis (see later section). Interstitial hemorrhage is unusual in acute cellular rejection and, if present, the pathologist should consider a more severe (acute, vascular or acute humoral) rejection process. Acute cellular (tubulointerstitial) rejection may also be combined with other types of rejections.

If acute cellular rejection occurs late (usually after 6 or 12 months) following transplantation, it is not uncommon to see large numbers of plasma cells infiltrating the interstitium. This form of rejection is best designated as plasma cell rich late acute rejection [14]. We commonly see this in patients with low immunosuppressive drug levels (noncompliant patients, primarily). The plasma cells are polyclonal and many times their presence is associated with prominent interstitial edema, as well as eosinophils. (Figure 16.9). In our experience, approximately 40 percent of the biopsies with plasma cell rich late acute rejection episodes also will display diffuse PTC C4d staining; such cases may represent a combination of acute cellular and humoral rejection [17]. The pathogenetic role of plasma cells in this form of acute rejection is unclear. Late, plasma cell rich acute rejection frequently does not respond well to antirejection treatment.

In acute cellular rejection, immunofluorescence findings are negative or nonspecific. However, in approximately 20–30 percent of biopsies, acute cellular rejection may be associated with diffuse PTC C4d staining. Such rejection cases represent a combination of cellular and antibody mediated rejection. If only mild focal PTC C4d staining occurs, it is usually irrelevant (see discussion of "Humoral Rejection").

Differential diagnosis

Borderline acute rejection. The diagnosis of borderline acute rejection is somewhat subjective and we try to refrain

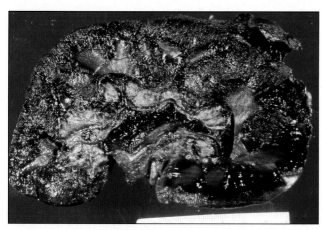

FIGURE 16.3: *This kidney was removed because of hyperacute rejection. Note the dark, dusky hemorrhagic cortex. The kidney underwent hemorrhagic necrosis.*

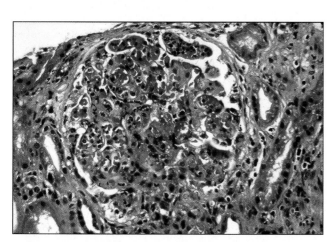

FIGURE 16.4: *A glomerulus in hyperacute rejection. Note the congested capillary loops with many red blood cells and polymorphonuclear leukocytes.*

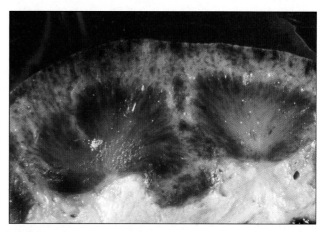

FIGURE 16.5: *An allograft nephrectomy with acute interstitial (cellular) rejection. Note the edematous renal cortex with patchy areas of hyperemia, particularly along the corticomedullary junction.*

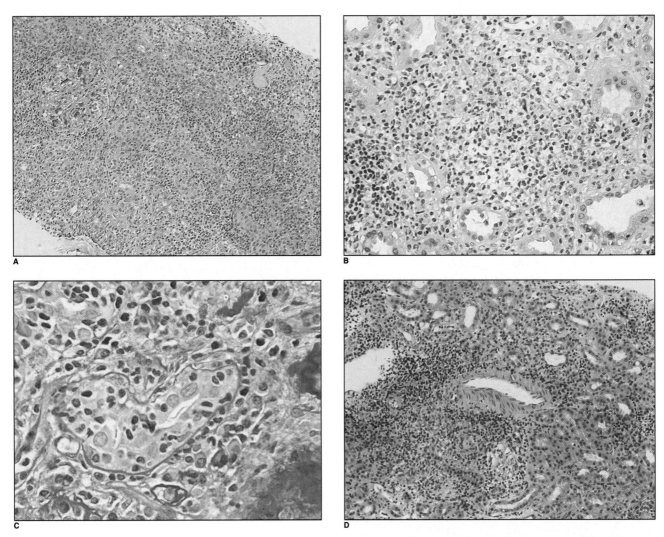

FIGURE 16.6: *Characteristic histologic findings in acute cellular (interstitial) rejection. A: prominent diffuse interstitial mononuclear cell infiltrate. H&E. B: Higher magnification reveals associated interstitial widening and destruction of tubules by the inflammatory cell infiltrate. H&E. C: The hallmark of acute interstitial (cellular) rejection is infiltration of the tubular epithelium by mononuclear cells (tubulitis). PAS. D: The arteries are usually unremarkable with no evidence of intimal arteritis. H&E× 200.*

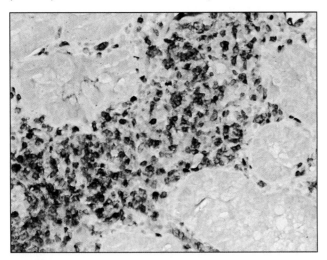

FIGURE 16.7: *In acute interstitial rejection the majority of the infiltrating inflammatory cells are T cells. Immunoperoxidase with an antibody to CD3.*

from making this diagnosis. However, there are biopsies where this diagnosis is appropriate. In such cases, the interstitial inflammatory cell infiltrate involves usually less than 25 percent of the renal cortex; it is not associated with relevant interstitial edema (Figure 16.10); tubulitis is mild and focal, and there is no evidence of vascular inflammation (intimal arteritis) [9]. One has to try to correlate graft function with histologic findings. If the mild interstitial inflammatory cell infiltrate does not explain the poor graft function, other etiologies (e.g., extrarenal factors or sampling error) should be considered.

Acute vascular rejection (i.e., acute cellular rejection with vascular involvement). This type of rejection is practically impossible to exclude in a small needle biopsy specimen because of the possibility of sampling error. This is particularly true if the biopsy contains none or only one arterial cross section. In cases of severe interstitial inflammation, edema, and/or interstitial hemorrhage, this possibility should be seriously considered, even if no vascular inflammation is evident.

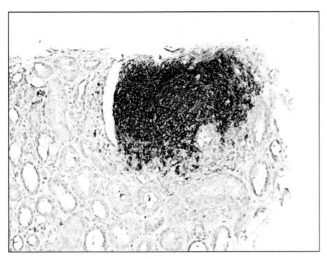

FIGURE 16.8: *A B cell cluster in a case of acute cellular rejection. Immunoperoxidase with an antibody to CD 20.*

Acute humoral rejection. As mentioned in an earlier section of the chapter, acute humoral rejection is frequently mixed with acute cellular rejection. PTC C4d staining is the most relevant finding for the pathologist to make this diagnosis (see later section).

Nonspecific inflammation. A common diagnostic error is to interpret scattered perivascular and subcapsular mononuclear cell infiltrates and mononuclear cells localized to fibrotic areas as signs of acute rejection (Figure 16.11). This can result in unnecessary immunosuppression with subsequent complications. If mononuclear cells are only localized to perivascular areas, fibrotic areas, or subcapsular zones, the diagnosis of acute rejection should not be made.

Acute pyelonephritis. There are many polymorphonuclears in the interstitium and, in particular, in the lumen of tubules. Neutrophilic tubulitis is evident. One has to keep in mind that the polymorphonuclear cell infiltrates in acute pyelonephritis may be missed in a renal biopsy specimen. In our experience, PTC margination of inflammatory cells is a frequent finding in acute pyelonephritis, but in such cases PTC C4d, staining is negative. It is common to see zones of normal renal parenchyma admixed with heavily inflamed areas in acute pyelonephritis; this is unusual in acute rejection.

Polyomavirus infection. The inflammatory cell infiltrate can be zonal, patchy, sometimes just encircling groups of tubules. Characteristic viral inclusions are usually, but not always present. A polyomavirus immunostain should be performed in every suspicious case.

Cytomegalovirus infection. In our experience, cytomegalovirus infection in the renal allograft is becoming quite rare, probably because of successful preventive treatments. Typical viral inclusions are evident, but an immunostain for cytomegalovirus should be performed in any suspicious biopsy.

Adenovirus infection. The histology represents extremely severe acute tubular necrosis with relatively mild interstitial

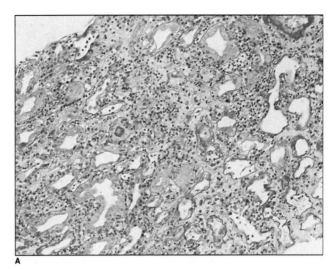

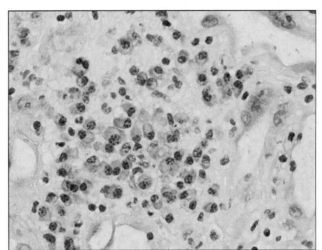

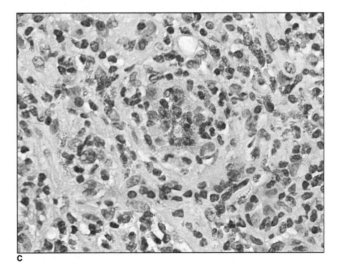

FIGURE 16.9: *Findings in late acute interstitial rejection. A: Prominent interstitial edema and inflammatory cell infiltrate. PAS. B: Higher magnification reveals that many of the inflammatory cells in the interstitium are plasma cells. H&E. C: Numerous eosinophils in a case of late acute rejection. In such instances, drug-induced interstitial nephritis is also a consideration. H&E.*

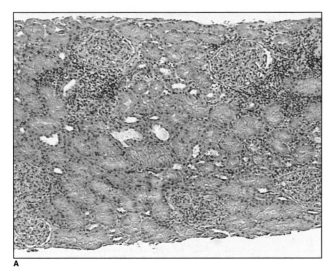
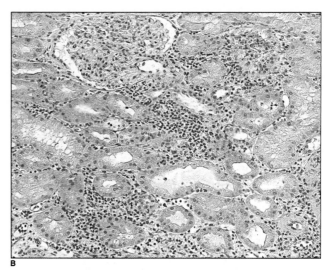

FIGURE 16.10: Borderline acute rejection. A: Patchy interstitial mononuclear cell infiltrate. H&E. B: Higher magnification reveals that the interstitial inflammatory cells do not cause obvious tubulitis in this area. The infiltrate is usually patchy and involves less than 25 percent of the renal cortex. H&E.

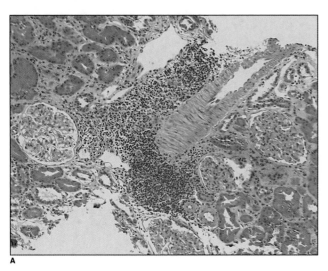
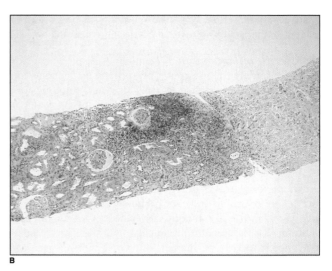

FIGURE 16.11: Nonspecific mononuclear cell infiltrates in renal allograft biopsies. A: Perivascular mononuclear cell infiltrate with no evidence of relevant interstitial inflammation and tubulitis in a protocol biopsy from a graft with normal function. H&E. B: Subcapsular area of fibrosis with some mononuclear cell infiltrate. H&E. Such focal mononuclear cell infiltrates in fibrotic areas should not be interpreted as acute rejection.

inflammation. Big smudgy nuclei are present in the tubular epithelial cells. An immunostain for adenovirus should be diagnostic.

Epstein–Barr virus infection/ posttransplant lymphoproliferative disorder. Over 90 percent of posttransplant lymphoproliferative disorders (PTLD) in renal allografts are associated with Epstein Barr virus (EBV). The infiltrate in the renal allografts in PTLD is bulky and lymphoma-like, but is not always monomorphic. Polymorphous infiltrates with many plasma cells may occur, which may resemble a late plasma cell rich acute rejection episode. In situ hybridization for EBV using the EBER probe can be very useful in the

differential diagnosis. Also, PTLD is usually a B cell lymphoproliferative process; therefore, most cells in the lymphomatous portion stain for B cells. One has to keep in mind, however, that PTLD and rejection may occur at the same time.

Drug-induced/hypersensitivity interstitial nephritis. This entity is practically impossible to differentiate with certainty from acute cellular rejection in a renal allograft biopsy. In drug-induced interstitial nephritis, tubulitis may not be as prominent as in an acute rejection episode, and in some cases, many eosinophils may be seen in the inflammatory cell infiltrate [18]. Still, these are very unreliable signs because eosinophils may also occur in acute rejection. If the suspicion emerges, the patient's medication should be reviewed. From the practical point of view, the inflammatory cell infiltrate should be considered acute rejection, until otherwise proven.

Etiology and pathogenesis

As indicated in the earlier part of the section of this chapter, acute cellular (interstitial) rejection is primarily associated with T-cell mediated alloimmune responses. Delayed type hypersensitivity may also be involved. It appears that CD4 positive, CD 25 positive regulatory T-cells (T regs) play an important role in controlling the rejection process.

Clinical course and outcome

Early acute cellular rejection, if not associated with vascular inflammation or humoral rejection, is almost always responsive to appropriate antirejection treatments and does not significantly affect long-term graft outcome unless it becomes a recurring event. The outcome of late acute cellular (interstitial) rejection is less favorable.

Acute Vascular Rejection

Acute vascular rejection, in fact, is frequently a more severe form of acute cellular rejection affecting the arteries (i.e., acute cellular rejection with vascular involvement). In approximately 30–40 percent of the cases, evidence of antibody mediated rejection is also present. It is worth discussing this form of rejection separately because of the distinctive morphology of the vasculature and the less favorable outcome.

Gross pathology

The kidney is somewhat swollen, usually congested with focal hemorrhages. Small, scattered subcapsular infarcts are common. (Figure 16.12).

Light microscopy

The hallmark of acute vascular rejection is inflammation of the arterial wall with or without fibrinoid necrosis. (Figure 16.13). In milder cases, the inflammatory cells infiltrate the arterial subendothelial space, the intima. (Figure 16.13A,B). This lesion is called intimal arteritis. The intimal inflammatory cell infiltrate is associated with variable degree of intimal edema and, depending on the amount of subendothelial inflammatory cell infiltrate; in some cases the intimal thickening can become quite prominent. In more severe forms of acute vascular rejection, the inflammatory cells are not only infiltrating the intima, but cause transmural inflammation, also involving the media. In severe cases, fibrinoid necrosis of the arterial wall is evident [19]. (Figure 16.13C). The Banff scoring system (see later section) is used to grade the severity of vascular lesions at acute vascular rejection [9]. The inflammatory cells in the intima are lymphocytes and macrophages [20,21]. In severe cases, the endothelial damage as well as the procoagulant activity of the macrophages can induce fibrinoid change

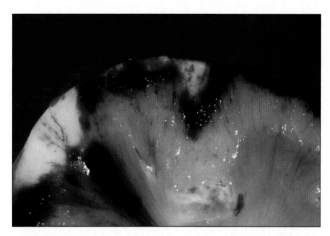

FIGURE 16.12: *Scattered anemic infarcts surrounded by a hyperemic zone in acute vascular rejection.*

and even fibrin thrombi. If vascular occlusion occurs, anemic infarcts can develop in the renal cortex. (Figure 16.12). One has to keep in mind that in acute vascular rejection, the lesion is not evident at every level of the artery and in every artery. Therefore, in a two dimensional tissue section, the lesion can be easily missed because of sampling error. As mentioned in the earlier part of this chapter, a variable degree of interstitial inflammatory cell infiltrate is almost always present. Interstitial hemorrhage is common in acute vascular rejection and most likely represents capillary injury and subsequent peritubular capillary disruption [19]. (Figure 16.14). Severe acute rejection with fibrinoid necrosis of the arteries used to be called humoral rejection in the older literature. This is incorrect because there is poor correlation between the severity of the vascular lesion and the presence of donor specific antibodies and subsequent antibody mediated rejection. In our experience, only about 50 percent of our Banff grade 3 vascular rejection cases display evidence of humoral rejection. In milder cases of acute vascular rejection, the prevalence of C4d staining in the PTC is not different from acute cellular rejection without vascular inflammation.

Differential diagnosis

Other forms of rejection. As discussed above, vascular lesions can be missed in the renal biopsy specimen because of sampling error.

Thrombotic microangiopathy. TMA can be quite difficult to differentiate from acute vascular rejection with fibrinoid necrosis and fibrin thrombi. In TMA, (unless associated with acute rejection) there is usually no inflammation within the vascular wall and glomerular microthrombi are common. Glomerular capillary thickening with widening of the subendothelial space on electron microscopy is a characteristic finding. In TMA, the interstitial inflammation is absent or mild (unless concomitant acute rejection is present). In certain stages and forms of TMA, fibrin thrombi are not seen, only subendothelial mucoid widening of the arterial/arteriolar wall is present, together with glomerular capillary subendothelial widening, resembling transplant glomerulopathy.

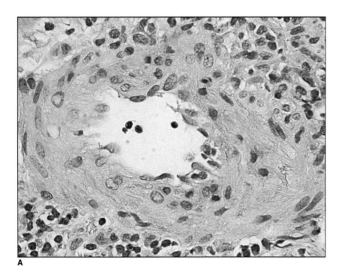

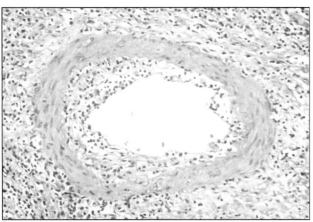

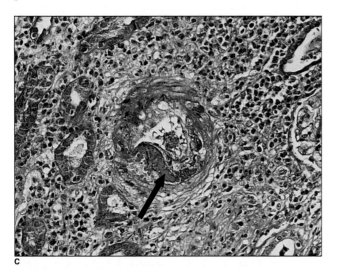

FIGURE 16.13: Vascular inflammation in acute vascular rejection. A: In mild intimal arteritis only a few inflammatory cells infiltrate the subendothelial space. H&E. B: Intimal arteritis with widespread inflammatory cell infiltrate in the subendothelial space. H&E. C: Fibrinoid necrosis in the wall of a small artery (arrow) in a case of severe acute vascular rejection. Trichrome.

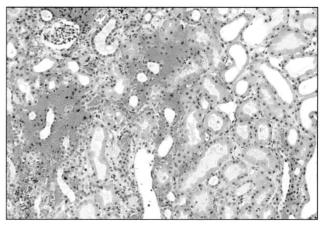

FIGURE 16.14: Interstitial hemorrhage in acute vascular rejection. H&E.

True vasculitis in the renal allograft. Theoretically, this could be a very difficult differential diagnostic problem; however, in practice, this is an exceptional situation. It could be an issue in a patient whose ESRD was secondary to vasculitis. Crescent formation in the glomerular capillaries, associated with vasculitis, should warn the pathologist about the possibility of a true vasculitis. We have seen a case of cryoglobulinemic vasculitis in an allograft.

Etiology and pathogenesis

Most cases of acute vascular rejection are mediated by T cell dependent alloimmune responses. However, there is evidence that in a substantial proportion of acute vascular rejection, particularly in severe cases associated with arterial wall necrosis, antibody-mediated immune responses also play an important role (see below).

Clinical course and outcome

Cases of severe acute vascular rejection with fibrinoid necrosis, transmural inflammation of the vascular wall or very prominent intimal arteritis usually have a poor long-term outcome and do not respond well to antirejection treatment [19,22].

Acute Humoral Rejection (Acute Antibody-Mediated Rejection, C4d Positive Humoral Rejection)

Introduction

Acute humoral rejection has been a recently emerging entity. Until the late 90's, most rejection episodes were thought to be the consequence of cellular immune responses. Therefore, practically all immunosuppressive regimens were aimed against the cellular branch of the immune response. In the 90's it became evident that certain patients with therapy resistant acute rejection have donor specific circulating antibodies and their allograft biopsies reveal complement deposition in the PTC [23,24]. Detecting complement deposition in the PTC with the conventional anticomplement antibodies was usually not successful;

however, with the introduction of antibodies to C4d, this became possible. C4d is a stable, split product of C4 that covalently binds to the endothelium where complement activation occurs. Since donor specific antibodies first react with the recipient's endothelium, complement fixing donor specific antibodies will activate the complement cascade and C4d will be detectable along the capillary endothelium; in particular, along the PTC endothelium. Several investigators proved that PTC C4d staining shows a very good correlation with the presence of circulating donor-specific antibodies [24–29]. However, this correlation is not perfect and different centers have slightly divergent experiences. These differences may be secondary to the various detection methods used to detect circulating donor-specific antibodies and to the possible presence of noncomplement fixing antibodies or non major histocompatibility complex (MHC) antibodies.

In recent years, C4d staining became a routine methodology in transplant biopsy evaluation. In our opinion, C4d deposition is best-detected using immunofluorescence on frozen sections because of the quick turnaround time. This is particularly relevant in transplant centers where presensitized recipients are transplanted following a desensitization protocol. We use indirect immunofluorescence to detect PTC C4d deposition providing results within 3 hours after the biopsy was taken. Antibodies that are applicable to paraffin sections are also available and results with C4d staining using immunoperoxidase methodology on paraffin sections are comparable to immunofluorescence on frozen sections [5]. However, using immunoperoxidase usually means next day result, which is clearly a disadvantage.

The current criteria for the diagnosis of acute humoral rejection were set by a national consensus conference [30]. These criteria include: (1) clinical evidence of graft dysfunction, (2) histologic evidence of tissue injury (margination of PMNs/monocytes in the PTC, vascular inflammation or necrosis, fibrin thrombi, acute tubular injury, and interstitial inflammation), (3) diffuse presence of C4d in PTC, (4) Serologic evidence of circulating donor specific antibodies. These are true in a classic case; however, as with other types of rejections, one can encounter subclinical or early cases where there is no clinical evidence of graft dysfunction [31,32]. Additionally, we keep encountering cases where PTC C4d staining is diffuse and obvious, but the patient does not have detectable donor specific antibodies. In rare cases, one may encounter patients with circulating donor specific antibodies, tissue injury, and graft dysfunction, but no obvious peritubular capillary C4d staining (perhaps because of noncomplement fixing antibodies). In such instances, in spite of the absence of all four criteria, the possibility of humoral rejection should be strongly considered. The consensus conference and Banff criteria [10,30] list acute tubular injury among the histologic changes associated with acute humoral rejection. In our experience, such cases should be handled with caution because acute tubular injury can be secondary to a variety of factors and if no inflammation or PTC margination of inflammatory cells is present in the biopsy specimen, we are reluctant to make the definitive diagnosis of acute humoral rejection, in spite of the presence of PTC C4d.

Acute humoral rejection occurs in approximately 30 percent of renal allograft biopsies with histologic evidence of acute cellular rejection and in approximately 6–9 percent of all allograft biopsies [2]. These patients develop de novo donor specific antibodies, usually within the first weeks or months after transplantation. Donor-specific antibodies and PTC C4d staining may occur, later following transplantation [33,34]. The significance of this so-called late or chronic humoral rejection is not entirely clear.

In the past, the presence of donor-specific antibodies (positive cross match) pretransplant was a contraindication for transplantation. Now, more and more transplant centers perform renal transplantation in such patients following a desensitization protocol. Obviously, the incidence of acute humoral rejection in the biopsy material of such transplant centers is higher than in transplant centers that do not perform transplantation in presensitized patients. Results with renal transplantation after desensitization are surprisingly good. PTC C4d staining is also common following transplantation of ABO incompatible renal allografts. Such patients also undergo desensitization and results are excellent. It is interesting that in ABO incompatible patients, PTC C4d staining is common in the absence of any graft damage and graft dysfunction. Several authors believe that in such recipients the C4d staining represents immunologic accommodation and not acute rejection [35].

Gross pathology

Renal allografts with antibody mediated rejection can have a variety of gross appearances depending on the severity of the rejection. From unremarkable grafts to slight swelling or hemorrhage and even necrosis.

Light microscopy

Light microscopic changes of acute humoral rejection are non-specific. The most characteristic finding is margination of inflammatory cells in the PTC [10,24–30,36,37]. (Figure 16.15). In early stages, many PMNs may be present in the PTC admixed with other mononuclear cells, mainly monocytes. In later stages, it appears that monocytes are the overwhelming cells in the PTC, admixed with lymphocytes. Gibson and coworkers [38] recently introduced a scoring for PTC margination of inflammatory cells, which is now incorporated into the 2007 update of the Banff classification [12] (See "Banff Scoring for Lesions in Acute Rejection"). In our experience, it is very unusual not to see PTC margination of inflammatory cells in a true acute humoral rejection; however, PTC margination of inflammatory cells is far from being specific and we have seen it in conditions such as pyelonephritis, acute tubular necrosis, and acute cellular rejection (without humoral component). Of course, inflammatory cells not only marginate in the PTC, but also in the glomerular capillaries (glomerulitis). (Figure 16.16). However, glomerulitis in acute humoral rejection may be less prominent than PTC margination of inflammatory cells. Vascular inflammation and/or necrosis may occur in severe forms of humoral rejection, but vascular inflammation and necrosis do not necessarily mean an underlying antibody mediated rejection process. As mentioned above, humoral rejection is frequently mixed with cellular rejection.

TMA is not an unusual finding in acute humoral rejection. In our experience, this is particularly common in patients who underwent desensitization, but subsequently develop a humoral

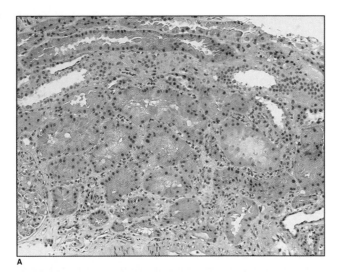

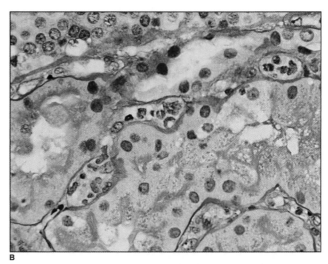

FIGURE 16.15: *Margination of inflammatory cells in the peritubular capillaries in acute humoral rejection. A: Low magnification appears to show mild interstitial inflammatory cell infiltrate. H&E. B. Higher magnification reveals that the inflammatory cells are localized to the peritubular capillaries. The inflammatory cells are usually a mixture of polymorphonuclears and mononuclear cells (monocytes/macrophages). PAS.*

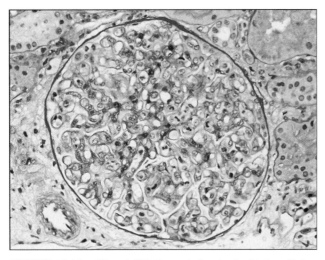

FIGURE 16.16: *Glomerulitis in acute humoral rejection. Note that the glomerular capillaries are filled with inflammatory cells resembling intracapillary proliferative glomerulonephritis. PAS.*

rejection episode. In such cases, arteriolar and glomerular microthrombi are evident, usually with variable degree of PTC margination of inflammatory cells. (Figure 16.17).

Immunofluorescence microscopy

The most important diagnostic finding is diffuse PTC C4d staining in the renal biopsies (Figure 16.18) [10,24–37]. As mentioned in the earlier part of this chapter, this can be detected using immunofluorescence or immunoperoxidase methodologies. In acute humoral rejection, the PTC staining should be diffuse and obvious. Focal mild PTC C4d staining may be clinically irrelevant, but the relevance of such staining is difficult to determine in individual cases (Figure 16.19). According to the most recent Banff update [12], focal PTC C4d staining is

defined as 10 percent to 50 percent C4d positive PTC. Minimal staining is defined as less than 10 percent PTC C4d staining. There are certain pitfalls that may influence the diagnosis. Scarred, poorly perfused areas of renal cortex may not stain very well; one should carefully look at the H&E section of the frozen tissue to make sure that appropriate nonscarred viable renal cortex is available for examination. If only a scarred piece of subcapsular cortex is available for C4d staining, the results should be evaluated with caution and immunoperoxidase stain for C4d on paraffin section should be performed, particularly if the paraffin sections contain better-preserved renal cortex. Also, if the renal parenchyma is necrotic, PTC C4d staining may be negative. However, in our experience, the PTC C4d staining may persist if the necrosis is not very advanced yet. Still, if the tissue is necrotic, negative PTC C4d staining has no diagnostic value. C4d is not only positive in the cortical PTC, but also in the vasa recta; therefore, if only renal medulla is available and the staining is strong and diffuse, we do not hesitate to consider the biopsy C4d positive. Still, in such cases we recommend repeating the C4d stain on paraffin sections, if they contain renal cortex. If one uses immunofluorescence, certain intrinsic staining can be useful as an internal positive control. The mesangium and arterioles do stain for C4d by immunofluorescence even in negative/normal cases. (Figure 16.20). Therefore, if a biopsy specimen is completely negative for C4d by immunofluorescence, one should think about technical error. Glomerular capillaries are usually also positive for C4d in acute humoral rejection; however, glomerular capillary staining in the absence of PTC C4d staining is not diagnostic of humoral rejection. One has to be careful not to interpret tubular basement membrane staining as PTC staining for C4d. (Figure 16.21). Although C4d usually does not stain normal tubular basement membranes, atrophic tubular basement membranes are commonly positive.

The C4d staining should be linear and circumferential in the PTC [10,24,26,30]. In our experience, this pattern of staining is only present in renal allograft rejection (humoral rejection).

C4d is obviously positive in immune complex deposits; therefore, it can be seen in tubulointerstitial immune complex deposits, such as in cases of lupus nephritis, but authors have not seen any native kidney biopsy yet that did show diffuse linear circumferential PTC staining. The best control tissue for C4d staining is an allograft nephrectomy specimen with proven peritubular capillary C4d. If such tissue is not available, immune complex glomerulonephritis, such as lupus nephritis can be used, but this control is less optimal. It is worth testing transplant nephrectomy specimens for C4d staining because usually the immunosuppression is discontinued prior to the nephrectomy and many of these kidneys display late acute rejection episodes, sometimes with diffuse PTC C4d staining.

Some transplant centers also use and advocate immunofluorescence with an antibody to C3d [39]. C3d is commonly positive in the PTC in a similar pattern as described for C4d. In authors' experience, there is no humoral rejection with positive C3d

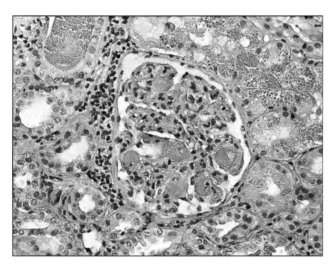

FIGURE 16.17: *Glomerular fibrin thrombi in a case of acute humoral rejection. Also, note the peritubular capillary margination of inflammatory cells. H&E.*

staining and negative C4d staining in the PTC. On the other hand, C4d staining in the absence of C3d staining may occur. In the past, we used to stain for both C3d and C4d every transplant biopsy, but failed to find any clinical advantage to adding C3d staining; therefore, we only use C4d staining currently.

Differential diagnosis

Is diffuse PTC C4d staining diagnostic of acute humoral rejection? This is a frequently asked question and the answer is no. As discussed above, in certain patients, PTC C4d staining may be evident without any inflammatory reaction or any renal pathology and normal renal function [31]. This is most commonly observed in patients who undergo ABO incompatible renal transplantation [35]. Very rarely, we have seen similar conditions even in patients who had preformed donor specific antibodies and underwent desensitization protocol. In such instances, the possibility of graft accommodation emerges. One has to keep in mind that C4d, covalently bound to the PTC endothelium, may remain there for quite some time after the humoral rejection was successfully treated. Although occasionally we have seen PTC C4d staining disappearing after one week in patients who underwent plasmapheresis, the staining can persist for months and sometimes even for years (obviously, persistence between biopsies years apart is impossible to prove to be continuous). Therefore, just the presence of diffuse PTC staining is not a good test to determine the end point of treatment protocols designed to fight acute humoral rejection.

Does the absence of PTC C4d staining exclude acute humoral rejection? In our experience, acute humoral rejection is almost always associated with diffuse PTC C4d staining. However, the possibility that noncomplement fixing antibodies may cause graft damage, exists. If the patient has donor specific antibodies, if the light microscopic histology shows the characteristic changes, and if there is graft dysfunction, this possibility can be raised. However, the diagnosis certainly cannot be made

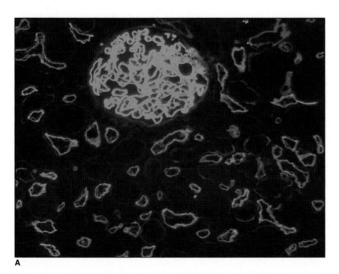
A

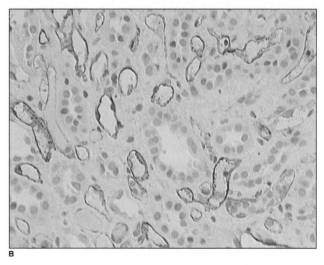
B

FIGURE 16.18: *A: Diffuse circumferential peritubular capillary C4d staining by immunofluorescence in a case of acute humoral rejection. Note that the glomerular capillaries also show diffuse linear staining. B: Immunoperoxidase stain reveals similar circumferential peritubular capillary staining in a case of acute humoral rejection.*

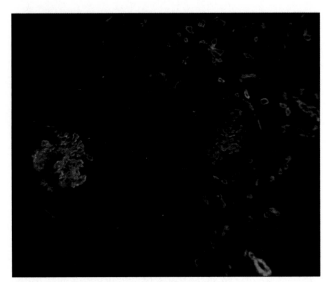

FIGURE 16.19: Focal peritubular capillary C4d immunofluorescence in an allograft with patchy cortical scarring.

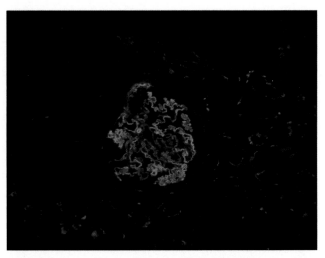

FIGURE 16.21: Focal tubular basement membrane fluorescence for C4d. This should not be confused with peritubular capillary fluorescence. The differentiation is usually quite easy. Some glomerular capillary staining is also present in this case with moderate chronic allograft nephropathy.

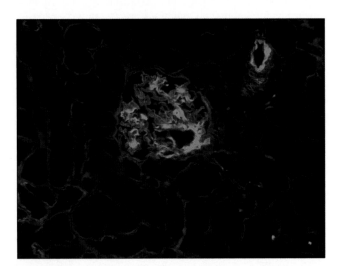

FIGURE 16.20: Mild to moderate smudgy mesangial fluorescence and some arteriolar fluorescence for C4d is almost always seen, even in normal kidneys. Note the absence of peritubular capillary and glomerular capillary C4d staining.

based on the renal biopsy findings alone. Other conditions, such as infection (pyelonephritis) should always be raised in such instances.

Acute tubular necrosis. Some degree of PTC margination of inflammatory cells, including PMNs and monocytes may occur in acute tubular necrosis (ATN), not related to a humoral rejection process. In ischemic or toxic ATN cases, PTC C4d staining is negative. However, one has to keep in mind that ATN may develop in the setting of PTC C4d positivity and may not necessarily indicate an acute humoral rejection process. However, it is truly difficult to decide whether diffuse PTC C4d staining in the setting of ATN means acute humoral rejection or clinically irrelevant or persistent C4d staining in a setting of

ATN for other reasons. Still, this constellation should always be a concern for the possibility of acute humoral rejection.

Acute pyelonephritis. In our experience, acute pyelonephritis can cause quite prominent PTC margination of inflammatory cells, including PMNs (see later section). The diagnostic lesions in acute pyelonephritis (microabscesses, PMNs filling and extending tubules, neutrophilic tubulitis) may not be evident because of sampling error. In such instances, the light microscopy may show changes that are characteristic of humoral rejection. In our experience, acute pyelonephritis is not associated with PTC C4d staining; therefore, the differential diagnosis is usually easy.

Thrombotic microangiopathy. It is not uncommon to see thrombotic microangiopathy (TMA) in acute humoral rejection. TMA in acute humoral rejection is most likely secondary to endothelial injury caused by donor specific antibodies. Therefore, TMA, in the setting of diffuse PTC C4d staining, is strongly suggestive of an underlying humoral rejection process. If TMA is evident, in the absence of PTC C4d staining, other etiologies, such as recurrent TMA or drug-induced TMA (such as calcineurin inhibitor-induced TMA) should be considered.

Etiology and pathogenesis

Acute humoral rejection is caused by donor specific antibodies that bind to the endothelium and activate the complement cascade [24,29,36,37]. As the consequence of capillary complement activation, inflammatory cells will attach to the endothelium. In some instances, severe peritubular capillary injury may occur with subsequent patchy interstitial hemorrhage and edema. Activation of the coagulation cascade with subsequent microthrombi may occur. It appears that complement activation is crucial in the pathogenesis; however, as indicated before, we cannot exclude the possibility that, occasionally, noncomplement fixing antibodies may play a role. Also, more and more evidence emerges that non MHC antibodies may cause graft injury. It is likely that different donor specific antibodies can induce acute humoral rejection with different pathology, clinical presentation, and clinical outcome.

Clinical course and outcome

Acute humoral rejection does not respond well to conventional antirejection treatment, which is aimed at the cellular branch of the immune response. Plasmapheresis, IVIG treatment, anti-CD20 antibodies, and immunoabsorption are used to treat acute humoral rejection. The treatment is fortunately successful in most patients; therefore, many transplant centers decided to introduce desensitization protocols (removing the preexisting donor specific antibodies) before transplanting patients with preexisting circulating donor-specific antibodies.

Chronic Rejection

During the last two decades, with the introduction of more potent immunosuppressive medications, one-year graft survival substantially improved and, in most centers, it is around 95 percent or above. However, long-term graft survival rates did not improve as much and chronic graft failure, and eventually graft loss, remains a major problem. Chronic injury in the renal allograft may develop because of chronic rejection or other injurious factors, not related to rejection. Chronic rejection is best- defined as chronic graft injury secondary to allospecific cellular and/or humoral immune responses. If a recipient has several acute cellular rejection episodes or has donor specific antibodies, we can safely conclude that, if chronic graft injury develops, it is secondary to chronic rejection. However, in many instances, chronic graft injury develops in the absence of obvious underlying alloimmune responses and it is impossible to determine how much of the chronic graft injury is secondary to true chronic rejection and how much of it is the consequence of other factors.

The issue of chronic allograft nephropathy (interstitial fibrosis/tubular atrophy)

A number of injurious agents and factors can be responsible for graft injury, including hypertension, diabetes, recurrent diseases, infections, obesity, drug toxicity, urinary tract obstruction, reflux nephropathy, dietary factors, hyperlipidemia, etc. In fact, anything that can cause chronic injury in the native kidney can cause graft injury as well. For example, it is extremely difficult to define how much of the chronic injury is secondary to rejection and how much of it is secondary to other factors in an allograft biopsy taken several years posttransplant, from a patient who is diabetic, hypertensive, obese with hyperlipidemia, has history of recurrent urinary tract infections, an early acute rejection episode and is immunosuppressed with calcineurin inhibitor. The term chronic allograft nephropathy (CAN) was introduced to indicate that the exact etiology of the chronic injury in a biopsy specimen cannot be determined

[10]. At the Banff 2005 meeting, however, the decision was made to eliminate the terminology of CAN and introduce the descriptive term "interstitial fibrosis/tubular atrophy" instead [30]. Participants at the conference were concerned that CAN is being considered as a specific disease entity by many.

In the later sections of the chapter, we will discuss chronic changes in transplant biopsies, which are associated with true chronic rejection (alloimmune responses).

Gross pathology

The kidney may be shrunken, but it may retain normal size. The surface can reveal scars, but not always. The renal surface is frequently uneven and the kidney is firm and pale. On cut surface, the corticomedullary junction is usually poorly demarcated. In nephrectomy specimens, hemorrhages and edema are common because of frequent superimposed acute rejection. This occurs because of tapering of immunosuppression before the transplant nephrectomy.

Light microscopy

The characteristic changes include interstitial fibrosis and tubular atrophy, obliterative transplant arteriopathy and transplant glomerulopathy [2,33]. Transplant glomerulopathy, because of its unique features, will be discussed under separate heading. Interstitial fibrosis and tubular atrophy are obviously nonspecific changes and can be seen in any chronic renal disease [Figure 16.22]. Therefore, if the biopsy specimen does not contain arteries with obliterative transplant arteriopathy, or glomeruli showing transplant glomerulopathy, the diagnosis of chronic rejection cannot be made with certainty. Some degree of interstitial inflammatory cell infiltrate is usually still present, although if chronic rejection is not associated with an acute rejection flare, those are usually just clusters of small lymphocytes, frequently localized to perivascular areas. Small lymphocytes in fibrotic interstitium or tubulitis involving atrophic tubules are common findings in chronic rejection and usually do not indicate an acute rejection episode [Figure 16.23]. To diagnose superimposed acute rejection, active inflammatory cell infiltrate between nonatrophic tubules should be present associated with tubulitis in nonatrophic tubules [14,17]. However, if much of the specimen contains only fibrotic parenchyma, an active appearing mononuclear cell infiltrate with interstitial edema and aggressive infiltration of atrophic tubules can be interpreted as probable superimposed acute rejection (or active chronic rejection). Large lymphoid aggregates, occasionally containing even germinal centers, may sometime be encountered (Figure 16.24). The relevance of these lymphoid nodules is unclear, but we have seen them in graft nephrectomies with evidence of chronic pyelonephritis/reflux nephropathy.

Obliterative transplant arteriopathy is a hallmark of chronic rejection. Arterial intimal thickening, by itself, is a nonspecific lesion and can be seen in almost any vascular disease, including hypertension. However, in a typical case of obliterative transplant arteriopathy, inflammatory cells are still present in the thickened intima. (Figure 16.25). Occasionally, intimal foam cells are evident (Figure 16.25C). In advanced cases, one may encounter the reorganization of intimal myofibroblasts as a new media around the narrowed lumen. This is the so-called vessel in vessel phenomenon (Figure 16.25D). The intrarenal distribution of obliterative transplant arteriopathy is uneven; certain arteries may show prominent intimal thickening with luminal narrowing; others show only mild intimal thickening (Figures 16.25A,B). The Banff scoring on the severity of arterial obliterative lesions is based on the percentage of luminal narrowing [9]. This can be quite difficult to determine and it is subjective. We prefer using a slightly different approach: we grade obliterative transplant arteriopathy as mild, if the intimal thickening does not exceed the thickness of the media. The grade of the intimal thickening is moderate if the intimal thickening is up to twice the thickness of the media. If the intimal thickening exceeds twice the thickness of the media, we grade it as severe. Since the media can show segmental atrophy in chronic obliterative arteriopathy, we take the thickest portion of the media into consideration where the artery is not tangentially sectioned. Arteriolar changes, such as arteriolar hyalin change are not considered to be characteristic of chronic rejection, but they can be seen, particularly if hypertension and/or metabolic disturbances (hyperlipidemia, hyperglycemia) are present.

Immunfluorescence microscopy

PTC C4d staining is not uncommon in a true chronic rejection (Figure 16.26). Various investigators report a prevalence of 25–80 percent [2]. These differences may be related to differences in the definition of chronic rejection and to individual interpretation of C4 staining and to the various methodologies used. In our experience, the prevalence of PTC C4d staining in chronic rejection is approximately 50 percent, if we define chronic rejection by the presence of obliterative transplant arteriopathy and/or transplant glomerulopathy and/or previous episodes of acute rejection. The presence of diffuse PTC C4d staining in the setting of chronic rejection indicates an antibody mediated chronic rejection process (chronic humoral rejection). The relevance of de novo appearing donor specific antibodies and PTC C4d staining in the chronic setting is not as clear as in the acute setting at the time of writing of this chapter.

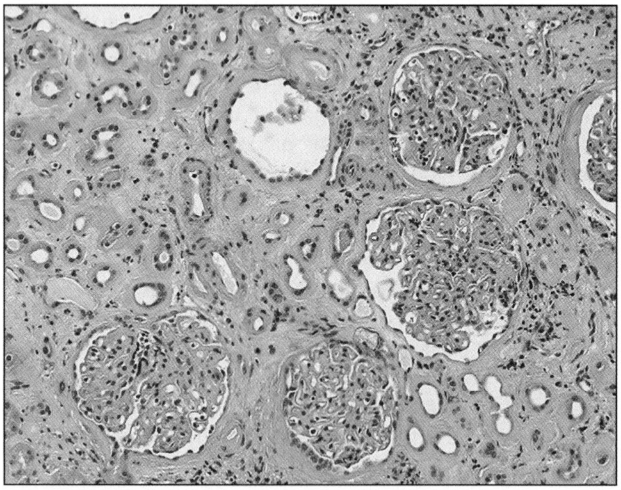

Electron microscopy

Several investigators reported lamellation of the peritubular capillary basement membrane in chronic rejection, particularly in biopsies with PTC C4d staining [34,40, 41] (Figure 16.27).

Differential diagnosis

Calcineurin inhibitor nephrotoxicity. This is perhaps the most common differential diagnostic dilemma in an allograft

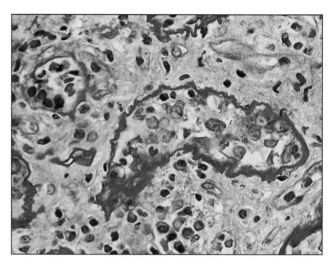

FIGURE 16.23: *Mononuclear cells infiltrate the epithelium of atrophic tubules. Tubulitis in atrophic tubules may be seen in the absence of obvious superimposed acute rejection. PAS.*

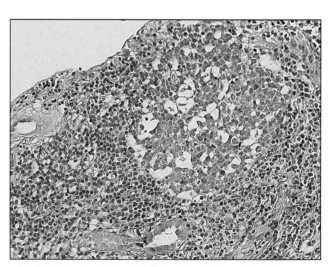

FIGURE 16.24: *A large lymphoid aggregate with a germinal center in a biopsy specimen with advanced chronic allograft nephropathy. H&E.*

FIGURE 16.22: *Interstitial fibrosis and tubular atrophy in a renal allograft. This is a non-specific finding, but the fact that the glomeruli show changes consistent with transplant glomerulopathy indicates that the chronic injury in this specimen is secondary to chronic rejection. H&E.*

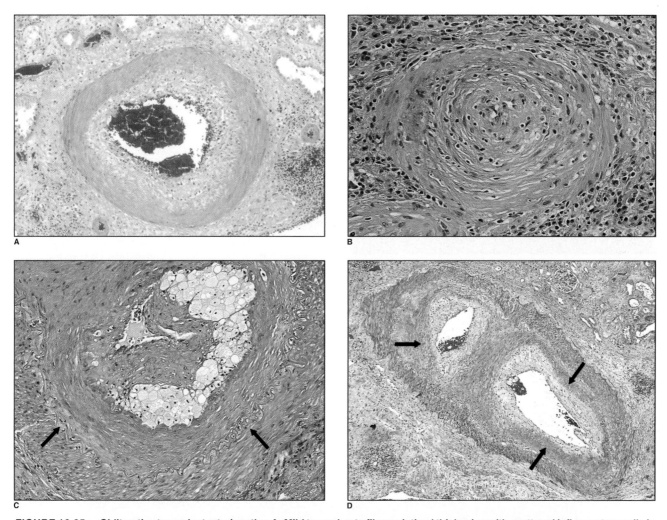

FIGURE 16.25: *Obliterative transplant arteriopathy. A: Mild to moderate fibrous intimal thickening with scattered inflammatory cells in the intima. The lumen is filled with red blood cells. H&E. B: Very prominent obliterative transplant arteriopathy with complete disappearance of the lumen. Note that inflammatory cells are still present in the fibrotic intima. H&E. C: Occasionally foam cells are present in the thickened intima. The arrows point the internal elastic membrane. H&E. D: Sometimes in advanced obliterative transplant arteriopathy, the intimal myofibroblasts reorganize as a "new media" around the narrow lumen (vessel in vessel phenomenon) (arrows). Masson's trichrome.*

biopsy with chronic injury taken from a patient on calcineurin inhibitor. The presence of arteriolar hyalin change, particularly if the hyalin change has the characteristic peripheral nodular pattern, indicates calcineurin inhibitor nephrotoxicity rather than chronic rejection. If arteries are present, in calcineurin nephrotoxicity the arteries are unremarkable or should only show mild fibrous intimal thickening. In chronic rejection, the situation is just the opposite; the arteries reveal prominent intimal thickening and the arterioles are relatively unremarkable. In calcineurin inhibitor nephrotoxicity, the glomeruli do not show evidence of transplant glomerulopathy; however, glomerular sclerosis, including focal segmental glomerular sclerosis can be seen. The pattern of interstitial fibrosis in calcineurin inhibitor nephrotoxicity is characteristically patchy, striped form. Many pathologists tend to rely on this so-called striped form of interstitial fibrosis in the diagnosis of calcineurin inhibitor nephrotoxicity, but in our opinion, this is a quite nonspe-

cific finding and is certainly not diagnostic. Striped form fibrosis may occur in chronic rejection, as well as nephrosclerosis secondary to hypertension.

Reflux nephropathy/chronic pyelonephritis. In our opinion, this is probably a commonly overlooked condition. The diagnosis can be quite difficult, particularly in a renal biopsy. Vesicoureteral reflux is not unusual in renal transplant patients and it can give rise to subsequent reflux nephropathy. Obvious episodes of acute pyelonephritis are not always evident. Interstitial fibrosis and tubular atrophy in reflux nephropathy can be quite zonal adjacent to normal appearing renal parenchyma. Such zonal, sharply demarcated areas of fibrosis are less common in chronic rejection. A mononuclear cell infiltrate in the fibrotic zones is usually present in chronic pyelonephritis and scattered polymorphonuclears may be seen in tubular lumina.

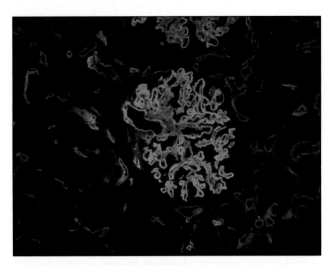

FIGURE 16.26: *Diffuse peritubular capillary and glomerular capillary C4d staining by immunofluorescence in a case of chronic rejection, complicated with transplant glomerulopathy.*

Hypertensive nephrosclerosis. One has to keep this condition in mind, particularly in patients who have suboptimally controlled blood pressure. The changes are not different from those seen in a native kidney. Changes in hypertensive nephrosclerosis can be very similar to those in calcineurin nephrotoxicity, but also to those in chronic rejection. Intimal thickening with lamellation of the elastic membrane is a common finding in the arteries in hypertensive nephrosclerosis, but if no rejec-

tion is associated with, the process, inflammatory cells are not present in the intima. Arteriolar hyalin change is common, but it is usually circumferential and nodular peripheral hyalin is rarely seen. Still, in many instances, hypertensive nephrosclerosis cannot be differentiated from chronic rejection and/or calcineurin inhibitor nephrotoxicity, particularly because there is frequent overlap with these conditions. Also, calcineurin inhibitors predispose to hypertension. Some degree of hypertensive nephrosclerosis is not unusual in deceased donor kidneys. Comparing allograft biopsy findings to a donor kidney biopsy (baseline biopsy) is important not to interpret changes of donor nephrosclerosis as chronic rejection or calcineurin inhibitor nephrotoxicity in a later allograft biopsy.

Polyomavirus nephropathy. The differential diagnosis relies on the detection of characteristic polyomavirus inclusions and positive immunostaining for polyomavirus in the biopsy specimen (see later section).

Other conditions. One could list any chronic condition affecting the kidney in the differential diagnosis of chronic rejection and this should be kept in mind. This includes recurrent diseases, such as recurrent diabetic nephropathy, recurrent glomerular diseases, recurrent thrombotic microangiopathies, etc. Frequently, the etiologies causing the chronic graft injury cannot be identified. In such cases, the terminology of chronic allograft nephropathy is appropriate to use; however, the 2005 revision of the Banff classification discourages the use of this term. The terminology "interstitial fibrosis/tubular atrophy" is now favored instead [11].

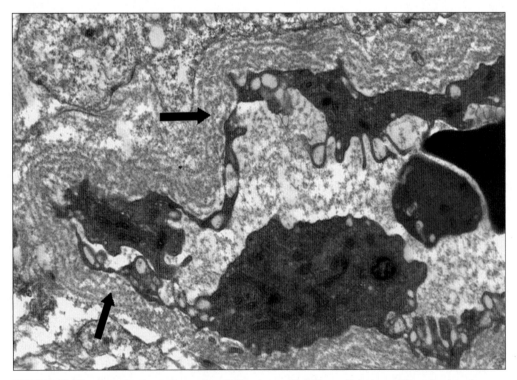

FIGURE 16.27: *Basement membrane lamellation (arrows) of the peritubular capillary in chronic rejection. Uranyl acetate and lead citrate.*

Etiology and pathogenesis

Both cellular and antibody mediated immune responses contribute to the development of chronic rejection. It is likely that nonimmune factors (e.g., hypertension, drug toxicity) contribute to the progression of chronic injury.

Clinical course and outcome

Appropriate therapeutic interventions in chronic rejection are still questionable and debated. For example, at this time there is no consensus whether removal of donor specific antibodies with plasmapheresis or other therapeutic interventions is necessary or truly beneficial in patients with chronic rejection who have circulating donor specific antibodies and PTC C4d staining in the biopsy. Unfortunately, most cases of true chronic rejection show a progressive disease course with poor response to therapeutic interventions.

Transplant Glomerulopathy

Transplant glomerulopathy develops in approximately 20–25 percent of long surviving renal allografts. If transplant glomerulopathy is evident, one can be quite certain that the patient has chronic rejection. It appears that transplant glomerulopathy is primarily the consequence of antibody mediated immune responses [33,34,42]. In our experience, approximately 50 percent of biopsies with transplant glomerulopathy also show concomitant diffuse PTC C4d staining [34]. Other patients who do not have concomitant PTC C4d staining at the time of the biopsy may have had previous biopsies with PTC C4d staining. Transplant glomerulopathy usually develops many years after transplantation, but in some patients with persistent humoral rejection, we have seen it developing within the first year of transplantation. Transplant glomerulopathy is the most common cause of severe proteinuria in renal allografts after the first year of transplantation.

Light microscopy

The glomeruli have thickened capillaries with frequent double contours on methenamine silver stain (Figure 16.28). Mesangial expansion is usually evident and slight mesangial hypercellularity and even some intracapillary hypercellularity may be present. According to the Banff scheme, transplant glomerulopathy is graded based on the percentage of glomeruli or capillary loops involved (see later section). Although it is true that not always all glomeruli are involved and different glomeruli may show lesions of different severity (e.g., more or less prominent capillary thickening), we always consider the degree of glomerular capillary thickening, in general, as an important change in grading the lesion.

Immunofluorescence microscopy

There is always strong linear to smudgy diffuse glomerular capillary C4d staining [33,34,42] (Figure 16.26). The remaining of the immunoreactants do not indicate specific immune com-

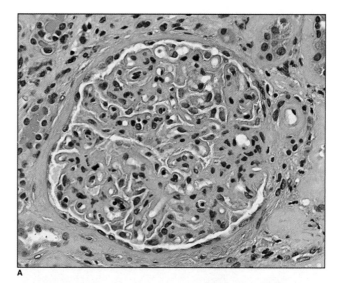

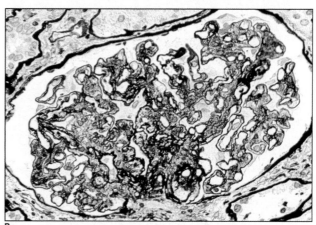

FIGURE 16.28: *Glomeruli in transplant glomerulopathy. A: H&E stain reveals thickened glomerular capillaries and expanded mesangium. B: Methenamine silver stain highlights double contours along the glomerular capillaries.*

plex deposition. One has to be careful with the evaluation because nonspecific staining patterns in transplant glomerulopathy are common (such as IgM, even some linear IgG staining, C3 staining).

Electron microscopy

Ultrastructurally, the characteristic finding is the widening of the subendothelial space along the glomerular capillaries [2,8,43] (Figure 16.29). The widened subendothelial space contains electron lucent "fluffy" material, but deposition of less electron lucent amorphous material, indistinct fibrillary material and even some dense deposits is common.

One has to be careful not to interpret these dense deposits as true discrete electron dense immune type deposits (Figure 16.29A). Mesangial cell interposition is a frequent finding (Figure 16.29B). Foot process effacement can be quite prominent, depending on the severity of proteinuria.

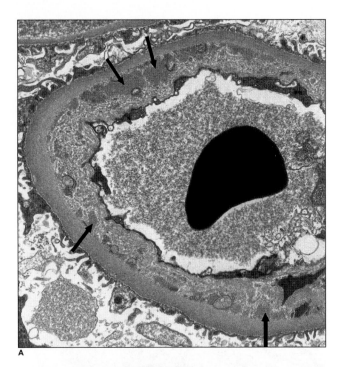

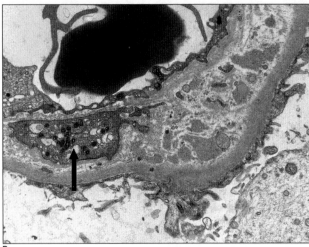

FIGURE 16.29: *Subendothelial widening of the glomerular capillaries in transplant glomerulopathy. A: note the prominent electron lucent widening of the subendothelial space. Occasional electron densities (arrows) are commonly seen in the widened subendothelial space. Such electron densities should not be interpreted as electron dense immune type deposits. Uranyl acetate-lead citrate. B: Mesangial cell interposition (arrow) in the widened subendothelial space. Uranyl acetate-lead citrate.*

Differential diagnosis

Thrombotic microangiopathy (TMA)/hemolytic uremic syndrome. It can be extremely difficult to differentiate transplant glomerulopathy from TMA because the glomerular morphology is quite similar. One should look for changes of TMA in arteries and, particularly in arterioles because those are usually missing in transplant glomerulopathy. Glomerular fibrin thrombi are usually not present in transplant glomerulopathy, but they are not always seen in TMA either. Also, the PTC

basement membrane lamellation on electron microscopy may not present in TMA and other recurrent or de novo glomerular diseases, whereas it is almost always seen in transplant glomerulopathy. Systemic clinical symptoms (such as inhemolytic uremic syndrome) of TMA are only present in approximately 50 percent of the renal allograft recipients who develop TMA [44], which make the differential diagnosis of transplant glomerulopathy also clinically difficult. Patients with TMA usually have less prominent proteinuria. In most cases, the differential diagnosis is possible, but in occasional biopsies, differentiating transplant glomerulopathy from TMA cannot be done with certainty.

Membranoproliferative glomerulonephritis (MPGN). Although there are many similarities, in our experience; this is not a common differential diagnostic problem in the everyday practice. Although MPGN type I may recur in renal allografts, in approximately 25–30 percent of the patients, this is a rare event in the everyday practice. Recurrent MPGN does have many similarities to transplant glomerulopathy, including the glomerular capillary thickening, double contours, and mesangial cell interposition. However, ultrastructurally, the differential diagnosis should be easy because of the presence of subendothelial electron dense deposits and the absence of prominent subendothelial widening of the glomerular capillaries in MPGN type I. Immunofluorescence shows the characteristic bright, coarsely granular subendothelial and mesangial C3 deposits in MPGN type I. MPGN Type II (dense deposit disease, [DDD]) almost always recurs in renal allografts, but it is easy to diagnose because of the diagnostic very electron dense intramembranous deposits within the glomerular and frequently also in the tubular basement membranes. Although recurrence of MPGN type III has been reported, this is a very rare event and the characteristic ultrastructure of MPGN type III and transplant glomerulopathy should make the differential diagnosis easy. The absence of PTC C4d staining in recurrent MPGN is also helpful, although it can be negative in cases of transplant glomerulopathy as well.

Cryoglobulinemic glomerulonephritis/hepatitis C-related glomerulonephritis. The differential diagnosis is easy if cryoglobulin deposits are present. If not, this could be problematic because the light microscopic histology may resemble transplant glomerulopathy. Ultrastructural examination usually does not reveal the characteristic subendothelial widening seen in transplant glomerulopathy.

Other glomerulonephritides. Other glomerulonephritides, including infection-related glomerulonephritis, recurrent fibrillary glomerulonephritis, and other recurrent de novo glomerulonephritides usually do not represent a serious differential diagnostic problem if tissue for immunofluorescence and electron microscopy is available.

Etiology and pathogenesis

As indicated above, it appears that transplant glomerulopathy is secondary to antibody mediated rejection and is considered to be a hallmark of chronic humoral rejection.

Clinical course and outcome

Patients develop worsening proteinuria, which, with disease progression, usually becomes nephrotic range. Unfortunately, no proven effective treatment exists and most patients with persistent heavy proteinuria develop progressive graft failure.

The Banff Schema for Diagnosing and Grading Renal Allograft Rejection

Banff 2007 Classification

In order to standardize the criteria for the diagnosis of renal allograft rejection, a group of pathologists, nephrologists and transplant surgeons held a meeting in Banff, Canada in 1991 and created a new classification system [6]. This Banff classification or Banff scheme for grading renal allograft rejection was modified later in 1997, in 2003, in 2005 and most recently in 2007 [9,10,11,12]. The most recent 2005 and 2007 update of the Banff diagnostic criteria includes the following:

1. Normal allograft.
2. Antibody mediated rejection
   a. Acute antibody mediated rejection
      I. ATN like, minimal inflammation, C4d positive.
      II. Capillary margination and/or thrombosis.
      III. Arterial-v3, C4d positive.
   b. Chronic active antibody mediated rejection C4d positive withtransplant glomerulopathy, interstitial fibrosis/tubular atrophy and/or fibrous intimal thickening in arteries.3.

   Borderline changes (suspicious for acute T cell mediated rejection)

4. T cell mediated rejection
   A. Acute T cell mediated rejection.

      Type (grade) 1A; acute T cell mediated rejection. Cases with significant interstitial inflammatory cell infiltrate (greater than 25 percent of the parenchyma involved, i2, or i3) and foci of moderate tubulitis (t2). Type 1B: Same as type 1A, but with severe tubulitis (t3). Type 2A: Cases with mild to moderate intimal arteritis (v1). Type 2B: Cases with severe intimal arteritis comprising more than 25 percent of the luminal area (v2). Type III: Cases with transmural arteritis and/or arterial fibrinoid change and necrosis of the medial smooth muscle cells (v3), with accompanying lymphocytic inflammation.
   B. Chronic active T cell mediated rejection (obliterative transplant arteriopathy, mononuclear cell infiltration in the fibrotic renal cortex).

5. Interstitial fibrosis and tubular atrophy, no evidence of any specific etiology.

   Grade I. Mild interstitial fibrosis and tubular atrophy, involving less than 25 percent of the cortical area.
   Grade II. Moderate interstitial fibrosis and tubular atrophy involving 26–50 percent of the cortical area.
   Grade III. Severe interstitial fibrosis and tubular atrophy, involving more than 50 percent of the cortical area.

6. Other changes not considered to be related to rejection.

Banff Scoring for Lesions in Acute Rejection

Interstitial inflammation (i)

i0: less than 10 percent of renal cortex involved by inflammation.

i1: 10–25 percent of renal cortex involved by inflammation.

i2: 26–50 percent of renal cortex involved by inflammation.

i3: more than 50 percent of the renal cortex involved by inflammation

Tubulitis (t)

t0: no tubulitis

t1: 1–4 inflammatory cells per tubular cross section

t2: 5–10 tubular epithelial cells per tubular cross section

t3: more than 10 inflammatory cells per tubular cross section

Glomerular inflammation (glomerulitis) (g)

g0: no glomerulitis

g1: less than 25 percent of glomeruli with glomerulitis

g2: 25–75 percent of glomeruli with glomerulitis

g3: more than 75 percent of glomeruli with glomerulitis.

(In our experience, glomerulitis is frequently diffuse and the degree of intracapillary hypercellularity should also be taken into consideration).

Arterial inflammation (v)

v0: no arterial inflammation

v1: intimal inflammation (intimal arteritis causing less than 25 percent luminal narrowing)

v2: intimal arteritis causing more than 25 percent luminal narrowing

v3: transmural inflammation or fibrinoid necrosis

Peritubular capillaritis (PTC) (introduced in the most recent Banff upgrade [12]

ptc0: No significant cortical ptc, or <10 percent of PTCs with inflammation

ptc1: ≥10 percent of cortical peritubular capillaries with capillaritis, with max 3 to 4 luminal inflammatory cells.

ptc2: ≥10 percent of cortical peritubular capillaries with capillaritis, with max 5 to 10 luminal inflammatory cells.

ptc3: ≥10 percent of cortical peritubular capillaries with capillaritis, with max >10 luminal inflammatory cells.

Banff Scoring for Chronic Lesions

Interstitial fibrosis (ci)

ci0: less than 5 percent of renal cortex involved by interstitial fibrosis

ci1: 6–25 percent of the cortex involved

ci2: 26–50 percent of the cortex involved.

ci3: more than 50 percent of the cortex involved

Tubular atrophy (ct)

ct0: no tubular atrophy

ct1: less than 25 percent of the cortex involved by tubular atrophy

ct2: 26–50 percent of the renal cortex involved by tubular atrophy

ct3: more than 50 percent of the renal cortex involved.

Allograft glomerulopathy (transplant glomerulopathy) (cg)

cg0: less than 10 percent of peripheral glomerular capillaries with double contours on methenamine silver stain

cg1: up to 25 percent of glomerular capillaries with double contours in the most affected glomeruli.

cg2: 26–50 percent of glomeruli with double contours in the most affected glomeruli.

cg3: more than 50 percent of glomeruli with double contours in the most affected glomeruli.

(We also take the degree of glomerular capillary thickness into consideration).

Mesangial Matrix increase (mm)

mm0: no mesangial matrix increase

mm1: less than 25 percent of nonsclerotic glomeruli with mesangial matrix increase

mm2: 26–50 percent of nonsclerotic glomeruli with mesangial matrix increase

mm3: more than 50 percent of nonsclerotic glomeruli with mesangial matrix increase.

(We also take the degree of mesangial expansion into consideration).

Arterial fibrointimal thickening (cv)

cv0: no fibrous intimal thickening

cv1: fibrous intimal thickening causing less than 25 percent luminal narrowing

cv2: 26–50 percent luminal narrowing

cv3: over 50 percent luminal narrowing

(we use a different approach – see text)

Arteriolar hyalinosis (ah)

ah0: no arteriolar hyalin

ah1: mild to moderate PAS positive arteriolar hyalin in at least one arteriole.

ah2: mild to moderate PAS positive hyalin thickening in more than one arteriole.

ah3: severe PAS positive arteriolar hyalin thickening in many arterioles.

This scoring system is a serious effort to standardize renal allograft biopsy evaluation among renal pathologists. Still, some interobserver variability is unavoidable and refining the scoring is an ongoing event. For example, the grading of arterial hyalin change is quite subjective (relying only on mild, moderate and severe, based on the observer's experience); a new modified scoring of arteriolar hyalin is now proposed according to the suggestion by Mihatsch [45]:

ah0: no arteriolar hyalin

ah1: one arteriole with noncircumferential hyalin change

ah2: more than one arteriole with non circumferential hyalin change

ah3: one or more arterioles with circumferential arteriolar hyalin change

The Chronic Allograft Damage Index and Banff Chronic Sum Score

For a pathologist who has only limited experience in renal allograft biopsy interpretation, the grading or determining the severity of chronic injury, in general, could be a challenge. Since the changes in chronic rejection and in chronic allograft nephropathy can be quite complex, we provide the chronic allograft image index (CADI) in our biopsy reports [46]. The CADI includes a variety of histologic variables, including the degree of glomerular sclerosis, mesangial expansion, interstitial inflammation, tubular atrophy, interstitial fibrosis, and arterial intimal thickening. These lesions are scored on a semiquantitative scale from 0–3. Therefore, the maximum score can be 15. The CADI scoring can be used to estimate the degree of chronic injury in chronic rejection, as well as chronic graft injury of other etiologies (chronic allograft nephropathy [interstitial fibrosis/tubular atrophy with no specific etiology]). Alternately, the sum score of the individual Banff chronic lesion scores (ci, ct, cg, mm, cv, ah) can be used. Neither the Banff sum score nor the CADI score is optimal in determining the degree of clinically relevant chronic injury [47].

PATHOLOGIC CHANGES NOT RELATED TO ALLOGRAFT REJECTION

Nearly every renal disease (except those few associated with genetic defects, which do not affect the donor kidney e.g. Alport syndrome) can occur in renal transplant specimens, particularly in long surviving renal allografts. Therefore, it is crucial that the pathologist examining renal allograft biopsies is also knowledgeable in general renal biopsy pathology. In this section of the chapter, we will discuss only the most common and relevant conditions that one can encounter during the evaluation of renal allograft biopsies.

Renal transplant patients are usually on a large number of medications, including immunosuppressive drugs, antimicrobial agents, and antihypertensive agents and so on. Because of space limitations, we cannot discuss all injuries secondary to drug toxicity. For example, interstitial nephritis may occur, secondary to a variety of medications, including antimicrobial medications. The reader is referred to other chapters in this book. We have briefly addressed the differential diagnosis of interstitial nephritis and acute rejection during the discussion of acute cellular rejection. In this chapter, we will focus on renal lesions that can be associated with immunosuppressive medications.

Renal Changes Associated with Immunosuppressive Medications

Calcineurin Inhibitor Nephrotoxicity

The two widely used calcineurin inhibitors are cyclosporine (cyclosporine A) and tacrolimus (FK506). Cyclosporine A is a lipophilic undecapeptide isolated from a fungus. FK506 is a macrolid antibiotic also isolated from a fungus. Cyclosporine and tacrolimus are structurally dissimilar but have similar therapeutic mechanisms, and toxic effects. While evaluating renal biopsy specimens, it is impossible to differentiate cyclosporine nephrotoxicity from FK506 (Tacrolimus) nephrotoxicity [48]; therefore, the toxic effects of these two immunosuppressive drugs will be discussed together.

Acute (Early) Calcineurin Inhibitor Nephrotoxicity

Acute calcineurin nephrotoxicity was not uncommon during the 80's and early 90's when cyclosporine was used in larger doses, frequently only in combination with steroids [48–51]. Now, with the use of multiple drug combinations, lower doses are administered and acute toxicity is less common. In a typical case, the proximal tubular epithelium shows isometric vacuolization (Figure 16.30). This change is histologically identical to osmotic nephrosis and can be seen in other conditions as well (e.g., in contrast media nephrotoxicity). Authors have encountered isometric vacuolization in occasional protocol biopsies from patients on calcineurin inhibitors with normal graft function.

Giant mitochondria are round or oval and could be as large as half of the nucleus in the tubular epithelial cells. This lesion is rarely seen nowadays with lower doses of calcineurin inhibitors.

Microcalcification of the tubular epithelium is another nonspecific finding and it is most likely merely the consequence of tubular epithelial necrosis with subsequent dystrophic calcification in a patient who has secondary hyperparathyroidism (Figure 16.31).

Peritubular capillary congestion was initially thought to be a characteristic finding, but most pathologists with expertise in renal allograft pathology would not rely on this in diagnosing acute calcineurin inhibitor nephrotoxicity.

In many cases, the main histologic finding is acute tubular necrosis with or without the presence of isometric vacuolization of the tubules. Calcineurin inhibitors are clearly toxic to the tubular epithelium and can cause ATN, particularly if other risk factors, such as poor perfusion of the graft are present or if tubular injury develops in the donor during preservation or before harvesting. The differential diagnosis of acute calcineurin inhibitor nephrotoxicity is quite difficult and involves any conditions that can cause early graft dysfunction. If acute tubular injury is associated with high calcineurin inhibitor levels

and isometric vacuolization of the tubules, this possibility should be raised in the renal biopsy report. Finally, we would like to note that graft dysfunction secondary to calcineurin inhibitors may occur without obvious morphologic changes in the biopsy (functional nephrotoxicity).

The exact pathogenesis of the toxic effect is not entirely clear, but there is some evidence that calcineurin inhibitors are directly toxic to the renal tubular epithelium. In addition, they also cause vasoconstriction that can further aggravate the tubular injury. It appears that calcineurin inhibitors can induce single cell necrosis of the smooth muscle cells in the arterioles and small arteries. They can also induce endothelial injury, and rarely, TMA can develop (see later section).

Acute calcineurin inhibitor nephrotoxicity is well-correlated with the blood levels of cyclosporine or tacrolimus. Most of the acute lesions are fortunately reversible and if the calcineurin inhibitor is discontinued or if the doses are substantially lowered, recovery of graft function is the rule. If extensive calcification develops, some degree of interstitial fibrosis will be left behind.

Chronic Calcineurin Inhibitor Nephrotoxicity

The development of chronic injury secondary to calcineurin inhibitor toxicity takes at least 6 months, usually several years. The diagnosis cannot be made clinically; the only clinical symptom is gradually worsening graft function.

The individual histologic changes are nonspecific, but the constellation of them can be characteristic [48–51]. The two major findings are interstitial fibrosis and arteriolar hyalin change (arteriolopathy). The interstitial fibrosis is characteristically patchy/zonal and is adjacent to areas of unremarkable tubulointerstitium (Figure 16.32). Many investigators use the term "striped interstitial fibrosis" to describe this patchy fibrosis because in the tissue section, it frequently appears as a longitudinal stripe of fibrotic zone. We would like to emphasize that the specificity of this lesion is quite low and striped patchy interstitial fibrosis can occur in a variety of chronic renal conditions.

Arteriolar hyalin change is another frequent and characteristic lesion in calcineurin inhibitor nephrotoxicity. In a typical case, the affected arterioles show peripheral nodular hyalin droplets with or without underlying subendothelial hyalin deposition (Figure 16.33). Subendothelial or circumferential arteriolar hyalin deposition is a common finding in numerous chronic conditions, including hypertension, diabetes, and hyperlipidemia, which are also quite common in the transplant population (Figure 16.34). Therefore, overlap of these patterns of arteriolar hyalin change is not unusual. Although the peripheral nodular hyalin in the arterioles is truly characteristic, this is not a specific lesion either and we have encountered it rarely even in native kidney biopsies. Also, the absence of the peripheral nodular arteriolar hyalin pattern does not mean that the arteriolar hyalin change is not related to calcineurin inhibitor nephrotoxicity. A scoring system for calcineurin inhibitor induced hyalin arteriolopathy was recently inducted [45] (see "Banff Chronic Lesion Scores"). In other instances, cyclosporine nephrotoxicity can cause mucoid subendothelial widening in the small arteries and mucoid, sometimes concentric thickening of the wall of arterioles (Figure 16.35). Since calcineurin inhibitors can cause vasoconstriction and can lead to worsening hypertension, some of these vascular lesions may at least partially be the result of high blood pressure.

Glomerular changes are not conspicuous; however, glomerular sclerosis, occasionally even focal and segmental glomerular sclerosis and hyalinosis, may occur in chronic calcineurin inhibitor nephrotoxicity (Figure 16.36).

Differential diagnosis. As discussed above, striped interstitial fibrosis is a nonspecific finding and, by itself, it does not warrant the diagnosis of cyclosporine nephrotoxicity. We also addressed the differential diagnosis of arteriolar hyalin change (hypertension, diabetes, and hyperlipidemia) at the discussion of chronic rejection. In our opinion, calcineurin inhibitor nephrotoxicity in a renal allograft biopsy specimen cannot be diagnosed with certainty. A diagnosis can only be made after careful correlation of the clinical data and the histologic findings. If the clinical course and the histology indicate that chronic calcineurin nephrotoxicity is the likely cause of the worsening graft function and switching the patient from calcineurin inhibitor to an alternative immunosuppressive treatment (or substantially reducing the calcineurin inhibitor doses) will result in the improvement of the renal function, the diagnosis of calcineurin inhibitor nephrotoxicity is very likely. If the graft function will not improve after adjusting the immunosuppression, the chronic injury was most likely not caused by chronic calcineurin inhibitor nephrotoxicity.

Etiology and pathogenesis. The changes are most likely related to chronic repeated subclinical toxic effects of the calcineurin inhibitor on the tubules, interstitium the vascular smooth muscle cells and the endothelium. It appears that the peripheral nodular hyalin change develops after single smooth muscle necrosis in the media of the small arteries and arterioles. As mentioned above, worsening high blood pressure, diabetes, hyperlipidemia will aggravate the changes.

Clinical course and outcome. The renal function usually improves, at least temporarily, if the calcineurin inhibitor treatment is stopped or the doses are lowered substantially. The long-term outcome depends on the degree of chronic injury at the time of diagnosis.

Calcineurin Inhibitor-Induced Thrombotic Microangiopathy

There is now overwhelming evidence that calcineurin inhibitors can induce TMA [44,52,53]. This form of TMA is not morphologically different from any other form of TMA; therefore, making the diagnosis of calcineurin inhibitor associated TMA can be difficult. This is particularly true because calcineurin inhibitors are used in most transplant centers; therefore, only few patients are not exposed to the effects of these medications.

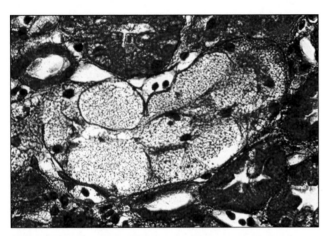

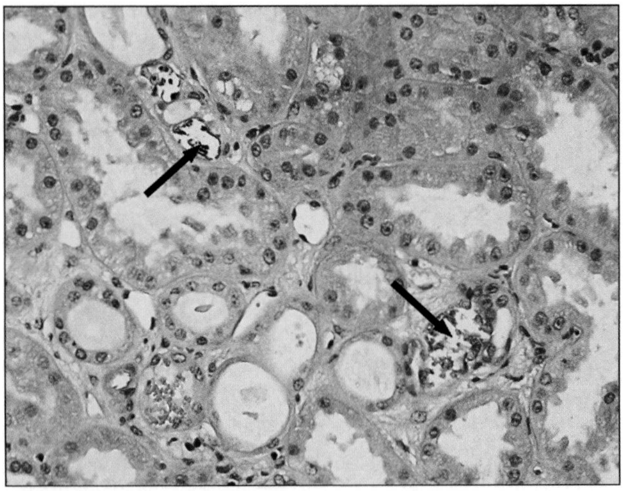

FIGURE 16.30: *Isometric fine vacuolization of the tubular epithelium in acute cyclosporine nephrotoxicity. H&E.*

FIGURE 16.31: *Acute tubular necrosis with tubular microcalcifications (arrows) in a patient treated with cyclosporine. Masson's trichrome.*

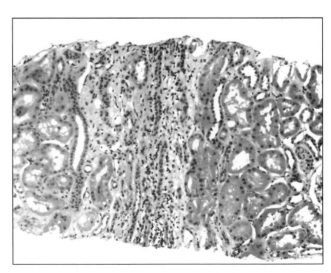

FIGURE 16.32: *Zonal, "striped" interstitial fibrosis in an allograft biopsy with chronic cyclosporine nephrotoxicity. H&E.*

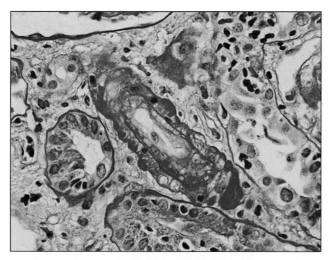

FIGURE 16.33: *Nodular peripheral hyalin deposits in an arteriole in chronic calcineurin inhibitor nephrotoxicity. Note that some subendothelial hyalin is also present. PAS.*

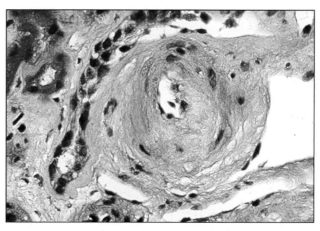

FIGURE 16.35: *Degenerated, thickened arteriolar wall with some mucoid change in a patient with chronic cyclosporine nephrotoxicity. H&E.*

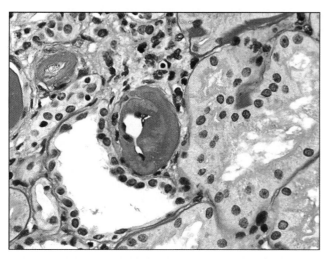

FIGURE 16.34: *Prominent circumferential arteriolar hyalin deposition in an allograft biopsy with presumed chronic calcineurin (cyclosporine) nephrotoxicity. PAS.*

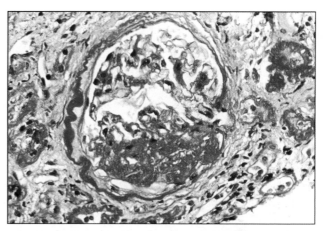

FIGURE 16.36: *A glomerulus with segmental sclerosis in a biopsy from a patient with chronic calcineurin inhibitor nephrotoxicity. PAS.*

In our opinion, we are now biased to make the connection between TMA and calcineurin inhibitor toxicity in most allograft biopsy specimens with evidence of TMA. The histology, as in most forms of TMA, reveals glomerular and/or arteriolar fibrin thrombi (Figure 16.37). The glomeruli, particularly in later stages, also display double contours and capillary thickening, similar to the changes seen in transplant glomerulopathy. Mucoid or concentric arteriolar thickening is also a common finding.

In spite of the above, we agree that, if an allograft biopsy of a patient on calcineurin inhibitor based immunosuppression displays TMA, the possibility that they are related should be raised. However, other etiologies have to be considered as well. If PTC C4d staining is evident, it is very likely that the TMA is

secondary to humoral rejection. If the patient's ESRD was secondary to TMA, a recurrent disease is a possibility. Other immunosuppressive medications, such as Rapamycin (see below) may perhaps also cause TMA.

The exact pathomechanism how calcineurin inhibitors induce TMA in a few transplant patients is unclear. It is most likely multifactorial and is probably only partially related to endothelial injury caused by the drug.

Nephrotoxic Effects of Rapamycin (Rapamune, Sirolimus)

Rapamycin is a macrolid antibiotic isolated from a fungus. It has an inhibitory effect on an intracellular FK binding protein, mammalian target of rapamycin (mTOR) that plays an important role in the regulation of cell proliferation. Therefore, rapamune has an antiproliferative effect and can inhibit the arterial proliferation of smooth muscle cells and intimal thickening.

One recognized form of nephrotoxicity related to rapamycin is ATN with many casts [54]. Most patients who develop this form of ATN are also on calcineurin inhibitors; therefore, some investigators named this condition "combined nephrotoxicity syndrome." We have recently proven that many of the casts in rapamune-induced ATN are myoglobin casts [55] (Figure 16.36). Therefore, it is possible that rapamycin, perhaps in combination with calcineurin inhibitors, may cause rhabdomyolysis and subsequent acute renal failure. Fortunately, if rapamycin is discontinued, the ATN is fully reversible.

Another more recently recognized toxicity of rapamune is heavy proteinuria. In rare patients, nephrotic range proteinuria may occur shortly after transplantation and it abruptly disappears after discontinuation of rapamycin [56]. In other patients, proteinuria will appear after switching them from other immunosuppressive medications (usually from calcineurin inhibitors) to Rapamune [57]. Renal biopsies usually do not reveal any specific glomerular lesions; foot process effacement may or may not be present. Recently rapamycin treatment has been associated with the development of de novo FSGS in renal allografts [58].

Some investigators believe that rapamycin may also induce TMA [59]. In our transplant center, rapamycin based immunosuppression protocol was introduced gradually from 2002 and we have not experienced an increased prevalence of TMA in our transplant patients.

Other Immunosuppressive Medications

TMA has been reported after anti-CD3 monoclonal antibody (OKT3) treatment. IVIG treatment rarely can cause acute tubular injury. Mycophenolate mofetil, and steroids are not associated with nephrotoxicity. There are numerous new immunosuppressive medications under clinical trials. With the introduction of these novel immunosuppressive medications, new pathologies in renal allograft biopsies may emerge.

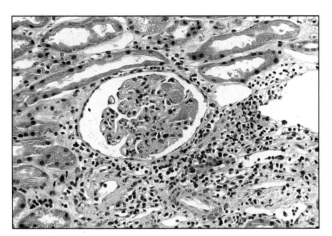

FIGURE 16.37: *Glomerular fibrin thrombi in a patient treated with cyclosporine. H&E.*

Infections of the Renal Allograft

Because transplant recipients are immunosuppressed, infections, including opportunistic infections, are much more common than in the general population. Many times, these infections involve the allograft.

Polyomavirus Infection (Polyomavirus Nephropathy, Polyomavirus Interstitial Nephritis)

Polyomavirus infection started to emerge as a relevant complication of transplantation towards the mid-90's when triple immunosuppressive therapy regimens, including mycophenolate mofetil, calcineurin inhibitors (usually tacrolimus) and steroid, were introduced [60–62]. The prevalence of polyomavirus infection of renal allografts (polyomavirus nephropathy) varies largely between transplant centers, probably depending on the immunosuppressive regimen used. In most transplant centers, the incidence is between 1–5 percent. The disease does not appear early; it usually takes at least a few months for clinical symptoms to develop. However, we have to admit that we do not truly know the natural history of the disease. Many cases are diagnosed years following transplantation.

Histologically, the renal cortex reveals variable degree of inflammatory cell infiltrate, which can be quite zonal. Normal areas of renal cortex may be juxtaposed to prominently inflamed zones (Figure 16.39). The inflammatory zones may contain fibrosis, depending on the stage of the disease. The inflammatory cells frequently abut individual tubules, but can cause tubulitis. The hallmark lesion is the presence of characteristic intranuclear viral inclusions (Figure 16.40). The nuclei are enlarged and contains amphophilic to basophilic smudgy inclusion with a dense basophilic chromatin rim around the periphery of the nucleus. However, these characteristic inclusions are not always present and infected nuclei can have variable morphology including homogenous or finely granular nuclear enlargement, vacuolization and, rarely, cytomegalovirus-like nuclear inclusions with a halo [60]. Sloughed off, necrotic/apoptotic, and infected epithelial cells are commonly seen filling tubular lumina. Zones of inflammation with viral inclusions in epithelial cells are commonly seen in the renal medulla as well. It is quite likely that polyomavirus infection is an ascending infection coming from the urinary tract. An immunoperoxidase stain for polyomavirus is essential for the diagnosis. An immunostain should always be performed if there is suspicion for polyomavirus nephropathy (Figure 16.41).

Immunofluorescence using the routine renal biopsy panel is somewhat useful in the diagnosis of polyomavirus nephropathy, because in several cases, small granular IgG deposits are present along the tubular basement membranes and occasionally along the glomerular capillary basement membrane [63] (Figure 16.42A). C4d staining reveals similar granular tubular basement membrane fluorescence (Figure 16.42B). Electron microscopy can be helpful if infected cells are present in the examined area. The viral particles may be arranged in a paracrystalline pattern within the nucleus (Figure 16.43A). Electron microscopy can also confirm the presence of electron dense deposits along the tubular basement membrane (Figure 16.43A).

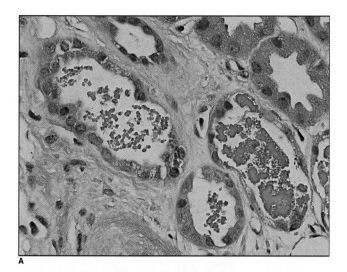

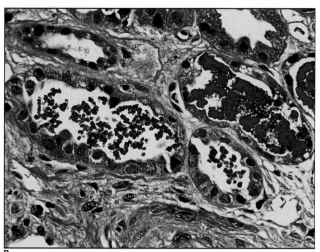

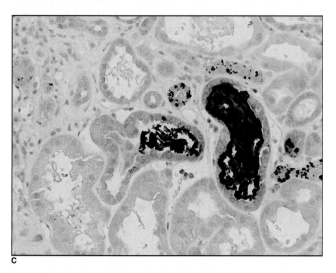

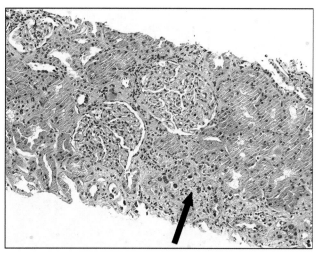

FIGURE 16.39: *Only a small portion of this renal biopsy specimen is involved by polyomavirus interstitial nephritis (arrow). H&E.*

FIGURE 16.38: *Myoglobin containing casts in a biopsy from a patient treated with sirolimus and cyclosporine. A: Note the globular bright eosinophilic casts, H&E. B: The globular cast material is brightly fuchsinophilic (red) on Masson's trichrome stain. C: An immunostain for myoglobin is strongly positive in the cast material.*

Urine cytology is a very useful tool for screening patients because, a negative urine cytology in a good sample practically excludes the possibility of polyoma virus nephropathy [60–62]. On the other hand, up to 50 percent of patients after renal transplantation may have decoy cells in the urine sediment in the absence of renal involvement (Figure16.44). Therefore, the recommended practice is to submit a blood sample for polyomavirus PCR if the urine cytology is positive [64]. If the blood sample is negative, polyomavirus infection is unlikely but cannot be excluded. If the blood sample is positive, a renal biopsy should be performed, even if the graft function is normal. If polyomavirus interstitial nephritis develops, the virus almost always can be detected in the peripheral blood by PCR. However, we have to emphasize that PCR positivity in the peripheral blood not necessarily equals polyomavirus interstitial nephritis and a negative PCR does not exclude it with absolute certainty. We recently encountered a patient with typical histologic findings in the graft biopsy, but negative polyoma virus PCR in the peripheral blood.

Differential diagnosis

The most important differential diagnostic dilemma is acute rejection. Although in most biopsies this is not a problem, occasionally acute rejection, and polyomavirus, nephropathy can coexist. As pointed out above, the inflammatory cell infiltrate in polyomavirus virus nephropathy is frequently zonal. If the inflammatory cell infiltrate appears to be diffuse with widespread tubulitis in tubules without viral inclusions, and in particular, if intimal arteritis is present, it is likely that the patient also has coexistent acute rejection. On the other hand, in acute rejection, regenerative tubular epithelial changes are common and regenerative nuclei can be large, vacuolated and sometimes resemble polyoma virus inclusions. Again, immunostain for polyomavirus is extremely helpful in making the correct diagnosis. In polyomavirus infection without rejection, PTC C4d

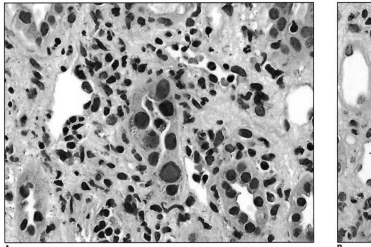
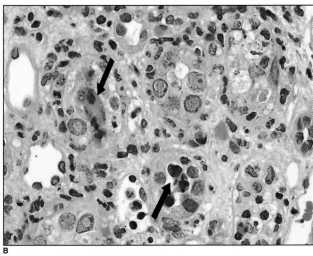
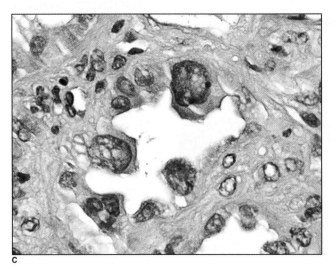

FIGURE 16.40: *Nuclear inclusions in polyomavirus infection. A: Enlarged dense basophilic smudgy nuclear inclusions in tubular epithelial cells. H&E. B: Finely granular amphophilic to basophilic intranuclear inclusions with a basophilic peripheral chromatin ring. Also note the mixed inflammatory cell infiltrate abutting the tubular basement membrane. Polymorphonuclears are also present. The tubular lumina frequently contain sloughed off necrotic end-stage infected cells (arrows). H&E. C: Large vesicular nuclei in tubular epithelial cells of a kidney with severe polyomavirus infection. H&E.*

staining is absent. If PTC C4d staining coexists with polyoma-virus infection, a concomitant humoral rejection process is likely.

Pyelonephritis could also be a differential diagnostic prob-lem. In polyomavirus nephropathy, polymorphonuclears are common in the interstitium and they may also be present within the tubules. Again, the characteristic viral inclusions and a positive immunostain for polyomavirus are helpful in the differ-ential diagnosis. If a biopsy specimen is small and the immu-nostain for polyomavirus is negative, the possibility of sampling error should be considered if the urine cytology reveals decoy cells and inflammatory cells.

Other conditions causing interstitial inflammation, such as rare other viral infection (cytomegalovirus, adenovirus) or drug-induced interstitial nephritides can be differentiated

using immunostains and detecting the characteristic viral inclusion.

Etiology and pathogenesis

As mentioned above, it appears that the disease is clearly related to the immunosuppressive regimen used; however, the infection cannot be safely avoided by any known immuno-suppressive regimen. The infection usually starts in the uri-nary tract, and urine cytology can be very helpful in detecting the infected cells (decoy cells) in the urine sediment (Figure 16.44). The distribution of polyoma virus infected cells in renal allografts also suggests an ascending infection [65]. How exactly the virus spreads to the kidney and why certain patients with positive urine cytology become severely affected and others not, is unclear. It appears that polyomavirus nephropathy is not closely associated with urinary reflux in the renal allograft.

Clinical course and outcome

Unfortunately, polyomavirus nephropathy is usually a progressive disease and resolution is rare. Treatment includes reduced immunosuppression, which in turn, can result in acute rejection. Certain medications, such as Cidofovir or leflunomide have some effect against polyomavirus, but in many patients, they are only capable of delaying the disease progression.

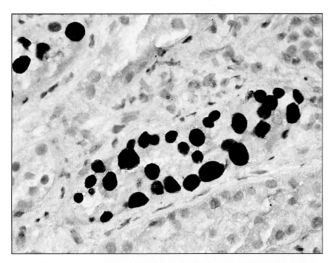

FIGURE 16.41: *An immunostain for polyomavirus is strongly positive in the infected nuclei. The immunostain is particularly helpful in milder and focal cases of polyomavirus nephropathy where typical intranuclear inclusions may not be always evident.*

Cytomegalovirus (CMV) Infection

CMV infection is one of the most common infections in renal allograft recipients, particularly in patients who were CMV negative before transplantation and received a CMV positive graft. However, the prevalence of the disease decreased after preventive treatment with Ganciclovir and its derivatives. Although systemic infection, manifested in fever, pneumonitis, and hepatitis is a life threatening condition, involvement of the renal allograft with productive CMV infection became extremely rare [66]. We have seen only two allograft biopsy specimens in the last four years with cytomegalovirus inclusions among approximately 1,500 renal allograft biopsy specimens. The most frequently infected cell in the renal allograft is the tubular epithelial cell. The affected tubules contain typical Cowdry-A type intranuclear inclusions with a clear halo around the periphery of the enlarged nucleus (Figure 16.45). The nuclear inclusions are so characteristic that the diagnosis can be made even without immunohistochemical stains. However, the infected cells with typical nuclear inclusions can be quite focal. Therefore, in any suspicious case, immunohistochemical stains or in situ hybridization for CMV is recommended (Figure 16.46). Certain tubules may contain numerous infected cells with typical intranuclear inclusions in the absence of any pathologic changes in the neighboring nephrons. Sometimes inflammatory cell infiltrate is associated with these inclusion bodies, but not necessarily. Occasionally even glomerular epithelial cells or endothelial cells can be infected by CMV. It is still a matter of debate whether active cytomegalovirus infection in the renal allograft can induce acute rejection [67]. With antiviral medications, the condition is reversible, but, occasionally, it can be fatal.

Adenovirus Infection

Adenovirus infection of the renal allograft is very rare, but it can cause graft failure. The characteristic histologic finding

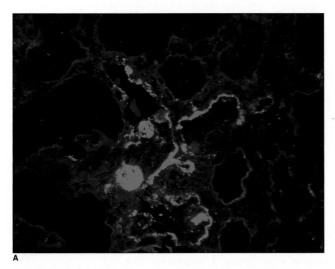
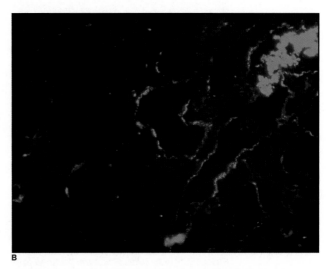

A   B

FIGURE 16.42: *Immunofluorescence finding in polyomavirus nephropathy. A: Focal granular tubular basement membrane staining for IgG. B: Focal granular staining for C4d along the tubular basement membrane corresponding to the IgG containing immune complex deposits.*

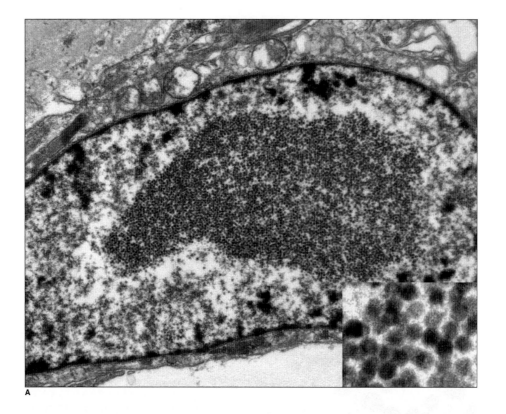

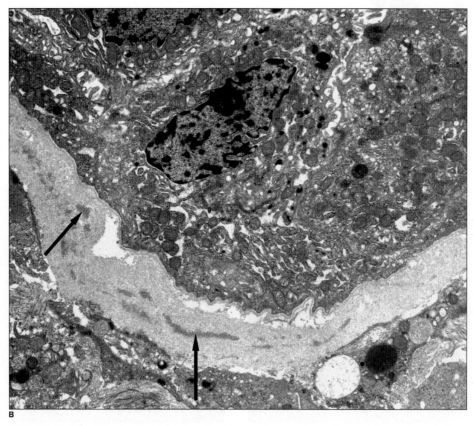

FIGURE 16.43: *Ultrastructural findings in polyomavirus nephropathy. A: Intranuclear viral particles in renal epithelial cells. The insert in the right lower corner shows the viral particles under higher magnification. Uranyl acetate, lead citrate. B: Electron dense deposits (arrows) along the tubular basement membrane. Uranyl acetate, lead citrate.*

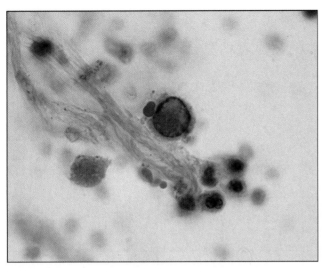

FIGURE 16.44: *A characteristic decoy cell in the urine sediment from a patient with polyomavirus nephropathy. Also, note the surrounding polymorphonuclears. Papanicolaou stain. (Courtesy of Dr. Paul Wakely).*

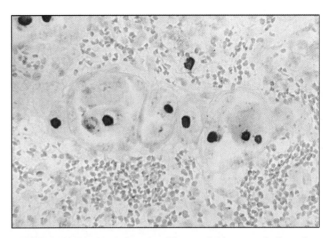

FIGURE 16.46: *Numerous positive nuclei in a renal allograft biopsy stained with an antibody to cytomegalovirus using immunoperoxidase methodology. Not all positive cells have typical intranuclear inclusions.*

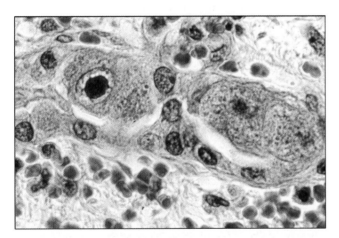

FIGURE 16.45: *Typical cytomegalovirus inclusions in enlarged tubular epithelial cells. Note the dense intranuclear inclusions with the clear halo around it. Basophilic dots, representing viral particles, are present in the cytoplasm of the enlarged infected cells. H&E.*

Epstein Barr Virus Infection and Post-Transplant Lymphoproliferative Disorder

EBV infection of allograft recipients may cause posttransplant lymphoproliferative disorder (PTLD), which may involve the renal allograft. Primary EBV infection of the recipient is a risk factor, but PTLD can also develop after reactivation of the EBV infection. PTLD became a serious clinical problem after the introduction of more aggressive immunosuppressive regimens including antilymphocyte antibodies, such as thyomoglobulin and OKT3. In recent years with preventive antiviral measures, the incidence of PTLD declined slightly and it involves approximately 1.4 percent of the renal transplant population in the US [70]. PTLD in most instances is a B cell lymphoproliferative disorder, which can be polyclonal or monoclonal, polymorphous or monomorphous. Most PTLDs are related to EBV infection, but occasionally, the EBV genome cannot be detected [71].

In approximately 30 percent of renal allograft recipients with PTLD, the disease involves the transplant kidney. In such cases, the renal allograft biopsy can provide the diagnosis. The appearance of the infiltrate in the kidney is usually that of a lymphoma with bulky lymphoid masses, pushing tubules apart without prominent tubulitis. The infiltrate can be monomorphic (these tend to behave as truly malignant lymphomas) or polymorphic with large lymphocytes and many plasmacytoid cells [72] (Figure 16.49). There are an unusually large number of B cells compared to acute cellular rejection. Particularly in the polymorphous form, the B cell infiltrate may not be monoclonal. In situ hybridization for EBV using the EBER probe is crucial in making the correct diagnosis (Figure 16.50). Immunophenotyping of the infiltrate is also helpful; most of the cells display B cell markers (e.g., CD20) (Figure 16.51).

Differentiating PTLD from acute rejection may occasionally be difficult [72]. Also, one has to keep in mind that PTLD and acute rejection may occasionally be present at the same time (Figure 16.51). As mentioned above, the bulky lymphoma like infiltrate with relatively mild tubulitis, the presence of atypical cells, many plasmacytoid lymphocytes should warn the

is severe necrotizing interstitial nephritis [68,69]. In fact, the tubular necrosis can be so prominent that it may resemble cortical necrosis (Figure 16.47A). Typically, many tubular epithelial cell nuclei have large smudgy intranuclear inclusions (Figure 16.47B). The intensity of interstitial inflammatory cell infiltrate is relatively mild. An immunostain for adenovirus is helpful to make the definitive diagnosis (Figure 16.48). The disease usually presents with high fever, malaise and generalized symptoms, followed by progressive graft dysfunction. In spite of the dramatic histologic changes in the renal biopsy, the condition can be reversible.

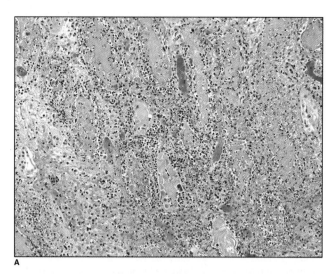

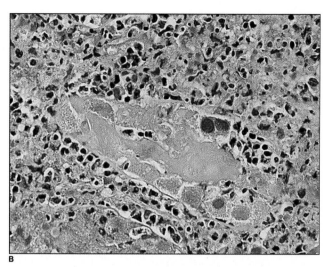

A   B

FIGURE 16.47: *Severe adenovirus interstitial nephritis in a renal allograft. A: Low magnification reveals widespread tubular necrosis and interstitial inflammation. The tubular necrosis is so prominent that cortical necrosis may emerge in the differential diagnosis. H&E. B: Higher magnification of a necrotic tubule reveals that some tubular epithelial nuclei are quite enlarged and smudgy. H&E.*

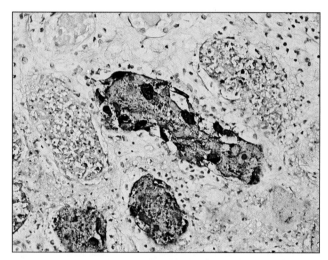

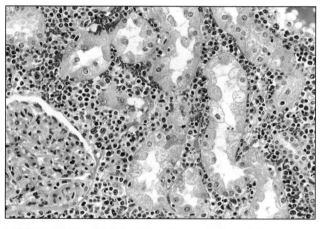

FIGURE 16.49: *PTLD involving the renal allograft. Note the bulky somewhat polymorphous appearing interstitial cellular infiltrate with occasional blast-like cells and several plasmacytoid cells. Tubulitis is very focal and mild. H&E.*

FIGURE 16.48: *An immunoperoxidase stain with an antibody to adenovirus reveals specific positive staining in the infected nuclei and in the cytoplasm.*

pathologist of the possibility of PTLD. In every suspicious case, EBV in situ hybridization and immunostains should be performed.

Reduced immunosuppression maybe sufficient to cause regression of PTLDs, particularly in the polymorphonuclear form. Monomorphic PTLDs can become quite aggressive and may have a poor outcome.

Bacterial and Fungal Infections (Pyelonephritis)

Acute pyelonephritis is not a rare complication of renal transplantation, but its recognition can be difficult both clinically and morphologically. We have seen several cases where urine cultures were repeatedly negative, in spite of the characteristic histologic findings. On the other hand, because of the focal nature of the lesion within the allograft, the biopsy needle may miss the diagnostic areas.

Transplant pyelonephritis is not different morphologically from pyelonephritis in the native kidney. The characteristic lesion is the presence of large numbers of polymorphonuclear leukocytes in the tubular lumina with destruction of the surrounding tubules and microabscess formation (Figures 16.52 and 16.53). Neutrophilic tubulitis is common and polymorphonuclears are also present in the interstitium [73]. In addition, polymorphonuclear leukocytes are frequently seen accumulating in the peritubular capillaries as well (Figure 16.54). Bacterial stains rarely will detect the pathogenetic bacteria in tissue

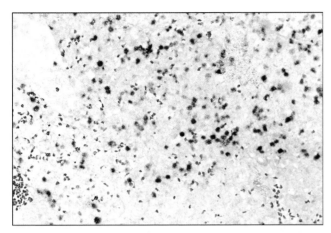

FIGURE 16.50: In situ hybridization using an EBER probe to detect EBV in PTLD. Note the large number of dark blue positive nuclei. ×200.

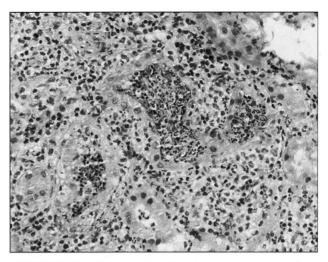

FIGURE 16.52: Polymorphonuclear leukocytes accumulating in the lumen of tubules with microabscess formation in a case of acute allograft pyelonephritis. H&E.

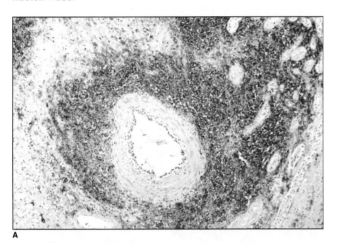

A

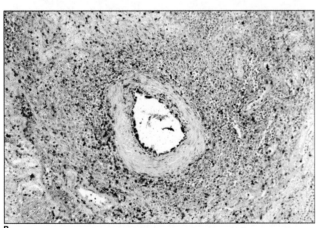

B

FIGURE 16.51: Graft infiltrating cells in PTLD. A: Most of the infiltrating cells in the perivascular interstitium and between the tubules are CD20 positive B cells. Note that there is intimal arteritis in the artery with CD20 negative inflammatory cells. Immunoperoxidase with an antibody to CD20. B: The same area stained with an antibody to CD3. Note that most of the inflammatory cells causing the intimal arteritis are CD3 positive T cells. This indicates a concomitant acute rejection process. There are relatively few CD3 positive T cells in the perivascular and peritubular interstitium.

sections. If transplant pyelonephritis becomes chronic, it may rarely turn into xanthogranulomatous pyelonephritis or malakoplakia. Occasionally, pyelonephritis can be caused by fungi. We routinely stain every renal biopsy with PAS, which is also a good fungal stain. One has to keep in mind that occasionally fungal infections, in particular cryptococcal infections, may not induce an inflammatory cell reaction (Figure 16.55). In many instances, fungal infection of the allograft is part of fungal sepsis.

As mentioned in the "differential diagnosis of chronic rejection," chronic pyelonephritis/reflux nephropathy may also involve the transplant kidney. This diagnosis cannot be made based on the renal biopsy findings alone and careful imaging studies of the allograft as well as studies for reflux are recommended.

The differential diagnosis of acute pyelonephritis involves acute rejection, including acute cellular and acute humoral rejection as well as acute tubular necrosis. In pyelonephritis, the inflammatory cell foci are usually patchy and zonal, adjacent to normal appearing renal parenchyma. This is uncommon in acute cellular rejection. Also, the large number of polymorphonuclear leukocytes, particularly if they are present in tubular lumina and within the tubular epithelium gives a helpful hint to make the diagnosis of pyelonephritis. If the biopsy needle does not hit an area with microabscess formation, the findings can resemble acute cellular rejection or acute humoral rejection with margination of polymorphonuclear leukocytes in the PTC. The absence of PTC C4d staining in such cases is important to exclude the possibility of underlying antibody-mediated rejection process. In severe acute tubular necrosis, and in any condition that is associated with severe acute tubular injury, (including acute rejection) apoptotic cell debris may be present in the tubular lumina. Such apoptotic cell debris may resemble polymorphonuclear leukocytes (Figure 16.57) and the erroneous diagnosis of pyelonephritis can be made.

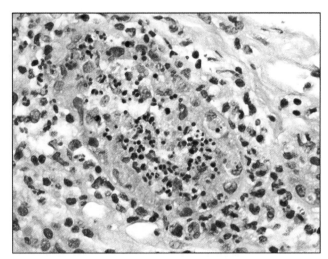

FIGURE 16.53: Large numbers of polymorphonuclear leukocytes filling the tubular lumen and infiltrating the tubular epithelium. Also note the interstitial edema and inflammation with several polymorphonuclears. This histology is highly characteristic of acute infection (pyelonephritis). Few polymorphonuclears in tubular lumina are not diagnostic of acute pyelonephritis and can be seen in acute rejection, in any condition causing renal inflammation, including glomerulonephritis, in ATN and in areas adjacent to infarcted zones. H&E.

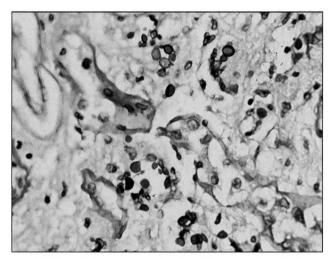

FIGURE 16.55: Cryptococcal infection of a renal allograft. Note the absence of surrounding inflammatory cell reaction. PAS.

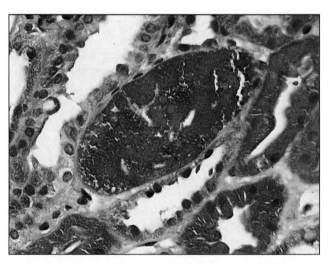

FIGURE 16.56: Prominent tubular protein resorption droplets in a proximal tubule from a patient with early recurrent focal segmental glomerular sclerosis. The glomeruli were normal in this biopsy specimen. Masson's trichrome.

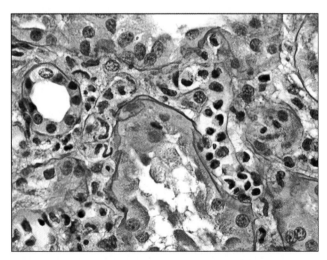

FIGURE 16.54: Peritubular capillary polymorphonuclear leukocytes in a case of acute pyelonephritis. The C4d stain was negative. H&E.

Recurrent Disease in Renal Allografts

A recurrent disease can be diagnosed only if the original disease in the native kidney is known. Both primary glomerular and systemic diseases may recur in renal transplant with variable frequency [76–78]. The morphology of the recurrent disease is not different from the native kidney disease, except that the changes may frequently be combined with features of acute or chronic rejection or other changes influencing allograft pathol-

ogy. Because of space limitation, only the most important or interesting recurrent diseases are discussed below, briefly.

Idiopathic Focal Segmental Glomerulosclerosis

The overall recurrence rate of focal segmental glomerular sclerosis (FSGS) is approximately 30 percent [79]. It appears that patients who have circulating permeability factor(s) are prone to recurrent disease and in such patients, the recurrence may occur within minutes in the form of heavy nephrotic range proteinuria. In spite of the frequently rapid recurrence, the characteristic changes of FSGS will not develop until approximately 4–6 weeks posttransplant, at the earliest. Proximal tubular epithelial cells frequently contain numerous protein resorption droplets (Figure 16.56).

Electron microscopy reveals diffuse foot process effacement, even in early stages, when the glomeruli are normal. One has to keep in mind that in rare instances, early heavy post-transplant proteinuria can be transient as occasionally reported with the use of sirolimus.

Membranous Glomerulopathy

Recurrent membranous glomerulonephritis may be a difficult diagnosis because membranous glomerulonephritis is the most common de novo glomerulonephritis in renal transplants. However, recurrent disease usually develops within the first few months following transplantation whereas de novo membranous glomerulonephritis usually appears after the first year (usually after many years).

Membranoproliferative Glomerulonephritis (MPGN) Type I

The recurrence rate is estimated to be around 30 percent but, as mentioned, at the differential diagnosis of transplant glomerulopathy, the diagnosis of membranoproliferative glomerulonephritis (MPGN) type I in renal allografts is not always straightforward. MPGN type I is becoming a rare disease and in the everyday practice, we rarely encounter recurrent MPGN type I. The detection of subendothelial discrete electron dense immune type deposits by electron microscopy and low complement levels are relevant to make the definitive diagnosis. Recurrent MPGN may be difficult to differentiate from transplant glomerulopathy.

MPGN Type II (Dense Deposit Disease)

Dense deposit disease (DDD) recurs in almost all allografts. The recurrence can be very rapid; however, the recurrent disease usually shows a slow progression and can be compatible with good graft function for several years.

IgA Nephropathy

The recurrence rate of IgA nephropathy is estimated to be around 50 percent. Early graft loss, because of recurrent IgA nephropathy is rare; however, after the first five years, recurrent IgA nephropathy can cause progressive graft failure.

Thrombotic Microangiopathy

Acquired *E. coli* infection-related hemolytic uremic syndrome does not recur in renal allografts. However, other forms, may recur, particularly the more and more recognized familial forms of thrombotic microangiopathy (TMA). Autoimmune disease related TMA also commonly recurs. The recurrence occurs frequently after the first couple of months following transplantation and in most cases, it is associated with progressive graft failure. The diagnosis can be difficult and it can be impossible to differentiate recurrent TMA from a de novo TMA. Knowledge of the native kidney disease leading to ESRD

is imperative for making the diagnosis of recurrent TMA. Unfortunately, in our experience, several patients with probable TMA in the native kidney carry the diagnosis of hypertensive nephrosclerosis.

Diabetic Nephropathy (Diabetic Glomerulosclerosis)

As renal allografts survive longer, recurrent diabetic nephropathy becomes more of a problem. Clinically relevant, recurrent diabetic glomerulosclerosis usually does not develop within the first five years following transplantation, but may cause progressive graft dysfunction and proteinuria after ten years. Optimal glucose control and metabolic control, blood pressure control and steroid free immunosuppressive regimens may prevent the recurrence of diabetic nephropathy.

Antineutrophil Cytoplasmic Antibody Associated Pauci-immune Crescentic and Necrotizing Glomerulonephritis

In one large study, the recurrence rate was estimated to be 17 percent [80]. The findings are histologically identical to those seen in the native kidney and recurrence can occur any time following transplantation.

Systemic Lupus Erythematosus (Lupus Nephritis)

Interestingly, lupus nephritis in a clinically relevant form recurs very rarely, in approximately 1–2 percent of allograft recipients. Although few mesangial immune complex deposits are not unusual in renal allografts of patients with systemic lupus erythematosus, these rarely cause progressive graft dysfunction or glomerulonephritis [81]. The reason for the rare recurrence of lupus nephritis, which is thought to be the prototype of immune complex glomerulonephritis secondary to the glomerular deposition of circulating immune complexes, is unclear but it may be secondary to the continuous immunosuppression from the beginning, or to the "burning out" of the lupus nephritis and probably to other factors.

Other Recurrent Diseases

A number of other renal glomerular tubulointerstitial and metabolic diseases may recur in allografts, including fibrillary glomerulonephritis, amyloidosis, monoclonal immunoglobulin deposition disease, antiglomerular basement membrane disease, primary or secondary oxalosis, cryoglobulinemia and rare other metabolic diseases, such as Fabry's disease.

De Novo Diseases in Renal Allografts

There is a wide array of diseases that may appear in a renal allograft de novo. This includes renal effects of systemic conditions, such as poor perfusion of the graft, hypertension, post-transplant diabetes, drug toxicities, and metabolic disorders that can all develop following transplantation. Rarely glomerular diseases can also occur de novo.

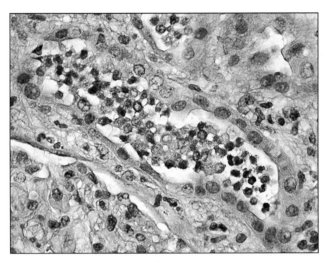

FIGURE 16.57: *Necrotic/apoptotic cells in the lumen of a tubule in a case of ATN. Such apoptotic/ necrotic cells should not be misinterpreted as polymorphonuclears. H&E.*

Acute Tubular Necrosis

ATN frequently occurs in renal allograft biopsies and is the most common finding in biopsies taken for delayed graft function. ATN is particularly common early post-transplant in deceased donor kidneys. Treatment with calcineurin inhibitors and Sirolimus may predispose some patients for the development of ATN (see appropriate sections in this chapter). The morphology of ATN in renal allografts is not substantially different from ATN in the native kidneys. Accumulation of necrotic/apoptotic cells in the tubular lumina is a common finding in ATN. One caveat is not to misinterpret these apoptotic cells as polymorphonuclears, which can lead to the erroneous diagnosis of acute pyelonephritis (Figure 16.57). ATN in renal allografts is most commonly secondary to poor graft perfusion (following ischemia reperfusion injury, tubular injury developing prior to death in a deceased donor kidney, preservation injury, technical issues during the transplant surgery, cardiac insufficiency in the recipient, etc.). However, several drugs, including calcineurin inhibitors and rapamycine (see earlier sections in this chapter) can cause tubular injury and ATN or can aggravate the preexisting tubular injury. One has to keep in mind that ATN in the allograft may commonly be associated with other pathologies, including acute rejection.

De Novo Membranous Glomerulopathy

De novo membranous glomerulonephritis is the most frequent de novo immune complex glomerulonephritis in renal transplants (Figure 16.58). Its prevalence shows a wide range between transplant centers up to 0.5 to 9 percent [82]. It usually appears after the first year of transplantation, is commonly associated with changes of chronic rejection, and occasionally with changes of transplant glomerulopathy. Interestingly, heavy proteinuria is not always evident in de novo membranous glomerulonephritis; some patients have very mild, or no proteinuria. Only approximately one-third of patients with de novo membranous glomerulonephritis have nephrotic range proteinuria.

De Novo Collapsing Glomerulopathy

Collapsing glomerulopathy is considered to be an aggressive variant of FSGS and is discussed in more detail in the appropriate chapter. Collapsing glomerulopathy can be idiopathic or secondary to HIV infection, pamidronate and perhaps to parvovirus B 19 infection. Recurrent collapsing glomerulopathy, although reported in renal allografts, is rare. In contrast, glomeruli with the characteristic changes of collapsing glomerulopathy, namely collapsing glomerular capillaries with large overlying podocytes filling the Bowman's capsule, are not unusual in a renal biopsy specimen [83,84] (Figure 16.59). Collapsing glomerular lesions, as most other glomerular lesions, merely represent a pattern of glomerular injury that can be secondary to a variety of etiologic agents. De novo collapsing glomerulopathy in renal allografts can be zonal in distribution [84]. It may be secondary to obliterative vascular changes and subsequent hemodynamic disturbances. Parvovirus B 19 infection or polyomavirus (SV 40) infection of the graft was implicated in the pathogenesis, but these are debated [85]. Some patients may develop heavy proteinuria; others have only non nephrotic or minimal proteinuria. Although, the clinical course of de novo collapsing glomerulopathy in renal allografts is different from that in native kidneys, it still represents a renal lesion indicating unfavorable graft outcome.

De Novo Focal Segmental Glomerulosclerosis

In contrast to recurrent FSGS, de novo FSGS usually develops years after transplantation. Many times, it is related to progressive nephron loss and is secondary to glomerular hyperperfusion/hyperfiltration injury (ablative nephropathy) (Figure 16.60). Recently de novo FSGS was described following rapamycin treatment [58].

Antiglomerular Basement Membrane Disease in Patients with Alport Syndrome

This is a very rare condition, but because of its interesting pathogenesis, it is worth mentioning. Patients with Alport syndrome may develop antibodies against the NC-1 globular domain of the alpha-3 subunit of type IV collagen, which is present in the normal donor kidney, but is absent in the recipient. However, one has to note that this type of antiglomerular basement membrane disease is very rare and affects approximately 2–5 percent of transplanted patients with Alport syndrome [86]. This is most likely related to the variable mutations in the gene responsible for Alport syndrome.

Other De Novo Diseases

As mentioned above, most renal conditions can develop in the renal allografts. Many of them were already addressed in this

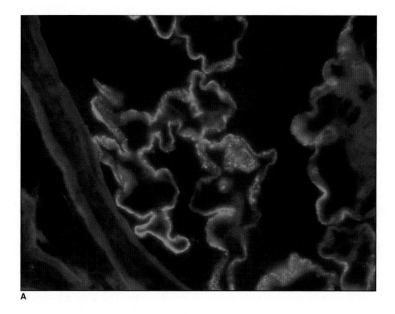

A

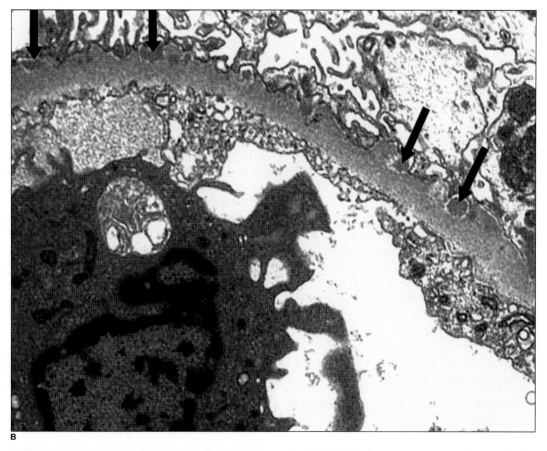

B

FIGURE 16.58: *A case of de novo membranous glomerulonephritis diagnosed four years post transplant. A: Finely granular diffuse peripheral glomerular capillary fluorescence for IgG. B: Small subepithelial electron dense deposits (arrows) on electron microscopy. Uranyl acetate, lead citrate. De novo membranous glomerulonephritis is less commonly associated with large subepithelial deposits and prominent spike formation, than recurrent membranous glomerulonephritis or membranous glomerulonephritis in native kidneys.*

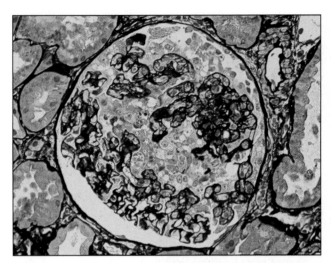

FIGURE 16.59: *A glomerulus with collapsed capillary loops and large podocytes filling the Bowman's space. Collapsing glomerulopathy in renal allografts is usually de novo and can be zonal in distribution. Jones methenamine silver.*

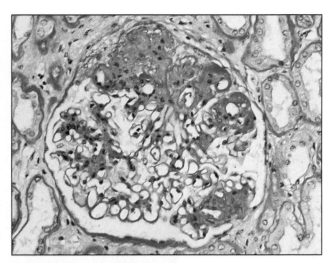

FIGURE 16.60: *A large glomerulus with segmental sclerosis and hyalinosis in a patient with advanced chronic allograft nephropathy. The large glomeruli and the segmental hyalin change indicate glomerular hyperperfusion/hyperfiltration injury. PAS.*

text, such as acute and chronic infections, hypertension, drug toxicities, metabolic disorders, etc.

Donor-Transmitted Renal Disease in the Allograft

Donor-transmitted renal disease may occur, particularly if a deceased renal allograft is transplanted. The most common transplanted condition is hypertensive nephrosclerosis and the outcome of it depends on the severity of the condition. We have seen examples where diabetic nephropathy was transplanted because the diagnosis was not made in the donor. Usually, such kidneys do not survive for very long; however, there are occasional reports describing the regression of diabetic changes in transplant recipients with a normal glucose metabolism [87].

IgA nephropathy is the most common transplanted immune complex glomerulonephritis because it can be subclinical in many patients. Interestingly, the IgA deposits almost invariably disappear within a few months following transplantation and they do not interfere with graft outcome.

Baseline Biopsy

The baseline biopsy is a very important tool to detect renal disease coming from the donor. There is a debate how reliable individual histopathologic changes in a baseline biopsy are to predict graft outcome. Unfortunately, many times the baseline biopsies are quite superficial, subcapsular wedge biopsies with no arteries present. Subcapsular scarring with numerous obsolescent glomeruli is not uncommon in such specimens and may give an erroneous impression of severe chronic injury in the entire renal cortex. This should be taken into consideration when evaluating a donor biopsy. Sometimes we encounter tubular epithelial cells in the glomerular capillary loops in baseline

wedge biopsies (Figure 16.61). These "tubular epithelial cell emboli" represent an artifact, which is not uncommon in wedge baseline biopsies, but is rare in needle biopsies taken later from the allograft. This peculiar artifact should not to be misinterpreted as fibrin thrombi. The differentiation is usually easy because they stain similarly to surrounding proximal tubular epithelial cells and are negative with fibrin stains. There is no consensus yet when a donor kidney should be discarded based on histologic changes. This is particularly difficult because the decision has to be made usually based on examination of frozen sections. A nephrosclerotic kidney can function adequately for many years and provide a good quality of life for a person who otherwise would not receive a living related donor kidney. In our experience, the donor kidney biopsy has limited informative value regarding graft outcome, unless the chronic injury is quite prominent and the vascular changes are striking. The decision is best made together with the transplant surgeons and by taking the gross appearance of the kidney and the perfusion pressure parameters into consideration.

CONCLUSION

The evaluation of renal transplant biopsies is a challenging task for the pathologist. The diagnosis should be made as soon as possible because of the urgent therapeutic considerations. False diagnosis can lead to inappropriate treatment, including too much or to too little immunosuppression and unwanted subsequent complications (e.g. infection or rejection). The optimal scenario for both the pathologist and the transplant team is to evaluate the biopsy specimens together in a form of a clinical pathology conference. Optimal evaluation of the renal transplant biopsy can be of immense help in the management of renal transplant patients.

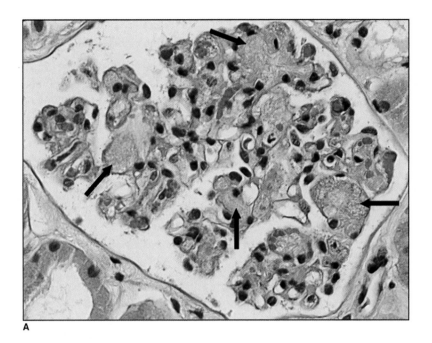

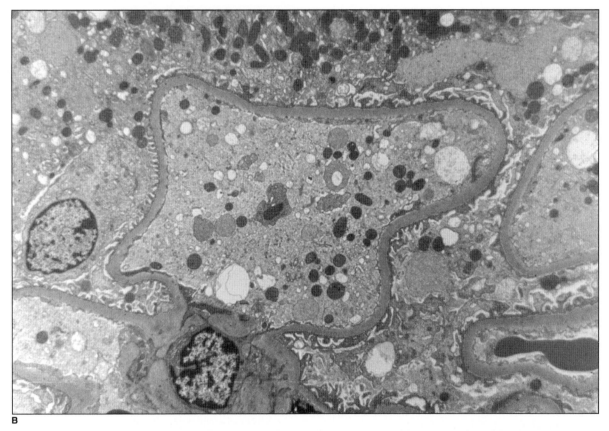

FIGURE 16.61: *Tubular epithelial cell emboli in glomerular capillaries. A: On H&E stain these tubular epithelial cell emboli (arrows) superficially resemble fibrin thrombi, but they have granular staining pattern similar to that of proximal tubules. H&E. On electron microscopy it is evident that the material in the glomerular capillary represents cytoplasm with lysosomes and mitochondria similar in appearance to the cytoplasm of renal tubular epithelial cells. Uranyl acetate, lead citrate.*

APPENDIX

Major Patterns of Injury Seen in Renal Allograft Biopsies

INTERSTITIAL INFLAMMATION IN THE ALLOGRAFT

Mononuclear Cells in Perivascular or Scarred Areas or in the Subcapsular Zone Only

– usually nonspecific

Inflammation between Tubules

1. Mononuclear cells with or without other inflammatory cells causing tubulitis.
   – Acute cellular rejection
   – Interstitial nephritis of other etiologies (less likely)

2. Many plasma cells admixed with other inflammatory cells
   – Late acute rejection
   – Consider PTLD (EBV stains positive, less tubulitis)

3. Many interstitial neutrophils and neutrophils in PTC
   – Acute rejection (could be humoral, C4d positive)
   – Pyelonephritis
   – Polyomavirus nephropathy
   – Adjacent infarcted area

4. Many neutrophils in the interstitium and tubules
   – Pyelonephritis
   – Consider polyomavirus nephropathy
   – Adjacent infarct
   – Severe acute rejection

5. Mixed inflammation with many eosinophils
   – Acute rejection
   – Hypersensitivity interstitial nephritis (drugs)

6. Bulky, monomorphic interstitial mononuclear cell infiltrate with disproportionately mild tubulitis
   – PTLD/lymphoma

7. Interstitial inflammatory cell infiltrate with disproportionately severe tubular necrosis
   – Adenovirus infection
   – Cortical necrosis (severe TMA– could be secondary to humoral rejection)

8. Inflammatory cell infiltrate with interstitial hemorrhage
   – Severe acute rejection (vascular and/or humoral)

   – Area adjacent to infarct
   – Rare viral infectious (Adenovirus, Hantavirus– unlikely).

9. Interstitial granulomas
   – Consider granulomatous interstitial nephritis not related to rejection (drugs, infection, etc.)

10. Many interstitial foam cells with a mixed inflammatory cell infiltrate
    – Xanthogranulomatous pyelonephritis
    – Exclude mycobacterial or fungal infections

11. Large macrophages with abundant PAS positive granular cytoplasm and PAS positive targetoid cytoplasmic inclusions.
    – Malakoplakia

INTERSTITIAL FIBROSIS IN THE ALLOGRAFT

1. Chronic rejection
   – Usually diffuse fibrosis with some inflammatory cell infiltrate
   – Commonly associated with transplant glomerulopathy and obliterative transplant arteriopathy
   – PTC C4d staining commonly present

2. Chronic calcineurin inhibitor nephrotoxicity
   – Frequently zonal (striped interstitial fibrosis)
   – Arteriolar hyalin is usually present; it may have a peripheral nodular pattern

3. Chronic pyelonephritis/reflux nephropathy
   – Usually patchy fibrosis
   – Mononuclear cell infiltrate is usually present but is localized to the fibrotic zones
   – PMNs may be found in rare tubules
   – Imaging studies usually reveal hydronephrosis and/or caliceal deformities

4. Hypertensive nephrosclerosis
   – Arteriolar hyalin and/or concentric or mucoid arteriolar / small arterial thickening
   – Intimal fibroelastosis in arteries
   – Usually patchy fibrosis

5. Advanced stage polyomavirus infection
   – Characteristic viral inclusions in tubular epithelial cells (immunostain helpful)
   – Some inflammation usually evident
   – Granular tubular basement membrane IgG deposits may be present on immunofluorescence
   – Can be zonal in distribution

6. Secondary to glomerular disease or diabetic nephropathy
   - Glomerular or diabetic changes predominate
   - Heavy proteinuria common

7. Secondary to progressive nephron loss (ablative nephropathy)
   - Many globally and segmentally sclerotic glomeruli
   - Large nonsclerotic glomeruli
   - Usually gradually worsening nonnephrotic proteinuria

INTERSTITIAL CHANGES OTHER THAN INFLAMMATION AND FIBROSIS

1. Interstitial edema in the absence of relevant inflammation
   - ATN
   - Vascular complications
   - Humoral rejection (PTC C4d staining)

2. Interstitial hemorrhage in the absence of relevant inflammation
   - Severe acute vascular and/or humoral rejection
   - Consider adjacent infarct
   - TMA (particularly if associated with cortical necrosis)
   - Vascular complications during or after the surgery

3. PTC margination of inflammatory cells in the absence of relevant interstitial inflammation
   - Humoral rejection (C4d positive)
   - Area adjacent to acute pyelonephritis or abscess
   - ATN
   - Rarely, with no apparent reason

4. Severe PTC congestion
   - ATN
   - Acute cyclosporine nephrotoxicity (in fact a form of ATN)
   - Vascular complications
   - Consider TMA
   - Humoral rejection (C4d positive)

TUBULAR CHANGES IN THE ALLOGRAFT

1. Tubulitis with mononuclear cells
   - Acute cellular rejection

2. Tubulitis with neutrophils
   - Pyelonephritis
   - Sometimes in polyoma virus infection

3. Isometric vacuolization of the epithelium
   - High calcineurin inhibitor levels
   - Diuretics
   - Hyperosmolar solutions

   - Contrast media
   - Intravenous immunoglobulin

4. Acute tubular necrosis (ATN)
   - Any ischemic or toxic etiology

5. Tubular calcification
   - Most commonly the consequence of secondary hyperparathyroidism
   - In calcineurin inhibitor nephrotoxicity
   - Other forms of tubular injury
   - Commonly seen in association with polyoma virus nephropathy

6. Oxalate Crystals
   - Common in transplant ATN
   - If many, consider metabolic problem (oxalosis)

7. Large, sometimes vacuolated epithelial nuclei, commonly with prominent nucleoli
   - Usually a regenerative change
   - Exclude viral infection, primarily polyoma virus

8. Multinucleated tubular epithelial cells with regular uniform round nuclei ("syncytial tubular giant cells")
   - Usually a regenerative, nonspecific change

9. Viral nuclear inclusions
   - Polyomavirus
   - Adenovirus
   - Cytomegalovirus

ARTERIAL CHANGES IN THE ALLOGRAFT

1. Intimal arteritis
   - Acute vascular rejection (v1 and v2)

2. Transmural arteritis
   - Acute vascular rejection (v3)

3. Arterial fibrinoid necrosis
   - With inflammation

     Acute vascular rejection (v3)
   - Without inflammation (rare)

     TMA, frequently with malignant hypertension

4. Arterial fibrin thrombi without necrosis
   - TMA
   - Coagulation abnormalities (localized clotting, thromboemboli)

5. Fibrous to mucoid intimal thickening with some intimal inflammation or intimal foam cells
   - Obliterative transplant arteriopathy in chronic rejection

6. Mucoid intimal thickening with no intimal inflammation
   - TMA – "chronic stage"
   - Severe hypertension

7. Concentric thickening of the wall
   - Poorly controlled hypertension
   - Chronic stage TMA

8. Fibrous intimal thickening with internal elastic membrane lamellation, no inflammation (intimal fibroelastosis)
   - Long-standing hypertension
   - "Burned out" inactive chronic rejection

9. Severely thickened intima with hemosiderin-laden macrophages, mucoid change and sometimes multiple lumens
   - Recanalized thrombus

10. Needle-shaped clefts in the occluded lumen
    - Cholesterol emboli

ARTERIOLAR CHANGES IN THE ALLOGRAFT

1. Circumferential arteriolar hyalin
   - Nephrosclerosis (donor transmitted or de novo in recipient)
   - Chronic calcineurin inhibitor nephrotoxicity
   - Diabetes and metabolic syndrome

2. Nodular peripheral arteriolar hyalin
   - Chronic calcineurin inhibitor nephrotoxicity

3. Mucoid arteriolar thickening
   - Poorly controlled hypertension
   - Chronic stage or subtle TMA
   - Calcineurin inhibitor nephrotoxicity

4. Concentric arteriolar thickening
   - Poorly controlled hypertension

5. Arteriolar fibrin thrombi without necrosis
   - TMA of any etiology

6. Arteriolar fibrin thrombi with necrosis
   - TMA, particularly forms with malignant hypertension
   - Severe acute vascular rejection and/or acute humoral rejection

MAJOR GLOMERULAR PATTERNS OF INJURY IN ALLOGRAFTS

1. Glomerular intracapillary hypercellularity (glomerulitis)
   - Acute humoral rejection (C4d positive)
   - Sometimes in acute rejection without PTC C4d staining
   - Rarely with no rejection and negative PTC C4d
   - Infection related glomerulonephritis

2. Thickened glomerular capillaries with double contours on methenamine silver stain
   - Transplant glomerulopathy
   - Later stages of TMA
   - Recurrent MPGN

3. Focal, global and segmental glomerular sclerosis
   - Usually secondary to nephron loss (ablative nephropathy) in chronic allograft damage (proteinuria usually non-nephrotic).
   - Recurrent FSGS if appears early with heavy proteinuria
   - Hemodynamic disturbances, such as poorly controlled hypertension and chronic calcineurin inhibitor nephrotoxicity.

4. Glomerular capillary collapse with hypertrophic glomerular epithelial cells.
   - De novo collapsing glomerulopathy (may be zonal, may not be associated with heavy proteinuria)
   - Recurrent collapsing glomerulopathy (rare)

5. Proteinaceous material occluding glomerular capillaries
   - Fibrin thrombi (TMA or donor DIC if seen in a baseline biopsy of a deceased donor kidney).
   - "Tubular epithelial cell emboli," an artefact, most commonly seen in baseline biopsies.
   - Cryoglobulin, large immune complexes, amyloid (all are rare)

6. Glomerular crescent and/or necrosis
   - Consider recurrent or de novo glomerulonephritis
   - Rarely, severe acute vascular rejection or TMA (usually only few glomeruli affected).

Most glomerular diseases may recur or appear de novo in an allograft.

REFERENCES

1. USRDS Annual Data Report, Chapter 7: Transplantation. www.usrds.org
2. Colvin RB, and Nickeleit V: Renal Transplant Pathology. In: Jennette, Olson, and, Schwarts, Silva (Eds.): *Heptinstall's Pathology of the Kidney*, Sixth Edition. Lippincott-Raven, 2006; pp. 1347–1490.
3. McCue PA, Santoianni RA: Expedited handling of transplant biopsies. *Am J Surg Pathol* 1988; 12: 155–157.
4. Lai F MM, Lai KN, Chew EC, Lee JC: Microwave fixation in diagnostic renal pathology. *Pathology* 1987; 19: 17–21.
5. Nadasdy GM, Bott C, Cowden D, Pelletier R, Ferguson R, Nadasdy T: Comparative study for the detection of peritubular capillary C4d deposition in human renal allografts using different methodologies. *Hum Pathol* 2005;36:1178–1185.
6. Solez K, Axelsen RA, Benediktsson H, Burdick JF, Cohen AH, Colvin RB, Croker BP, Droz D, Dunnill MS, Halloran PF, et al: International standardization of criteria for the histologic diagnosis of renal allograft rejection; the Banff working classification of kidney transplant pathology. *Kidney Int* 1993; 411–422.
7. Sorof JM, Vartanian RK, Olson JL, Tomlanovich SJ, Vincenti FG, Amend WJHistopathological concordance of

paired renal allograft biopsy cores. Effect on the diagnosis and management of acute rejection. *Transplantation*1995; 60: 1215–1219.

8. Porter KA, and: Renal transplantation. In Heptinstall RH (ed): *Pathology of the Kidney*. 4th edition. Little, Brown, Boston, 1992; pp 1799–1933.

9. Racusen LC, Solez K, Colvin RB, Bonsib SM, Castro MC, Carallo T, et al: The Banff 97 working classification of renal allograft pathology. *Kidney Int* 1999; 55: 713–723.

10. Racusen LC, Colvin RB, Solez K, Mihatsch MJ, Halloran PF, et al: Antibody-mediated rejection criteria – an addition to the Banff 97 classification of renal allograft rejection. *Am J Transplant* 2003; 3: 704–714.

11. Solez K, Colvin RB, Racusen LC, Sis B, Halloran PF, Bink PE, et al: Banff 2005 meeting report: differential diagnosis of chronic allograft injury and elimination of chronic allograft nephropathy ('CAN'). *Am J Transplant* 2007; 7: 518–526.

12. Solez K, Colvin RB, Racusen LC, Haas M, Sis B et al: Banff 2007 Classification of renal allograft pathology: updates and future directions. *Am J Transplant* 2008; 8:753–760.

13. Bishop GA, Hass BM, Duggin GG, Horvath JS, SHeil AG, Tiller DJ: Immunopathology of renal allograft rejection analyzed with monoclonal antibodies to mononuclear cell markers. *Kidney Int* 1986; 29: 708–717.

14. Charney DA, Nadasdy T, Lo AW, Racusen LC: Plasma cell rich acute renal allograft rejection. *Transplantation* 1999; 68: 791–797.

15. Nadasdy T, Krenacs T, Kalmar N, Csajbok E, Boda K, Ormos J: Importance of plasma cells in the infiltrate of renal allografts. An immunohistochemical study. *Pathol Res Pract*1991;187: 178–183.

16. Sarwal M, Chua MS, Kambham N, Hsieh SC, Satterwhite T, Masek M, Salvatierra O: Molecular heterogeneity in acute renal allograft rejection identified by DNA microarray profiling. *N Eng J Med* 2003; 349: 125–128.

17. Satoskar AA, Lehman AM, Nadasdy GM, Sedmak DD, Pesavento TE, et al: Peritubular capillary C4d in late acute allograft rejection- Is it relevant? *Clin Transplant* 2008; 22:61–67.

18. Josephson MA, Chiu MY, Woodle ES, Thistlewaite JR, Haas M: Drug-induced acute interstitial nephritis in renal allografts: histopathologic features and clinical course in six patients. *Am J Kidney Dis* 1999; 34: 540–548.

19. Nickeleit V, Vamvakas EC, Pascual M, Poletti BJ, Colvin RB: The prognostic significance of specific arterial lesions in acute renal allograft rejection. *J Am Soc Nephrol* 1998; 9: 130–138.

20. Tauzon TV, Schneeberger EE, Bhan AK, McClusky RT, Cosimi AB, Schooley RT, Rubin RH, Colvin RB: *Mononuclear cells in acute allograft glomerulopathy*. 1987; 129: 119–132.

21. Alpers CE, Gordon D, Gown AM: Immunophenotype of vascular rejection in renal transplants. *Mod Pathol* 1990; 3: 198–203.

22. Haas M, Kraus ES, Samaniego-Picota M, Racusen LC, Ni W, Eustace JA: Acute renal allograft rejection with intimal arteritis: Histologic predictors of response to therapy and graft survival. *Kidney Int* 2002; 61: 1516–1526.

23. Feucht HE, Schneeberger H, Hillebrand G, Burkhardt K, Weiss M, et al: Capillary deposition of C4d complement fragment and early renal graft loss. *Kidney Int* 1993; 43: 1333–1338.

24. Collins AB, Schneeberger EE, Pascual MA, Saidman SL, Williams WW, et al: Complement activation in acute humoral renal allograft rejection: diagnostic significance of C4d deposits in peritubular capillaries. *J Am Soc Nephrol* 1999; 10: 2208–2214.

25. Crespo M, Pascual M, Tolkoff-Rubin N, Mauiyyedi S, Collins AB, et al: Acute humoral rejection in renal allograft recipients: I. Incidence, serology and clinical characteristics. *Transplantation* 2001; 71: 652–658.

26. Mauiyyedi S, Crespo M, Collins AB, Schneeberger EE, Pascual MA, et al: Acute humoral rejection in kidney transplantation: II. Morphology, immunopathology, and pathologic classification. *J Am Soc Nephrol* 2002; 13: 779–787.

27. Nickeleit V, Zeiler M, Gudat F, Theil G, Mihatsch MJ: Detection of the complement degradation product C4d in renal allografts: diagnostic and therapeutic implications. *J Am Soc Nephrol* 2002; 13: 242–251.

28. Bohmig GA, Exner M, Habicht A, Schillinger M, Lang U, et al: Capillary C4d deposition in kidney allografts: a specific marker of alloantibody-dependent graft injury. *J Am Soc Nephrol* 2002; 13: 1091–1099.

29. Herzenberg AM, Gill JS, Djurdjev O, Magil AB: C4d deposition in acute rejection: an independent long-term prognostic factor. *J Am Soc Nephrol* 2002; 13: 234–241.

30. Takemoto SK, Zeevi A, Feng S, Colvin RB, Jordan S, et al: National conference to assess antibody mediated rejection in solid organ transplantation. *Am J Transplant* 2004; 4: 1033–1041.

31. Dickenmann M, Steiger J, Descoeudres B, Mihatsch M, Nickeleit V: The fate of C4d positive kidney allografts lacking histologic signs of acute rejection. *Clin Nephrol* 2006; 65: 173–179.

32. Haas M, Montgomery RA, Segev DL, Rahman MH, Racusen LC, et al: Subclinical acute antibody-mediated rejection in positive crossmatch renal allografts. *Am J Transplant* 2007; 3: 576–85.

33. Mauiyyedi S, Pelle PD, Saidman S, Collins AB, Pascual M, et al: Chronic humoral rejection: identification of antibody mediated chronic renal allograft rejection by C4d deposits in peritubular capillaries. *J Am Soc Nephrol* 2001; 12: 574–582.

34. Regele H, Bohmig GA, Habicht A, Gollowitzer D, Schillinger M, et al: Capillary deposition of complement split product C4d in renal allografts is associated with basement membrane injury in peritubular and glomerular capillaries: a contribution of humoral immunity to chronic allograft rejection. *J Am Soc Nephrol* 2002; 13: 2371–2380.

35. Haas M, Rahman MH, Racusen LC, Kraus ES, Bagnasco SM, et al: C4d and C3d staining in biopsies of ABO- and HLA- incompatible renal allografts: correlation with histologic findings. *Am J Transplant* 2006; 6: 1753–1754.

36. Magil AB, Tinckam K: Monocytes and peritubular capillary C4d deposition in acute renal allograft rejection. *Kidney Int* 2003; 63: 1888–1893.

37. Fahim T, Bohmig GA, Exner M, Huttary N, Kerschner H: The cellular lesion of humoral rejection: predominant recruitment of monocytes to peritubular and glomerular capillaries. *Am J Transplant* 2007; 7: 385–393.

38. Gibson IW, Gwinner W, Bröcker V, Sis B, Riopel J, Roberts ISD et al: Peritubular capillaritis in renal allografts: prevalence, scoring system, reproducibility and clinicopathological correlates. *Am J Transplant* 2008; 8:819–825.

39. Kuypers DR, Lerut E, Evenepoel P, Maes B, Vanrenterghem Y, Van Damme B: C3d deposition in peritubular capillaries indicates a variant of acute renal allograft rejection characterized by a worse clinical outcome. *Transplantation* 2003; 76: 102–108.

40. Mazzucco G, Motta M, Segoloni G, Monga G: Intertubular capillary changes in the cortex and medulla of transplanted kidneys and their relationship with transplant glomerulopathy: an ultrastructural study of 12 transplantectomies. *Ultrastruct Pathol* 1994; 18: 533–537.

41. Ivanyi B, Fahmy H, Brown H, Szenohradszky P, Halloran PF, Solez K: Peritubular capillaries in chronic renal allograft rejection: a quantitative ultrastructural study. *Hum Pathol* 2000; 31: 1129–1138.

42. Sijpkens YW, Joosten SA, Wong MC, Dekker FW, Benediktsson H, Bayema EM, et al: Immunologic risk factors and glomerular C4d deposits in chronic transplant glomerulopathy. *Kidney Int* 2004; 65: 2409–2418.

43. Habib R, Zurowska A, Hinglais N, Gubler MC, Antignac C, Niaudet P, et al: A specific glomerular lesion of the graft: allograft glomerulopathy. *Kidney Int Suppl* 1993; 42: S104–111.

44. Schwimmer J, Nadasdy TA, Spitalnik PK, Kaplan KL, Zand M S: De novo thrombotic microangiopathy in renal transplant recipients: a comparison of hemolytic uremic syndrome with localized renal thrombotic microangiopathy. *Am J Kidney Dis* 2003; 41: 471–479.

45. Sis B, Dadras F, Khoshjou F, Cockfield S, Mihatsch MJ, Solez K: Reproducibility studies on arteriolar hyaline thickening scoring in calcineurin inhibitor-treated renal allograft recipients. *Am J Transplant* 2006; 6: 1444–1450.

46. Isoniemi HM, Krogerus L, von Willebrand E, Taskinen E, Ahonen J, Häyry P: Histopathological findings in well-functioning, long-term renal allografts. *Kidney Int* 1992; 41: 155–160.

47. Colvin RB: *CADI, Canti, Cavi: Transplantation* 2007; 83: 677–678.

48. Randhawa PS, Shapiro R, Jordan ML, Starzl TE, Demetris AJl: The histopathological changes associated with allograft rejection and drug toxicity in renal transplant recipients maintained on FK 506. Clinical significance and comparison with cyclosporine. *Am J Surg Pathol* 1993; 17: 60–68.

49. Mihatsch MJ, Thiel G, Basler V, Ryffel B, Landmann J, von Overbec J, Zollinger HUl: Morphologic patterns in cyclosporine-treated renal transplant recipients. *Transplant Proc* 1985; 17 (Suppl 1): 101–116, 1985.

50. Sibley RK, Rynasiewicz J, Ferguson RM, Fryd D, Sutherland DR, Simmons RL, Najarian JS: Morphology of cyclosporine nephrotoxicity and acute rejection in patients immunosuppressed with cyclosporine and prednisone. *Surgery* 1983;94: 225–234.

51. Bergstrand A, Bohman SO, Farnsworth A, Gokel JM, Krause PH, Lang W, et al: Renal histopathology in kidney transplant recipients immunosuppressed with Cyclosporine A: results of an international workshop. *Clin Nephrol* 1985; 24: 107–119.

52. Randhawa PS, Tsamandas AC, MAgnone M, Jordan M, Shapiro R, Starlz TE, Demetris AJ: Microvascular changes in renal allografts associated with FK506 (Tacrolimus) therapy. *Am J Surg Pathol* 1996; 20: 306–312.

53. Remuzzi G, Bertani T: Renal vascular and thrombotic effects of cyclosporine. *Am J Kidney Dis* 1989;13: 261–272.

54. Smith KD, Wrenshall LE, Nicosia RF, Pichler R, Marsh CL, Alpers CE, et al: Delayed graft function and cast nephropathy associated with tacrolimus plus Rapamycin use. *J Am Soc Nephrol* 2003; 14: 1037–1045.

55. Pelletier R, Nadasdy T, Nadasdy G, Satoskar A, Tewari AK, Cotrill J: Acute renal failure following kidney transplantation associated with myoglobinuria in patients treated with Rapamycin. *Transplantation* 2006; 82: 645–650.

56. Straathof-Galema L, Wetzels JF, Dijkman HB, Steenbergen EJ, Hilbrands LB: Sirolimus-associated heavy proteinuria in a renal transplant recipient: evidence for a tubular mechanism. *Am J Transplant* 2006; 6: 429–433.

57. van den Akker JM, Wetzels JF, Hoitsma AJ: Proteinuria following conversion from azathioprine to sirolimus in renal transplant recipients. *Kidney Int* 2006; 70: 1355–1357.

58. Letavernier E, Bruneval P, Mandet C, Doung van Huyen J-P, Peraldi M-N, Helal I, Noel L-H, Legendre C: High sirolimus levels may induce focal segmental glomeruloslerosis de novo. *Clin J Am Soc Nephrol* 2007; 2: 326–333.

59. Sartelet H, Toupance O, Lorenzato M, Fadel F, Noel LH, Lagonotte E, Birembaut P, Chanard J, Rieu P: Sirolimus-induced thrombotic microangiopathy is associated with decreased expression of vascular endothelial growth factor in kidneys. *Am J Transplant* 2005; 5: 2441–2447.

60. Nickeleit V, Hirsch HH, Binet IF, Gudat F, Prince O: Polyomavirus infection of renal allograft recipients: from latent infection to manifest disease. *J Am Soc Nephrol* 1999; 10: 1080–1089.

61. Randhawa P, Brennen DC: BK virus infection in transplant recipients: an overview and update. *Am J Transplant*: 2006; 6: 2000–2005.

62. Drachenberg CB, Papadimitriou JC: Polyomavirus-associated nephropathy: update in diagnosis. *Transpl Infect Dis* 2006; 8: 68–75.

63. Bracamonte E, Leca N, Smith KD, Nicosia RF, Nickeleit V, Kendrick E, et al: Tubular basement membrane immune deposits in association with BK polyoma virus nephropathy. *Am J Transplant* 2007; 7: 1552–1560.

64. Nickeleit V, Klimkait T, Binet IF, Dalquen P, Del Zenero V, Theil G, et al: Testing for polyomavirus type BK DNA in plasma to identify renal-allograft recipients with viral nephropathy. *N Engl J Med* 2000; 342: 1309–1315.

65. Meehan SM, Kraus MD, Kadambi PV, Chang A: Nephron segment localization of polyoma virus large T antigen in renal allografts. *Hum Pathol* 2006; 37: 1400–1406.

66. Kashyap R, Shapiro R, Jordan M, Randhawa PS: The clinical significance of cytomegalovirus inclusions in the allograft kidney. *Transplantation* 1979; 67: 98–103.

67. Sagedal S, Hartmann A, Rollag H: The impact of early cytomegalovirus infection and disease in renal transplant recipients *Clin Microbiol Infect* 2005; 11: 518–1530.

68. Mathur SC, Squiers EC, Tatum AH, Szmalc FS, Daucher JW, Welker DM, Shanley PF: Adenovirus infection of the renal allograft with sparing of pancreas graft function in the recipient of a combined kidney-pancreas transplant. *Transplantation* 1998; 65: 138–141.

69. Lim AK, Parsons S, Ierino F: Adenovirus tubulointerstitial nephritis presenting as a renal allograft space occupying lesion. *Am J Transplant* 2005; 5: 2062–2066.

70. Caillard S, Dharnidharka V, Agodoa L, Bohen E, Abbot K: Posttransplant lymphoproliferative disorders after renal transplantation in the United States in era of modern immunosuppression. *Transplantation* 2005; 80: 1233–1243.

71. Nalesnik MA: The diverse pathology of post-transplant lymphoproliferative disorders: the importance of a standardized approach. *Transpl Infect Dis* 2001; 3: 88–96.

72. Randhawa PS, Magnone M, Jordan M, Shapiro R, Demetris AJ, Nalesnik MA: Renal allograft involvement by Epstein-Barr virus associated post-transplant lymphoproliferative disease. *Am J Surg Pathol* 1996; 20: 563–571.

73. Fonseca LE, Shapiro R, Randhawa PS: Occurrence of urinary tract infection in patients with renal allograft biopsies showing neutrophilic tubulitis. *Mod Pathol* 2003; 16: 281–285.

74. Scarpero HM, Copley JB: Xanthogranulomatous pyelonephritis in a renal allograft recipient. *Am J Kidney Dis* 1997; 30: 846–848.

75. Pusl T, Weiss M, Hartmann B, Wendler T, Parhofer K, Michaely H: Malacoplakia in a renal transplant recipient. *Eur J Intern Med* 2006; 17: 133–135.

76. Denton MD, Singh AK: Recurrent and de novo glomerulonephritis in the renal allograft. *Semin Nephrol.* 2000; 20: 164–175.

77. Couser W: Recurrent glomerulonephritis in the renal allograft: an update of selected areas. *Exp Clin Transplant* 2005; 3: 283–288.

78. Choy BY, Chan TM, Lai KN: Recurrent glomerulonephritis after kidney transplantation. *Am J Transplant* 2006; 6: 2535–2542.

79. Vincenti F, Ghiggeri GM: New insights into the pathogenesis and the therapy of recurrent focal glomerulosclerosis. *Am J Transplant* 2005; 5: 1179–1185.

80. Nachman PH, Selegelmark M, Westman K, Hogan SL, Satterly KK, Jennette JC, Falk R: Recurrent ANCA-associated small vessel vasculitis after transplantation: a pooled analysis. *Kidney Int* 1999; 56: 1544–1550.

81. Ponticelli C, Moroni G: Renal transplantation in lupus nephritis. *Lupus* 2005; 14: 95–98.

82. Monga G, Mazzucco G, Basolo B, Quaranta S, Motta M, Segoloni G, Amoroso A: Membranous glomerulonephritis (MGN) in transplanted kidneys: Morphologic investigation on 256 renal allografts. *Modern Pathol* 1993; 6: 249–258.

83. Meehan SM, Pascual M, Williams WW, Tolkoff-Rubin N, Delmonico FL et al: De novo collapsing glomerulopathy in renal allografts. *Transplantation* 1998; 65: 1192–1197.

84. Nadasdy T, Allen C, Zand MS: Zonal distribution of glomerular collapse in renal allografts: possible role of vascular change. *Hum Pathol* 2002; 33: 437–441.

85. Sundararaman S, Lager DJ, Qian X, Stegall MD, Larson TS, Griffin MD: Collapsing and non-collapsing focal segmental glomerulosclerosis in kidney transplants. *Nephrol Dial Transplant* 2006; 21: 2607–2614.

86. Byrne MC, Budisavljevic MN, Fan Z, Self SE, Ploth DW: Renal transplant patients with Alport Syndrome. *Am J Kidney Dis.* 2002; 4: 769–775.

87. Abouna GM, Adnani MS, Kumar MS, Samhan SA: Fate of transplanted kidneys with diabetic nephropathy. *Lancet* 1986; 1: 622–623.

CHAPTER 17

Tumors of the Kidney

Satish K. Tickoo, MD, Pedram Argani, MD, and Mahul B. Amin, MD

ADULT RENAL TUMORS

Introduction

Renal epithelial tumors constitute approximately 3 percent of all malignant tumors in humans, and are the third most common malignancies of the genitourinary tract [1]. In the United States, approximately 51,200 new cases and 12,890 deaths due to kidney and renal pelvis cancer were expected in 2007 [1]. Although majority of the tumors are now detected incidentally [2] and at a small tumor size [3,4], the mortality (particularly in larger-sized tumors) has continued to rise [5]. Up to 30 percent of patients with renal cell carcinoma (RCC) present with metastatic disease, and recurrence develops in approximately 40 percent of patients treated for a localized tumor. The median overall survival in patients with metastatic disease is approximately twelve months [6]. Clear cell RCC represents about 70 percent of the primary and 90 percent of the metastatic renal cell tumors [7].

Before 1985, RCCs were primarily grouped as clear cell, granular cell, papillary, and sarcomatoid. The first reports of chromophobe RCC and its eosinophilic variant in humans in mid-1980s by Thoenes et al. [8,9] were instrumental in the reevaluation and better understanding of the clinicopathological features of renal tumors. It was thus recognized that each of the pre-1985 entities consist of different tumors with varying pathologic features and biological behaviors (Table 17.1). The resultant classification system, which is now even adopted by the WHO in its 2004 classification of tumors of the kidney (Figure 17.1) [10], stands validated by a number of molecular studies [11–13]. The clinical implications of this now universally accepted classification suggest that publications about clinicopathological aspects of renal tumors in pre-1985 era may not correspond to the current knowledge about these tumors.

Our better understanding of the molecular aspects of renal tumors in the recent past has resulted in the realization that different renal tumors involve different molecular pathways, resulting in the development and usage of multiple targeted therapies, particularly for advanced clear cell RCC, with promising initial results [6].

Grading and Staging of Renal Tumors

Amongst the several grading systems proposed for renal tumors over the years, Fuhrman's system is the most widely used. This system uses nuclear grades based on nuclear size, irregularity of the nuclear membrane, and nucleolar prominence. However for practical purposes, easily identifiable nucleoli, at low-power (10×) examination, are characteristic of nuclear grade 3 or 4, with grade 4 nuclei also showing marked pleomorphism and/or

Table 17.1 Comparison of "Pre-1985" Classification of Renal Epithelial Tumors in Adults with the Current Classification System Indicating the Multiple Tumor Types within Each of the Older Groups

Pre-1985	Modern Classification Groups
Clear cell RCC	Clear cell RCC
	Chromophobe RCC
	Translocation-associated RCC
	RCC, unclassified
Granular cell RCC	Clear cell RCC
	Chromophobe RCC
	Renal oncocytoma
	Papillary RCC
	Epithelioid angiomyolipoma
	RCC, unclassified
Papillary/Tubulopapillary RCC	Papillary RCC
	Collecting duct carcinoma
	Translocation-associated RCC
	Mucinous tubular and spindle cell carcinoma
	RCC, unclassified
Sarcomatoid RCC	Clear cell RCC
	Chromophobe RCC
	Papillary RCC
	Collecting duct carcinoma
	RCC, unclassified

RCC, renal cell carcinoma.

multilobulation. Grade 1 or 2 nuclei generally require examination at high magnification (40×) to identify and evaluate the level of prominence of the nucleoli (Figures 17.2A–D). Although the utility of Fuhrman grading system in clear cell RCC is well established, its value in papillary and chromophobe RCC remains controversial. There is no reason to grade renal oncocytomas since these are benign tumors.

The TMN classification of the American Joint Committee on Cancer (AJCC) and Union Internationale Contre le Cancer (UICC) is the most widely used, and clinically relevant, staging system for renal tumors [14]. Over the years it has been modified and improved multiple times; the latest modifications were made in 2002. Although it cannot be claimed to be a perfect staging system, at present the latest TMN classification is recommended in the hopes of establishing uniformity in reporting, while future AJCC staging criteria will certainly correct the deficiencies in the present system.

Recently, a series of publications have highlighted the importance of the renal sinus and sinus veins in the staging of RCC [15,16], the factors first included in the AJCC staging system in 2002. Therefore, we recommend a careful gross examination and adequate sampling of the renal sinus–tumor interface, especially in larger tumors (Figure 17.3).

Malignant Tumors

Clear Cell (Conventional) Renal Cell Carcinoma

Clear cell carcinoma comprises approximately 60–70 percent of all RCCs and is characterized primarily by tumor cells with clear cytoplasm and an acinar growth pattern invested by an intricate, arborizing vasculature. The "clearing" typically involves the entire cytoplasm, particularly in low-grade tumors, whereas higher grade lesions may have a combination of clear cells and cells with eosinophilic cytoplasm, or may be purely eosinophilic. Figures 17.4 and 17.5 depict an algorithmic approach to the differential diagnostic considerations for tumors with clear or eosinophilic cytoplasm. The intricate vasculature tends to be retained in most clear cell RCCs, except in the very high-grade areas with solid or sarcomatoid differentiation. Sarcomatoid or spindle cell differentiation occurs in approximately 5 percent of these tumors (Figure 17.6), and like in other subtypes of RCC, is an indicator of Fuhrman grade 4 tumor, with ominous prognosis [13,17,18]. Diagnostically, it is important to search for transition(s) to lower grade areas, thereby establishing the correct diagnosis. Clear cell RCC may take on a focal papillary or pseudopapillary appearance, which often (but not always) is due to cellular dyscohesion secondary to degenerative changes rather than true papillae formation.

Clear cell RCCs are characterized by the loss of genetic material of the short arm of chromosome 3 (3p) and mutations in *von Hippel Lindau (VHL)* gene. In patients with VHL syndrome, such losses and mutations are described in virtually all cases. Somatic mutations/hypermethylations in the same region can be found in 75–80 percent of the more common sporadic, unilateral, and unifocal tumors, as well [10,13,19]. The normal *VHL* gene product, pVHL, is required to target and degrade hydroxylated hypoxia inducible factor (HIF) in normoxemic states. In cells that are hypoxic, or lack pVHL (as in most cases of clear cell RCC), HIF escapes degradation and activates many

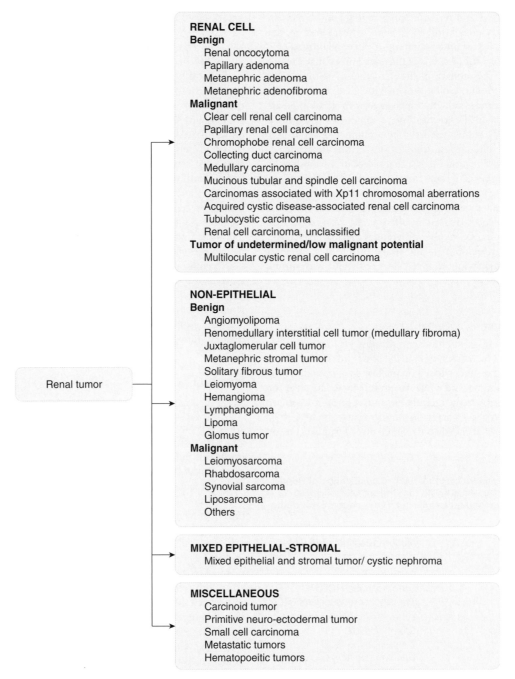

RENAL CELL
Benign
    Renal oncocytoma
    Papillary adenoma
    Metanephric adenoma
    Metanephric adenofibroma
Malignant
    Clear cell renal cell carcinoma
    Papillary renal cell carcinoma
    Chromophobe renal cell carcinoma
    Collecting duct carcinoma
    Medullary carcinoma
    Mucinous tubular and spindle cell carcinoma
    Carcinomas associated with Xp11 chromosomal aberrations
    Acquired cystic disease-associated renal cell carcinoma
    Tubulocystic carcinoma
    Renal cell carcinoma, unclassified
Tumor of undetermined/low malignant potential
    Multilocular cystic renal cell carcinoma

NON-EPITHELIAL
Benign
    Angiomyolipoma
    Renomedullary interstitial cell tumor (medullary fibroma)
    Juxtaglomerular cell tumor
    Metanephric stromal tumor
    Solitary fibrous tumor
    Leiomyoma
    Hemangioma
    Lymphangioma
    Lipoma
    Glomus tumor
Malignant
    Leiomyosarcoma
    Rhabdosarcoma
    Synovial sarcoma
    Liposarcoma
    Others

MIXED EPITHELIAL-STROMAL
    Mixed epithelial and stromal tumor/ cystic nephroma

MISCELLANEOUS
    Carcinoid tumor
    Primitive neuro-ectodermal tumor
    Small cell carcinoma
    Metastatic tumors
    Hematopoeitic tumors

Renal tumor

FIGURE 17.1: Classification of adult renal tumors and tumor-like conditions.

downstream molecules, including vascular endothelial growth factor (VEGF), glucose transporter 1 (GLUT1), and carbonic anhydrase IX (CA-IX), among others. The diffuse (and not only perinecrotic) expression of these downstream products at the immunohistochemical level may be used as markers of clear cell RCC or as targets for novel targeted therapies. Phase III trials of agents that target these molecules are underway, with encouraging survival results for patients with metastatic RCC [6].

Multilocular cystic RCC is considered to be a variant of clear cell. It is composed of usually a well-circumscribed lesion with variably sized fibrous-walled cysts that are lined by clear cells

with low nuclear grade. By definition, the septa contain small clusters of clear cells with similar low-grade cytology. There should be no expansile nodules that alter the general cystic outlines. Although regarded as a variant of clear cell RCC, none of the reported cases of multilocular cystic RCC has recurred, and no metastases have been reported.

Papillary Renal Cell Carcinoma

Papillary RCC constitutes up to 15 percent of all renal cortical neoplasms. Architecturally, most of these tumors have a papillary,

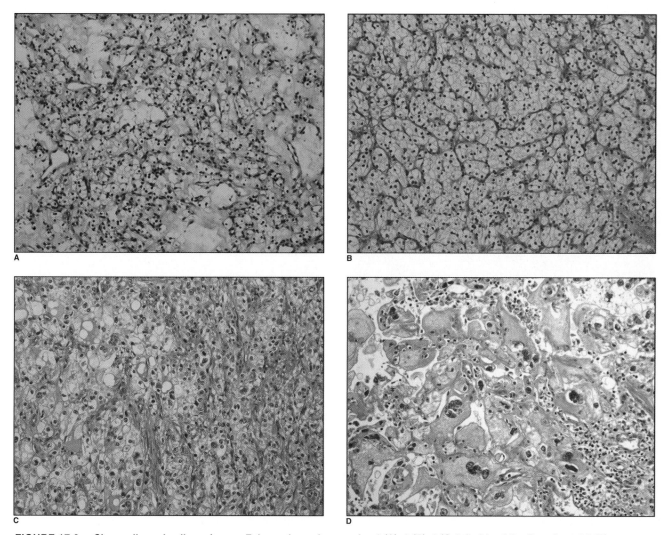

FIGURE 17.2: *Clear cell renal cell carcinoma, Fuhrman's nuclear grades 1 (A), 2 (B), 3 (C, left side of the figure), and 4 (D).*

tubular, or tubulopapillary growth pattern (Figures 17.7–17.9). Some tumors have a "solid" growth pattern due to compression of the papillary structures, whereas other tumors show a "glomeruloid" appearance (Figure 17.10) [7,20,21]. The cytoplasm may be amphophilic, eosinophilic, or even partially clear. Papillary RCCs are often multifocal, are frequently associated with other minute papillary tumors (so-called papillary adenomas, if they are less than 5 mm in size, by definition) (Figure 17.11) and are the most common RCC type with bilateral disease. Classically, papillary tumors display abundant lipid-laden, "foamy" macrophages within fibrovascular cores, a feature helpful in establishing the correct diagnosis.

Although many experts feel that the Fuhrman grading scheme is well suited for papillary RCC, others disagree. In the late 1990s, Delahunt and Eble suggested a two-tier system based on nuclear features and growth pattern characteristics: type 1 tumors as those with thin papillae, basophilic to amphophilic cytoplasm, and generally low nuclear grade (Figure 17.8), and type 2 as those with larger papillae with abundant eosinophilic cytoplasm, nuclear pseudostratification, and higher grade

nuclei (Figure 17.9) [22]. This classification system is now incorporated in the 2004 WHO classification system. Many cytogenetic and molecular studies have revealed distinct findings in papillary RCC that distinguish them from other renal epithelial tumors. Nearly 10 percent of sporadic papillary RCC show somatic mutations in *c-MET* gene, a genetic abnormality commonly seen as a germline mutation in familial cases. The majority of sporadic papillary RCC are characterized by trisomy of chromosomes 7 and 17 (type 1 tumors), as well as loss of chromosome Y [10,12]. However, controversy remains about grading of papillary RCC, for example in cases showing mixed type 1 and 2 features. Recently, Yang et al. have attempted a molecular classification of papillary RCC [23]. They propose a two-class system with class 1 tumors encompassing a range of morphology – from WHO type 1 tumors to lesions with eosinophilic cytoplasm but low nuclear grade to combinations of the two – and displaying a distinct molecular and immunohistochemical profile. Molecular class 2 tumors in their work correspond to some of the WHO type 2 tumors with high nuclear grade, and are associated with vastly different expression signature and topoisomerase IIα immunoreactivity. Some published series have shown that type 1 tumors have a better prognosis than type 2 tumors [24].

We believe that papillary RCC still remains a not very well-defined subtype of RCC. Among its differential diagnostic considerations are collecting duct carcinoma, clear cell RCC with

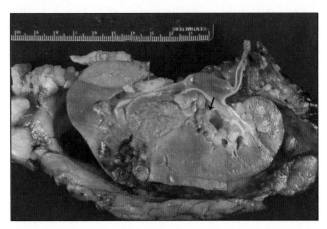

FIGURE 17.3: *Clear cell renal cell carcinoma. The tumor is grossly closely associated with renal sinus (arrow). Extensive sampling of renal sinus to evaluate renal sinus fat or large vein invasion is strongly recommended.*

focal papillary architecture, translocation-associated RCC, and mucinous tubular and spindle cell carcinoma (see later). Papillary RCC is usually well circumscribed, and in most cases with a prominent pseudocapsule. Collecting duct carcinoma and other related distal nephron carcinomas are multinodular, show prominent desmoplasia, with or without a prominent papillary architecture, and often with other architectural patterns including solid, tubular, micro- and macrocystic, yolk sac tumor–like, or adenoid cystic–like. It is important that all tumors with prominent papillary architecture, but with other features not characteristic of papillary RCC (e.g., prominent desmoplasia, multinodularity, solid architecture) are not included among papillary RCC, as it may artifactually dilute the reported biologic behavior and prognosis of papillary RCC. In most large well-studied series, papillary RCC is a less aggressive tumor than clear cell RCC, with five-year survival rates of 80–85 percent [13,21,25,26].

Chromophobe Renal Cell Carcinoma

Chromophobe RCC, first described in 1985 by Thöenes et al. [8], constitutes approximately 6 percent of renal cortical neoplasms. Many of these tumors may have previously been classified under the clear cell or granular RCC category (Table 17.1). The morphologic features include a solid growth pattern with sheets of cells separated by incomplete fibrovascular septations.

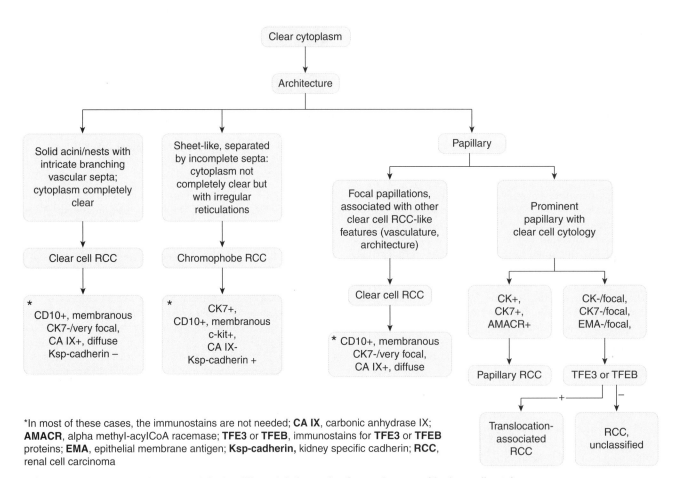

*In most of these cases, the immunostains are not needed; **CA IX**, carbonic anhydrase IX; **AMACR**, alpha methyl-acylCoA racemase; **TFE3** or **TFEB**, immunostains for **TFE3** or **TFEB** proteins; **EMA**, epithelial membrane antigen; **Ksp-cadherin,** kidney specific cadherin; **RCC**, renal cell carcinoma

FIGURE 17.4: *Algorithmic approach in the differential diagnosis of a renal tumor with clear cell cytology.*

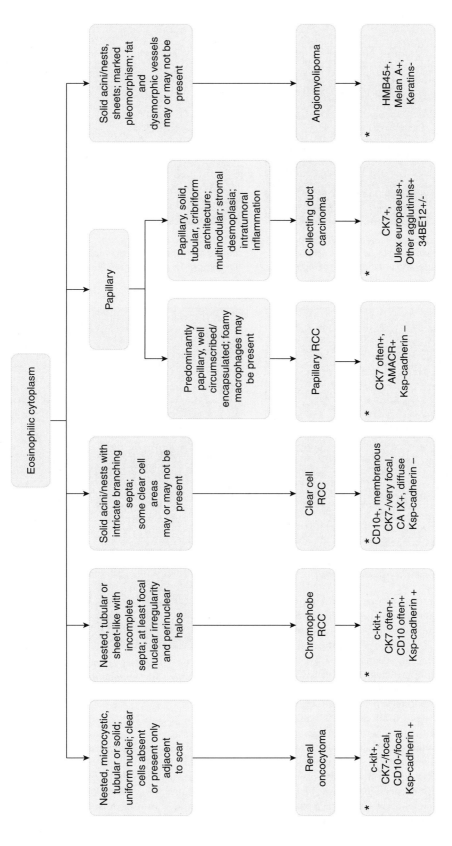

*In most cases, the immunostains are not needed; **CA IX**, carbonic anhydrase **IX**; **AMACR**, alpha methyl-acyl CoA racemase; **34BE12**, high molecular weight cytokeratin; **HMB45**, melanocyte marker; **Ksp-Cadherin**, Kidney specific cadherin

FIGURE 17.5: *Algorithmic approach in the differential diagnosis of a renal tumor with eosinophilic cytology.*

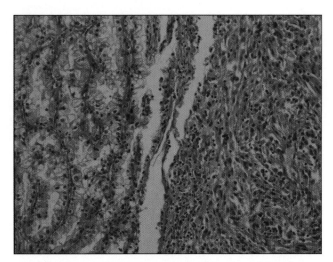

FIGURE 17.6: *Clear cell renal cell carcinoma with sarcomatoid differentiation. Sarcomatoid features can be seen in any of the subtypes of renal cell carcinoma, and are indicative of high-grade (Fuhrman's grade 4) tumors.*

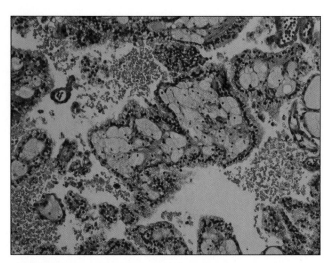

FIGURE 17.8: *Papillary renal cell carcinoma, type 1. Type 1 tumors have basophilic to amphophilic cytoplasm, generally low nuclear grade, and high nucleus-to-cytoplasm ratio.*

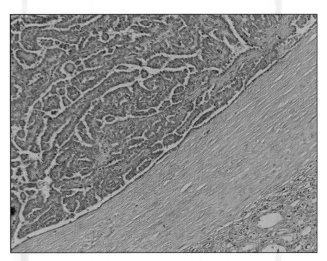

FIGURE 17.7: *Papillary renal cell carcinoma. Most tumors are well circumscribed, with a prominent pseudocapsule.*

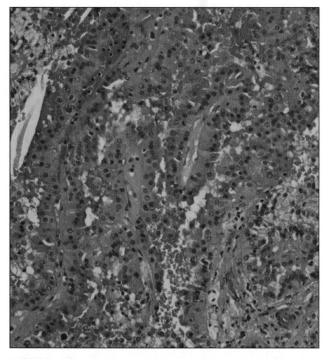

FIGURE 17.9: *Papillary renal cell carcinoma, type 2. Type 2 tumors usually show abundant eosinophilic cytoplasm, nuclear pseudostratification and high-grade nuclei.*

Occasionally, tubular, nested, or cord-like growth, mimicking renal oncocytoma, may be present. The cells may be predominantly clear (with finely reticulated cytoplasm), eosinophilic, or most often with a mixture of clear and eosinophilic cell features (Figure 17.12). Nuclei are centrally located, often hyperchromatic, and show nuclear membrane irregularity, usually widespread but sometimes only focal. Binucleate cells are a common finding. Classically, one sees perinuclear clearing (perinuclear "halo"), corresponding to distended microvesicles seen ultrastructurally in this region. At the periphery of the tumor cells, pushing and aggregation of other organelles in the cytoplasm may result in an apparent thick cell wall or "plant cell"–like appearance. Thöenes et al. also described an eosinophilic variant that may be confused with oncocytoma (Figure 17.13) [9]. As in other RCC types, chromophobe RCC with sarcomatoid features is a highly aggressive variant (Figure 17.14).

As opposed to clear cell RCC, the cytoplasm of chromophobe RCC stains for Hale's colloidal iron but contains sparse

amounts of lipid or glycogen. These tumors exhibit genetic losses of chromosomes 1 and Y as well as combined chromosomal losses, usually affecting chromosomes 1, 6, 10, 13, 17, and 21. Loss of multiple chromosomes leads to hypodiploid tumor cells, a unique feature seen in many of these tumors.

Overall, chromophobe RCCs have a much better prognosis than clear cell tumors, with five-year disease-free survival of more than 90 percent [13,21]. Except for the series published

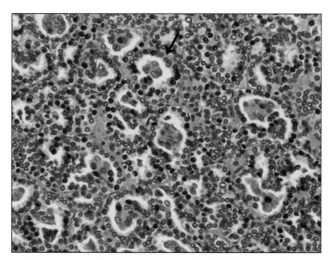

FIGURE 17.10: *Papillary renal cell carcinoma, with glomeruloid features (arrow).*

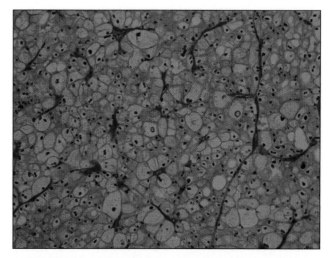

FIGURE 17.12: *Chromophobe renal cell carcinoma. Most tumors have a mixture of cells with clear (finely reticulated) and eosinophilic cytoplasm.*

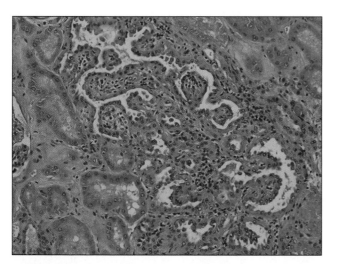

FIGURE 17.11: *Papillary adenoma. By definition, these are less than 5 mm in size, and should not show any clear cell carcinoma–like features.*

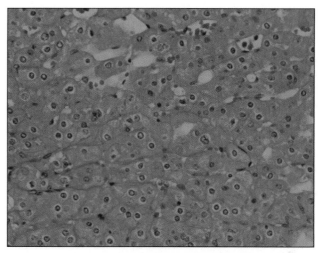

FIGURE 17.13: *Chromophobe renal cell carcinoma, eosinophilic variant. Note the nuclear irregularities with perinuclear "halos," a characteristic of all chromophobe renal cell carcinomas.*

by Cheville et al. [26], most series also suggest that they have a better prognosis than papillary RCC. Motzer et al. demonstrated that even metastatic chromophobe carcinomas progressed more indolently than metastatic disease from other RCC types [27].

Renal Cell Carcinoma, Unclassified

This diagnostic category includes the renal carcinomas that do not fit into any of the usual subtypes of renal cortical tumors [10]. Thus, tumors of unrecognizable cell or architectural types, or those with apparent composites of the recognized types are all included in this category. These make up to 6 percent of all renal epithelial tumors [13,21]. Although many of the tumors from this category are of high cytomorphological grade (Figures 17.15 and 17.16) and aggressive clinical behavior, by definition, they are not a pure entity limited to only such aggressive tumors, and include many other less aggressive tumors (Figures 17.17 and 17.18).

It is expected that with accumulation of tumors, and the experience gained therefrom, we would be in a better position to recognize tumors with similar features in this category. This would enable us to extract such tumors from the unclassified group and reclassify them as distinct entities, as is exemplified by the next few tumor types.

Mucinous Tubular and Spindle Cell Carcinoma

This recently described tumor is unique among renal epithelial neoplasms; in spite of showing a spindle cell (low-grade sarcomatoid) component, it usually does not behave in an aggressive manner [28,29]. Of the nearly 100 reported cases in the literature, only 1 has had local lymph node metastasis. Most tumors have been reported in females, with age ranges of 17 and 78 years (average 53 years). Grossly, it is a well-circumscribed

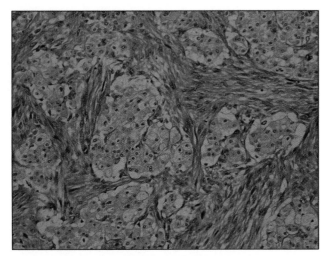

FIGURE 17.14: *Chromophobe renal cell carcinoma with sarcomatoid differentiation. Biphasic histology of chromophobe carcinoma with sarcomatoid component is evident.*

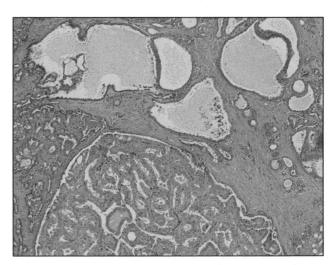

FIGURE 17.16: *Renal cell carcinoma, unclassified. Another high-grade tumor in which the tumor morphology does not resemble any of the known subtypes of renal cell carcinoma.*

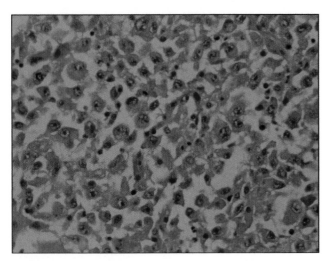

FIGURE 17.15: *Renal cell carcinoma, unclassified. A high-grade carcinoma with rhabdoid features.*

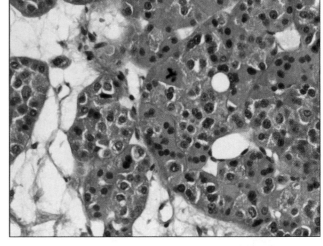

FIGURE 17.17: *Renal cell carcinoma, unclassified. This example shows superficial resemblance to a renal oncocytoma. However, nuclear variability and the presence of atypical mitosis mitigates against the diagnosis of an oncocytoma.*

tumor with the epicenter usually located in the renal medulla. Microscopically, the tumor is composed of elongated, interconnected tubules, many appearing straight and with slit-like lumina, solid compressed cords, and prominent low-grade spindle cell areas (Figure 17.19). The cells, other than in the spindled areas, are low cuboidal with small amount of amphophilic to eosinophilic cytoplasm, and with low-grade bland-appearing nuclei. Occasionally, tumors show some uncommon features, including the presence of foamy macrophages, papillations, and focal clear cells in tubules, necrosis, and oncocytic tubules [30]. Myxoid stroma is present in virtually all cases, although in "mucin-poor" rare cases this may require alcian blue stain for confirmation [30]. Foci resembling mucinous tubular and spindle cell carcinoma (MTSC) may be found in low-grade papillary RCCs, although such changes are only focal. Because of such morphological and some immunohistochemical observations [31], it has recently been suggested that

MTSC may be a variant of papillary RCC with spindle cell features [32].

Ultrastructural evaluation done on a few cases shows close resemblance to the normal loop of Henle [28,29]. Comparative genomic hybridization (CGH) data available on a few cases shows frequent losses at chromosomes 1, 4q, 6, 8p, 11q, 13, 14, and 15, with gains at 11q, 16q, 17, and 20q. No evidence of VHL deletions was found by fluorescent in situ hybridization (FISH) analysis [29].

Acquired Cystic Disease of Kidney-associated Renal Cell Carcinoma

This recently described RCC is associated with end-stage kidneys with acquired cystic disease (ACD) [33]. Most, but not all, of the reported cases occurred in patients on dialysis. The tumors characteristically are composed of large eosinophilic

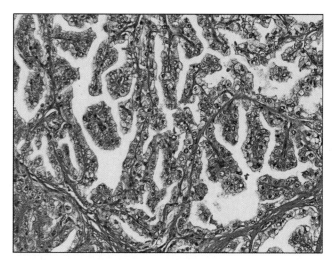

FIGURE 17.18: *Renal cell carcinoma, unclassified. A tumor with papillary architecture and extensive clear cell cytology. Although this may raise the possibility of a translocation-associated carcinoma, the morphologic features, as well as the absence of immunoreactivity for TFE3 and TFEB, argue against such a diagnosis.*

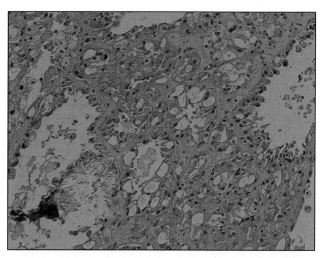

FIGURE 17.20: *Acquired cystic disease of the kidney (ACD)-associated renal cell carcinoma. The tumor characteristically has high-grade eosinophilic cytology, tubular, microcystic, papillary, or solid architecture with intracytoplasmic lumina ("holes"), and frequent intratumoral oxalate crystals.*

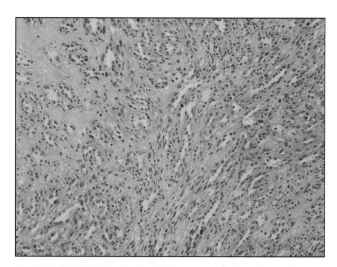

FIGURE 17.19: *Mucinous tubular and spindle cell carcinoma. A combination of myxoid stroma, elongated, interconnected tubules lined by cuboidal cells, and low-grade spindle cell areas are characteristic and are present in almost all tumors, though in variable proportions.*

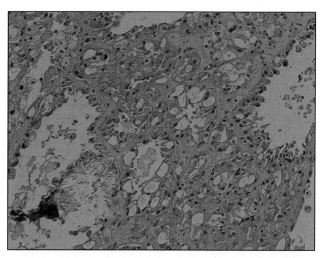

FIGURE 17.21: *Acquired cystic disease of the kidney (ACD)-associated renal cell carcinoma, seen under partially polarized light. Prominent papillary architecture in some tumors may have resulted in these being considered as papillary RCC in the past.*

cells with prominent nucleoli, inter- and intracellular vacuoles (holes), resulting in a vaguely cribriform architecture, and intratumoral oxalate crystals in majority of the cases (Figure 17.20). Foci with clear or amphophilic cytoplasm may also be present. Architecture is variable and there may be papillary, acinar, tubular, and sheet-like areas in variable proportions (Figure 17.21). Such architectural features may have led in the past to many of these being considered papillary, clear cell, or even unclassified RCC [34]. Immunohistochemical staining for alpha methylacyl-CoA racemase (AMACR) is strongly positive, whereas cytokeratin 7 (CK7) is mostly negative [33]. Some of these tumors behave aggressively, metastasize, and may cause death.

The other group of tumors that, because of their prominent clear cell cytology and often a papillary architecture, might sometimes have been considered as unclassified RCCs is the translocation-associated RCC. It is described later in detail under pediatric renal tumors.

Collecting Duct Carcinoma

Collecting duct carcinoma (CDC)/Bellini duct carcinoma is rare, comprising approximately 1 percent of renal epithelial tumors. Although earlier cases had been reported, it was first recognized as a separate clinicopathologic entity only in 1986 [35]. In general, the tumors are centered in the renal medulla, particularly when small, show marked invasive multinodular growth pattern with desmoplasia, highly atypical cytological features, and papillary, tubular, solid, and/or microcystic architecture (Figures 17.22 and 17.23) [36]. The papillae rarely, if ever, contain foamy macrophages, but acute or chronic inflammatory cells may be abundant within the tumor. Characteristically, dysplastic or neoplastic cells may be present within adjacent renal tubules. Cytoplasmic and luminal mucin is frequent. Most show immunoreactivity for carcinoembryogenic antigen (CEA), peanut lectin agglutinin (PNA), and Ulex europaeus agglutinin (UEA) [37,38]. High-molecular-weight cytokeratin and CK7 may be positive, as well.

CDC may occur at any age, the mean age at presentation approximating 53 years with a range of 13–83 years. Nevertheless, the overall impression of most experts is that they tend to present in younger patients, with the mean ages described as 34–58 years [37,39]. More than 50 percent of the patients present with metastatic disease. In a large Japanese series of eighty-one cases, regional lymph node metastasis was detected in 44 percent, and distant metastasis in another 32 percent [39].

Relatively few tumors have been studied by cytogenetic analysis, most are hypodiploid with losses involving chromosomes 1, 13, 22, X, and Y [10,13]. Less frequently, additional abnormalities in chromosomes 3, 14, and 21 are also reported. Importantly, of all the tumors studied, none has shown trisomy 7/17 or losses of chromosome 3, features seen in papillary and clear cell RCC, respectively.

The differential diagnoses include papillary RCC, medullary carcinoma, and more commonly, urothelial carcinoma. Papillary RCC is rarely associated with desmoplastic stroma and the papillae are more likely to contain foamy macrophages. Histochemical, immunohistochemical, and genetic features can also aid in classifying these tumors. Distinguishing between high-grade urothelial carcinoma and CDC may present a more formidable problem since both may be associated with an inflamed, fibrotic, or desmoplastic stroma and may contain neoplastic cells within the renal tubules (see section on the "Tumors of the Renal Pelvis"). In addition, both may have a tubular or tubulopapillary pattern of growth and a similar immunophenotype. Intracytoplasmic mucin may be seen in urothelial tumors, as well. In our experience, the best way to resolve this differential diagnosis is by sampling the renal pelvis well, looking for in situ urothelial carcinoma. Molecular studies may also be of diagnostic utility.

Tubulocystic Carcinoma

In the not-so-distant past, the morphologic spectrum of CDC was expanded to include some "low-grade" tumors characterized by a tubulocystic pattern of growth, tumor cells with low-grade nuclei, and mucin production [40]. More recently, Amin et al. proposed the terminology of "tubulocystic carcinoma of the kidney" for these tumors [41]. All their twenty-nine tumors were grossly well circumscribed. Microscopically, besides the tubulocystic growth pattern, the tumor cells showed abundant eosinophilic cytoplasm, and usually round nuclei with prominent nucleoli (Figure 17.24). In another molecular profiling study, they demonstrated marked molecular differences between these tumors and clear cell and chromophobe RCC [42]. However, not only do tumors with such pure morphologic features exist, but

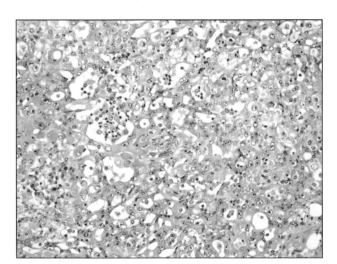

FIGURE 17.22: *Collecting duct carcinoma. The tumors typically show multinodular growth pattern, tubular, solid, cribriform, or papillary architecture, and desmoplastic stromal response.*

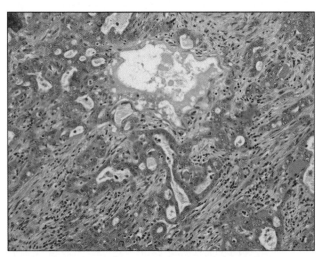

FIGURE 17.23: *Collecting duct carcinoma, with intratumoral inflammatory cell infiltrates, another characteristic feature of the tumor.*

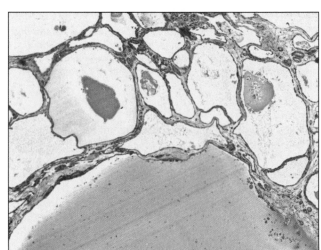

FIGURE 17.24: *Tubulocystic carcinoma. The tumors are well circumscribed, composed of tubules, and cysts lined by eosinophilic cells with round nuclei and prominent nucleoli.*

other tumors showing similar morphologic features admixed with otherwise high-grade CDC-like areas can be observed. Therefore, further evidence to show that they are a distinct entity or tumors of true collecting duct origin is awaited. Two recent, large studies of more than forty cases have been reported and although these tumors appear to be distinctive entities, their relationship to CDC remains to be established [43,44].

Medullary Carcinoma

First reported in 1995, this unique group of tumors predominantly, though not exclusively, afflicts young patients of African-American descent [45]. These tumors are usually centered in the renal medulla, have distinctive morphological features, and follow a very aggressive clinical course. They are believed to arise from the distal portions of the collecting ducts. Almost all patients have sickle cell trait, with rare cases showing hemoglobin SC disease, or even more rarely sickle cell (SS) disease [45,46]. Its association with young patients with sickle cell trait, whether of African-American, Mediterranean, or other ancestry, has been confirmed in other reports [10,13]. Other characteristic genetic abnormalities have not been defined yet. Morphologically, these tumors share many features with CDC and, in fact may be a particularly virulent variant of that entity. Tumors are composed of cells with high-grade nuclei and prominent nucleoli arranged in solid nests or irregular tubules. Microcystic or reticular growth reminiscent of yolk sac tumors is also common. Areas resembling adenoid cystic carcinoma have also been described. The surrounding stroma is usually fibrotic or desmoplastic and infiltrated by abundant inflammatory cells, mostly polymorphonuclear cells. Sickled and deformed red blood cells are easily identified within the vessels (Figure 17.25).

Most reported cases had metastatic disease at the time of presentation. In the series reported by Davis et al., mean survival was fifteen weeks [45], and in a more recent series by Swartz et al. it was four months [46]. Differential diagnosis includes CDC and high-grade urothelial carcinoma. Careful sampling and attention to the clinical features of the case may be needed to accurately classify the tumor. In our experience, the immunohistochemical features of all three tumor types overlap significantly, nullifying its diagnostic utility.

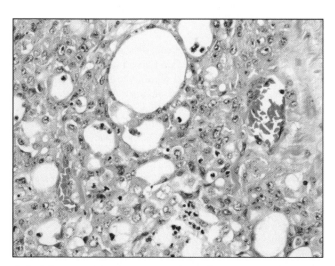

FIGURE 17.25: *Medullary carcinoma. Sickled red blood cells are easily identified in the tumoral, as well as nontumoral vessels.*

Renal Oncocytoma

Oncocytomas of the kidney also constitute approximately 6–9 percent of renal cortical neoplasms. They are benign neoplasms that require distinction from a number of malignant renal epithelial neoplasms with eosinophilic cytoplasm (Figure 17.5). Histologically, oncocytomas are characterized by cells with deeply eosinophilic cytoplasm arranged in nests, cords, or tubules and with round, vesicular nuclei often with prominent central nucleoli (Figures 17.26 and 17.27) [47,48]. Electron microscopy reveals cytoplasm loaded with mitochondria, which is responsible for the cytoplasmic eosinophilia and a mahogany brown gross appearance [49,50]. Uniformity of nuclear features is the rule, although occasional isolated or groups of cells may exhibit marked degenerative-appearing hyperchromasia and pleomorphism (Figure 17.28). Prominent papillary growth and extensive tumor necrosis are not the features of renal oncocytoma. Likewise, mitotic activity

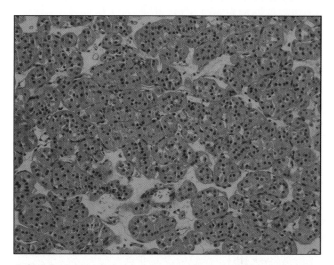

FIGURE 17.26: *Renal oncocytoma. The characteristic nested growth pattern. Note the uniform, round nuclear contours, a prerequisite for the diagnosis of renal oncocytoma.*

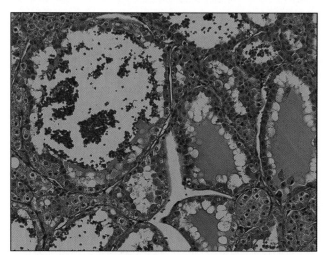

FIGURE 17.27: *Renal oncocytoma with predominantly microcystic growth pattern.*

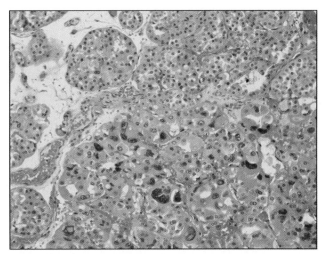

FIGURE 17.28: *Renal oncocytoma. Focal, nuclear hyperchromasia, pleomorphism, and multilobulation are quite common in these tumors. These atypical nuclei almost never show immunoreactivity for proliferation markers like Ki-67.*

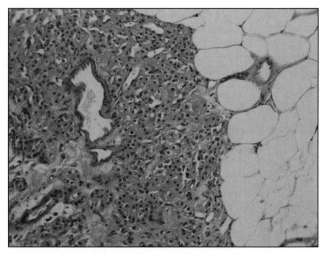

FIGURE 17.30: *Renal oncocytoma with extension into perinephric fat. This is not associated with desmoplasia, and does not influence the benign biological behavior of the tumor.*

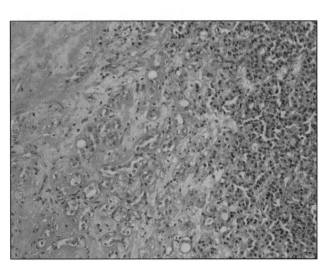

FIGURE 17.29: *Renal oncocytoma. Clear cell change adjacent to a scar.*

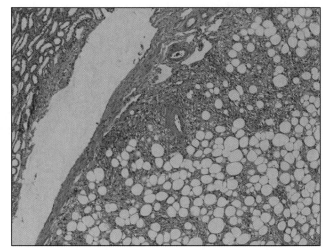

FIGURE 17.31: *Angiomyolipoma, triphasic. This represents the typical histology with the vascular, smooth muscle, and adipocytic components.*

is rarely noted. A central, stellate scar has been considered characteristic of this neoplasm, but can be seen in other low-grade renal epithelial neoplasms. Microscopically, the scar is composed of loose or dense hyalinized connective tissue containing occasional entrapped tumor cells, which may exhibit focal cytoplasmic clearing (Figure 17.29). Other than in this scenario, clear cells are not a feature of renal oncocytoma. Tumor cells may permeate perirenal soft tissue (Figure 17.30), and may occasionally be present within small and even the larger vessels. None of these features, however, affect its benign clinical behavior. Although rare questionable reported cases have metastasized [48], no known case has died of disease.

Genetically, oncocytomas do not exhibit 3p-, trisomy 7/17, or multiple combined chromosomal losses. They commonly exhibit loss of chromosomes Y and 1 and a few cases have been described with translocation involving chromosome 11. In the past few years, a group of patients with multiple oncocytic lesions ("renal

oncocytosis") has been described. Among several characteristic morphologic features, some have tumors with hybrid morphology between oncocytoma and chromophobe RCC, suggesting that these tumors may etiopathogenetically be related [51]. Indeed, it has been hypothesized that chromophobe RCC may represent a genetic/morphologic progression from oncocytoma. It is very likely that many if not all of those patients belonged to Birt-Hogg-Dubé syndrome families (see later).

Angiomyolipoma

Angiomyolipomas (AML) are distinctive neoplasms composed of smooth muscle, adipose tissue, and vasculature in variable combinations (Figure 17.31). Though most commonly found in the kidneys, they may occur at extrarenal sites including liver, lungs, lymph nodes, and retroperitoneal soft tissues [13,52,53]. Although fewer than half of all cases occur in patients with tuberous sclerosis, approximately 80 percent of patients with tuberous sclerosis develop an AML. AML is related to a family of mesenchymal tumors that include lymphangioleiomyomatosis, clear cell "sugar" tumors of the lung, pancreas and uterus, and cardiac rhabdomyomas [54]. All these are immunoreactive with the melanocytic marker antibody HMB-45 [10,13].

Tumors composed predominantly of adipose tissue may be confused with well-differentiated liposarcoma (Figure 17.32), whereas smooth muscle–dominant tumors may be mistaken for leiomyosarcoma or sarcomatoid RCC (Figure 17.33). The majority are unilateral and unifocal. The presence of bilateral or multifocal tumors strongly suggests the diagnosis of tuberous sclerosis. Microscopically, greater than 90 percent of tumors contain at least focal areas of mature adipose tissue [55]. The smooth muscle cells often appear to originate and radiate from vessel walls. The morphology of the vascular component is variable. Thickened and hyalinized vessels with eccentric lumens are seen in most cases. Mitotic activity is rare.

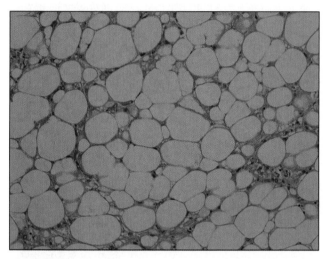

FIGURE 17.32: *Angiomyolipoma, fat predominant. Because of occasional nuclear atypia and cells mimicking lipoblasts, these tumors sometimes may be mistaken for well-differentiated liposarcoma.*

The epithelioid variant of AML is composed either exclusively or predominantly of polygonal cells with densely eosinophilic cytoplasm. Variable degrees of nuclear atypia are seen, including cells with multilobulated nuclei and multinucleated forms (Figure 17.34). Extensive intratumoral hemorrhage and necrosis are more common in the epithelioid variant than in others. Rare examples of AML composed predominantly of epithelioid cells with densely eosinophilic cytoplasm reminiscent of oncocytoma have been recently described under the rubric of renal epithelioid oxyphilic neoplasm (REON) [56] or oncocytoma-like AML [57]. We also believe that the tumors classified as "renal capsulomas," the spindle cell tumors arising from the renal capsule and frequently showing HMB 45 immunoreactivity, are smooth muscle–predominant AMLs.

Immunostains for antibodies to several melanoma-related antigens, including HMB-45 and A-103 (melan-A/MART-1), are positive, usually focally, in the majority of cases. Ultrastructural examination reveals spherical structures with internal lamellations, consistent with aberrant melanosomes, in a subset of cases. Rare type-2 premelanosomes and rhomboid crystals may also be seen [13].

The overwhelming majority of AML behave in a benign fashion. The primary complication is retroperitoneal hemorrhage, mostly associated with large tumors usually greater than 4 cm, which rarely can be fatal [13]. Renal failure may complicate massive bilateral disease, particularly in patients with tuberous sclerosis [58]. Invasion of contiguous organs occurs rarely and has resulted in death. Some patients with AML of the kidney also have AML involving noncontiguous sites, particularly regional lymph nodes. Most consider these cases to represent multifocal rather than metastatic disease. Rare acceptable examples of "sarcomatous transformation," as well as malignant AMLs with subsequent distant metastases, have been reported [59,60]. All cases with epithelioid histology should be considered potentially malignant especially in tumors with nuclear anaplasia, atypical mitotic activity, and geographic necrosis.

Recently, AMLs containing cuboidal- to hobnail-type cell-lined cysts, and presenting as cystic mass have been described, and these tumors have been designated as AML with epithelial cysts (AMLEC) [61].

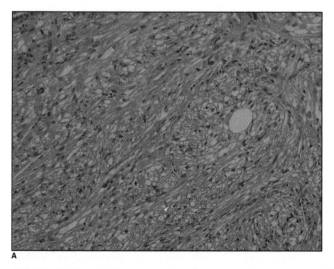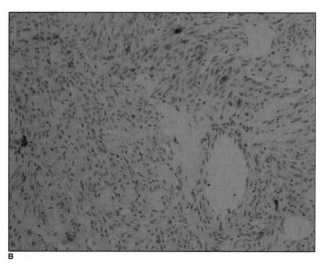

FIGURE 17.33: *Angiomyolipoma, smooth muscle predominant (A), with focal immunoreactivity for HMB-45 (B).*

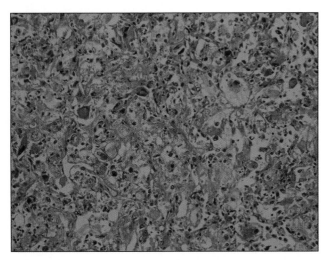

FIGURE 17.34:   Angiomyolipoma, epithelioid variant, marked nuclear pleomorphism.

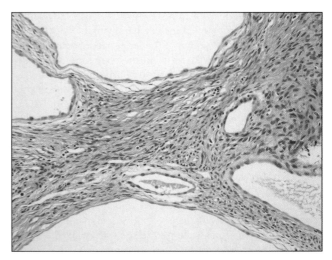

FIGURE 17.35:   Mixed epithelial and stromal tumor. Tubules are lined by hobnail cells and are intermixed with an ovarian-like stroma.

Mixed Epithelial and Stromal Tumor/Cystic Nephroma

These are multicystic to solid and cystic biphasic tumors that likely represent a morphologic spectrum of the same or similar entities; an encompassing name "renal epithelial and stromal tumor (REST)" has recently been proposed for both [62,63].

At one end of the morphologic spectrum of this entity is the mixed epithelial and stromal tumor (MEST). It is composed of mesenchymal (stromal) and epithelial components with a combination of solid and cystic areas in variable proportions. Females outnumber males by a ten to one margin. The stromal component most often resembles the classical form of pediatric mesoblastic nephroma or fibromatosis. In some cases, the mesenchymal component resembles ovarian stroma [62,63]. Mitotic figures, hemorrhage, and necrosis are uncommon. Mature adipose tissue and smooth muscle bundles have rarely been described in the mesenchymal component. The epithelial components vary from round and regular tubules to more complex structures that show papillations and cystic dilatation. They are lined by cuboidal to flattened epithelium that may show clear cell change or have a hobnail appearance (Figure 17.35). Positive reactions with antibodies to estrogen and progesterone receptors (ER and PR) in the mesenchymal component are common [62–64].

All reported cases of adult mixed epithelial and stromal tumors have behaved in a benign manner following surgical excision, though one recurred locally 21 years after resection [65]. The recurrent tumor invaded the liver and was composed exclusively of spindle cells.

Cystic nephroma, which forms the other end of the morphologic spectrum of these tumors, is composed of multiple, noncommunicating cysts of variable size, containing clear fluid, with relatively thin cyst walls. Definitionally, solid expansile areas or mural nodules are not found. The majority of affected adults with adult cystic nephroma are females, although some report an almost equal female to male occurrence [62,63]. Microscopically, the cysts are lined by flattened, cuboidal, or hobnail cells (similar to those in MEST) and the septa are composed of fibrous tissue of variable cellularity, at times having the appearance of ovarian-type stroma. The ovarian-type stroma frequently shows positive immunohistochemical reac-

tion for ER and PR. The fibrous septa may contain microscopic cysts lined by bland, cuboidal cells reminiscent of renal tubules. Sarcomas have been known to arise from cystic nephromas, although this is a rare occurrence. Most are undifferentiated embryonal-type tumors [66]. Recently, embryonal sarcomas arising in the background of cystic nephroma were found to have the SYT-SSX gene fusion resulting from the t(X;18), a characteristic of synovial sarcoma. These tumors have been redesignated as "primary renal synovial sarcomas" [67].

Metanephric Adenoma and Related Tumors

Metanephric adenoma and the closely related metanephric adenofibroma and metanephric stromal tumor (metanephric stromal tumor is described later in more detail) are recently characterized benign renal cortical neoplasms. Affected patients range in age from the first through the ninth decades of life with a female to male ratio of 2:1. Presenting signs and symptoms are similar to those associated with other renal mass lesions, but polycythemia has been reported in approximately 12 percent of the patients [68–71]. Cytogenetic studies have shown variable results, including normal karyotypes, trisomies of chromosomes 7 and 17, and loss of sex chromosomes, and more recently 2p losses [72].

Metanephric adenoma and metanephric adenofibroma are well-circumscribed cortical neoplasms that are most often not encapsulated, but are sharply demarcated from the surrounding renal parenchyma. On microscopic evaluation, metanephric adenoma is characterized by tightly packed small tubules separated by a modest amount of stroma (Figure 17.36). Papillary or glomeruloid components are seen in roughly half of the cases and are often associated with microcalcifications including psammoma bodies. Cytoplasm is scant and nuclei are small, round to ovoid, and may overlap. Nucleoli are typically inconspicuous and mitotic figures are rare. Multifocal tumors are rare and bilateral tumors have not been reported. Secondary changes including hyalinization, hemorrhage, and necrosis may be present. Metanephric adenofibroma is a biphasic neoplasm composed of an epithelial component identical to that of metanephric adenoma and a mesenchymal component consisting of bland,

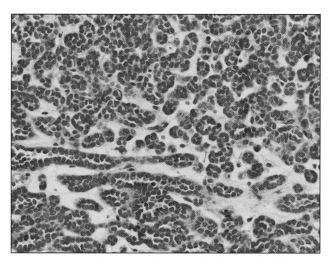

FIGURE 17.36: *Metanephric adenoma showing the characteristic tightly packed small tubules separated by a modest amount of stroma. The nuclei are uniform, without any prominent nucleoli.*

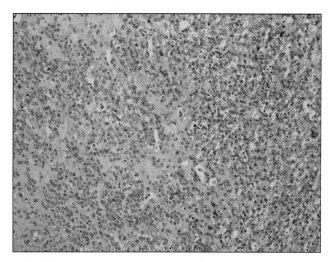

FIGURE 17.37: *Juxtaglomerular cell tumor with uniform cells resembling a glomus tumor, prominent vascularity, and dispersed lymphoplasmacytic infiltrates.*

fibroblast-like cells arranged in interlacing fascicles with focal hyalinization and myxoid change [71].

On immunohistochemical staining, epithelial components of metanephric adenoma and adenofibroma are positive for pancytokeratin and CD57, and Wilms tumor 1 antibody (WT-1) in some cases [73]. Positive reactions with epithelial membrane antigen (EMA) are uncommon and usually confined to papillary/cystic areas. Stromal component in each is positive for vimentin, and is CD34-positive in metanephric stromal tumor. Electron microscopy shows variable numbers of microvilli and few cytoplasmic organelles consisting mainly of free ribosomes and mitochondria in the epithelial components.

Wilms tumor and papillary renal carcinoma are important considerations in the differential diagnosis. In contrast to Wilms tumor, metanephric adenoma shows minimal mitotic activity, and is composed of bland cells with small nuclei. No blastemal elements or nephrogenic rests are present. Metanephric adenoma is often CD57-positive, whereas Wilms tumor is negative. Distinguishing some cases of papillary RCC from metanephric adenoma may pose a more difficult diagnostic challenge. Unlike metanephric adenoma, papillary RCC frequently contains numerous foamy histiocytes, and is multifocal in up to half of the cases. Nuclear atypia, prominent nucleoli, and well-formed capsule are not the features of metanephric adenoma. On immunohistochemical staining, papillary RCC is usually AMACR- and CK7-positive, whereas metanephric adenoma is usually diffusely positive for CD57, and usually negative or only focally positive for AMACR and CK7 [73].

Juxtaglomerular Cell Tumor

Juxtaglomerular cell tumor is an extremely uncommon renal tumor of young adults (in second and third decades of life); very few cases have been described in the sixth and seventh decades [10,13]. Signs and symptoms of hyperreninism are the hallmark of juxtaglomerular cell tumor and include hypertension, hyperaldosteronism, and hypokalemia. Females outnumber males by a roughly 1.5:1 margin. Juxtaglomerular cell tumors are well-encapsulated, light tan to yellow, unilateral, and solitary tumors.

Most are solid though small cysts may be present. The majority of the tumors are relatively small, ranging in diameter from 2 to 3 cm. The histologic appearance is variable. The classical examples have a glomus tumor–like appearance and are composed of sheets of homogeneous round to polygonal cells with clear to slightly eosinophilic cytoplasm and distinct cell borders (Figure 17.37). Others consist of sheets or irregular cords of polygonal to spindle cells with indistinct cell borders. Numerous capillaries and branching blood vessels and sinusoids similar to those of hemangiopericytoma are typically found. The stroma may be scanty or consist of large areas of hyalinized or myxoid fibrous tissue and often contains a scattered lymphoplasmacytic infiltrate. Some tumors contain well-developed tubules. A papillary pattern has been described in which the neoplastic cells form papillary fronds lined by cuboidal cells [74]. Pleomorphism and mitotic activity are uncommon.

Periodic acid-Schiff (PAS) stain reveals cytoplasmic granules in a subset of cells. Immunohistochemistry (IHC) shows diffuse positive staining with antibodies to renin and vimentin. Variable number of common muscle actin (HHF-35)-, and smooth muscle actin-positive cells may be found, whereas neuroendocrine markers are negative. Cytokeratin stains label the cuboidal epithelium of the tubules but not the polygonal or spindle cells. Recently, Kim et al. reported CD34 and CD117 to be diffusely positive in five of five tumors they stained [75]. Electron microscopy shows distinctive membrane-bound rhomboid and polygonal granules that are immunoreactive with antibodies to renin.

Juxtaglomerular cell tumors are benign neoplasms. Surgical resection of the affected kidney cures systemic hypertension in most patients.

Medullary Fibroma (Renomedullary Interstitial Cell Tumor)

Medullary fibroma (renomedullary interstitial cell tumor) is most often an incidental finding in nephrectomies performed for other reasons, or at autopsy [10,13,76]. An association between multiple medullary fibromas and systemic hypertension has been reported. Grossly, they are well circumscribed, tan to white,

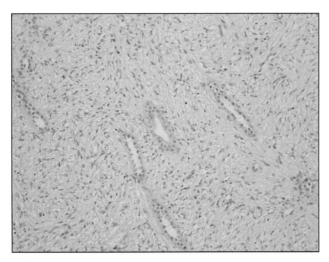

FIGURE 17.38: *Medullary fibroma/renomedullary interstitial cell tumor.*

and found within the renal medulla. Most measure fewer than 5 mm in greatest dimension. Microscopically, they consist of bland stellate cells set within a loose to densely sclerotic collagenous background (Figure 17.38). Entrapped tubules may be seen at the periphery of the nodules.

Miscellaneous Tumors

Carcinoid Tumor

Carcinoid tumor of the kidney is a very rare tumor and fewer than eighty cases have been described in the literature [10,13]. Before accepting a tumor as primary carcinoid tumor of the kidney, it is imperative to exclude the possibility of a metastasis from other sources. In a case of renal carcinoid tumor with vascular invasion, such a possibility is more likely, and the primary source may become apparent only after prolonged follow-up. Most cases are discovered incidentally following radiological investigation for other diseases; overt endocrine disturbances, including the carcinoid syndrome, are uncommon. Morphologically, they are similar to carcinoids found at other sites, with nested or trabecular architecture supported by a well-vascularized stroma, and the characteristic "salt and pepper" appearance of generally uniform, round nuclei. Though focal pleomorphism may be seen, mitotic figures and vascular invasion are uncommon. Diffuse infiltration of renal parenchyma is not a feature of renal carcinoid, though invasion of perinephric adipose tissue and renal vein have been described. Interestingly, a number of examples have been described in horseshoe kidneys. Rare cases have been described as components of cystic teratoma of the kidney [77]. By IHC, renal carcinoids show positive reactions to neuron-specific enolase (NSE), chromogranin, synaptophysin, serotonin, somatostatin, pancreatic polypeptide, and glucagon. Like hindgut carcinoids, positive reactions to prostatic acid phosphatase (PSAP) have been reported [78]. Electron microscopy confirms the presence of dense core granules. In the largest series to date of twenty-one cases, fifteen cases had metastases to regional lymph nodes, liver, lung, and bone at presentation

[79]. However, only one patient died of disease within eight months of diagnosis. Like carcinoids found elsewhere, histologic features do not predict outcome. However, rare studies show that mitotic activity and pleomorphism may be associated with an aggressive behavior [13].

Other Neuroendocrine Neoplasms

Primary renal small cell carcinoma, pheochromocytoma, and neuroblastoma have been described. Small cell carcinomas are large, locally invasive neoplasms that often present with regional or distant metastases. Before accepting a tumor as a primary small cell carcinoma of the kidney, the possibility of a metastasis must be excluded [10,13].

Hematologic Malignancies

Malignant lymphoma rarely presents as a primary extranodal renal neoplasm. More often, renal involvement is secondary and seen as a component of late-stage, generalized malignant lymphoma. However, even in the setting of generalized disease, clinical manifestations referable to renal involvement are exceptional. This is remarkable given that autopsy confirmation of renal parenchymal extension is seen in as many as 50 percent of patients with non-Hodgkin's lymphomas [13]. Grossly, primary renal lymphoma most often consists of a solitary, large, well-circumscribed intrarenal or hilar mass, and less often of diffuse parenchymal infiltration. Histologically, the majority are either large-cell or small, noncleaved-cell type. Examples of renal plasmacytoma have also been described [10,13]. Renal involvement by leukemia is most often bilateral and diffuse and only rarely results in renal failure or is the presenting site of disease [13].

Hereditary Forms of Renal Tumors

The majority of renal neoplasms are sporadic, although a small percentage may be hereditary, such as clear cell RCC associated with VHL disease. In all forms of inherited renal neoplasms, tumors are more likely to be diagnosed at an earlier age and are more likely to be multifocal and bilateral. VHL disease is an autosomal dominant syndrome characterized by retinal hemangiomas, clear cell (conventional) RCCs, multiple renal cysts, cerebellar and spinal hemangioblastomas, pheochromocytomas, endocrine pancreatic tumors, and epididymal cystadenomas. The tumor suppressor *VHL* gene is located at chromosome 3p25, and can be inactivated by various mutations, loss of heterozygosity, hypermethylation, or alterations in *VHL* modifier genes. Lack of normal VHL protein increases HIF-1α levels resulting in overexpression of endothelial growth factors and culminating in a hypervascular state seen in most VHL-related tumors, and possible tumorigenesis. Other familial non-VHL clear cell (conventional) RCCs have been reported, most of which involve translocations of chromosome 3 including 3p14 (fragile histidine triad, FHIT), 3q13.3, and 3q21 genes, whereas a few others do not involve chromosome 3.

Hereditary forms of papillary RCC are sometimes associated with tumors of the breast, pancreas, lung, skin, and stomach. The syndrome is associated with activating mutations of *c-MET* proto-oncogene at chromosome 7q34. Upregulation of the gene results in the activation of a heterodimeric membrane-spanning tyrosine kinase involved in angiogenesis, cellular motility, growth, invasion, and cellular differentiation.

The renal tumors with trisomy 7 in this syndrome have been shown to harbor *c-MET* mutations in 2 of the chromosome copies.

Birt-Hogg-Dubé syndrome (BHD) is another syndrome recently recognized to be related to multifocal and bilateral renal tumors. This autosomal dominant syndrome is characterized by cutaneous lesions (fibrofolliculomas, trichodiscomas, and acrochordons), spontaneous pneumothorax, bronchiectasis, bronchospasms, colonic neoplasms, and lipomas, which occur in conjunction with the renal tumors. The associated renal tumors have been variably reported as renal oncocytomas, chromophobe RCC, hybrid oncocytic tumors with features of both oncocytoma and chromophobe RCC, or tumors with some unusual morphologic features. The *BHD* gene has been mapped to chromosome 17p12-q11.2, and the exact mode of tumorigenesis is not yet elucidated. Of families identified with familial renal oncocytoma, a number of these have been subsequently found to have BHD syndrome. Rarely a constitutional reciprocal translocation between 8q24.1 and 9q34.3 has been reported in cases of bilateral, multifocal renal oncocytoma.

PEDIATRIC RENAL TUMORS

Staging

Table 17.2 presents the staging system currently used by the Children's Oncology Group (COG) for the vast majority of pediatric renal neoplasms (Wilms tumor, clear cell sarcoma of the kidney, and rhabdoid tumor of the kidney). This system is very similar to that used in National Wilms Tumor Study-5 (NWTS-5) (1995–2002) [80,81]. Two relatively minor changes distinguish the current COG staging criteria from the prior NWTS-5 criteria. First, localized spillage or rupture, or any form of biopsy before removal of the kidney, is no longer considered stage II but instead is considered stage III. Second, several protocols that reduce therapy for stage I tumors require that regional nodes are examined microscopically. These protocols allow avoidance of adjuvant chemotherapy for young patients (<2 years) with small (<550g nephrectomy weight) stage I favorable histology Wilms tumor, and no radiation therapy for stage I clear cell sarcoma of the kidney. If lymph nodes are not identified by the pathologist, children who would otherwise qualify for these protocols will be ineligible.

Table 17.3 lists the most common renal neoplasms of childhood, along with their prevalence.

Wilms Tumor (Nephroblastoma)

Wilms tumor (WT) is the most common pediatric renal neoplasm. Its peak incidence is between 2 and 5 years. Several dysmorphic syndromes predispose to the development of WT; these are listed in Table 17.4. The most common sites of metastases are regional lymph nodes, lungs, and liver ("the three Ls"). Overall survival has progressively improved and now exceeds 90 percent.

WT typically forms a unicentric, spherical mass that is sharply demarcated from the renal parenchyma [82]. Approximately 5 to 6 percent of WT are bilateral at presentation. The cut surface of WT frequently shows prominent septa that impart a multinodular appearance. Scattered cysts are commonly encountered in conventional WT, but rarely the encapsulated, well-delineated neoplasm is composed entirely of cystic spaces and delicate septa, without an expansile solid component. For neoplasms that are entirely composed of mature cells, the term

Table 17.2 Staging of Pediatric Renal Neoplasms (Children's Oncology Group)

Stage	
Stage I	*Tumor is limited to kidney and is completely resected* Renal capsule intact, not penetrated by tumor No tumor invasion of veins or lymphatics of renal sinus No nodal or hematogenous metastases No prior biopsy Negative margins
Stage II	*Tumor extends beyond kidney but completely resected* Tumor penetrates renal capsule Tumor in lymphatics or veins of renal sinus Tumor in renal vein with margin not involved No nodal or hematogenous metastases Negative margins
Stage III	*Residual tumor or nonhematogenous metastases confined to abdomen* Involved abdominal nodes Peritoneal contamination or tumor implant Tumor spillage of any degree occurring before or during surgery Gross residual tumor in abdomen Biopsy of tumor (including fine needle aspiration) prior to removal of kidney Resection margins involved by tumor
Stage IV	*Hematogenous metastases or spread beyond abdomen*
Stage V	*Bilateral renal tumors* Each side's tumor should be substaged separately according to the above criteria [e.g., stage V, substage II (right), substage I (left)]

Table 17.3 Primary Renal Neoplasms of Childhood

Tumor	Frequency
Wilms tumor	
Favorable histology	80%
Anaplastic	4%
Congenital mesoblastic nephroma	3%
Clear cell sarcoma of the kidney	3%
Rhabdoid tumor of the kidney	2%
Miscellaneous	8%
Lymphoma, angiomyolipoma, renal cell carcinoma, Ewing's sarcoma/primitive neuroectodermal tumor, metanephric stromal tumor, etc.	

Table 17.4 Congenital Syndromes Associated with Wilms Tumor (From NEJM 331;586–590, 1991)

Syndrome	Characteristics	Chromosome Locus	Genetic Alteration	Risk of Wilms tumor
WAGR	Wilms tumor, aniridia, genitourinary malformations, and mental retardation	11p13	Monoallelic 11p13 deletion involving *WT-1* gene	>30%
Denys-Drash	Intersexual disorders, nephropathy, and Wilms tumor	11p13	*WT-1* point mutation	>90%
Beckwith-Wiedemann	Macroglossia, organomegaly, hemihypertrophy, neonatal hyperglycemia, and several embryonal tumors	11p15	Duplication of paternal allele	<5%

is "cystic nephroma" (CN). These CNs in children, although bearing some morphologic resemblances, clinicopathologically show significant differences from those in the adults. If the septa contain embryonal-cell types, the designation cystic partially differentiated nephroblastoma (CPDN) is appropriate. In contrast, cystic WT is distinguished by the presence of solid, expansile regions that replace or distort the cystic spaces, rather than being passively molded by the cysts. CPDN may be a transitional stage in the development of pediatric CN, and these lesions seem to represent a cystic, highly favorable end of the WT spectrum [83].

Most WTs exhibit, at least focally, the triphasic appearance, including cells of blastemal, stromal, and epithelial lineage (Figure 17.39). However, monophasic and biphasic WTs are relatively common, consisting of only one or two of these cell lineages. Each of the three major cell types can demonstrate a spectrum of patterns and degrees of differentiation.

The blastemal cells of WT are small, tightly packed, round blue cells with a high nucleus-to-cytoplasm ratio. Their nuclei have moderately coarse chromatin, and the nucleoli are relatively inconspicuous. Blastemal cells form several distinctive aggregation patterns, which can be divided into two broad categories, diffuse and nested, based on their structure and degree of invasiveness. The diffuse blastemal pattern is the most consistently aggressive pattern of WT; the majority of diffuse blastemal WTs present at advanced stage, stage III or IV [84]. The diffuse blastemal pattern can be readily confused with other small, blue cell tumors of childhood and ultrastructural or other special studies may be required to establish the correct diagnosis (Figure 17.40). Nested blastemal patterns refer to sharply outlined clusters of blastemal cells in a myxoid mesenchymal background. They usually lack the invasive behavior seen with the diffuse blastemal pattern, and these neoplasms have sharply defined margins.

Epithelial differentiation in WT produces a variety of cell types and degrees of differentiation. Most of these recapitulate events in normal nephrogenesis (homologous differentiation), such as tubular or glomerular differentiation. Others, such as squamous differentiation or mucinous differentiation, do not occur in the normal kidney at any stage of development (heterologous differentiation). Immature myxoid and spindled mesenchymal cells are the most common stromal-cell types seen in WTs. Skeletal muscle is the most common heterologous-cell

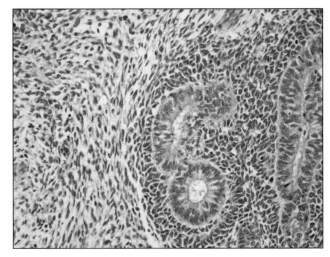

FIGURE 17.39: *Wilms tumor, favorable histology, triphasic pattern. Epithelial, stromal, and blastemal components are evident.*

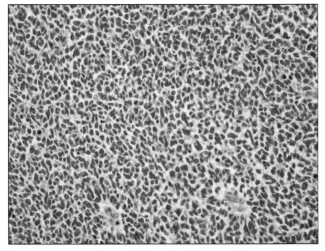

FIGURE 17.40: *Wilms tumor, favorable histology, diffuse blastemal pattern. The tumor shows the predominant component of primitive blastemal tissue.*

type. In fact, the presence of skeletal muscle in a pediatric renal neoplasm is very strong evidence supporting the diagnosis of WT.

Approximately 5 percent of WTs demonstrate anaplasia, the only criterion of "unfavorable histology" [85]. All WTs lacking this feature are designated as having "favorable histology." Anaplastic nuclear change reflects extreme polyploidy and is usually apparent under low magnification (10× objective). The features of anaplasia include: (a) markedly enlarged tumor-cell nuclei with increased chromatin content (hyperchromasia), and (b) multipolar mitotic figures (Figure 17.41). The former criteria reflect polyploidy, whereas the latter criterion helps exclude degenerative nuclear changes, as are commonly seen in cells showing skeletal muscle differentiation, from the anaplastic category. Anaplasia is tightly correlated with the presence of *p53* gene mutations [86]. At a practical level, p53 protein overexpression by IHC correlates well but not perfectly with morphologically defined anaplasia [87].

The definition of focal anaplasia (FA) includes only those WTs meeting all of the following criteria:

1. Anaplasia is confined to one or more discrete sites within the primary tumor and not present in extrarenal sites. This emphasizes the importance of mapping the sections taken from a WT, best done on a photograph of a cut section of the tumor.

2. Tumor cells outside anaplastic foci show no "nuclear unrest" (nuclear or mitotic abnormalities that approach, but do not quite attain the severity required for a designation of anaplasia).

Any WT not meeting this definition of FA is designated as having diffuse anaplasia (DA) [88].

Chemotherapy usually results in massive necrosis of immature and actively proliferating cell types in WT, whereas slowly replicating and differentiated cell types are usually unaffected. The presence of actively proliferating tumor (particularly blastema) after chemotherapy indicates resistance and indicates a diminished prognosis. Cells with anaplasia are generally unaffected by chemotherapy and have the same significance as in untreated WT [89].

Ultrastructural study is rarely necessary to establish a diagnosis of WT but can occasionally be very helpful in distinguishing blastemal WT from other undifferentiated neoplasms [90]. The diversity of differentiation in WT creates a correspondingly varied immunohistochemical profile. Blastemal cells may or may not label for vimentin and cytokeratin, whereas various differentiating elements will label according to their patterns of differentiation. WT blastemal cells characteristically label for desmin but not for actin, myogenin, or other muscle markers [91]. Immunoreactivity for WT-1 protein is typically limited to the blastemal and epithelial components of WT, with the stroma being negative [92]. The tumors are usually positive for PAX-2.

In more than 30 percent of kidneys resected for WT, the renal parenchyma contains one or more regions of persistent embryonal tissue [nephrogenic rests (NRs)] that represent potential precursors of WT [93]. The presence of multiple or diffusely distributed NRs is termed nephroblastomatosis. Two fundamental categories of NRs are recognized, based on their topographic relation to the renal lobe. These are designated perilobar nephrogenic rests (PLNRs) and intralobar nephrogenic rests (ILNRs). ILNRs may occur anywhere in the renal lobe, including the peripheral cortex. ILNR are often stroma-rich but have a more varied structure than do PLNRs and typically intercolate between nephrons (Figure 17.42), whereas PLNRs are usually composed of blastemal and primitive tubular cells that are well delineated from adjacent nephrons (Figure 17.43). These features are summarized in Table 17.5. Rests of either major category may be further classified based on their developmental fates. An individual NR may remain dormant, undergo sclerosis/obsolescence, hyperplasia, or neoplastic transformation of WT. Very rarely, anaplasia may develop in nephrogenic rests [94]. An individual rest commonly progresses through several of these processes sequentially.

The presence of NRs in a kidney removed for WT is correlated with an increased risk for subsequent WT formation in the remaining kidney. The type of rest and age of the patient

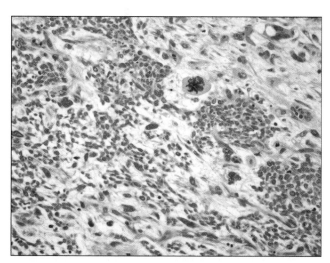

FIGURE 17.41: *Wilms tumor, anaplastic. Pleomorphism, atypical mitosis, and nuclear enlargement are noted.*

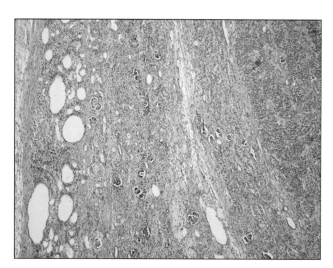

FIGURE 17.42: *Intralobar nephrogenic rest (ILNR) with interstitial location and intermingling with normal nephronic elements.*

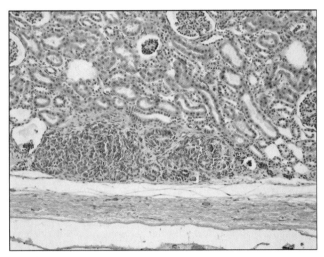

FIGURE 17.43: *Perilobar nephrogenic rest (PLNR) is noted at the periphery of the renal lobule, hence, located on the surface.*

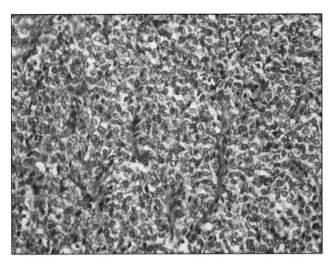

FIGURE 17.44: *Clear cell sarcoma of the kidney (CCSK). Neoplastic cells are separated by clear spaces and contain nuclei with finely dispersed chromatin and regularly spaced fibrovascular septae.*

Table 17.5 Nephrogenic Rests

	Perilobar Nephrogenic Rests	Intralobar Nephrogenic Rests
Site	Peripheral	Random, often deep
Margins	Sharp	Indistinct, entraps nephrons
Predominant composition	Blastema, tubular epithelium	Stroma
Number	Often multiple	Often single
Syndromic association	Beckwith-Wiedemann	WAGR, Denys-Drash

modify this risk [95]. When a carefully sampled kidney is free of rests, the risk of contralateral WT is extremely low.

Clear Cell Sarcoma of the Kidney

Clear cell sarcoma of the kidney (CCSK) comprises about 3 percent of pediatric renal tumors, and is included in the "unfavorable histology" category. CCSK metastases occur in a variety of sites that would be unusual for WT, including bone, brain, and soft tissue. Recurrences may be delayed, occurring decades after diagnosis. Prognosis has been improved by the addition of doxorubicin to chemotherapy regimens [96].

CCSK is always unicentric. The cut surface is often glistening and gelatinous. Under low magnification, most CCSKs appear monomorphous, without the prominent lobulation usually seen in WT. CCSK usually has a scalloped border that appears fairly sharp under low power. Under higher magnification, the neoplastic cells penetrate a short distance into the surrounding kidney, surrounding and isolating individual single nephrons. The entrapped tubules are usually confined to the peripheral 2–3 cm of a CCSK. Their epithelium commonly shows cystic change or embryonal metaplasia, with the resultant basophilic epithelium creating confusion with WT.

The hallmark of the classic pattern of CCSK is an evenly distributed network of vascular *septa*, which has a branching, "chicken-wire" pattern similar to that seen in myxoid liposarcoma or oligodendroglioma. These fibrovascular septa subdivide the tumor into a pattern of *cords* or nests, averaging six to ten cells in width, composed of polygonal cells. Nuclear chromatin is usually finely granular, with inconspicuous nucleoli (Figure 17.44). In well-fixed specimens, the fine nuclear chromatin pattern is the most helpful clue to the diagnosis. The cytoplasm usually lacks distinct borders and is surrounded by extracellular mucopolysaccharide, which creates the illusion of clear cytoplasm.

CCSK is easily confused with other neoplasms because the classic pattern is often modified. Fortunately, the classic pattern of CCSK predominates in most specimens and is present at least focally in greater than 90 percent of tumors. These variant patterns are described in the following discussion. Condensation of cord cells of the classic CCSK pattern creates striking *epithelioid* arrangements. These condensations usually form trabeculae or rosettes. In all of the examples analyzed by IHC, these epithelioid formations have been negative for epithelial markers, in contrast to the epithelial cells of WT. *Spindle* cell patterns often resemble the storiform patterns seen with fibrohistiocytic neoplasms. In the *myxoid* pattern of CCSK, mucopolysaccharide occupies more volume than the neoplastic cells themselves and forms large pools. In time, the mucoid material becomes denser, eosinophilic, and hyaline in appearance. Hyaline *sclerosis* surrounding individual tumor cells may create an osteosarcoma-like appearance. Dense stromal sclerosis is relatively uncommon in untreated WT, and this finding can be a clue to the diagnosis of CCSK or rhabdoid tumor in limited biopsy material. Nuclear *palisading* may resemble schwannoma. Unlike schwannomas, these areas are not immunoreactive for S-100 protein. Rarely, CCSK have an *anaplastic* pattern, consisting of foci with enlarged, pleomorphic nuclei and bizarre mitotic figures, resembling the appearance of anaplastic WTs. This is the only pattern of CCSK that frequently overexpresses p53 protein [96].

Recurrences of CCSK after therapy may have a deceptively hypocellular and bland appearance, suggesting low-grade fibromatosis or myxoma. A lump appearing anywhere in a child with a history of CCSK should be viewed as a potential metastasis until proven otherwise.

Ultrastructurally, CCSK [97] tumor cells are characterized by a high nucleus-to-cytoplasm ratio. The cytoplasm is usually tenuous, with elongated, irregular processes surrounding abundant intercellular matrix. This latter feature is responsible for the vacuoles often seen with the light microscope. IHC helps exclude various potential lines of differentiation for CCSK. Vimentin is positive in nearly all specimens and bcl-2 in some, but other markers are consistently negative. These include stains for epithelial markers (cytokeratins and EMA), neural markers (S100 protein), neuroendocrine markers (chromogranin, synaptophysin), muscle markers (desmin), CD34, and CD99 (MIC2).

Congenital Mesoblastic Nephroma

Congenital mesoblastic nephroma (CMN) is the most common pediatric renal neoplasm in the first three months of life: 90 percent are diagnosed in the first year of life. Most cases are cured by nephrectomy alone; however, recurrences and/or metastases occur in 5 percent of cases. CMN is usually unicentric and located deep within the medial parenchyma, near the renal sinus. The renal sinus and adjacent structures on the medial side of the kidney are major sites of extrarenal spread of CMN. Surgeons and pathologists must pay particular attention to the medial margin of the CMN resection specimen. The appearance of the sectioned surface of CMN is variable and depends upon the subtype. Classic CMNs have a tough, whorled appearance resembling leiomyoma, but cellular CMNs may be soft, friable tumors.

CMNs are low-grade fibroblastic sarcomas of the infantile kidney. Morphologically, classic CMN is identical to infantile fibromatosis; it is composed of bland fibroblastic/myofibroblastic cells, arranged in fascicles that dissect into the native kidney (Figure 17.45) [98]. Mitoses are usually rare, and necrosis is absent. Entrapped renal tubules may acquire a primitive appearance (embryonal metaplasia). In contrast, the cellular variant of CMN is identical to infantile fibrosarcoma (IFS) [99]. Compared to the classic variant, cellular CMNs more often have a "pushing" border, demonstrate sheet-like growth patterns, are less often fascicular, are more cellular, and have a higher mitotic rate (Figure 17.46). Tumor cells may be polygonal with well-demarcated pink cytoplasm and nuclei with vesicular chromatin and prominent nucleoli; this raises the differential diagnosis of rhabdoid tumor of the kidney. Alternatively, the tumor cells may be thinner, primitive, and spindled, yielding a more embryonal "blue cell" appearance. Mixed CMNs have areas identical to both cellular and classic CMN in varied proportions.

By IHC, the cells of CMN label in a fashion consistent with fibroblasts or myofibroblasts. Although actin may be focally positive, desmin and CD34 are typically negative (P. Argani, unpublished observations). INI1 protein is retained. Ultrastructural studies also reveal features consistent with fibroblasts or myofibroblasts [100]. Most CMN cells show abundant rough endoplasmic reticulum (RER) with branching and anastomosing profiles, and primitive cell junctions are often found.

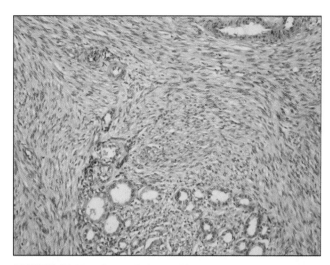

FIGURE 17.45: *Congenital mesoblastic nephroma, classic type. Renal elements are entrapped by interlacing bundles of spindle cells.*

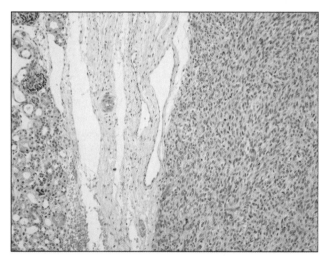

FIGURE 17.46: *Congenital mesoblastic nephroma, cellular type. There is increased cellular density by clumped cells with vesicular nuclei and scant to moderate amount of cytoplasm.*

IFS and cellular CMN are characterized by a specific t(12;15)(p13;q25). The t(12;15) results in fusion of the *ETV6* gene on chromosome 12 with the *NTRK3* gene on chromosome 15 [101–103]. The chimeric ETV6-NTRK3 protein is postulated to be constitutively dimerized and therefore affects constitutively active tyrosine kinase growth pathway signaling. Importantly, infantile fibromatosis, classic CMN, or adult type fibrosarcomas do not contain this gene fusion. Hence, one may consider cellular CMN to be essentially an IFS of the renal sinus. Additionally, these data highlight the fact that classic and cellular CMN are molecularly distinctive neoplasms. An analogy between infantile fibroblastic tumors of the soft tissue and kidney may be drawn (Table 17.6) [103].

Table 17.6 Analogous Infantile Fibroblastic Neoplasms of Kidney and Soft Tissue

Kidney	Soft Tissue
Classic congenital mesoblastic nephroma	Infantile fibromatosis
Cellular congenital mesoblastic nephroma	Infantile fibrosarcoma
Mixed congenital mesoblastic nephroma	Composite fibromatosis

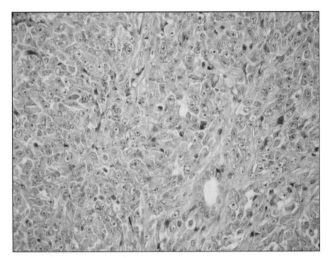

FIGURE 17.47: *Rhabdoid tumor of the kidney (RTK). The tumor cells are large with occasional pale cytoplasmic inclusions and large nuclei containing prominent nucleoli.*

Rhabdoid Tumor of the Kidney

Rhabdoid tumor of the kidney (RTK) comprises 2 percent of pediatric renal neoplasms. RTK tends to affect infants (median age is thirteen months), and, typically proves to be lethal despite all therapy in greater than 80 percent of cases. Fifteen percent of the cases are associated with primitive neuroectodermal tumor (PNET) of the posterior fossa midline of the central nervous system. Most RTKs are relatively small, because metastasis occurs early in the neoplasm's evolution. On gross examination, RTK is a typically fleshy or hemorrhagic neoplasm, with ill-defined borders and frequent satellite nodules that reflect the tumor's highly invasive nature [104].

Microscopically, RTK typically engulfs native renal elements at its periphery, and demonstrates extensive vascular invasion. RTK classically consists of sheets of monotonous cells featuring a characteristic cytologic triad: vesicular chromatin, prominent nucleoli, and hyaline cytoplasmic inclusions (Figure 17.47). These features are variably well developed within a given tumor, so that one may need to examine multiple microscopic fields from many sections to find them.

Ultrastructurally, the cytoplasmic inclusions correspond to whorled intermediate filaments [105]. The whorled filaments may trap antibodies used for IHC, yielding a nonspecific poly-phenotypic pattern. With this caveat, strong vimentin and focal EMA labeling are characteristic. Recently, an immunohisto-chemical assay for INI1 protein has become available. Loss of INI1 protein expression reflects *INI1* genetic status and is a sensitive and specific marker for RTK [106].

The diagnosis of RTK is often challenging because a wide variety of renal and extrarenal tumors of adult and children may feature fully developed "rhabdoid" cytology, at least focally [107,108]. In general, thorough sampling of such tumors is most helpful, as it typically reveals specific differentiation that excludes RTK. Additionally, the age of the patient is very helpful, since RTK is seen within early childhood. Finally, loss of INI1 protein expression by IHC is highly specific for RTK.

Metanephric Stromal Tumor

Many tumors previously considered to be CMNs in children above the age of three are in fact distinct from CMN, and represent the newly recognized entity, metanephric stromal tumor (MST) [109]. MST is identical to the stromal component of metanephric adenofibroma (MAF) [110] (previously known as nephrogenic adenofibroma) [71], a biphasic tumor containing an epithelial component that is identical to metanephric adenoma (MA). MST is a benign lesion composed of spindled to stellate cells featuring thin hyperchromatic nuclei, and thin indistinct cytoplasmic extensions. Several of the characteristic features of MST distinguish it from CMN. MST characteristically surrounds and entraps renal tubules and blood vessels to form concentric "onionskin" rings or collarettes around these structures. Most MSTs induce angiodysplasia of entrapped arterioles, consisting of epithelioid transformation of medial smooth muscle and myxoid change. One-fourth of MSTs feature juxtaglomerular cell hyperplasia within entrapped glomeruli, which may occasionally lead to hypertension associated with hyperreninism. Finally, unlike CMN, MSTs are typically immunoreactive for CD34, but labeling may be patchy.

Pediatric Renal Cell Carcinoma

Most pediatric RCCs correspond to the distinctive neoplastic entities described below.

Xp11.2 Translocation Renal Cell Carcinomas

RCCs with chromosome translocations involving Xp11.2 and resulting gene fusions involving the *TFE3* transcription factor gene were officially recognized in the 2004 WHO renal tumor classification [111]. One distinctive subtype bears a t(X;17)(p11;q25), which results in the identical *ASPL-TFE3* gene fusion as was initially identified in alveolar soft part sarcoma (ASPS), and has been designated the *ASPL-TFE3* RCC [112]. Other subtypes are listed in Table 17.7. Approximately 10–15 percent of children with translocation RCC have previously been exposed to chemotherapy [113].

A papillary carcinoma comprised of clear cells with prominent psammoma bodies is the most distinctive histopathologic appearance of Xp11.2 translocation RCC (Figure 17.48), since this combination is uncommon in other defined types of renal carcinomas. However, the Xp11.2 translocation RCCs often have nested architecture, and often contain cells with granular eosinophilic cytoplasm [114]. Xp11.2 translocation RCC

Table 17.7 MiTF/TFE Translocation Neoplasms

Gene Fusion	Chromosome Translocation	Age (Years)	Tumor
ASPL-TFE3	der(17)t(X;17)(p11.2;q25)	5–40	ASPS
ASPL-TFE3	t(X;17)(p11.2;q25)	2–68	RCC
PRCC-TFE3	t(X;1)(p11.2;q21)	2–70	RCC
PSF-TFE3	t(X;1)(p11.2;p34)	5–68	RCC
NoNo-TFE3	inv(X)(p11;q12)	39	RCC
CLTC-TFE3	t(X;17)(p11.2;q23)	14	RCC
Alpha-TFEB	t(6;11)(p21;q12)	6–53	RCC

ASPS, alveolar soft part sarcoma; RCC, renal cell carcinoma; ASPL, alveolar soft part sarcoma locus; CLTC, clathrin heavy chain gene.

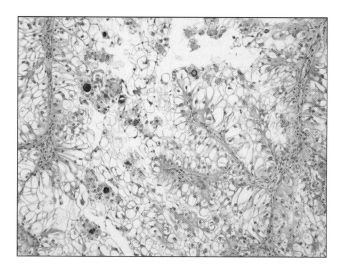

FIGURE 17.48: *Xp11.2 translocation renal cell carcinoma. The cytoplasm is voluminous pale to clear. Calcifications are noted.*

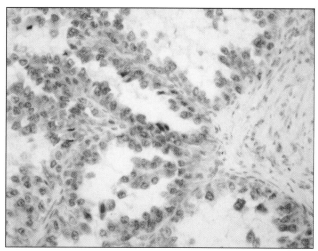

FIGURE 17.49: *Xp11.2 translocation renal cell carcinoma, TFE3 immunohistochemistry. Immunoreactivity is nuclear in location.*

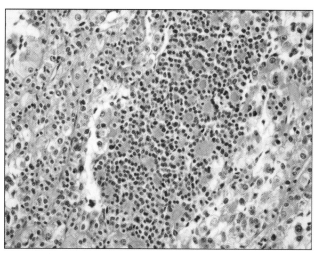

FIGURE 17.50: *Renal cell carcinoma with t(6;11) (p12;q12) translocation. Nests of tumor show two cell types, the larger at the periphery and the smaller cells in the center surrounding the hyaline material.*

characteristically underexpresses epithelial immunohistochemical markers such as cytokeratin and EMA. Only approximately one-half of cases will be positive with these markers, and the labeling is often focal. Rare Xp11.2 translocation carcinomas, specifically ones with variant gene fusions such as *PSF-TFE3* and *CLTC-TFE3* [115], have labeled for melanocytic markers HMB45 and melan A, creating confusion with epithelioid AML. The most distinctive immunohistochemical feature of these neoplasms is nuclear labeling for TFE3 protein using an antibody to the C-terminal portion of TFE3, which is retained in the gene fusions. Nuclear labeling for TFE3 is a common feature of all Xp11.2 translocation RCCs and ASPSs but does not occur in other RCCs (Figure 17.49). Since native TFE3 is known to be ubiquitously expressed but is not detectable in normal tissues by IHC, it is postulated that the different *TFE3* gene fusions consistently lead to overexpression of the fusion protein relative to native TFE3, such that the protein becomes detectable by this assay [116].

t(6;11)(p21;q12) Renal Cell Carcinomas

Another distinctive type of RCC bears a t(6;11)(p21;q12) [117]. On microscopic examination, these neoplasms usually feature nests and tubules of polygonal epithelioid cells, separated by thin capillaries. Some cases have had papillary formations. The majority of the tumor cells have abundant clear to granular eosinophilic cytoplasm, well-defined cell borders, and round nuclei with small nucleoli. However, a second population of smaller epithelioid cells is also characteristic, typically (but not always) clustered around the nodules of the hyaline basement membrane material within larger acini (Figure 17.50). The cases examined have generally been negative for cytokeratins by IHC, but all have labeled at least focally for HMB45 and melan A, again creating confusion with epithelioid AML.

The t(6;11)(p21;q12) has been shown to result in a fusion of the intronless, untranslated *Alpha* gene with *TFEB*, a gene belonging to the same transcription factor family as *TFE3* [118,119]. The consequence of the *Alpha-TFEB* fusion is the

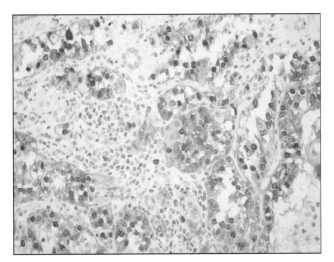

FIGURE 17.51: Renal cell carcinoma with t(6;11) (p12:q12) translocation, TFEB immunohistochemistry. Immunoreactivity is nuclear and cytoplasmic.

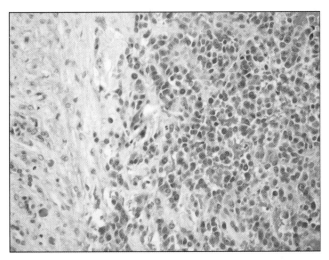

FIGURE 17.52: Primitive neuroectodermal tumor (PNET) with patternless proliferation of round blue cells.

dysregulated expression of the normal full-length TFEB protein. Along these lines, the t(6;11) RCC (also known as *Alpha-TFEB* RCC) demonstrates specific nuclear labeling for TFEB protein by IHC, whereas other neoplasms and normal tissues do not (Figure 17.51). Hence, nuclear labeling for TFEB is a sensitive and specific diagnostic marker for this neoplasm with a *TFEB* gene fusion, just as nuclear labeling for TFE3 is a sensitive and specific marker for neoplasms bearing *TFE3* gene fusions [120]. It is now thought that the t(6;11) RCCs are related to the Xp11 translocation RCCs based on their similar clinical predilection to affect young patients, similar morphology, similar immunohistochemical profiles, and related molecular pathology [121].

Oncocytic Renal Carcinomas in Neuroblastoma Patients

Meideros et al. [122] have described the oncocytic renal carcinomas arising in children who had previously had neuroblastoma. The genetic alterations identified in these lesions did not match those of known renal carcinomas, suggesting that these are another distinctive entity.

Miscellaneous Renal Neoplasms

Primitive Neuroectodermal Tumor of Kidney

Primary renal PNET is encountered mainly in adolescent and young adult patients, tends to present at advanced stage, and is associated with a poor prognosis [123,124]. Tumors consist of sheets of undifferentiated small blue cells with frequent necrosis and occasional rosettes (Figure 17.52). Renal PNET are frequently mistaken for blastemal WT of adolescent or adult patients and might account for some of the adverse prognosis attributed to "adult WT." Compared to WT, the tumor cell nuclei are less hyperchromatic and more evenly placed. Molecular detection of the *EWS-FLI1* gene fusion that results from the characteristic and specific t(11;22)(q24;q12) chromosome translocation is a useful way to confirm the diagnosis of PNET.

Also helpful is immunohistochemical labeling for CD99; the characteristic membrane-staining pattern observed in PNETs is rarely, if ever, observed in WT blastemal cells or cellular clear cell sarcoma of the kidney, which are the main differential diagnosis.

Synovial Sarcoma of the Kidney

Like renal PNET, primary renal synovial sarcoma has been established as a distinctive neoplastic entity by demonstration of its specific chromosome translocation and gene fusion [125,126]. Genetically confirmed cases have affected young adults. Many have previously been misclassified as adult blastemal WT, embryonal sarcoma of the kidney, adult cellular mesoblastic nephroma, or sarcoma arising in cystic nephroma. Renal synovial sarcomas are typically large, often cystic, and present at advanced stage. The typical appearance is that of a monomorphic, highly cellular neoplasm composed of plump, spindled cells growing in short fascicles. Tumor cells have ovoid nuclei and minimal cytoplasm, and may be associated with sclerosis. Grossly identified cysts are lined by mitotically inactive, polygonal eosinophilic cells with apically oriented nuclei ("hobnailed epithelium"), and the cellularity of their walls may be deceptively low, creating confusion with cystic nephroma in limited biopsy samples. Overall, the appearances are best conceptualized as monophasic spindle cell synovial sarcoma encircling native renal collecting ducts. True epithelial differentiation yielding a biphasic synovial sarcoma may occur, but is less common. Immunohistochemically, tumor cells label focally for epithelial markers (EMA more likely than cytokeratin), but many cases are completely negative for all epithelial markers. Many cases have labeled for CD99. The diagnosis can be confirmed in such cases by molecular demonstration of the *SYT-SSX* gene fusion that results from the t(X;18)(p11;q11) that is characteristic of this neoplastic entity. As with renal PNET, renal synovial sarcoma is more aggressive than WT, and also may account for some of the adverse prognosis attributed to "adult WT."

TUMORS OF THE RENAL PELVIS

Tumors of the renal pelvis are relatively uncommon and account for approximately 7–8 percent of all renal malignancies, although the incidence appears to be increasing [127,128]. Tumors affect 0.7–1.1 per 100,000 individuals with a male to female incidence of 1.7:1 [129,130]. The tumors are more common in older individuals with the mean age of incidence of 70 years [128–132]. Most patients present with flank pain or hematuria [132]. Imaging studies reveal a filling defect or an obstructive mass often associated with hydronephrosis, hydroureter, or renal stones. Greater than 90 percent of the tumors of the renal pelvicalyceal system are of urothelial (transitional cell) origin; however, these constitute only 5 percent of all the urothelial tumors [128–131].

Urothelial (Transitional Cell) Neoplasms

Urothelial carcinoma of the renal pelvis accounts for 0.1 and 0.07 percent of all cancers in men and women respectively in North America [128]. Tobacco smoking is an important risk factor for these tumors; the lifetime risk increases with increased consumption and intensity of smoking [132,133]. Long-term use of analgesics, especially phenacetin has also been implicated as an independent risk factor [132,134,135]; it increases the risk of renal pelvis tumors by 4–8 times in men and 10–13 times in women [136,137]. Other risk factors include Balkan nephropathy, papillary necrosis, stones, and occupational exposures to petrochemicals, plastic materials, coal, asphalt, tar, and thorium-containing contrast media [128,132,138]. History of previous lower urinary tract carcinoma is also a well-known predisposing factor and is noted in nearly 80 percent of the patients [139]. Suspected upper tract urothelial carcinomas are usually evaluated with retrograde uteropyelography, upper urinary tract cytology, and cystourethroscopy with biopsy. The sensitivity of cytology is related to the degree of tumor differentiation, poor in low grade but significantly better in high-grade tumors [140,141]. The molecular and genetic basis of upper tract urothelial carcinoma appears to be similar to that of the urothelial carcinomas of the bladder and involves tumor suppressor genes such as p53 gene locus and several gene foci on chromosome 9 (50–75 percent of the patients). Amongst these, chromosome 9 abnormalities are noted early in the development of the carcinoma and p53 mutation is associated with dysplasia and higher grade. Microsatellite instability and loss of the mismatch repair proteins MSH2, MLH1, or MSH6 may be noted in 20–30 percent of the cases [142]. These are more commonly observed in females or patients with low tumor stage and grade or inverted tumor growth pattern [143]. The presence of upper urinary tract tumor also progressively increases the risk of bladder cancer from 15 to 75 percent over a five-year period thus mandating routine bladder surveillance in these patients [144–146]. The tumors are also known for multicentricity and high incidence of recurrence [129,132,139,146–149].

The gross appearance of the tumors is variable and may range from a papillary, polypoid, or infiltrative mass to an ulcerative lesion with thickening of the pelvic wall (Figure 17.53). The tumors may extensively involve the renal parenchyma, thus mimicking a primary renal tumor. On occasion, equivocal radiographic localization may warrant intraoperative assessment of whether the tumor is of urothelial origin versus renal parenchymal primary for decision to preserve the ureter. Although this

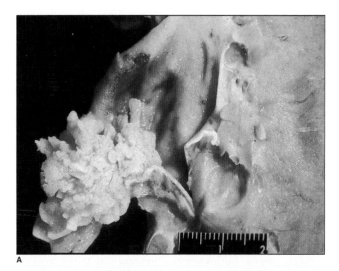

A

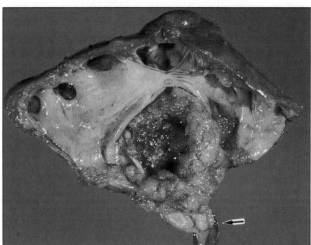

B

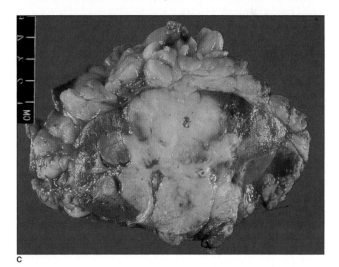

C

FIGURE 17.53: *Gross appearance of urothelial carcinoma of pelvicalyceal system. (A) Papillary tumor protruding into and expanding the renal pelvis. (B) Large tumor associated with hydronephrosis and extending into proximal ureter (arrow). (C) Infiltrative mass that extensively involves the renal parenchyma and may mimic a primary renal tumor.*

distinction commonly may be achieved with gross evaluation, difficulty arises especially when extensive invasion by poorly differentiated neoplasm is present (poorly differentiated urothelial carcinoma vs. RCC, not otherwise specified [RCC, NOS] discussed in the following section).

Urothelial carcinomas involving the renal pelvis have two major forms of presentation each necessitating a different approach to prosection [150]. They may present as papillary/polypoid tumors expanding the pelvicalyceal system or large invasive cancers involving the kidney and centered on the pelvicalyceal system and renal medulla. Tumors primarily appearing as papillary or polypoid type, which expand and fill the pelvicalyceal system, tend to be noninvasive or are associated with limited invasion such that systematic sampling after fixation and maintaining relationship to underlying structures is important for accurate pathologic staging [150]. Extensive sampling may be needed to comfortably exclude invasion and for accurate staging [150]. Tumors presenting as large invasive carcinomas in the region of the renal medulla need meticulous examination to determine relationship of the tumor to the pelvicalyceal mucosa including appropriate sampling of transition areas for documentation of origin [150].

The basic histopathology of upper tract tumors is similar to those of the urothelial neoplasia of the urinary bladder (Table 17.8) [128]. The histopathologic diversity of the urothelial neoplasia with morphologic variants and aberrant differentiations that are well described in the literature of bladder tumors are also largely applicable in this region (Table 17.9) [128,151-163]. The wide histologic range seen in the bladder can be encountered in tumors of the pelvicalyceal system; aberrant patterns such as micropapillary areas, lymphoepithelioma-like carcinoma, sarcomatoid carcinoma, squamous differentiation and squamous cell carcinoma, clear cells, glandular differentiation, rhabdoid, signet-ring or plasmacytoid cells, and pseudosarcomatous stromal changes occur more commonly in pelvicalyceal system [158,161].

Urothelial carcinoma that presents as a highly infiltrative neoplasm extensively involving the renal parenchyma may be diagnostically straightforward in terms of histologic categorization or may mimic a high-grade RCC, NOS, a CDC, or a metastasis. Urothelial carcinoma overlaps, considerably in many aspects, with CDC in that both show highly infiltrative carcinoma with desmoplastic response in the renal medullary region. Features in favor of urothelial carcinoma include: history of bladder cancer, carcinoma in situ or papillary tumor involving the pelvicalyceal system, or predominantly nested or solid architecture with variable squamous or glandular differentiation (in contrast to CDC that is primarily an adenocarcinoma with an established glandular architecture). Features that favor metastatic carcinoma over urothelial carcinoma include: histology not conforming to any of the known subtypes of RCC or typical urothelial carcinoma, extensive interstitial growth, multifocality both grossly and microscopically, and extensive vascular-lymphatic invasion.

In most cases, careful microscopic and gross examination, and clinicopathologic correlation will help resolve the differential diagnosis, although IHC may play an ancillary role. Figure 17.54 outlines the algorithmic approach and the expected immunoprofile for each of the three major differential diagnostic categories.

Table 17.9 Classification of Urothelial Neoplasia of the Upper Urinary Tract

Benign
Transitional papilloma [WHO (2004)/ISUP, 1998; WHO 1973, grade 0]
Inverted papilloma

Papillary urothelial neoplasm of low malignant potential [WHO (2004)/ISUP; WHO 1973, grade I]

Malignant
A. Papillary
   a. Typical [low grade or high grade, WHO (2004)/ISUP; WHO 1973, grade I, II, and III]
      Variant–with squamous or glandular differentiation
   b. Micropapillary
B. Nonpapillary
   a. Carcinoma in situ
   b. Frankly invasive carcinoma
      Variants containing or exhibiting
      (a) Deceptively benign features
         • Nested pattern (resembling von Brunn's nests)
         • Small tubular pattern/glandular pattern
         • Microcystic pattern
         • Inverted pattern
      (b) Squamous differentiation
      (c) Glandular differentiation
      (d) Micropapillary histology
      (e) Sarcomatoid foci (sarcomatoid carcinoma)
      (f) Urothelial carcinoma with unusual cytoplasmic features
         • Clear cell (glycogen rich)
         • Plasmacytoid
         • Rhabdoid
         • Lipid rich
      (g) Urothelial carcinoma with syncytiotrophoblasts
      (h) Unusual stromal reactions
         • Pseudosarcomatous stroma
         • Stromal osseous or cartilaginous metaplasia
         • Osteoclast-type giant cells
         • With prominent lymphoid infiltrate
      (i) Urothelial carcinoma with multiple patterns of divergent differentiation

Table 17.8 Histologic Classification of Tumors of the Upper Urinary Tract

I. Urothelial carcinoma (see Table 17.9)
II. Squamous cell carcinoma
III. Adenocarcinoma
IV. Undifferentiated carcinoma
   Small cell carcinoma
   Large cell neuroendocrine carcinoma
   Lymphoepithelioma-like carcinoma
   Osteoclast-rich carcinoma
   Giant cell carcinoma
   Not otherwise specified
V. Metastatic carcinoma
VI. Mesenchymal tumors
VII. Rare entities
   Lymphoma
   Plasmacytoma
   Melanoma

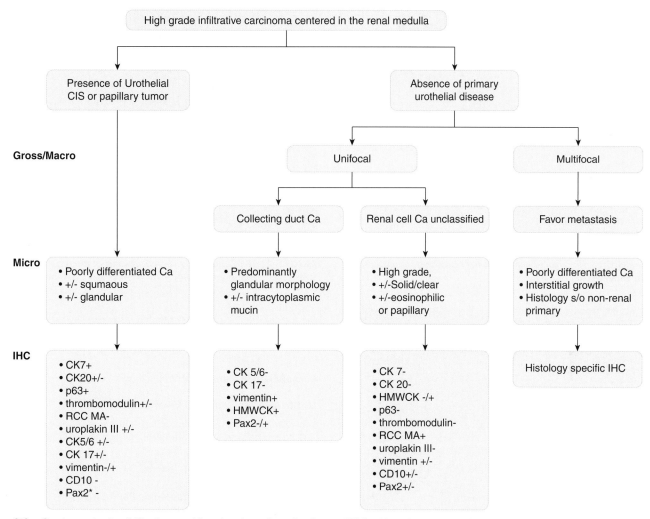

High grade infiltrative carcinoma centered in the renal medulla

Presence of Urothelial CIS or papillary tumor

Absence of primary urothelial disease

Gross/Macro

Unifocal

Multifocal

Collecting duct Ca

Renal cell Ca unclassified

Favor metastasis

Micro

- Poorly differentiated Ca
- +/- squmaous
- +/- glandular

- Predominantly glandular morphology
- +/- intracytoplasmic mucin

- High grade,
- +/-Solid/clear
- +/-eosinophilic or papillary

- Poorly differentiated Ca
- Interstitial growth
- Histology s/o non-renal primary

IHC

- CK7+
- CK20+/-
- p63+
- thrombomodulin+/-
- RCC MA-
- uroplakin III +/-
- CK5/6 +/-
- CK 17+/-
- vimentin-/+
- CD10 -
- Pax2* -

- CK 5/6-
- CK 17-
- vimentin+
- HMWCK+
- Pax2-/+

- CK 7-
- CK 20-
- HMWCK -/+
- p63-
- thrombomodulin-
- RCC MA+
- uroplakin III-
- vimentin +/-
- CD10+/-
- Pax2+/-

Histology specific IHC

CIS = Carcinoma in situ; **IHC** = Immunohistochemistry; **Ca** = Carcinoma; **NOS** = Not otherwise specified; **RCC MA** = Renal Cell Carcinoma Marker; **CK** = Cytokeratin; **HMWCK** = High Molecular Weight Cytokeratin

FIGURE 17.54: Approach to the diagnosis of high-grade infiltrative carcinoma in the renal medulla.

The grading system employed for upper tract neoplasms is identical to that employed for vesical tumors and urothelial tumors: noninvasive papillary urothelial neoplasms of low malignant potential (PUNLMP), and a two-tier system for carcinomas – low and high grade [128]. The distinction is based on architectural and cytologic abnormalities such as loss of polarity, lack of differentiation from the base to the surface, and nuclear anaplasia and is assigned by the grade in the worst area [164]. Very few studies have evaluated the importance of grading in urothelial neoplasms of the renal pelvis [165]. A nephrectomy is commonly performed in these cases and therefore more subtle prognostic differences among PUNLMP, low-grade carcinoma, or high-grade carcinoma may not be apparent between noninvasive and minimally invasive tumors. Grade may be an independent prognostic factor in papillary pT1 tumors; however, most pT2 and higher stage tumors tend to be nonpapillary and of higher grade [128] and in these cases, grade is not a significant prognostic factor on multivariate analysis. For squamous cell carcinoma and adenocarcinoma, histologic grading has no known prognostic significance but is traditionally assigned using criteria applied at other sites.

The pathologic stage is the single most important prognostic factor for urothelial carcinomas of the upper urinary tract (Figures 17.55–17.57) [131,132,154,156,157,166]. Surveillance, epidemiology, and end results program (SEER) data from 9,072 of reported cases to the registry has demonstrated a five-year overall survival rate that is significantly different among the stage groupings (95.1 percent for noninvasive, 88.9 percent for localized disease, 62.6 percent for regional disease, and 16.5 percent for patients with distant metastasis) [130]. In another series, five-year survival was 100 percent for Ta and

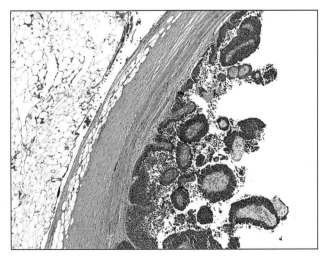

FIGURE 17.55: *Noninvasive papillary urothelial carcinoma of the renal pelvis.*

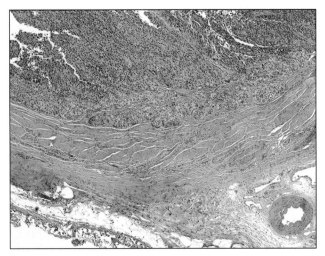

FIGURE 17.56: *Papillary urothelial carcinoma of the renal pelvis invading the muscularis.*

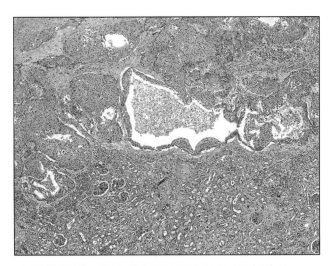

FIGURE 17.57: *Urothelial carcinoma of the renal pelvis infiltrating the renal parenchyma.*

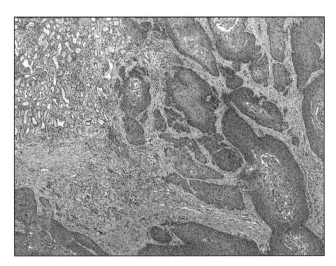

FIGURE 17.58: *Squamous cell carcinoma of the renal pelvis with keratinization and obvious invasion of renal parenchyma.*

in situ disease, 91.7 percent for T1, 72.6 percent for T2, and 40.5 percent for T3 tumors [167].

Miscellaneous Tumors of the Renal Pelvis

Urothelial Papilloma and Inverted Papilloma

Both the lesions may be incidentally noted and are extremely rare. These are twice as common in the ureter as the renal pelvis. The renal pelvic mucosa has a greater predilection to have von Brunns nests than bladder mucosa [168].

Villous Adenoma and Squamous Papilloma

Both these neoplasms are very rare. The diagnosis of a villous adenoma is nearly impossible in a limited sample as an adeno-carcinoma in the vicinity cannot be excluded. Thus, complete excision of the entire clinically visible lesion is mandatory.

Squamous Cell Carcinoma

Squamous cell carcinoma is the second most common tumor in this region, more commonly seen in the renal pelvis as compared to the ureter. They generally occur on the background of neph-rolithiasis presumably from a precarcinogenic sequence of squa-mous metaplasia to dysplasia, carcinoma in situ, and invasive carcinoma. These tumors tend to be high grade, high stage, and frequently invade the kidney (Figure 17.58). The prognosis of these tumors is extremely poor and survival for 5 years is rare [169].

Adenocarcinoma

Adenocarcinoma of the upper tract also occurs on a background of nephrolithiasis and repeated infections. Intestinal metaplasia is a putative precursor as it may be seen in the nonneoplastic mucosa. Pure adenocarcinomas (Figure 17.59) are rare and sev-eral phenotypes such as mucinous, signet-ring and, enteric type may be noted together [170,171]; a case of hepatoid pattern con-taining bile pigments has been reported. The differential diagno-sis includes metastatic colonic carcinoma, lung adenocarcinoma, and other carcinomas, such as carcinomas from the pancreas,

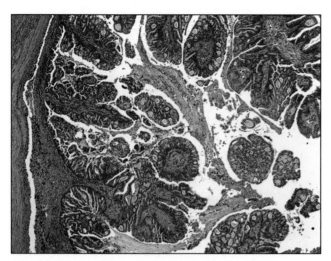

FIGURE 17.59: *Adenocarcinoma of the renal pelvis. Low power of a high-grade adenocarcinoma lining calyceal mucosa.*

breast, or gynecologic tract. Clinicopathologic correlation and history are key factors. Multifocal lesions, lack of mucosal involvement, and lack of hydronephrosis or stones should at least raise the possibility of a metastasis from another site.

Stromal Tumors

A wide range of stromal tumors, as seen in the bladder or any visceral organ has been documented in the upper tract including leiomyoma, neurofibroma, hibernoma, hemangioma, and peri-ureteric lipoma [172–176]. The most common primary mesen-chymal malignancy of the upper tract is leiomyosarcoma; its overall incidence is very low. The other documented entities include rhabdomyosarcoma, angiosarcoma, fibrosarcoma, Ewing's tumor, and malignant peripheral nerve sheath tumor [177–179].

A spectrum of miscellaneous other rare malignant tumors including neuroendocrine carcinoma, small cell carcinoma, lym-phoma, plasmacytoma, melanoma, choriocarcinoma, etc. have all been anecdotally documented in the renal pelvis [180–182].

REFERENCES

1. Jemal A, Siegel R, Ward E, Murray T, Xu J, Thun MJ. Cancer statistics. *CA Cancer J Clin.* 2007;57:43–66.
2. Lee CT, Katz J, Fearn PA, Russo P. Mode of presentation of renal cell carcinoma provides prognostic information. *Urol Oncol.* 2002;7:135–40.
3. Hollingsworth JM, Miller DC, Daignault S, Hollenbeck BK. Rising incidence of small renal masses: a need to reas-sess treatment effect. *J Natl Cancer Inst.* 2006;98:1331–4.
4. Volpe A, Panzarella T, Rendon RA, Haider MA, Kondylis FI, Jewett MA. The natural history of incidentally detected small renal masses. *Cancer.* 2004;100:738–45.
5. Hollingsworth JM, Miller DC, Daignault S, Hollenbeck BK. Five-year survival after surgical treatment for kidney cancer: a population-based competing risk analysis. *Cancer.* 2007;109:1763–8.
6. Motzer RJ, Hutson TE, Tomczak P, Michaelson MD, Bukowski RM, Rixe O, Oudard S, Negrier S, Szczylik C,

7. Kim ST, Chen I, Bycott PW, Baum CM, Figlin RA. Suni-tinib versus interferon alfa in metastatic renal-cell carci-noma. *N Engl J Med.* 2007;356:115–24.
7. Reuter, VE. The pathology of renal epithelial neoplasms. *Semin Oncol.* 2006;33:534–43.
8. Thoenes W, Storkel S, Rumpelt HJ. Human chromophobe cell renal carcinoma. *Virchows Arch B Cell Pathol Incl Mol Pathol.* 1985;48:207–17.
9. Thoenes W, Storkel S, Rumpelt HJ, Moll R, Baum HP, Werner S. Chromophobe cell renal carcinoma and its variants – a report on 32 cases. *J Pathol.* 1988;155:277–87.
10. Eble JN, Sauter G, Epstein JI, Sesterhenn IA, eds. World Health Organization Classification of Tumours, Pathology and Genetics. *Tumours of the Urinary System and Male Gen-ital Organs.* Lyon: IARC Press, 2004.
11. Kovacs G, Wilkens L, Papp T, De Riese W. Differentiation between papillary and nonpapillary renal cell carcinomas by DNA analysis. *J Natl Cancer Inst.* 1989;81:527–30.
12. Linehan WM, Walther MM, Zbar B. The genetic basis of cancer of the kidney. *J Urol.* 2003;170:2163–72.
13. Reuter VE, Tickoo SK. Adult renal tumors. In: *Sternberg's Diagnostic Surgical Pathology.* Mills, Carter, Greenson, Oberman, Reuter, Stoler, eds. 4th ed. Philadelphia: Lippin-cott Williams & Wilkins; 2004, pp.1955–99.
14. Green F, Page D, Fleming I, et al. *AJCC Cancer Staging Manual.* Berlin: Springer, 2002.
15. Bonsib SM. The renal sinus is the principal invasive path-way: a prospective study of 100 renal cell carcinomas. *Am J Surg Pathol.* 2004;28:1594–1600.
16. Bonsib SM. T2 clear cell renal cell carcinoma is a rare entity: a study of 120 clear cell renal cell carcinomas. *J Urol.* 2005;174:1199–1202.
17. Tickoo SK, Alden D, Olgac S, Fine SW, Russo P, Konda-gunta GV, Motzer RJ, Reuter VE. Immunohistochemical expression of hypoxia inducible factor-1alpha and its down-stream molecules in sarcomatoid renal cell carcinoma. *J Urol.* 2007;177:1258–63.
18. De Peralta-Venturina M, Moch H, Amin M, Tamboli P, Hailemariam S, Mihatsch M, Javidan J, Stricker H, Ro JY, Amin MB. Sarcomatoid differentiation in renal cell carci-noma. *Am J Surg Pathol.* 2001;25:275–84.
19. Zbar B. Von Hippel-Lindau disease and sporadic renal cell carcinoma. *Cancer Surv.* 1995;25:219–32.
20. Amin MB, Corless CL, Renshaw AA, Tickoo SK, Kubus J, Schultz DS. Papillary (chromophil) renal cell carcinoma: histomorphologic characteristics and evaluation of conven-tional pathologic prognostic parameters in 62 cases. *Am J Surg Pathol.* 1997;21:621–35.
21. Amin MB, Amin MB, Tamboli P, Javidan J, Stricker H, De Peralta-Venturina M, Deshpande A, Menon M. Prognostic impact of histologic subtyping of adult renal epithelial neo-plasms: an experience of 405 cases. *Am J Surg Pathol.* 2002;26:281–91.
22. Delahunt B, Eble JN. Papillary renal cell carcinoma: a clin-icopathologic and immunohistochemical study of 105 tumors. *Mod Pathol.* 1997;10:537–44.
23. Yang XJ, Tan MH, Kim HL, Ditlev JA, Betten MW, Png CE, Kort EJ, Futami K, Furge KA, Takahashi M, Kanayama HO, Tan PH, Teh BS, Luan C, Wang K, Pins M, Tretia-kova M, Anema J, Kahnoski R, Nicol T, Stadler W,

Vogelzang NG, Amato R, Seligson D, Figlin R, Belldegrun A, Rogers CG, Teh BT. A molecular classification of papillary renal cell carcinoma. *Cancer Res.* 2005;65:5628–37.

24. Delahunt B, Eble JN, McCredie MR, Bethwaite PB, Stewart JH, Bilous AM. Morphologic typing of papillary renal cell carcinoma: comparison of growth kinetics and patient survival in 66 cases. *Hum Pathol.* 2001;32:590–5.

25. Tickoo SK, Reuter VE. Subtyping papillary renal cell carcinoma: a clinicopathologic study of 103 cases. *Mod Pathol.* 2001;14:124A.

26. Cheville JC, Lohse CM, Zincke H, Weaver AL, Blute ML. Comparisons of outcome and prognostic features among histologic subtypes of renal cell carcinoma. *Am J Surg Pathol.* 2003;27:612–24.

27. Motzer RJ, Bacik J, Mariani T, Russo P, Mazumdar M, Reuter V. Treatment outcome and survival associated with metastatic renal cell carcinoma of non-clear-cell histology. *J Clin Oncol.* 2002;20:2376–81.

28. Parwani AV, Husain AN, Epstein JI, Beckwith JB, Argani P. Low-grade myxoid renal epithelial neoplasms with distal nephron differentiation. *Hum Pathol.* 2001;32:506–12.

29. Srigley JR, Kapusta L, Reuter V, Amin M, Grignon DG, Eble JN, Weber A, Moch H. Phenotypic, molecular and ultrastructural studies of a novel low grade renal epithelial neoplasm possibly related to the loop of Henle. *Mod Pathol.* 2002;12:182A.

30. Fine SW, Argani P, DeMarzo AM, Delahunt B, Sebo TJ, Reuter VE, Epstein JI. Expanding the histologic spectrum of mucinous tubular and spindle cell carcinoma of the kidney. *Am J Surg Pathol.* 2006;30:1554–60.

31. Paner GP, Srigley JR, Radhakrishnan A, Cohen C, Skinnider BF, Tickoo SK, Young AN, Amin MB. Immunohistochemical analysis of mucinous tubular and spindle cell carcinoma and papillary renal cell carcinoma of the kidney: significant immunophenotypic overlap warrants diagnostic caution. *Am J Surg Pathol.* 2006;30:13–19.

32. Shen SS, Ro JY, Tamboli P, Truong LD, Zhai Q, Jung SJ, Tibbs RG, Ordonez NG, Ayala AG. Mucinous tubular and spindle cell carcinoma of kidney is probably a variant of papillary renal cell carcinoma with spindle cell features. *Ann Diagn Pathol.* 2007;11:13–21.

33. Tickoo SK, De Peralta-Venturina MN, Harik LR, Worcester HD, Salama ME, Young AN, Moch H, Amin MB. Spectrum of epithelial neoplasms in end-stage renal disease: an experience from 66 tumor-bearing kidneys with emphasis on histologic patterns distinct from those in sporadic adult renal neoplasia. *Am J Surg Pathol.* 2006;30:141–53.

34. Sule N, Yakupoglu U, Shen SS, et al. Calcium oxalate deposition in renal cell carcinoma associated with acquired cystic kidney disease: a comprehensive study. *Am J Surg Pathol.* 2005;29:443–51.

35. Fleming S, Lewi HJ. Collecting duct carcinoma of the kidney. *Histopathology.* 1986;10:1131–41.

36. Srigley JR, Eble JN. Collecting duct carcinoma of kidney. *Semin Diagn Pathol.* 1998;15:54–67.

37. Amin MB, Varma MD, Tickoo SK, et al. Collecting duct carcinoma of the kidney. *Adv Anat Pathol.* 1997;4:85–94.

38. Rumpelt HJ, Storkel S, Moll R, Scharfe T, Thoenes W. Bellini duct carcinoma: further evidence for this rare variant of renal cell carcinoma. *Histopathology* 1991;18:115–22.

39. Tokuda N, Naito S, Matsuzaki O, Nagashima Y, Ozono S, Igarashi T. Collecting duct (Bellini duct) renal cell carcinoma: a nationwide survey in Japan. *J Urol* 2006;176:40–3.

40. MacLennan GT, Farrow GM, Bostwick DG. Low-grade collecting duct carcinoma of the kidney: report of 13 cases of low-grade mucinous tubulocystic renal carcinoma of possible collecting duct origin. *Urology.* 1997;50:679–84.

41. Amin MB, MacLennan GT, Paraf F, Cheville JC, Vieillefond A, Radhakrishnan A, Che M, Srigley JR, Grignon DJ. Tubulocystic carcinoma of the kidney: clinicopathologic analysis of 29 cases of a distinctive rare subtype of renal cell carcinoma (RCC). *Lab Invest.* 2004; 84(Suppl. 1):137A.

42. Young AN, Paner GP, MacLennan GT, Cheville JC, Vieillefond A, Hes O, McKenney JK, Paraf F, Grignon DJ, Epstein JI, Srigley JR, Amin MB. Molecular profiling of the novel thyroid-like renal cell carcinoma and tubulocystic RCC by high-density oligonucleotide microarrays. *Mod Pathol.* 2007;20(Suppl. 2):185A.

43. Yang XJ, Zhou M, Hes O, et al. Tubulocystic carcinoma of the kidney: clinicopathologic and molecular characterization. *Am J Surg Pathol.* 2008;32:177–187.

44. Azoulay S, Viellefond A, Paraf F, et al. Tubulocystic carcinoma of the kidney: a new entity among renal tumors. *Virch Arch.* 2007;451:905–9.

45. Davis CJ, Mostofi FK, Sesterhenn IA. Renal medullary carcinoma. The seventh sickle cell nephropathy. *Am J Surg Pathol.* 1995;19:1–11.

46. Swartz MA, Karth J, Schneider DT, Rodriguez R, Beckwith JB, Perlman EJ. Renal medullary carcinoma: clinical, pathologic, immunohistochemical, and genetic analysis with pathogenetic implications. *Urology.* 2002;60:1083–9.

47. Amin MB, Crotty TB, Tickoo SK, Farrow GM. Renal oncocytoma: a reappraisal of morphologic features with clinicopathologic findings in 80 cases. *Am J Surg Pathol.* 1997;21:1–12.

48. Perez-Ordonez B, Hamed G, Campbell S, Erlandson RA, Russo P, Gaudin PB, Reuter VE. Renal oncocytoma: a clinicopathologic study of 70 cases. *Am J Surg Pathol.* 1997; 21:871–83.

49. Tickoo SK, Lee MW, Eble JN, Amin M, Christopherson T, Zarbo RJ, Amin MB. Ultrastructural observations on mitochondria and microvesicles in renal oncocytoma, chromophobe renal cell carcinoma, and eosinophilic variant of conventional (clear cell) renal cell carcinoma. *Am J Surg Pathol.* 2000;24:1247–56.

50. Erlandson RA, Shek TW, Reuter VE. Diagnostic significance of mitochondria in four types of renal epithelial neoplasms: an ultrastructural study of 60 tumors. *Ultrastruct Pathol.* 1997;21:409–17.

51. Tickoo SK, Reuter VE, Amin MB, Srigley JR, Epstein JI, Min KW, Rubin MA, Ro JY. Renal oncocytosis: a morphologic study of fourteen cases. *Am J Surg Pathol.* 1999;23:1094–101.

52. Fegan JE, Shah HR, Mukunyadzi P, Schutz MJ. Extrarenal retroperitoneal angiomyolipoma. *South Med J.* 1997;90:59–62.

53. Guinee DG, Jr., Thornberry DS, Azumi N, Przygodzki RM, Koss MN, Travis WD. Unique pulmonary presentation of an angiomyolipoma: analysis of clinical, radiographic, and histopathologic features. *Am J Surg Pathol.* 1995;19:476–80.

54. Bonetti F, Pea M, Martignoni G, Doglioni C, Zamboni G, Capelli P, Rimondi P, Andrion A. Clear cell *("sugar") tumor of the lung is a lesion strictly related to angiomyolipoma-the concept of a family of lesions characterized by the presence of the perivascular epithelioid cells (PEC). Pathology.* 1994;26:230–6.

55. Bryant DA, Gaudin PB, Hutchinson B, Erlandson RA, Reuter VE. Angiomyolipoma of the kidney: a histologic and immunohistochemical study of 39 cases. *Mod Pathol.* 1998;11:77A.

56. Martignoni G, Pea M, Bonetti F. Renal epithelioid oxyphilic neoplasms (REON): a pleomorphic variant of renal angiomyolipoma. *Int J Surg Pathol.* 1995;2(Suppl):539.

57. Martignoni G, Pea M, Bonetti F, Brunelli M, Eble JN. Oncocytoma-like angiomyolipoma: a clinicopathologic and immunohistochemical study of 2 cases. *Arch Pathol Lab Med.* 2002;126:610–2.

58. Kalra OP, Verma PP, Kochhar S, Jha V, Sakhuja V. Bilateral renal angiomyolipomatosis in tuberous sclerosis presenting with chronic renal failure: case report and review of the literature. *Nephron.* 1994;68:256–8.

59. Eble JN, Amin MB, Young RH. Epithelioid angiomyolipoma of the kidney: a report of five cases with a prominent and diagnostically confusing epithelioid smooth muscle component. *Am J Surg Pathol.* 1997;21:1123–30.

60. Ferry JA, Malt RA, Young RH. Renal angiomyolipoma with sarcomatous transformation and pulmonary metastases. *Am J Surg Pathol.* 1991;15:1083–8.

61. Fine SW, Reuter VE, Epstein JI, Argani P. Angiomyolipoma with epithelial cysts (AMLEC): a distinct cystic variant of angiomyolipoma. *Am J Surg Pathol.*2006;30:593–9.

62. Antic T, Perry KT, Harrison K, Zaytsev P, Pins M, Campbell SC, Picken MM. Mixed epithelial and stromal tumor of the kidney and cystic nephroma share overlapping features: reappraisal of 15 lesions. *Arch Pathol Lab Med.* 2006;130:80–5.

63. Turbiner J, Amin MB, Humphrey PA, Srigley JR, De Leval L, Radhakrishnan A, Oliva E. Cystic nephroma and mixed epithelial and stromal tumor of kidney: a detailed clinicopathologic analysis of 34 cases and proposal for renal epithelial and stromal tumor (REST) as a unifying term. *Am J Surg Pathol.* 2007;31:489–500.

64. Pierson CR, Schober MS, Wallis T, Sarkar FH, Sorensen PH, Eble JN, Srigley JR, Jones EC, Grignon DJ, Adsay V. Mixed epithelial and stromal tumor of the kidney lacks the genetic alterations of cellular congenital mesoblastic nephroma. *Hum Pathol.* 2001;32:513–20.

65. Levin NP, Damjanov I, Depillis VJ. Mesoblastic nephroma in an adult patient: recurrence 21 years after removal of the primary lesion. *Cancer.* 1982;49:573–7.

66. Antonescu CR, Bisceglia M, Reuter V, et al. Sarcomatous transformation of cystic nephroma in adults. *Mod Pathol.* 1997;10:69A.

67. Argani P, Faria PA, Epstein JI, Reuter VE, Perlman EJ, Beckwith JB, Ladanyi M. Primary renal synovial sarcoma: molecular and morphologic delineation of an entity previously included among embryonal sarcomas of the kidney. *Am J Surg Pathol.* 2000;24:1087–96.

68. Davis CJ, Jr., Barton JH, Sesterhenn IA, Mostofi FK. Metanephric adenoma: clinicopathological study of fifty patients. *Am J Surg Pathol.* 1995;19:1101–14.

69. Jones EC, Pins M, Dickersin GR, Young RH. Metanephric adenoma of the kidney: a clinicopathological, immunohistochemical, flow cytometric, cytogenetic, and electron microscopic study of seven cases. *Am J Surg Pathol.* 1995;19:615–26.

70. Gatalica Z, Grujic S, Kovatich A, Petersen RO. Metanephric adenoma: histology immunophenotype, cytogenetics, ultrastructure. *Mod Pathol.* 1996;9:329–33.

71. Hennigar RA, Beckwith JB. Nephrogenic adenofibroma. A novel kidney tumor of young people. *Am J Surg Pathol.* 1992;16:325–34.

72. Stumm M, Koch A, Wieacker PF, Phillip C, Steinbach F, Allhoff EP, Buhtz P, Walter H, Tonnies H, Wirth J. Partial monosomy 2p as the single chromosomal anomaly in a case of renal metanephric adenoma. *Cancer Genet Cytogenet.* 1999;115:82–5.

73. Olgac S, Hutchinson B, Tickoo SK, Reuter VE. Alpha-methylacyl-CoA racemase as a marker in the differential diagnosis of metanephric adenoma. *Mod Pathol.* 2006;19:218–24.

74. Tetu B, Vaillancourt L, Camilleri JP, Bruneval P, Bernier L, Tourigny R. Juxtaglomerular cell tumor of the kidney: report of two cases with a papillary pattern. *Hum Pathol.* 1993;24:1168–74.

75. Kim HJ, Kim CH, Choi YJ, Ayala AG, Amirikachi M, Ro JY. Juxtaglomerular cell tumor of kidney with CD34 and CD117 immunoreactivity: report of 5 cases. *Arch Pathol Lab Med.* 2006;130:707–11.

76. Lerman RJ, Pitcock JA, Stephenson P, Muirhead EE. Renomedullary interstitial cell tumor (formerly fibroma of renal medulla). *Hum Pathol.* 1972;3:559–68.

77. Kojiro M, Ohishi H, Isobe H. Carcinoid tumor occurring in cystic teratoma of the kidney: a case report. *Cancer.* 1976;38:1636–40.

78. Azumi N, Traweek ST, Battifora H. Prostatic acid phosphatase in carcinoid tumors. Immunohistochemical and immunoblot studies. *Am J Surg Pathol.* 1991;15:785–90.

79. Hansel DE, Epstein JI, Berbescu E, Fine SW, Young RH, Cheville JC. Renal carcinoid tumor: a clinicopathologic study of 21 cases. *Am J Surg Pathol.* 2007;31:1539–44.

80. Beckwith JB. National Wilms tumor study: *an update for pathologists. Pediatr Dev Pathol.* 1998;1:79–84.

81. Perlman EJ. Pediatric renal tumors: practical updates for the pathologist. *Pediatr Dev Pathol.* 2005;8:320–38.

82. Argani P, Beckwith JB, . Renal neoplasms of childhood. In: Mills SE, ed. *Sternberg's Diagnostic Surgical Pathology.* 4th ed. Philadelphia: Lippincott Williams & Wilkins; 2004, pp. 2001–33.

83. Joshi VV, Beckwith JB. Multilocular cyst of the kidney (cystic nephroma) and cystic, partially differentiated nephroblastoma: terminology and criteria for diagnosis. *Cancer.* 1989;64:466–79.

84. Beckwith JB, Zuppan CE, Browning NG, et al. Histological analysis of aggressiveness versus responsiveness in Wilms tumor. *Med Pediatr Oncol.* 1996;27:422–8.

85. Zuppan CW, Beckwith JB, Luckey DW. Anaplasia in unilateral Wilms' tumor: a report from the National Wilms' Tumor Study pathology center. *Hum Pathol.* 1988;19:1199–209.

86. Bardeesy N, Beckwith JB, Pelletier J. Clonal expansion and attenuated apoptosis in Wilms' tumors are associated with *p53* gene mutations. *Cancer Res.* 1995;55:215–9.

87. Govender D, Harilal P, Hadley GP, Chetty R. p53 protein expression in nephroblastomas: a predictor of poor prognosis. *Br J Cancer.* 1998;77:314–8.

88. Faria P, Beckwith JB, Mishra K, et al. Focal versus diffuse anaplasia in Wilms tumor – new definitions with prognostic significance: a report from the National Wilms Tumor Study Group. *Am J Surg Pathol.* 1996;20:909–20.

89. Zuppan CW, Beckwith JB, Weeks DA, et al. Effect of preoperative therapy on Wilms' tumor histology: analysis of cases from the third National Wilms' Tumor Study. *Cancer.* 1991;68:385–94.

90. Weeks DA, Mierau GW, Malott RL, Beckwith JB. Practical electron microscopy of pediatric renal tumors. *Ultrastruct Pathol.* 1996;20:31–3.

91. Folpe AL, Patterson K, Gown AM. Antibodies to desmin identify the blastemal component of nephroblastoma. *Mod Pathol.* 1997;10:895–900.

92. Grubb GR, Yun K, Williams BRG, Eccles MR, Reeve AE. Expression of WT1 protein in fetal kidneys and Wilms tumors. *Lab Invest.* 1994;71:472–9.

93. Beckwith JB. Precursor lesions of Wilms tumor: clinical and biological implications. *Med Pediatr Oncol.* 1993;21:158–68.

94. Argani P, Collins MH. Anaplastic nephrogenic rest. *Am J Surg Pathol.* 2006;30:1339–41.

95. Coppes MJ, Arnold M, Beckwith JB et al. Factors affecting the risk of contralateral Wilms tumor development. *Cancer.* 1999;85:1616–25.

96. Argani P, Perlman EJ, Breslow NE, et al. Clear cell sarcoma of the kidney: a review of 351 cases from the National Wilms Tumor Study Group Pathology Center. *Am J Surg Pathol.* 2000;24:4–18.

97. Haas JE, Bonadio JF, Beckwith JB. Clear cell sarcoma of the kidney with emphasis on ultrastructural studies. *Cancer.* 1984;54:2978–87.

98. Bolande RP. Congenital mesoblastic nephroma of infancy. *Perspect Pediatr Pathol.* 1973;1:227–50.

99. Pettinato G, Manivel JC, Wick MR, Dehner LP. Classical and cellular (atypical) congenital mesoblastic nephroma: a clinicopathologic, ultrastructural, immunohistochemical, and flow cytometric study. *Hum Pathol.*1989;20:682–90.

100. O'Malley DP, Mierau GW, Beckwith JB, Weeks DA. Ultrastructure of congenital mesoblastic nephroma. *Ultrastruct Pathol.*1996;20:417–27.

101. Knezevich SR, McFadden DE, Tao W, Lim JF, Sorensen PH. A novel *ETV6-NTRK3* gene fusion in congenital fibrosarcoma. *Nat Genet.* 1998;18:184–7.

102. Knezevich SR, Garnett MJ, Pysher TJ et al. *ETV6-NTRK3* gene fusions and trisomy 11 establish a histogenetic link between mesoblastic nephroma and congenital fibrosarcoma. *Cancer Res.*1998;58:5046–8.

103. Argani P, Fritsch M, Kadkol SS et al. Detection of the *ETV6-NTRK3* chimeric RNA of infantile fibrosarcoma/cellular congenital mesoblastic nephroma in paraffin-embedded tissue: application to challenging pediatric renal stromal tumors. *Mod Pathol.* 2000;13:29–36.

104. Weeks DA, Beckwith JB, Mierau GW, Luckey DW. Rhabdoid tumor of kidney: a report of 111 cases from the National Wilms' Tumor Study Pathology Center. *Am J Surg Pathol.*1989;13:439–58.

105. Haas JE, Palmer NF, Weinberg AG, Beckwith JB. Ultrastructure of malignant rhabdoid tumor of the kidney: a distinctive renal tumor of children. *Hum Pathol.* 1981;12:646–57.

106. Hoot AC, Russo P, Judkins AR, Perlman EJ, Biegel JA. Immunohistochemical analysis of hSNF5/INI1 distinguishes renal and extra-renal malignant rhabdoid tumors from other pediatric soft tissue tumors. *Am J Surg Pathol.* 2004;28:1485–91.

107. Weeks DA, Beckwith JB, Mierau GW, Zuppan CW. Renal neoplasms mimicking rhabdoid tumor of kidney: a report from the National Wilms' Tumor Study Pathology Center. *Am J Surg Pathol.* 1991;15:1042–54.

108. Parham DM, Weeks DA, Beckwith JB. The clinicopathologic spectrum of putative extrarenal rhabdoid tumors. *Am J Surg Pathol.* 1994;18:1010–29.

109. Argani P, Beckwith JB. Metanephric stromal tumor: report of 31 cases of a distinctive pediatric renal neoplasm. *Am J Surg Pathol.* 2000;24:917–26.

110. Arroyo MR, Green DM, Perlman EJ, Beckwith JB, Argani P. The spectrum of metanephric adenofibroma and related lesions. Clinicopathologic study of 25 cases from the National Wilms Tumor Study Group Pathology Center. *Am J Surg Pathol.* 2001;25:433–44.

111. Argani P, Ladanyi M, . Renal carcinomas associated with Xp11.2 translocations/*TFE3* gene fusions. In: Eble JN, , Sauter G, Epstein J, Sesterhenn I, eds. *Pathology and Genetics of Tumors of the Urinary System and Male Genital Organs.* Lyon: IARC Press; 2003, pp. 37–8.

112. Argani P, Antonescu CR, Illei PB, et al. Primary renal neoplasms with the *ASPL-TFE3* gene fusion of alveolar soft part sarcoma. A distinctive tumor entity previously included among renal cell carcinomas of children and adolescents. *Am J Pathol.* 2001;159:179–92.

113. Argani P, Lae M, Ballard ET, et al. Translocation carcinomas of the kidney after chemotherapy in childhood. *J Clin Oncol.* 2006;24:1529–34.

114. Argani P, Antonescu CR, Couturier J, et al. *PRCC-TFE3* renal carcinomas. Morphologic, immunohistochemical, ultrastructural, and molecular analysis of an entity associated with the t(X;1)(p11.2;q21). *Am J Surg Pathol.* 2002;26:1553–66.

115. Argani P, Lui MY, Couturier J, et al. Cloning of a novel *CLTC-TFE3* gene fusion in pediatric renal adenocarcinoma with t(X;17)(p11.2;q23). *Oncogene.* 2003;22:5374–8.

116. Argani P, Lal P, Hutchinson B, et al. Aberrant nuclear immunoreactivity for TFE3 in neoplasms with *TFE3* gene fusions: a sensitive and specific immunohistochemical assay. *Am J Surg Pathol.* 2003;27:750–61.

117. Argani P, Hawkins A, Griffin CA, et al. A distinctive pediatric renal neoplasm characterized by epithelioid morphology, basement membrane production, focal HMB45 immunoreactivity, and t(6;11)(p21.1;q12) translocation. *Am J Pathol.* 2001;158:2089–96.

118. Davis IJ, His BL, Arroyo JD, et al. Cloning of a novel *Alpha-TFEB* fusion in renal tumors harboring the t(6;11)(p21;q12) chromosome translocation. *Proc Natl Acad Sci USA.* 2003;100:6051–6.

119. Kuiper RP, Schepens M, Thijssen J, et al. Upregulation of the transcription factor TFEB in t(6;11)(p21;q13)-positive renal cell carcinomas due to promoter substitution. *Hum Mol Genet*. 2003;12:1661–9.

120. Argani P, Lae M, Hutchinson B, et al. Renal carcinomas with the t(6;11)(p21;q12): clinicopathologic features and demonstration of the specific *Alpha-TFEB* gene fusion by immunohistochemistry, RT-PCR, and DNA PCR. *Am J Surg Pathol*. 2005;29:230–40.

121. Argani P, Ladanyi M. Translocation carcinomas of the kidney. *Clin Lab Med*. 2005;25:363–78.

122. Meideros LJ, Palmedo G, Krigman HR, et al. Oncocytoid renal cell carcinoma after neuroblastoma: a report of four cases of a distinct clinicopathologic entity. *Am J Surg Pathol*. 1999;23:772–80.

123. Parham DM, Roloson GJ, Feely M, et al. Primary malignant neuroepithelial tumors of the kidney: a clinicopathologic analysis of 146 adult and pediatric cases from the National Wilms Tumor Study Group Pathology Center. *Am J Surg Pathol*. 2001;25:133–46.

124. Jimenez RE, Folpe AL, Lapham RL, et al. Primary Ewing's sarcoma/primitive neuroectodermal tumor of the kidney: a clinicopathologic and immunohistochemical analysis of 11 cases. *Am J Surg Pathol*. 2002;26:320–7.

125. Argani P, Faria PA, Epstein JI, et al. Primary renal synovial sarcoma. Morphologic and molecular delineation of an entity previously included among embryonal sarcomas of the kidney. *Am J Surg Pathol*. 2000;24:1087–96.

126. Kim D-W, Sohn JH, Lee MC, et al. Primary synovial sarcoma of the kidney. *Am J Surg Pathol*. 2000;24:1097–104.

127. Gupta R, Paner GP, Amin MB. Neoplasms of the upper urinary tract: a review with focus on urothelial carcinoma of the pelvicalyceal system and aspects related to its diagnosis and reporting. *Adv Anat Pathol*. 2008 (in press).

128. Delahunt B , AM, Hofstadter F, et al. Tumors of the renal pelvis and the ureter. In: Eble JN , SG, Epstein JI, Sesterhenn IA, eds. *World Health Organization Classification of Tumors: Tumors of the Urinary System and Male Genital Organs*. Lyon, France: IARC Press; 2004, pp. 150–3.

129. Guinan P, Vogelzang NJ, Randazzo R, et al. Renal pelvic cancer: a review of 611 patients treated in Illinois 1975–1985. Cancer Incidence and End Results Committee. *Urology*. 1992;40:393–9.

130. Munoz JJ, Ellison LM. Upper tract urothelial neoplasms: incidence and survival during the last 2 decades. *J Urol*. 2000;164:1523–5.

131. Olgac S, Mazumdar M, Dalbagni G, Reuter VE. Urothelial carcinoma of the renal pelvis: a clinicopathologic study of 130 cases. *Am J Surg Pathol*. 2004;28:1545–52.

132. Wein. *Campbell-Walsh Urology*. 9th ed. Philadelphia: Saunders, 2007.

133. McLaughlin JK, Silverman DT, Hsing AW, et al. Cigarette smoking and cancers of the renal pelvis and ureter. *Cancer Res*. 1992;52:254–7.

134. McLaughlin JK, Blot WJ, Mandel JS, Schuman LM, Mehl ES, Fraumeni JF, Jr. Etiology of cancer of the renal pelvis. *J Natl Cancer Inst*. 1983;71:287–91.

135. Bringuier PP, McCredie M, Sauter G, et al. Carcinomas of the renal pelvis associated with smoking and phenacetin abuse: p53 mutations and polymorphism of carcinogen-metabolising enzymes. *Int J Cancer*. 1998;79:531–6.

136. McCredie M, Ford JM, Taylor JS, Stewart JH. Analgesics and cancer of the renal pelvis in New South Wales. *Cancer*. 1982;49:2617–25.

137. McCredie M, Stewart JH, Mahony JF. Is phenacetin responsible for analgesic nephropathy in New South Wales? *Clin Nephrol*. 1982;17:134–40.

138. Jensen OM, Knudsen JB, McLaughlin JK, Sorensen BL. The Copenhagen case-control study of renal pelvis and ureter cancer: role of smoking and occupational exposures. *Int J Cancer*. 1988;41:557–61.

139. Sanderson KM, Roupret M. Upper urinary tract tumour after radical cystectomy for transitional cell carcinoma of the bladder: an update on the risk factors, surveillance regimens and treatments. *BJU Int*. 2007;100:11–6.

140. Konety BR, Getzenberg RH. Urine based markers of urological malignancy. *J Urol*. 2001;165:600–11.

141. Lodde M, Mian C, Wiener H, Haitel A, Pycha A, Marberger M. Detection of upper urinary tract transitional cell carcinoma with ImmunoCyt: a preliminary report. *Urology*. 2001;58:362–6.

142. Blaszyk H, Wang L, Dietmaier W, et al. Upper tract urothelial carcinoma: a clinicopathologic study including microsatellite instability analysis. *Mod Pathol*. 2002;15:790–7.

143. Hartmann A, Dietmaier W, Hofstadter F, Burgart LJ, Cheville JC, Blaszyk H. Urothelial carcinoma of the upper urinary tract: inverted growth pattern is predictive of microsatellite instability. *Hum Pathol*. 2003;34:222–7.

144. Hisataki T, Miyao N, Masumori N, et al. Risk factors for the development of bladder cancer after upper tract urothelial cancer. *Urology*. 2000;55:663–7.

145. Miyake H, Hara I, Arakawa S, Kamidono S. A clinicopathological study of bladder cancer associated with upper urinary tract cancer. *BJU Int*. 2000;85:37–41.

146. Kang CH, Yu TJ, Hsieh HH, et al. The development of bladder tumors and contralateral upper urinary tract tumors after primary transitional cell carcinoma of the upper urinary tract. *Cancer*. 2003;98:1620–6.

147. Kauffman EC, Raman JD. Bladder cancer following upper tract urothelial carcinoma. *Expert Rev Anticancer Ther*. 2008;8:75–85.

148. Sved PD, Gomez P, Nieder AM, Manoharan M, Kim SS, Soloway MS. Upper tract tumour after radical cystectomy for transitional cell carcinoma of the bladder: incidence and risk factors. *BJU Int*. 2004;94:785–9.

149. Tran W, Serio AM, Raj GV, et al. Longitudinal risk of upper tract recurrence following radical cystectomy for urothelial cancer and the potential implications for long-term surveillance. *J Urol*. 2008;179:96–100.

150. Amin MB, Srigley JR, Grignon DJ, et al. Updated protocol for the examination of specimens from patients with carcinoma of the urinary bladder, ureter, and renal pelvis. *Arch Pathol Lab Med*. 2003;127:1263–79.

151. Jewett MA. Upper tract urothelial carcinoma. *J Urol*. 2006;175:12–13.

152. Murphy WM GD, Perlman EJ. Tumors of the ureters and the renal pelvis. *AFIP Atlas of Tumor Pathology: Tumors of the Kidney, Bladder and Related Urinary*

*Structures*Washington DC: American Registry of Pathology, 2004, pp. 375–82.

153. Kvist E, Lauritzen AF, Bredesen J, Luke M, Sjolin KE. A comparative study of transitional cell tumors of the bladder and upper urinary tract. *Cancer*. 1988;61:2109–12.

154. WM M, . Disease of the urinary bladder, urethra, ureters and renal pelvis. In: WM M, ed. *Urologic Pathology*. Philadelphia: WB Saunders, 1997, pp. 127–31.

155. Pusztaszeri M, Hauser J, Iselin C, Egger JF, Pelte MF. Urothelial carcinoma "nested variant" of renal pelvis and ureter. *Urology*. 2007;69:778 e15–17.

156. Korkes F, Silveira TS, Castro MG, Cuck G, Fernandes RC, Perez MD. Carcinoma of the renal pelvis and ureter. *Int Braz J Urol*. 2006;32:648–53; discussion 653–5.

157. Melamed MR, Reuter VE. Pathology and staging of urothelial tumors of the kidney and ureter. *Urol Clin North Am*. 1993;20:333–47.

158. Perez-Montiel D, Hes O, Michal M, Suster S. Micropapillary urothelial carcinoma of the upper urinary tract: clinicopathologic study of five cases. *Am J Clin Pathol*. 2006;126:86–92.

159. Canacci AM, MacLennan GT. Sarcomatoid urothelial carcinoma of the renal pelvis. *J Urol*. 2006;175:1906.

160. Thiel DD, Igel TC, Wu KJ. Sarcomatoid carcinoma of transitional cell origin confined to renal pelvis. *Urology*. 2006;67:622 e9–11.

161. Perez-Montiel D, Wakely PE, Hes O, Michal M, Suster S. High-grade urothelial carcinoma of the renal pelvis: clinicopathologic study of 108 cases with emphasis on unusual morphologic variants. *Mod Pathol*. 2006;19:494–503.

162. Leroy X, Leteurtre E, De La Taille A, Augusto D, Biserte J, Gosselin B. Microcystic transitional cell carcinoma: a report of 2 cases arising in the renal pelvis. *Arch Pathol Lab Med*. 2002;126:859–61.

163. Lopez-Beltran A, Escudero AL, Cavazzana AO, Spagnoli LG, Vicioso-Recio L. Sarcomatoid transitional cell carcinoma of the renal pelvis: a report of five cases with clinical, pathological, immunohistochemical and DNA ploidy analysis. *Pathol Res Pract*. 1996;192:1218–24.

164. Holmang S, Johansson SL. Urothelial carcinoma of the upper urinary tract: comparison between the WHO/ISUP 1998 consensus classification and WHO 1999 classification system. *Urology*. 2005;66:274–8.

165. Genega EM, Kapali M, Torres-Quinones M, et al. Impact of the 1998 World Health Organization/International Society of Urological Pathology classification system for urothelial neoplasms of the kidney. *Mod Pathol*. 2005;18:11–18.

166. Racioppi M, D'Addessi A, Alcini A, Destito A, Alcini E. Clinical review of 100 consecutive surgically treated patients with upper urinary tract transitional tumours. *Br J Urol*. 1997;80:707–11.

167. Hall MC, Womack S, Sagalowsky AI, Carmody T, Erickstad MD, Roehrborn CG. Prognostic factors, recurrence, and survival in transitional cell carcinoma of the upper urinary tract: a 30-year experience in 252 patients. *Urology*. 1998;52:594–601.

168. Volmar KE, Chan TY, De Marzo AM, Epstein JI. Florid von Brunn nests mimicking urothelial carcinoma: a morphologic and immunohistochemical comparison to the nested variant of urothelial carcinoma. *Am J Surg Pathol*. 2003;27:1243–52.

169. Blacher EJ, Johnson DE, Abdul-Karim FW, Ayala AG. Squamous cell carcinoma of renal pelvis. *Urology*. 1985;25:124–6.

170. Hes O, Curik R, Mainer K, Michal M. Urothelial signet-ring cell carcinoma of the renal pelvis with collagenous spherulosis: a case report. *Int J Surg Pathol*. 2005;13:375–8.

171. Takehara K, Nomata K, Eguchi J, et al. Mucinous adenocarcinoma of the renal pelvis associated with transitional cell carcinoma in the renal pelvis and the bladder. *Int J Urol*. 2004;11:1016–8.

172. Gulmez I, Dogan A, Balkanli S, Yilmaz U, Karacagil M, Tatlisen A. The first case of periureteric hibernoma. Case report. *Scand J Urol Nephrol*. 1997;31:203–4.

173. Le Cheong L, Khan AN, Bisset RA. Sonographic features of a renal pelvic neurofibroma. *J Clin Ultrasound*. 1990;18:129–31.

174. Smith EM, Resnick MI. Ureteropelvic junction obstruction secondary to periureteral lipoma. *J Urol*. 1994;151:150–1.

175. Tamboli P, Mohsin SK, Hailemariam S, Amin MB. Colonic adenocarcinoma metastatic to the urinary tract versus primary tumors of the urinary tract with glandular differentiation: a report of 7 cases and investigation using a limited immunohistochemical panel. *Arch Pathol Lab Med*. 2002;126:1057–63.

176. Varela-Duran J, Urdiales-Viedma M, Taboada-Blanco F, Cuevas C. Neurofibroma of the ureter. *J Urol*. 1987;138:1425–6.

177. Coup AJ. Angiosarcoma of the ureter. *Br J Urol*. 1988;62:275–6.

178. Charny CK, Glick RD, Genega EM, Meyers PA, Reuter VE, La Quaglia MP. Ewing's sarcoma/primitive neuroectodermal tumor of the ureter: a case report and review of the literature. *J Pediatr Surg*. 2000;35:1356–8.

179. Fein RL, Hamm FC. Malignant schwannoma of the renal pelvis: a review of the literature and a case report. *J Urol*. 1965;94:356–61.

180. Acikalin MF, Kabukcuoglu S, Can C. Sarcomatoid carcinoma of the renal pelvis with giant cell tumor-like features: case report with immunohistochemical findings. *Int J Urol*. 2005;12:199–203.

181. Zettl A, Konrad MA, Polzin S, et al. Urothelial carcinoma of the renal pelvis with choriocarcinomatous features: genetic evidence of clonal evolution. *Hum Pathol*. 2002;33:1234–7.

182. Molinie V, Pouchot J, Vinceneux P, Barge J. Osteoclastoma-like giant cell tumor of the renal pelvis associated with papillary transitional cell carcinoma. *Arch Pathol Lab Med*. 1997;121:162–6.

Index

O